Essentials of Pediatric Neurology

Third Edition

Editor

Dr. Bibek Talukdar

DCH, MD

Former Director-Professor, Pediatrics
Maulana Azad Medical College (MAMC) and associated
Chacha Nehru Bal Chikitsalaya (CNBC), New Delhi
Former Head, Department of Pediatrics, CNBC
Former Chief, Section of Pediatric Neurology, MAMC and
Section of Pediatric Neurology and Development, CNBC
Currently Visiting Professor, CNBC

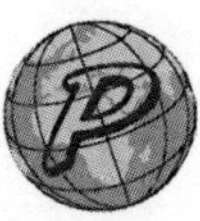

Peepee Publishers and Distributors (P) Ltd.®

Essentials of Pediatric Neurology

Published by:
Pawaninder P. Vij and Anupam Vij

Peepee Publishers and Distributors (P) Ltd.
Head Office: 160, Shakti Vihar, Pitam Pura, Delhi-110 034 (India)

Correspondence Address:
7/31, First Floor, Ansari Road, Daryaganj
New Delhi-110 002 (India)
Ph: 41512412, 23246245, 9811156083
e-mail: *peepee160@yahoo.co.in*
e-mail: *peepee160@gmail.com*
www.peepeepub.com
join us on facebook.com/pp.publishers

Third Edition: 2022

ISBN: 978-81-9523-440-0

Preface

This edition of the book **'Essentials of Pediatric Neurology'**, the first edition of which was published in 1997 with the objective of highlighting the basics of diagnosis and treatment of common and important neurological disorders in pediatric age group in India and also to make pediatric neurology a subject of interest amongst Indian physicians, is an attempt to continue with the same goal. Large number of children in our country are victims of neurological disorders many of which are associated with significant morbidity and mortality. Many children suffering from such disorders are afflicted with a variety of disabilities and handicaps, often life-long.

Advancement in Pediatric Neurology has been tremendous in recent years. The chapters in this edition of the book have been updated to accommodate the current knowledge in diagnosis and management of the of the common and important neurological disorders. Few earlier chapters have been deleted while several new chapters have been added. Special emphasis has been given to the topics of clinical evaluation, congenital malformations, neurodevelopmental disorders, neurobehavioural problems, seizures and epilepsies, important encephalopathies, CNS infections, neuromuscular disorders and neurodegenerative disorders, so common and often problematic in our country. The primary objective of the book however remains same as before – a comprehensive and clinically oriented approach to the common neurological disorders in pediatric age group in our country. Despite a comprehensive approach, there is no compromise however in addressing the basics and fundamentals, relevant investigative tools and techniques currently in vogue and also recent advances.

The contributing authors, faculty in different institutions across India having expertise and also research contribution in the field of pediatric neurology, took out their valuable time for writing the chapters. The editor expresses heartfelt thanks to all the authors.

The editor expresses his thanks to Dr. Vinod Puri, former Director-Professor and Head, Department of Neurology, GB Pant Hospital (GIPMER), New Delhi for the valuable assistance rendered by him. The editor is also thankful to Dr. Devendra Mishra, Professor, Pediatrics, Maulana Azad Medical College, New Delhi, for his valuable assistance.

The publication of the book has been delayed due to the prolonged lock-down and other restrictions in connection with the Covid 19 pandemic in the counrty. The editor expresses his heartfelt thanks to Mr. P. P. Vij, Director, Peepee Publishers for completing the work with perfection despite all odds.

The editor hopes that the treatise will be useful to doctors, medical students and other medical professionals interested in Padiatric Neurology.

Dr. Bibek Talukdar

New Delhi

Contributors

Dr. Ajay Garg, MD
Eur. Dip. in Neuroradiology (EDiNR), Eur. Dip. in Pediatric Neuroradiology (EDiPNR), Professor, Department of Neuroimaging and Interventional Neuroradiology
All India Institute of Medical Sciences, New Delhi

Dr. AK Gupta, MD
Professor and Head
Department of Radiology
All India Institute of Medical Sciences, New Delhi

Dr. Arushi Gahlot Saini, MD, DM
Associate Professor, Department of Pediatrics
Postgraduate Institute of Medical Education and Research
Chandigarh

Dr. Arvind K Rathi, MD
Former Professor and Head, Department of Pediatrics
BRD Medical College, Gorakhpur

Dr. Ashish Kumar Duggal, MD, DM
Associate Professor
Department of Neurology
GB Pant Hospital, GIPMER, New Delhi

Dr. Ashok K Patwari, MD
Former Director-Professor
Department of Pediatrics
Lady Hardinge Medical College, New Delhi

Dr. Atin Kumar, MD
Professor, Department of Radiology
All India Institute of Medical Sciences, New Delhi

Dr. Bibek Talukdar, DCH, MD
Former Director-Professor, Pediatrics
Maulana Azad Medical College and associated
Chacha Nehru Bal Chikitsalaya, New Delhi
Currently Visiting Professor, Pediatrics, Chacha Nehru Bal Chikitsalaya, Delhi

Dr. Bina Ahuja, MD
Former Senior Specialist in Pediatrics
Kalawati Saran Children's Hospital, New Delhi

Dr. Biswaroop Chakravarty, MD, DM
Additional Professor, Department of Pediatrics
All India Institute of Medical Sciences, New Delhi

Dr. C. Leema Pauline, MD, DM
Professor of Pediatric Neurology
Madras Medical College, Institute of Child Health, Chennai

Dr. Chandrakanta, MD
Professor, Department of Pediatrics
King George Medical University, Lucknow

Dr. Devendra Mishra, MD
Professor, Department of Pediatrics
Maulana Azad Medical College, New Delhi

Dr. D Meikandan, MD, DM
Former Professor of Pediatrics and Incharge
Pediatric Neurology, Institute of Child Health
Government Rajaji Hospital, Madurai

Dr. Kausik Mandal, MD, DM
Additional Professor, Department of Medical Genetics
Sanjay Gandhi Postgraduate Institute of Medical Sciences
Lucknow

Dr. Mahesh Kamate, MD, DM
Professor, Pediatric Neurology
JN Medical College, Belgaum, Karnataka

Dr. Mahima Mittal, MD
Professor and Head, Department of Pediatrics
AIIMS, Gorakhpur

Dr. Manisha Jana, MD
Additional Professor, Department of Radiology
All India Institute of Medical Sciences, New Delhi

Dr. Medha Mittal, MD
Associate Professor of Pediatrics
Chacha Nehru Bal Chikitsalaya, Delhi

Dr. Monica Juneja, MD
Director-Professor, Pediatrics
Maulana Azad Medical College, New Delhi

Dr. MS Bhatia, MD
Director Professor and Head
Department of Psychiatry
University College of Medical Sciences, Delhi

Dr. Naveen Sankhyan, MD, DM
Professor, Head, Pediatric Neurology
Department of Pediatrics
Postgraduate Institute of Medical Education and Research
Chandigarh

Dr. Neera Chaudhry, MD, DM
Professor and Head, Department of Neurology
Vardhaman Mahavir Medical College and Safdarjung Hospital, New Delhi; Former Professor, Department of Neurology, GB Pant Hospital, GIPMER, New Delhi

Dr. N Thilothammal, DCH, MD, DM, MPH (USA)
Former Professor and Head
Department of Pediatric Neurology
Madras Medical College
Institute of Child Health, Chennai

Dr. Prarthana Kharod
Associate Professor
Department of Pediatrics
GCS Medical College, Ahmedabad

Dr. Pratibha Singhi, MD
Former Professor & Head and Chief, Pediatric Neurology and Neurodevelopment, Department of Paediatrics
Advanced Pediatrics Centre, Post Graduate Institute of Medical Education and Research, Chandigarh, India
Currently Director, Pediatric Neurology and Neurodevelopment, Medanta, The Medicity, Gurgaon
Haryana, India

Dr. Puneet Jain, MD, DM
Former Assistant Professor, Department of Pediatrics
Lady Hardinge Medical College, New Delhi
Currently Epilepsy Program, Division of Neurology
Department of Pediatrics, The Hospital for Sick Children
Toronto, Ontario, Canada

Dr. Rahul Jain
Associate Professor, Department of Pediatrics
Maulana Azad Medical College, New Delhi
Formerly Assistant Professor, Pediatrics
Chacha Nehru Bal Chikitsalaya, Delhi

Dr. Rajeev Kulshrestha, MS, MCh
Former, Senior Specialist and Head of the Department of Pediatric Surgery, Safdarjang Hospital, New Delhi
Currently Senior Consultant, Department of Pediatric Surgery, Sir Ganga Ram Hospital, New Delhi

Dr. Rashmi Kumar, MD
Professor of Pediatrics and Former Head
Department of Pediatrics
King George Medical University, Lucknow

Dr. R Ramesh Kumar, MD, DNB, DM
Associate Professor
Division of Pediatric Critical Care
Department of Pediatrics
Jawaharlal Institute of Medical Education and Research (JIPMER), Puducherry

Dr. Sangeeta Sharma, MD
Professor and Head, Department of Neuropharmacology
Institute of Human Behaviour and Allied Sciences, Delhi

Dr. Satinder Aneja, MD
Former Director-Professor and Head
Department of Pediatrics
Lady Hardinge Medical College, New Delhi
Currently Professor, Department of Pediatrics School of Medical Sciences and Research Sharda University, Noida

Dr. Shahzadi Malhotra, M.Phil, Ph.D
Assistant Professor, Clinical Psychology
Chacha Nehru Bal Chikitsalaya, Delhi

Dr. Sharmila B Mukerjee, MD
Professor, Department of Pediatrics
Lady Hardinge Medical College, New Delhi

Dr. Sheffali Gulati, MD
Professor, Coordinator
DM Paediatric Neurology Programme
Faculty Incharge, Center of Excellence and Advanced Research on Childhood Neurodevelopmental Disorders
Chief, Child Neurology Division, Department of Pediatrics
All India Institute of Medical Sciences, New Delhi, India

Dr. Sheweta Tandon, M.Phil, Ph.D
Assistant Professor, Clinical Psychology
Chacha Nehru Bal Chikitsalaya, Delhi

Dr. Shivanand Gamanagatti, MD, FICR
Professor, Department of Radiology
All India Institute of Medical Sciences, New Delhi

Dr. Shruti Jain, MD, DM
Neurology Resident, Department of Neurology
GB Pant Hospital, New Delhi

Dr. Shruti Srivastava, DNB
Professor, Department of Psychiatry
University College of Medical Sciences, Delhi

Dr. S Mahadevan, MD, PhD
Senior Professor and Head
Division of Pediatric Critical Care
Department of Pediatrics
Jawaharlal Institute of Medical Education and Research (JIPMER), Puducherry

Dr. Sujata Kanhere, DCH, DNB, FRCPCH, PhD
Fellowship in Pediatric Neurology (U.K.)
Professor and HOD, Incharge, Pediatric Neurology
Department of Pediatrics and Neonatology
KJ Somaiya Medical College, Hospital and Research Centre
Mumbai

Dr. Suvasini Sharma, MD, DM, FRCPCH
Professor, Department of Pediatrics
Lady Hardinge Medical College, New Delhi

Dr. Vinod Puri, MD, DM
Former Director-Professor and Head
Department of Neurology
GB Pant Hospital, GIPMER, New Delhi
Currently Head, Department of Neurology
National Heart Institute, New Delhi

Dr. V Viswanathan, DCH, MRCP, PhD
Consultant Pediatric Neurologist
Kanchi Kamakoti Child's Trust Hospital, Chennai
Currently Consultant Paediatric Neurologist
Apollo Children's Hospitals, Chennai

Contents

INFECTIONS

MISCELLANEOUS DISORDERS

1 Chapter

NEUROLOGICAL EXAMINATION: INFANCY AND CHILDHOOD

Bibek Talukdar

Neurological examination of a child specially the young ones, is often a challenging task. The technique of eliciting various signs in pediatric neurology is greatly influenced by the level of development of the child. The methods of examinations, thus, have to be modified according to the age of the child. The developmental approach has led to the exploration of many newer areas in the child's neurologic functioning in recent times. Excellent works by several researchers in last two decade have given new direction to pediatric neurologic examination (Paine, 1960, Oppe, 1966, Amiel-Tison, 1986, Grenier, 1986).

Neurological examination in pediatrics is aimed at detecting the presence of neurologic disease, site of lesion, nature of lesion and possible etiologic diagnosis. History and clinical findings are mainstay in neurologic diagnosis. Systematic examination gives a definite shape to the process of diagnosis and also proper direction to investigations. Examination of the nervous system has two main components, observation and passive elicitation of signs. In infants and young children, elicitation of signs in response to specific maneuvers is often difficult as obtaining cooperation is often difficult; observation, therefore, is an extremely important tool in this age group.

INITIATION OF THE EXAMINATION

Children, specially the infants and young ones often become frightened when doctors start examining them. Crying and turning away is a frequent initial response. Cooperation is the centre point of a fruitful neurological examination. The examiner should approach the child with a smile and a 'hello'. He should start talking to the child asking his name, names of his brothers, sisters or parents, who are his friends, what did he take in the morning and so on. Children like shaking hands. These measures usually make the child comfortable, relaxed and cooperative. In case of infants, a smiling 'hello', whistling, showing objects like a toy, a torch light or pen, letting him handle a toy, pen, stethoscope or examiner's finger usually make him comfortable and co-operative.

The approach should be slow and gentle. Abrupt undressing and commanding him to carry out something usually frightens the young child and he resists examination. A few minutes should be spent taking measures as detailed above to make him cooperative before touching him. Undressing, which is important for a good neurological examination, is disliked and even resisted by most children. This should be done in stages and as necessary. Many areas of examination can be carried out without undressing or with partial undressing. It is also important to see that the infant is not hungry or sleepy. If satisfactory examination is not possible at the initial contact, the examination should be repeated at another sitting; by that time, the child is likely to be more cooperative as he will be more familiar with the examiner and the environment.

Position in which the child is examined also needs flexibility. A large part of the examination in the infant and the young child is better and easily carried out in the parents' lap in the sitting position or lying. Young ones are often more comfortable in the mother's lap. Examination in standing position is done to see the child's abilities of locomotion. Examination in supine or prone position is done as necessary.

Attempts should be made to complete the examination while the child is cooperative and is in good mood. Those examinations that are painful and are likely to upset the mood of the child should be left to the end.

Besides usual equipments like stethoscope, reflex hammer, measuring tape, pen torch, tongue depressor and ophthalmoscope, some others are needed to suit the developmental approach to the examination. Some such equipments are coloured toys, pen, pencil, paper, crayon, one-inch-cube, plastic ball with and without a string, rattle and some toffees or biscuits.

Order of Examination

The neurological examination of the child is carried out in the order given below:

1. General observation.
2. Station and gait.
3. Head, neck and spine.
4. Mental status / Higher mental function.
5. Cranial nerves.
6. Motor system.
7. Reflexes.
8. Sensory system.
9. Development.

The order, however, may be changed according to clinical situation, mood and cooperation of the child. The important pediatric aspects of examinations are detailed below. Details of the basic methods for example how to test the cranial nerves or how to elicit the reflexes or how to test muscle power have however been omitted as these are available in any book on clinical method. Some common and classic clinical signs and their interpretations have been shown in insets.

GENERAL OBSERVATION

As soon as the child enters the room, the examiner should note his *appearance, behaviour and activity.* A dull and blank look often suggests intellectual deficiency. Undue lethargy, hyperactivity, inattentiveness, undue anxiety, obvious congenital malformations should be noted. Tell-tale squint, facial palsy, monoplegia, hemiplegia, abnormal posture due to hypertonia and hypotonia may be obvious. Ataxia and imbalance and in-coordination are excellent observational findings specially in infants and young children.

STATION AND GAIT

Station, as envisaged by Paine (1960), refers to static posture and to standing and sitting. Abnormality in station can be due to ataxia, muscular weakness and skeletal deformities like kyphosis, scoliosis and lordosis. The child's gait should be observed during natural walking and/or stimulated walking. Common and clinically useful gait abnormalities in children are *waddling gait* (with broadbase) seen in muscular dystrophies, *hemiplegic gait* (circumduction with dragging of one foot) seen in hemiplegia and *ataxic gait* seen in disorders involving cerebellum and spinal cord. While examining station and gait, age of the child be kept in mind as development of these skills are related to age.

MENTAL STATUS/HIGHER MENTAL FUNCTION

Mental status examination includes consciousness, orientation in time, place and person, memory – immediate, recent and past, intelligence and speech. In children, emotional state and dominance should also be tested.

In the infant, examination of mental status is usually limited to assessment of consciousness and behaviour. The normal infant responds to stimuli by looking around, looking at the examiner or the parents, crying, expressing pleasure or displeasure, making withdrawal movements etc. according to the nature of the stimulus. The baby with normal mental functioning is usually, alert, active, playful and interested in the surrounding.

Consciousness that implies wakefulness and awareness of self and surrounding is assessed by response to stimuli, usually verbal, visual and tactile. If there is altered consciousness, often stated as altered sensorium, it is useful to qualify further in terms of confusions, lethargy, delirium, stupor and coma. In *confusion,* the patient is not fully oriented but is able to maintain arousal. *Delirium* is an agitated form of confusion. In *lethargy*, the patient is not fully oriented as well as unable to maintain arousal fully. In *stupor*, the patient is unconscious at rest but is arousable to a verbally responsive state by stimulus but drifts back to the state of unconscious quickly when the stimulus is withdrawn. In *coma,* the patient is unarousable and does not respond to stimuli of any kind, verbal, visual, tactile or other; vigorous stimulation may lead to decorticate or decerebrate posture. One of the children's coma scale may be used for assessing the depth of coma. Glasgow Coma Scale is commonly used. Some common causes of altered consciousness that we commonly see are shown in Inset 1.1.

Inset 1.1: Common Causes of Coma/Altered Sensorium in Children

CNS infections–meningitis, encephalitis, *severe septicemia, severe dehydration, encephalopathies*–hepatic, uremic, hypoxic, metabolic and toxic, *poisoning/toxicity*–opiates, organophosphorus, sedatives, tranquilizers, anticonvulsants, *Inborn errors of metabolism*–organic acidemias, *endocrine disorder*–diabetic ketoacidosis *head trauma, ICSOL.*

While testing orientation, memory and intelligence, the questions put to the child should be graded according to his age and maturity. *Orientation* can be tested by asking questions like what is his name, where he is now and what is the time. *Immediate memory* can be tested by asking the child to repeat something uttered by the examiner (commonly numbers). *Past memory* can be tested by asking about an event in the family in the past, which is verified, from the parents. *Intelligence* can be tested at bed-side by using tests like counting of numbers, forward and backward, solving arithmetical problems and response to problem-solving questions. More accurate assessment of intelligence will, however, need formal psychometric testing.

Speech is assessed by listening to conversation with the child and also listening to his reading. Note should be made of any *stammering* (interruption of the normal rhythm of speech by involuntary repetition, prolongation or arrest of sound), *dysphonia* (altered loudness, tone, pitch and vibration of the sound), often seen in bulbar poliomyelitis, laryngitis and other laryngeal and pharyngeal involvement, *aphonia* usually due to same causes as of dysphonia, *dysarthria* (difficulty in articulation), often seen following stroke involving Broca's area, in Bell's palsy, spastic C.P., myotonic dystrophy and Wilson's disease and *dysphasia*, that may be receptive, expressive or global. Global aphasia can be developmental or acquired and is often associated with intellectual deficiency disorder, hearing defect, brain damage and autism. Delay in speech development is often seen following prematurity, birth anoxia, CNS infections, encephalopathies. Isolated non-development of speech is often idiopathic, although perinatal insult can be the cause in many.

The **emotional state** of the child also should be noted. Older children can often express their mental conflict and disturbances quite well given the opportunity. The lack of attention, abnormal behaviour, hyperactivity, emotional lability, undue anxiety, fear etc. should be noted.

Dominance should be assessed by history and by observing during examination which hand the child prefers to use. Left-handedness, although familial at times, can have pathological basis like hemiplegia. Left handedness is common in infants born preterm, children with intellectual deficiency and learning disability.

HEAD, NECK AND SPINE

The *shape, size, fontanelles, sutures and rate of growth* of **head** should be examined routinely and any abnormality noted. Head growth should be correlated to established standards (Inset 1.2). Abnormalities in *shape, size and rate of growth* of the head are associated with many CNS disorders, often developmental in origin. The *head circumference,* the maximum occipitofrontal circumference, should be measured with an inelastic fiber glass or steel tape measure. Slipping of the tape from the occiput while measuring, is common that may result in erroneous reading and it is always better to repeat the measurement in case of doubt. Common abnormal findings on examination of the head circumference are unusually large head or macrocephaly and unusually small head or microcephaly. In infants, the size and tension of the *fontanelle* should be noted; wide open fontanelle often indicate raised intracranial pressure, most commonly seen in hydrocephalus meningitis. The size of the anterior fontanelle is quite variable, mostly however, it measures about 2 × 2 cms. The fontanels are closed by about 18 months. The *sutures* should be palpated for evidence of separation that indicates intracranial hypertension or for premature closure (craniostenosis) where the sutures feel like a ridge, often associated with microcephalopathy. The skull should also be *palpated* for fractures in cases of suspected head trauma and this may at times give clue to unexplained coma. *Percussion of the skull* may be done in suspected intracranial hypertension as in hydrocephalus to elicit the cracked-pot sign (Macewen sign), that occurs due to sutural separation. *Transillumination* may be useful in diagnosis of hydrocephalus, porencephaly, hydranencephaly and subdural hematoma. *Auscultation of the skull* may reveal loud bruit suggesting intracranial aneurysm or arteriovenous malformation. *Signs of rickets* may be found like craniotabes, delayed closure of fontanelle, frontal and parietal prominence. Midline *swellings* often indicate encephalocele and dermoid cyst. Swelling with firm margin and relatively soft center, often parietal and occipital, is usually seen in cephalhematoma. Some common abnormalities related to head circumference are shown in Inset 1.3.

Inset 1.2: Rate of Head Growth and Head Circumference

Age	Rate of growth
0-3 months	2 cms / month
3-6 months	1 cm / month
6-9 months	0.5 cm / month
9-12 months	0.5 cm / month
1-3 years	0.25 cm / month
4-6 years	1 cm / year

Inset 1.3: Findings on Examination of the Head in Common Neurological Disorders

Microcephaly–genetic/familial, craniostenosis, congenital infections, *Large head*–hydrocephalus, megalencephaly, familial large head, ICSOL, leukodystrophy, storage disorders, *Wide open fontanelle*–raised ICP commonly due to hydrocephalus,

Contd.

Contd.

meningitis, subdural effusion and hygroma, ICSOL like AVM or abscess. *Engorged scalp veins*–hydrocephalus, raised ICP, sagittal sinus thrombosis. *Premature closure of fontanelle*–craniostenosis. *Craniotabes*–rickets, prematurity. *Proptosis*–cavernous sinus thrombosis, tumour. *Scalp swellings*–abscess, inflamed lymph nodes, trauma, cephalhematoma, encephalocele, dermoid cyst, osteomyelitis, histiocytosis, metastatic lesion.

The **face** and head should be examined for *dysmorphic features* and other craniofacial abnormalities like abnormal hair, prominent epicanthus, hypertelorism, depressed bridge of the nose, low-set malformed ears and abnormal lips and palate. These anomalies have been shown to be associated with conduct problems, mainly hyperactivity and also many systemic and genetic disorders. Neurocutaneous stigmata like adenoma sebaceum, hypopigmented macules, angiomatosis, should be looked for.

The **neck** should be examined for midline swelling (meningocele or meningomyelocele) and signs of meningeal irritation like neck stiffness, Kernig's sign and Brudzinski's sign specially in presence of fever and altered sensorium presence of which suggests meningitis. Neck stiffness may also be seen in presence of subarachnoid hemorrhage. The **spine** should be examined for undue shortening (platybasia), midline defect like meningocele, meningomyelocele, cutaneous abnormalities, i.e., like tuft of hair, pilonidal sinus and gibbus (often seen in tuberculosis of the spine).

CRANIAL NERVES

First Cranial Nerve (Olfactory): It is tested by presenting to each nostril in turn common odours like that of banana, orange and noting the response. First cranial nerve involvement is seen after head injury with fracture of the cribriform plate, following meningitis, frontal lobe tumour and also in functional disorders.

Second Cranial Nerve (Optic): It is tested by examining the field of vision, colour vision and acuity of vision. *Visual field* is tested by the standard confrontation test. While testing an eye, the other eye should be covered by the examiner's hand or an index card; in case of infant and young children it may be done more comfortably by the mother's hand since covering of an eye often upsets the child. The examiner should keep talking to the infant so that he keeps looking at the examiner or a target in the front. The object brought from the periphery should be bright and dangling for the young ones so as to attract attention. As soon as the object is in the field of vision of the infant, he looks at it quickly. Visual field defect is common in tumour involving the optic chiasma, i.e., pituitary tumour.

Colour vision testing at bedside by colour matching or by Ishihara chart is possible in older children.

Visual acuity in older children is tested by usual bedside finger counting test and Snellen's chart. In infants it is tested by visual fixation and pursuit. Any object like torch, pen, stethoscope or toy can be used to attract attention of the baby. Good visual fixation and following usually indicates good visual acuity in an infant. A blind infant does not have visual fixation; he also exhibits roving, aimless and wandering eye movement. Covering the normal eye in a child with unilateral visual loss also helps in bringing out the defect; when the good eye is covered, the infant, who was otherwise playing, becomes irritable, often starts screaming and tries to move his head away from the cover. Some important causes of visual loss are shown in Inset 1.4.

Inset 1.4: Important Causes of Neurogenic Visual Loss
Congenital amblyopia, Sequelae of congenital infections (TORCH), Sequelae of head trauma, meningitis, encephalitis and brain abscess, Hydrocephalus, Brain tumour specially involving optic nerve and pathway like pituitary tumour, optic glioma, Sequelae of chronic intracranial hypertension.

Eliciting *optokinetic nystagmus* (railroad nystagmus) is a useful test in detecting/confirming visual field defect and cortical blindness in infant and uncooperative child. It is elicited by moving a succession of stripes across the child's visual field. A large rotating drum, the surface of which is painted with black and white stripes in succession, is kept in the child's visual field. The rotation of the drum, on which the infant is fixing, produces nystagmus. The response can be obtained horizontally as well vertically. This optokinetic nystagmus tests the intactness of the visual pathway and the ocular muscles.

The *fundus* can give vital clues to many neurological abnormalities (see Inset 1.5). Mydriatics should not be used as far as possible, specially in children with altered sensorium since papillary signs are extremely important in diagnosis and monitoring of a comatose child; if at all needed it should be used at the end after completing the neurologic examination. Papilledema and optic atrophy are common ophthalmoscopic abnormalities seen in pediatrics. Papilledema is manifested by fullness of the optic up, engorgement of the veins, blurring of the disc margin and presence of exudates. Hemorrhage can sometimes associated with papilledema often in cases of hypertensive encephalopathy. Retinal bleed is seen in bleeding disorder; in newborn it is often normal.

Inset 1.5: Common and Important Abnormalities in Fundus and Causes

Papilledema–intracranial hypertension, as in meningitis, encephalitis, brain tumour, benign intracranial hypertension, hypertensive encephalopathy. *Optic atrophy*–primary optic atrophy, sequelae of meningitis commonly tuberculous and encephalitis, neurodegenerative disorders. *Bleed*–severe papilledema, bleeding diathesis, stroke, infective endocarditis. *Chorioretinitis* – congenital infections. *Choroid tubercles* – CNS tuberculosis.

Optic atrophy is characterised by marked pallor of the disc and attenuation of the vessels. In primary optic atrophy, the disc is uniformly pale, often white with clear regular margin and in secondary optic atrophy, usually following papilledema, the disc is pale, dirty white and the margin is irregular. Optic atrophy is usually associated with blindness; in cortical blindness, commonly seen in tuberculous meningitis, however the disc may be normal. Choreoretinitis is seen in cases of congenital CNS infections. Macular cherry red spot is suggestive of neurodegenerative disorders, commonly GM_1 and GM_2 and gangliosidoses. Temporal pallor is commonly seen in multiple sclerosis. Pigmentary disorders of the retina are seen in several heredofamilial disorders and syndromes like Lawrence Moon-Biedl syndrome.

Third (Oculomotor), Fourth (Trochlear) and Sixth (Abducent) Cranial Nerves: The standard tests used to examine these nerves are examining the *movements of the eyeballs* and examination of the *pupils* and also looking for *ptosis*. Other abnormalities related to movement of the eyeballs that should also be noted are *nystagmus* and *opsoclonus*.

The *eye movements* are tested in all the standard directions of gaze in each eye separately. In infants and young children the eye movement can be elicited by the method of visual fixation and following as discussed above, by moving the target object in the desired direction. Conjugate gaze should also be observed simultaneously. Tests for eye movements are directed at bring out paralysis of extraocular muscles and also paralysis of conjugate gaze (gaze palsy). Abnormal gaze like skew deviation resulting from vertical displacement of the eyes may also be seen.

Clinical examination of the *pupils* should include size, shape and light reflex, both direct and consensual, as usual. In internuclear ophthalmoplegia, on looking up at an object, there is adduction defect on one eye due to paralysis of medial rectus and nystegmus on the other eye that is abducting; this usually results from brainstem lesion in the medial lemniscus. In internal ophthalmoplegia there is dilatation of the affected pupil with loss of all pupillar reflexes but the extraocular muscles are normal. In external ophthalmoplegia all extraocular muscles are paralysed and there is ptosis but pupillary response is normal.

Strabismus or squint, resulting from paralysis or malfunctioning of the extraocular muscles needs careful evaluation. Eyes looking at different directions while focusing at an object may be obvious on observation of the eye movements spontaneous or elicited. Paralytic squint is associated with paresis or paralysis of one of the extra-ocular muscles and concomitant strabismus is without it. Paralytic squint becomes worse when the direction of gaze is towards the field of the affected muscle; diplopia is often in the older children. In concomitant squint, which is more common in children, there is no paresis of extra-ocular muscles and the defect is usually equal in all directions of gaze. Strabismus is detected by:

(a) Observation of eye movements, spontaneous or elicited.

(b) Symmetry of the corneal light reflex when a light is flashed on the eyes, and

(c) **Cover/uncover test:** In the cover/uncover test, the eyes are alternately covered with an index card with the child fixing at a target in the front and the eyes are observed for re-fixation movement. In the presence of strabismus, the deviating eye will move outwards or inwards as the fixing eye is occluded. No movement occurs in the uncovered eye if there is no nystegmus. Red glass test is also useful for examining extraocular palsies and diplopia; on following a white light in different directions with a red glass on one eye, the child sees maximum separation of red and white lights in the direction of the affected muscle.

Ptosis resulting from 3rd nerve palsy, is often associated with dilatation of the pupils and loss of accommodation reflexes. To examine the degree of ptosis it is important to push the frontalis muscles down to negate the effect of this muscle in closing the eyelids.

While examining for *nystagmus* the patient's eye and the examiner's eyes should be at the same level. Spontaneous nystagmus if present should be examined for the type, i.e., horizontal, vertical or rotatory and also the fast and slow component in relation to the direction of gaze.

Opsoclonus is characterized by chaotic, jerky movements of the eyeballs. It is commonly seen in neuroblastoma and also in encephalitis. Some findings related to eye movements and their causes are shown in Inset 1.6.

Inset 1.6: Findings Related to Eye Movement Disorders and Causes
Paralysis of 3rd, 4th, 6th cranial nerves–meningitis specially TBM, encephalitis, encephalopathies like ADEM, tumour, trauma, stroke, intracranial hemorrhage, intracranial hypertension commonly affecting the 6th nerve (often false localizing sign), multiple sclerosis, diphtheria (paralysis of accommodation), myasthenia (commonly ptosis), botulism, intracranial structural lesions (cyst, hydrocephalus, gliosis) and congenital nuclear agenesis. *Ptosis* – congenital, myasthenia, botulism. *Gaze palsy* –encephalitis, hydrocephalus (upward gaze), hypothalamic tumour, vascular lesions, Perinaud syndrome (upward gaze). *Skew deviation*–diseases of labyrinth, 8th nerve and of cerebellum. *Nystegmus*–congenital, decreased visual acuity, albinism, aniridia, congenital cataract, congenital macular lesions, congenital optic atrophy, amblyopia (usually pendular), vestibular lesions (usually jerky and horizontal), labyrinthine lesions (usually horizontal) lesions, cerebellar lesions (usually horizontal), toxic effects of drugs like phenytoin (usually horizontal), brainstem lesions (usually vertical). *Small/constricted pupil*–pontine lesion like hemorrhage, opiate poisoning, organophosphorus poisoning, Horner's syndrome. *Dilated pupil*–third nerve palsy often associated with midbrain lesion, use of mydriatics, toxic as in case of atropine poisoning. *Internuclear ophthalmoplegia*–brainstem lesion, *Internal ophthalmoplegia*–mid brain lesion, *External ophthalmoplegia*–myasthenia, Kearns Sayre syndrome.

Fifth Cranial Nerve (Trigeminal): The motor function (mandibular division) in infants and young children is examined by:

(a) Observing chewing and sucking movement, which is good in normal situation.

(b) Observing opening and closing of the mouth on stimulation, request or during crying; the jaw will deviate to the affected side in case of unilateral paralysis; and

(c) Feeling for the strength of the masseter and temporalis muscles on biting a tongue spatula or clenching the teeth. The sensory function is examined by testing the sensation in the appropriate dermatome and also the corneal and conjunctival reflexes. 5th cranial nerve lesion is uncommon except rarely in trauma.

Seventh Cranial Nerve (Facial): The facial nerve is easily examined by observing the muscles of the face in action. The most striking sign of facial palsy is 'facial asymmetry', due to lack of contraction of facial muscles on the affected side, which becomes more prominent when the infant or the young one cries or the older child smiles or shows his teeth on asking to do so. Other signs are:

(a) Flattening of the nasolabial fold.

(b) Drooling of saliva.

(c) Defective eye closure; and

(d) Absence of wrinkling of the forehead on looking up, frowning or crying, all on the affected side in lower motor neuron type of facial palsy. In upper motor neuron type of facial palsy, wrinkling of the forehead is preserved due to bilateral innervation of the muscles of the forehead. It is also worth observing the emotional smile which is spared in supranuclear facial palsy.

The sensory function of the facial nerve can be tested by using salt and sugar solutions in the anterior two third of the tongue in older children, usually above 4 years of age. Some important causes of 7th nerve palsy are shown in Inset 1.7.

Inset 1.7: Important Causes of 7th Nerve Palsy
Meningitis commonly TBM, Encephalitis, Trauma, Bell's palsy, Stroke, Tumour, Abscess, Intracranial structural lesions–developmental and acquired, Congenital nuclear agenesis.

Eighth Cranial Nerve (Auditory): Hearing in infant is tested by response to sound/noise. On making a loud sound like ringing a bell or clapping behind the ears and out of vision, the infant turns his head towards the sound indicating normal hearing. Similar response can be obtained by calling the infant loudly by his name from behind. In older children observing response to sound like calling by name, whispering and finger rustling can be used to test hearing, the response being gauzed by facial expression and/or answer from the child. Rinne's and Weber's test can be employed in older children. Some important causes of 8th nerve palsy are shown in Inset 1.8.

Inset 1.8: Important Causes of 8th Cranial Nerve Palsy
Sequelae of meningitis and encephalitis, tumour, abscess and congenital infections, Sequel of neonatal sepsis, bilirubin encephalopathy and HIE, Diseases of the middle and internal ear, Intracranial structural lesions–developmental and acquired.

9th Cranial Nerve (Glossopharyngeal): It is tested by observing the contraction of the pharynx by eliciting the gag reflex (opening the mouth by tongue depressor and tickling the back of the pharynx) and testing the sensation in posterior one-third of the tongue.

10th Cranial Nerve (Vagus): The tenth cranial nerve which is motor to palate, pharynx and larynx is tested by:

(a) Observing the movement of the palate elicited in the infant by opening the mouth with a tongue depressor or asking the older child to say 'Ah', sometimes it can be observed when the child cries.

(b) Observing the contraction of the pharynx while eliciting gag reflex; and

(c) Noting the character of the voice, i.e., nasal twang or hoarseness. Paralysis of 9th and 10th cranial nerves frequently result in accumulation of secretion in the throat. This is often seen in respiratory involvement in poliomyelitis and Guillain-Barré syndrome. It is seen in diphtheria as well.

11th Cranial Nerve (Accessory): It is tested by observing the elevation or shrugging movement of the shoulder, against resistance when possible and assessing the power of the sternocleidomastoid muscle. The younger child may be made to turn his head laterally by attracting his attention to a target object while giving resistance to the movement at the chin to test the sternocleidomastoid muscles in action.

12th Cranial Nerve (Hypoglossal): It is tested by:

(a) Looking for atrophy and fasciculation of the tongue (in lower motor neuron palsy); and

(b) Observing the position of the tongue during protrusion (in lower motor neuron palsy the tongue deviates or is pushed out, to the paralysed side). Lower motor neuron type of 12th nerve palsy is commonly seen in SMA. In supranuclear palsy (pseudo bulbar palsy), commonly seen in spastic cerebral palsy, the tongue is small and spastic producing difficulty in speech and in controlling salivation. The jaw jerk is also exaggerated. Some important causes of paralysis of the bulbar nerves are shown in Inset 1.9.

Inset 1.9: Important Conditions Associated with Lower Cranial Nerve Palsies (9th-12th) Bulbar Palsy

Lower motor neuron type–poliomyelitis, GBS, diphtheria, botulism, myasthenia, tumour commonly brainstem tumours, brainstem encephalitis, Arnold Chiary malformation.

Upper motor neuron type (Pseudo bulbar palsy)–vascular lesions, demyelinations, spastic CP.

Supranuclear Control of Cranial Nerves

It is important to take note of supranuclear control of certain cranial nerves that gives important clinical findings. The 7th cranial nerve supplies the face including the forehead. The upper part of forehead is bilaterally innervated. The lower part of the face receives control only from the opposite hemisphere's facial motor cortex (This probably helps in better control of facial expression). Cranial nerves 3rd, 4th and 6th are controlled by the hemispheres via the horizontal and vertical gaze centers in the brainstem. Lesions of cerebral hemispheres can produce gaze palsies, like some lesions of the brainstem.

Cranial nerves 5th and 9th-12th are bilaterally innervated, like the forehead. Because of these the tongue and palate and muscles of mastication and swallowing move as a whole, both sides moving at the same time together.

MOTOR SYSTEM

Muscle Bulk: It is tested as usual by observation of muscle size and palpating for the feel.

Tone: Tone is examined as usual, by passive movements at joints. It is important to see that while examining the tone, the child is not putting up voluntary resistance. In fretful infants and young children, one must wait for the moment when he is relatively relaxed and not putting up any voluntary resistance. Hypertonia, commonly spastic type, is seen in upper motor type of lesions. Hypotonia, classically seen in lower motor neuron type of lesions, is however found to occur in a wide variety of disorders in children as shown in Inset 1.10.

Inset 1.10: Some Common and Important Causes of Hypotonia

Central–diffuse intracranial pathology like coma, meningo-encephalitis, intracranial structural lesion – congenital and acquired, neurodevelopmental abnormalities and mental retardation, toxic and metabolic encephalopathies, cerebellar disease,

Peripheral–lower motor neuron disorders–like motor neuron disease, peripheral neuropathies, neuromuscular disorders like SMA, congenital myopathies, myasthenia.

Miscellaneous PEM, hypokalemia, certain metabolic disorders specially IEM, some cases with congenital malformation and many genetic / chromosomal disorders like Down syndrome, Prader-Willi syndrome.

Power: In older children and even the younger ones muscle power is tested by the standard *pull-push* technique. This technique measures the kinetic power of the muscle. In younger children it is often easier to measure the static power of muscles by asking the child to hold a limb still after steadying it in a particular position and the examiner attempting to move it in the desired direction. The ability of the child to resist the movement indicates the power of the muscles concerned. The muscle power thus assessed may be graded according to MRC scale, i.e., 0=no detectable contraction, 1=some muscle contraction but no movement at joint, 2=active movement with gravity eliminated, 3=active movement against gravity but not resistance, 4=active movement against gravity and resistance simultaneously, 5=normal power.

In infants and young children, *observation of movements*, spontaneous or stimulated, is a useful way of assessing gross muscle power. Good active movement of the body and the extremities suggest good muscle power. During such active movements the examiner may catch hold of a limb and feel the resistance and even exert force; this way reasonable grading of muscle power is also possible. By asking, the child to sit down and then get up, the examiner can have fair idea of the power of muscles of the hip, thighs and legs. Power of shoulder girdle muscles can be tested by holding up the infant or the young child by the axillae, if the shoulder girdle muscles are weak the infant tends to slip or even slips down. The power of the muscles of the hands as a whole can be tested by letting the infant grasp the examiner's fingers tightly and then the examiner trying to pull out his finger.

Good examination of muscle bulk, tone and power along with reflexes (described below) guides to the correct detection of various disorders namely monoplegia, hemiplegia, paraplegia, quadriplegia and a large number of neuromuscular disorders. Tone and reflexes help in determining whether the muscular weakness is of lower motor neuron type (having hypotonia and hyporeflexia) or upper neuron type (hypertonia and hyperreflexia). Upper motor neuron type of weakness implicates some pathology in the brain and spinal cord, lower motor neuron type of weakness implicates some pathology in the cranial nerve nuclei, and the peripheral nerves (Inset 1.11).

Inset 1.11: Important Causes of Muscular Weakness

(a) Upper Motor Neuron Type:

Intracranial lesions–trauma, infections like meningitis, encephalitis, ICSOL-like brain abscess, brain tumour, AVMs, stroke, other intracranial structural lesions–congenital and acquired like gliosis, cysts, atrophy, cerebral palsy, certain neurometabolic and neurodegenerative disorders.

Spinal cord lesions–commonly trauma, infections like transverse myelitis, tuberculosis of spine, syringomyelia, AVM and CV anomaly, abscess, tumour.

(b) Lower Motor Neuron Type:

Poliomyelitis, GBS, peripheral nerve injury, Erb's palsy, lumbar myelomeningocele.

(c) Primarily Muscular:

A wide variety of neuromuscular disorders.

In practice, however, many acute intracranial and even spinal cord disorders in children initially have lower motor neuron type of weakness; it needs careful evaluation and consideration several facts and findings together before coming to a conclusion. Thus hypotonia and hyporeflexia of extremities are common in meningitis and encephalitis. In stroke with acute onset hemiplegia there is often hypotonia and hyperreflexia, but the plantar reflex may be extensor; at times the plantar reflex also may be flexor. In established upper motor neuron diseases, also the classic findings may not be seen at times due to disuse muscular atrophy and contractures.

If neurogenic muscular weakness is found on examination, *localization* of the pathology/lesion has to be done and this involves consideration of:

(a) Finding accurately the muscles that are weak and what are their nerve supplies.

(b) Reflexes that are lost that tells the spinal segment involved.

(c) The area/level of sensory loss that tells the cutaneous innervation of the sensory roots / the dermatome; and

(d) The relation between the spinal segment and the vertebrae since spinal segments do not correspond numerically to the overlying vertebrae because of disproportionate differential growth of the spine and the spinal cord (the spinal cord ends at the level of the lower border of the first lumbar vertebra. Muscular weakness can be in the form of hemiplegia, paraplegia or monoplegia that can be brachial (upper extremity) or crural (lower extremity) or patchy (as seen in poliomyelitis).

Coordination

In the upper extremities, it is easily tested by the standard finger-nose-finger test. The examiner's finger should be within the field of vision of the child and within easy range of his outstretched arm. The test should be done rapidly testing each upper limb in turn. The examiner's finger may be shifted with each repetition to increase the difficulty.

Dysdiadochokinesis is also frequently used to test the coordination in upper limb. It is however not easy for young children to perform the rapid pronation-supination movement required and a verity of techniques have been used to elicit these movements like:

(a) Tapping on the examiner's hand or on some surface or on the child's own knee with the palm and then the dorsum of his hand alternately.

(b) Clapping hands with alternating movements of the palms, right upon left and then left upon right (simulating chapati making in India).

(c) Child tapping on the examiner's palm and then the examiner tapping on the child's palm.

(d) Child holding an object like a reflex hammer and turning it back and forth in a rhythmic manner; and

(e) Examiner himself doing pronation-supination of his hand and asking the child to mimic it simultaneously with his hand. Whatever is the technique, the rapidity of the movement should be increased gradually, and both the hands should be tested individually and/or together.

Coordination in the lower limb is tested by the standard heel-knee-shin test. Other tests that are often useful and easily performed by the young child are standing erect with feet together first with eyes open then eyes closed, standing on one leg, hopping on one leg, walking in straight line, walking heel to toe in one line (tandem walking), walking on inside or outside of the sole (Fog test*).* Important disorders associated with in-coordination are shown in Inset 1.12.

Inset 1.12: Common Disorders Associated with In-coordination
Cerebellar disorders – acute cerebellar ataxia, congenital anomalies, i.e., hypoplasia, aplasia, tumour, abscess, metastatic lesions, ataxia telangiectasia, *posterior column lesions, clumsy child.*

In infants and young children coordination can be tested by offering an object and observing the approach and manipulation. If gross in-coordination is present the infant shows tremulous movements of the hands and distractions as he approaches the object. Such movements can also be seen during other manipulatory activities like picking up objects, holding a spoon or a toy and manipulating buttons. Gross intention tremor may be observed while an infant brings his hand to his mouth. Ataxia is well observed during movement and even standing.

Involuntary Movements

Abnormal involuntary movements like chorea, athetosis, dystonia, tetany, ticks, tremor, convulsions, myoclonus and fasciculations should be looked for during examination. Fasciculations are commonly seen in SMA frequently in the tongue. Contractions of the tongue on percussion, is characteristically seen in myotonia. In infants and children with seizures Chvostek's sign and Erb's sign should be elicited specially if there are signs of rickets where positive tests may suggest hypocalcemia as the cause.

It is also worthwhile noting *associated movements* and *mirror movements*. Associated movements like swinging of the arm while walking are lost in cases of hemiplegia. In mirror movement, a movement made on one side of the body is simultaneously reproduced on the other side; for example while performing dysdiadochokinesis test with one hand, a preschooler often exhibit marked mirroring of the movement on the other hand as well, the significance of mirror movement is however not very clear. Strong mirror movements may cause disability in play activities of the child. Mirror movements usually disappear by about 10 years of age.

SENSORY SYSTEM

In infants and young children the examination of the sensory system, that involves clear expression of certain feelings and accurate response to commands, is difficult and results have to be interpreted with caution. Pain is the only modality that can be tested reliably in infants and young children. The child shows the response by withdrawal, change in facial expression and even crying. The stimulus should be such as to just elicit the response and not to hurt the child.

The examination where possible, should include tests for *spinothalamic tract* (touch, pain, temperature and pressure), *posterior column* (sense of position, sense of vibration) and *cortical sensation* (steriognosis, graphesthesia, two-point discrimination and double simultaneous stimulation). Romberg's sign should be attempted in all cases of ataxia. It is positive (ataxia develops on closure of the eyes) in disorders involving the posterior column.

Autonomic dysfunctions like excessive sweating, as seen in familial dysautonomia should also be looked for. While testing for pain one may come across with cases of congenital insensitivity to pain; it is usually associated with anhidrosis. Common sensory abnormalities are shown in Inset 1.13.

Inset 1.13: Common Sensory Abnormalities in Children
Localised/segmental hypoesthesia/anesthesia/hyperalgesia–post traumatic, burn, leprosy, various peripheral neuropathy (lead, diphtheria, leucodystrophy) spinal cord lesion like trauma, tumour, tuberculosis, transverse myelitis, syringomyelia (dissociated sensory loss, usually segmental).
Generalised–congenital insensitivity to pain.

REFLEXES

All the superficial and deep tendon reflexes should be elicited in standard way. While eliciting reflexes it is important to see that the child is relatively comfortable and relaxed and not putting up any voluntary resistance. In fretful young infants and children one may have to wait to have the child in such a state. The result of testing reflexes should be recorded in one of the five categories: exaggerated, normal, diminished, absent or doubtful as the case may be. The cranial nerves and spinal segments responsible for the reflexes and the common pathologies encountered are shown in Inset 1.14 and Inset 1.15.

Inset 1.14: Reflexes and Nerve Supply

Superficial reflexes dependent on cranial nerves:

Conjunctival (5th cranial as afferent and 7th cranial nerves as efferent), Corneal (5th cranial nerve as afferent and 7th cranial nerve as efferent), Palatal (5th and 9th cranial nerves as afferents and 10th cranial nerve as efferent), Pupillary (3rd cranial nerve, sympathetic and parasympathetic), Clio-spinal (cervical sympathetic), Jaw jerk (5th nerve).

Superficial reflexes dependent on spinal segments:

Plantar (L-5 and S-1), Anal (S-3 and S-4), Bulbocavernosus (S-3 and S4), Cremasteric (L1 and L2), Abdominal (7th–12th thoracic segment), Scapular (5th cervical to 1st thoracic segment).

Deep tendon reflexes and spinal segments:

Biceps jerk (5th and 6th cervical), Triceps (6th and 7th cervical), Radial supinator (5th and 6th cervical), Knee jerk (2nd, 3rd, 4th lumbar), Ankle jerk (1st and 2nd sacral).

Inset 1.15: Abnormalities of Reflexes and Diagnostic Clue

(a) Superficial reflexes:

Loss of corneal reflex–5th nerve palsy.

Loss of conjunctival reflex–5th nerve palsy.

Exaggerated jaw jerk–supranuclear 5th nerve palsy resulting in pseudobulbar palsy characterized by small and spastic tongue.

Loss of abdominal reflex–pyramidal tract lesion.

Scapular reflex–spinal cord lesion.

Loss of para spinal reflex–spinal cord disorder.

Loss of cremasteric reflex–spinal cord disorder, upper motor neuron lesions.

Loss of anal reflex–spinal cord disorder, paraplegia, meningomyelocele, sacrococcygeal.

Extensor plantar reflex–suggests upper motor neuron diseases except in the infants and some toddlers where the diagnosis may not be authentic since plantar reflex may be physiologically extensor at this age group.

Contd.

Contd.

(b) Deep tendon reflexes:

Loss of / weak deep tendon reflexes–lower motor neuron diseases, neuromuscular disorders.

Exaggerated deep tendon reflexes–upper motor neuron diseases.

Pendular jerks, often observed clearly while eliciting knee jerk–cerebellar disorder

In infants and very young children, certain neonatal reflexes also should be examined, since persistence or untimely disappearance or appearance of these may indicate pathological states like cerebral palsy. These reflexes should include moro, rooting and sucking, grasp, tonic neck reflex, placing and stepping and parachute reflex.

DEVELOPMENTAL EXAMINATION

Developmental examination, aimed at physical verification of status of neurodevelopment of the child, should be done as usual and routine examination should include at least the areas of motor, adaptive (fine motor), language, social and general understanding. The norms of normal development are available in standard pediatric textbooks and also in a few classic monograms on child development. Table 1.1 shows some important developmental landmarks (milestones) that should be useful for a clinician in assessing the neurodevelopment of the child during routine neurologic examination (Gesell and Amatruda, ′47, Illingworth, ′74 Developmental examination is done in children till 5 years of age. In infants and young children, developmental examination is extremely useful in detecting/suspecting cognitive disorders and also other neurological disorders in which neurodevelopmental delay is a common association like cerebral palsy and degenerative brain diseases and many neurometabolic disorders. Developmental examination remains the most valuable tool for diagnosing intellectual deficiency disorder in infants and young children till about 3 years of age.

Table 1.1: Some Common and Important Developmental Landmarks (Milestones) and Their Age at Attainment

Motor Development		Language Development	
Head holding (complete)	3 months	Vocalizes (mostly vowels)	8 weeks
Sitting	6-9 months	Repetitive vowels	6-6.5 months
Pulls self to sitting	10 months	Consonants (repetitive) and Bi-Syllables	9-10 months
Rolls over	5-6 months		
Prone to supine	6 months	1-2 words with meaning	1 year
Creeping and crawling	9-10 months	Jargon	18 months
Standing	11-12 months	3 words with pronoun, verb and object	2 years

Contd.

Contd.

Cruising holding railing	12 months	Almost normal speech	3 years
Walking one hand held	12 months		
Creeps upstairs	15 months		
Creeps downstairs	18 months		
Walks up/downstairs (2 feet/step)	2 years		
Walks downstairs (1feet/step)	3 years		
Runs stiffly	18 months		
Runs well	2 years		
Kicks a ball	2 years		
Jumps	2-2.5 years		
Hops on one foot	4 years		
Skips	5 years		
Adaptive (Fine Motor) Development		**Social Development**	
Palmer grasp	6-7 months	Social smile	6-8 weeks
Grasp – radial digital	9 months	Laughs aloud	16 weeks
Transfer	6 months	Prefers mother	7 months
Index finger approach	9-10 months	Separation anxiety	6-8 months
Pincer grasp	10-12 months	Waves 'by - by'	9 months
Release object	10-12 months	Peek-a- boo	10 months
		Toilet habits:	
		• Indicates wet pants	15 months
		• Partial regulation	15 months
		• Bowel control	15 months
		• Regulated day time	18 months
		• Complete control	2-2.5 years
		Self feeding starts	15 months
		Plays simple games	3 years
		Dressing and undressing self reasonably well	5 years

Certain objective tests are useful in developmental diagnosis in clinical setting. Some of these are shown below:

Builds tower of	2 cubes	15 months
	3 cubes	18 months
	6 cubes	2 years
	9 cubes	3 years
Draws	Circle	3 years
	Cross	4 years
	Square	4 years
	Triangle	5 years
	Diamond	6 years
Draws a man with 2-4 parts		4 years

LOCALIZATION OF PATHOLOGY IN NEUROLOGICAL DISORDERS

Good neurologic examination often helps in pinpointing the site of lesions in many neurological disorders that result from focal pathology. This is because different areas of the brain carry out different/specific functions like speech, cognition and memory, behaviour, vision, hearing, emotion, perception of special sensation and a variety of motor functions. Abnormalities seen in cognitive functions, behaviour, speech, hearing and vision may suggest lesions in cortex. *Cranial nerves* have important localizing value. *Type of lesion*, whether upper motor neuron (UMN) or lower motor neuron (LMN), is extremely valuable in localizing a lesion, upper motor neuron lesion suggesting pyramidal tract lesion and lower motor neuron suggesting nuclear or nerve lesion. Unilateral lesion above foramen magnum results in UMN signs on opposite half of body. Unilateral lesion below the foramen magnum results in UMN signs on same side of the body. The localizing values of some common and important neurologic findings are shown in Table 1.2.

Table 1.2: Diagnostic Value of Some Common Neurologic Findings	
Finding	**Common Diagnostic Clue**
Symptomatic and Observational	
Aphasia, visual field defect, apraxia, neglect	Cortical lesion
Intelligence and memory abnormality	Cortical lesion/HSV/SSPE
Behaviour abnormality	Drug toxicity, Frontal lobe lesion
Headache	SOL, stroke, inf, trauma
Blurred vision/diplopia	Brainstem lesion
Speech arrest/difficulty	Broca's area lesion
Seizure	Diffuse cerebral involvement, SOL, stroke, seizure disorders
Gait, balance, posture disturbance	Cerebellar lesion, posterior column lesion, SOL, cerebral palsy
Tingling numbness	Sensory cortex lesion
Mood disorders	CNS toxicity, psychiatric/psychologic disorders
Cranial Nerve Palsy Related	
1st cranial nerve	Trauma, trigeminal ganglion/nerve lesion, SOL
2nd cranial nerve	Trauma, SOL, stroke
3rd cranial nerve	Mid brain lesion–trauma, SOL, stroke, infection
4th cranial nerve	Pontine lesion–trauma, SOL, stroke, infection
5th cranial nerve	Pontine lesion–trauma, SOL, stroke, infection
6th cranial nerve	Lesion in brainstem/medulla
7th cranial nerve	Pontine lesion–facial palsy LMN type, unilateral facial numbness, unilateral deafness
8th cranial nerve	Trauma, SOL
9th, 10th,11th,12th cranial nerve	Bulbar palsy–poliomyelitis, GBS, botulism
Motor System Related	
Monoplegia of UL (UMN type)	Contralateral hemispheric lesion usually motor cortex
Monoplegia of LL (UMN type)	Contralateral hemispheric lesion usually motor cortex
Hemiplegia with facial nerve involvement	Contralateral hemispheric lesion above pons
Hemiplegia (Rt) with aphasia	Broca's area lesion on left side (with normal dominance)
Hemiplegia (Lt) with neglect, apraxia, cortical sensory loss	Right cortex involvement
Homonymous hemianopia	Vascular lesion–MCA territory, SOL
Hemiplegia with arms and legs affected more severely, no cortical sign, rarely hemianopia	Internal capsular lesion
Hemiplegia with UMN facial palsy	Lesion above brainstem–Usually in internal capsule
Hemiplegia with LMN cranial nerve palsy	Brainstem lesion
Bulbar palsy LMN	Medullary lesion, poliomyelitis, GBS, botulism
Bulbar palsy UMN (Pseudobulbar palsy)	Commonly seen in spastic cerebral palsy
Nystegmus	Brainstem lesion ~ medullo-pontine junction
Cerebellar sign	Cerebellar lesion on same side/damage to crus cerebri
Horner's syndrome–Ipsilateral	Thalamic lesion, medullary lesion, lesion of C8 and T1 roots or a lesion of sympathetic fibers as they climb up the carotid and pass through the cavernous sinus on their way to the eye
Horners's syndrome–Bilateral	Pontine bleed: Pinpoint pupils
Paraplegia or unilateral paresis of lower half of body with sensory level	Spinal cord lesion
Paresis/paralysis of one half of body with cranial nerve palsy	Lesion above cervico-medullary junction (contralateral lesion)
Paresis/paralysis of one half of body without cranial nerve palsy	Lesion below cervico-medullary junction (ipsilateral lesion)
Peripheral weakness of extremities or trunk but no sensory loss	Lesions in anterior horn cell, motor nerve roots or motor nerve
Distal weakness with sensory loss	Peripheral nerve disease
Limb weakness, proximal weakness > distal, no sensory loss	Myopathy

Suggested Reading

- Amiel-Tison C. Grenier A. Neurologic Assessment During the First Year of Life. New York. Oxford University Press. 1986.
- Annett M. Left. Right. Hand and Brain: The Right Shift Theory. Hillsdale. NJ. Erlbaum Associates. 1985.
- Bodensteiner J. Coma. In: Pediatric Neurology for the Clinician. David RB (ed) Norwalk. Connecticut. Appleton and Lange 1992:537-45.
- Berger JR. Stupor and Coma. In: Neurology in Clinical Practice. 5th Edition. Eds: Bradley WG. Daroff RB. Fenichel GM. Jancovic J. Butterworth Heineman. Philadelphia 2008: 39-58.
- Connoly K. Stration P. Developmental Changes in Associated Movements. Dev Med Child Neurol 1968:49-56.
- Glynn M. Walker. RWH. In: Hutchinson's Clinical Method. 23rd Edition. Eds: Glynn M. Drake W Saunders. Edinburgh 2012:283-329.
- Gesell A and Amatruda CS. Developmental Diagnosis. Hoeber. New York. 1947.
- Glaser JS. Neuro-ophthalmology. New York. Harper and Row. 1978.
- Illingworth RS. Normal Development. In: Development of the Infant and Young Child Normal and Abnormal. 5th Edition. Edinburg. Churchill Livingstone 1974:137-76.
- Kirkham TH. Neuro-ophthalmology. In: Pediatric Neurology. Rose FC (Ed). Oxford. Blackwell Scientific Publications 1979:425-37.
- Paine RS. Neurologic Examination of Infants and Children. Pediatric Clin North America 1960:7:471-510.
- Paine RS. Oppe TE. Neurologic Examination of Children. In: Clinics in Developmental Medicine. Nos 20/21. London SIMP/Heinemann. 1966.
- Ross G. Lipper E. Auld P. Hand Preference in 4-Year-Old Children: Relation to Prematurity. Dev. Med. Child Neurol 1987:26:615-22.
- Swaiman KF. Brown LW. Neurologic Examination After the Newborn Period Until 2 Years of Age. In: Swaiman's Pediatric Neurology Principles and Practice. 5th Edition. Ed: Swaiman KF. Ashwal S. Ferrerio DM. Schor NE. Elsevier. 2012.
- Touwen BCL. Prechtl HFR. The Neurologic Examination of the Child with Minor Central Nervous System Dysfunction. London. Spastic International. 1970.
- Taylor D. Hoyt CS. Pediatric Ophthalmology and Strabismus. 3rd Edition. Elsevier Saunders. Edinburgh. 2005.

2 Chapter

IMAGING IN DEVELOPMENTAL ANOMALIES OF BRAIN AND SPINE

Arun Kumar Gupta, Shivanand Gamanagatti, Atin Kumar, Manisha Jana

NEUROIMAGING IN DEVELOPMENTAL ANOMALIES OF BRAIN AND SPINE

The appearance of congenital brain anomalies is best understood in context of normal fetal brain development. At approximately 20 days' gestation, the neural tube is formed with the coaptation of the primitive neural folds. Progressive closure of the tube ensues in a bi-directional fashion, both craniad and caudad. By 25 days, the anterior end closes, and by 28 days, the caudal or posterior end closes. Subsequent development of 3 components (vesicles) at the cranial portion of the neural tube constitutes formation of the prosencephalon, mesencephalon and the rhombencephalon. Between 5 and 10 weeks, there is further differentiation of these structures. The prosencephalon will eventually develop into the telencephalon (the precursor of the cerebrum) and the diencephalon. The rhombencephalon differentiates into the myelencephalon (which forms the pons and medulla) and the metencephalon, which forms the cerebellum. At 7 weeks, the germinal matrix forms, and during the second through the fifth month cellular proliferation and migration occur. After the fifth month, cortical organization and myelination transpire, and continue postpartum. Any insult, which affects the brain during the crucial period of neuronal differentiation, migration and organization, will have a relatively predictable impact on subsequent brain development. In fact, the timing of the insult, rather than the type of insult (vascular, infectious, traumatic, etc.) primarily determines the subsequent malformation.[1,2] Imaging studies have tremendous role in diagnosis of developmental disorders.

EMBRYOLOGY

Neurulation

Dorsal induction is the first stage in the formation and closure of the neural tube. This occurs at weeks 3-4 gestation. The first phase of neurulation leads to the formation of the neural tube, which will be the foundation for the brain and spinal cord. The second phase and third phase of dorsal induction involving canalization and retrogressive differentiation leads to the formation of the caudal part of the neural tube and subsequent defects with these two phases lead to such things as sacral agenesis, caudal regression syndromes, lipomas and tethered cords.

During **neurulation (phase 1)**, there is formation of embryonic ectoderm dorsal to the node cord, and this thickens to form a neural plate. The neuro ectoderm will invaginate along its central axis to form the neural groove with neural folds on either side. This will then close like a zipper to form the neural tube. With abnormal closure of the neural tube, problems such as cephaloceles and spinal dysraphisms as well as anencephaly can easily occur (details of spinal anomalies discussed later in this chapter).

In **stage 2 of ventral induction**, there is formation of the brain and face by the formation of vesicles. Three main vesicles form. These are the prosencephalon (which eventually forms the cerebral hemispheres) and the thalamus, the mesencephalon (which forms the mid-brain), and the Rhombencephalon (which will form the pons, cerebellum and medulla). During this time, the face also develops such that facial anomalies may accompany brain anomalies during ventral induction. These anomalies include the holoprosencephalies, corpus callosal agenesis and Dandy-Walker.[3,4]

Stage 3 (Migration and Histiogenesis)

These two processes occur about the same time between two to five months of gestation. Neuronal migration proceeds from the germinal matrix to the cortex. Disorders of migration include the heterotopias, agyria-Pachygyria, polymicrogyria. Disorders of histiogenesis include the phakomatosis. It should be noted that often phakomatosis may also involve certain gray matter heterotopias (e.g., Tuberous sclerosis have a subependymal tumors that most likely represent failure of n euronal migration). In addition, vascular malformations and teratomas may also form at this time.

Stage 4 (Myelination)

This is the formation of white matter which generally proceeds from more primitive areas to more advanced areas of the brain. Thus one might see this occurring from an inferior to a superior direction and from a posterior to anterior direction. This occurs between approximately five and fifteen months and should be mature by three years of age. Failure of myelination would lead to developmental delay as well as to demyelinating diseases.[3,4]

Imaging Techniques

Magnetic resonance imaging has supplanted computed tomography (CT) as the modality of choice for most categories of central nervous system (CNS) pathology. The multiplanar capabilities of MRI provide unsurpassed visualization of brain structures. Its superior contrast resolution provided by the multiple sequences, which are available exploit the various tissue characteristics of normal and pathologic structures. MR is exquisitely sensitive for the detection of both solid and cystic lesions within the brain, and for depicting aberrant anatomic structures. This allows accurate assessment of congenital malformations, which affect the CNS.[3]

Routine MR Imaging Sequences: Sagittal T1-weighted sequence should be performed in all patients, which allows assessment of the midline structures. After obtaining sagittal images, axial T1 and T2 weighted (T2W) images should be obtained in all patients. Three-dimensional gradient echo (GE) techniques using either SPGR or 3D-FLASH can also be used to acquire T1W images. These gradient sequences have the ability to acquire very thin (<1mm) contiguous images in a relatively very short imaging time. Fluid attenuated inversion recovery (FLAIR) sequence should be used as a secondary sequence in patients with focal neurological deficits but normal looking standard sequences because of high sensitivity of FLAIR for subtle lesions. After the sagittal and axial images have been obtained, coronal FSE-T2W images may be obtained. T2W GE images are useful in the evaluation of vascular malformations and hemorrhage because they are sensitive to the magnetic susceptibility changes and local heterogeneity of magnetic fields.[3,5]

Diffusion Tensor Imaging and Fiber Tractography

- Data processing done by using the Fiber Assignment by Continuous Tracking (FACT) method to achieve 3-dimensional FT images.
- Image acquisition time 7-9 minutes.
- Post-processing time < 5 minutes.
- Excellent demonstration of white matter architecture.
- May be useful in describing the aberrant fiber connections and provides a better understanding of the pathogenetic mechanisms.
- **Caveats:** Fiber tracking technique is quite operator dependent. DTI-FT depends considerably on a qualitative visual analysis by the radiologist.

Classification

Stage 1	**Dorsal Induction: Formation and Closure of the Neural Tube** Weeks 3-4 Three phases: Neurulation, canalization, retrogressive differentiation Failure: Anencephaly Cephalocele Chiari Spinal dysraphism
Stage 2	**Ventral Induction: Formation of the Brain Segments and Face** Weeks 5-10 Three vesicles (prosencephalon, mesencephalon and rhombencephalon) form the cerebrum, mid-brain, cerebellum, and lower brainstem. Division into two hemispheres Failure: Holoprosencephalies Corpus callosum agenesis Dandy-Walker Facial anomalies
Stage 3	**Migration and Histogenesis** Neuronal migration from germinal matrix to the cortex. Cellular differentiation Months 2-5 Disorders: Heterotopias, agyria-pachyria, polymicrogyria, vascular malformations, teratomas, phakomatosis
Stage 4	**Myelination** Inferior to superior; posterior to anterior 5-15 months; matures by 3 years Failure: Developmental delay, dysmyelinating disease

1. DISORDERS RELATED TO DORSAL INDUCTION (NURULATION STAGE 1)

Encephalocele

An encephalocele is a developmental abnormality in which part of the CNS herniates through a cranial defect. Encephaloceles can be classified as containing only CSF and meninges (meningocele), neural tissue and meninges (meningoencephalocele), or neural tissue, meninges, and ventricle (hydroencephalomeningocele). Encephaloceles represent approximately 10-15% of all neural tube defects (NTD). Of all encephaloceles, those located in the occipital region (~80%) are the most common (Fig. 2.1) in North America, and are easily diagnosed at birth. While routine use of ultrasound has been helpful in the prenatal diagnosis, maternal alpha-fetoprotein levels are often normal since the lesions are usually completely epithelialized and hence do not leak AFP. Upon delivery diagnosis, further imaging is critical for treatment planning regardless of the size of the defect. MRI and MRA have become the standard in pre-operative evaluation. MRI/A is critical in determining the extent of neural tissue herniation into the defect, a factor which is generally considered one of the most important prognostic indicators. In addition, operative planning with regards to venous sinus drainage can be determined.

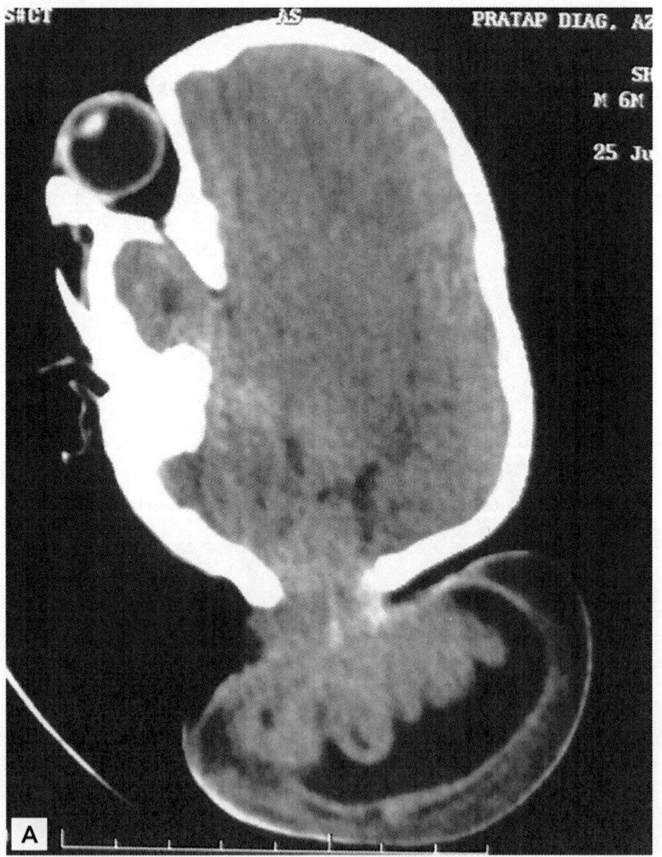

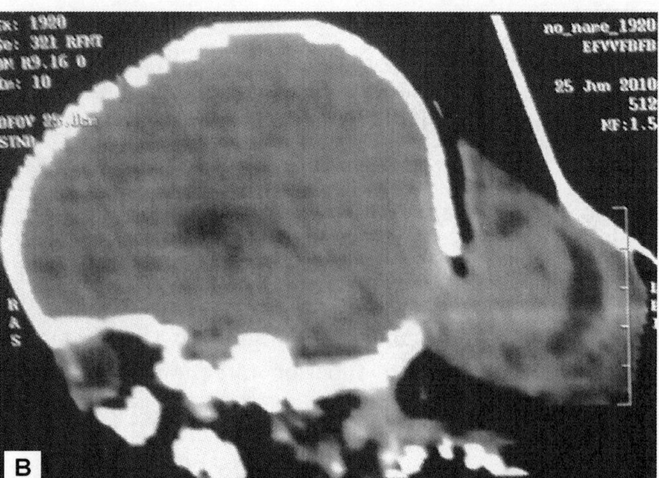

Fig. 2.1: Occipital meningoencephalocele: Axial (A) and sagittal reformatted NCCT image showing herniation of neural tissue and meninges through occipital defect (B)

Complete CNS imaging is important since 15-20% of children have additional severe CNS defects including NTDs, Dandy-Walker, Chiari II/III, hydrocephalus and optic nerve malformations, all of which can decrease long-term functional status and overall operative success.[6,7]

Arnold-Chiari Malformation (ACM)

A malformation of the brainstem that may or may not be associated with hydrocephalus, described by Chiari in 1891. Four different forms were identified by Chiari, according to the degree of severity of the developmental anomaly of the hindbrain.

Chiari I malformation involves caudal displacement of the cerebellar tonsils, and sometimes the inferior vermis, through the foramen magnum into the rostral cervical spinal canal. The amount of normal extension below the foramen magnum varies with age. The maximum normal level for the cerebellar tonsils to extend below the foramen magnum in the first decade of life is 6 mm, the second and third decade of life 5 mm, and the fourth through eighth decades of life 4 mm, and the ninth decade and beyond 3 mm. The fourth ventricle is usually normal in position but attenuated in shape. The cisterna magna is usually small or absent.

The Chiari II malformation involves displacement of the brainstem and lower cerebellum into the cervical spinal canal (Fig. 2.2). In such cases, the fourth ventricle is caudally displaced and extends below the foramen magnum. Type II abnormality is nearly always associated with lumbar myelomeningoceles.

Chiari III malformation involves downward displacement of the medulla with herniation of the cerebellum initially through the foramen magnum, then

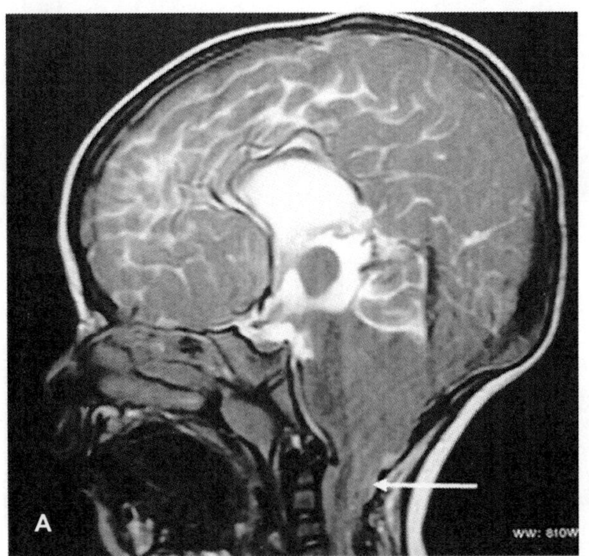

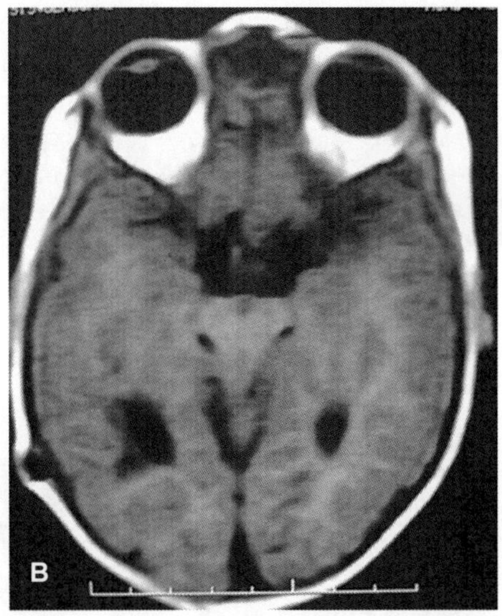

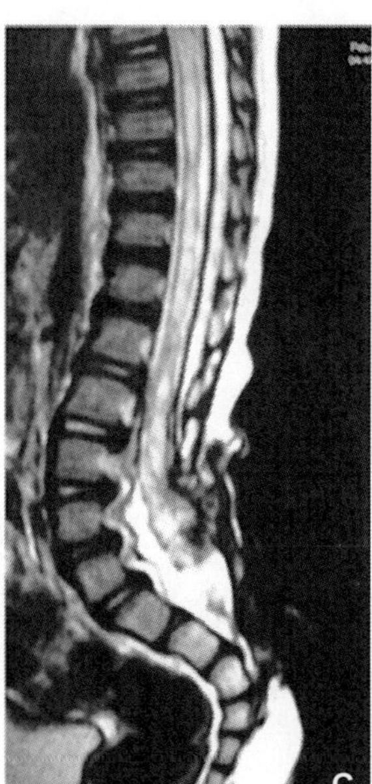

Fig. 2.2: Type II Chiari malformation: Sagittal T2W (A), axial T1W (B) MR image showing herniation of cerebellar tonsils through foramen magnum, small posterior fossa. The patient has lumbosacral meningomyelocele which was operated at birth. Sagittal T2WI of the lumbar spine (C) shows the open spina bifida

dorsally through a cervical spina bifida, resulting in a cervical encephalocele.

Chiari IV malformation is a severe cerebellar hypoplasia without displacement of brain through the foramen magnum.

MR clearly shows all the features of the different types of Chiari anomaly, particularly on sagittal T1-weighted image, but coronal views may also be useful. Since the advent of MR it has become apparent that Chiari I anomaly is more frequently found than expected, mainly asymptomatic; it is not always easy to distinguish this condition from the even more frequent mild cerebellar ectopia, a condition in which the tonsils may be positioned low, although by not more than 3 mm, below the inferior border of the foramen magnum.[8,9,10] The pointed morphology of the cerebellar tonsils is also helpful in distinguishing Chiari I malformations from low-lying tonsils.

CSF flow at the level of the foramen magnum may be disturbed by tonsillar ectopia; according to some author, this may cause hydrosyringomyelia, frequently associated with Chiari anomaly. According to other pathogenetic theories *hydrosyringomyelia* is only part of a more complex dysraphic pattern such as mesencephalic beaking, or the frequently associated bony anomalies at the level of the craniovertebral junction.[3]

2. DISORDERS RELATE TO VENTRAL INDUCTION (NURULATION STAGE 2)

Holoprosencephaly

Holoprosencephaly results from failure of anatomic division of the primitive forebrain. The prosencephalon fails to divide and form the diencephalon and telencephalon. The cerebral hemispheres do not form due to failure of cleavage of the telencephalon. This results in a grossly dysmorphic brain which is variable in severity. There are variable degrees of differentiation and division of the primitive brain structures, which are encountered. A classification system proposed by DeMyer allows a general categorization of this entity, although these abnormalities describe spectrum of severity. Thus, a given patient may not display all of the characteristics of a single form of holoprosencephaly.

Alobar holoprosencephaly is the most severe form. There is complete failure of telencephalon cleavage to form the cerebral hemispheres. Thus the falx and interhemispheric fissure are absent. The thalami are fused, and therefore there is no intervening third ventricle. A holoventricle is seen adjacent to the small, deformed cerebrum. Severe midline facial anomalies accompany this form of holoprosencephaly.[11]

Semilobar holoprosencephaly is a less severe cleavage deformity in which the dorsal portion of the cerebrum is divided into distinct hemispheres with an intervening fissure and falx. Likewise, there is partial separation of the thalami, between which there is usually a small, malformed third ventricle. The dorsal portion of the corpus callosum may be present as well.

Lobar holoprosencephaly is the least severe form of this group of anomalies. All but the most anterior portion of the interhemispheric fissure is present, where there is continuity of the frontal lobes. The septum pellucidum is absent, and there is variable formation of the anterior portion of the callosum. Patients with this mild form of holoprosencephaly may have normal facial features[3,8] (Fig. 2.3).

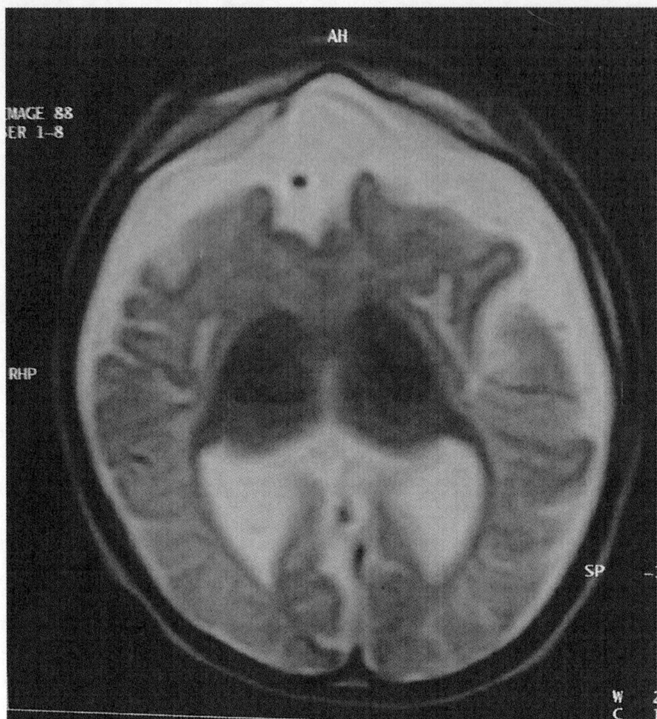

Fig. 2.3: Lobar holoproscencephaly: Axial MR image showing, presence of most anterior portion of the interhemispheric fissure, absence of septum pellucidum, and there is variable formation of the anterior portion of the callosum

Corpus Callosal Agenesis (ACC)

The corpus callosum develops from the lamina reuniens in the telencephalon, and it begins to appear between the anterior and hippocampal commissures at about 10.5 weeks. The adult form of the corpus callosum is achieved by 17 weeks' gestational age. Initial formation of the corpus callosum occurs in the genu and the body, progressing posteriorly. The anterior genu and rostrum develops last, folding back under the genu. The callosum thickens with increasing myelination.

ACC can be complete (Fig. 2.4), partial, or atypical. With complete agenesis, the corpus callosum is totally absent.

With partial agenesis (hypoplasia), the anterior portion (posterior genu and anterior body) is formed, but the posterior portion (posterior body and splenium) is not formed. The rostrum and the anterior/inferior genu are also not formed.

Secondary destruction of corpus callosum occurs when the genu and anterior body are destroyed, leaving the posterior portion of the corpus callosum intact. This can occur secondary to porencephaly or schizencephaly, in transcallosal surgical approaches to the lateral and third ventricle, and with hemisection of the callosum for the treatment of seizures.

Other cerebral malformations may coexist with callosal dysgenesis. Examples of these include inter-

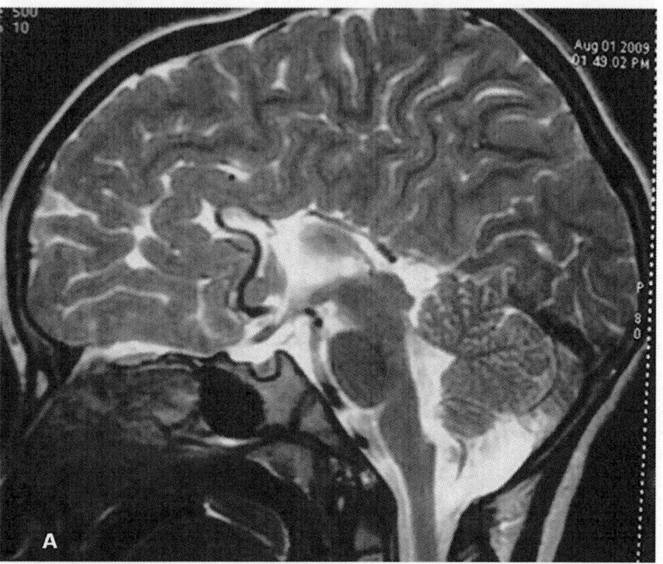

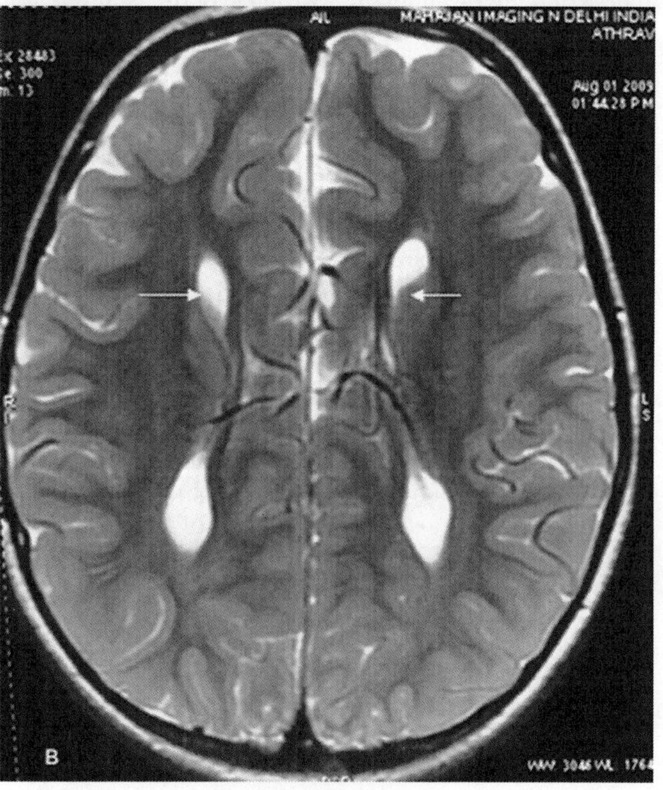

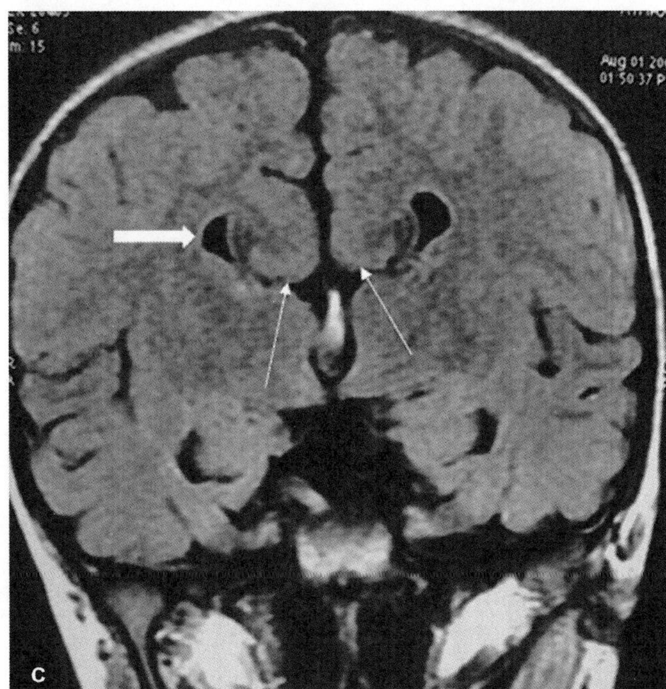

Fig. 2.4: Corpus Callosal Agenesis: Sagittal T2W MR image (A) showing absence of corpus callosum, axial T2W image (B) showing parallel lateral ventricles, coronal FLAIR image (C) shows viking-head appearance of frontal horns (black arrow), and the Probst bundles (arrow)

hemispheric cysts; intracranial lipomas (Fig. 2.5); and disorders of neuronal migration, such as schizencephaly, neuronal heterotopias, lissencephaly, and pachygyria. CNS anomalies (85%), Dandy-Walker cyst (11%), Interhemispheric cysts, Hydrocephalus (30%), Midline lipoma of corpus callosum (10%), Arnold-Chiari malformation (7%), Midline encephalocele, Porencephaly, Holoprosencephaly.[12,13]

Imaging Features: When the corpus callosum is absent, the third ventricle is often high riding, extending superiorly between the lateral ventricles. On coronal imaging, a candelabra appearance occurs, with the third ventricle forming the central vertical portion and the lateral ventricles the peripheral arms of the candelabra. On axial imaging, the lateral ventricles are parallel. The occipital horns of the lateral ventricles are dilated in patients with ACC, probably because of a deficiency of peritrigonal white matter fibers. This anatomic finding is known as colpocephaly (Fig. 2.4).

Medial to the lateral ventricles, longitudinal bundles of white matter are present. These are known as Probst bundles and presumably would have formed a normal corpus callosum. Probst bundles are seen best on coronal or axial T1-weighted MRIs (Fig. 2.4). When the corpus callosum is absent, the cingulate gyrus is inverted, the

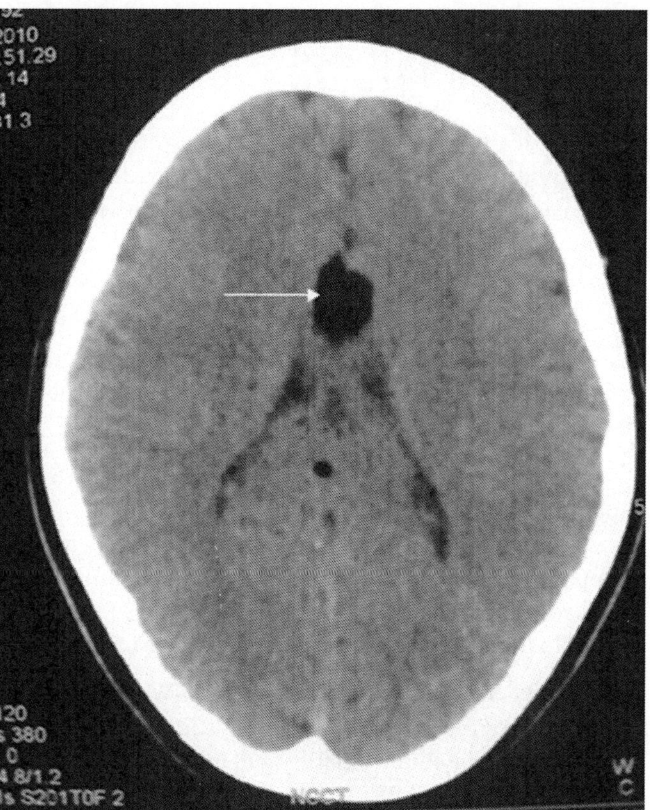

Fig. 2.5: Corpus Callosal Lipoma. Axial NCCT image of brain shows hypodense lesion in anterior interhemispheric location (arrow)

normal cingulate sulcus is absent, and the medial cerebral sulci radiate toward the midline in a radial configuration. This finding is especially helpful in evaluating newborns in whom the corpus callosum is normally thin.

The hippocampal formations are frequently hypoplastic in patients with ACC, with resulting mild dilatation of the temporal horns. Associated midline cysts are noted in some cases. The exact origin and nature of these cysts is controversial. While some of these cysts represent a dilated superiorly migrated third ventricle, others represent true midline cysts that may be lined by ependymal cells or by arachnoid membranes.

Dandy-Walker Malformation

Dandy-Walker malformation is a rare congenital malformation and involves the cerebellum and fourth ventricle. The condition is characterized by agenesis or hypoplasia of the cerebellar vermis, cystic dilatation of the fourth ventricle, and enlargement of the posterior fossa. A large number of concomitant problems may be present, but the syndrome exists whenever these 3 features are found. Approximately 70-90% of patients have hydrocephalus, which often develops postnatally. Dandy-

Walker malformation may be associated with atresia of the foramen of Magendie and, possibly, the foramen of Luschka.

Classically, posterior fossa cystic malformations have been divided into Dandy-Walker malformation, Dandy-Walker variant, mega cisterna magna, and posterior fossa arachnoid cyst. Precisely differentiating the malformations may be possible using imaging methods.

Dandy-Walker malformation, variant, and mega cisterna magna currently are believed to represent a continuum of developmental anomalies on a spectrum that has been termed the Dandy-Walker complex.[14]

Dandy-Walker complex is characterized by an enlarged posterior fossa, high position of tentorium with upward displacement of the lateral sinuses, torcular herophili associated with varying degrees of vermian aplasia or hypoplasia, and a cystic dilatation of the fourth ventricle that nearly fills the entire posterior fossa.

Dandy-Walker Variant: Dandy-Walker variant consist of vermian hypoplasia and cystic dilatation of the fourth ventricle without enlargement of the posterior fossa.

Mega Cisterna Magna

The mega cisterna magna consist of an enlarged posterior fossa, secondary to an enlarged cisterna magna, but a normal cerebellar vermis and fourth ventricle.

Arachnoid Cyst

Retrocerebellar arachnoid cysts of developmental origin are uncommon but clinically important. True retro-cerebellar arachnoid cysts displace the fourth ventricle and cerebellum anteriorly and show significant mass effect. Differentiation of posterior fossa arachnoid cyst from Dandy-Walker malformation is essential as surgical therapy differs between the two entities.

Imaging Features of Dandy-Walker Malformation (Fig. 2.6)

- Enlarged posterior fossa.
- Varying degrees of cerebellar and vermian hypoplasia or complete vermian absence.
- Cyst formation in the posterior fossa.
- Vermian remnant is everted above the posterior fossa cyst.
- Hypoplastic cerebellar hemispheres winged antero-laterally (outward) in front of the cyst.
- Obstructive hydrocephalus secondary to cystic dilatation of the fourth ventricle (70-90%).
- Abnormally high position of the straight sinus, torcular herophili and tentorium.
- Sinus confluence and lateral sinuses elevated above the lambdoid sutures (high tentorial insertion = lambdoid-torcular inversion).
- Aqueductal obstruction is an important component since it may affect the need for supratentorial decompression.
- If callosal agenesis coexists (20-25%), development of dilatation of the occipital horns (colpocephaly).
- Brainstem possibly compressed and hypoplastic; degree of pontine hypoplasia related directly to degree of cerebellar hypoplasia.
- Thinning and bulging of occipital bones.

Associated central nervous system (CNS) abnormalities of Dandy-Walker malformation are reported

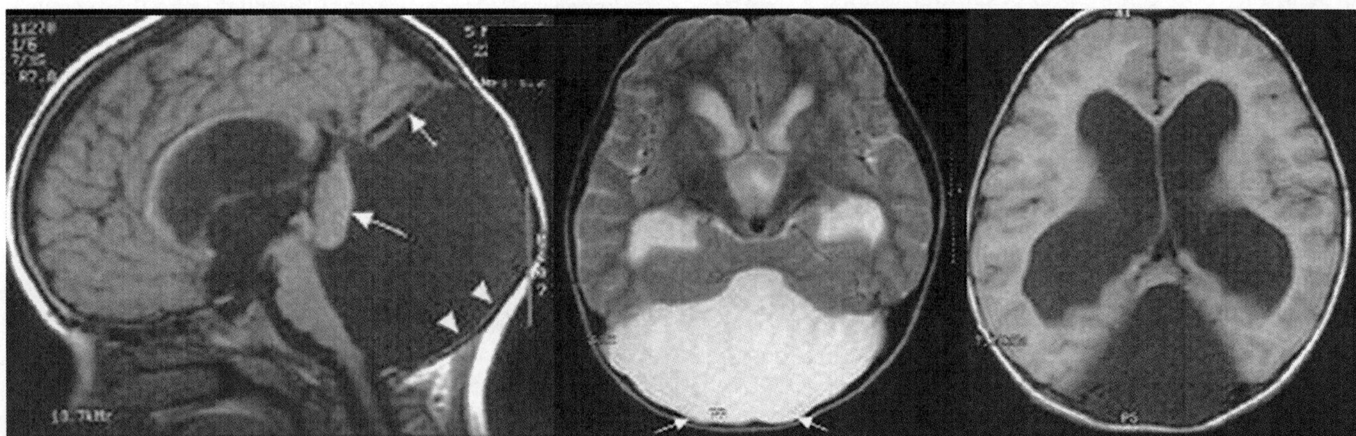

Fig. 2.6: Dandy-Walker malformation: MR images showing, enlarged posterior fossa, posterior fossa cyst, cerebellar hypoplasia and hydrocephalus

in 70% of children. Dysgenesis of corpus callosum, Lipoma of corpus callosum, Holoprosencephaly (25%), Porencephaly, Dysplasia of cingulate gyrus (25%), Schizencephaly, Polymicrogyria/gray matter heterotopia (5-10%), Cerebellar heterotopia, Occipital encephalocele (7%), Microcephaly, Dermoid cysts, Malformation of cerebellar folia (25%), Malformation of inferior olivary nucleus, Hamartoma of tuber cinereum, Syringomyelia, Klippel-Feil deformity.[14,15]

3. DISORDERS RELATED TO MIGRATION AND HISTIOGENESIS (NURULATION STAGE 3)

Agyria/Pachygyria (Lissencephaly)

These are severe migration anomalies. Agyria (complete lack of cortical sulcation) and pachygyria (broad, flat gyri with shallow sulci) often coexist, and represent a spectrum of anomalous brain development. When they are both present, pachygyria is most commonly located in the frontotemporal distribution, while agyria is more commonly encountered in the posterior frontal and parietal lobes. Clinically, patients present with seizures, motor and developmental retardation and coexistent extra-CNS anomalies.[16]

Imaging studies reveal smooth, thick gyri with no or sparse, shallow sulci (Fig. 2.7). The Sylvian fissure is shallow. The brain essentially has the appearance of that of a second trimester fetus. Associated features include a hypoplastic brainstem and occasionally a small dorsal corpus callosum.

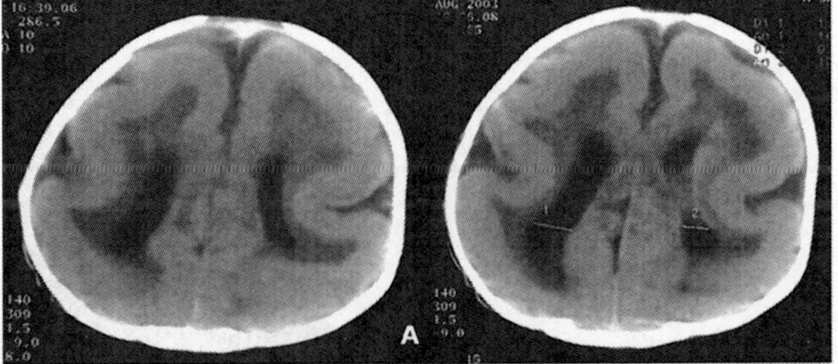

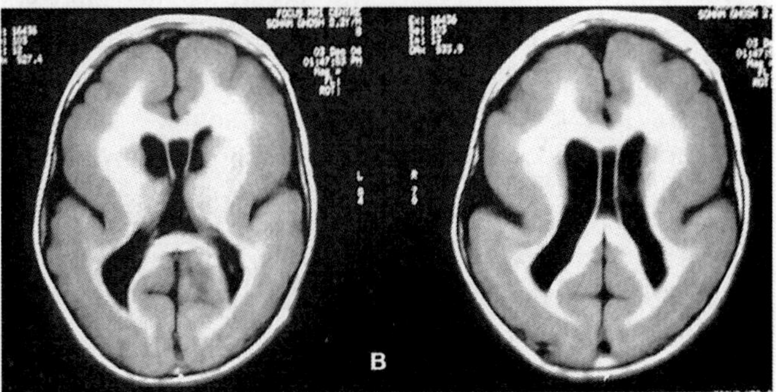

Fig. 2.7: Agyria/Pachygyria: CT (A) and MR (B) images showing thick gyri with no or sparse, shallow sulci

Polymicrogyria

This most often occurs in the middle cerebral artery territory near the posterior aspect of the Sylvian fissure (Fig. 2.8). Grossly, it may appear similar to pachygyria, due to aggregation of small, malformed gyri at the brain surface. This imparts a thickened appearance to the cortical mantle. The presence of gliosis in the subjacent white matter may differentiate it from pachygyria which is not associated with this finding. Prominent vessels may be seen in conjunction with polymicrogyria, usually in the form of large, anomalous draining veins.[15]

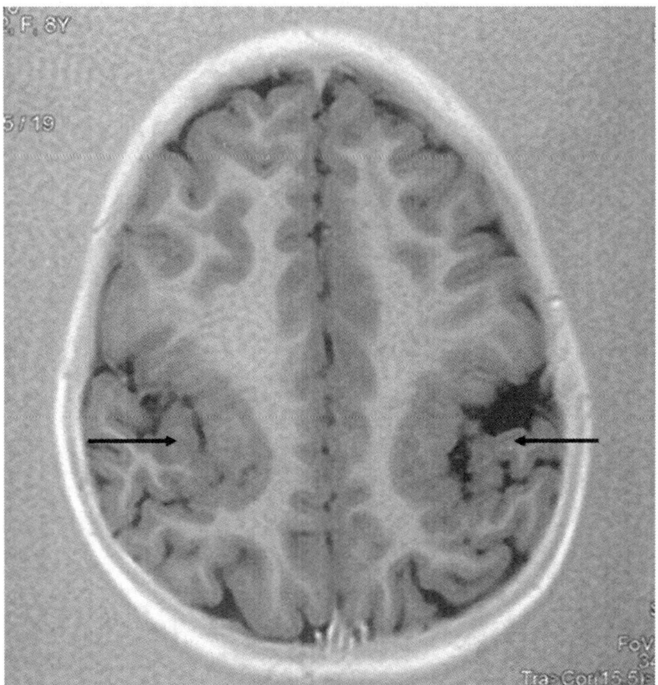

Fig. 2.8: Polymicrogyria: Axial T1W IR MR image shows multiple bilateral small gyri in parasylvian locations (arrows)

Unilateral Megalencephaly

This may include localized regions of both polymicrogyria and pachygyria. In this condition, complete or partial hamartomatous overgrowth of a cerebral hemisphere is accompanied by migration defects, heterotopias and gliotic white matter changes. The involved cortex is nonfunctional, and unfortunately serves as a seizure focus in most patients. In addition to seizures, patients may present with hemiplegia (with or without hemihypertrophy). On imaging studies, the enlarged hemisphere demonstrates morphologic and signal abnormalities such that dysplastic cortex is relatively isointense with the abnormal underlying white matter. The lateral ventricle within the involved hemisphere is enlarged, with abnormal configuration of the frontal horn[17] (Fig. 2.9).

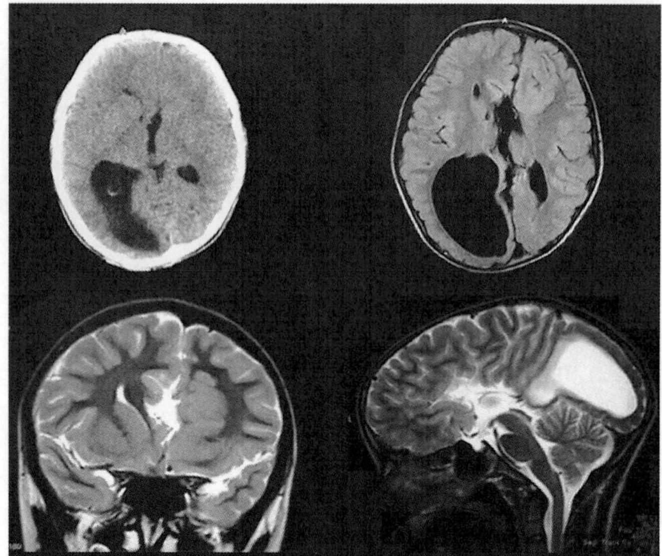

Fig. 2.9: Unilateral hemimegalencephaly: MR images showing enlarged right cerebral hemisphere, lateral ventricle within the involved hemisphere is enlarged, with abnormal configuration of the frontal horn

Schizencephaly

This describes a cleft in the brain, which extends through one or both hemispheres from the lateral ventricle to the cortical surface. The fissure is lined with abnormal gray matter, and there may be close apposition of the bordering parenchyma (closed-lip schizencephaly). If there is intervening CSF between the gray matter-lined margins, it is termed open-lip schizencephaly. Bilateral involvement and an increase in volume of involved parenchyma portend a worse prognosis. Seizures and developmental delay are characteristic clinical features. On imaging studies, the gray matter lined cleft may show evidence of polymicrogyria or other morphological abnormalities. A small dimple in the lateral margin of the ventricle may provide a clue to an otherwise subtle close-lip defect. The septum pellucidum is usually absent[18] (Fig. 2.10).

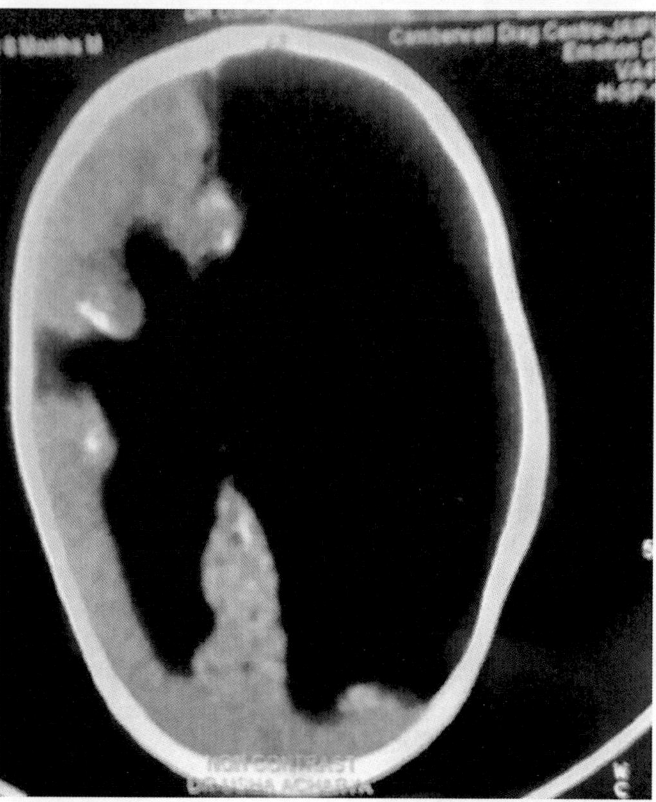

Fig. 2.10: Schizencephaly: Axial NCCT image showing CSF filled cavities bilaterally extending from the lateral ventricle to the cortical surface. Open lip schizencephaly. Note the periventricular calcifications suggestive of perinatal TORCH infection

Heterotopias

Greek word means "ectopic grey matter", i.e., collections of normal neurons in an abnormal location, outside the cortex. Heterotopia is classified as a neuronal migration anomaly and is due to an arrest or damage of migration of the primitive neuroblasts from the germinal matrix to the forming cortex, along the radial glioneuronal fibres. Heterotopia almost always produces seizure disorders, with some variability in clinical presentation.

The anomalies may be focal or diffuse, and subependymal, cortical or mixed in location. For clinical and prognostic purposes they are divided into:

1. Subependymal heterotopia.
2. Subcortical heterotopia.
3. Diffuse grey matter heterotopia, also called band heterotopia or "double cortex" heterotopia.

MR is superior to CT scan in the detection and definition of this kind of anomaly. Heterotopic grey matter appears as round or oval masses that indent the adjacent ventricles and grow into them. Characteristically heterotopia parallels the signal of the cortex in all MR imaging sequences, does not enhance after contrast and lacks surrounding edema.[19,20]

Subependymal heterotopia: The lesions differ from the subependymal hamartomas of tuberous sclerosis which are more irregular in shape, often calcified, not precisely isointense with cortical grey matter and sometimes show contrast enhancement (Fig. 2.11).

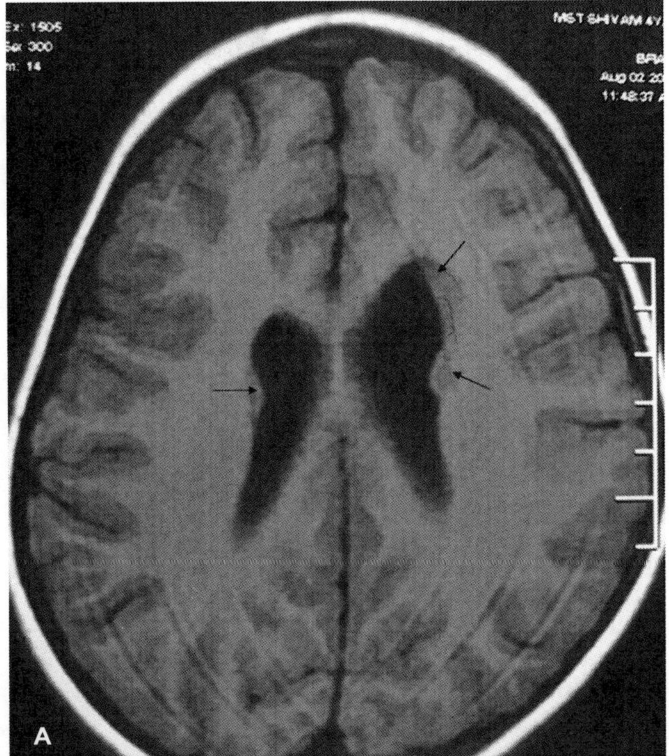

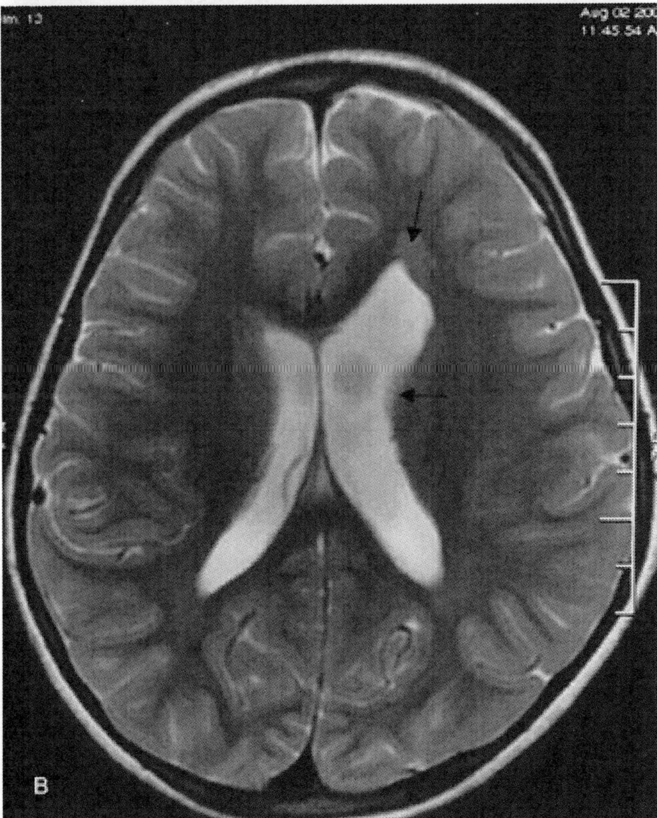

Fig. 2.11: Subependymal heterotopia: Axial T1W (A) and T2W (B) MR image showing, round or oval hypointense masses indenting the adjacent lateral ventricles (arrows) and growing into them

Band heterotopia is a rare type of neuronal migration disorders. A ribbon of heterotopic neurons is located circumferentially beneath the cerebral cortex. Incomplete types of band heterotopia can also occur. On imaging, the overlying cortex may appear normal, atrophic or it may show dysplastic areas.

Subcortical heterotopias may appear as multinodular, swirling or curvilinear masses of grey matter. The overlying cortex is often abnormal with thin cortex and shallow sulci. Associated congenital malformations such as agenesis of the corpus callosum are frequent. The affected hemisphere may also be small. The clinical manifestations of grey matter heterotopia is very variable.

Focal Cortical Dysplasias

There is a range of MR abnormalities associated with this type of abnormality: focal thickening of the cortex, loss of differentiation between cortical and subcortical regions and increased T2 signal within the dysplastic cerebral cortex or no MR change (Fig 2.12). Thin section three-dimensional volumetric MR imaging is extremely useful in evaluating these anomalies. Some centres have the

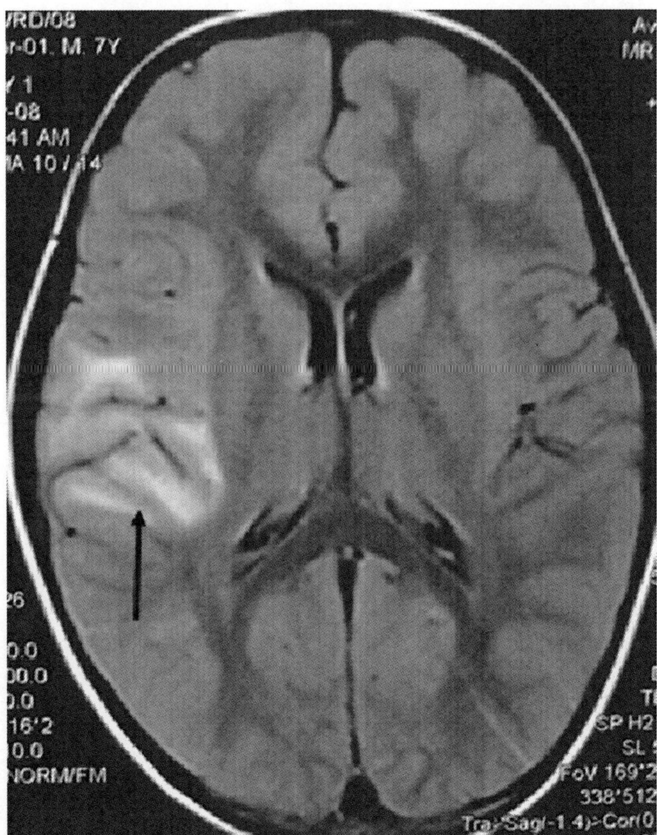

Fig. 2.12: Focal cortical dysplasia. Axial FLAIR image showing focal area of hyperintensity involving the right perisylvian grey matter and adjacent subcortical white matter (arrow)

capability of processing images so that 3D images of the cortical surface can be seen. Reformatted images which show incremental peeling off of the cortical surface. It is difficult to assess cortical mantle thickness with 2D images because of volume averaging across gyri and sulci. As such this technique helps visualize some cortical dysplasias. It is important to realize that some cortical dysplasias are MR visible. These may sometimes be visualized by ictal SPECT or PET.[20] Focal cortical dysplasias are the most often considered for surgical resection and perhaps the only lesion in this group other than hemimegalencephaly, which is amenable to surgery.

CONGENITAL DEVELOPMENTAL ANOMALIES OF THE SPINE

Embryology

The development of the spinal canal can be divided into different stages similar to the development of brain; the neurulation, canalization and retrogressive differentiation, and the formation of the vertebral column. The closure of the neural tube (neurulation) begins separately at different levels.[21] Immediately after the closure, the edges of the neural ectoderm meet at the centre and fuse, separating the overlying ectoderm from the neural tissue. The separation of the neural ectoderm from cutaneous ectoderm is called disjunction. Complete non-disjunction results into myelomeningocele, whereas focal non-disjunction gives rise to dorsal dermal sinus. Premature disjunction gives rise to spinal lipomas.

Canalization (or secondary neurulation) is a process in which there is development of caudal cell mass develops caudal to the posterior neuropore or the caudal most part of the developing spinal cord. Caudal cell mass is composed of pleuripotential stem cells. Eventually cysts develop within the caudal cell mass which coalesce to form an ependymal-lined tubular structure, which then fuses with the neural tube above.

Retrogressive differentiation is the process of apoptosis by which the cells of the caudal cell mass and central lumen of the caudal neural tube decrease in size. Caudal cell mass gives rise to the caudal most part of the conal medullaris, the filum terminale, and the ventriculus terminalis.[22-23]

Classification

Abnormalities of neurulation

1. *Disorders resulting from non-disjunction*
   - Myelocele and myelomeningocele.
   - Dorsal dermal sinus.
   - Cervical myelocystocele.
2. *Disorders resulting from premature disjunction*
   - Intradural lipomas.
   - Lipomyeloceles.
   - Lipomeningomyelocele.
   - Terminal lipoma.

Abnormalities of caudal cell mass

- Filum terminale lipoma.
- Caudal regression syndrome.
- Terminal myelocystocele.
- Anterior sacral meningocele.
- Sacrococcygeal teratoma.

Abnormalities of notochordal development

- The split notochord syndrome.
- The split cord malformation (diastematomyelia).

Malformations of unknown etiology

- Segmental spinal dysgenesis.
- Dorsal meningocele.
- Lateral meningocele.

Myelocele and Meningomyelocele

Myelocele and meningomyelocele develop from focal non-disjunction, resulting in open spinal dysraphism. The open neural tissue located at the skin surface posteriorly is termed neural placode. In myelocele the ventral CSF space does not show expansion, whereas in meningomyelocele, the ventral CSF space is expanded. Both are open defects in which the neural placode is open in the absence of overlying skin covering. The vertebral bodies can be normal or can have segmentation anomalies. The diagnosis in a newborn is made clinically and imaging is rarely performed. It can be detected prenatally on fetal MRI (Fig. 2.13). Neuroimaging is indicated when the child deteriorates after surgery and adequate treatment of hydrocephalus, or if the child has unusual neurologic examination. Imaging of the brain is indicated because of high incidence of association of Arnold-Chiari II malformation with these anomalies.

Hemimyelocele

In this anomaly, myelomeningocele is associated with diastematomyelia. It can be observed in about 10% of patients with myelomeningocele. There is splitting of the cord with two separate dural coverings, a bony

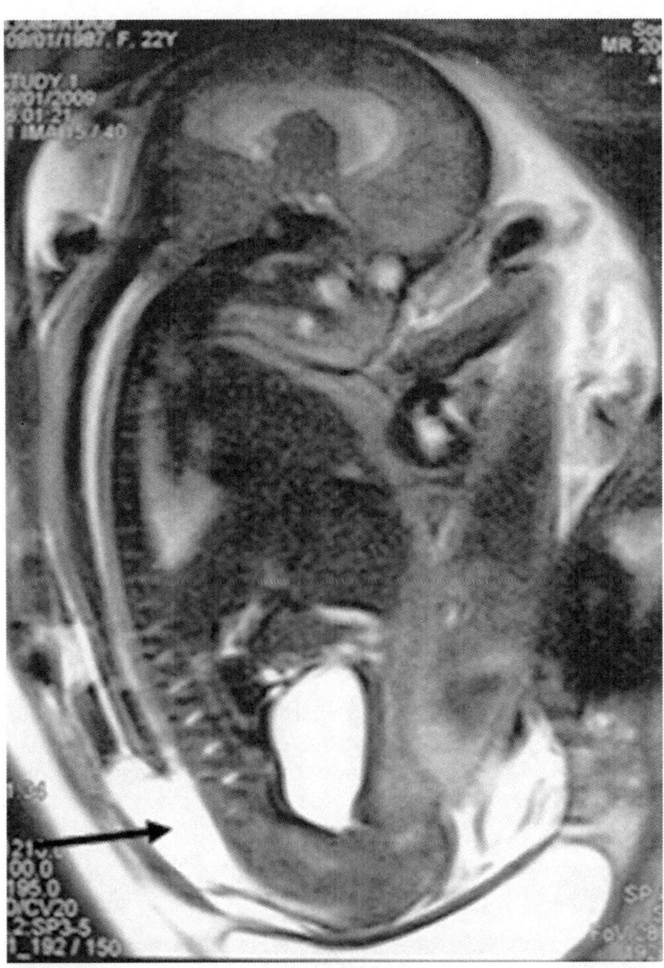

Fig. 2.13: Lumbosacral myelomeningocele detected prenatally on fetal MRI. Sagittal TruFISP image of the fetus showing open neural tube defect at the lumbosacral region with herniation of the meninges and neural elements (arrow)

or fibrous spur. One of the hemicord shows a small myelomeningocele, and the other can either be normal. Tethered or can have a small myelomeningocele at a much lower level. If one of the hemicords is normal, the patient shows neurological abnormalities on the side of the myelomeningocele.[24,25]

Dorsal Dermal Sinus

Dorsal dermal sinuses are epithelium-lined tracts extending from the skin surface inwards for varying distance. They result from focal incomplete disjunction of cutaneous ectoderm. They are commonly found in the lumbar and lumbosacral location. Physical examination reveals a midline pit, often associated with hyperpigmented patch or tuft of hair. Symptoms are usually due to infection or compression of neural tissues by associated dermoid or epidermoid tumor.[26,27] MRI demonstrates the tract as a hypointense line both on T1WI as well as T2WI. Associated lesions (dermoids, epidermoids) are also detected by MRI.

Cervical Myelocystocele

Cervical myelocystocele is the protrusion of the dilated central canal through a bony spinal bifida. They are different from a terminal myelocystocele, which are anomalies of the caudal cell mass. It is a skin covered spinal dysraphism in which a dilated central canal is protruded in the dorsal subcutaneous tissues, though the communication with the central canal is not always visible.

Spinal Lipomas

Spinal lipomas result from premature disjunction of the cutaneous ectoderm from neural ectoderm. Once the mesenchymal tissue comes in contact with the primitive ependymal lining along the neural ectoderm, it evolves into fat. Spinal lipomas can be divided into three major types:[28,29]

1. Intradural lipomas.
2. Lipomyelocele/lipomyelomeningocele.
3. Lipomas of caudal call mass.

Intradural lipomas are intradural juxtamedullary masses, commonly located in cervical and thoracic region. Common location is dorsal to the cord. Intradural lipomas are seen as well defined masses dorsal to the cord (hyperintense on T1WI as well as T2WI, and low attenuation on CT). The bony spinal canal may be expanded, may show a localized spinal bifida, but segmentation anomalies are usually absent.[30]

Lipomyelocele and lipomyelomeningocele are skin covered spinal dysraphisms, often presenting with back masses located in lumbosacral area. They are anatomically similar to myelocele and meningomyelocele; differing from them in the following aspects:

- Lipomyelocele and lipomyelomeningocele are skin covered lesions (c.f. myelocele and myelomeningocele).
- Lipoma seen attached to the dorsal surface of the placode.

In lipomyelocele, the placode-lipoma interface lies within the bony spinal canal and the ventral CSF space is not enlarged; whereas in lipomyelomeningocele (Fig. 2.14) there is expansion of ventral CSF space and the placode-lipoma interface lies outside the bony spinal canal. On imaging, the lipoma extends through the open spina bifida and seen continuous with the subcutaneous fat. The bony spinal canal is expanded and there is association with segmentation anomalies.[31,32] Dura is attached at the lateral margins of the placode and the dorsal surface of the placode lies in contact with the lipoma.

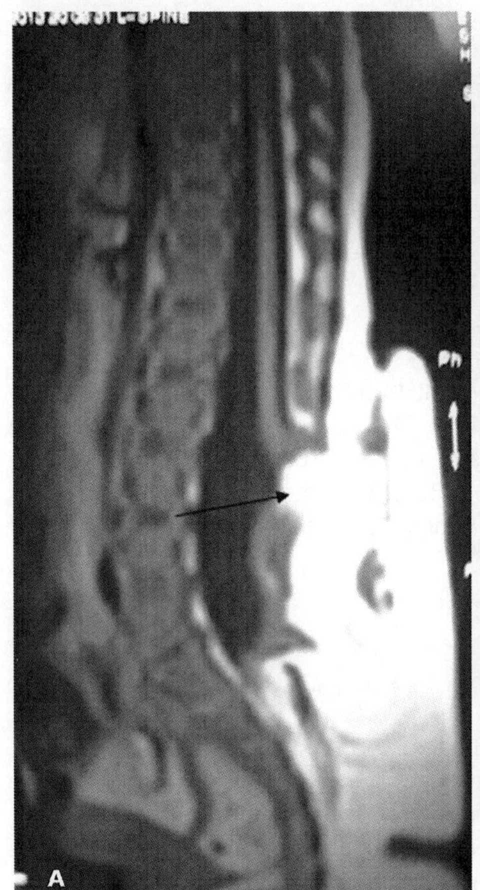

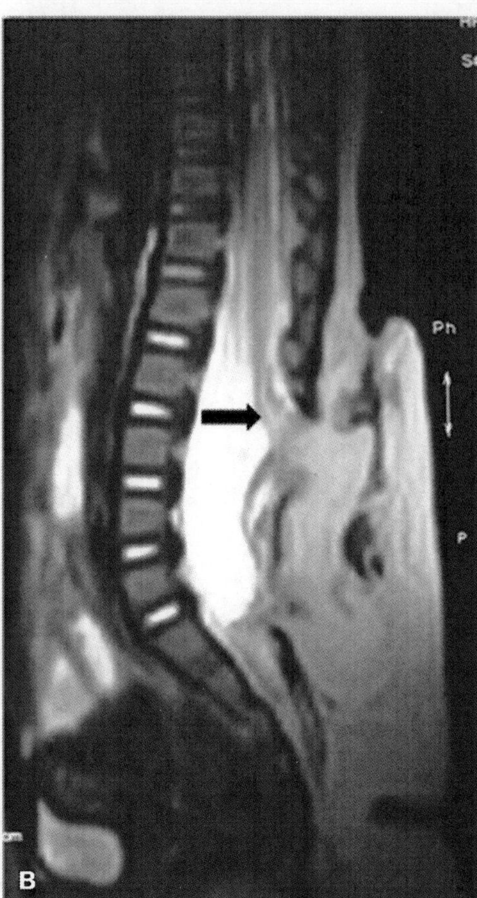

Fig. 2.14: Lipomyelomeningocele. Sagittal T1W (A) and T2W (B) MR image of the spine show a skin covered spinal dysraphism with lipoma (arrow) and placode (black arrow), lipoma–placode interface lying outside the bony spinal canal

Lipomyelocele and lipomyelomeningocele are commonly associated with sacral dysgenesis, anorectal malformation, genitourinary abnormalities; and less commonly with terminal diastematomyelia, epidermoid, dermoid, dorsal dermal sinus, angioma and arachnoid cysts.[33]

Anomalies of the Caudal Cell Mass

The conus medullaris, the filum terminale, lower lumbar and sacral nerve roots develop from the caudal cell mass. Anomalies of the caudal cell mass are commonly associated with anorectal and genitourinary anomalies.

Fibrolipoma of Filum Terminale/Tight Filum Terminale

Normal filum terminale is a thin fibrous structure extending from the tip of conus medullaris to the dorsal aspect of first coccygeal vertebra. Fibrolipomas are a result of minor abnormality in canalization and retrogressive differentiation. Fibrolipoma may involve intradural filum, extradural filum or both. Normal filum is 1 mm thick at L5- S1 level.[34] Lipoma is seen as an area of hyperintensity on T1WI and T2WI at the caudal end of filum (Fig. 2.15). The conus medullaris is commonly low lying, tethered by a tight filum.

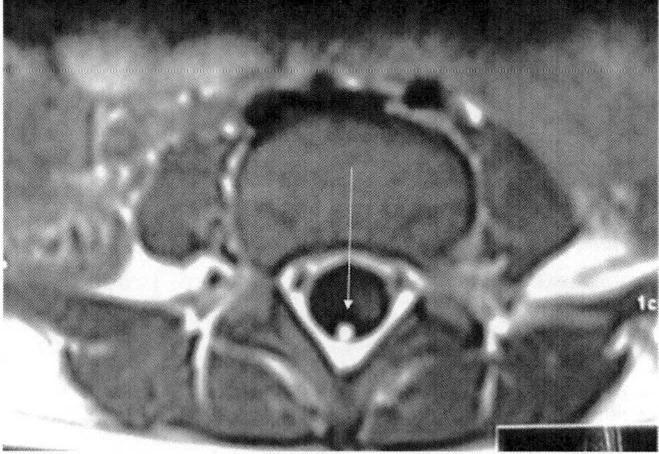

Fig. 2.15: Lipoma of filum terminale. Axial T1W MR image shows hyperintense fatty signal at the thickened filum terminale (arrow)

Caudal Regression Syndrome

The syndrome of caudal regression results from abnormal development of the caudal cell mass and cloaca and describes a complete spectrum of distal spinal cord and vertebral maldevelopment and genitourinary and gastrointestinal abnormalities. The anatomical abnormalities may be sirenomelia, complete sacral agenesis, sacral hypogenesis, anal atresia, exstrophy of urinary bladder, malformed external genitalia etc.[35] The caudal regression syndrome is seen with an incidence of approximately 1 in 7500 births. Infants of diabetic mothers are at an increased risk.[36] There is an association of lumbosacral hypogenesis with OEIS complex (omphalocele, exstrophy, imperforate anus and spinal anomalies) and VACTERL anomalies (vertebral anomalies, anorectal malformations, cardiac malformations, tracheoesophageal fistulae, renal anomalies and limb anomalies). The major neural abnormality is hypoplasia is the distal spinal cord, with abrupt termination of the conus medullaris giving a truncated appearance.[37] The spinal cord may be tethered when the conus ends below the L1 level; whereas in severe sacral agenesis the conus ends above L1 level with no cord tethering.[38] On imaging, the sacrum shows variable degrees of hypogenesis. The conus gives a truncated appearance with termination higher than L1 level (Fig. 2.16); whereas it is tapered when terminates below L1 level. Other associated imaging findings include fatty filum terminale, terminal hydromyelia, lipomyelocele, terminal lipoma or bony spinal stenosis.[37]

Terminal Myelocystocele

It is the least common form of spinal dysraphism. It is a closed spinal dysraphism where the spinal cord with dilated central canal herniates through a posterior spinal bifida (Fig. 2.17).[38] Patients present with a skin covered back mass and there is association with lower genitourinary anomalies and gastrointestinal abnormalities. In this anomaly, the spinal cord with the dilated central canal traverses the meningocele and inserts at its posterior wall.

Anterior Sacral Meningocele

This includes a spectrum of anomalies where the CSF filled meningeal sac herniates anteriorly into the pelvis through a defect in the sacral or coccyx. They can present as pelvic retrorectal cystic masses in children.

Split Cord Malformation (Diastematomyelia)

It is the sagittal division of the spinal cord into two hemicords. Developmentally, it results from splitting of the notochord when any obstacle comes in the path of the

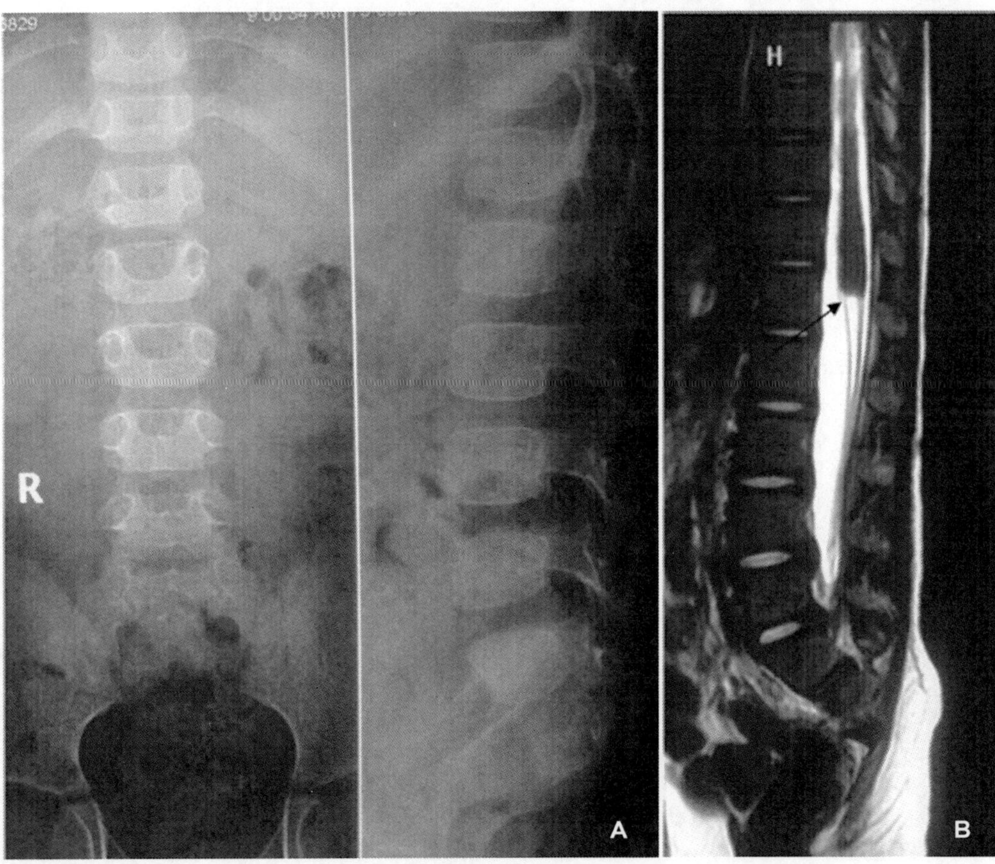

Fig. 2.16: Caudal regression syndrome. Lumbar spine radiograph (A) (AP and lateral) shows hypogenesis of sacrum, with absent S3-5 sacral segments. Sagittal T2W MR image (B) shows truncated appearance of conus medullaris (arrow) with double bundle appearance of the filum

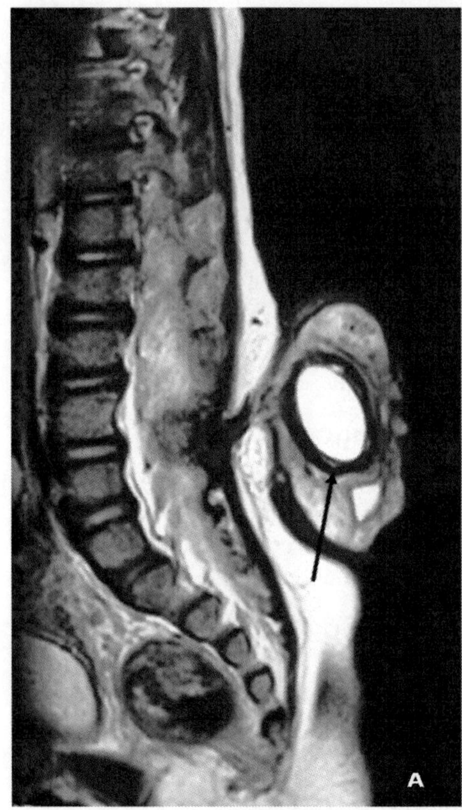

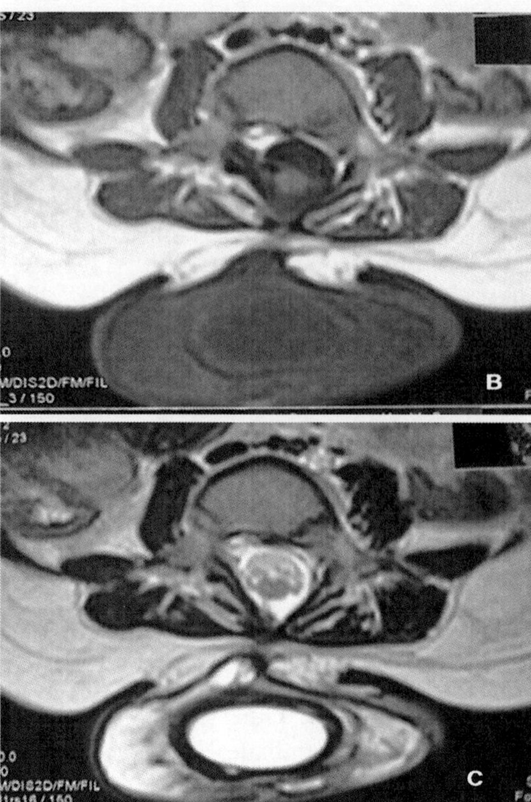

Fig. 2.17: Terminal myelocystocele. Sagittal T2W (A), Axial T1W (B) and axial T2W (C) MR images show herniation of the distal spinal cord with dilated spinal canal (arrow) through a posterior spina bifida

growing notochord. As the development of the vertebral bodies is dependent on the notochordal development, there is frequent association of this anomaly with vertebral body segmentation anomalies like butterfly vertebra and hemivertebra.[39] The patients can be symptomatic from tethering of cord, low back pain, sciatica, or may have associated scoliosis and clubfoot. The level of split is most commonly located in the lumbar region, less commonly in thoracic and very rare in cervical location. Two types have been described.[40] In type I diastematomyelia, two hemicords are covered in two separate dural sheaths, separated by a fibrous or bony spur. In type II diastematomyelia, they are enclosed in a single dural covering. Usually the two cords unite caudal to the level of the split; but very rarely, they may extend caudally as two conus medullaris and two fila.

On imaging (Fig. 2.18), the vertebral segmentation anomalies, widening of the bony spinal canal are visualized on plain radiograph. Bony spur may be visualized on plain radiographs. MRI sequences should include T1WI, T2WI and gradient echo sequences to help visualize the bony or fibrous spur.

Segmental Spinal Dysgenesis

It is a malformation of unknown origin, which shows focal hypoplasia of the vertebral column, thecal sac and

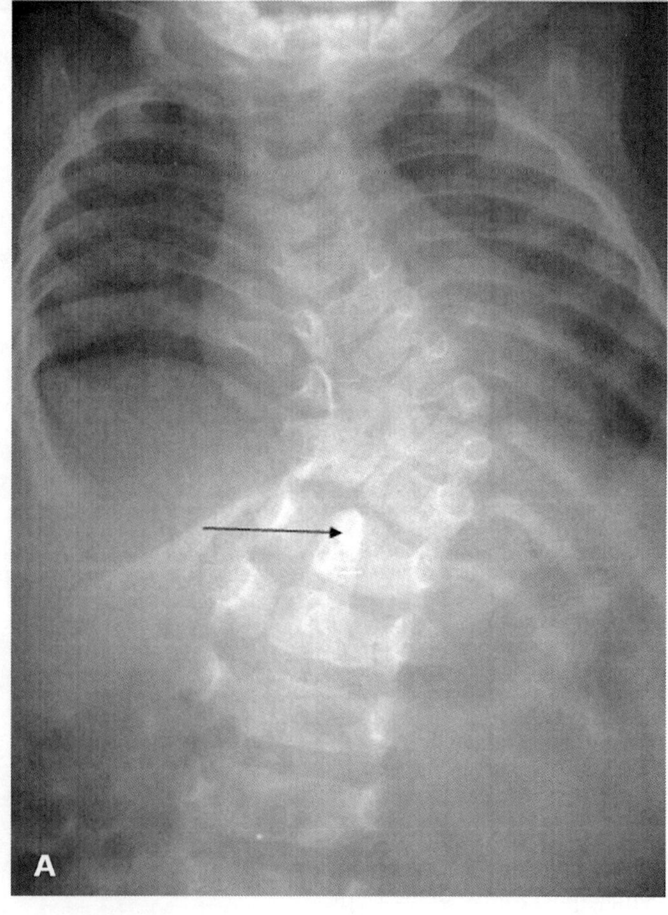

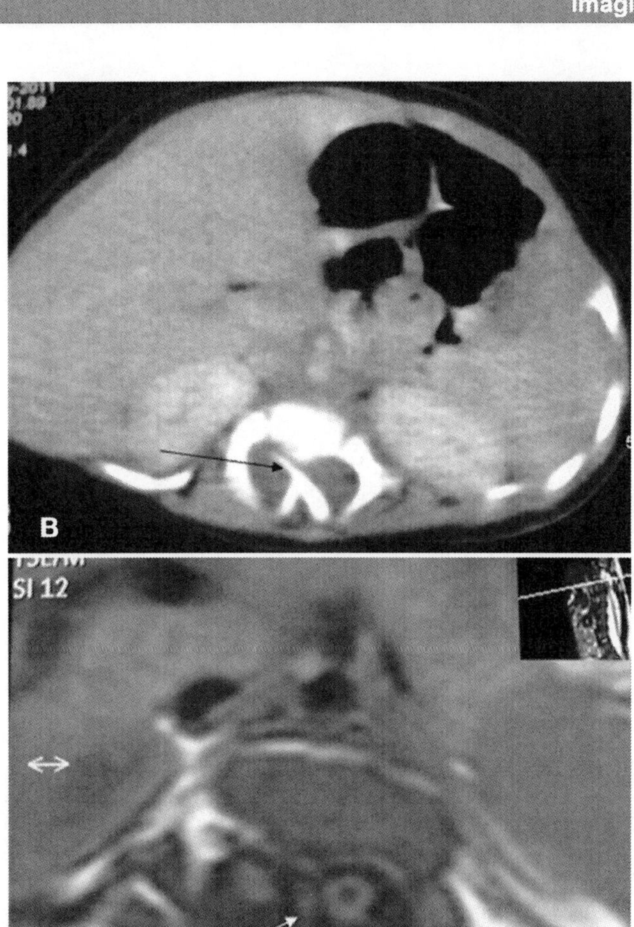

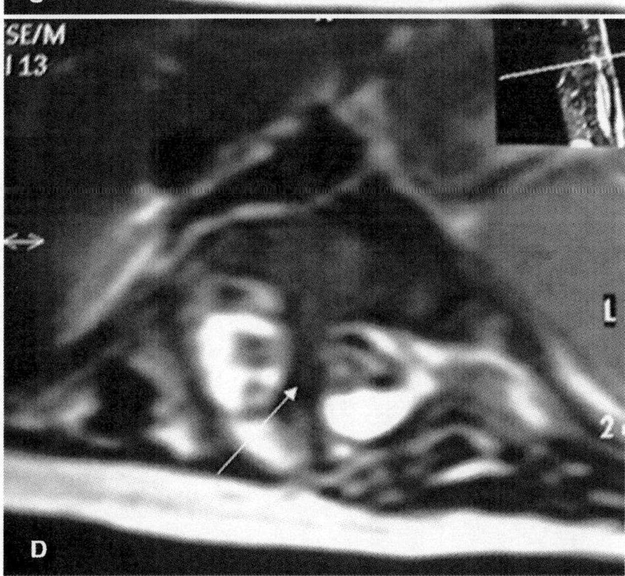

Fig. 2.18: Diastematomyelia. Frontal radiograph of the dorsolumbar spine (A) shows vertebral segmentation anomalies, focal widening of the bony spinal canal and a bony spur (arrow). Axial CT (B), axial T1W (C) and T2W (D) MR image show two hemicords with separate dural coverings and a bony spur (arrow)

spinal cord. The patients have sharply angulated hyphotic deformity, usually at dorsolumbar junction; and lower limb abnormalities like talipes equinovarus, flexion contractures at hips and knees.[41,42]

On imaging, there is tapered narrowing of the spinal cord to a thin hypoplastic cord or focal absence; caudal to which the lower spinal cord segments are visualized. The termination of the cord may be abrupt also in some cases.

SUMMARY

Familiarity with brain development and the imaging manifestations of the anomalies, which result when an insult occurs during formation of the brain and spine (or on a genetic basis), is critical for the imager. This allows the accurate description of morphologic abnormalities and guides the acquisition and evaluation of imaging studies. The multiplanar capabilities and superior contrast resolution of MRI provide the best noninvasive means for evaluating the anatomic features of these anomalies.

References

1. Norman MG, McGillivray BC, Kalousek DK, Hill A, Poskitt KJ. Congenital Malformations of Brain: Pathologic, Embryologic, Clinical, Radiologic and Genetic Aspects. Oxford: Oxford University 1995:223-307.
2. Muuler F, O' Rahilly R. The First Appearance of the Human Nervous System at Stage 8, Anat Embryol 1981;163:1-13.
3. Barkovich AJ. Pediatric Neuroimaging. Raven Press, New York, 1990.
4. Barkovich AJ, Gressens P., *et al.* Formation, Maturation, Disorders of the Brain Neocortex. AJNR 1992;13:423-46.
5. Zimmerman RA and Bilaniuk LT. Applications of Magnetic Resonance Imaging in Diseases of the Pediatric Central Nervous System, Magn Reson Imaging 1986;4:11.
6. Simpson DA, David DJ, White J. Cephaloceles: Treatment, Outcome and Antenatal Diagnosis. Neurosurgery 1984;15: 14-21.
7. Mealey J. Dzenitis AJ, Hockey AA. The Prognosis of Encephaloceles, J, Neurosurgery 1970;32:209-18.
8. Taveras JM. Brain Congenital Anomalies, Neuroradiology, Taveras JM, Williams and Wilkins, Baltimore 1996:166-75.
9. Mikulis DG, Diaz O, Egglin TK, Sanchez R, *et al.* Variance of the Position of the Cerebellar Tonsils with Age: Preliminary Report. Radiology 1992;183:725-28.
10. Woodruff WW. Pediatric Neuroimaging, Fundamentals of Neuroimaging, Woodruff WW, WB Saunders Co., Philadelphia 1993:513-17.
11. Castillo M, Bouldin TW, *et al.* Radiologic Pathologic Correlation Allobar Holoprosencephaly. AJNR 1993;14: 1151-56.

12. Barkovich AJ. Norman D. "Anomalies of the Corpus Callosum." AJNR 1988;9:493-501.

13. Raybaud CA. Girad N. Etude Anatomique par IRM des Agenesies et Dysplasies Commissurales Telencephaliques. Neurochirurgie 1198;44(suppl 1):38-60.

14. Altman NR. Naidich TP and Braffman BH. Posterior Fossa malformations. Am J Neuroradiol 1992:13:691.

15. Kollias S. Ball W. *et al.* Cystic Malformations of the Posterior Fossa Differential Diagnosis Clarified through Embryologic Analysis. Radiographics 1993:13:1211-31.

16. Barkovich AJ. Chuang SH and Norman D. MR of Neuronal Migration Anomalies. Am J Neuroradiol 1987:8:1009.

17. Barkovich AJ and Chuang SH. Unilateral Megalencephaly: Correlation of MR Imaging and Pathologic Characteristics. Am J Neuroradiol 1990;11:523.

18. Barkovich AJ, Kjos BO. Skizencephaly: Correlation and Clinical Findings with MR Characteristics. AJR 1992;13: 85-94.

19. Barkovich AJ, Kjos BO. Grey Matter Heterotopias: MR Characteristics and Correlation with Developmental and Neurologic Manifestations. Radiology 1992;182:493-99.

20. Raymond AA. Fish DR. Sisodiya SM. Alsanjari N. Stevens JM. Shorvon SD. Abnormalities of Gyration. Heterotopias. Tuberous Sclerosis. Focal Cortical Dysplasia. Microdysgenesis. Dysembryoplastic Neuro-epithelial Tumor and Dysgenesis of the Archicortex in Epilepsy: Clinical. EEG and Neuroimaging Features in 100 Adult Patients. Brain 1995;118:629-60.

21. Golden J, Chernoff G. Intermittent Pattern of Neural Tube Closure in Two Strains of Mice. Teratology 1993:47:73-80.

22. Nievelstein RAJ. Hartwig NG. Vermeij-Keers C. Valk J. Embryonic Development of the Mammalian Caudal Neural Tube. Teratology 1993;48:21-31.

23. Naidich TP. Mcleone DG. Harwood–Nash DC. Spinal dysraphism. In: Newton TH. Potts DG. eds. Modern Neuroradiology. Vol I:C Computed Tomography of the Spine and Spinal Cord. San Anselmo. CA: Clavadel 1983:299-353.

24. Emery JL. Lendon RG. The Local Cord Lesion in Neurospinal Dysraphism (Meningomyelocele). J Pathol 1973:110:83-96.

25. Duckworth T. Sharrad WJ. Lister J. Seymour N. Hemimyelocele. Dev Med Child Neurol 1968;10 (suppl16):69-75.

26. Haworth JC. Zachary RB. Congenital Dermal Sinuses in Children: Their Relation to Pilonidal Sinuses. Lancet 1955: 2:10-14.

27. Walker AE. Bucy PC. Congenital Dermal Sinuses: Source of Spinal Meningeal Infection and Subdural Abscesses. Brain 1934:57:401-21.

28. Arai H. Sato K. Okuda O. *et al.* Surgical Experience of 120 Patients with Lumbosacral Lipomas. Acta Neurochir (Wien) 2001:143:857-64.

29. Chapman PH. Congenital Intraspinal Lipomas: Anatomic Consideration and Surgical Treatment. Child's Brain 1982:9: 37-47.

30. Fujiwara F. Tamaki N. Nagashima T. Nakamura M. Intradural Spinal Lipomas not Associated with Spinal Dysraphism: A Report of Four Cases. Neurosurgery 1995;37:1212-15.

31. Leveuf JB. Spina Bifida Avec Tumeur. In: Leveuf J. Ed Etudes Sur Le Spina Bifida. Paris:Masson 1937;93-106.

32. Gold LH. Kieffer SA. Peterson HO. Lipomatous Invasion of the Spinal Cord Associated with Spinal Dysraphism: Myelographic Evaluation. AJR Am J Roentgenol 1969;107:479-85.

33. Pierre-Kahn A. Zerah M. Renier D. *et al.* Congenital Lumbosacral Lipomas. Child Nerv Syst 1997;13:298-335.

34. Naidich P. McLone DG. Harwood-Nash DC. Spinal Dysraphism. In: Newton TH. Potts DG. eds. Modern Neuroradiology. Vol 1: Computed Tomography of the Spine and Spinal Cord. San Anselmo. CA:Clavadel 1983;299-353.

35. Kallen B. Winberg J. Caudal Mesoderm Pattern of Anomalies: From Renal Agenesis to Sirenomelia. Teratology 1974;9: 99-112.

36. Passarge E. Congenital Malformations and Maternal Diabetes. Lancet 1965;1:324-25.

37. Barkowich AJ. Raghavan N. Chuang SH. MR of Lumbosacral Agenesis. AJNR AM J Neuroradiol 1989;10:1223-31.

38. Pang D. Scaral Agenesis and Caudal Spinal Cord Malformations. Neurosurgery 1993:32:755-79.

39. Pang D. Dias MS. Ahab-Barmada M. Split Cord Malformation: Part I: A Unified Theory of Embryogenesis for Double Spinal Cord Malformations. Neurosurgery 1992:31:451-80.

40. Guthkelch AN. Diastematomyelia with Median Septum. Brain 1974;97:729-42.

41. Scott RM. Wolpert SM. Bartoshesky LE. Zimbler S. Karlin L. Segmental Spinal Dysgenesis. Neurosurgery 1988;22:739-43.

42. Mamelak AN. Cogen PH. Barkowich AJ. The "Filum Intermedium" Sign: Focal in Utero Spinal Cord Infarct and Extraspinal Thecal Sac. J Neurosurg 1994;81:941-46.

3 Chapter

PEDIATRIC CEREBROVASCULAR DISEASES AND STROKE

Ajay Garg

Pediatric cerebrovascular diseases and stroke have been increasingly recognized in children in recent years. The symptoms tend to appear rather abruptly and the condition can be alarming and potentially life-threatening. Their treatment often requires the expertise of several specialists as well as advanced diagnostic and treatment approaches. Modern imaging techniques often enable the clinician to quickly confirm the diagnosis of cerebrovascular disease. In some cases, appropriate imaging also establishes stroke etiology.

In this chapter, imaging finding in various cerebrovascular diseases and stroke is described.

PEDIATRIC CEREBROVASCULAR DISEASES

Cerebrovascular disease includes a large group of conditions in which the arteries in the brain, or those connected to the brain, are defective. These conditions are rare in children and generally not considered childhood ailments.

1. Developmental Venous Malformation (DVA)

DVA is the most common type of vascular malformation found at autopsy, with a prevalence of 2%.[1] DVAs, formerly known as venous angiomas, represent an arrest during the development of the venous system which results in the retention of primitive embryological medullary veins draining into a single collector vein.[2]

DVA is characterized by a caput medusae or an umbrella-like convergence of multiple venules on a single, or occasionally multiple, enlarged parenchymal or medullary veins, like the trunk of a tree or the shank of an umbrella.[3] This dilated terminal vein penetrates the cortex to drain either superficially to cortical veins or sinuses; or deeply to subependymal veins of the lateral ventricle and then into the galenic venous system. In DVAs normal cerebral tissue intervenes between the dilated veins. About one-third of the DVAs are located in the posterior fossa, and the remaining two-thirds in a supratentorial location.[4] DVAs don't exist in the diencephalon, brainstem or spinal cord. In general, these anomalies are incidentally found and of no consequence to the patient. The brain surrounding the DVA is nearly always normal, and histologically the anomaly is limited to the venous structures, without involvement of capillaries or arteries. DVA is essential for the venous drainage of the brain and that surgical resection or radiotherapy should generally be avoided.[2,5]

DVAs have a characteristic appearance on CT and MR studies, and angiography is seldom needed for diagnosis. On CT they are rarely detectable without contrast enhancement. After administration of contrast medium, the draining veins appear as a linear focus of enhancement (Fig. 3.1). Most of the DVAs and draining veins cannot be appreciated on the unenhanced T1-WI unless they are large.[6] Some of the DVAs and draining veins can also be seen on T2-WI as flow voids or as flow

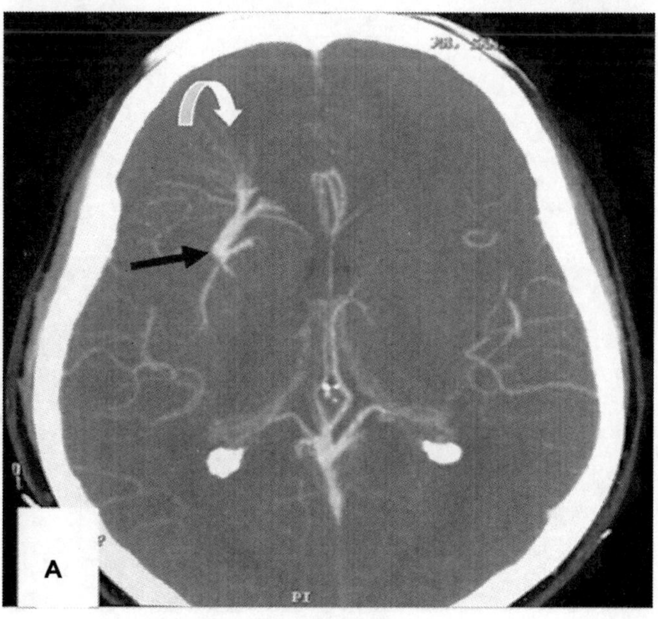

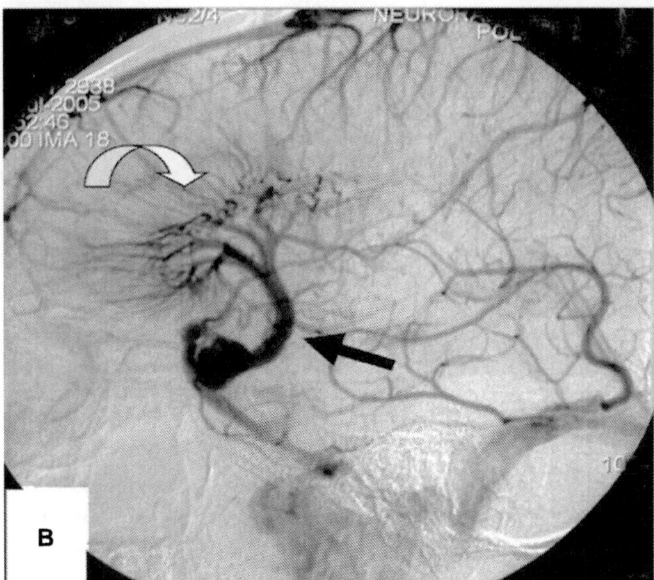

Fig. 3.1: DVA. Contrast-enhanced CT image (A) shows a stellate collection (curved arrow) of venous tributaries that drain into a prominent collector vein (arrow). Venous phase of right internal carotid angiogram (B) shows multiple enlarged medullary veins converging to a dilated "collector" vein (arrow)

phase-shift artifacts. Generally, the draining vein was seen more often than the caput on T2-WI. Small DVAs are not seen as easily. Some of the draining veins appear hyperintense on the T2-WI because of slow flow and even-echo rephasing (Fig. 3.2).[6] Both the caput medusae

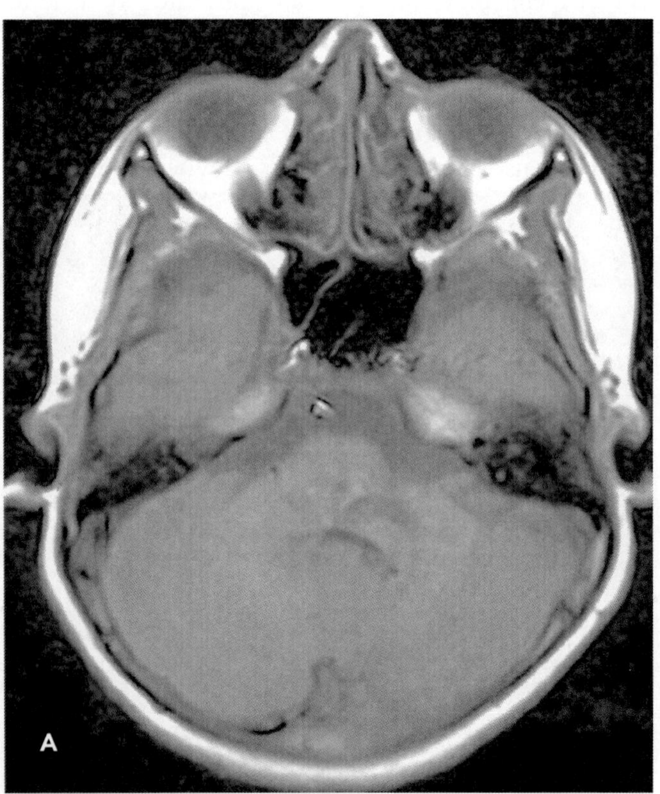

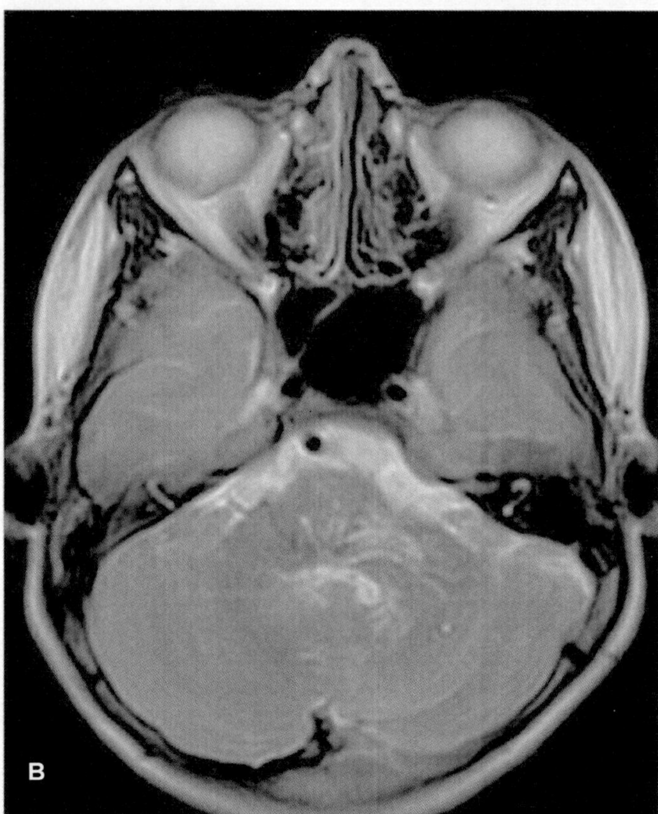

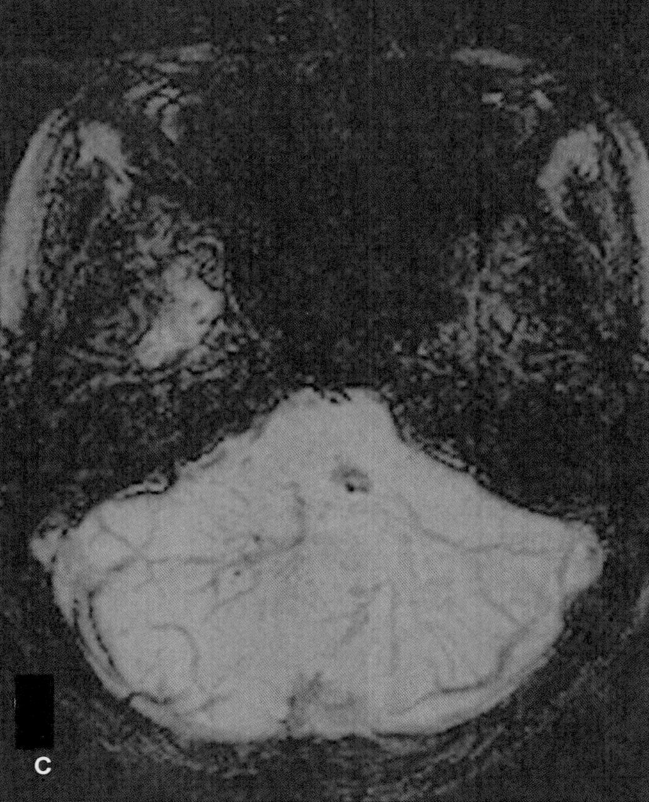

Fig. 3.2: DVA. Axial T1 (A), T2 (B) and SWI (C) show cerebellar DVA which appear hypointense on T1-WI, hyperintense on T2-WI and marked hypointense on SWI

and the draining veins are seen best on contrast-enhanced T1-WI. On cerebral angiography they present typically as deep, medullary veins during the early or middle venous phase accompanied by a single large draining vein. A DVA is typically not seen on 3D-TOF or PC-MR angiography (MRA). Susceptibility-weighted imaging (SWI) shows low signal intensity for DVA due to the blood oxygen level-dependent (BOLD) effect in the abnormal medullary and draining veins (Fig. 3.2).[7] DVAs are typically not associated with imaging findings. However, a subset of DVAs has been associated with findings such as cavernous malformations (CMs),[3,8] thrombosis with subsequent venous infarction,[9] lobar atrophy,[10] T2 and FLAIR signal-intensity abnormalities,[10,11] and SWI hypointensities.[12] Signal abnormalities on MR imaging are more common in DVAs with deep venous drainage, associated with cavernous malformation and parenchymal atrophy, and younger subject age.[13] The pathophysiology of these signal-inten-sity abnormalities remains unclear but may represent effects of delayed myelination and/or alterations in venous flow within the DVA drainage territory.[13]

2. Cerebral Cavernous Malformations

Cerebral cavernous malformations (CCMs) are a heterogeneous group of lesions mostly described as a mulberry like assembly of vascular sinusoids with varying vessel diameter and wall thickness, lined by a thin endothelium lacking smooth muscle and elastin, surrounded by hemosiderin deposits and gliosis. Unlike DVA or AVMs, no intervening neural tissue is present. On occasion they are intimately associated with a DVA, in which case they are known as mixed vascular malformations.

Most CCMs (75%) occur as solitary sporadic lesions. There is a familial form of CCMs (10%–30%) in which lesions are often multiple and prone to repeated spontaneous hemorrhages. CCMs tend to be supratentorial (~80% cases) but can be found anywhere including the brainstem (Fig. 3.3). The most frequent symptoms at the time of diagnosis are seizures, hemorrhage, focal neurologic signs and headaches.[14,15] However, affected patients may be entirely asymptomatic.[14,15] The risk of hemorrhage is 1% per year for familial cases, and somewhat less for sporadic lesions.

MR imaging is the most sensitive modality for the diagnosis of CCM.[14,16] CCMs that have previously bled are usually detectable on routine MR imaging due to the prominent signal intensity of hemorrhagic products. With T2-weighted sequences, the lesion is typically characterized by an area of mixed signal intensity, with a central reticulated core and a peripheral rim of decreased signal intensity related to deposition of hemosiderin ("popcorn" or "berry" appearance) (Fig. 3.3). Gradient Echo or T2* sequences are able to delineate these lesions better than T1 or T2 weighted images. SWI may have sensitivity better than that of GRE in detecting these CCMs in brain. Familial CCMs are seen as multiple area of punctate-macro hemorrhages in both supratentorial and infratentorial compartment (Fig. 3.4). CCMs may also develop dystrophic calcifications that can be detected

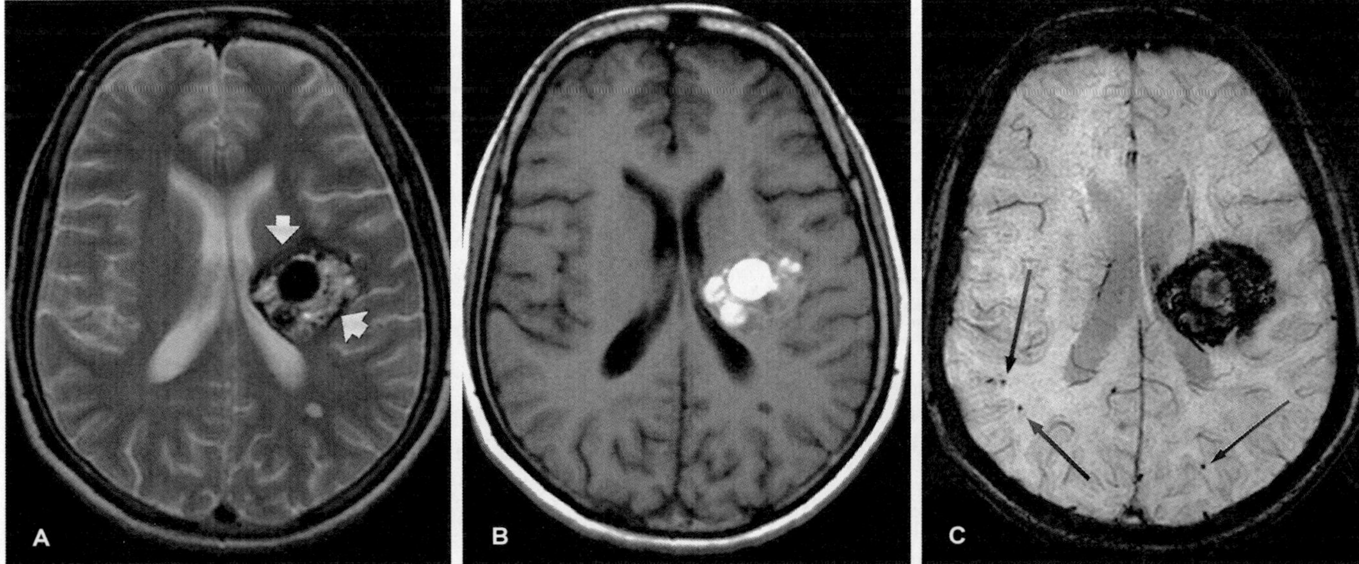

Fig. 3.3: Cerebral cavernous malformation (CCM). Axial T1 (A), Ax T2 (B) and Axial SWI (C) images show classic "popcorn ball" configuration in CCM. Note the multiple locules filled with blood products of different ages and fluid level surrounded by a hypointense hemosiderin rim (arrow) which blooms in SWI

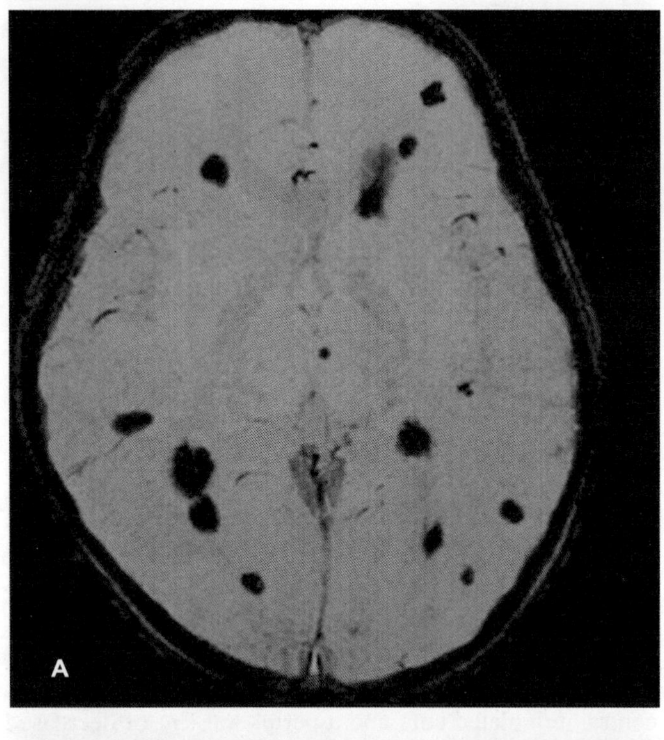

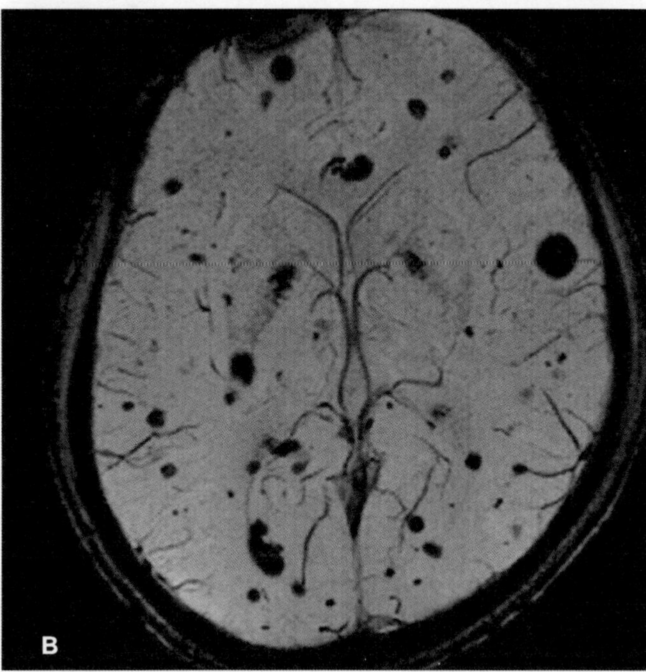

Fig. 3.4: Familial CCMs. Ax SWI images show multiple hypointense CCMs in both cerebral hemispheres in 6-year-old boy (A) and his father (B). Note increase in lesion load in the father

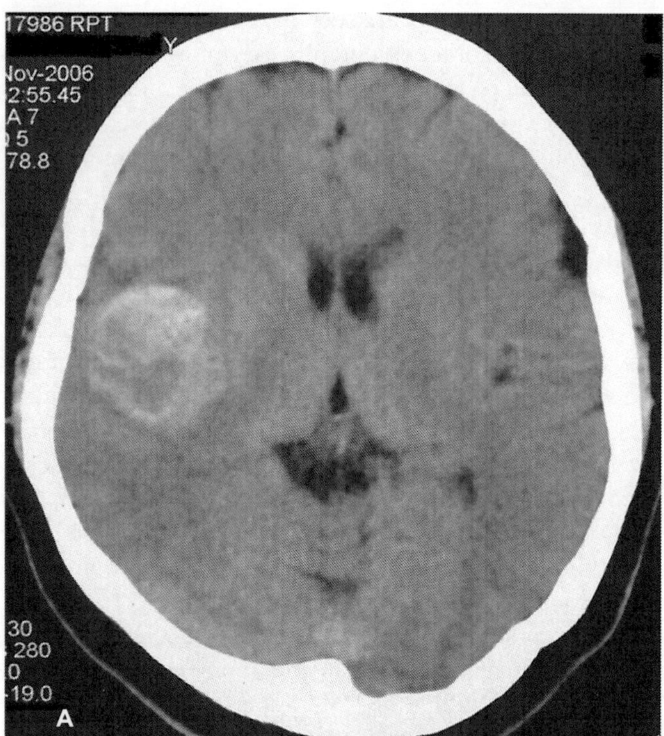

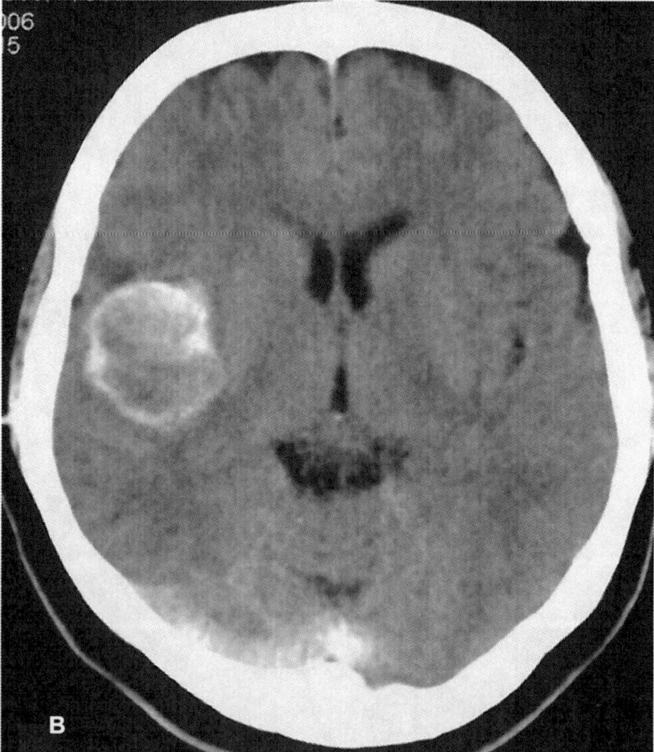

Fig. 3.5. CCM. NCCT (A) shows a hyperdense lesion in right temporal lobe which show mild peripheral enhancement following contrast administration (B)

on CT (Fig. 3.5). CCMs lesions, which are intact and have not bled may be almost invisible on CT except for a faint or ill-defined blush of enhancement after contrast administration. However, contrast enhancement is inconsistent and often nonspecific. CCMs become very dark on the SWI images, even if not bled.

3. Capillary Telangiectasia

Capillary telangiectasia is a small slow-flow vascular malformation that is typically asymptomatic and usually occult on MRA. It can be seen as a contrast blush on T1-weighted imaging, occurring in characteristic locations, most often in the central pons. SWI has recently been reported to be helpful in depicting the microvascular characteristics of capillary telangiectasia, thereby confirming the lesion and eliminating more ominous differential considerations.

4. Intracranial Aneurysms

Cerebral aneurysms are pathologic focal dilatations of the cerebral vasculature that are prone to rupture. Intracranial aneurysms in children are rare; only 0.5% to 4.6% of intracranial aneurysms occur in patients aged 18 years or younger.[17-19]

Childhood cerebral aneurysms are morphologically different from their saccular counterparts in adults, including a high number of fusiform shape, giant size, and *de novo* formation. Patients with cerebral aneurysms in childhood also have a high risk for developing new and recurrent aneurysms ~up to 41% in one series especially if they start to smoke as adults.[20]

In children, most of the risk factors associated with intracranial aneurysms in adults do not exist; therefore, the pathogenesis is thought to be different. Multiple conditions have been associated with cerebral aneurysms, which include autosomal dominant inherited polycystic kidney disease, fibromuscular dysplasia, Osler-Weber-Rendu syndrome, coarctation of the aorta, moyamoya syndrome, Marfan syndrome, Ehlers-Danlos syndrome, bacterial endocarditis, fungal infections, Neurofibromatosis type 1 and tuberous sclerosis.[21]

Aneurysm Features

Dissecting aneurysms are dominant during the first 5 years of life, whereas saccular aneurysms are more common in children older than 6 years.

(a) Saccular Aneurysms

Saccular aneurysms are the most common type of aneurysm occurring in the pediatric population (between 50-70%).[21] The cause of saccular aneurysms is unknown. They usually occur at bifurcation points of vessels, suggesting hemodynamic factors (Fig. 3.6). Giant aneurysms (diameter > 2.5 cm) are found in 20-40% of affected pediatric patients (Fig. 3.7).[22,23]

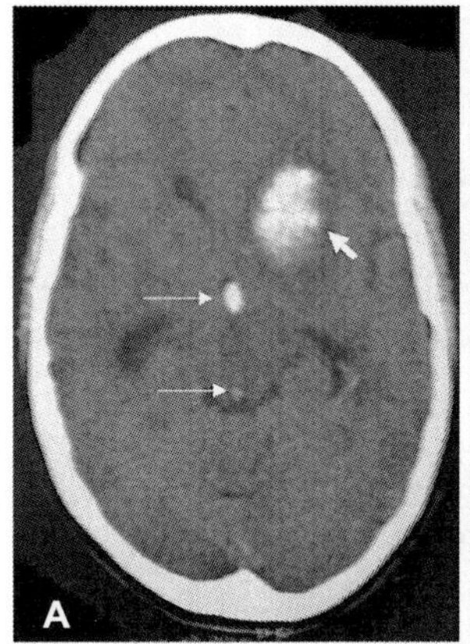

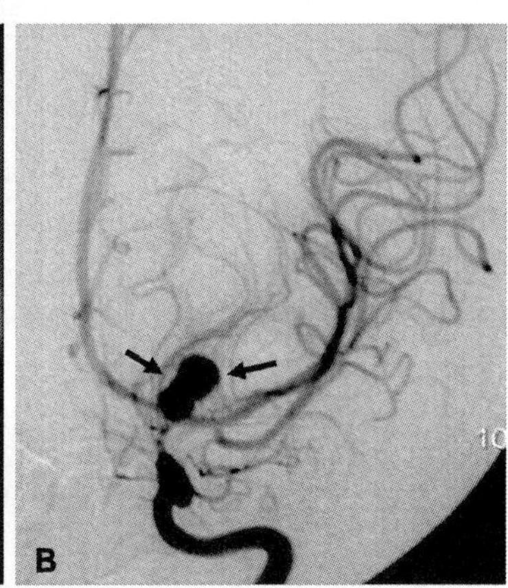

Fig. 3.6: ICA bifurcation aneurysm. A 12-year-old girl presented with sudden onset severe headache. NCCT scan (A) shows an acute hyperdense hematoma in left caudate and anterior limb of internal capsule (small arrow) with intraventricular extension (long arrows). Digital subtraction left internal carotid angiogram (B) reveals an ICA-bifurcation aneurysm (arrows)

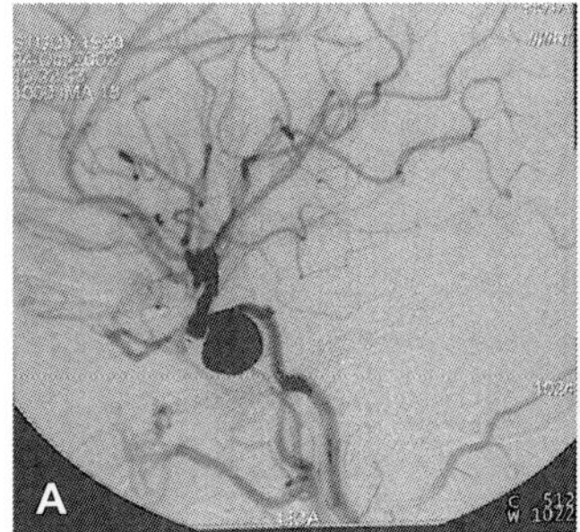

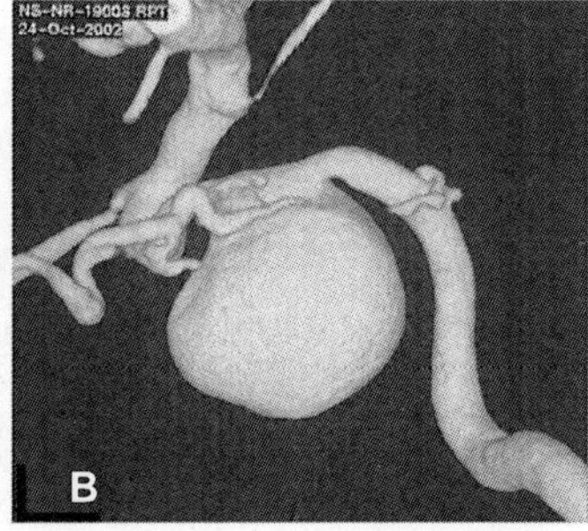

Fig. 3.7: Giant aneurysm. Digital subtraction right internal carotid angiogram (A) reveals a giant cavernous ICA aneurysm (arrows). The aneurysm morphology is better appreciated in 3D DSA (B)

Most studies indicate that the internal carotid artery bifurcation is the most common location for aneurysms in children (Fig. 3.6).[23-26] In addition, 15% of pediatric aneurysms arise from the posterior circulation compared with 5-10% in adults.[23-26] Other studies show a high incidence of intracavernous internal carotid artery aneurysms in children (Fig. 3.7).[23] The multiplicity of saccular aneurysms in children is low compared with adults, except in children with aneurysms of infectious origin.[27,28]

Clinical Presentation

Approximately 70% of children with aneurysms present with subarachnoid hemorrhage (SAH).[21] About 20% of patients have a history of recurrent headaches. Children tend to present with better clinical grades than those of adults.[22] Children who have giant aneurysms often present with mass effect and only 35% of the time with SAH.[22,27,29]

Neuroimaging

In a child with suspected SAH, the diagnosis begins with a non-contrast computed tomography (NCCT) scan of the head (Fig. 3.8). If this study is normal and the clinical history is strongly suspicious for SAH, then a lumbar puncture is required. The presence of xanthochromia or blood in CSF requires additional imaging in the form of a Digital subtraction angiography (DSA) or CT angiogram (CTA). The choice of imaging modality is made on a case-by-case basis with an effort to reduce unnecessary radiation exposure while obtaining the necessary data to plan treatment and postoperative management. DSA is still the gold standard for the diagnosis of cerebral aneurysms. For patients with unruptured aneurysms who may present with headache, seizures, or mass effect, MR imaging of the brain with an MR angiogram (MRA) of the circle of Willis is valuable to limit radiation exposure.

The presence of subarachnoid, intraventricular, intraparenchymal, or subdural hemorrhage with or without hydrocephalus should alert the physician to the possibility of an intracranial aneurysm. Although aneurysms can sometimes be detected by CT and MR as blood-filled saccular dilatations arising from major intracerebral vessels, DSA is essential to study precise anatomy (location and size of the neck of the aneurysm, precise size and orientation of the sac) and to locate additional aneurysms.

Management

Surgical treatment includes direct clipping, clip reconstruction, and aneurysm trapping with or without bypass procedures. In recent years there has been a shift toward the use of endovascular intervention with a strong desire to avoid open surgery in young children. Platinum detachable coils can be navigated into the aneurysm and electrolytically detached to occlude the aneurysm. Broad neck aneurysms may be occluded with coils using neck-remodelling techniques.

Fusiform aneurysm can be treated with surgical bypass with vessel occlusion or reconstruction. Alternatively, a balloon test occlusion of the parent vessel can be performed in an awake patient. If the test occlusion is tolerated, the parent artery and the aneurysm are permanently occluded with coils or detachable balloons.

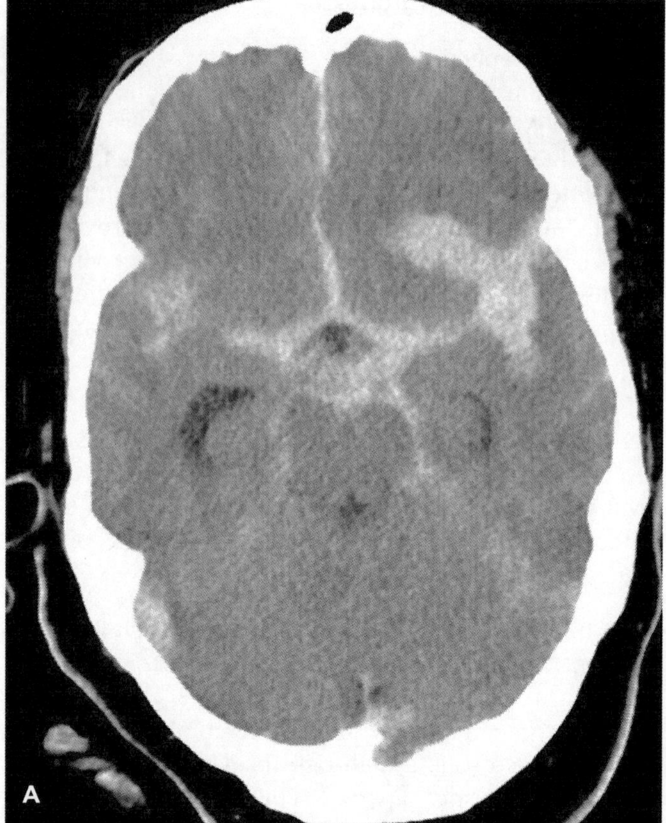

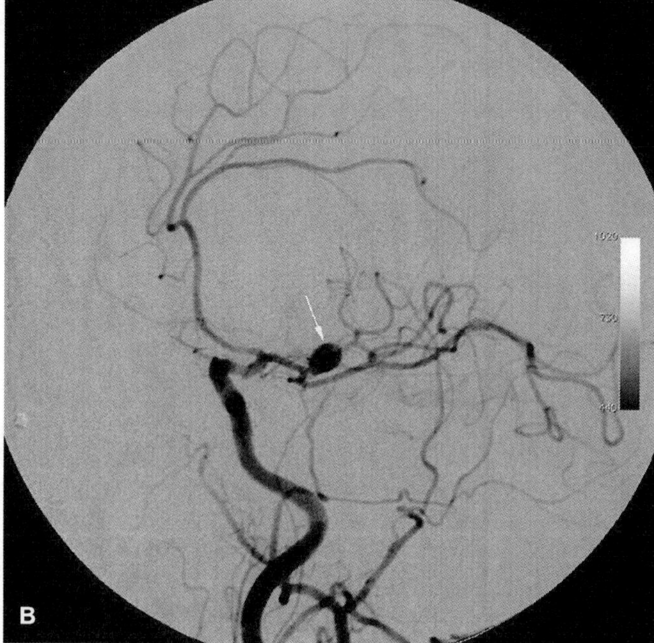

Fig. 3.8: SAH. NCCT shows diffuse hyperdensity in the basal and sylvian cisterns suggestive of SAH. IADSA (B) shows a left MCA bifurcation aneurysm (white arrow)

(b) Mycotic Aneurysm

The term "mycotic" aneurysm refers to those aneurysms resulting from any infectious process and includes bacterial, fungal and protozoan infections. Infectious or mycotic aneurysms are situated peripherally and accounts for about 15% of pediatric aneurysms.[30] The most common cause of mycotic aneurysms is an underlying bacterial endocarditis from which infectious thromboemboli cause a focal arteritis with degeneration of the elastic lamina and muscularis, resulting in a fusiform aneurysmal dilatation (Fig. 3.9). Another important cause of mycotic aneurysms in children is invasion of intracranial vessels by adjacent infections (i.e., middle ear/sinus infection, meningitis, osteomyelitis of the skull, septic cavernous thrombophlebitis). In these patients, the adventitia is involved first, followed by the muscularis and finally, the internal elastic lamina.

Clinical Presentation

When mycotic aneurysms are caused by bacterial endocarditis, the most common presenting symptom is subarachnoid or intracerebral hemorrhage resulting from aneurysmal rupture.[31] Less commonly, symptoms of cerebral ischemia may precede hemorrhage. Those patients with mycotic aneurysm within the cavernous sinus present with symptoms of septic cavernous sinus thrombophlebitis, including fever, orbital edema, venous engorgement, proptosis, chemosis and ophthalmoplegia.

Neuroimaging

CT or MRI may help to localize the aneurysm by demonstrating adjacent intraparenchymal hemorrhage (Fig. 3.9) or by directly visualizing the lesion, especially in the case of intracavernous aneurysms. Associated cerebritis, abscess, edema or infarction may be identified. Cerebral DSA is necessary for definitive diagnosis. On angiograms, mycotic aneurysms appear as fusiform dilatations of the affected vessel. They tend to be located peripherally (Fig. 3.9), most frequently in the distribution of the middle cerebral artery, in contrast to the saccular congenital aneurysms, which tend to be located on the circle of Willis.

Management

Following appropriate antimicrobial therapy, endovascular occlusion of the aneurysm can be considered. The decision regarding when to treat a mycotic aneurysm depends upon the size and location of the aneurysm, the clinical presentation, and observed changes in the patient and the aneurysm over time. Because mycotic aneurysms are typically fusiform, aneurysm treatment often necessitates occlusion of the involved vessel segment immediately proximal to the aneurysm origin. Collateral flow may preserve perfusion of parenchyma distal to the aneurysm. Surgical bypass (either entirely intracranial or extra-cranial to intracranial) with surgical interruption of the vessel proximal to the aneurysm may be indicated to preserve perfusion of eloquent cerebrovascular territory.

(c) Traumatic Aneurysm

Traumatic aneurysms account for about 5-15% of pediatric aneurysms, of which 40% involve distal anterior cerebral artery, 35% involve major vessels along the skull base and 25% are cortical in location.[21] They are most commonly caused by penetrating injuries, although blunt trauma, even seemingly mild concussive injury, may also result in damage to the craniocervical vessels. Penetrating injuries in children are often related to intraoral trauma, when the child falls on a stick or a pencil held in the mouth.

Unlike berry aneurysms, traumatic aneurysms tend to be peripheral, irregular and without necks. They also lack an endothelial lining, making them effectively

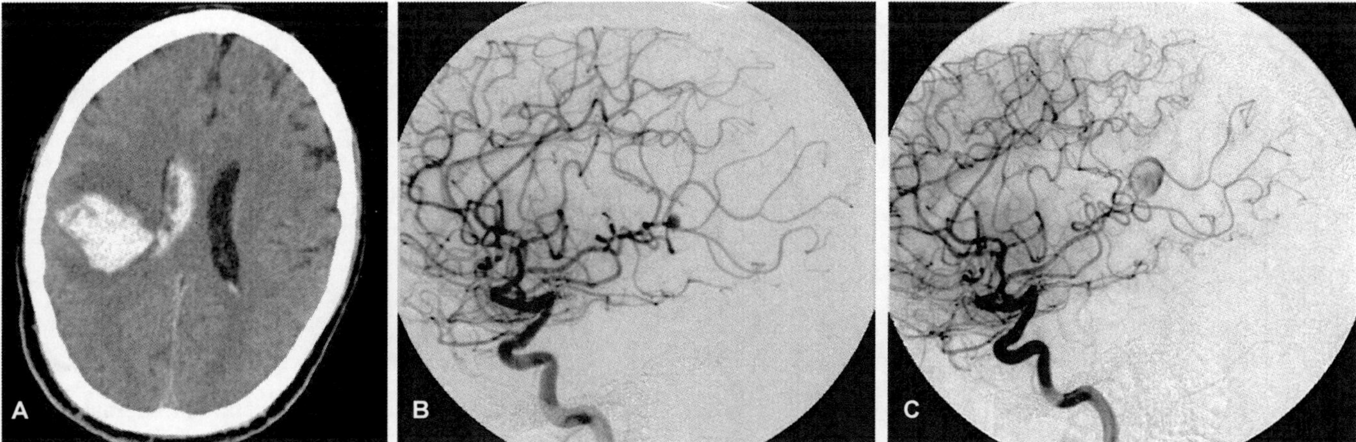

Fig. 3.9: Mycotic aneurysm CT scan. NCCT shows acute hyperdense hematoma in right frontal region with intraventricular extension. A 12-year-old boy with infective endocarditis presented with sudden onset left hemiparesis. NCCT (A) shows right frontal hematoma. Lateral view of right ICA angiogram (B) reveals a small aneurysm (arrow) in distal branches of right MCA. This patient was managed conservatively. Repeat angiogram (C) after 6 weeks shows increase in the size of aneurysm (arrow in C)

pseudoaneurysms and have a high risk of rupture or re-bleeding. When they are discovered, careful observation or treatment may be required. Once they are enlarged, they have a high risk of rupture, and immediate treatment is essential.

Clinical presentation may be significantly delayed with respect to the traumatic event, and a high index of clinical suspicion is warranted if these lesions are to be identified prior to catastrophic hemorrhage. Immediate arteriographic evaluation has been recommended, and arteriographic re-evaluation is suggested if no lesion is identified or after treatment is completed. Historically, the surgical approach has been difficult because disruption of the tenuous pseudocapsule may result in massive hemorrhage before vascular control can be established. More recently, endovascular occlusion of the feeding vessel or endovascular trapping of inflow and outflow to the aneurysm has proven effective.

(d) Dissecting Aneurysm (Nontraumatic)

Dissecting aneurysms are fusiform in appearance and has preaneurysmal or postaneurysmal narrowing. They occur 4 times more often in the pediatric population than in the adult population.[27,32] This type of aneurysm can occur in the anterior or posterior circulation, especially the P1 and P2 segments of the posterior cerebral artery, supraclinoid ICA, and middle cerebral artery (Fig. 3.10).[27,29] There are reports of dissecting aneurysms in children healing spontaneously with occlusion of the parent artery.

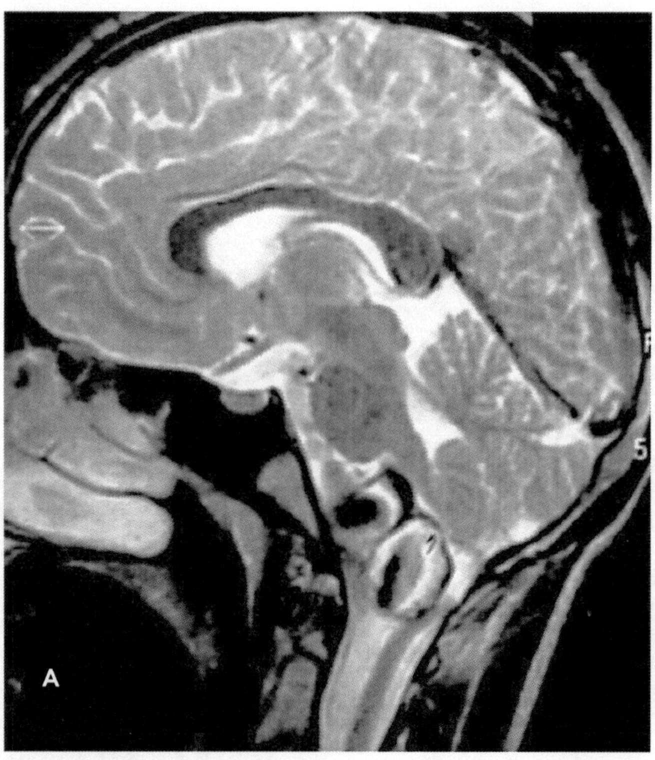

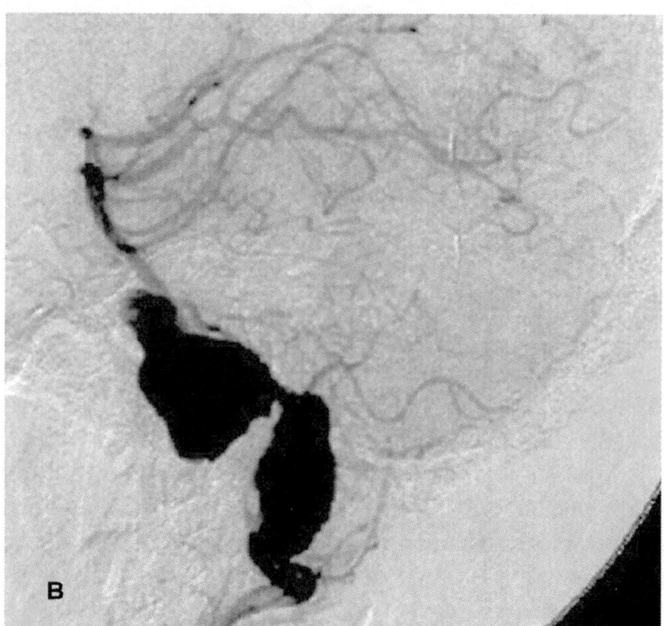

Fig. 3.10: HIV vasculopathy. A 14-year-old boy (seropositive for HIV) presented with sudden onset severe headache. CECT (A) shows acute right frontal hematoma with intraventricular extension. Axial T2-weighted image (B) reveals multiple aneurysms involving circle of Willis. Lateral view of left ICA angiogram (C) shows multiple dysplastic aneurysms involving ICA and its branches Dissecting aneurysm. Vertebral artery angiogram shows a dissecting aneurysm in the distal vertebral artery

5. Arteriovenous Malformations and Fistulas

Cerebral arteriovenous malformations (AVMs) are the most common and readily recognizable vascular malformations with a prevalence of roughly 0.2% to 0.8% of general population per year.[33] AVMs are congenital lesions composed of a complex tangle of arteries and veins connected by fistulae (Fig. 3.11).[34] In a certain group of

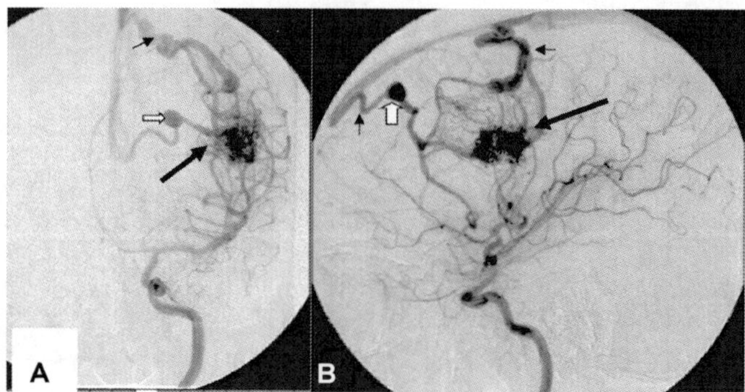

Fig. 3.11: AVM DSA. Digital subtraction left internal carotid angiogram, anteroposterior (A) and lateral views (B) show enlarged MCA branches feeding the AVM nidus (large arrows). Arteriovenous shunting is seen as early appearance of contrast in enlarged cortical veins (small arrows). Flow-related venous angiopathic change is illustrated by venous aneurysm (open arrow) in the one of the draining cortical veins

patients (up to 20%) the angioarchitectural abnormality is a direct arteriovenous fistula without an intervening angiomatous complex (Fig. 3.12).

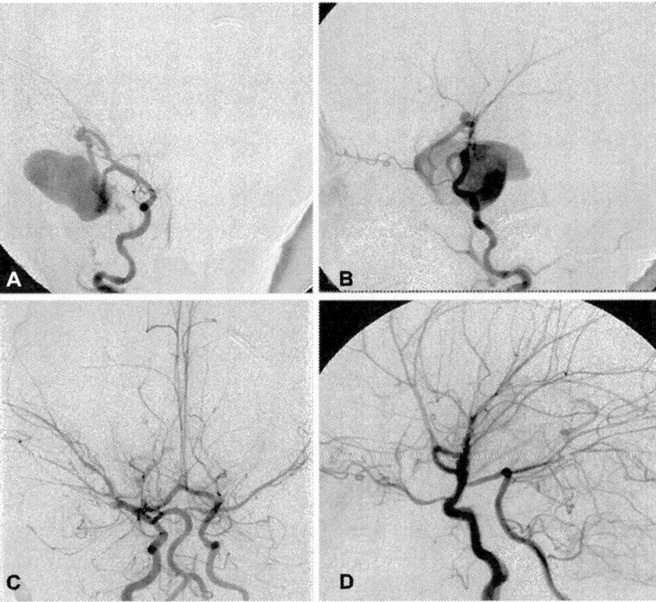

Fig. 3.12: AVM. A 3-year-male presented with right temporal hematoma. Digital subtraction right internal carotid angiogram, anteroposterior (A) and lateral view (B) show a pial arteriovenous fistula fed by right middle cerebral artery. Large venous pouch is present with no intervening nidus. Following embolization with glue, the fistula is completely occluded (C and D)

Cerebral AVMs have different characteristics in children than in adults, such as multifocal lesions, induced remote AV shunts, large venous ectasia, high flow lesions, venous thrombosis, brain atrophy and systemic phenomenon. Conversely, high flow angiopathic changes and flow related arterial aneurysms are extremely rare in children.[35]

More than 50% of cerebral AVMs present with intracranial hemorrhage (Fig. 3.13).[36] Other common presentations are seizure (20% to 25%), headaches (15%), focal neurological deficit (< 5%) and pulsatile tinnitus. In children younger than 2 years of age, presentation can include congestive heart failure, large head due to hydrocephalus and seizures.

Management

Management of intracranial AVMs is a multidisciplinary effort. Management strategies include single or combined therapy applying micro-neurosurgery, endovascular techniques, or radiosurgery (focused radiation) (Fig. 3.12). The lesion can be monitored expectantly with the understanding that the patient would have some risk of

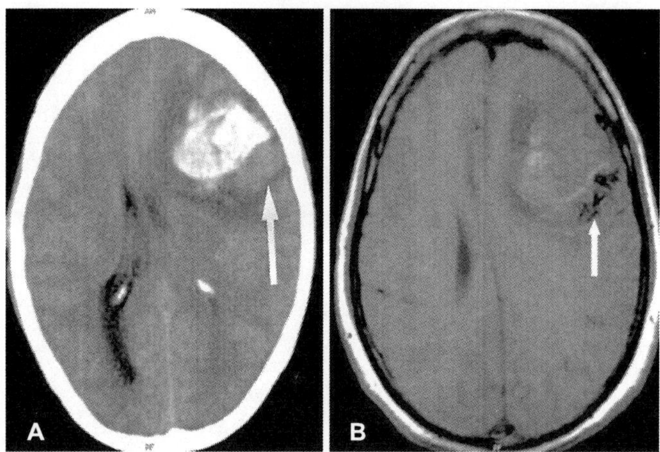

Fig. 3.13: AVM. A 12-year-old girl presented with acute onset headache. NCCT (A) reveals left frontal acute hematoma, which is iso-hyperintense on T1-WI (B). The posterior portion of hematoma is isodense on NCCT (arrow in A), which shows vascular flow-voids on T1-W1 (arrow in B), suggesting AVM with bleed

hemorrhage or other neurological symptoms such as seizures or focal deficit.

6. Complex Cranio-Facial Vascular Lesions

Complex cranio-facial vascular diseases are rare disease constituting 0.5% of all cerebral vascular malformations, without sex dominance.[37] It is nonhereditary and is believed to be caused by somatic mutation in neural crest or adjacent cephalic mesoderm prior to migration. It include two recently recognized forms of presentation, both carrying an underlying metameric linkage between the intracranial and facial vascular territories:

(1) Cerebrofacial arteriovenous metameric syndrome (CAMS); and

(2) Cerebrofacial venous metameric syndrome (CVMS). CAMS corresponds to Wyburn-Mason or Bonnet-Dechaume-Blanc syndromes, whereas CVMS to Sturge-Weber syndrome (SWS). According to the involved metamere (hypothalamonasal, prosencephalo-orbito-maxillary, or rhombencephalo-mandibular), these lesions are named CAMS-1, CAMS-2, CAMS-3 and CVMS-1, CVMS-2 or CVMS-3 respectively.[38] Each group can be expected to be inhomogeneous.[39]

CAMS-1/CVMS-1	Medial prosencephalic group with involvement of nose and hypothalamus
CAMS-2/CVMS-2	Lateral prosencephalic group with involvement of occipital lobe, optic chiasma, optic tract, thalamus, retina and maxilla
CAMS-3/CVMS-3	Rhombencephalic group with involvement of cerebellum, pons and mandible

Clinical Presentation

The age at presentation of the patients with CAMS is much younger than in sporadic AVMs.[38] The clinical presentation of patients with CAMS varies according to the spectrum of organ involvement in this metameric disease. But in general, the most common presenting symptom is progressive visual loss, followed by neurological deficit with or without hemorrhagic event.[38] Seizures are infrequent presenting features.

Neuroimaging

The cerebral AVMs in CAMS could evolve continuously from the optic chiasm, hypothalamus, thalamus and cortical lesion around the calcarine fissure or even cerebellum depending on the 1, 2 or 3 subtype of CAMS, mostly presenting in contiguous scattered fashion; but could infrequently present as isolated multiple lesions.[38] AVM nidi in CAMS patient are usually described as a cluster or bunch of smoke-like, small fine nidi intervening with normal brain tissue and optic pathways with some degree of angiogenesis. Usually lesions are localized in one hemisphere, but there are a few reports of bilateral involvement, crossing the midline.

The appropriate investigations for patients suspected of harboring CAMS vary, due to different clinical manifestations and revealing lesions in their spectrum.[40] The patients suspected of CAMS 1 with hypothalamic AVMs should be investigated in detail for nasal AVMs and orbital AVMs by physical examination and detailed ophthalmological examination.[40] For CAMS 2, patients with mesencephalic lesions such as chiasmatic or optic nerve AVMs with progressive visual loss, should be investigated for maxillary vascular lesions including AVMs or metameric proximal dysplastic aneurysm within the nasal or pterygopalatine fossa. This could prevent life-threatening epistaxis from the asymptomatic aneurysm.[40] For CAMS 3, patients with cerebellar AVMs should be investigated for mandibular lesions such as high flow mandibular AVMs; those could lead to severe bleeding after tooth extraction in the adolescent.[40] Conversely, the presence of maxillary or mandibular AVM should raise the possibility of intracranial AVM, in the related metameric area.

(a) Wyburn-Mason Syndrome

Wyburn-Mason syndrome (WMS) is a distinct congenital neurocutaneous entity comprising ipsilateral AVMs of the midbrain, vascular abnormalities affecting the visual pathway, and facial nevi. The presence of all three is not required for the diagnosis, and there are numerous reports of patients in whom one or more characteristics are absent. WMS usually belongs to the CAMS 2 group originating from the lateral prosencephalon.

Clinical Presentation

WMS usually presents in childhood, occasionally at birth. Specific symptoms and signs vary with location and size of the AVM.

The facial nevi are vary from faint discolorations to extensive angiomatous nevi. They are usually unilateral, infrequently bilateral, and may conform to the distribution of the trigeminal nerve.

Ocular features include decreased visual acuity, proptosis (occasionally pulsatile), pupillary defects, optic atrophy, congestion of bulbar conjunctiva, and visual field defects.

CNS symptoms include headache or retro-orbital pain and hemiparesis and subarachnoid hemorrhage. Other presentations include mental retardation, irritability, cerebellar dysfunction, and Parinaud's syndrome.[41] In one-third of the patients, intracranial AVM may be asymptomatic.[41]

Neuroimaging

The imaging findings reflect the primary vascular lesions and any secondary complications. MR imaging of the brain and orbit, as well as MR angiography should also be considered (Fig. 3.14). MR imaging and CT are helpful in delineating the extent and the precise location of vascular lesions affecting the brain and orbit, and their relationship to neighboring structures (Fig. 3.14).[41] Cerebral angiography can provide further information about the hemodynamics and the arterial supply of such lesions, and is used to confirm the diagnosis.[41] Cerebral angiography, however, is typically reserved for symptomatic patients, given the significant risks associated with the procedure.[41]

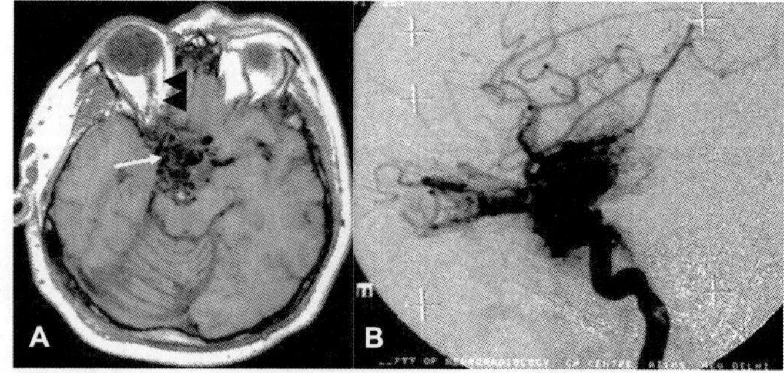

Fig. 3.14: Wyburn Mason syndrome. T1-weighed MR scan (A) reveals vascular flow-voids in the right orbit (black arrowhead) and optic chiasm (arrow). Lateral (B) right internal carotid artery angiograms show arteriovenous malformation involving the right optic nerve and optic chiasma

The retinal AVMs vary from tiny angiographically occult lesions to large, tortuous, and dilated vessels covering much of the retina. Arterial supply to the AVMs arises from the internal carotid artery more often than from the vertebrobasilar arteries or the external carotid artery. Venous drainage is primarily via the cavernous sinus or the vein of Galen.

(b) Sturge-Weber Syndrome (Encephalotrigeminal Angiomatosis)

Sturge-Weber syndrome (SWS) is a rare, sporadic neurocutaneous syndrome characterized by a classical triad of facial port wine nevus involving the first sensory branch of trigeminal nerve, ipsilateral leptomeningeal angiomatosis, and choroidal angioma.[42] Sporadic cases of SWS without facial nevus (SWS type III) have been rarely reported. It has been postulated that venous stasis results in hypoperfusion of the subjacent brain parenchyma, progressively insufficient to meet metabolic demands, particularly in the presence of seizures.

Clinical Presentation

The facial angioma has a predilection for the distribution of the first division of the trigeminal nerve. The disease process is usually unilateral. Progressive neurologic symptoms, including epilepsy (80%), visual field defects, and hemiparesis, are often present in children with SWS and are probably the result of hypoxia-induced cortical injury.

Neuroimaging

Imaging studies are useful for confirming the diagnosis of Sturge-Weber syndrome and evaluating the extent of intracranial involvement and may be important when clinical stigmata are atypical or not yet developed.

CT scans show the tramline gyriform calcification of apposing gyri that underlies the contrast-enhancing leptomeningeal angiomatosis (Fig. 3.15). The subjacent white matter may be hypodense on CT scans. The choroid plexus may be enlarged ipsilateral to the angiomatosis with enlarged transcortical (medullary) veins. Other features on CT scans include ipsilateral cortical atrophy, enlargement of the ipsilateral ventricle, and loss of volume of the ipsilateral cranial cavity (Fig. 3.15).

MRI demonstrates atrophy of the cerebral hemisphere subjacent to the leptomeningeal angioma, with small gyri and enlarged adjacent sulci. Subtle atrophy is frequently more obvious on MRIs than on CT scans. On T2-weighted images, the angioma appears as a hyperintense leptomeningeal thickening. Contract-enhanced MRI reveals a pial, enhancing, angiomatous malformation, often in the occipital or posterior temporoparietal region ipsilateral to the facial angioma (Fig. 3.16). The subcortical white matter underlying the area of leptomeningeal angiomatosis shows decreased T2 signal intensity. Calcification in the underlying cortex is not as evident as on CT scans (Fig. 3.15), but it does not mask enhancement of the underlying angiomatous malformation, which can be a problem with CT. As in contrast-enhanced CT, the glomus of the choroid plexus may be enlarged, and enlarged draining transcortical veins may be present in the involved cerebral hemisphere. The overlying superficial cortical veins are reduced in size and number, with a prominent deep collateral venous system.

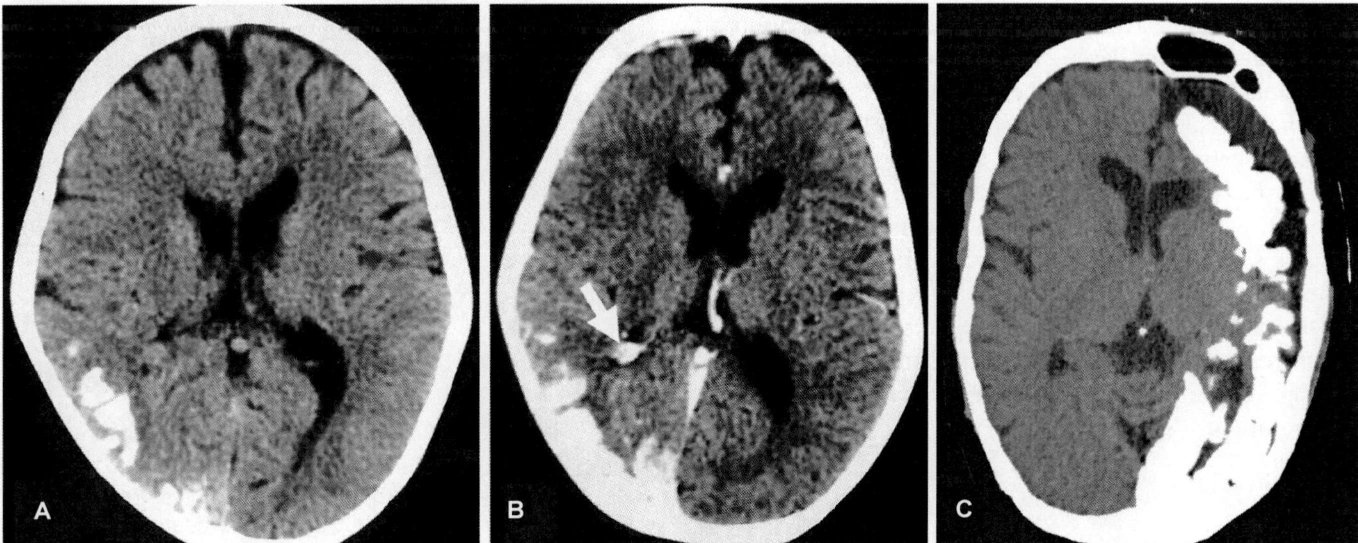

Fig. 3.15: Sturge-Weber syndrome. NCCT (A) and CECT (B) reveal gyriform calcification and enhancement in the right occipital lobe and enlargement of left choroids plexus (arrow in B). NCCT (C) shows advanced SWS with hemispheric calcification and atrophy

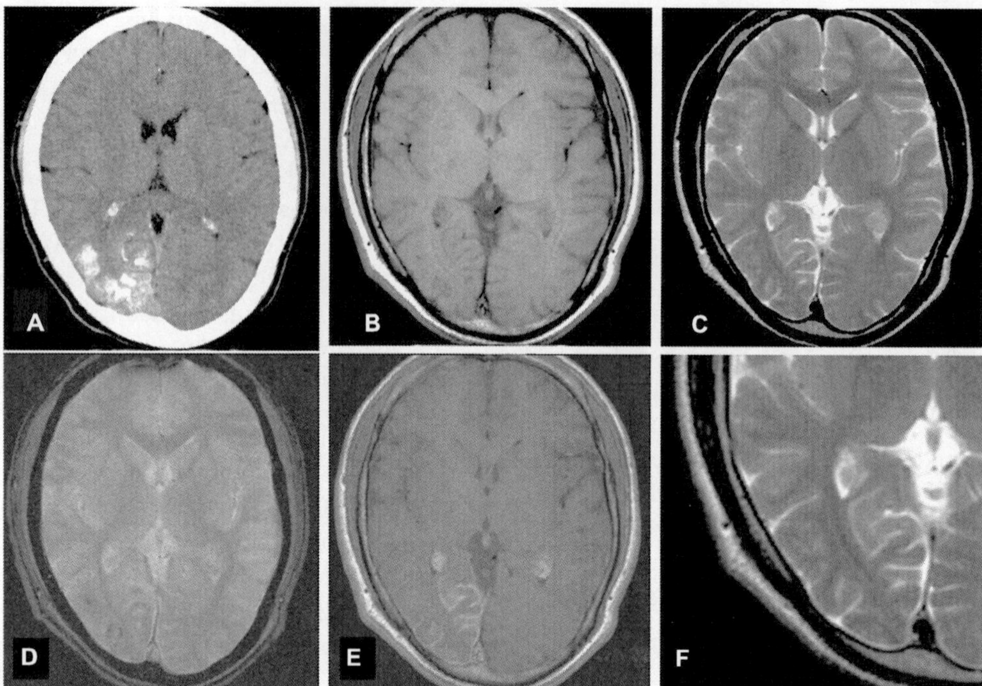

Fig. 3.16: Sturge-Weber syndrome

Perfusion-weighted MRI is a helpful technique to quantitatively evaluate blood flow abnormalities at different stages of evolution of SWS.[43] Increased perfusion in mostly younger patients may represent a transient phenomenon, before severe brain atrophy occurs in the affected brain regions. Decreased perfusion is associated with high seizure frequency, long epilepsy duration, and brain atrophy, suggesting a detrimental effect of chronic seizures on brain structure and function.[43]

7. Carotid Cavernous Fistula

Carotid cavernous fistulas (CCFs) are abnormal communications between the carotid arterial system and the venous cavernous sinus. CCFs can be spontaneous, secondary to trauma, or associated cavernous sinus pathology. Typically they are seen in adults and have been classified according to their hemodynamic properties.[44-45] They rarely occur in children with connective tissue disorders such as Ehlers-Danlos syndrome. These fistulas can often present to the ophthalmologist with eyelid fullness, proptosis, dilated episcleral vessels, chemosis, bruit, increased intraocular pressure, and decreased visual acuity. Initially, these signs may be subtle, and early suspicion by the eye care provider is paramount.

Neuroimaging

Initial imaging often consists of a CT scan. An asymmetrically enlarged cavernous sinus or superior ophthalmic vein is suggestive of a CCF and should prompt a call to the referring physician for further clinical information (Fig. 3.17). DSA is essential in confirming the diagnosis and delineating exact venous drainage patterns (Fig. 3.18). To accurately identify a CCF, selective catheterization of the right and left external and internal carotid arteries and the vertebral arteries is necessary.

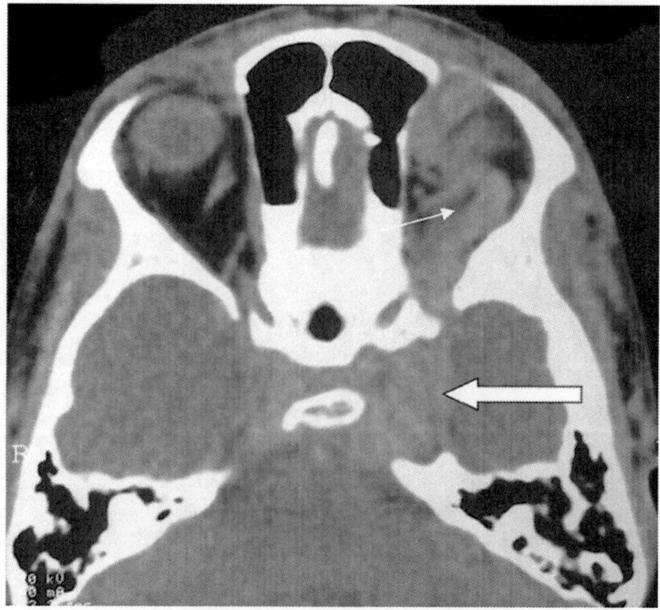

Fig. 3.17: CCF CT. A 9-year-old boy had head injury 6 months back and presented with left eye proptosis, redness and diplopia for last 4 months. CECT shows dilated left superior ophthalmic vein (thin arrow) and left cavernous sinus (thick arrow), suggesting left carotid cavernous fistula in view of clinical presentation

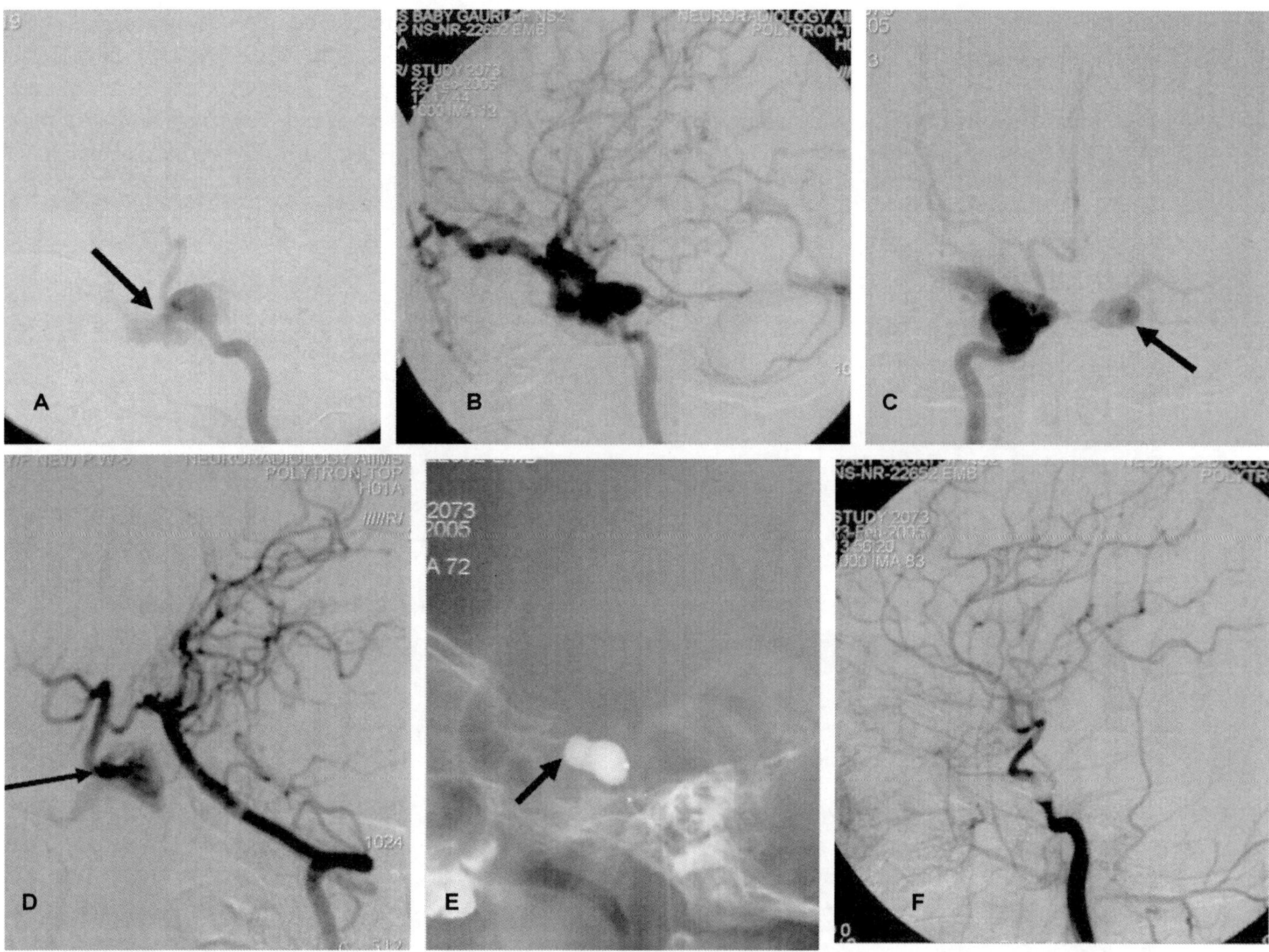

Fig. 3.18 (A-F): CCF DSA. A 5-year-old girl, known case of Down syndrome, developed a spontaneous direct carotid-cavernous fistula during an episode of dengue hemorrhagic fever. Right ICA angiogram (A and B) shows the probable site of fistula (arrow in A) and the venous drainage into ophthalmic and cortical veins. Right ICA angiogram in AP view (C) shows that the fistula was also draining into contralateral cavernous sinus (arrow). The site of fistula (arrow) is better visualized in vertebral artery injection during carotid compression (D). The fistula was embolized with detachable balloon (E) with complete closure of the shunt (F)

Management

Most direct CCFs can be effectively treated by occluding the fistula with transarterially deployed detachable balloons, with preservation of the internal carotid artery (Fig. 3.18). In the event that the balloon cannot be fed through the fistula via a transarterial approach, electrolytically detachable platinum coils are often deployed via a transarterial route. In the event that a transarterial route is impossible or ineffective, a transvenous approach using platinum coils may be warranted. This can be achieved either via the femoral route or surgically via the superior ophthalmic vein.

8. Vein of Galen Malformations

Vein of Galen aneurysmal malformations (VGAMs) are rare congenital malformations arising from fistulous communication with the median vein of the prosencephalon, a primitive precursor of midline cerebral venous structures. VGAMS constitute 1% of all intracranial vascular malformations. However, they represent 30% of vascular malformations presenting in the pediatric age group.[46] Most of these malformations present in early childhood, often causing congestive heart failure in the neonate.

VGAM is caused by persistence of the 'median prosencephalic vein of Markowski', the precursor of the true vein of Galen, which normally disappears by 6-11 weeks (21-50 mm) stage.[47,48] The aetiology of VGAMs is unknown; however, an early insult, perhaps resulting in a somatic mutation in neural crest and/or adjacent cephalic mesoderm in the early embryo, could be expected to cause such vascular abnormalities.[49]

According to angioarchitecture, two forms of VGAM exist, i.e., choroidal and mural.[50] The choroidal type corresponds to a very primitive condition, with a contribution of several choroidal arteries and an interposed network before the opening into the large venous pouch (Fig. 3.19). Mural lesions, by contrast, are characterized by a fistula or fistulae in the wall of the median prosencephalic vein, often located laterally. They typically have fewer feeding arteries and do not have a complex arterial maze (Fig. 3.20).[35,51,52] Mixed forms may occur, such as those with a choroidal nidus and high-flow fistulas located in the wall of the venous pouch.

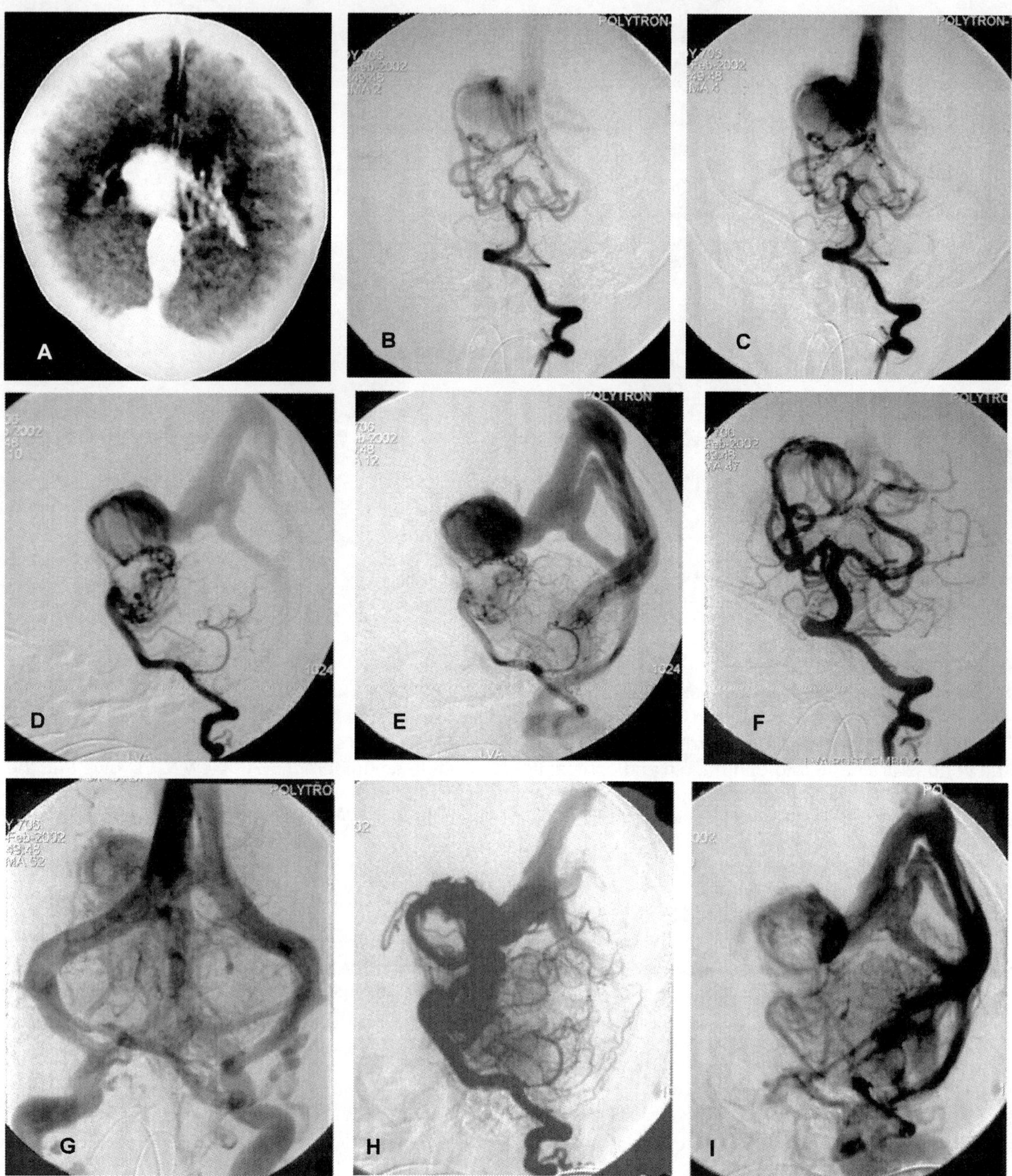

Fig. 3.19: Choroidal VGAM. A 6-month-old girl child presented with congestive cardiac failure. CECT (A) revealed a VGAM. Anteroposterior (B,C) and lateral (D,E) left vertebral angiogram show a choroidal (subarachnoid) arteriovenous shunt of the vein of Galen fed by posterior choroidal arteries (single arrows) and draining into the embryonic precursor to the vein of Galen (double white arrow). There is presence of falcine sinus (black arrow). Following embolization with glue, Anteroposterior (F, G) and lateral (H, I) left vertebral angiogram show reduced shunt through the fistula

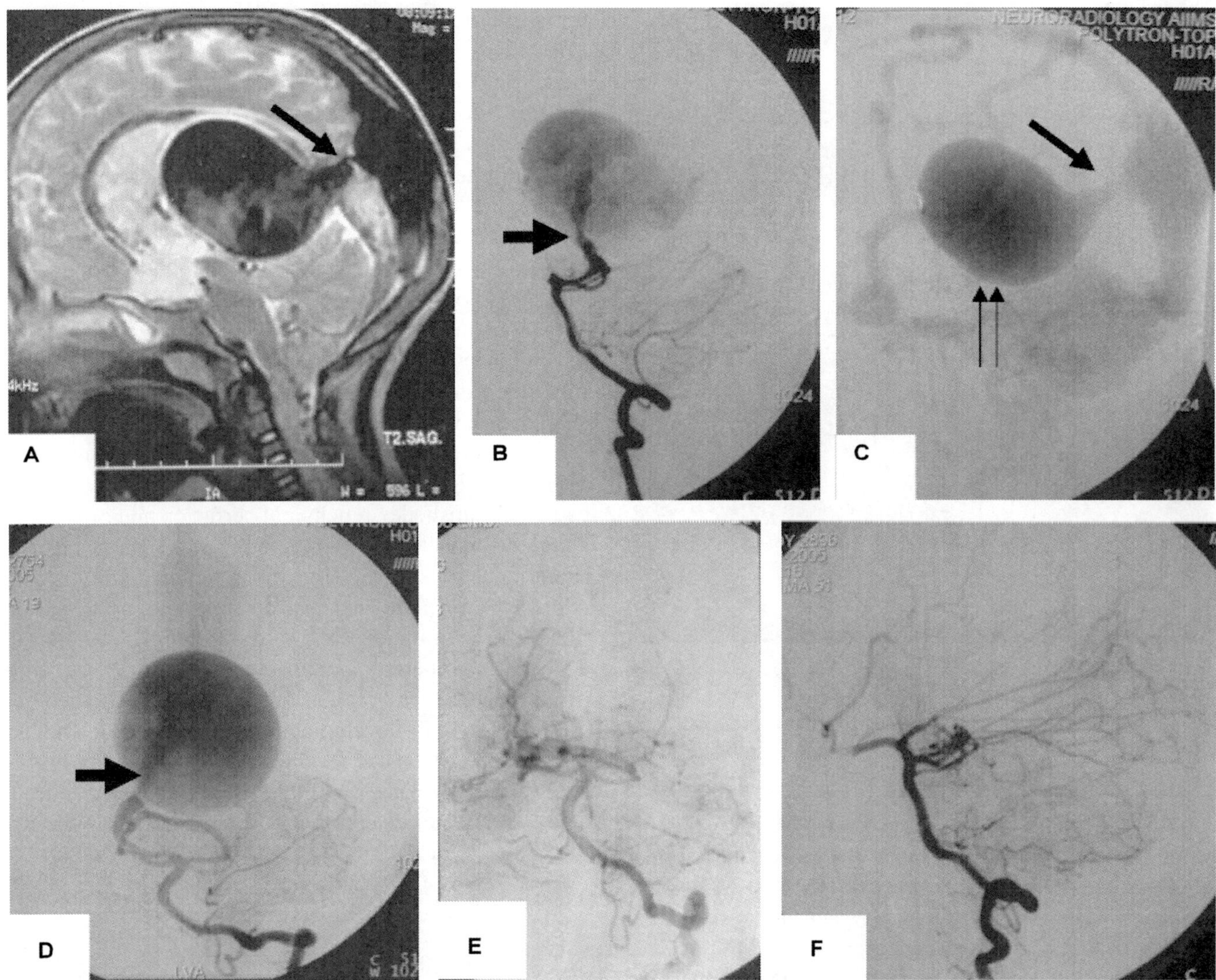

Fig. 3.20: Mural VGAM. An 8-month-old boy presented with increasing head size and inability to walk. On MRI (A), there is evidence of vein of Galen aneurysmal malformation associated with persistent falcine sinus (arrow). Left vertebral artery (LVA) lateral (arterial phase B, venous p C) angiograms shows a large arteriovenous fistula (AVF; thick arrow in B) with a large venous pouch (double arrow), persistent falcine sinus and atresia of straight sinus. LVA AP (D) angiograms shows fistula (arrow) with large venous pouch. The AVF was embolized with almost pure glue. Post embolisation LVA AP (E) and lateral (F) angiograms show complete closure of fistula

Clinically, the choroidal type is more common and usually present in neonates with congestive cardiac failure. The mural type presents in infants with macrocephaly, asymptomatic cardiomegaly, or mild heart failure. Macrocrania and hydrocephalus result from abnormal hemodynamic conditions present in torcular sinus confluence and the immaturity of the arachnoidal granulation.

Neuroimaging

VGAMs are occasionally detected on antenatal ultrasound scans (from about 25 weeks gestation) as apparently cystic midline brain lesions, colour flow Doppler then suggesting a VGAM. Antenatal MR imaging will confirm the diagnosis.

Calcifications are related to slow, relentless insults to the brain and can be seen in CT scan in:

(1) Mural (i.e., in the lesion itself), secondary to partial or complete thrombosis.

(2) In the subcortical white matter, reflecting deep watershed failure.

(3) In the striatum bilaterally and symmetrically, as a result of striatal congestion (venous ischemia) (Fig. 3.21).

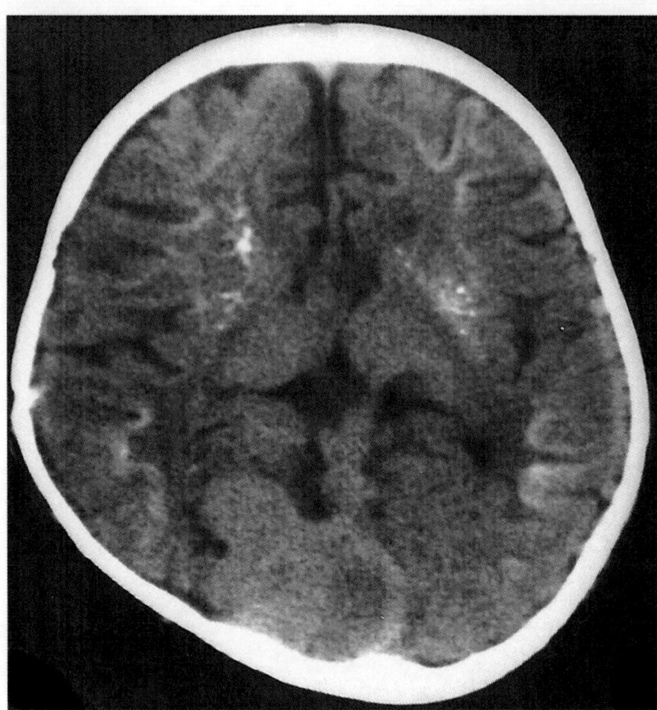

Fig. 3.21: VGAM CT scan. A 12-year-girl was referred to us because of seizure disorder in a neglected VGAM. NCCT demonstrates bilateral symmetrical calcifications in subcortical region and putamino-caudate region, indicating transcerebral venous collateral circulation in the brain

The exquisite soft tissue contrast of MRI makes it the modality of choice in the evaluation of the ventricular system and cerebral parenchymal changes. MR angiography is being increasingly used as a non-invasive alternative to diagnostic angiographic studies in the initial evaluation of these lesions.[53] MR angiography can demonstrate the location of fistula, presence of any nidus, the arterial components, the venous sac as well as the status of venous drainage.

Catheter angiography remains the gold standard for the evaluation of VAGMs (Figs. 3.19 and 3.20). It scores over non-invasive modalities such as CT angiography and MR angiography in demonstrating small feeders supplying the fistula, as well as the dynamic aspects of the venous drainage of the normal brain, and hemodynamic relationships with the venous drainage of the arteriovenous shunt.[53]

Management

Endovascular management is a suitable method of treatment and results in cure or stabilization of the shunt.

The timing of endovascular management is determined by the clinical presentation. Congestive cardiac failure in a neonate that is refractory to medical treatment is an indication for emergency embolization. Embolization is then performed after the first week of life to allow the infant's circulatory system to adapt to its new postnatal requirements. At this time, the goal of therapy in such patients would be to arrest the congestive cardiac failure rather than to achieve complete obliteration of the shunt so even partial embolization is acceptable. Afterward, embolization may be completed at 5 months of age. If embolization is still incomplete at that time, other sessions may be scheduled depending on the clinical evolution. In neonate apart from heart failure, the development of hydrocephalus is generally an indication for urgent embolization. Ventricular shunt procedure should be avoided as far as possible as CSF diversion results in a reversal of flow in the medullary veins from a cerebrofugal direction to a cerebripetal one which, in turn, causes diminished parenchymal perfusion and progressive deterioration;[54] only after embolization can ventricular shunting be contemplated for nontolerated hydrocephalus cases. In an infant who has not presented with cardiac failure or decompensated hydrocephalus, the aim of endovascular therapy would be to prevent consequences of chronic cerebral venous hypertension and to promote normal cerebral development.[55] Treatment at the age of 5 months balances the benefits of safe embolization against the risk of cerebral damage. Imaging evidence of encephalomalacia is considered a relative contraindication to endovascular therapy.[50]

The choice of the specific endovascular approach depends on the angioarchitecture of the malformation. Arteriovenous fistulas are occluded on the arterial side, using embolic agents such as coils, cyanoacrylates and detachable balloons. This route is preferred for embolization by most authors. Transvenous and transtorcular coil embolization of the venous sac have been used to achieve flow reduction in selected cases with high-flow fistulas. Venous embolization may be reserved for patients in whom arterial route embolization is impossible or unsuccessful.

Spontaneous thrombosis of a VGAM is rare (2.5%)[56] and only one half of them are neurologically normal, which is less than what can be accomplished with proper treatment. Spontaneous thrombosis should not be considered a favorable outcome, and expecting it to occur does not represent an acceptable therapeutic strategy.[56]

PEDIATRIC STROKE

Stroke is defined as the sudden occlusion or rupture of cerebral arteries or veins resulting in focal cerebral damage and neurological deficits. Forms of stroke resulting from vascular occlusion are arterial ischemic stroke (AIS) and sinovenous thrombosis (SVT) and those resulting from vascular rupture are called hemorrhagic stroke. The International Pediatric Stroke Study (IPSS) group defines AIS as neurological deficit of acute onset, or seizures alone in neonate, and MRI or CT demonstrating cerebral parenchymal infarct(s) corresponding to known arterial territory(ies). Neuroimaging is therefore included in the definition and is now a necessary part of the diagnosis of pediatric stroke.[57]

Neuroimaging should be done early in the diagnostic evaluation to confirm the stroke diagnosis, to assess for intracranial hemorrhage, and to evaluate both the stroke type (arterial vs venous distribution) and pattern (multifocal embolic, border-zone, large-vessel, etc.). The choice of imaging modality in pediatric stroke depends on many factors including availability, sensitivity, potential risks, and the need for sedation. Magnetic resonance imaging provides a non-invasive method of investigating childhood stroke, aiding in both better diagnosis and management of this problem.[58]

Pediatric stroke can be segregated in perinatal or neonatal and childhood subtypes as they have different etiologies and management.

1. Perinatal or Neonatal Stroke

Neonatal stroke encompasses both ischemic and hemorrhagic events resulting from disruption of either arteries or veins from early gestation through the first month of life. The term perinatal stroke describes cerebrovascular lesions that occur from 28 weeks' gestation through the first 7 days of life, although some authors broaden this range from 20 weeks' gestation to 28 days after birth, and lesions occurring even before 20 weeks have been documented.[59,60] Approximately 80% of these are ischemic, and the remainder are due to CVST or hemorrhage. Risk factors for neonatal stroke include cardiac disorders, coagulation disorders, infection, trauma, drugs, maternal and placental disorders, and perinatal asphyxia.[60] Suspected maternal risk factors for perinatal arterial ischemic stroke include a history of infertility, chorioamnionitis, premature rupture of membranes, and preeclampsia.[61] Perinatal/neonatal strokes are increasingly recognized, although the exact incidence is unknown because of variations in presentation, evaluation and criteria for diagnosis.

Both neonatal arterial and venous strokes often present with seizures, typically focal motor seizures involving only 1 extremity. Stroke accounts for an estimated 10% of the seizures in term neonates.[62]

The majority of infarcts occur in full-term infants who present with neonatal encephalopathy and seizures in the first few days of life. The infarcts may be in the distribution of an arterial territory or in a border-zone distribution. Most frequently, the infarcts involve the middle cerebral artery territory and its branches, with the left hemisphere more frequently affected than the right. Although the reported causes of neonatal stroke include cardiac disorders, emboli, infection, coagulation abnormalities and/or perinatal events (birth asphyxia), the cause of a large number of cases remain undetermined.

The optimal imaging study is somewhat dependent on the child's clinical stability. Cranial ultrasound is safe and readily available, but it may miss superficial and ischemic lesions.[63] CT is relatively quick, accurately depicts superficial or hemorrhagic lesions, and confirms the lesion location. However, venous thrombosis and early arterial ischemic stroke (AIS) are easily missed with CT.

Like ultrasound, MRI techniques do not expose the neonate to the potentially harmful effects of ionizing radiation. MRI, magnetic resonance angiography (MRA), and magnetic resonance venography (MRV) may more accurately define the site of an arterial or venous occlusion. Additionally, MR studies often demonstrate associated parenchymal abnormalities more clearly, including non-ischemic lesions that clinically mimic arterial or venous stroke. Diffusion-weighted imaging can confirm the presence and location of an infarction earlier than other MRI sequences or CT.[64] CT angiography (CTA) is an accurate means of identifying primary vascular abnormalities when there is an unexplained hemorrhagic lesion. Catheter angiography (CA) is technically more difficult in babies and tends to be done only when endovascular surgical intervention is anticipated.

Similar to adult strokes, DWI, by demonstrating cytotoxic edema, has been found to increase the sensitivity and conspicuity of detecting neonatal strokes compared with conventional MRI. It has, however, been found that the normalization of restricted diffusion may occur earlier than in adult strokes (about 2 weeks) and DWI may be falsely negative after 1 week. T2-weighted sequences therefore should supplement DWI to reliably detect subacute ischemic lesions.

2. Childhood Stroke

Stroke in children is relatively rare and frequently results in a lack of recognition and delay in diagnosis. Reported incidence of pediatric stroke outside the neonatal period is estimated between 2.3 and 13 per 100,000 per year.[65,66]

The incidence is slightly higher in boys and those of black ethnicity, which is not fully explained by the increased prevalence of sickle cell disease in this population.[67,68] Patterns of stroke vary from adults, with ischemic strokes accounting for only approximately 55% of childhood strokes, versus 80-85% in adults.

Infants and older children present in a similar manner to adult stroke, however the multitude of risk factors, which often act synergistically, may compound the clinical findings, which may be more subtle and less specific. Heart disease whether congenital or acquired, malformations, metabolic and hematological disorders and vasospastic conditions like migraine are seen more often in childhood strokes. Cardiac disorders and hemoglobinopathy are the most common causes of ischemic infarction in children, whereas various congenital anomalies of the blood vessels or defects in coagulation or platelet function often are found in children with parenchymal hemorrhage.

Imaging in Childhood Stroke

The role of imaging is to establish the diagnosis, exclude stroke mimics, investigate the cause of the stroke and to guide and monitor treatment. MRI is the modality of choice due to its greater sensitivity and specificity compared to CT. DWI sequences are mandatory in all stroke imaging as it allows detection of a hyperacute infarct prior to changes on T2W sequences. If MRI is not available within 48 hours then a CT is acceptable as a suitable alternative. MR angiography has been shown to be as effective as conventional angiography (CA) in diagnosing most of the cerebrovascular disorders in children,[69-72] although CA should be performed for cases where the diagnosis remains unclear. It should also be considered in suspected cases of small vessel arteriopathy and vasculitis.[70] Imaging with fat suppression sequences (short tau inversion recovery (STIR) with fat suppression inversion time or fat-saturated T1W imaging) through the neck increases conspicuity of the intramural hematoma in cases of arterial dissection.[73]

Treatment options include aspirin and anticoagulation, surgical revascularisation procedures and management of risk factors.[62] As data regarding the safety and efficacy of thrombolysis are lacking in children, thrombolysis is not recommended for children with AIS outside a clinical trial.[62]

CAUSES OF CHILDHOOD STROKE

Below are the more common conditions associated with AIS.

1. Arteriopathy

(a) Focal Cerebral Arteriopathy of Childhood

The most common type of arteriopathy associated with AIS is a focal cerebral arteriopathy (FCA).[74] The arteriopathy is often monophasic and non-progressive (i.e., it does not progress or recur but the arterial stenosis often persists), and if this can be demonstrated then it may be termed transient cerebral arteriopathy (TCA). There is typical involvement of proximal vessels around the circle of Willis, mostly the M1, A1 and P1 segments (Fig. 3.22). The stenosis can be multifocal and may also affect more distal intracranial arterial branches. It is best demonstrated on CA, but MRA can also show the areas. Multifocal stenosis is seen as beading on vascular imaging. It usually presents as infarction of the anterior circulation, typically in the MCA territory (Fig. 3.22).

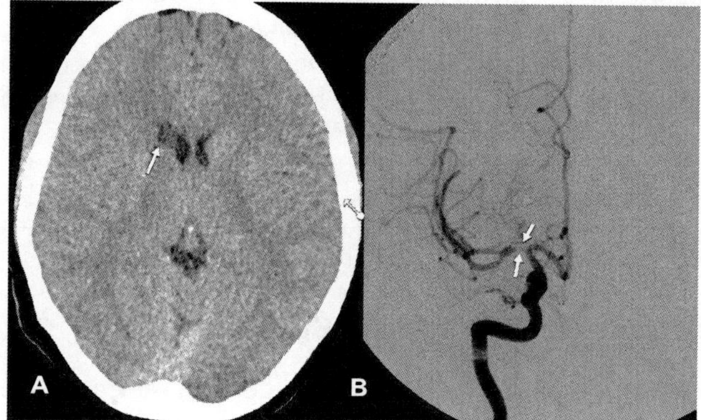

Fig. 3.22: Focal cerebral arteriopathy. NCCT (A) shows a hypodense chronic infarct (arrow) in right caudate head. IADSA of Right ICA (B) shows focal stenosis of proximal middle cerebral artery (arrows)

The cause of FCA is unknown. The pathophysiology is thought to be inflammation of the blood vessels induced by infection. There have been numerous studies demonstrating an association between AIS and a preceding varicella zoster infection in the 12 months prior to the stroke.[57,75] This has been termed 'post varicella angiopathy'.[76] A recent upper respiratory tract infection was the only significant univariate predictor of FCA in the IPSS, suggesting that infections other than varicella zoster may also play a role in the pathophysiology of this disease.[74] However, trauma and non-infectious inflammation can also result in the same angiographic appearance and FCA may therefore represent the end angiographic appearance of multiple pathologies.

(b) Infectious Vasculitis

Secondary vasculitis due to infection is a well-recognized cause pediatric stroke; many different agents have been implicated. It is important to have a high index of suspicion for infection as the cause of vasculitis and stroke, because treatment can be directed at the underlying organism. General clues to infectious vasculitis are associated fever, abnormality of the peripheral leukocyte count, and recent or current extraneural infection.

Mycobacterium tuberculosis is the most common cause of chronic meningitis. The thick gelatinous inflammatory exudate that typically contains organisms, mononuclear cells, tubercles, and caseation necrosis, settles at the base of the brain along basal cisterns where arteritis can form along traversing blood vessels. Resultant ischemic infarction occurs in up to 41% of patients[77] particularly in the basal ganglion and deep white matter region (Fig. 3.23).

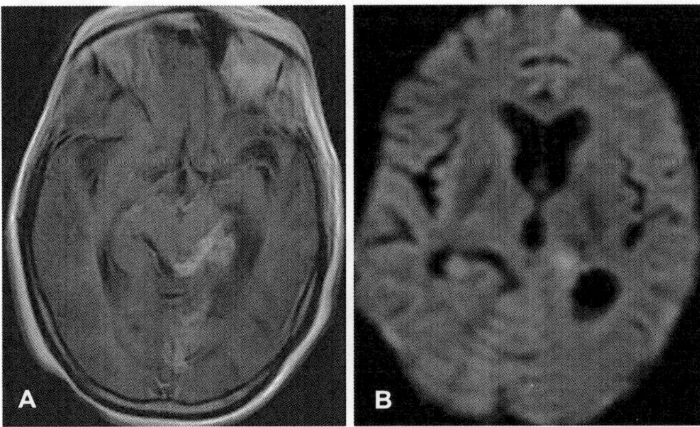

Fig. 3.23: Tuberculous vasculitis with infarct. Contrast enhanced axial T1-weighted image shows enhancing exudates in left perimesencephalic cistern. Axial diffusion-weighted MR image (B) shows an acute infarct in left posterior thalamus

Four fungal agents, aspergillus,[78] candida, coccidioides[79] and mucormycetes are important CNS pathogens and all have the capacity to invade arteries of the CNS in the course of disseminated infection and meningitis. Cerebral infarction results from direct vascular injury leading to aneurysm formation, vascular thrombosis, endarteritis, and cerebral hemorrhage, or results from microabscesses, or extension along contiguous sites of infection. Mucormycosis may be particularly aggressive in poorly controlled diabetes. There may be associated spread from sites of nasopharyngitis, oropharyngitis and sinusitis to the cavernous sinus and ICA, leading to focal thrombosis and cerebral infarction, detectable by imaging studies (Fig. 3.24).

VZV vasculopathies can complicate zoster (secondary VZV infection) or varicella (primary VZV infection). The spectrum of VZV vasculopathy is widening and includes ischemic infarction of the brain and spinal cord, aneurysm formation,[80] subarachnoid and cerebral hemorrhage, carotid dissection and rarely, peripheral arterial disease.[81] VZV vasculopathy in immunocompetent or immunocompromised individuals can be unifocal or multifocal with both deep-seated and superficial infarctions. Lesions at the grey-white matter junction on brain imaging are a clue to diagnosis.[81] Angiography

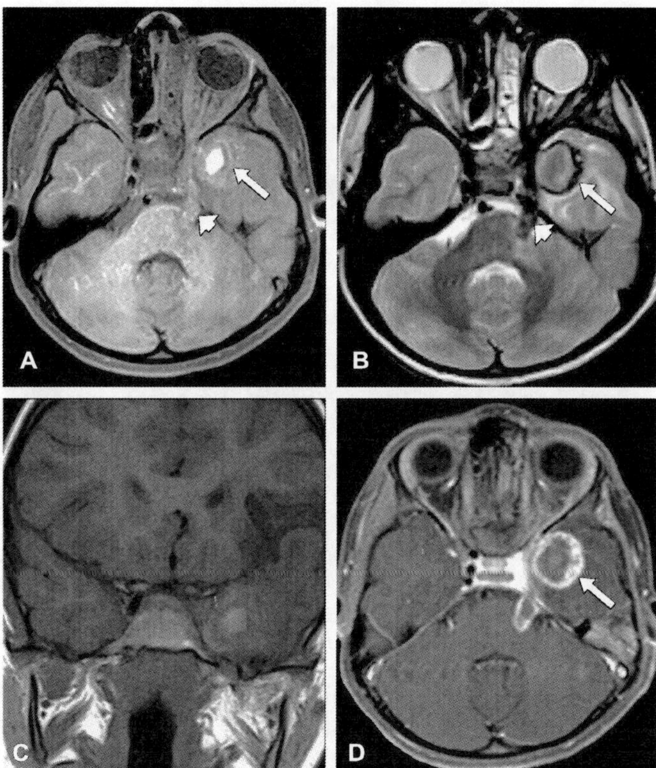

Fig. 3.24: Mucormycosis with angioinvasion. Axial fat-saturated T1-weighted image (A), T2-weighted image and coronal T1-Wi (C) show T2-hypointense and T1-hyperintense lesions in sphenoid sinus, left cavernous sinus (CS) and extending posteriorly along the left trigeminal nerve suggestive of fungal sinusitis with involvement of left CS and left trigeminal nerve (arrowheads). The left cavernous ICA flow-void is not seen. In addition, a globular lesion (arrows) with T2-hypointense rim and core of T1- hyperintensity and T2 hypointensity is present in left CS suggestive of thrombosed aneurysm. The wall of the aneurysm, sphenoid sinusitis, left CS and left trigeminal nerve enhance following intravenous gadolinium administration (D)

reveals segmental narrowing, thrombosis, and beading along proximal branches of the anterior and middle cerebral arteries.

HIV-infected children have an increased incidence of cerebrovascular disease that is associated with severe immune suppression and with vertically acquired HIV infection or exposure to the virus in the neonatal period. Both medium-size arteries and veins are involved with the development of aneurysms, vessel occlusion, embolic disease and venous thrombosis. The aneurysms tend to be fusiform in shape and involve both major arteries of the circle of Willis and second- and third-order branches, which differentiates these aneurysms from berry aneurysms[82-83] (Fig. 3.25). Vasculopathy often remains asymptomatic until a complication, such as the rupture of an aneurysm or a stroke occurs. Vasculopathy can be identified both on MR and digital angiography as calibre variation and irregularity of vessels (Fig. 3.13). Early

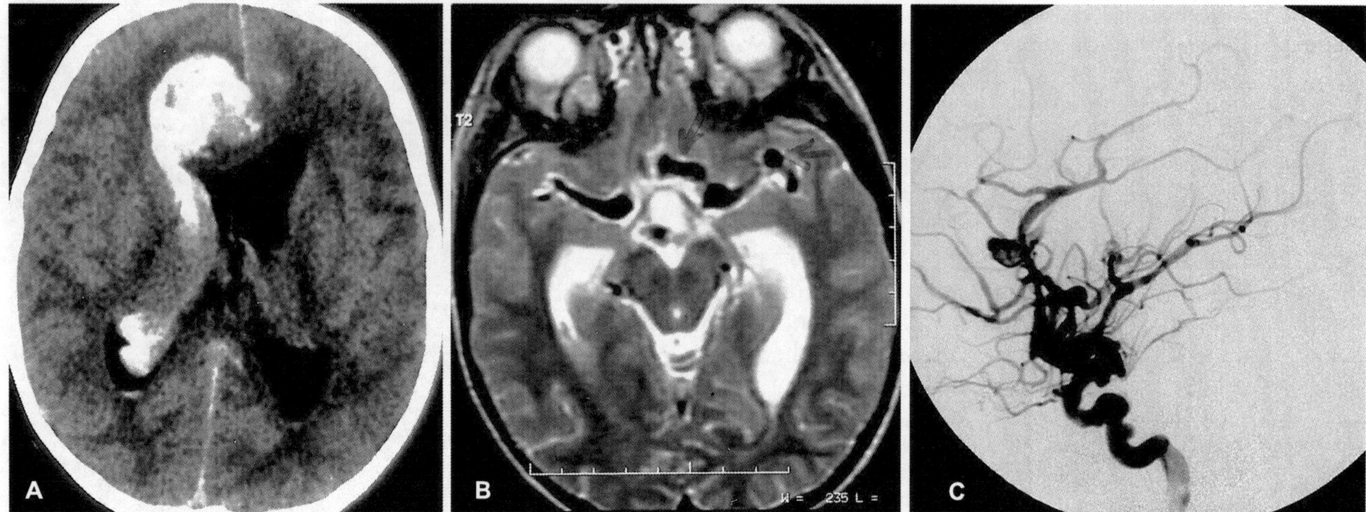

Fig. 3.25: HIV vasculopathy. A 14-year-old boy (seropositive for HIV) presented with sudden onset severe headache. CECT (A) shows acute right frontal hematoma with intraventricular extension. Axial T2-weighted image (B) reveals multiple aneurysms involving circle of Willis. Brain parenchyma appears normal. Lateral view of left ICA angiogram (C) shows multiple dysplastic aneurysms involving ICA and its branches

diagnosis is important because treatment with highly active antiretroviral therapy (HAART) and corticosteroids may stop disease progression or even induce regression of the vasculopathy.[84]

Cerebrovascular complications of neurocysticercosis include lacunar infarction or large-vessel disease, progressive midbrain syndrome, transient ischemic attacks and brain hemorrhage.[85, 86] Mechanisms of cerebrovascular complications include luminal narrowing due to subintimal cushions, vasospasm due to arteritis in midsized and small perforating vessels of the brain and fresh thrombi.[85] Vasculitis must be suspected when segmental narrowing, a beaded appearance, or an abrupt or tapered area of vascular obstruction is noted at angiography.[87] On the basis of angiographic criteria, arteritis is seen in up to 53% of patients with subarachnoid neurocysticercosis, including asymptomatic patients, with the middle and posterior cerebral arteries being most commonly affected.[87] Multivessel involvement is noted in nearly 50% of cases, and infarction associated with arteritis is seen in 2%-12%.[87] Neuroimaging studies reveal cysts, mural nodules, basilar meningitis, hydrocephalus, and vascular lesions (Fig. 3.26).

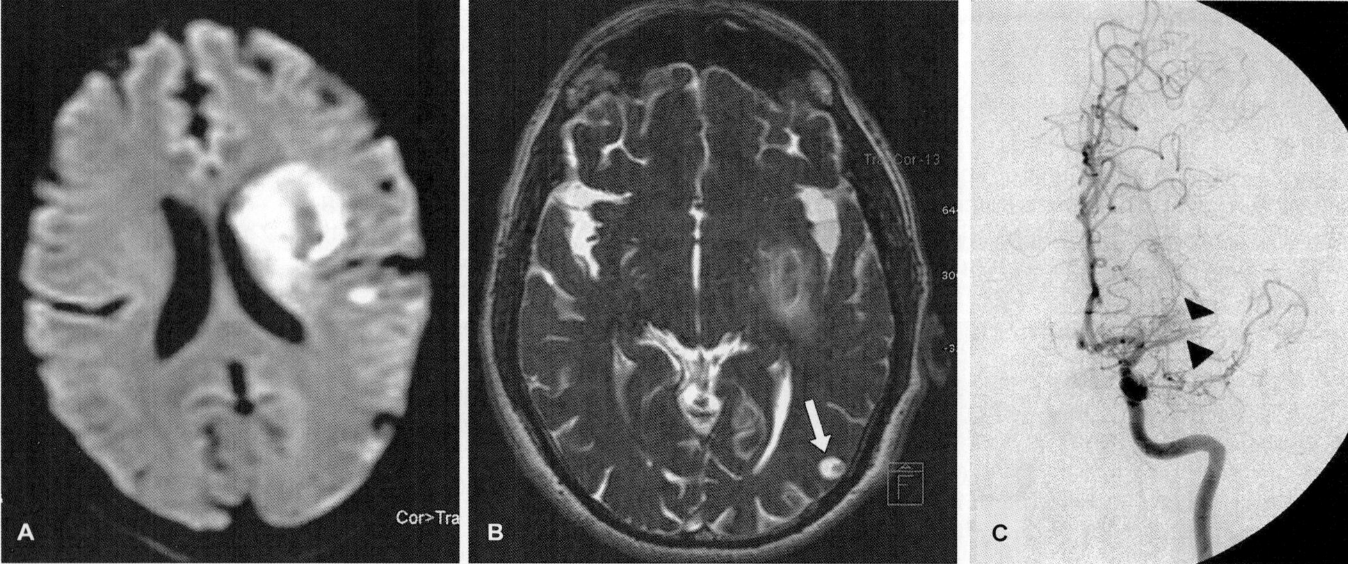

Fig. 3.26 Neurocysticercosis vasculitis. Axial diffusion – weighted image (A) shows an acute infarct in left corona radiata. Axial constructive interference in steady state (CISS) image (B) shows racemose neurocysticercosis in left sylvian fissure. Another cysticercus with scolex is present in left occipital lobe (arrow). AP projection of left ICA angiogram (C) shows stenosis and irregularity of proximal left MCA (arrowheads) and non-visualization of distal left MCA branches

(c) Moyamoya Disease and Moyamoya Syndrome

Moyamoya disease (MMD) is an uncommon cerebrovascular disease characterized by steno-occlusive changes in the terminal internal carotid arteries (ICA) which may progress to the proximal middle, anterior and posterior cerebral arteries, in decreasing order of frequency. The term moyamoya comes from "a Japanese expression for something hazy just like a puff of cigarette smoke drifting in the air" which describes the appearance on catheter angiography of the abnormal collateral vessels adjacent to the stenotic vessels.[88] Moyamoya disease refers to the primary form of the condition, whereas moyamoya syndrome refers to the secondary form in association with other risk factors, most commonly trisomy 21, neurofibromatosis type 1, sickle cell disease, Marfan's syndrome, tuberous sclerosis, Turner's syndrome, tuberculous meningitis and previous irradiation. This wide spectrum of associations suggests multiple mechanisms are implicated in the genesis of the arteriopathy.

Symptoms

Moyamoya disease accounts for approximately 6% of childhood strokes in western countries. The pattern of stroke varies with age. Children are more likely to present with ischemic stroke or transient ischemic attack, whereas adults are more likely to develop hemorrhage from rupture of the friable collateral vessels or the associated flow related aneurysms, which may develop at the bifurcations of major vessels, particularly within the posterior circulation. The ischemic strokes are often multiple and recurrent, and involve the superficial and deep watershed territories. Transient ischemic attacks are often associated with hyperventilation in children with moyamoya, suggesting hypoperfusion rather than thrombotic vasoocclusion as a prominent mechanism.

A Japanese research committee issued the following guidelines for the diagnosis of moyamoya:

(1) Stenosis involving the region of the distal ICA bifurcation (C1) and proximal portions of the ACA (A1) and MCA (M1).

(2) Appearance of dilated basal collateral arteries; and

(3) Bilateral abnormalities. If any of the conditions listed above is present and the angiographic pattern is found on 1 side only, the diagnosis is probable.

Neuroimaging

The workup of a patient in whom the diagnosis of moyamoya syndrome is suspected typically begins with either an MRI study or CT scan of the brain. On CT, small areas of hypodensity suggestive of stroke are commonly observed in cortical watershed zones, basal ganglia, deep white matter watershed zones, or periventricular regions.[89-90] Although rare in children, hemorrhage from moyamoya vessels can be readily diagnosed on head CT with the most common sites of hemorrhage being the basal ganglia, ventricular system, medial temporal lobes and thalamus.

Patients with these findings on CT are often subsequently evaluated with MRI/magnetic resonance angiography (MRA). Acute infarcts are well seen using diffusion-weighted imaging (DWI) as areas with restricted diffusion (Fig. 3.27); chronic infarcts are better delineated

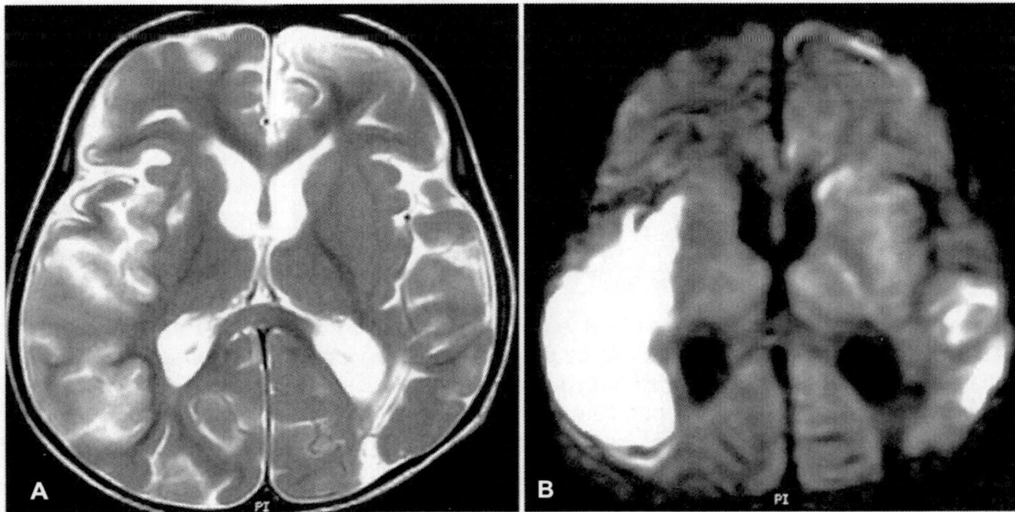

Fig. 3.27: Moyamoya disease. T2-WI (A) show focal area of hyperintensity in right temporo-occipital lobe, which shows evidence of restricted diffusion on diffusion-weighted image (B), suggesting acute infarct. (B) On DWI, another lesion is seen in left posterior temporal lobe, which is not appreciated on T2-WI

with T1 and T2 imaging and cortical ischemia may be inferred from fluid attenuated inversion recovery (FLAIR) sequences, which demonstrate linear high signal following a sulcal pattern, felt to represent slow flow in poorly perfused cortical circulation (the so-called ivy sign) (Fig. 3.28).[91,92] Most suggestive of moyamoya on MRI is the finding of diminished flow voids in the internal carotid and middle and anterior cerebral arteries coupled with prominent collateral flow voids in the basal ganglia and thalamus (Fig. 3.28). These imaging findings are virtually diagnostic of moyamoya syndrome.[89,93,94]

Because of the excellent diagnostic yield and non-invasive nature of MRI, it has been proposed that MRA be used as the primary diagnostic imaging modality for moyamoya syndrome instead of conventional CA (Fig. 3.28).[94-96] CT and MR perfusion studies give a measure of resting perfusion and blood flow reserve and can help determine the extent of improvement in perfusion post therapy (Fig. 3.29).

Definitive diagnosis is based on a distinct arteriographic appearance characterized by bilateral stenosis of the distal intracranial ICA extending to the proximal anterior (ACA) and middle (MCA) arteries (Fig. 3.30). MMD is a progressive cerebrovascular disorder whose vascular changes are divided into the six stages described below:[88,97,98]

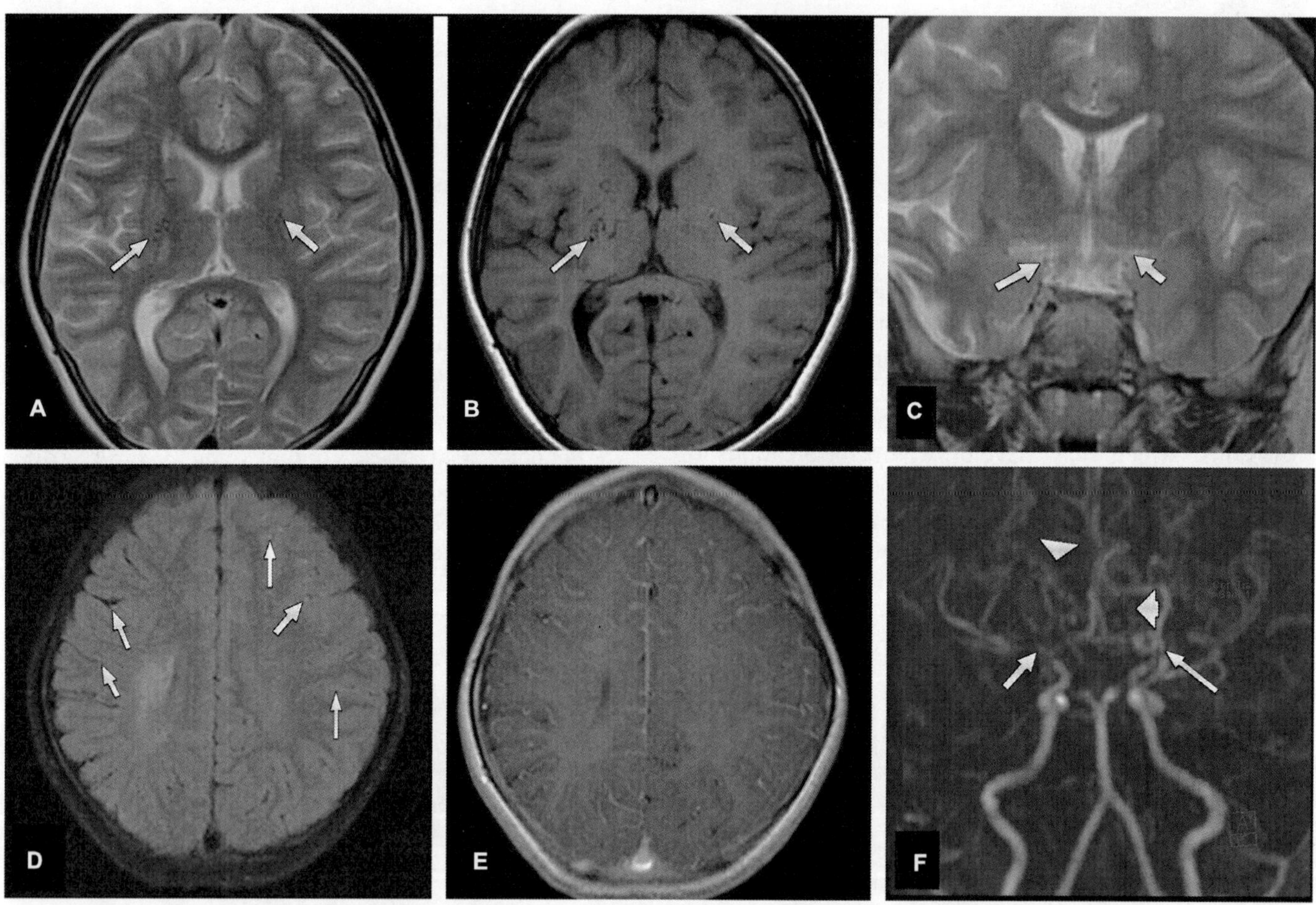

Fig. 3.28: An 8-year-old girl presented with sudden onset left hand weakness 3-month back. Her weakness gradually improved. MR scans, Axial T2-WI (A) and T1-WI (B) show the dilated basal moyamoya vessels in the basal ganglia (arrows). (C) Coronal T2-WI shows multiple serpiginous flow-voids (small arrows) in suprasellar cistern suggestive of moyamoya disease. (D) Axial FLAIR image shows leptomeningeal linear and punctate high intensity along sulci in bilateral frontal and parietal lobes. (E) Contrast-enhanced T1-WI show diffuse leptomeningeal enhancement. (F) MRA shows stenosis or occlusion in the terminal ICA, proximal ACA and MCA (arrows), and moyamoya vessels in the basal ganglia (bold arrows)

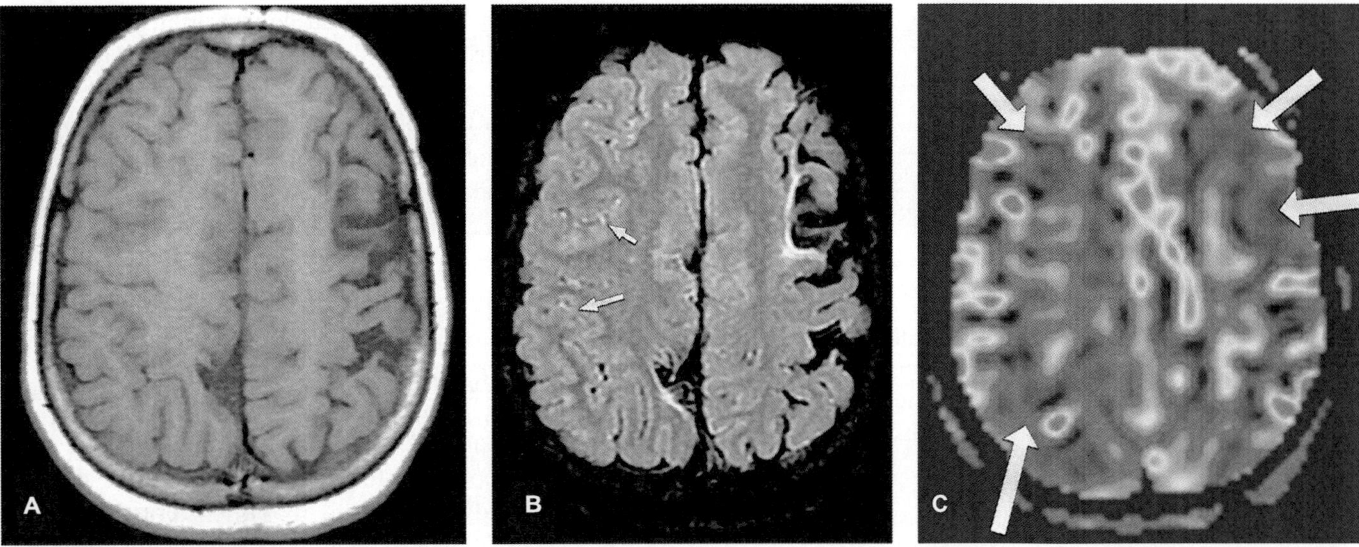

Fig. 3.29: Perfusion MRI in moyamoya. (A) T1 WI show chronic infarcts in left frontal convexity region. (B) Ax FLAIR image show prominent leptomeningeal linear and punctate high intensity along sulci (arrows in B). (C) ASL perfusion images show areas of hypoperfusion in bilateral anterior watershed and right posterior watershed region (arrows)

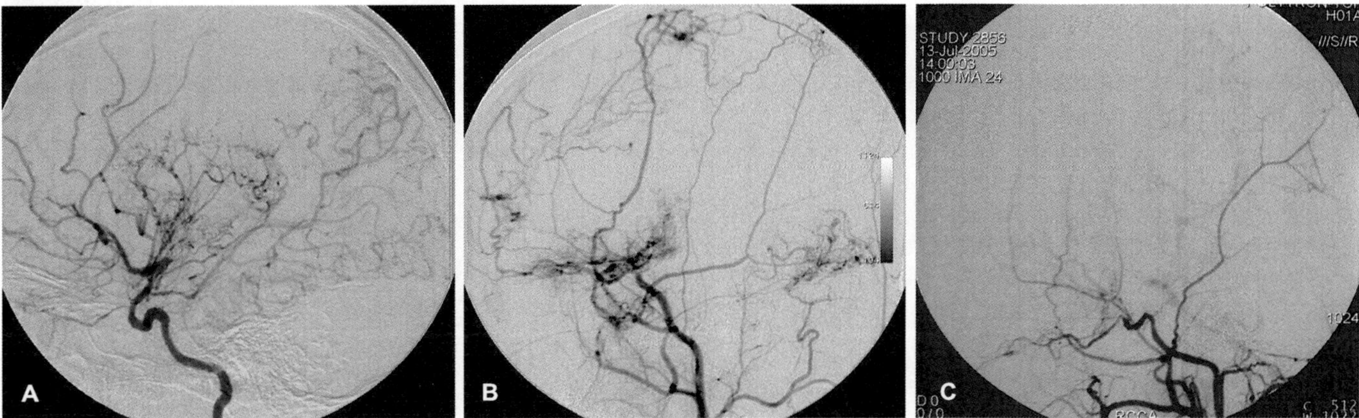

Fig. 3.30: Moyamoya. Angiographic findings in different stages of moyamoya. (A) shows Suzuki grades I to II, with stenosis of terminal ICA with development of basal and pial collaterals. (B) shows Suzuki grades III to IV, with significant narrowing of the internal carotid artery and characteristic "puff-of-smoke" collaterals. There is diminished cortical perfusion. (C) shows Suzuki grades V to VI, with obliteration of the internal-carotid-artery distal to origin of ophthalmic artery with concomitant disappearance of the puff-of-smoke collaterals

Table 3.1: ICA angiographic staging of moyamoya[88]

Stage 1	Narrowing of terminal ICA. Only terminal ICA stenosis is observed.
Stage 2	Initiation of basal moyamoya. Appearance of moyamoya vessels with dilated ACA, MCA and narrowed ICA bifurcation.
Stage 3	Intensification of moyamoya. Remarkable moyamoya vessels at the base of the brain and narrowed ACA and MCA.
Stage 4	Minimization of moyamoya. Decrease of moyamoya vessels with occlusive changes in ICA and tenuous ACA and MCA.
Stage 5	Reduction of moyamoya. Further decrease of moyamoya vessels with occlusion of ICA, ACA and MCA.
Stage 6	Disappearance of moyamoya. Moyamoya vessels disappear and the cerebral blood supply is only from the external carotid arteries.

Table 3.2: PCA angiographic staging[99]	
Stage 1	No occlusive changes in PCA
Stage 2	Stenosis in PCA with or without slightly developed PCA moyamoya
Stage 3	Severe stenosis or virtually complete occlusion of PCA with well-developed PCA moyamoya
Stage 4	Occlusion of PCA with decreased PCA moyamoya

Suzuki's angiographic staging[88,100] represents the natural course of the angio-architecture in moyamoya patients by physiological reorganization system and does not reflect the severity of MMD, while it explains how 'moyamoya disease' compensates its ischemic condition by physiological process.[101]

Moyamoya like very distinctive radiological phenotype of cerebral arteriopathy is associated with mutations in the alpha-actin-2 (ACTA2) gene. Unlike moyamoya, these patients have several distinctive radiological features, namely proximal ectasia, distal occlusive disease, absence of basal collaterals, and an unusually straight morphology of the intracranial arteries. Because this mutation is dominantly inherited and predisposes to aortic aneurysms, it is an important condition to identify by the radiological signature. Therefore, to confirm the diagnosis of moyamoya syndrome and to visualize the anatomy of the vessels involved and the patterns of flow through the hemispheres, conventional cerebral angiography is typically required.

Treatment

There are no effective medical therapies for moyamoya disease. Surgical revascularization is thought to improve cerebral perfusion, and to reduce the risk of subsequent stroke in both pediatric and adult patients. The need for revascularization surgery in children with moyamoya is dependent on the extent and type of ischemic infarction (bilateral and multiple strokes), the presence of advanced vascular stage and poor cerebrovascular reserve (as indicated by the ivy sign on MRI brain FLAIR and contrast-enhanced T1-weighted sequences) and cerebrovascular reserve mapping studies including single-photon emission computerized tomography (SPECT) and perfusion scans (CT/MRI) and progression of the disease. In pediatric patients, the incidence of TIA rapidly decreases after surgery.

Surgical procedures are classified into three categories, direct bypassing including superficial temporal artery to MCA (STA-MCA) anastomosis, indirect bypassing including encephaloduroarteriosynangiosis (EDAS) and encephalomyosynangiosis (EMS), and combined bypassing. Direct bypassing can be technically challenging in some pediatric patients with cortical arteries of smaller diameter, but can improve cerebral hemodynamics immediately after surgery. Indirect bypass surgery that induces spontaneous angiogenesis between the brain surface and the vascularised donor tissues is technically simple, but requires 3-4 months for the collaterals to develop. Indirect surgery can provide extensive collaterals in almost all pediatric patients, but only around half of adult patients.

(d) Cerebral Arterial Dissection

Cerebral arterial dissection (CAD) is an important cause for stroke, accounting for up to 20% of stroke cases in some series and increasing to 50% of posterior circulation strokes.[102,103] Trauma is the most common cause of a dissection.[102] In contrast to adults, very few children have an underlying vasculopathy, such as Ehlers-Danlos syndrome, that can predispose to dissections. CAD most commonly affects the extracranial vessels but intracranial CAD is more common than in adults, accounting for up to 60% of anterior circulation dissections.[102,103] The most common location for a posterior CAD, however, was extracranially at the level of C1/C2. Children are more likely to present with signs of neurological deficit than local symptoms of dissection, such as neck pain.

Confirmation of the diagnosis of intracranial or cervical arterial dissection requires MRI/MRA or CA with one of the following three patterns:

(1) Angiographic findings of a double lumen, intimal flap, or pseudo aneurysm, or, on axial T1 fat saturation MRI images, a 'bright crescent sign' in the arterial wall.

(2) The sequence of cervical or cranial trauma, or neck pain, less than six weeks preceding angiographic findings of segmental arterial narrowing (or occlusion) located in the cervical arteries; and

(3) Angiographic segmental narrowing (or occlusion) of the vertebral artery at the level of the C2 vertebral body, even without known traumatic history.[57]

2. Cardiac Disease

Congenital heart disease, valvular heart disease, cardiac arrhythmias, and cardiomyopathy are also risk factors for childhood AIS.[62,104] Up to a third of childhood AIS are associated with cardiac disease, most of which have a known pre-existing cardiac lesion at the time of the stroke.[105]

Congenital heart disease is the most common cardiac disorder that causes stroke. Patent foramen ovale and atrial septal defect, relatively mild forms of congenital heart disease, have both been correlated with an increased risk of embolic stroke. Cardiac procedures, including catheterization, extracorporeal membrane oxygenation, and surgery, are all considered risk factors for childhood AIS.[62] In pediatric patients with cardiomyopathy, congestive heart failure or other end-stage cardiac disease, especially when complicated by pulmonary problems, episodes of bradycardia, hypotension, or hypoxia, lead to watershed infarction in the parasagittal distribution between anterior and middle and posterior and middle cerebral arteries. Acutely, these are best demonstrated by DWI. Infarcts associated with cardioembolic disease frequently have a hemorrhagic component.

3. Sickle Cell Disease

Sickle cell disease (SCD) is one of the most common causes for AIS in childhood. The highest risk for stroke is between the ages of 2 and 5 years of age.[106,107] The annual risk of initial stroke in sickle cell disease is estimated to be 0.7%/year. Subsequent infarction, after the first stroke, occurs in 50%-75% of untreated patients (not transfused), with 80% having a second infarction within 36 months.

The type and pattern of AIS depends on the underlying pathophysiological mechanism, in addition to the patient's age. These patients have both small vessel hypoperfusion disease causing lesions within the white matter of the centrum semiovale, and stenoses and/or occlusions of the more proximal major vessels, leading to infarctions within vascular territories[108] (Fig. 3.31). Occlusive disease in the terminal ICA/proximal MCA/ACA may progress to moyamoya syndrome and ICH may also occur from rupture of the moyamoya type collaterals or flow related aneurysms. Approximately 20% of children with SCD have 'silent' brain lesions on MRI, defined as increased signal intensity on T2-weighted MR images predominantly in frontal and parietal cortical, subcortical, and border-zone locations and no history of physical findings of a focal neurologic deficit lasting more than 24 hours.[109,110] These so-called "silent infarcts" are important because they are associated with deterioration in cognitive function with effects on learning and behaviour.[111]

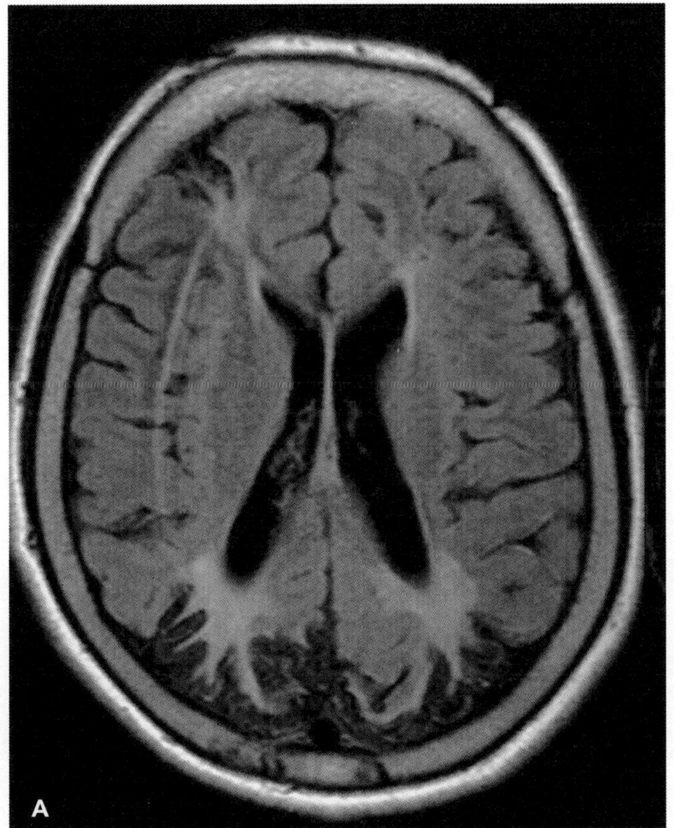

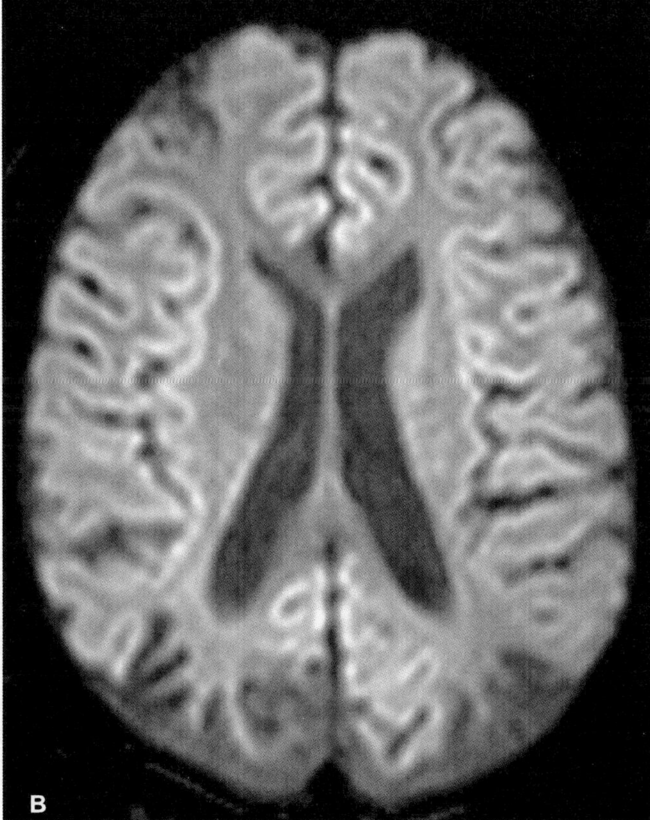

Fig. 3.31: Sickle cell anemia. Axial FLAIR (A) and Diffusion WI (B) show chronic infarcts in bilateral posterior watershed and right anterior watershed territories

CT scan is generally performed without contrast in patients with SCD, as hypertonic contrast agents may precept sickling.[112] Small amount of paramagnetic contrast is probably safe during MR scanning but use of MR contrast is rarely necessary; it should only be used if absolutely essential and the patient should be well hydrated before and during the examination.[112] CA should be restricted to those patients who have hemorrhage, and should be performed only after patient is transfused and well hydrated.[62] The osmolality of the contrast should be as low as possible for a diagnostic study.[112]

Blood transfusion, aiming to reduce the circulating level of Hemoglobin S (HbS) below 20% and correct anemia sufficiently to suppress bone marrow production of HbS, is extremely effective in both primary and secondary prevention of AIS.[113] The standard of care in many countries is now to institute screening for cerebrovascular disease in children with SCD using transcranial Doppler ultrasound from the age of 2 years, at annual intervals, and instituting blood transfusion for those with abnormally elevated velocity above 200 cm/sec in the middle cerebral arteries.[114] Blood transfusion is also recommended for children who have had clinical AIS, for secondary prevention. The rate of stroke in children with positive MRI (silent infarcts) but TCD findings that do not reach current treatment guidelines is not clear, and regular blood transfusions are not recommended on the basis of MRI alone.[62]

4. Hypercoagulable States with Thrombosis

There are a large number of etiologies of hypercoagulable states, both primary and secondary, many quite rare (i.e., homocystinuria) and some thought previously to be rare (i.e., protein C deficiency), but more recently recognized with increasing frequency as a cause of stroke in pediatric patients. Imaging findings in most of the ischemic infarcts due to hypercoagulability do not reveal the underlying disorder, and are thus nonspecific. However, their presence necessitates that hypercoagulable states be excluded as part of the clinical diagnostic workup of pediatric stroke when more obvious etiologies (i.e., presence of a dissection) are not present.

5. Genetics and Pediatric Stroke

A number of single gene disorders can cause vasculopathy leading to small and large vessel disease.

Col4A1is a gene encoding the type IV collagen alpha 1 chain, which is a basement membrane protein expressed in vessels. Mutations in this gene cause sporadic and hereditary porenchephaly and infantile hemiparesis.[115,116] Col4A1mutations are also associated with small vessel disease with a radiological pattern of lacunar infarcts, leukoariosis, micro and macrohemorrhages.[117]

Alpha actin-2 is a protein found in smooth muscle cells throughout the arterial system. Mutations in its encoding ACTA2 gene cause a variety of vascular conditions such as aortic dissection, aortic aneurysms, coronary artery disease and strokes, including moyamoya disease.[118] Munot *et al.* describe a distinct cerebrovascular radiological phenotype of dilatation of the internal carotid artery to the terminal portion, occlusive disease of distal intracranial circulation, an abnormally straight course of intracranial arteries and absence of 'moyamoya', other basal and leptomeningeal collaterals.[119]

Cerebral autosomal dominant arteriopathy with subcortical infarcts and leukoencepahlopathy (CADASIL) is the most common cause of hereditary stroke disorder and is caused by mutations on the Notch 3 gene on chromosome.[120] The key features are of recurrent subcortical ischemic events and vascular dementia with diffuse white matter abnormalities on imaging. Typical age at presentation is 30-50 years, but can present at childhood from as young as three years old.[121]

Mitochondrial dysfunctions are one of the genetic causes of stroke in children. These include mitochondrial encephalomyopathy, lactic acidosis and stroke-like episodes (MELAS); myoclonic epilepsy with ragged red-fibers (MERRF); MERFF/MELAS overlap syndrome; and Kearns-Sayre syndrome. Mitochondrial encephalopathies are suspected when lactic acidosis (diagnosed by serum, CSF analysis, or MRS) occurs in association with seizures, recurrent strokes, and respiratory failure. DNA classification of these disorders is now possible in many instances. The proposed mechanism of stroke is regional failure to produce sufficient energy to maintain cell function. Sites of normal high energy metabolism appear to be at greatest risk when attacks occur. MRI, DWI and MRS provide the imaging information for diagnostic workup. MRA is useful to exclude other vascular diseases that might mimic mitochondrial disease, such as basilar artery stenosis.

6. Cerebral Sinovenous Thrombosis

Cerebral sinovenous thrombosis (CSVT) is becoming increasingly diagnosed in children due to the recognition of the associated subtle clinical symptoms and improved cerebrovascular imaging. Two types of CSVT disease present as neurologic compromise with acute onset of symptoms.[122] These are:

(1) Superficial dural sinus thrombosis with or without cortical vein thrombosis; and

(2) Deep venous thrombosis. The superficial venous system is more frequently involved than the deep system, and the most common sites of CSVT are the transverse, superior sagittal, sigmoid, and straight sinuses. The setting for deep venous thrombosis is the very young age of patients, often newborns or young infants, and significant dehydration.[123] Superficial dural sinus thrombosis tends to occur in older patients (not exclusively) and to have a wide variety of etiologies, including dehydration, sepsis, and hypercoagulable states.[123] Superior sagittal sinus thrombosis may be relatively asymptomatic if only that structure is involved; however, with the frequent involvement of transverse sinuses and cortical veins, cerebral infarction, often hemorrhagic, becomes more frequent and acutely symptomatic.[123] Superior sagittal sinus thrombosis may present with chronic symptoms, such as papilledema with pseudotumor cerebri, and given that clinical diagnosis, imaging evaluation is required. Between one- and two-thirds of children with CSVT may have parenchymal brain lesions such as venous infarction and hemorrhage.[124]

Neuroimaging

Non-contrast CT is often the initial diagnostic study in the patient with sinovenous occlusion. Acute blood clot or thrombus within the dural sinus or cortical vein can be identified as an elongated hyperdense lesion on NCCT (Fig. 3.32). Unfortunately, infants tend to have normally relatively large dense dural venous sinuses that can be misdiagnosed as thrombosed by the less experienced. The presence of hemorrhage and edema secondary to venous infarct and/or thrombosed cortical veins make the diagnosis easier (Fig. 3.33). On contrast administration, CVT appear as a central intraluminal filling defect (empty delta sign) that represents a thrombus surrounded by contrast-enhanced dural collateral venous channels and cavernous spaces within the dural envelope (Fig. 3.33).

MRI and MRV are now the gold standards in diagnosis of sinovenous thrombosis. Conventional arteriography is almost never used. On MRI, the thrombus is readily recognizable in the subacute phase, when it is of high signal on a T1-weighted scan, and MRV may not be required. In the acute phase, the thrombus is isointense with brain on T1-weighted imaging and of low signal on T2-weighted imaging. This appearance can be mistaken for flowing blood, but MRV will demonstrate an absence of flow in

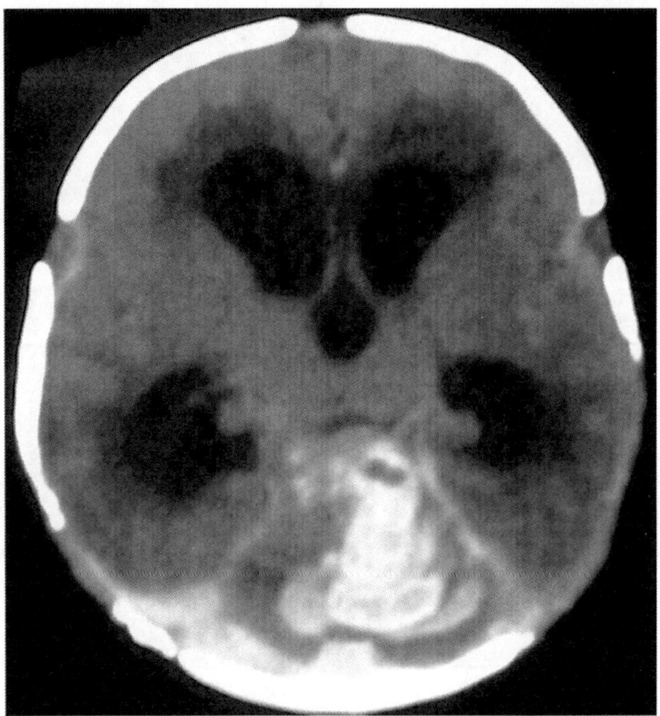

Fig. 3.32. A 6-day-old child presented in the emergency with failure to thrive. NCCT shows acute hematoma (straight arrow) in the left cerebellum causing compression of fourth ventricle and resultant hydrocephalus. Both transverse sinuses are hyperdense (curved arrow), suggesting thrombosis

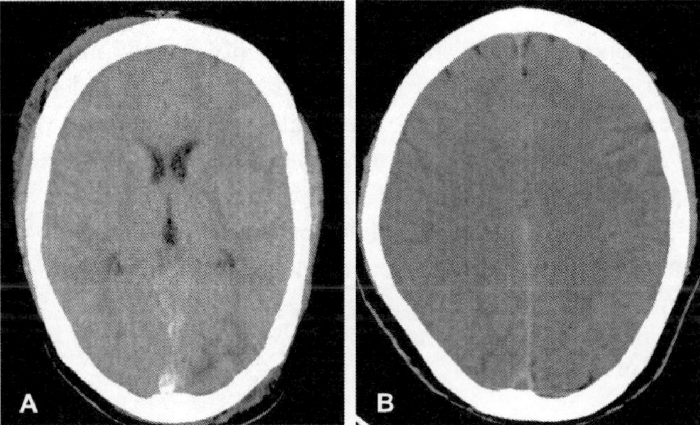

Fig. 3.33: CT in cerebral venous thrombosis. (A) NCCT head shows hyperdense superior sagittal sinus (arrow) suggesting thrombosis. (B) CECT shows filling defect (arrowhead) within posterior superior sagittal sinus (empty delta sign)

the thrombosed sinus. T2*-weighted MRI seems to be more sensitive than T1- or T2-weighted or fluid-attenuated inversion recovery (FLAIR) imaging in demonstrating venous thrombosis and associated hemorrhage[125-126] (Fig. 3.34). On MR imaging, FLAIR and T2-WI show cortical and subcortical high-signal-intensity lesions.[127] DWI reveals mixed signal intensity and relates to both cytotoxic and vasogenic edema.[127,128] An infarction not conforming

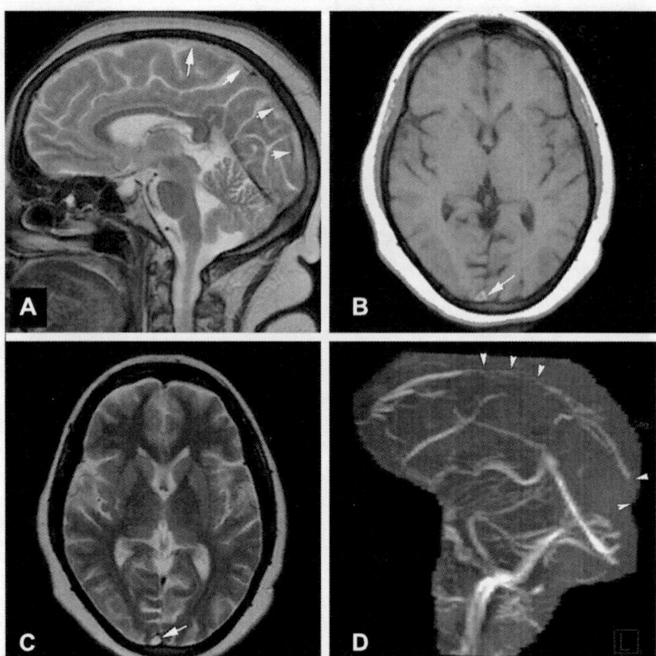

Fig. 3.34: Superior sagittal sinus thrombosis. (A-C) Sagittal T2-WI (A), axial T1- (B) and axial T2-WI (C) show loss of flow-void in superior sagittal sinus (arrows). (D) TOF-MRA shows non-visualization of posterior superior sagittal sinus (arrows) confirming thrombosis

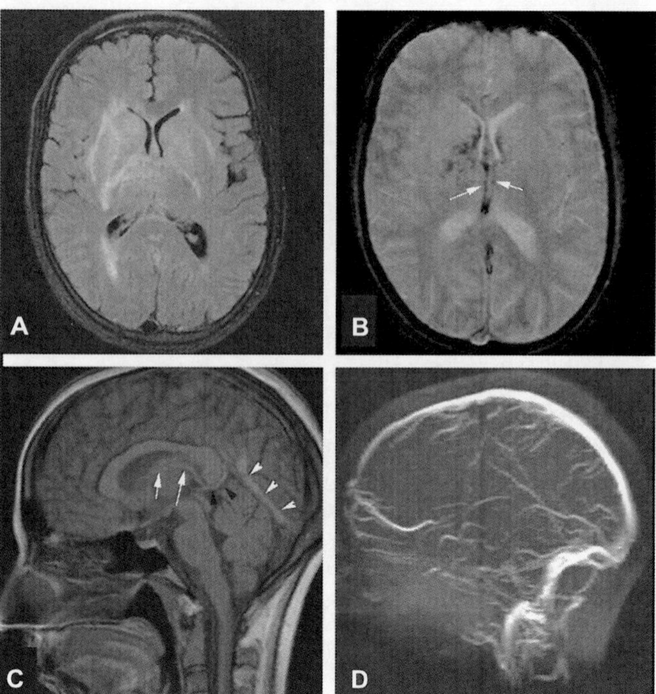

Fig. 3.35: Deep venous sinus thrombosis. (A) Axial FLAIR MR image shows hyperintensity in bilateral corpus striatum and thalami. (B) Axial T2-WI demonstrates hemorrhages in bilateral basal ganglia. Both internal cerebral veins are hypointense (white arrows). (C) Sagittal T1-WI shows hyperintensity in region of internal cerebral veins (white arrows), veins of Galen (black arrowhead) and straight sinus (white arrowheads) suggestive of subacute thrombosis. (D) MR venography shows non-visualization of deep venous system

to a major arterial vascular territory, such as the presence of multiple isolated lesions, involvement of a subcortical region with sparing of the cortex, and extension over more than one arterial distribution, is highly suspicious for a venous cause.[129] Bilateral parasagittal hemispheric lesions are suggestive of superior sagittal sinus thrombosis (Fig. 3.34). Ipsilateral temporo-occipital and cerebellar lobe lesions can be found in transverse sinus thrombosis. Bilateral or unilateral infarction in the thalami, basal ganglia, and internal capsule is typically seen in deep venous thrombosis (Fig. 3.35).

CONCLUSION

The imaging diagnostic workup of the pediatric patient with cerebrovascular disease and stroke depends to a large extent on the neuroradiologists and their ability to perform and interpret correctly the appropriate studies. There is now a wide array of studies with varying specificity and some pitfalls. However, it has never been easier than now to obtain the important information. CT remains the initial screening test for most acute events occurring beyond early infancy, but while it is good for SAH, ICH and IVH, it is often less informative regarding etiology of bleeds and in the demonstration of acute ischemic infarction and hypoxia. MRI with T1, T2, FLAIR, DWI, susceptibility scanning, MRA and MRV have revolutionized the capability of the neuroradiologists to provide diagnostic information to the clinician. Despite the imaging advances, arriving at the etiology of ischemic stroke is still mostly dependent on the history and laboratory findings. Conventional arteriography has been relegated to a limited, but important, role in providing definitive information in specific circumstances (aneurysm, AVM, vasculitis, etc.).

References

1. Garner TB, Del Curling O, Kelly DL, Laster DW. The Natural History of Intracranial Venous Angiomas. J Neurosurg 1991 November:75(5):715-22.
2. Lasjaunias P, Burrows P, Planet C. Developmental Venous Anomalies (DVA): The So-called Venous Angioma. Neurosurg Review 1986:9(3):233-42.
3. Abe T, Singer RJ, Marks MP, Norbash AM, Crowley RS, Steinberg GK. Coexistence of Occult Vascular Malformations and Developmental Venous Anomalies in the Central Nervous System: MR Evaluation. AJNR Am J Neuroradiol 1998 January;19(1):51-57.
4. Töpper R, Jürgens E, Reul J, Thron A. Clinical Significance of Intracranial Developmental Venous Anomalies. J Neurol Neurosurg Psychiatry 1999 August;67(2):234-38.

5. Konan AV, Raymond J, Bourgouin P, Lesage J, Milot G, Roy D. Cerebellar Infarct Caused by Spontaneous Thrombosis of a Developmental Venous Anomaly of the Posterior Fossa. AJNR Am J Neuroradiol 1999 February;20(2):256-58.

6. Lee C, Pennington MA, Kenney CM. MR Evaluation of Developmental Venous Anomalies: Medullary Venous Anatomy of Venous Angiomas. AJNR Am J Neuroradiol 1996 January;17(1):61-70.

7. Reichenbach JR, Barth M, Haacke EM, Klarhöfer M, Kaiser WA, Moser E. High-resolution MR venography at 3.0 tesla. J Comput Assist Tomogr 2000;24(6):949-57.

8. Perrini P, Lanzino G. The Association of Venous Developmental Anomalies and Cavernous Malformations: Pathophysiological, Diagnostic and Surgical Considerations. Neurosurg Focus, 2006;21(1):e5.

9. Kiroglu Y, Oran I, Dalbasti T, Karabulut N, Calli C. Thrombosis of a Drainage Vein in Developmental Venous Anomaly (DVA) Leading Venous Infarction: A Case Report and Review of the Literature. J Neuroimaging 2011 April;21(2):197-201.

10. San Millán Ruíz D, Delavelle J, Yilmaz H, Gailloud P, Piovan E, Bertramello A, *et al.* Parenchymal Abnormalities Associated with Developmental Venous Anomalies. Neuroradiology 2007 December;49(12):987-95.

11. Santucci GM, Leach JL, Ying J, Leach SD, Tomsick TA. Brain Parenchymal Signal Abnormalities Associated with Developmental Venous Anomalies: Detailed MR Imaging Assessment. AJNR Am J Neuroradiol 2008 August;29(7): 1317-23.

12. Takasugi M, Fujii S, Shinohara Y, Kaminou T, Watanabe T, Ogawa T. Parenchymal Hypointense Foci Associated with Developmental Venous Anomalies: Evaluation by Phase-Sensitive MR Imaging at 3T. AJNR Am J Neuroradiol 2013 October;34(10):1940-44.

13. Linscott LL, Leach JL, Zhang B, Jones BV. Brain Parenchymal Signal Abnormalities Associated with Developmental Venous Anomalies in Children and Young Adults. AJNR Am J Neuroradiol 2014 August;35(8):1600-07.

14. Zabramski JM, Wascher TM, Spetzler RF, Johnson B, Golfinos J, Drayer BP, *et al.* The Natural History of Familial Cavernous Malformations: Results of an Ongoing Study. J Neurosurg 1994 March;80(3):422-32.

15. Rigamonti D, Hadley MN, Drayer BP, Johnson PC, Hoenig-Rigamonti K, Knight JT, Spetzler RF. Cerebral Cavernous Malformations. Incidence and Familial Occurrence. N Engl J Med 1988 August;11;319(6):343-47.

16. Rigamonti D, Drayer BP, Johnson PC, Hadley MN, Zabramski J, Spetzler RF. The MRI Appearance of Cavernous Malformations (Angiomas). J Neurosurg 1987 October; 67(4): 518-24.

17. Huang J, McGirt MJ, Gailloud P, Tamargo RJ. Intracranial Aneurysms in the Pediatric Population: Case Series and Literature Review. Surg Neurol 2005 May;63(5):424-32; Discussion 432-33.

18. Meyer FB, Sundt TM, Fode NC, Morgan MK, Forbes GS, Mellinger JF. Cerebral Aneurysms in Childhood and Adolescence. J Neurosurg 1989 March;70(3):420-25.

19. Ostergaard JR, Voldby B. Intracranial Arterial Aneurysms in Children and Adolescents. J Neurosurg 1983 June;58(6): 832-37.

20. Koroknay-Pál P, Niemelä M, Lehto H, Kivisaari R, Numminen J, Laakso A, Hernesniemi J. De Novo and Recurrent Aneurysms in Pediatric Patients with Cerebral Aneurysms. Stroke 2013 May;44(5):1436-39.

21. Lasjaunias P. Vein of Galen Aneurysmal Malformation. In: Lasjaunias P, Editors. Vascular Diseases of Neonates, Infants and Children, Berlin: Springer-Verlag; 1997n.

22. Kanaan I, Lasjaunias P, Coates R. The Spectrum of Intracranial Aneurysms in Pediatrics. Minim Invasive Neurosurg 1995 March;38(1):1-9.

23. terBrugge KG. Neurointerventional Procedures in the Pediatric Age Group. Childs Nerv System 1999 November;15(11-12): 751-54.

24. Heiskanen O, Vilkki J. Intracranial Arterial Aneurysms in Children and Adolescents. Acta Neurochir (Wien) 1981;59 (1-2):55-63.

25. Allison JW, Davis PC, Sato Y, James CA, Haque SS, Angtuaco EJ, Glasier CM. Intracranial Aneurysms in Infants and Children. Pediatr Radiol 1998 April;28(4):223-29.

26. Patel AN, Richardson AE. Ruptured Intracranial Aneurysms in The First Two Decades of Life. A Study of 58 Patients. J Neurosurg 1971 November; 35(5):571-76.

27. Agid R, Souza MP, Reintamm G, Armstrong D, Dirks P, TerBrugge KG. The Role of Endovascular Treatment for Pediatric Aneurysms. Childs Nerv System 2005 December; 21(12):1030-36.

28. Lasjaunias PL, Campi A, Rodesch G, Alvarez H, Kanaan I, Taylor W. Aneurysmal Disease in Children. Review of 20 Cases with Intracranial Arterial Localisations. Interv Neuroradiol 1997 September;30;3(3):215-29.

29. Hetts SW, Narvid J, Sanai N, Lawton MT, Gupta N, Fullerton HJ, *et al.* Intracranial Aneurysms in Childhood: 27-Year Single-Institution Experience. AJNR Am J Neuroradiol 2009 August; 30(7):1315-21.

30. Krings T, Geibprasert S, terBrugge KG. Pathomechanisms and Treatment of Pediatric Aneurysms. Childs Nerv System 2010 October;26(10):1309-18.

31. Chukwudelunzu FE, Brown RD, Wijdicks EF, Steckelberg JM. Subarachnoid Hemorrhage Associated with Infectious Endocarditis: Case Report and Literature Review. Eur J Neurol 2002 July;9(4):423-27.

32. Lasjaunias P, Wuppalapati S, Alvarez H, Rodesch G, Ozanne A. Intracranial Aneurysms in Children Aged Under 15 years: Review of 59 Consecutive Children with 75 Aneurysms. Childs Nerv System 2005 June;21(6):437-50.

33. Lasjaunias P, Berenstein A. New York: Springer-Verlag; 1992r.

34. Arteriovenous Malformations of the Brain in Adults. N Engl J Med 1999 June;10;340(23):1812-18.

35. Lasjaunias P. Intracranial Aneurysms in Children. In: Lasjaunias P, Editors. Vascular Diseases of Neonates, Infants and Children. Berlin: Springer-Verlag;1997t.,373-92.

36. Brown RD, Wiebers DO, Torner JC, O'Fallon WM. Frequency of Intracranial Hemorrhage as a Presenting Symptom and Subtype Analysis: A Population-Based Study of Intracranial Vascular Malformations in Olmsted Country, Minnesota. J Neurosurg 1996 July;85(1):29-32.

37. Willinsky RA, Lasjaunias P, Terbrugge K, Burrows P. Multiple Cerebral Arteriovenous Malformations (AVMS). Review of Our Experience from 203 Patients with Cerebral Vascular Lesions. Neuroradiology 1990:32(3):207-10.

38. Bhattacharya JJ, Luo CB, Suh DC, Alvarez H, Rodesch G, Lasjaunias P. Wyburn-Mason or Bonnet-Dechaume-Blanc as Cerebrofacial Arteriovenous Metameric Syndromes (CAMS). A New Concept and a New Classification. Interv Neuroradiol 2001 March:30:7(1):5-17.

39. Bergwerff M, Verberne ME, DeRuiter MC, Poelmann RE, Gittenberger-de Groot AC. Neural Crest Cell Contribution to the Developing Circulatory System: Implications for Vascular Morphology? Circ Res1998 February:9:82(2):221-31.

40. Jiarakongmun P, Alvarez A, Rodesch G, Lasjaunias P. Clinical Course and Angioarchitecture of Cerebrofacial Arteriovenous Metameric Syndromes. Three Demonstrative Cases and Literature Review. Interv Neuroradiol 2002 September:30; 8(3):251-64.

41. Dayani PN, Sadun AA. A Case Report of Wyburn-Mason Syndrome and Review of the Literature, Neuroradiology 2007 May;49(5):45-56.

42. Griffiths PD. Sturge-Weber Syndrome Revisited: The Role of Neuroradiology. Neuropediatrics 1996 December:27(6): 284-94.

43. Miao Y, Juhász C, Wu J, Tarabishy B, Lang Z, Behen ME, *et al.* Clinical Correlates of White Matter Blood Flow Perfusion Changes in Sturge-Weber Syndrome: A Dynamic MR Perfusion-Weighted Imaging Study. AJNR Am J Neuroradiol 2011 August;32(7):1280-85.

44. Debrun GM, Viñuela F, Fox AJ, Davis KR, Ahn HS. Indications for Treatment and Classification of 132 Carotid-Cavernous Fistulas Neurosurgery 1988 February:22(2):285-89.

45. Barrow DL, Spector RH, Braun IF, Landman JA, Tindall SC, Tindall GT. Classification and Treatment of Spontaneous Carotid-Cavernous Sinus Fistulas. J Neurosurg 1985 February: 62(2):248-56.

46. Casasco A, Lylyk P, Hodes JE, Kohan G, Aymard A, Merland JJ. Percutaneous Transvenous Catheterization and Embolization of Vein of Galen Aneurysms. Neurosurgery 1991 February; 28(2):260-66.

47. Jones BV, Ball WS, Tomsick TA, Millard J, Crone KR. Vein of Galen Aneurysmal Malformation: Diagnosis and Treatment of 13 Children with Extended Clinical Follow-up. AJNR Am J Neuroradiol 2002;23(10):1717-24.

48. Raybaud CA, Strother CM, Hald JK. Aneurysms of the Vein of Galen: Embryonic Considerations and Anatomical Features Relating to the Pathogenesis of the Malformation. Neuroradiology 1989;31(2):109-28.

49. Bhattacharya JJ, Thammaroj J. Vein of Galen Malformations. J Neurol Neurosurg Psychiatry 2003 March: 74 Suppl 1:i42-44.

50. Lasjaunias P, Rodesch G, Terbrugge K, Pruvost P, Devictor D, Comoy J, Landrieu P. Vein of Galen Aneurysmal Malformations. Report of 36 Cases Managed between 1982 and 1988. Acta Neurochir (Wien) 1989;99(1-2):26-37.

51. Mitchell PJ, Rosenfeld JV, Dargaville P, Loughnan P, Ditchfield MR, Frawley G, Tress BM. Endovascular Management of Vein of Galen Aneurysmal Malformations Presenting in the Neonatal Period. AJNR Am J Neuroradiol 2001 August;22(7):1403-39.

52. Garcia-Monaco R, Lasjaunias P, Berenstein A. Therapeutic Management of Vein of Galen Aneurysmal Malformations. In: Viñuela F, Halbach VV, Dion JE, Editors. Interventional Neuroradiology: Endovascular Therapy of the Central Nervous System, New York 1992u;113-27.

53. Horowitz MB, Jungreis CA, Quisling RG, Pollack I. Vein of Galen Aneurysms: A Review and Current Perspective. AJNR Am J Neuroradiol 1994 September:15(8):1486-96.

54. Zerah M, Garcia-Monaco R, Rodesch G, Terbrugge K, Tardieu M, de Victor D, Lasjaunias P. Hydrodynamics in Vein of Galen Malformations. Childs Nerv System 1992 May;(3):111-7; discussion 117.

55. Unknown Publication Type for: terBrugge 2001.

56. Alvarez H, Garcia Monaco R, Rodesch G, Sachet M, Krings T, Lasjaunias P. Vein of Galen Aneurysmal Malformations. Neuroimaging Clin N Am 2007 May;17(2):189-206.

57. Sébire G, Meyer L, Chabrier S. Varicella as a Risk Factor for Cerebral Infarction in Childhood: A Case-Control Study. Ann Neurol 1999 May;45(5):679-80.

58. Hunter JV. Magnetic Resonance Imaging in Pediatric Stroke. Top Magn Reson Imaging 2002 February;13(1):23-38.

59. Ozduman K, Pober BR, Barnes P, Copel JA, Ogle EA, Duncan CC, Ment LR. Fetal Stroke. Pediatr Neurol 2004 March; 30(3):151-62.

60. Nelson KB, Lynch JK. Stroke in Newborn Infants. Lancet Neurol 2004 March;3(3):150-58.

61. Lee J, Croen LA, Backstrand KH, Yoshida CK, Henning LH, Lindan C, *et al.* Maternal and Infant Characteristics Associated with Perinatal Arterial Stroke in the Infant. JAMA 2005 February;9;293(6):723-29.

62. Roach ES, Golomb MR, Adams R, Biller J, Daniels S, Deveber G, *et al.* Management of Stroke in Infants and Children: A Scientific Statement from A Special Writing Group of the American Heart Association Stroke Council and the Council on Cardiovascular Disease in the Young. Stroke 2008 September; 39(9):2644-91.

63. Golomb MR, Dick PT, MacGregor DL, Armstrong DC, DeVeber GA. Cranial Ultrasonography has a Low Sensitivity for Detecting Arterial Ischemic Stroke in Term Neonates. J Child Neurol 2003 February;18(2):98-103.

64. Wu YW, Miller SP, Chin K, Collins AE, Lomeli SC, Chuang NA, *et al.* Multiple Risk Factors in Neonatal Sinovenous Thrombosis. Neurology 2002 August;13;59(3):438-40.

65. Giroud M, Lemesle M, Gouyon JB, Nivelon JL, Milan C, Dumas R. Cerebrovascular Disease in Children Under 16 Years of Age in the City of Dijon, France: A Study of Incidence and

Clinical Features from 1985 to 1993. J Clin Epidemiol 1995 November;48(11):1343-48.

66. Fullerton HJ, Wu YW, Zhao S, Johnston SC. Risk of Stroke in Children: Ethnic and Gender Disparities. Neurology 2003 July: 22;61(2):189-94.

67. Earley CJ, Kittner SJ, Feeser BR, Gardner J, Epstein A, Wozniak MA, *et al.* Stroke in Children and Sickle-Cell Disease: Baltimore-Washington Cooperative Young Stroke Study. Neurology 1998 July;51(1):169-76.

68. Golomb MR, Fullerton HJ, Nowak-Gottl U, Deveber G, International Pediatric Stroke Study Group. Male Predominance in Childhood Ischemic Stroke: Findings from the International Pediatric Stroke Study. Stroke 2009 January: 40(1):52-57.

69. Chabrier S, Rodesch G, Lasjaunias P, Tardieu M, Landrieu P, Sébire G. Transient Cerebral Arteriopathy: A Disorder Recognized by Serial Angiograms in Children with Stroke. J Child Neurol 1998 January;13(1):27-32.

70. Husson B, Lasjaunias P. Radiological Approach to Disorders of Arterial Brain Vessels Associated with Childhood Arterial Stroke–A Comparison between MRA and Contrast Angiography. Pediatr Radiol 2004 January;34(1):10-15.

71. Ganesan V, Savvy L, Chong WK, Kirkham FJ. Conventional Cerebral Angiography in Children with Ischemic Stroke. Pediatr Neurol 1999 January;20(1):38-42.

72. Husson B, Rodesch G, Lasjaunias P, Tardieu M, Sébire G. Magnetic Resonance Angiography in Childhood Arterial Brain Infarcts: A Comparative Study with Contrast Angiography. Stroke 2002 May;33(5):1280-85.

73. Ganesan V, Chong WK, Cox TC, Chawda SJ, Prengler M, Kirkham FJ. Posterior Circulation Stroke in Childhood: Risk Factors and Recurrence. Neurology 2002 November 26;59(10): 1552-56.

74. Amlie-Lefond C, Bernard TJ, Sébire G, Friedman NR, Heyer GL, Lerner NB, *et al.* Predictors of Cerebral Arteriopathy in Children with Arterial Ischemic Stroke: Results of the International Pediatric Stroke Study. Circulation 2009 March; 17;119(10):1417-23.

75. Askalan R, Laughlin S, Mayank S, Chan A, MacGregor D, Andrew M, *et al.* Chickenpox and Stroke in Childhood: A Study of Frequency and Causation. Stroke 2001 June;32(6):1257-62.

76. Sébire G, Fullerton H, Riou E, deVeber G. Toward the Definition of Cerebral Arteriopathies of Childhood. Curr Opin Pediatr 2004 December;16(6):617-22.

77. Leiguarda R, Berthier M, Starkstein S, Nogués M, Lylyk P. Ischemic Infarction in 25 Children with Tuberculous Meningitis. Stroke 1988 February;19(2):200-04.

78. Martins HS, da Silva TR, Scalabrini-Neto A, Velasco IT. Cerebral Vasculitis Caused by Aspergillus Simulating Ischemic Stroke in An Immunocompetent Patient. J Emerg Med 2010 June;38(5):597-600.

79. Blair JE. Coccidioidal Meningitis: Update on Epidemiology, Clinical Features, Diagnosis and Management. Curr Infect Dis Rep 2009 July;11(4):289-95.

80. Gürsoy G, Aktin E, Bahar S, Tolun R, Ozden B. Post-herpetic Aneurysm in the Intrapetrosal Portion of the Internal Carotid Artery. Neuroradiology 1980;19(5):279-82.

81. Gilden D, Cohrs RJ, Mahalingam R, Nagel MA. Varicella Zoster Virus Vasculopathies: Diverse Clinical Manifestations, Laboratory Features, Pathogenesis and Treatment. Lancet Neurol 2009 August;8(8):731-40.

82. Shah SS, Zimmerman RA, Rorke LB, Vezina LG. Cerebrovascular Complications of HIV in Children. AJNR Am J Neuroradiol 1996;17(10):1913-17.

83. Dubrovsky T, Curless R, Scott G, Chaneles M, Post MJ, Altman N, *et al.* Cerebral Aneurysmal Arteriopathy in Childhood AIDS. Neurology 1998 August;51(2):560-65.

84. Berkefeld J, Enzensberger W, Lanfermann H. MRI in Human Immunodeficiency Virus–Associated Cerebral Vasculitis. Neuroradiology 2000 July;42(7):526-28.

85. Rodriguez-Carbajal J, Del Brutto OH, Penagos P, Huebe J, Escobar A. Occlusion of the Middle Cerebral Artery Due to Cysticercotic Angiitis. Stroke 1989 August;20(8):1095-99.

86. terPenning B, Litchman CD, Heier L. Bilateral Middle Cerebral Artery Occlusions in Neurocysticercosis. Stroke 1992 February;23(2):280-83.

87. Barinagarrementeria F, Cantú C. Frequency of Cerebral Arteritis in Subarachnoid Cysticercosis: An Angiographic Study. Stroke 1998 January;29(1):123-25.

88. Suzuki J, Takaku A. Cerebrovascular "moyamoya" disease. Disease Showing Abnormal net-like Vessels in Base of Brain. Arch Neurol 1969 March;20(3):288-99.

89. Fujita K, Shirakuni T, Kojima N, Tamaki N, Matsumoto S. Magnetic Resonance Imaging in Moyamoya Disease. No Shinkei Geka 1986 March;14(3 Suppl):324-30.

90. Shin IS, Cheng R, Pordell GR. Striking CT Scan Findings in a Case of Unilateral Moyamoya Disease–A Case Report. Angiology 1991 August;42(8):665-71.

91. Fujiwara H, Momoshima S, Kuribayashi S. Leptomeningeal High Signal Intensity (Ivy sign) on Fluid-attenuated Inversion-Recovery (FLAIR) MR Images in Moyamoya Disease. Eur J Radiol 2005 August;55(2):224-30.

92. Chabbert V, Ranjeva JP, Sevely A, Boetto S, Berry I, Manelfe C. Diffusion–and Magnetisation Transfer-weighted MRI in Childhood Moyamoya. Neuroradiology 1998 April;40(4): 267-71.

93. Brady AP, Stack JP, Ennis JT. Moyamoya Disease–Imaging with Magnetic Resonance. Clin Radiol 1990 August;42(2):138-41.

94. Yamada I, Matsushima Y, Suzuki S. Moyamoya Disease: Diagnosis with Three-dimensional Time-of-flight MR Angiography. Radiology 1992 September;184(3):773-78.

95. Yamada I, Suzuki S, Matsushima Y. Moyamoya Disease: Comparison of Assessment with MR Angiography and MR Imaging Versus Conventional Angiography. Radiology 1995 July;196(1):211-18.

96. Takanashi JI, Sugita K, Niimi H. Evaluation of Magnetic Resonance Angiography with Selective Maximum Intensity Projection in Patients with Childhood Moyamoya Disease. Eur J Paediatr Neurol 1998;2(2):83-89.

97. Suzuki J, Kodama N. Moyamoya disease–A Review. Stroke 1983;14(1):104-09.

98. Kuroda S, Houkin K. Moyamoya Disease: Current Concepts and Future Perspectives. Lancet Neurol 2008 November; 7(11):1056-66.

99. Mugikura S, Takahashi S, Higano S, Shirane R, Kurihara N, Furuta S, *et al.* The relationship between Cerebral Infarction and Angiographic Characteristics in Childhood Moyamoya Disease. AJNR Am J Neuroradiol 1999 February;20(2): 336-43.

100. Health Labour Sciences Research Grant for Research on Measures for Infractable Diseases. Guidelines for Diagnosis and Treatment of Moyamoya Disease (Spontaneous Occlusion of the Circle of Willis). Neurol Med Chir (Tokyo) 2012;52(5): 245-66.

101. Fujimura M, Tominaga T. Lessons Learned from Moyamoya Disease: Outcome of Direct/Indirect Revascularization Surgery for 150 Affected Hemispheres. Neurol Med. Chir (Tokyo) 2012;52(5):327-32.

102. Rafay MF, Armstrong D, Deveber G, Domi T, Chan A, MacGregor DL. Craniocervical Arterial Dissection in Children: Clinical and Radiographic Presentation and Outcome. J Child Neurol 2006 January;21(1):8-16.

103. Fullerton HJ, Johnston SC, Smith WS. Arterial Dissection and Stroke in Children. Neurology 2001 October 9;57(7):1155-60.

104. Lo W, Stephens J, Fernandez S. Pediatric Stroke in the United States and the Impact of Risk Factors. J Child Neurol 2009 February;24(2):194-203.

105. Mackay MT, Wiznitzer M, Benedict SL, Lee KJ, Deveber GA, Ganesan V, International Pediatric Stroke Study Group. Arterial Ischemic Stroke Risk Factors: The International Pediatric Stroke Study. Ann Neurol 2011, January;69(1): 130-40.

106. Ohene-Frempong K, Weiner SJ, Sleeper LA, Miller ST, Embury S, Moohr JW, *et al.* Cerebrovascular Accidents in Sickle Cell Disease: Rates and Risk Factors. Blood 1998 January;1;91(1):288-94.

107. Prengler M, Pavlakis SG, Prohovnik I, Adams RJ. Sickle Cell Disease: The Neurological Complications, Ann Neurol 2002 May;51(5):543-52.

108. Kandeel AY, Zimmerman RA, Ohene-Frempong K. Comparison of Magnetic Resonance Angiography and Conventional Angiography in Sickle Cell Disease: Clinical Significance and Reliability, Neuroradiology 1996 July;38(5): 409-16.

109. Miller ST, Macklin EA, Pegelow CH, Kinney TR, Sleeper LA, Bello JA, *et al.* Silent Infarction as a Risk Factor for Overt Stroke in Children with Sickle Cell Anemia: A Report From the Cooperative Study of Sickle Cell Disease, J Pediatr 2001 September;139(3):385-90.

110. Moser FG, Miller ST, Bello JA, Pegelow CH, Zimmerman RA, Wang WC, *et al.* The Spectrum of Brain MR Abnormalities in Sickle-cell Disease: A Report from the Cooperative Study of Sickle Cell Disease. AJNR Am J Neuroradiol 1996, May; 17(5):965-72.

111. Armstrong FD, Thompson RJ, Wang W, Zimmerman R, Pegelow CH, Miller S, *et al.* Cognitive Functioning and Brain Magnetic Resonance Imaging in Children with Sickle Cell Disease. Neuropsychology Committee of the Cooperative study of Sickle Cell disease. Pediatrics 1996 June;97(6 Pt 1): 864-70.

112. Meyers PM, Halbach VV, Barkovich JA. Anomalies of Cerebral Vascular: Diagnostic and Endovascular Considerations. In: Barkovich JA, Raybaud C, Editors. Pediatric Neuroimaging. Philadelphia: Lippincott Williams and Wilkins 2012av., 1051-108.

113. Adams RJ, McKie VC, Hsu L, Files B, Vichinsky E, Pegelow C, *et al.* Prevention of A First Stroke by Transfusions in Children with Sickle Cell Anemia and Abnormal Results on Transcranial Doppler Ultrasonography, N Engl J Med 1998 July;2;339(1):5-11.

114. Wang WC, Gallagher DM, Pegelow CH, Wright EC, Vichinsky EP, Abboud MR, *et al.* Multicenter Comparison of Magnetic Resonance Imaging and Transcranial Doppler Ultrasonography in the Evaluation of the Central Nervous System in Children with Sickle Cell Disease. J Pediatr Hematol Oncol 2000;22(4): 335-39.

115. Breedveld G, de Coo IF, Lequin MH, Arts WF, Heutink P, Gould DB, *et al.* Novel Mutations in Three Families Confirm a Major Role of COL4A1 in Hereditary Porencephaly. J Med. Genet 2006 June;43(6):490-95.

116. Gould DB, Phalan FC, Breedveld GJ, van Mil SE, Smith RS, Schimenti JC, *et al.* Mutations in Col4a1 Cause Perinatal Cerebral Hemorrhage and Porencephaly. Science 2005 May; 20;308(5725):1167-71.

117. Lanfranconi S, Markus HS. COL4A1 Mutations as A Monogenic Cause of Cerebral Small Vessel Disease: A Systematic Review, Stroke 2010 August;41(8):e513-18.

118. Guo DC, Papke CL, Tran-Fadulu V, Regalado ES, Avidan N, Johnson RJ, *et al.* Mutations in Smooth Muscle Alpha-actin (ACTA2) Cause Coronary Artery Disease, Stroke and Moyamoya Disease, along with Thoracic Aortic Disease. Am J Hum Genet 2009 May;84(5):617-27.

119. Munot P, Saunders DE, Milewicz DM, Regalado ES, Ostergaard JR, Braun KP, *et al.* A Novel Distinctive Cerebrovascular Phenotype is Associated with Heterozygous arg179 ACTA2 Mutations. Brain 2012 August;135(Pt 8):2506-14.

120. Joutel A, Corpechot C, Ducros A, Vahedi K, Chabriat H, Mouton P, *et al.* Notch3 Mutations in CADASIL, A Hereditary Adult-onset Condition Causing Stroke and Dementia. Nature 1996 October; 24;383(6602):707-10.

121. Benabu Y, Beland M, Ferguson N, Maranda B, Boucher RM. Genetically Proven Cerebral Autosomal-dominant Arteriopathy with Subcortical Infarcts and Leukoencephalopathy (CADASIL) in a 3-year-old, Pediatr Radiol 2013 September;43(9): 1227-30.

122. Wong I, Kozak FK, Poskitt K, Ludemann JP, Harriman M. Pediatric Lateral Sinus Thrombosis: Retrospective Case Series and Literature Review. J Otolaryngol 2005 April;34(2):79-85.

123. Zimmerman RA, Larissa TB. Cerebraovascular Disease in Infants and Children. In: Tortori-Donati P, Rossi A, Editors. Pediatric Neuroradiology Brain, Head, Neck and Spine, Berlin: Springer; 2010ax.

124. Teksam M. Moharir M. Deveber G. Shroff M. Frequency and Topographic Distribution of Brain Lesions in Pediatric Cerebral Venous Thrombosis. AJNR Am J Neuroradiol 2008 November;29(10):1961-65.

125. Dormont D. Anxionnat R. Evrard S. Louaille C. Chiras J. Marsault C. MRI in Cerebral Venous Thrombosis. J Neuroradiol 1994 April:21(2):81-99.

126. Dormont D. Sag K. Biondi A. Wechsler B. Marsault C. Gadolinium-enhanced MR of Chronic Dural Sinus Thrombosis. AJNR Am J Neuroradiol 1995;16(6):1347-52.

127. Forbes KP. Pipe JG. Heiserman JE. Evidence for Cytotoxic Edema in the Pathogenesis of Cerebral Venous Infarction. AJNR Am J Neuroradiol 2001 March:22(3):450-55.

128. Ducreux D. Oppenheim C. Vandamme X. Dormont D. Samson Y. Rancurel G. *et al.* Diffusion-weighted Imaging Patterns of Brain Damage Associated with Cerebral Venous Thrombosis. AJNR Am J Neuroradiol 2001 February:22(2):261-68.

129. Poon CS. Chang JK. Swarnkar A. Johnson MH. Wasenko J. Radiologic Diagnosis of Cerebral Venous Thrombosis: Pictorial Review. AJR Am J Roentgenol 2007 December; 189(6 Suppl):S64-75.

4 Chapter

EEG IN CLINICAL PRACTICE

Vinod Puri, Neera Chaudhry

The first recording of human epileptic activity was published by Gibbs *et al.* in 1935[1] and one year later Grey Walter localized the tumor by EEG which was confirmed on surgery.[2] However, Hans Berger, a German psychiatrist was the first person to record EEG in man and coined the term electroencephalogram in 1929. But it was Mr. Caton, a physiologist who had first recorded EEG in animals in 1875.

After the invention, EEG became important tool of investigation and research in the neurology and neurosurgical practice. But with the advent of CT scan and MRI, the role EEG has witnessed a sea change. Radio imaging is now the modality of investigation of structural lesion while EEG being used for cerebral functional disorders.

In pediatric clinical practice EEG is of great value in evaluating patients with epilepsy, coma, infections, etc.

EPILEPSY

EEG is an important test in the evaluation of patient with epilepsy. It contributes significantly to establish the diagnosis as the clinician rarely gets the opportunity to observe the patient during seizure. But, one must remember that epilepsy is a clinical diagnosis where EEG is a complement and epileptiform pattern can be seen, though with a low frequency, in non-epileptic persons as well. Various contributions of EEG in patients with epilepsy could be as follows:

1. Confirmation of epilepsy.
2. Classification of epilepsy.
3. Location of focus or foci.
4. Presence or absence of underlying lesion.
5. Presence of trigger factors, i.e., reflex epilepsies.
6. Suitability of patient for surgical treatment.
7. To direct and monitor medication.

Confirmation of Diagnosis

Epileptiform activity in EEG consists of paroxysmal waveforms of cerebral origin that have a distinct morphologic appearance and clearly distinguishable from the ongoing background activity. The main form of epileptiform discharge are spikes, sharp waves, spike and wave paroxysm. Most of the discharges seen in the EEG represent interictal activity. When an ictal discharge occurs, the EEG manifestation consist of repetitive or rhythmic waveforms that have an abrupt onset, a characterstic pattern of evolution, and an abrupt termination.[3]

More than 90% of patients with epilepsy eventually have abnormal EEG recordings when multiple recordings, non-invasive activation techniqes and sleep recordings are used.[4] The frequency of false negative EEG can be further reduced by prolonged recordings techniques. However, 0.4 to 1.7% of normal non-epileptic population may have epileptiform pattern in EEG recordings.[5,6] Spikes in the central, mid temporal or occipital area is not uncommon in normal children without epilepsy.[7] Such spikes are usually

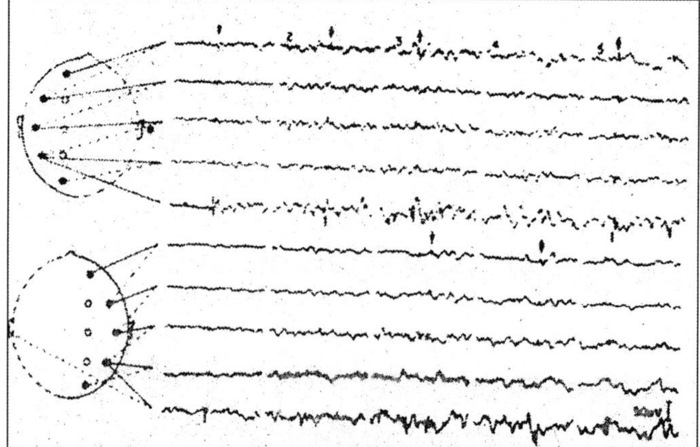

Fig. 4.1: Benign epileptiform transient of sleep (BET) or small sharp spikes (SSS) occurring independently in the temporal regions during sleep. The amplitude of the spikes (arrows) is gently increased in montage between temporal electrodes to opposite ear

benign and disappear in teenage period. Epilepsy should not be diagnosed in patients with such spikes unless there is equivalent clinical evidence of seizure disorder. In clinical practice one should be cautious not to[3] misinterpret normal EEG pattern as epileptiform discharge and[4]/or incidental or irrelevant EEG abnormality as epileptiform.

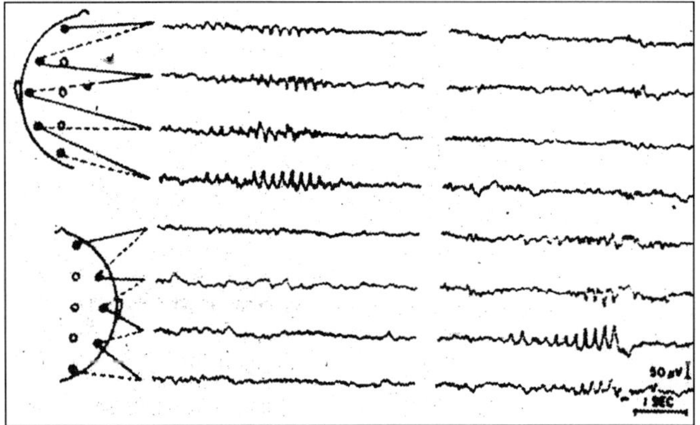

Fig. 4.2: Rhythmical mid-terminal discharge (RMTD) at about 6 Hz occurring independently on either side during drowsiness. This 12 years old girl had headache and no seizure

Classification of Epilepsy

The international classification of epileptic seizure is based on clinical and EEG pattern.[8] Thus EEG assumes importance in the evaluation of epilepsy. On the basis of distribution of epileptiform activity, it may be generalized or focal.

Generalized Epileptiform Patterns

The main types of these epileptiform discharges are:

1. 3 Hz spike and wave.
2. Slow spike and wave.
3. Atypical spike and wave.
4. Hypsarrhythmia; and
5. Paroxysmal rhythmic; fast activity.

1. *3 Hz Spike and Wave Discharge*

The typical, stereotyped, generalized, synchronous, symmetric, spike and wave burst occurring at a rate of 3 per second is the classic pattern associated with absence seizures.[9,10] There may be some variability in the typical pattern. Although the frequency is usually 3 Hz, the rate may be faster, i.e., 4 Hz at the beginning of discharge and slower, i.e., 2.5 Hz at the end of discharge. The inter-ictal period is normal. Some patients with 3 Hz spike wave pattern may demonstrate rhythmic synchronous delta slow waves over the posterior head regions.[10] During sleep, the morphological pattern of spike-wave discharge is altered, the discharges becoming more fragmented and multiple spike wave burst may occur. This EEG pattern resolve often after adolescence and the children with this pattern are normal mentally and neurologically and have no underlying organic disease.

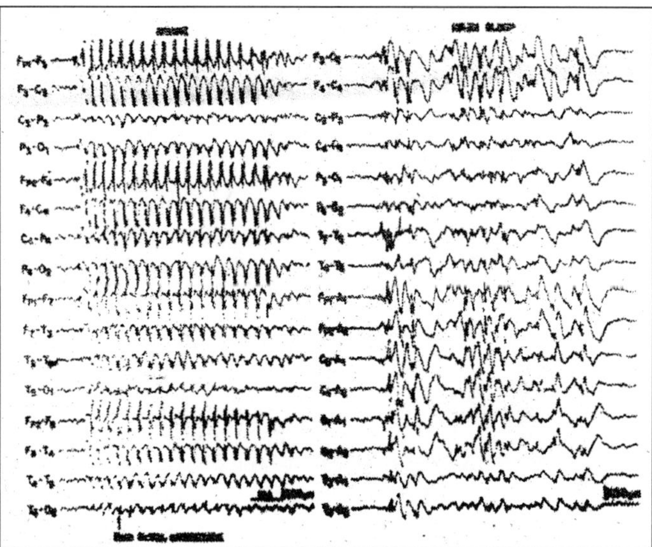

Fig. 4.3: Hz spike and slow wave complexes. This eight years old girl had absence seizures. Left: While awake, she had a spontaneous absence (arrow). Right: During stage II NREM sleep

2. *Slow Spike and Wave*

This pattern consists of spike and wave discharge occurring with a frequency of 1.5 to 2.5 Hz. This pattern is also referred to as generalized sharp and slow wave complex or petitmal variant.[11]

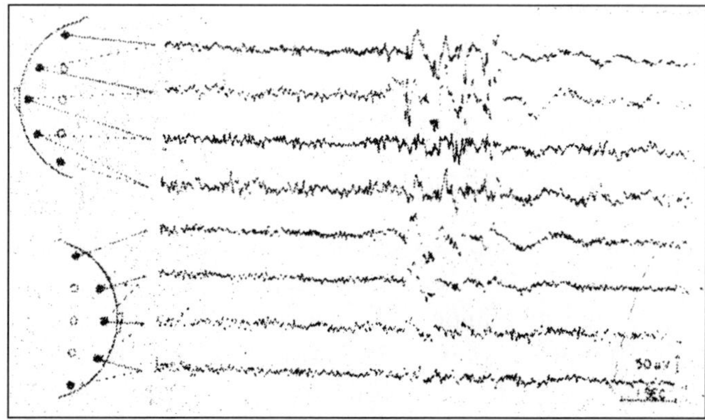

Fig. 4.4: Slow spike and waves at 1.5-2 Hz maximal over the anterior region. This 8 years old boy had a history of generalized seizures of many types since birth; he was mildly retarded but without other neurological abnormalities

These discharges may be diffuse, synchronous or asymmetric with shifting lateralized or focal emphasis. The interictal background is often abnormal. Drowsiness tends to enhance the occurrence of the slow spike and wave pattern. During sleep, the EEG often shows generalized spikes and multiple spike and wave discharge or burst of generalized paroxysmal fast activity. This pattern on EEG is usually seen in children with some type of organic or diffuse encephalopathy who have sign of cerebral damage.

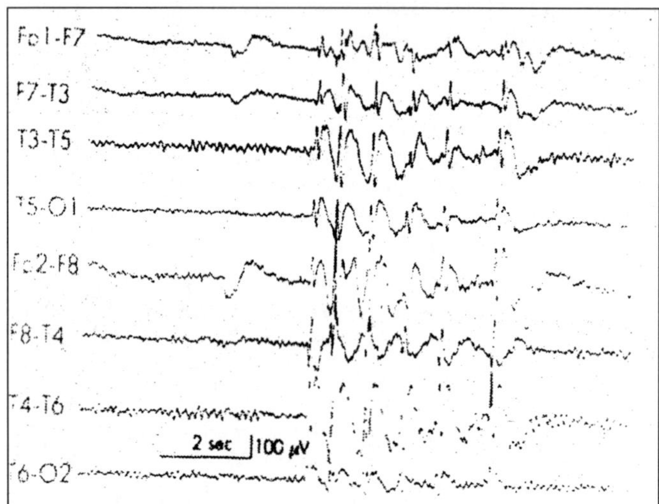

Fig. 4.5: Burst of bilaterally synchronous 1.5 Hz slow spike wave complexes with greater amplitude over right hemisphere

3. *Atypical or Irregular Spike and Wave*

There is no regular repetition or stereotyped appearance of 3 Hz spike and wave or the slow spike and wave pattern. The spike and wave complexes occur with varying frequencies, usually ranging between 2.5 and 5 Hz. There may be admixed polyspike component. The expression of this pattern is variable from asymmetric to localized. The interictal background may be normal or abnormal depending on the underlying cause of the seizures disorder. Sleep potentiates the presence of spike and wave bursts.[12]

4. *Hypsarrhythmia*

This refers to a high voltage arrhythmic and disorganized EEG pattern with a chaotic admixture of continuous, multifocal, high amplitude spike and sharp wave discharges and arrhythmic slow waves. This EEG pattern occurs in response to a severe insult or a diffuse or multifocal disease process occurring usually before one year of age. This pattern is age related and resolves after therapy or spontaneously after 4 or 5 years of age.

5. *Generalized Paroxysmal Fast Activity*

The characteristic features are repetitive serial spike discharges or fast activity in the range of 10-20 Hz. This pattern is also referred a grandmal pattern because of its frequent association with grandmal seizures. Such paroxysm can also occur during sleep recording of patients with generalized seizures and patients with slow spike and wave pattern.[9]

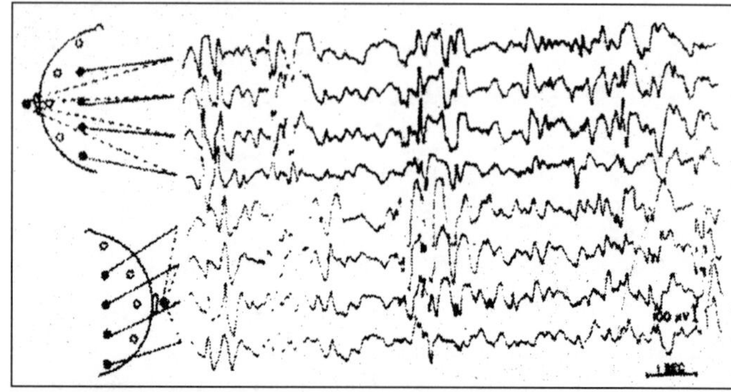

Fig. 4.6: Hypsarrhythmia. Interictal continuous spikes and slow wave of high amplitute in a distribution. This 6-month-old baby had infantile spasms

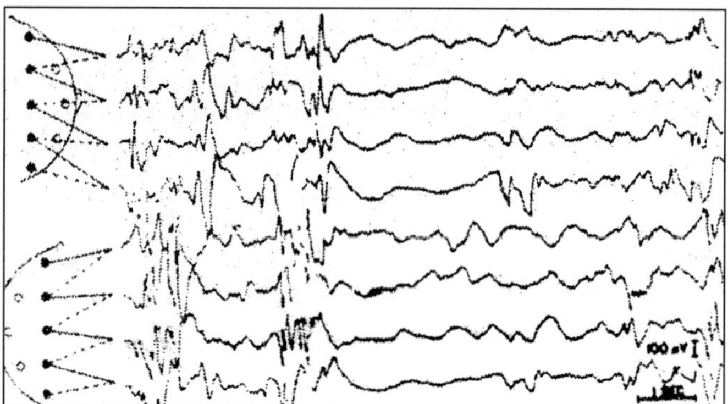

Fig. 4.7: Hypsarrhythmia interrupted by an electrodecremental seizure

Focal Patterns

The main focal pattern are:

(a) Occipital spikes.

(b) Centroparietal spikes (Rolandic spikes).

(c) Centromidtemporal spike discharge.

(d) Anterior temporal spikes.

(e) Frontal spike discharge.

(f) Midline epileptiform discharge; and

(g) Periodic lateralized epileptiform discharge.

(a) **Occipital spikes:** The spikes occur as a single or multiple spike discharge in a unilateral or bilateral fashion over the occipital region (Fig. 4.8). Occipital spikes may be a benign phenomenon in children (50-60%) while in adults it is often related to underlying infarct, tumour, trauma or vascular malformation. However, a number of children with this phenomenon have visual difficulty such as amblyopia, cataracts etc. A rapid spike discharge referred to as needle sharp has been seen in congenitally blind children without a seizure disorder.[9]

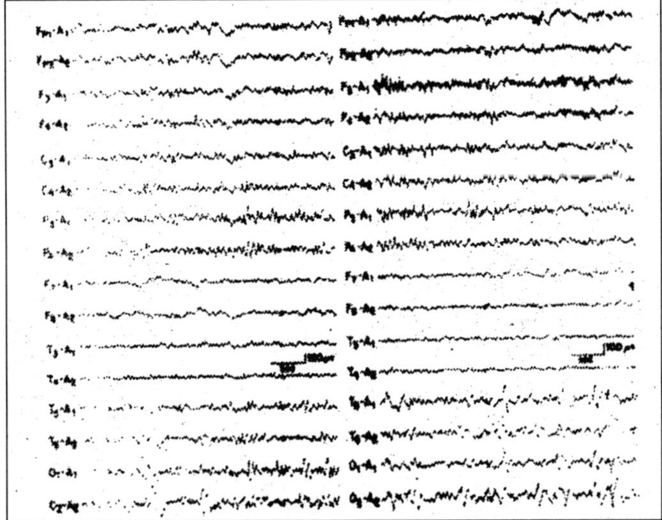

Fig. 4.8: Independent bioccipital foci of spikes. Left: The child had generalized tonic-clonic seizure. The spike generator extending into posterior temporal and parietal regions. Right: Another child with no seizure but having temper tantrums

(b) **Centroparietal spikes:** Centroparietal spike discharge occurs in children between 4 and 10 years of age. About 38 to 50% of children with this type of discharge have seizure. A number of patients with this type of spike discharge have cerebral palsy or some type of motor dysfunction or mental retardation.

(c) **Centromidtemporal spike discharge (Rolandic spike):** This discharge is seen in the central and mid temporal leads. The discharge may be unilateral (Figs. 4.9 and 4.10) or bilateral (Fig. 4.11) or may shift from one side to another. About 60% to 85% of children with such spikes have seizure.

(d) **Anterior temporal spikes:** The anterior temporal spike discharge is one of the most epileptogenic of all spike discharge, more than 90% of patients with this pattern have seizure. Drowsiness and sleep potentiates the presence of temporal discharge (Figs. 4.12 and 4.13). This pattern is more commonly seen in adolescent and adult age.

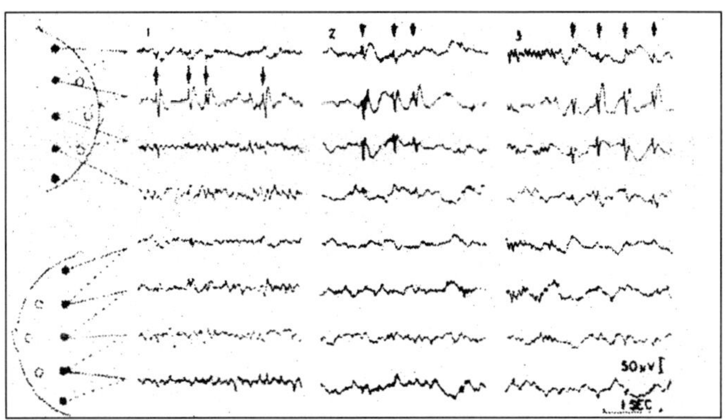

Fig. 4.9: Spike in right fronto-central region (Rolandic spikes).1. Awake: Spikes limited to region between frontal and central region. 2. Sleep (stage 1: Slightly wilder distribution and occasional polyphasic spike. 3. Sleep (stage 2): Wider distribution

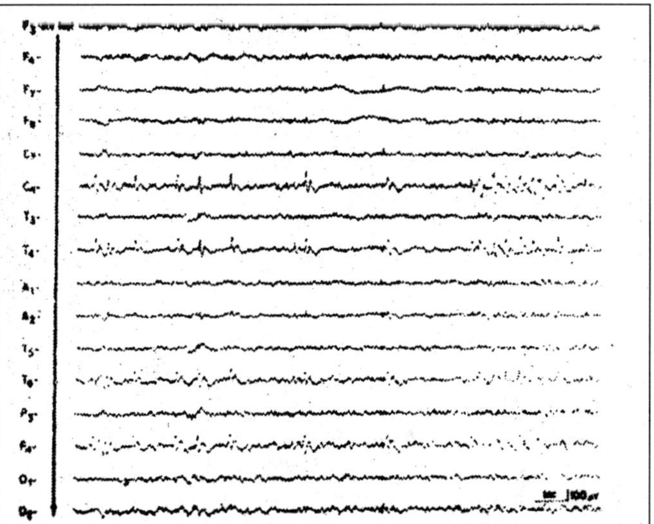

Fig. 4.10: Rolandic focus of sharp waves. This 12 years old boy had benign Rolandic epilepsy

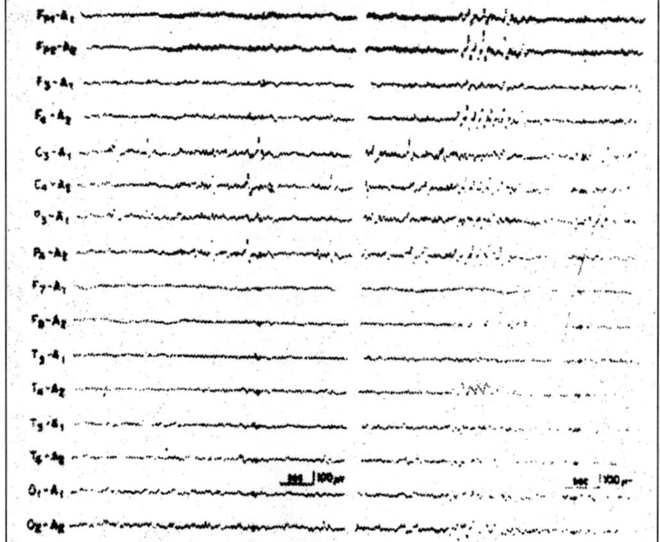

Fig. 4.11: Independent asymmetric Rolandic foci

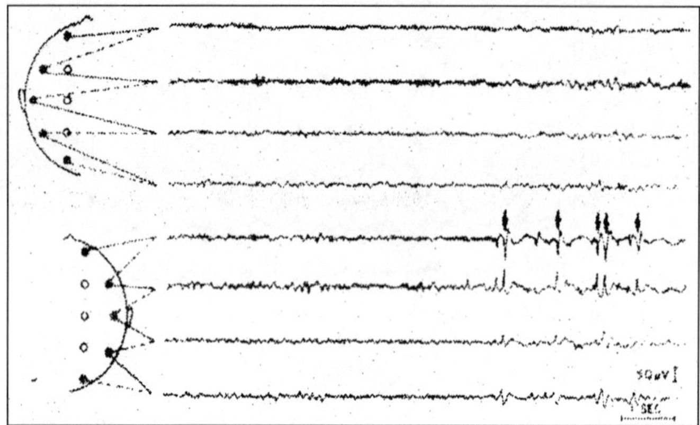

Fig. 4.12: Sharp waves in right anterior temporal region. This 10 years old boy had complex partial seizure

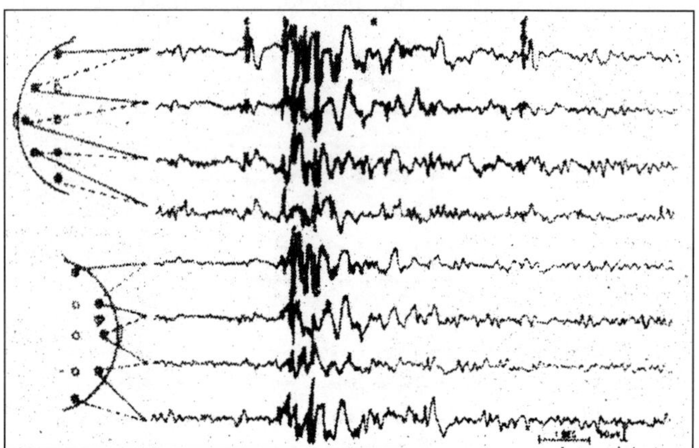

Fig. 4.13: Generalized spike and wave discharge. (a) Preceded (b, c) and followed (d) by left temporal spikes. This 10 years old boy had complexes partial seizure with secondary generalization

(e) Frontal spike discharge: These spike are highly epileptogenic, with approximately 80% of patients who have such pattern suffering from seizure. This pattern is more common with underlying pathology such as head trauma, tumor, vascular lesion, scarring or encephalitis.

(f) Midline epileptiform discharge: They arise from midline or central vertex region and may not be apparent unless midline leads are employed.

(g) Periodic lateralized epileptiform discharge: PLED consist of unilateral sharp waves (Fig. 4.14) that occur in a periodic or quasiperiodic fashion of 1 per second. The sharp wave complexes have a variable morphologic appearance and vary in duration and amplitude. PLEDs may occur with a widespread distribution over one hemisphere or in a more focal fashion, also vary in the morphologic appearance, and even shift in area of maximal emphasis. The background activity is attenuated or slowed on this side of PLEDs.

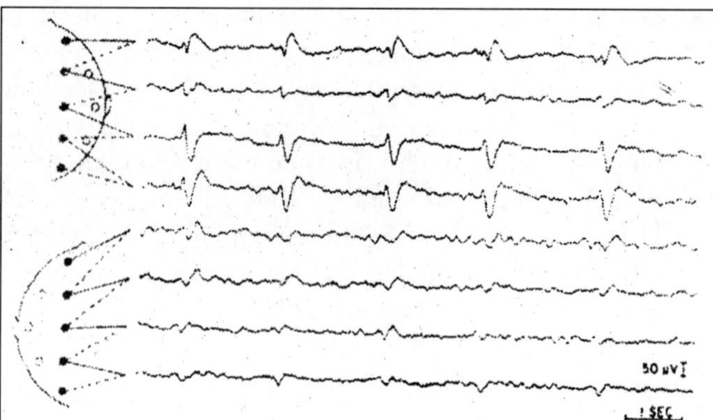

Fig. 4.14: Periodic lateralizing epileptiform discharges (PLEDs) on right side. This 11 years old girl had cerebral infarct

PLEDs usually occur as a result of an acute or subacute disturbance of cerebral function due to vascular insult, herpes simplex encephalitis, tumor, abscess, trauma or subdural hematoma. Bilateral PLEDs (Fig. 4.15) are more commonly seen with herpes simplex encephalitis or vascular disease.

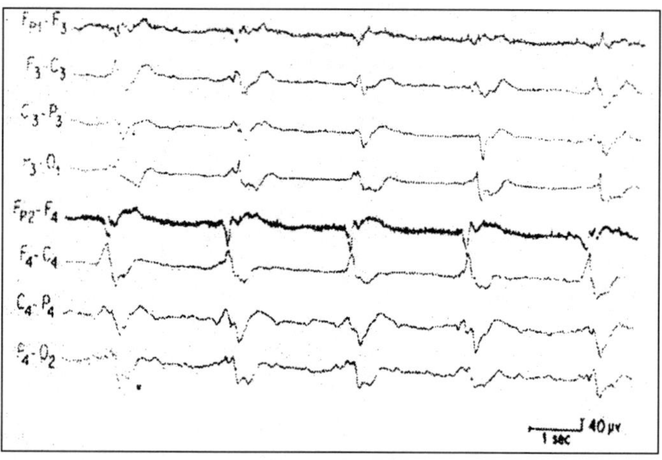

Fig. 4.15: Bilateral asynchronous periodic sharp wave complexes in 13 years old boy with herpes simplex encephalitis

Localization of Focus

The major responsibility of the electroencephalographer interpreting the EEG is not only to recognize the presence of abnormal pattern but also to localize them to a certain area of the brain (Fig. 4.16). In referential recording, this is accomplishment by simply noting the electrode, which records the highest amplitude of the abnormal pattern, while in bipolar recordings this is done by observing the presence of phase reversal (Fig. 4.17). The magnetoencephalogram is perhaps more sensitive than EEG for the location of focus or foci.

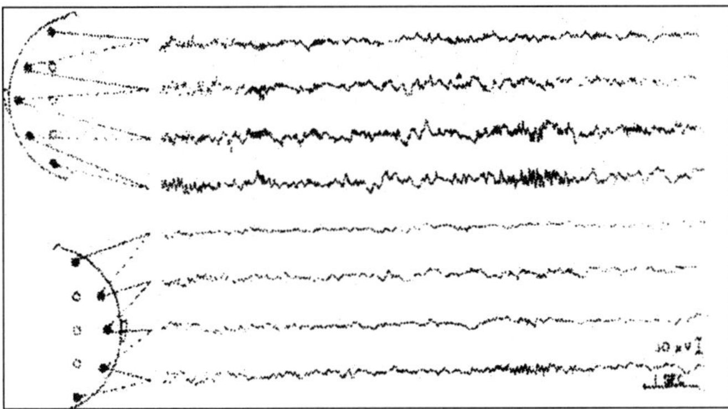

Fig. 4.16: Asymmetry of normal background activity, sleep spindles and slow waves of sleep are attenuated over the right side. This 6 years old boy had Sturge-Weber syndrome

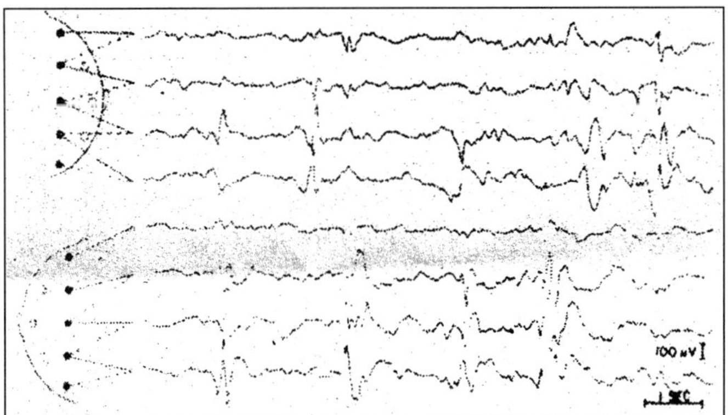

Fig. 4.17: Multifocal independent spikes. This 1 year old girl had hypsarrhythmia on EEG at 6 months of age

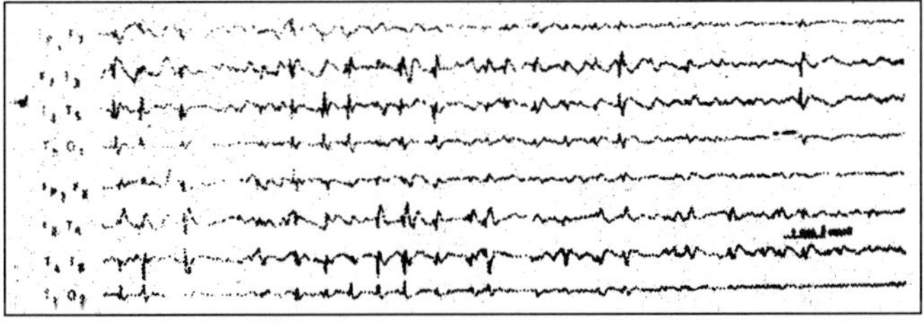

Fig. 4.18: Multifocal spikes and slow spikes and wave activity in an 8 years old boy with suspected neurodegenerative disorder

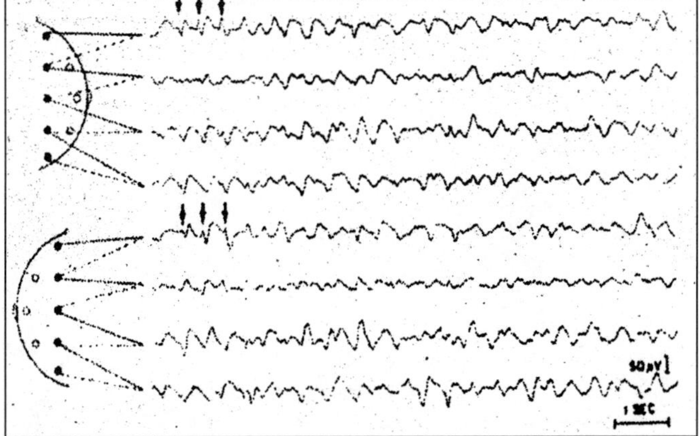

Fig. 4.19: Continuous bisynchronous slow waves mixed with sharp waves (arrows). This 12 years old boy was in delirium and had hyponatremia

Presence or Absence of Underlying Brain Disease

The EEG can be helpful in the evaluation of patients (Figs. 4.18 and 4.19) with altered states of consciousness. Diffuse slowing of background rhythms and the presence of triphasic wave suggest metabolic dysfunction, particularly hepatic coma. Generalized fast activity may be seen in patient with drug intoxication. Abnormalities such as PLEDs or focal continual polymorphic delta activity support a diagnosis of supratentorial lesion, while a normal appearing EEG in a comatose patient suggest a brainstem lesion.

Reflex Epilepsis

Predisposition to seizure, a facilitation of seizure through moment to moment change in the threshold and the presence of specific stimuli are the factors consistently present in all sensory-precipitated seizure. A propensity from certain EEG features elicited by specific types of stimuli is characteristic of reflex epilepsies. Visual induced seizure are the largest category. Various visual related seizure are: photosensitive epilepsy, pattern eye closure, induced by eye movement, reading and television epilepsy. Other reflex epilepsies are eating, musicogenic, hot water bath, tactile epilepsy.

Suitability of Patients for Surgical Treatment

The localization of focus on EEG is a must before considering any patients for surgery in epilepsy. The focus must be located in cortex, which could be dispensable and accessible. Depth electrode recording is also indicated before surgery in some case. A minimum of at least 3 ictal recordings are made to ensure the seizure origin focus.

To Direct and Monitor Treatment

The value of EEG in directing management of absence seizure is well established. The control of spike-wave paroxysms on EEG can be equated with the clinical control of the seizure. The value of EEG in guiding medication is less certain Rowan *et al.*[13,14] demonstrated that suppression of EEG spikes on long recording correlated with improved seizure control and increased blood levels of anti-epileptic drugs.

A well recognized EEG sequence occurs with increasing drug intoxication. The most obvious feature is appearance of excessive beta activity. Then this diminishes somewhat as the background rhythm slow into the low end of alpha range/upper end of theta range. This rhythmic activity is rather persistent and unresponsive to eye opening. Bursts of generalized delta activity with frontal emphasis may also occur. In an epileptic patient presenting with behavior retardation where drug toxicity is suspected EEG can be helpful in such a situation if series of previous recordings are available. EEG will show progressive slowing of background frequencies.

The EEG can aid in making the decision of whether or not to discontinue antiepileptic medication. In several studies[15,16], where antiepileptic drugs were discontinued after 4 years on medication without seizures. Seizures recorded in 30-50% of the children whose EEGs were abnormal at the time of discontinuation of medication and in 13-19% of those where EEGs were normal at the time medication was stopped.

COMA

EEG is of great help in evaluating patients of coma. Although EEG changes are non-specific (Fig. 4.20) but it provides clues to various diagnostic possibilities. Depending upon the background activity of alpha or beta range the coma may be classified as alpha or beta. Alpha coma carries a bad prognosis and is seen with brainstem lesion while the beta coma should raise the suspicion of drug intoxication especially barbiturates or benzodiazepines.

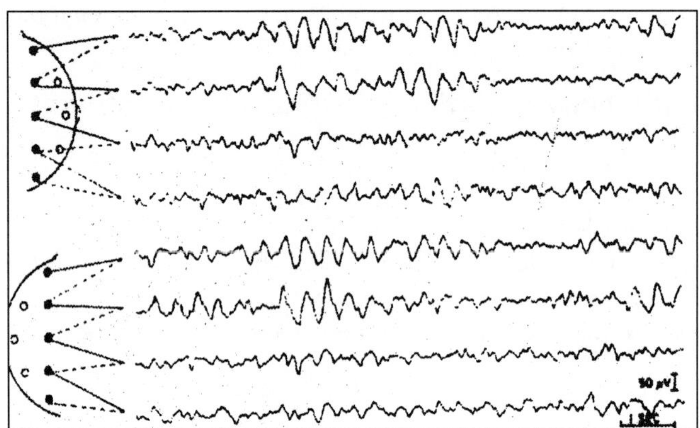

Fig. 4.20: Frontal intermittent rhythmical delta activity (FIRDA). Trains of bisynchronous slow waves of 2-3 Hz and high amplitude with a maximum in the frontal regions. This 13 years old girl had head injury and was confused

With impairment of consciousness, the EEG becomes slow. The slow activity may be episodic or continuous usually with frontal emphasis. With deepening coma the EEG amplitude diminishes, slowing more marked, unreactive and eventually it becomes flat.

Presence of typical triphasic waves are suggestive of hepatic encephalopathy. However, triphasic waves are also seen in hypernatremia, uremia etc.

In hypoxic encephalopathy, EEG becomes progressively slower with decline in amplitude and depending upon severity the activity may be altogether suppressed.

INFECTIONS

Presence of slowing (Fig. 4.21) or PLEDs in the temporal region in the clinical setting of encephalitis is suggestive of underlying herpes encephalitis. Early treatment with acyclovir is the key to good recovery of herpes encephalitis.

Periodic discharges are seen in chronic infective disorders as SSPE (Figs. 4.22 and 4.23).

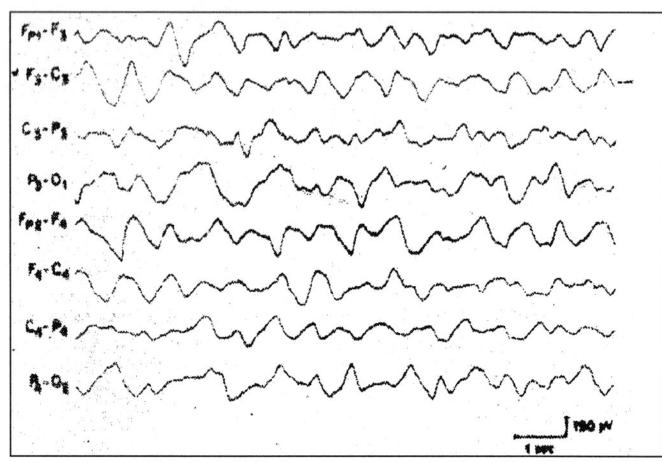

Fig. 4.21: Generalized slow waves abnormality in a 10 years old girl with encephalitis

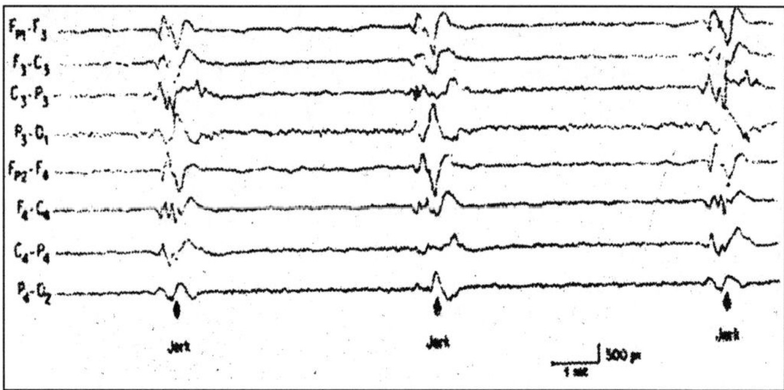

Fig. 4.22: Periodic sharp and slow wave complexes associated with generalized jerks of the body in a 5 years old boy with SSPE

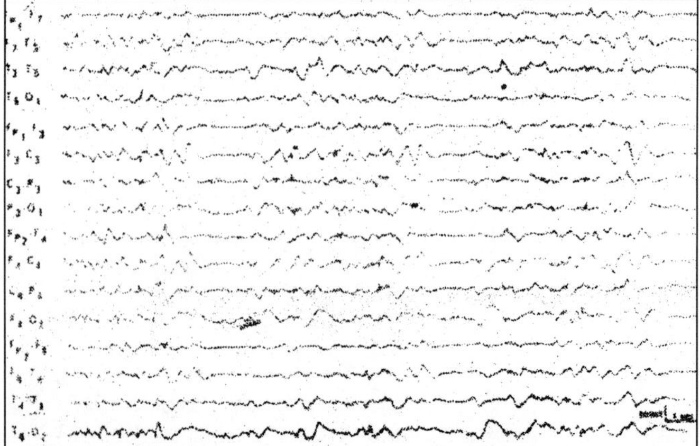

Fig. 4.23: Hypsarrhythmia pattern alternating with periods of flattening during sleep EEG in a 2 years old boy with SSPE

References

1. Gibbs FA. Davis H and Lennox WG. The Electroencephalogram in Epilepsy and in Conditions of Impaired Consciousness. Arch. Neuro. Psych 1935:34:1133.
2. Walter WG. The Location of Cerebral Tumors by Electroencephalography Lancet 1936:2:305.
3. Cheitrian GE. Bergamine L. Dondey M *et al.* Appendix B. A glossary of terms most commonly used by electroencephalographers. electroencephalogr. Clin. Neurophysiol 1974: 37:538-48.
4. Aird RB. Woodbury OM. The Management of Epilepsy. Springfield III. Thomas 1974.
5. Gastaut H. Tassinari CA. Epilepsies. In A Remand (ed) Handbook of EEG and Clinical Neuro Physiol YOL 13 Part A. Amsterdam: Elsevier. 1975.
6. Zivin I. Ajmone Marsan C. Incidence and Prognostic Significance of Epileptiform Activity in the EEG of Nonepileptic Subjects. Brain 1968;81:751.
7. Lerman P. Kiviti Ephraim S. Focal Epileptic EEG Discharges in Children not Suffering from Clinical Epilepsy: Etiology. Clinical Significance and Management. Epilepsy 1981:22:551.
8. Dreifuss RE. Proposal for Revised Clinical and Electroencephalographic Classification of Epileptic Seizure. Epilepsia 1981;22:489.
9. Gibbs FA and Gibbs EL. Atlas of Electroencephalograph. Yol 2 ED 2 Cambridge Massachusetts. Addison–Wesley Press 1952:422.
10. Dalby MA. Epilepsy and 3 per Second Spike and Wave Rhythm. Acta Neurol. Scand (Suppl. 40) 1969:45:1-180.
11. Gastaut H. Roger J. Soulayrol R *et al.* Childhood Epileptic Encephalopathy with Diffuse Slow Spike Waves (otherwise known as petit mal variant) or Lennox syndrome. Epilepsia 1966:7:139-79.
12. Pedlay TA. Interictal Epileptiform Discharges. Discriminating Characteristics and Clinical Correlations. Am J. Electroencephalogr. Technol 1980:20:101-19.
13. Rowan AI. Protass LM. Transient Global Amnesia: Clinical and Electroencephalographic Findings in 10 Cases.
14. Rowan AI. Binnie CD. De-Beer Pawlikowski NKB Geodgart OM. Gutter T *et al.* Sodium Valproate: Serial Monitoring of EEG and Serum Levels. Neurology 1979:29:1450.
15. Thurston JH *et al.* Prognosis in Childhood Epilepsy. Additional Follow-up of 148 Children 15 to 23 Years After Withdrawal of Anticonvulsant Therapy. N. Eng J Med 1982;306:831.
16. Emerson R *et al.* Stopping Medication in Childhood Epilepsy. Predictors of Outcome. N. Eng J Med 1981:304:1125.

5 Chapter NERVE CONDUCTION AND ELECTROMYOGRAPHY IN CLINICAL NEUROLOGIC PRACTICE

Vinod Puri, Neera Chaudhry

The electromyography/nerve conduction study (EMG/NCS) is an extension of the neurologic examination for the diagnosis of neuromuscular disorders. The EMG/NCS findings must be interpreted in their clinical context. They are of immense value for the pathophysiological classification of neuropathies and may be the only laboratory means of determining the site of focal peripheral nerve abnormality. Histologic evaluation of nerve is limited because biopsy is restricted to small sensory nerve branches, which are not involved in many disorders and moreover biopsy may leave a permanent sensory deficit. Needle EMG helps differentiate between neuropathic and myopathic affliction and provides strong evidence for disorders as myotonic dystrophy.

NERVE CONDUCTION STUDIES

NCS provide a reliable assessment of motor and sensory peripheral nerve function.[1] All NCS require stimulation of peripheral nerve using cathode (negative) and anode (positive). After stimulation, motor conduction studies are obtained by recording a compound muscle action potential (CMAP), which is the summation of action potentials for all muscle fibers depolarized by the nerve. The CMAP latency is the time from stimulus onset to the baseline deflection and represents the time required for propagation of the fastest conducting fibers to the nerve terminal, neuromuscular transmission and depolarisation of muscle fibers. CMAP amplitude is directly proportional to the number and synchrony of muscle fibers depolarized by the nerve. Sensory fibers are assessed in two ways, sensory nerve is stimulated distally and compound sensory nerve action potential (SNAP) recorded orthodromically over the proximal portion. Alternatively, antidromic SNAPs are obtained by stimulation at a proximal site over the nerve and recording the response over distal sensory branches. The SNAP amplitude is a measure of the number of axon and their firing synchrony.[2,3]

Motor or sensory conduction velocity is calculated by dividing the measured distance between two sites of stimulation by their latency difference.

Several technical factors affect NCS results. Incorrect measurement of nerve length is the most common error, but other sources include improper sweep, incorrect stimulus, inaccurate instruments calibration, failure to recognize anatomic and physiological variants. Skin temperature, height, age profoundly affect the NCS.[4,5,6,7]

Pathological afflictions of peripheral nerves are divided into those of axon, myelin or both. Abnormalities can be either focal or diffuse and affect selective nerve fiber populations. The routine NCS measure conduction in the fast conducting fibers, however, with collision techniques one can study the small as well as intermediate sized fibers.

Demyelination has several characteristics:

(i) Block of action potential conduction will produce a reduced CMAP or SNAP.

(ii) Slowing of conduction velocity with prolonged latencies occur presumably when continuous conduction is established by redistribution of sodium ion channels. One must remember that sparing of a few conduction fibers from the process of demyelination will result in conduction velocities within the entire nerve increase. Since individual axons vary in the extent of conduction slowing, with remylination these physiological measures become normal, however, the conduction may continue slow because of increased number of nodes of Ranvier. Examples of demyelinating neuropathy include acute and chronic forms of inflammatory demyelinating polyradiculoneuropathy, hereditary motor and sensory neuropathies type I (Charcot-Marie-Tooth).

(iii) Dejerine–Sottas.

(iv) Refsum, Metachromatic leucodystrophy.

Axonal disruption that has been present for 5 days or longer produce low amplitude CMAPs and SNAPs.[8] Conduction velocity remains greater than 70% of normal with axonal loss alone. The causes of axonal neuropathies are frequently toxic, metabolic, nutritional including for example thiamine deficiency, pyridoxine deficiency or excess, uremia, vincristine, cisplastin, collagen vascular disease, amyloid etc. Axonal neuropathies must be differentiated from low amplitude motor responses on NCS in cases of Myasthenic syndrome and botulism, both of which have weakness and preserved sensation.

Many patients with a generalised neuropathy will demonstrate features of combined axonal loss and demyelination on NCS/EMG. In addition, patients with generalised neuropathies are more susceptible to compression neuropathies at common sites such as carpal tunnel etc. The earliest feature on electrophysiology of axonal polyneuropathy may be reduced or absent sural sensory potentials with fibrillations in the distal muscles while conduction block is the first feature of demyelination.

The NCS findings of focal neuropathy depend on the cause, duration and severity of the injury.[9] Acute injury may cause conduction block from metabolic factors, such as ischemia. Chronic injury may produce intussusception of myelin with disruption of the nodes of Ranvier and longer lasting block.[10] Slowed conduction across the nerve segment arises from loss of salutatory conduction and axonal narrowing thereby producing prolonged latencies and waveform dispersion. Axonal disruption with wallerian degeneration can be present with injuries of greater severity.

NCS are routinely performed on easily accessible nerves. In the arm this includes median and ulnar motor and sensory, and in the leg, tibial and peroneal motor and sural sensory. After stimulation of motor nerves, an impulse will be antidromically conducted to the motor neuron which will then discharge an orthodromic response of F wave (Fig. 5.1). F wave latencies are used for detecting abnormalities in conditions that affect proximal nerves, such as inflammatory demyelinating polyradiculo-neuropathies.[11] Another measure of proximal conduction is the H reflex (Fig. 5.2). The characteristic features of demyelination Vs axonal injury are as in Table 5.1.

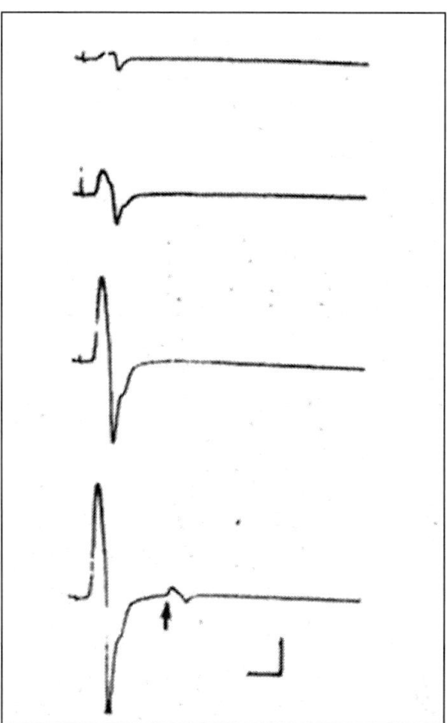

Fig. 5.1: F wave, increasing stimulus strength from top to bottom trace. Note the appearance of F. Response (arrow) with the supra maximal shock

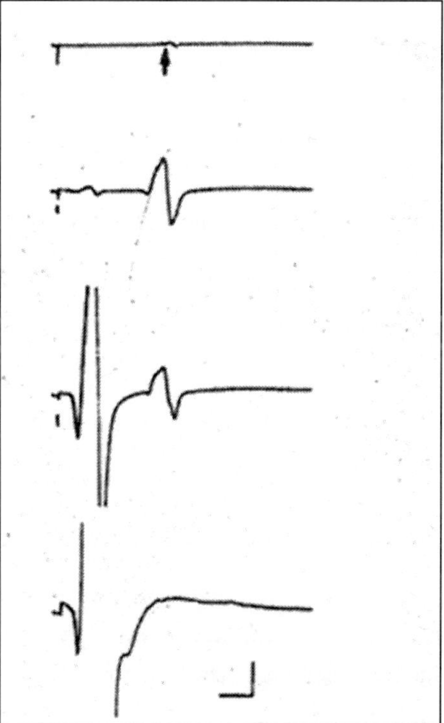

Fig. 5.2: H reflex, increasing stimulus strength from top to bottom trace. Note the appearance of H reflex (arrow) before that of the direct M response

Table 5.1: EMG/NCS Finding of Neuropathies

	Demyelination	Axonopathy
CMAP	Low amplitude with conduction block and or wave-form dispersion	Low amplitude
Conduction velocity	< 70% of normal with prolonged distal latencies	>70% of normal
Needle	No fibrillation	Normal latencies
EMG	Normal MUP morphology Normal MUP recruitment Reduced MUP recruitment with conduction block	Normal MUP Morphology Reduced MUP recruitment

ELECTROMYOGRAPHY

The electrical activity of muscle is studied by using EMG needle electrodes. The action potentials are acquired from single muscle fibers or summated from several fibers while recording motor unit potential (MUP). Concentric or monopolar electrodes are the most commonly used for EMG.

The EMG examination for a muscle is comprised two phases:

(1) Activity at rest.

(2) During contraction. At least 10 to 20 MUPs for each muscle should be examined. The examination is systematized for the presence and extent of insertional activity, spontaneous activity, MUP and recruitment or interference pattern.

Insertional Activity

The activity related to mechanical stimulation or injury of muscle fiber usually lasts less than 500 msecs in normal muscle (Fig. 5.3). Prolonged insertional activity can be an early indication of denervation myotonic disorders.[12] Reduced insertional activity most often occur with infiltration of muscle by fat or from fibrosis but may be observed during an episode of hypokalemic periodic paralysis.[13]

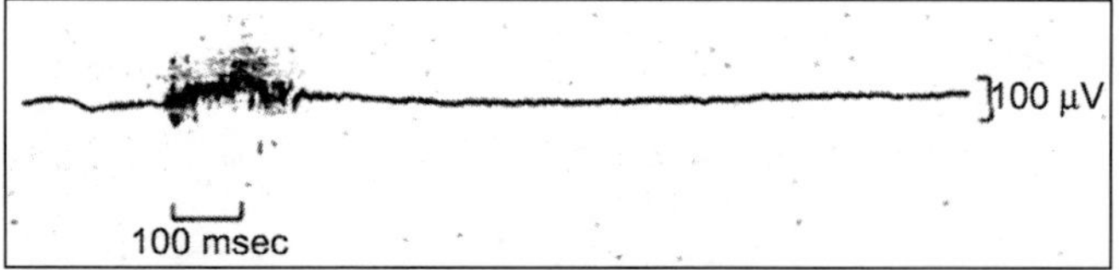

Fig. 5.3: Insertional activity in normal muscle

Spontaneous Activity

Spontaneous activity is observed when both the needle and muscle are at rest. This is a quiet period in normal muscle unless the electrode is near nerve or neuromuscular junction.

End plate Noise[14] produce a sound reminiscent of seashell roar, is derived from miniature end plate potentials (MEEP), while end plate spikes which fire irregularly originate from muscle fibre.

The various spontaneous activity are:

1. **Fibrillations (Fig. 5.4):** These are action potentials of fibre whose membrane potentials is unstable because of a loss of innervation. They may take 1-3 weeks to appear and are seen in addition to denervation in variety of muscle disease as: polymyositis, dystrophies, etc.

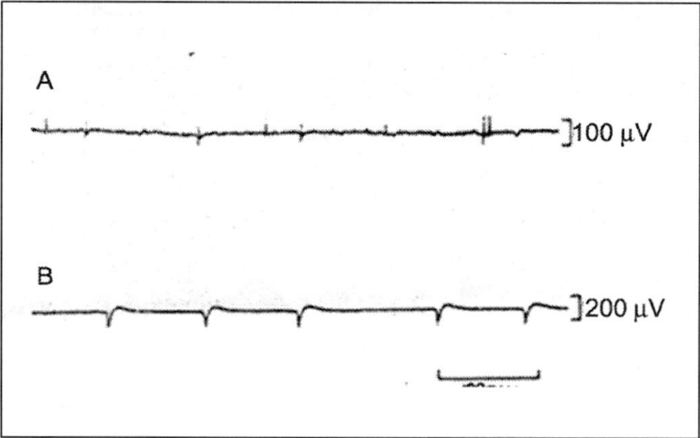

Fig. 5.4: Spontaneous activity recorded in denervated muscle (a) Fibrillation potentials (b) Positive sharp waves

2. **Positive sharp waves:** They appear early to fibrillations and carry the same significance as of fibrillations.

3. **Fasciculation:** These discharges are similar to MUP and range in their morphology from elementary triphasic potentials to complex waveforms. They are present in normal and many disorders with denervation or degeneration of the muscle fibres.

4. **Myotonic discharges** are single muscle fibre action potentials with a distinct firing pattern that waxes and wanes. Myotonic discharges are activated by needle

movement, voluntary contraction, muscle percussion and enhanced by cold. Myotonic discharges are seen in myclonic dystrophy, myotonia congenita, acid maltase deficiency[15] hyperthyroidism.[16]

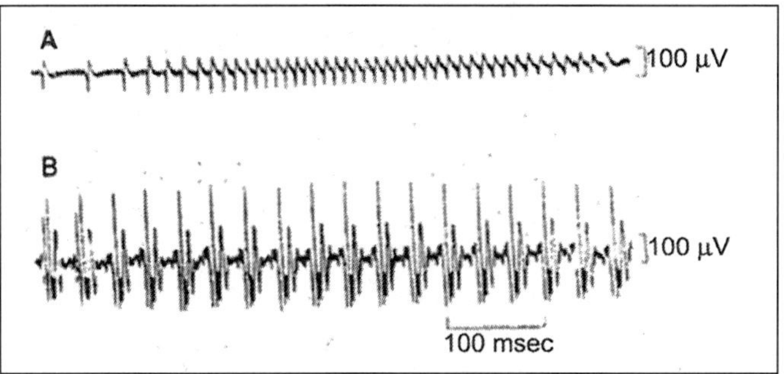

Fig. 5.5: Spontaneous high frequency activity (A) myotonic discharge, (B) complex repetitive discharge

5. **Myokymia:** They are seen in multiple sclerosis, brainstem gliomas, radiation injury,[17] snake bite.[18]

6. **Neuromyotollia:** They are high frequency discharges of up to 300 Hz, that occur in short bursts or long trains. It is common with continuous motor unit activity.[19,20]

7. **Complex repetitive discharges:** These are summation of action potentials for several muscle fibres and are believed to be propagated by ephatic transmission from a pacemaker fibre.[21] They are seen in chronic denervation.

8. **Cramps:** They are seen with pregnancy, uremia, dehydration, hypothyroidism.

The characteristics of various spontaneous discharges are given in Table 5.2.

Table 5.2: Characteristics of Various Spontaneous Discharges

	Potential	Rhythm	Frequency	Morphology	Pattern
Endplate Activity					
(i)	Endplate noise	Seashell roar	> 500 Hz	Monophasic 10-50 µV 1-2 msec. duration	Persistent
(ii)	Endplate spikes	Irregular	05-50 Hz	Biphasic, 100-200 µV 3-4 msec. duration	Persistent
Spontaneous Activity					
(i)	Positive sharp waves	Regular	10 Hz	(i) Positive spike (ii) Negative wave 20-200 µV 10-30 msec.	Variable
(ii)	Fibrillations	Regular	1-30 Hz	(i) Positive spike (ii) Negative wave 20-200 µV 1.5 msec.	Variable
(iii)	Fasciculation	Irregular	0.1-10 Hz	MUP	Variable
(iv)	Complex repetitive discharges	Regular	5-100 Hz	Complex, polyphasic 25-1000 µV 50-100 msec	Abrupt onset and cessation
(v)	Cramp	Irregular	10-150 Hz	MUP	Gradual onset and cessation
(vi)	Myotonia	Wax and Wane	10-80 Hz	(i) Biphasic (ii) Positive wave 20-500 µV	Wane
(vii)	Myokymia	Regular	Bursts of 2-10 potentials Recur at interval of 0.1 to 10 secs	MUP	Rhythmic bursts of MUP discharges
(viii)	Neuromyotoni	Regular	100-300 Hz	MUP	Abrupt onset and cessation

DURING ACTIVITY

Motor Unit Potential (Fig. 5.6)

Short duration MUPs indicate a loss of muscle fibres and such MUPs are often of low amplitude. Brief MUPs are typically present in primary disorders of muscle.[22] Myasthenic syndrome or botulism.[23] Long duration MUPs are often of high amplitude, in part from increased fibre density and represent fibre type grouping. Such MUPs are seen with reinnervation and are a feature of neurogenic type of muscle disorders.[24] Polyphasia signify desynchronization of muscle fibre action potentials and are a feature of both myopathic and neuropathic disorders.[25] The number of polyphasic units of more than four phases normally constitute only 5-15% or less of all motor unit potentials. The percentage increase with

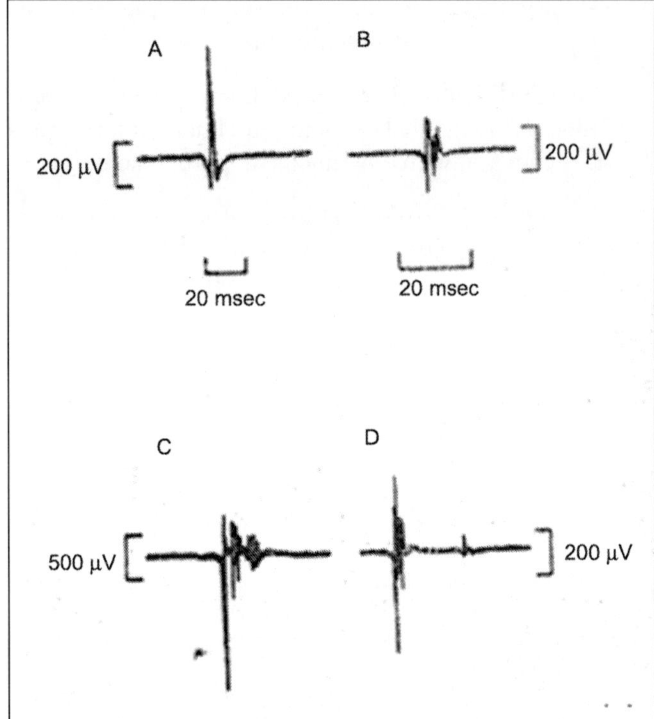

Fig. 5.6: Motor unit action potentials (A) Normal potentials (B) Low amplitude, short duration, polyphasic potential (C) Maximal voluntary contraction of muscle

decreasing synchrony in the firing of individual muscle fibres. Many biologic factors influence MUP parameters, e.g., temperature aging etc. and must be taken into consideration while interpreting MUP.

RECRUITMENT

A mild voluntary contraction of the muscle normally results in up to 5 Hz discharge of one motor unit. Increasing muscle force brings about a higher rate of firing for the already active unit and addition of new units or recruitment (Fig. 5.7). The recruitment frequency, the rate of discharge just before the next unit begins to fire, normally ranges between five and ten impulses per second. The recruitment, i.e., the ratio of average unit firing rate to the number of firing units should not exceed five. A ratio greater than ten indicates a loss of motor units.[26]

INTERFERENCE PATTERN

Full activation of the muscle normally fills the oscilloscope screen, precluding the recognition of individual motor unit potentials. The interference pattern may be graded from mild decrease (–1) or 1 moderate decrease in firing units (–2), a single unit firing (–3) or no motor unit firing with effort (–4).

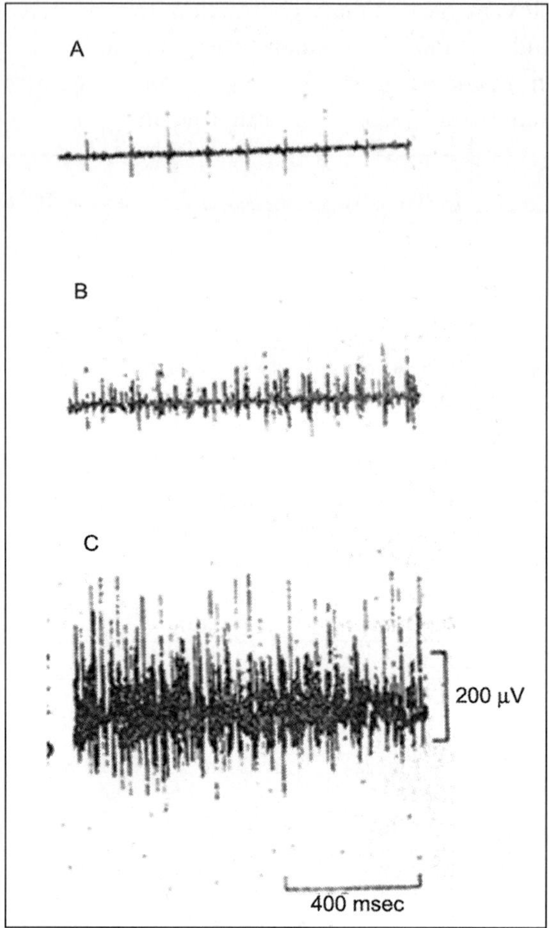

Fig. 5.7: Motor unit action potentials recorded during (A) Slight (B) Moderate and (C) Maximal voluntary contraction of muscle

INTERPRETATION

The abnormalities may be divided into two major categories:

(1) **Neurogenic**

(2) **Myogenic**

One must remember that these findings overlap among different conditions, e.g., MUPs consistent with myopathic pattern can occur with chronic denervation.

Patients with upper motor neuron lesions have normal insertional activity and normal motor unit potentials in size and morphology and spontaneous activity may[27] or may not[28] occur. The only abnormality observed is reduced interference pattern with slow firing rate.

Lower motor neuron lesions show increased insertional activity. Spontaneous commonly consists of fibrillations potentials, positive sharp waves. Complex repetitive discharges occur in chronic lower motor neuron disorder, e.g., SMA. Post polio etc. MUPs are of long duration, polyphasic with increased recruitment frequency and ratio. In extreme case, only a single motor unit fires rapidly.

Myopathies characteristically show normal insertional activity usually absent spontaneous activity. MUP shave reduced amplitude and duration due to random loss of fibres. Motor units often show no abnormality in mild abnormality in mild metabolic or endocrine myopathies. Early recruitment occurs in myoptahy disorders because efforts to maintain given force must bring more motor units to play earlier to compensate for the smaller size of motor units. These patients cannot recruit only one or two single motor units. The interference is full but of low amplitude.

Myotonic disorders have myotonic discharge with early recruitment.

Inflammatory myopathies, e.g., polymyositis, dermatomyositis, infectious myositis typically show increased insertional activity, fibrillation potentials, positive sharp wave. The MUPs are of low amplitude polyphasic, brief duration, with early recruitment. The spontaneous activity is polymyositis disappear in a few weeks with steroid therapy.

References

1. Gilliatt R. Electrophysiology of Peripheral Neuropathies–An Overview. Muscle Nerve 1982;5:S108-16.
2. Kimura J. Electrodiagnosis in Diseases of Nerve and Muscle: Principles and Practices. Philadelphia: FA Davis 1989;31-34.
3. Kimura J, Machida M, Ishida T *et al.* Relation Between Size of Compound Sensory or Muscle Action Potentials and Length of Nerve Segment. Neurology 1986;36:647-52.
4. Halar EM, De Lisa JA, Saine TL. Nerve Conduction Studies in Upper Studies. Skin Temperature Corrections. Arch. Phys. Med. Rehabilitation 1986;64:412-16.
5. Rivner MH, Swift TR, Crout 80, Rhodes KP. Toward More Rational Nerve Conduction Interpretations: The Effect of Height: Muscle Nerve 1990.
6. Miller RG, Kuntz NL. Nerve Conduction Studies in Infants and Children. J. Child Neurol 1986;1:19-26.
7. Mayer RF. Nerve Conduction Studies in Maatn. Neurology 1963:13:1021-30.
8. Gilliat RW, Hjorth RJ nerve conduction during Wallerian Degeneration in the baboon J. Neurol, Neurosurg. Psychiatry 1972;35:335-41.
9. Thomas PK. Focal Nerve Injury: Guidance Factors during Axonal Regeneration, Muscle Nerve 1989:12:796-802.
10. Ocha J Fowler TJ, Gilliat RW. Anatomical Changes in Peripheral Nerve Compressed by a Pneumatic Tourniquet. J. Anat 1972;35:335-41.
11. Gilmore RG, Nelson KR SSEP and F Wave Studies in Acute Inflammatory Demyelinating Polyradiculo Neuropathy. Muscle Nerve 1989:12:538-43.
12. Wilbourn AJ. An Unreported Distinctive Type of Increased Insertional Activity. Muscle 1982:5:S101-05.
13. Engel AJ, Lambard EH, Rosevar JW, Tauxe WN. Clinical and Electromyogrpahic Studies in Patient with Primary Hypokalemic Periodic Paralysis AM J Med 1965:38:626-40.
14. Wiederholt We. Endplate Noise in Electromyography. Neurology 1970:20:214-24.
15. Okuno T, Mori K, Furomi K. *et al.* Myotonic Dystrophy and Hyperthyroidism Neurology 1981:31:91-93.
16. Engle AG, Gomez MR, Seybold ME, Kambert EH. The Spectrum and Diagnosis of Acid Maltase Deficiency. Neurology 1973:23:95-106.
17. Albers JW, Allen AA, Bastrom JA, Daube JR, Limb Myokymia. Muscle Nerve 1981:4:494-504.
18. Brick JF, Gutman L, Birck J *et al.* Timber Rattle Snake Venom Induced Myokymia. Evidence for Peripheral Nerve Origin. Neurology 1987;37:1545-46.
19. LK, Appenzeller O, Bichnell JM. Peripheral Neuropathy with Myokymia. Sustained Muscle Contraction and Continuous Motor Unit Activity. Neurology 1972:22:161-69.
20. Molts JR, Mendell JR. Neurotonia: Impulse Induced Repetitive Discharges in Motor Nerves in Peripheral Neuropathy. Neurol 1980;7:245-50.
21. Stalberg E. Bizarre Repetitive Discharges Recorded with Single Fibre EMG J. Neurol. Neurosurg. Psychiatry 1983;46:310-16.
22. Buchal F. Electrophysiological Signs of Myopathy as Related with Muscle Biopsy. Acta Neurol (Napoli) 1977;32:1-29.
23. Comblath DR, Sladky JT. Sumner AJ, Clinical Electrophysiology of Infantile Botulism. Muscle Nerve 1983;6: 448-52.
24. Buchthal F, Kamieniecka Z. The Diagnostic Yield of Quantified Electromyography and Quantified Muscle Biopsy in Neuromuscular Disorders. Muscle Nerve 1982;92:5:265-80.
25. Stewart CR, Nandedkar SD, Massey JM *et al.* Evaluation of An Automatic Method of Measuring Features of Motor Unit Action Potentials. Muscle Nerve 1989;12:141-48.
26. Daube JR. Principles and Practice of Electromyography. In: Kimura J Director. Clinical EMG Course # 209, Chicago, American Academy of Neurology 1987;63:98.
27. Johnson EW, Denny ST, Kelly JP. Sequence of Electromyography Abnormalities in Stroke Syndromes. Arch. Phys. Med. Rahabil 1975:56:468-73.
28. Chokroverty S, Medina J. Electrophysiological Study of Hemiplegic. Arch. Neurol 1978;35:360-63.

6 Chapter

EVOKED POTENTIALS IN CLINICAL PRACTICE

Vinod Puri, Neera Chaudhry

The cortical responses to sensory stimuli can be recorded readily and these provide data that is a quantitative extension of the neurological examination. The clinical utility of evoked potentials (EPs) is as follows:

1. Demonstrate abnormal sensory system conduction, when the history and/or neurological examination is equivocal.
2. Delineate sub-clinical involvement of a sensory system ("silent" lesions), particularly when demyelination is suggested by symptoms and/or signs in another area of the central nervous system.
3. Define the anatomic distribution and give some insight into pathophysiology of a disease process.
4. Detect and monitor changes in a patient's neurological status.

Almost any sensory modality may be tested, although in routine clinical practice visual evoked potentials (VEPs), somatosensory evoked potentials (SSEPs), and brainstem auditory evoked potentials (BSAEPs) are tested most frequently.

EPs have an advantage of providing an objective analysis and are often more sensitive than detailed neurological examination. These can be recorded in patients who are anesthetised or comatose and so have newer applications in the operating theatre and intensive care units. However, the major disadvantages are that they are rarely disease specific and can be confounded by end organ disease (for example, VEPs may be abnormal in ocular disease, SSEPs in patients with peripheral neuropathy, and BSAEPs in conductive and sensorineural deafness), are affected by age, and require a degree of patient cooperation to obtain artifact-free recordings.

VISUAL EVOKED POTENTIALS

Visual evoked potentials (VEP) are electrical potential differences recorded from scalp in response to visual stimuli. The functional integrity of the visual pathways can be evaluated by VEPs.[1,2] Furthermore, manipulation of visual stimuli permits the preferential evaluation of the various segments of the visual pathways.[3]

Normal VEP is present if the entire visual system is intact and disturbances anywhere in the visual system can produce abnormal VEP, thereby restricting the localizing value of VEP. It is most useful when they detect clinically silent abnormalities that might otherwise go unrecognized or when it assists in resolving vague or equivocal symptoms and findings.

Pathway of VEP

The optic nerve and chiasma are arbitrarily included in the definition of anterior visual pathways for the purpose of this review. The optic nerve from the eye to the chiasm is about 50 mm long and comprises nerve fibers originating in the ganglion cells. Nerve fibers from ganglion cells in the macula constitute the papillomacular bundle that occupies the entire temporal side of the optic disc. This bundle of fibers then moves toward the center of the optic nerve as it approaches the chiasma. Fibers from peripheral ganglion cells occupy less central positions in the optic disc and optic nerve.[4,5] The optic nerve fibers are small myelinated fibers; 92% of the axons are 2μ or less in diameter, 6% have a diameter around 4μ and only 2% have a large axon (> 4μ).[6] Calculated conduction velocities range from 1.3 to 20 m/sec.[7]

The human retina projects to both ipsilateral and contralateral sides of the cortex. Fibers from the nasal retina cross in the chiasma; crossed and uncrossed fibers begin to separate at the termination of the optic nerve. Macular fibers also are subdivided into crossed and uncrossed fibers; the macular fibers from the nasal portion of the macula cross in the chiasma into the contralateral optic tract, whereas the macular temporal fibers travel into the ipsilateral optic tract. The optic tract ends in lateral geniculate body from where the optic radiation emerges and ends in the primary visual area, area 17, which are interlinked with secondary visual association areas 18 and 19

About 80% of VEP response occurs from central 8° although the peripheral 8°-32° also contribute to the amplitude of VEP. The waveform of VEP, i.e., P100 is generated in the striate and peristriate occipital cortex not only due to activation of primary cortex but also due to thalamocortical volleys. On giving pattern/flash stimulation not only there is increased metabolism[8] in primary visual area but also in visual association areas (area 18 and 19). The regional cerebral blood flow increases with stimulation up to 8 Hz and gradually declines thereafter.[9]

Stimulus type and method of generation: The visual stimulus can be either patterned or unpatterned. The patterned visual stimuli elicit responses that have far less intra- and inter-individual variability than responses to unpatterned stimuli. Checkerboard pattern reversal is the most widely used pattern stimulus because of its relative simplicity and reliability. Unpatterned stimuli are generally reserved for patients who are unable to fixate or attend to the stimulus, and also for study of steady state VEP.

In pattern stimulation, the selection of check size, field size and field location allow selective testing for specific segments of the visual pathway. The visual stimulus is a high contrast black and white checkerboard composed of squares subtending a visual angle of 1° and span the central 20°–30° of the visual field. Responses to smaller checks are more sensitive to disorders of the visual pathway but they are also more affected by defocusing and amblyopia. The use of the larger check size minimizes these problems. The black and white squares periodically exchange places. One cycle/sec equals two reversals/second, and a reversal rate of 4/sec or less is used. The VEP is the averaged response to this reversal.

The brightness of the dark and bright elements of a pattern directly affects the amplitude and latency of the VEP waveform. They must be calibrated and be kept constant as the stimulating equipment ages. A high contrast (> 50%) is usually used. It is essential to specify whether the pattern stimulus is presented to one or to both eyes at a time. Clinical testing usually requires monocular "full field" stimulation. The subject should be placed no closer than 70 cm to the stimulus screen. Visual fixation should be at the center of the stimulus screen.

Full field testing is most sensitive in detecting lesions of the visual system anterior to the optic chiasm. The majority of the P 100 response arises in the neural elements of the eye sub serving the central 8° to 10° of the visual field. Lesions which produce half or partial visual field deficits but spare much of central vision will usually not produce significant changes in P 100 response latency or amplitude. Such partial lesions in prechiasmal, postchiasmal or chiasmal locations may produce changes in response to topography, but are best tested for using partial visual field stimulation.

Stimulation of one-half of the visual field gives rise to excitation in the contralateral occipital lobe. P 100 might therefore be expected to appear at the electrode contralateral to the half field stimulated. In practice, P 100 is usually seen over the lateral electrode ipsilateral to the half field stimulated. The paradoxical topography of the response is attributed to the oblique orientation of the cortex at the occipital pole, the area serving the central areas of the visual field. Stimulation of the peripheral field evokes a later positive VEP component, P 135. The lateralization of this component is orthodox and it can be seen at the electrode contralateral to the stimulated half field. The half field responses therefore allow responses to central and peripheral stimuli to be distinguished. Moreover, inclusion of the half field responses enables lesions affecting the retro chiasmal part of the pathway to be detected more reliably.

The responses are recorded from three electrodes spanning the occipital region with a mid-frontal electrode as the reference. Standard disk EEG electrodes are suitable.

Electrode placement: Both the Queen Square System of placement and the International 10/20 system placement (leads O_1, Oz and O_2) have been used for routine testing.

In the Queen Square System, the electrodes are labeled and positioned as follows:

MO – Mid occipital, in midline 5 cm above inion.

LO and RO – Lateral occipital, 5 cm to left and right of MO.

MF – Mid frontal, in midline 12 cm above nasion.

A1/A2 – At ear or mastoid, left and right.

Ground – At vertex.

These additional leads may also be useful:

MP – Mid parietal, in midline 5 cm above MO.

I – Inion, in midline at the inion.

Recording montage: At least 4 channels should be recorded. In routine testing the following montage and derivations have been recommended.

Channel 1: Left occipital to mid frontal = LO-MF.

Channel 2: Mid occipital to mid frontal = MO-MF.

Channel 3: Right occipital to mid frontal = RO-MF.

Channel 4: Mid frontal to ear/mastoid = MF-A1.

In situations where the P100 is low in amplitude or apparently absent, the following montage should be used to ensure that the peak is not displaced above or below the usual MO electrode site.

Channel 1: Inion to ear/mastoid = $I - A_1 + A_2$.

Channel 2: Mid occipital to ear/mastoid = $MO - A_1 + A_2$.

Channel 3: Mid parietal to ear/mastoid = $MP - A_1 + A_2$.

Channel 4: Mid frontal to ear/mastoid = $MF - A_1 + A_2$.

VEP in Children

The VEP protocol for children of 5 years or above is similar to that of adults. The latency of PSVEP is maximum at birth and reaches the adult value by the age of 5 years. In the children below 5 years, the PSVEP is first carried out; if the potentials are unrecordable then a flash VEP should be undertaken. The PSVEP are useful as these assess the visual acuity, and flash VEP only determines the presence or absence of light perception. The room should be dark and child should not be able to see anything other than the screen. During the first six months of life, the optimal check size to elicit VEP varies. It is recommended to use 120 min check at 1 month, 60 min at 2 months or older. In infants younger than 6 months of age, it is usually binocular vision which is of interest. Monocular VEP testing is usually needed after 6 months. In an uncooperative child, or if the question is regarding the integrity of visual pathways especially during anesthesia or coma, flash VEP is used.

Analysis of Results

The signal at the midline occipital electrode normally contains a prominent positive component which occurs approximately 100 ms after the pattern reversal (called P100). It is usually preceded by a smaller negative component with a latency of about 75 ms (N75) (Fig. 6.1). The waveforms at the lateral electrodes are rather variable and so the latency of P100 at the midline electrode is taken as the measure of retina-striate conduction time. The latency of P100 appears to vary little with age from childhood through adult life. However, its latency begins to increase in the over 60s.

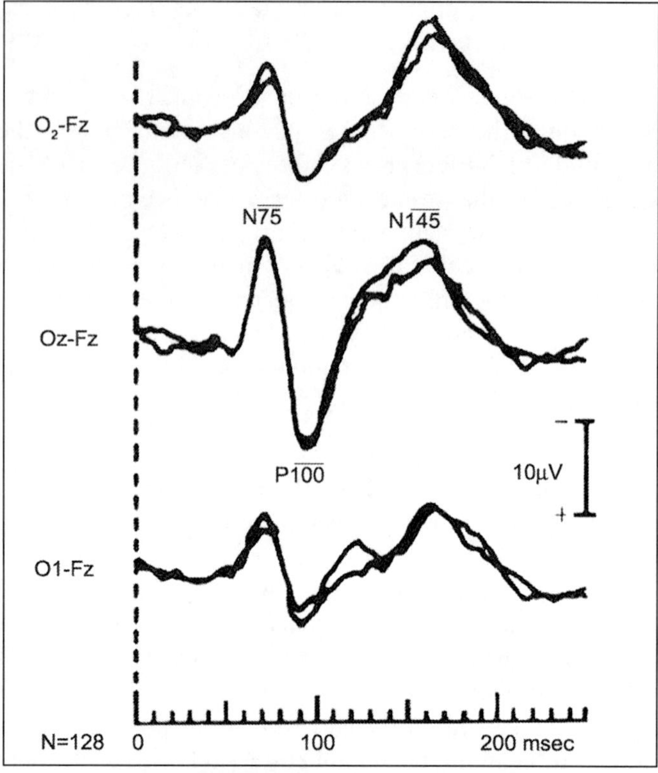

Fig. 6.1: Full field stimulation showing the rostral caudal extent of the occipital components N75, P100 and N145. These may be maximal above or below the mid occipital site in normal individuals with a minimal amplitude response at the mid occipital lead

The most clinically useful measurements on the responses to monocular Full Field stimulation are:

1. P100 latency at the MO site.
2. Amplitude of the P100 component at all three occipital sites.

Amplitude may be measured from baseline to peak, or peak to peak of the N75-P100 component or the P100-N145 component or both, depending on the VEP waveform.

The following derived measurements are also useful:

1. The difference in P100 latency measured at the MO site to left and right eye stimulation, i.e., the interocular latency difference.
2. The ratio of P100 amplitude measured at the LO and RO sites on stimulation of each eye individually, i.e., the interhemisphere amplitude ratio.

   (Amplitude ratios are usually calculated as the quotient of the larger over the smaller value.)

Criteria for Clinically Significant Abnormality

Abnormality may present as changes in latency, amplitude, topography and waveform. P100 latency prolongation is the most reliable indicator of clinically significant abnormality, being least affected by technical factors and degree of patient cooperation. Amplitude and topographic measures are closely related and may be indicators of clinically significant abnormality. However, they are more prone to alteration with technical factors and changes in patient cooperation, fixation and alertness.

Each laboratory performing VEP testing should either collect its own normative data, using its own stimulating and recording equipment. VEP normative data are not routinely interchangeable between laboratories. Normative data vary with age and gender. The apparent effects of gender on latency values may actually be determined by head size.

Latency Criteria

1. Abnormally prolonged P100 peak latency.
2. Abnormally prolonged P100 interocular latency difference, with the longer latency eye being abnormal.
3. Most laboratories regard as abnormal P100 latencies and interocular latencies, if the absolute value differences are exceeding 2.5 or 3 standard deviations above the mean of an age matched control sample from the normal population.

Latency abnormalities are indicative of visual pathway dysfunction only when ocular and retinal disorders have been excluded by appropriate examination. When these factors have been excluded, a monocular latency abnormality indicates a unilateral optic nerve dysfunction. Bilateral latency abnormality suggests bilateral visual pathway dysfunction. This cannot be localized to pre or post chiasmatic sites without further evaluation of amplitude and topographic features.

Amplitude Criteria

1. Absence of any response when recording from multiple midline and lateral occipital sites, with prolonged analysis times as long as 500 msec.
2. Absence of an identifiable P100 when recording from multiple midline and lateral occipital sites, other positive peaks may be present.
3. Abnormally low amplitude of the P100.
4. Abnormally high P100 interocular amplitude ratio.

Amplitude and amplitude ratio values are not normally distributed in control populations so it is inappropriate to use the mean value plus standard deviations to determine the limits of the normal control population. The 99% upper tolerance limit for the interocular amplitude ratio usually lies within the range of 2:1 to 2.5:1 when large field stimulation is used.

Causes of Abnormal Visual Evoked Potentials

- **Ocular disease**
  - Major refractive error.
  - Lens and media opacities.
  - Glaucoma.
  - Retinopathies.
- **Compressive lesions**
  - Extrinsic tumors.
  - Optic nerve tumors.
- **Non compressive lesions**
  - Demyelinating disease.
  - Ischemic optic neuritis.
  - Nutritional and toxic amblyopias (including pernicious anemia).
  - Leber's hereditary optic atrophy.
- **Diffuse central nervous system disease**
  - Adrenoleukodystrophy.
  - Spinocerebellar degenerations.
  - Parkinson's disease.

For convenience, abnormal VEP can be considered under the following sections as retinopathies and maculopathies, disorders of optic nerve and chiasm and retro chiasmatic lesions.

Retinopathies and Maculopathies

Diseases of the retina, especially affecting the macular regions, are associated with abnormal VEP. Simultaneous recording the pattern electroretinogram (ERG) and VEP is diagnostically useful in differentiating between involvement of the macula and the optic nerve. In maculopathies and retinopathies, the ERG is abnormal and in optic nerve diseases, VEP is abnormal. Abnormalities of VEP in patients with a normal funduscopic examination (including a normal macula) suggest dysfunction in the optic nerve or visual pathways.

Disorders of the Optic Nerve (Especially Multiple Sclerosis) and Chiasm

Pattern reversal VEP are most sensitive in the diagnosis of demyelination of optic nerve. It has been calculated that a demyelinating plaque of 10 mm size would result in VEP delay of 25 ms. The ability of VEP to detect clinically silent optic nerve lesions remains a very useful tool for the diagnosis of multiple sclerosis. By using more than one stimulus parameter in optic nerve function assessment, one can test more than one "parallel information processing channel" and more accurately detect abnormalities. Pathological processes can affect these channels differentially. For instance, patients with suspected MS have been found to have delayed VEPs only when the stimulus pattern was presented in a specific orientation or with a specific spatial frequency. A pattern presented in a different orientation or specific frequency often evoked normal potentials.[10]

Several studies have compared VEP and MRI of the optic nerve in optic neuritis. MRI demonstrated high signal lesions in 84-88% of symptomatic patients, where as VEP were abnormal in 100% of cases. Thus, VEP are more sensitive than MRI in detecting lesions and are still the investigation of choice in suspected demyelinating diseases involving the optic nerve. The sensitivity of VEP in detecting or becoming positive in demyelinating disease of brain (MS) with or without clinical optic nerve involvement is shown in Table 6.1. If a patient has normal PSVEP, invariably the neuro-ophthalmologic examination is also normal, however, normal, neuro-ophthalmologic examination may have abnormal PSVEP. Chiappa reported, with abnormal PSVEPs, normal visual fields in 96%; normal formal fields in 55%; normal papillary responses in 74%; normal fundus appearance in 39%; no red color desaturation in 27% of cases.

The overall sensitivity of PSVEP vs. other evoked potentials is as follows: VEP 80-85%; BAEPs 50-65%; SSEP 65-80%. However, various studies have concluded that there is no specific differential susceptibility to demyelination in the systems involved in the test. Rather, it is the length and amount of myelinated tract being tested which determine the likelihood of detection of a lesion in a given system.

In a prospective 12 months study of optic neuritis, visual field, visual acuity, contrast sensitivity, color vision, and VEP to 15' and 30' checks, were evaluated.[11] Visual fields, color vision and VEPs to 15' checks were initially abnormal in all patients. Contrast sensitivity was abnormal in 95% and visual acuity and VEPs to 30' in 90% of patients. Recovery of vision occurred in 80% of patients. It was rapid and complete in the majority of cases within the first 2 months. VEPs latency, however, remained prolonged in 19 (95%) patients, even when their vision had returned to normal. VEPs are a reliable indicator of resolved optic neuritis and can be useful to verify a past episode of optic neuritis.[12]

A delayed P100 or absent VEP has been reported in many other disorders involving the optic nerve:

- Systemic lupus erythematosus.
- Sarcoidosis.
- Vitamin B_{12} deficiency.
- Neurosyphilis.
- Tropical spastic paraparesis.
- Spinocerebellar ataxia.

In vitamin B_{12} deficiency, the P100 improves with treatment. Abnormal VEP also occur in ischemic optic neuropathy and in toxic optic neuropathy. The amplitude is more disturbed in ischemic optic neuropathy than the latency of P100. No consistent correlation exists between improvement in visual acuity and VEP but the prolonged VEP latency persists for long time in optic neuritis even when the vision has returned to normal. Even the absence of VEP and pattern ERG in acute optic neuritis is compatible with full visual recovery. No prospective study has determined whether VEP can be used in patients with chiasmatic and perichiasmatic lesions as a prognostic indicator for the risk of visual impairment.

Table 6.1: Abnormal PSVEP in Multiple Sclerosis and Optic Neuritis

	Definite	Probable	Possible	Total
MS patients with a history of optic neuritis	90.36%	75%	52.94%	82%
MS patients without a history of optic neuritis	67.85%	44.70%	20%	42%
All patients with MS	81%	52%	26%	56%
Pure optic neuritis group	–	–	–	96%
All patients with a past history of optic neuritis				88%

Retrochiasmatic Disorders

The retrochiasmal pathways including optic tracts, lateral geniculate bodies, optic radiations, and visual cortex are evaluated by hemi field pattern stimulation; pattern reversal hemi field stimulation activates the hemi macula. However, the value of VEPs in retrochiasmatic lesion diagnosis remains highly controversial. Part of the difficulty relates to the complex topographical distribution of VEPs and their variations in normal subjects.[13,14] Hemi field stimulation (Fig. 6.2) with checks greater than 50' of arc is recommended for studying retrochiasmatic function by the American Electroencephalographic Society in its Guidelines for Clinical Potential Studies.[15]

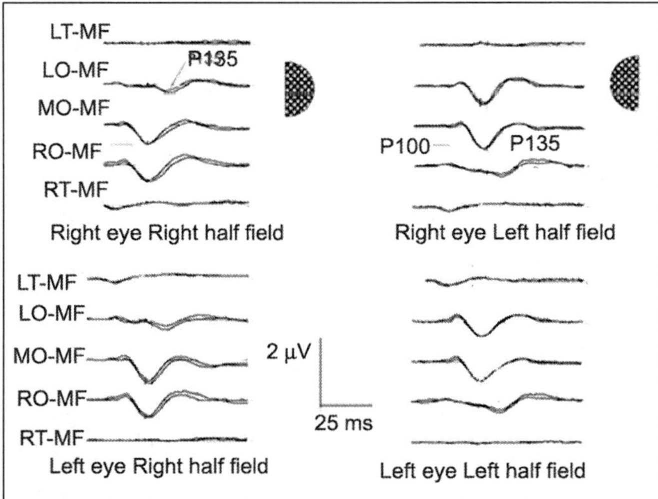

Fig. 6.2: Half field stimulation. The central half field components N75, P100 and N145 are most consistently recorded over the lateral occipital lead ipsilateral to the half field stimulated. The peripheral half field components P75, N105 and P135 are most consistently recorded over the lateral temporal lead contralateral to the half field stimulated. If the central half field P100 peak is lost, the peripheral half field P75 and P135 may be apparent in all occipital leads. They may then be mistakenly identified as the P100

Hemi field stimulation evokes asymmetrical amplitude responses in 64% of cases, with usually higher amplitude potentials ipsilateral to the hemi field stimulated. The greater amplitude of P100 over the scalp ipsilateral to the stimulated hemi field has been explained by the mesial location of the generators in the hemisphere contralateral to the stimulated hemi field.[16]

VEPs to hemi field pattern-reversal stimulation detect 75-85% of patients with known visual pathway lesions and homonymous field defects.[17] VEPs to hemi field stimulation are considered abnormal when there is no response to stimulation of the appropriate hemi field.

VEP to full field pattern stimulation are usually normal in patients with unilateral hemispheric lesions, even in the presence of dense homonymous hemianopia. Even in severe cortical blindness, the VEP may be preserved because it is proposed that VEP in cortically blind subjects originate in remnants of area 17.

Special Applications of VEPs

VEP abnormalities have been reported abnormal in disorders affecting neurotransmitters and specifically the dopaminergic and cholinergic systems. Parkinson's disease is the prototype of a disorder caused by neurotransmitter dysfunction and specifically related to dopamine depletion. Abnormalities of VEPs in Alzheimer's disease are attributed to impairment of the cholinergic system.

VEPs have been used to study congenital abnormalities of the retino geniculostriate projections. Albinism is characterized by hypomelanosis and by aberrant retinal projections. Albinos have crossing fibers arising from the temporal retina near the vertical meridian, while the more peripheral temporal retina projects non-decussating projections. This disorganization alters the orderly representation within the lateral geniculate body and the striate cortex. Abnormal topographic distribution of VEPs reflecting anomalous visual projections have been demonstrated.

VEPs have also been used to study amblyopia exanopsia. Abnormal latencies of pattern VEPs have been noted in about one-half of the patients studied.

VEPs to flashes and LEDs have been used to monitor visual function during pituitary tumor surgery. The aim of intraoperative monitoring is to prevent excessive manipulation of the optic nerve and chiasma and to prevent visual loss. Unfortunately, complete absence of VEPs to flashes or LEDs does not preclude the possibility of severe post-surgical visual impairment. The visual stimuli used in the operating room are too crude to permit satisfactory monitoring of visual function. Better technology is needed to improve the sensitivity and reliability of operative VEP monitoring.

Role of VEP in Malingering

VEP may be helpful in distinguishing hysteria or malingering from blindness. A normal pattern reversal VEP is strong evidence of psychogenic illness. However, rare cases have been reported in which essentially normal VEP were present in cortical blindness because of bilateral destruction of area 17, with preservation of areas 18 and

19 or bilateral occipital infarcts with preservation of area 17.

Somatosensory Evoked Potentials

Somatosensory evoked potentials (SSEPs) is an important tool for unfolding the fundamental aspects of central sensory physiology and has an application in evaluation of various neurological disorders.

The mixed nerve is most commonly stimulated to evoke SSEPs. After peripheral nerve stimulation both group Ia muscle afferents and group II cutaneous afferent fibers contribute to the resultant responses. The ascending axons continue rostrally to form the cuneate and gracilis funiculus and synapse with the second order neurons in the dorsal column nuclei of the medulla. The axons of these second order neurons cross the midline and ascend the brainstem on the contralateral side as the medial lemniscus. These lemniscal pathways terminate in the thalamus and synapse with third order neurons that project to their relative somatosensory cortex in the parietal lobe. On the scalp the cortical median N20 (Fig. 6.3) and tibial P37 (Fig. 6.4) responses are recorded from the contralateral hand area and the vertex, respectively, reflecting the cutaneous input to the primary somatosensory cortex (Brodmann area 3b). The number of axons that are activated synchronously is large, so the response is relatively large and easy to record. A short duration stimulus (200-300 μsec) at a repetition rate of 3 Hz with a stimulus intensity that induces a slight twitch of the muscle is popularly used for stimulating the mixed nerve.

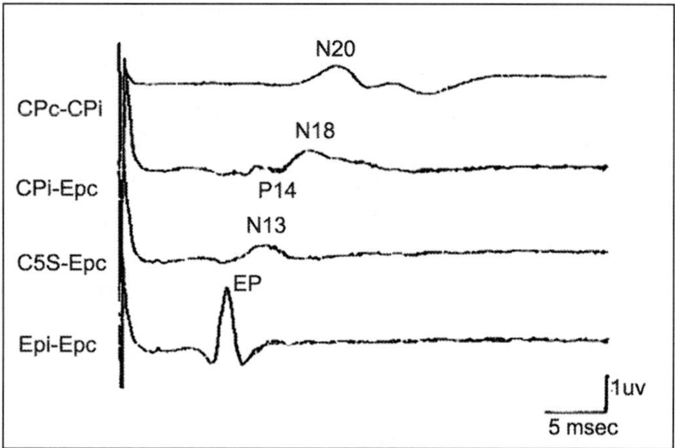

Fig. 6.3: SSEP on median nerve stimulation showing the different waveforms

- **EP (N9)**–Propagated volley passing under Erb's point
- **N13**–Post synaptic activity in cervical cord
- **P14**–Activity in caudal medial leminiscus
- **N18**–Post synaptic activity in brainstem, perhaps thalamus
- **N20**–Activation of primary cortical somatosensory area

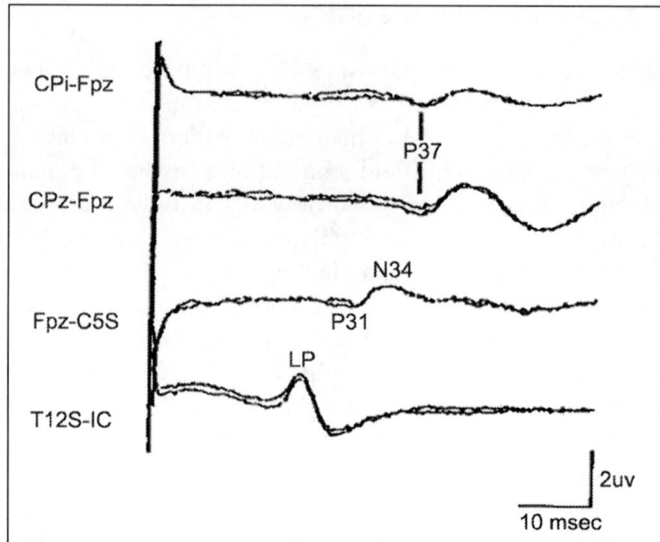

Fig. 6.4: SSEP on tibial nerve stimulation showing the different waveforms

- Popliteal (N7)
- LP (N17)–Post synaptic activity in the lumbar cord
- N34–Analogous to N18 of median nerve, post synaptic activity from multiple generator sources in brainstem, perhaps thalamus
- P37–Activation of primary cortical somatosensory area

Recording SSEP

Surface or needle electrodes can be used for recording SSEPs. Recording montage can be either cephalic bipolar in which both electrodes are placed on the head or referential in which the reference electrode is placed at a non-cephalic site. A cephalic bipolar montage has the advantage of being relatively free from noise and is preferred for routine clinical use. However small amplitude far field potentials, which reflect activity within subcortical structures, are largely cancelled. The non-cephalic reference electrode can be placed on the opposite mastoid, shoulder, arm, hand or knee.

Measurement of SEP

Several characteristics of the SSEP which can be measured are: onset latency, interpeak latency, amplitude, morphology (presence or absence of components), and dispersion of the SSEP, and side to side comparisons. The onset latency is the easiest SSEP feature to measure and standardize, it however gives limited information. It also varies with the limb length. The interpeak latency on the other hand is not affected by limb length, is a reliable parameter and usually independent of peripheral nerve disease.

Adult values of conduction are reached by 7-8 years of age, and aging is associated with prolongation of latencies.[18,19,20] Latency or interpeak conduction times are considered abnormal when they are more than 3 SD above the normal mean. The absolute amplitude of SSEP components is quite variable, but a side to side difference exceeding 50% is regarded as abnormal. A difference of this extent may be indicative of either central conduction block or considerable neuronal loss. SSEP amplitude increases with age and giant potentials are seen in patients with hereditary myoclonic epilepsy.

Neural Generators of SSEP

The different SSEP components are designated by their polarity and latency. Polarity at the active electrode is indicated as either positive (P) or negative (N). The origin of the specific early latency SSEP components elicited by median (Fig. 6.3) and tibial nerve (Fig. 6.4) stimulation are summarized in the following Table:

ORIGIN OF SOMATOSENSORY POTENTIAL COMPONENTS

Component	Generator
Median Nerve	
N9	Brachial plexus
N11	Cervical dorsal root entry pre synaptic
N13	Cervical, post synaptic
N18	Ipsilateral brainstem, thalamus
N20	Contalateral somatosensory area
Tibial Nerve	
LP	Lumbar cord, post synaptic
N34	Ipsilateral brainstem, thalamus
P37	Primary somatosensory cortex

Clinical Utility of SSEP

1. Diagnosis
2. Prognosis

1. **Diagnosis**
   a. Disorders of peripheral nerves
   b. Plexus lesions
   c. Radiculopathy
   d. Myelopathy
   e. Multiple sclerosis
   f. Thoracic outlet syndrome
2. **Prognostic Guide**
   a. Coma
   b. Brain death
   c. Spinal injurie

Disorders of Peripheral Nerve

SSEP have a definite role in evaluation of peripheral nerve lesions when conventional techniques cannot be used as in:

- Proximal site of pathology.
- Monitor patients of complete section of nerve.
- Entrapment neuropathies as Carpal tunnel syndrome, lateral femoral cutaneous nerve, saphenous and antebrachial cutaneous nerve.

Plexus Lesions

SSEP studies help to differentiate a preganglionic from a postganglionic lesion, the importance of which lies in the poor prognosis of a preganglionic (root avulsion) lesion. The SNAPs are preserved in preganglionic lesions despite clinical sensory loss. However, recording SSEP over the scalp and spine following stimulation of median nerve shows an attenuation of N13 [cervical potential], which relates to total proportion of damaged fibers, while that of N9 [plexus potential] reflects proportion of fibers damaged postganglionically and hence enhances accuracy of electrophysiological assessment. Intraoperative SEP recording can be used when ruptured nerves are to be grafted. The presence of a cortical response to stimulation of the proximal stump makes a second more rostral lesion unlikely; whereas lack of a response is usually associated with a poor outcome.

SSEPs obtained after dermatomal stimulation is of help in localization of root lesions. Medial side of 1st metatarsophalangeal joint on dorsal aspect can be stimulated for L5 root and lateral side of 5th metatarsophalangeal joint for S1 root. In "MRI negative" nerve root lesions isolated cervical and lumbar radiculopathies may be detected by a modified recording technique of the dermatomal SSEPs.

Multiple Sclerosis

With the advent of magnetic resonance imaging (MRI) the clinical diagnosis and monitoring of multiple sclerosis patients no longer requires EP studies for the detection of silent lesions. Nonetheless, they may be requested in patients with equivocal diagnostic evaluation such as a "negative" MRI (either abnormalities are too few or do not satisfy specific radiological criteria). With demyelination within the central fibers of the dorsal column–medial lemniscal pathways, there occurs delay or even an absence of the SSEPs. Such findings are said to be present in about 80% of patients with multiple sclerosis who do not have sensory symptoms or signs.[21] There is an increase in the diagnostic yield in those patients with sensory involvement, particularly from the SSEPs following stimulation of the lower limbs, which is probably due to the longer length of white matter that is being assessed. When the responses from the lower limbs are normal, the upper limb responses will only show additional abnormalities in less than 10% of the patients studied. It is, however, worth stimulating all four limbs, as the abnormalities may only affect one side in a third of the patients studied.

Unfortunately, abnormalities are not always pathognomic of demyelination and as with all laboratory investigations, these must be analyzed in the context of the clinical findings and other test results. SSEPs are also abnormal in a variety of other conditions and therefore sometimes used in their diagnosis, these include neurogenic thoracic outlet syndrome, myeloradiculopathies, Friedreich's ataxia, hereditary spastic paraplegia, and leucodystrophies, together with infarctions and tumors of the spinal cord, brainstem and thalamus.[22]

Myoclonus

SSEPs have been widely used for supporting the diagnosis and therapeutic management of cortical myoclonus. The later components of the cortical potential may be enlarged by more than 10 times reflecting cortical hyperexcitability. These "giant" potentials can be seen in a group of disorders known as the progressive myoclonic epilepsies, as well as juvenile myoclonic epilepsy, post-anoxic myoclonus (Lance-Adams syndrome), Alzheimer's disease, advanced Creutzfeldt-Jacob disease, metabolic encephalopathies, olivopontocerebellar atrophy (OPCA) and Rett's syndrome.[23]

Coma

Loss of cortical N20-P22 responses in a comatosed patient implies a poor prognosis. The absence of these responses bilaterally, suggest a fatal outcome. While responses that are consistently asymmetric in amplitude and latency or absent over one hemisphere are suggestive of the probable development of a severe residual deficit such as hemiplegia.

Brain Death

SSEP help to evaluate brain death. N13-N14 components are recorded over neck while there is lack of later components, reflecting absence of cerebral activity more rostrally.

Spinal Injury

Numerous studies have documented changes in SEP with spinal injury.[24,25,26] It was initially hoped that presence or absence of responses over that scalp to stimulation of nerve below the level of lesion would provide a reliable guide to completeness of a cord lesion, however that response is commonly not elicitable in the acute stage even in an incomplete lesion. Although preserved responses or their early return implies a good prognosis.

Intraoperative or post-operative improvement in SEPs following surgical decompression in patients with cord injury may be followed by clinical improvement, moreover the normalization of a previously abnormal or absent response may precede clinical change implying a better prognosis.

SSEPs have been used intraoperatively to monitor cord function, but overall utility of this approach has been controversial. It has been used to monitor corrective surgery for scoliosis, however, post-operative clinical deficits may occur despite preservation of SSEPs during intraoperative monitoring. Such false negative results may occur because of:

1. Operative procedure leading to a lesion not involving somatosensory pathway.
2. Pre-existing abnormalities may preclude further monitoring.
3. Peri-operative complications might develop after discontinuation of the monitoring procedure.

4. Interpretation may be confounded by factors like hypotension or general anesthesia.

BRAINSTEM AUDITORY EVOKED POTENTIALS

Brainstem auditory evoked potentials (BAEPs) are a set of seven waves recorded from the scalp during the first 12 msecs following a click stimulus. They represent far field potentials originating in the brainstem and are labeled I to VII. BAEPs are used to study the functional integrity of the central auditory pathways.

Stimulation

Brief acoustics click stimuli, delivering monophasic square pulses of 100 msec duration to head phones at a rate of about 10 Hz with a stimulus intensely of 60-65 dB is commonly used. To prevent a response developing from the contralateral year stimulation via bone conduction, the contralateral ear is masked with continuous white noise at an intensity of 30-40 dB below that of BAEP stimulus.

Recording

Recording electrodes are typically placed at vertex (Cz of International 10-20 system) and at both ears, (Ai [ipsilateral] and Ac [contralateral] ear to site of stimulation) or mastoids (Mi and Mc).

BAEPs should be recorded between Cz and Ai or Mi. A minimum of a two recording channel system with Cz-Ac or Cz-Mc in second channel has been recommended[27] the contralateral side recording helps in identification of waves III and V. The neural generators of these waves (Fig. 6.5) are as follows:

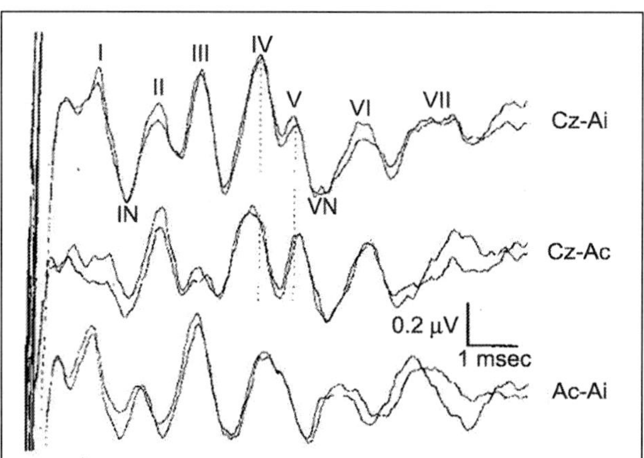

Fig. 6.5: BAER showing waveforms from I-VII

- Wave I–Auditory nerve
- Wave II–Cochlear nucleus
- Wave III–Superior olivary nucleus
- Wave IV–Lateral lemniscus
- Wave V–Inferior colliculus
- Wave VI–Medial geniculate body
- Wave VII–Auditory radiations

Wave I is the first major upgoing peak of Cz-Ai, and is markedly attenuated in Cz-Ac. This is contributed by cochlea. A bifid wave I is occasionally present and represents contributions from different portions of the cochlea. The earlier of the two peaks, which reflects activation of the base of the cochlea, corresponds to the single wave I that is typically present in the Cz-Ai waveform. Reversal of stimulus polarity can be used to distinguish a bifid wave I from a cochlear microphonic followed by a single wave I.

Wave II is usually of similar amplitude in the Cz-Ai. However, wave II may be small and difficult to identify in some normal subjects.

Wave III is usually present in both the Cz-Ai and Cz-Ac channels. However, it is substantially smaller in Cz-Ac channel than that in the Cz-Ai. A bifid wave III is occasionally observed as a normal variant; the wave III latency in such waveforms can be scored as midway between the peak latencies of the two subcomponents.

Waves IV and V are often fused into a IV/V complex, whose morphology varies from one subject to another, and may differ between the two ears in the same subject. The IV/V complex is often the most prominent component in the BAEP waveform. It is usually followed by a large negative deflection that lasts several milliseconds and brings the waveform to a point below the pre stimulus baseline.

When wave IV and V overlap in the Cz-Ai waveform, the wave V latency measurement used for BAEP interpretation should be taken from the second subcomponent of the IV/V complex even if this is not the highest peak in contrast to the amplitude measurement used to calculate the IV/V: I amplitude ratio, which is taken from the highest point in the complex. Measurement of the peak latency of wave V may be inaccurate if V appears only as an inflection on the falling edge of wave IV and impossible if they are smoothly fused. However, measurement of wave V latency in a CZ-Ac recording channel helps in differentiating wave IV and V as the overlapping peaks are more clearly separated there because the latency of wave IV is typically early and that of wave V is later than in the Cz-Ai. It is important to distinguish wave V from wave IV. If wave V were abnormally delayed but an earlier and larger wave IV that dominated the IV/V complex was mistaken for wave V, the BAEP abnormality might be missed. If the latency of an apparent wave V is abnormally short, efforts should be made to determine whether this peak is in fact a dominant wave IV.

Stimulation at Several Intensities

In a patient with conductive hearing loss, the stimulus intensity reaching the cochlea is less than that delivered to the external ear, and an abnormal BAEP with a delayed or absent wave I may result. If the stimulus intensity is increased to compensate for the conductive hearing loss and no co-existing sensorineural hearing loss is present, a normal BAEP will be recorded. In contrast, BAEPs that are delayed as a result of abnormally slowed neural conduction do not normalize when the stimulus intensity is increased. Thus increasing the stimulus intensity can help to differentiate peripheral from neural abnormalities, especially when wave I is not clear.

CLINICAL INTERPRETATION OF BAEPS

Waves II, IV, VI and VII are sometime not identifiable in normal individuals[28,29] and their peak latencies display more inter individual variability than do the peak latencies of waves I, III and V. Amplitude measurements of the individual components are also highly variable across subjects,[30] but the ratio between the amplitude of the IV/V complex and that of wave I has proved to be a clinically useful measure. Clinical interpretation of a patient's BAEPs is based primarily on the presence or absence of waves I, III and V and on the measurements of wave I latency, the I-V interpeak interval, the I-III and III-V interpeak intervals, the right-left differences in these values, and the IV/V:I amplitude ratios. Measurement of right-left differences, increases test sensitivity because the inter subject variability of these measures is less than that of the absolute component latencies and interpeak intervals from which they were derived.

SIGNIFICANCE OF SPECIFIC BAEP ABNORMALITIES

Abnormalities of Wave I

Because wave I originates in the distal portion of the auditory nerve, abnormalities (delay or absence) of wave I usually reflect peripheral auditory dysfunction, either conductive or cochlear, or pathology involving the most distal portion of the eighth nerve. An audiogram is useful to identify and quantitate the degree of hearing loss; a BAEP waveform with a poorly formed or absent wave I but a well-formed wave V, may reflect high-frequency hearing loss.

Cochlear dysfunction may reflect intracranial pathology because the cochlea receives its blood supply from the intracranial circulation via the internal auditory artery.[31-34] This vessel, which is usually a branch of the anterior inferior cerebellar artery, passes through the internal auditory canal alongside the eighth nerve. Cochlear ischemia or infarction may result from compression of the internal auditory artery within the canal or from occlusion of its parent vessel. Thus, wave I may be delayed or absent in patients with basilar artery thrombosis or other posterior circulation vascular disease, acoustic nerve tumors, or brain death due to interference with the blood supply of the cochlea.

With mild cochlear ischemia, BAEPs may be normal to standard high-intensity stimuli but become abnormally delayed or absent as the stimulus intensity is lowered.

Abnormalities of the I-III Interpeak Interval

Prolongation of the I-III interpeak interval, either absolute (in comparison to normal limits) or relative (excessive right-left difference), in the presence of a prolonged I-V interpeak interval, reflects an abnormality within the neural auditory pathways between the distal eighth nerve on the stimulated side and the lower pons. Absence of waves III and V carries the same significance. However, the rare absence of wave III in the presence of a clear wave V with a normal I-V interpeak interval should not be interpreted as an abnormality. Abnormality of the I-III interpeak interval is the characteristic BAEP finding in eighth nerve lesions such as acoustic neuromas, although there may also be a simultaneous peripheral abnormality, if the internal auditory artery has been compromised. Abnormal I-III interpeak intervals can also result from other processes such as demyelinating disease, brainstem tumors, or vascular lesions of the brainstem. In a patient with unilateral auditory nerve pathology, prolongation of the I-III interpeak interval will be found on stimulation of the ear on the side of the lesion. In patients with unilateral brainstem lesions and unilateral I-III abnormalities (abnormal BAEPs to stimulation of one ear and normal BAEPs to stimulation of the other), the ear in which stimulation produces the abnormal BAEP waveform is most often ipsilateral to the lesion, but there are rare exceptions.

Abnormalities of the III-V Interpeak Interval

Prolongation of both the I-V and III-V interpeak intervals, or complete absence of the IV/V complex in the presence of a wave III, reflects an abnormality within the neural auditory pathways between the lower pons and the mesencephalon. Prolongation of the III-V interpeak interval is best not interpreted as an abnormality if the I-V interpeak interval is normal.

Abnormalities in the III-V interpeak interval are seen in a variety of disease processes involving the brainstem, including demyelination, tumor and vascular diseases. If the disease process also involves the lower pons or eighth nerve, both the I-III and the III-V interpeak intervals may be prolonged.

RELATIONSHIP BETWEEN BAEPS AND HEARING: CATEGORIZATION OF ABNORMALITIES

BAEP abnormalities can be divided into a central pattern, in which the III-V interpeak interval is prolonged, and a peripheral pattern, in which wave I is delayed. A single tracing of waveforms may contain both of these abnormalities.

Although much of the I-III interpeak interval represents the conduction time of the afferent volleys along the auditory nerve, abnormalities of the I-III interpeak interval are common in patients with multiple sclerosis (MS). This observation is not surprising in light of the histological structure of the auditory nerve. Most of the cranial nerves, with the exception of I and II (which are actually central nervous system tracts) are histologically peripheral nerves, their myelin is produced by Schwann cells, except for a short segment at the nerve root. In contrast, eighth nerve fibers are unsheathed along most of their length by central type myelin produced by oligodendrogliocytes; the transition to peripheral type myelin produced by Schwann cells occurs near the distal end of the nerve. Therefore, in MS the eighth nerve is vulnerable to demyelination along most of its length. While it might at first glance seem inappropriate to include the conduction time along the eighth cranial nerve in the "central" conduction time (I-V interpeak interval), it is actually reasonable to do so because most of that conduction is through fibers with central type myelin.

PERIPHERAL HEARING LOSS

The BAEP waveform to a click predominantly reflects activity originating in the base of the cochlea. It is mediated by neurons with characteristic frequencies in the 2,000 to 4,000 Hz range. Thus, significant high-frequency hearing losses in this frequency band typically produce BAEP abnormalities, whereas BAEPs are relatively insensitive to isolated low-frequency hearing losses.

In patients with peripheral auditory dysfunction, high stimulus intensities can partially or completely correct BAEP abnormalities that become obvious at lower stimulus intensities. Thus, BAEP studies used to screen for hearing loss should be performed with multiple stimulus intensities, and latency-intensity curves should be constructed. BAEP studies intended to diagnose conduction abnormalities within the neural auditory pathways can be performed with a single, relatively high (60 to 65 dB n HL), stimulus intensity.

CENTRAL AUDITORY PATHWAY ABNORMALITIES

Because BAEPs reflect activity in only a subset of the auditory pathways, dysfunction in another portion of the auditory system can affect hearing without altering the BAEPs. For example, patients with bilateral temporal lobe infarctions involving the auditory cortex may be deaf and yet have completely normal BAEPs.

Conversely, BAEPs may be abnormal in patients with brainstem disease who have normal hearing. Unilateral brainstem lesions only rarely cause hearing loss because the ascending projections from each ear are bilateral. In addition, lesions (whether unilateral or bilateral) that affect the short-latency, highly synchronized subsystem involved in sound localization may spare other portions of the brainstem auditory pathways that are sufficient to maintain normal perception.

The possibility of normal hearing in the presence of abnormal BAEPs, enhances their clinical utility and is an addendum to the clinical evaluation of patients with suspected neurologic disease.

In patients with auditory symptoms that are suspected of being functional, an abnormal BAEP study demonstrates the existence of pathology within the auditory system. However, a normal study does not prove that the symptoms are psychogenic.

BAEPS IN SPECIFIC NEUROLOGIC CONDITIONS

Acoustic Neuroma

Acoustic neuromas typically originate from the distal vestibular nerve at the vestibular ganglion, and the auditory portion of the nerve may be unaffected early in the course of the disease.

As acoustic neuroma enlarges, it begins to compress the auditory nerve. Such compression produces prolongation of the I-III interpeak interval and eventually complete absence of wave III and subsequent BAEP components.

Simultaneous with I-III interpeak interval abnormalities, wave I may become delayed as the degree of cochlear ischemia increases. Infarction of the cochlea may cause elimination of all BAEPs, a common finding with large tumors in patients who have major hearing loss or are completely deaf. As acoustic neuromas expand within the posterior fossa, they begin to compress the brainstem. Prolongation of the III-V interpeak interval in response to stimulation of the ear contralateral to the tumor is indicative of brainstem compression by a large tumor.

The pattern of BAEP abnormality on the side of the tumor can be used to predict the likelihood of hearing preservation during surgical resection of the tumor.

Other Posterior Fossa Tumors

BAEPs are almost always abnormal in brainstem gliomas and other intrinsic brainstem tumors. Exceptions are tumors that are located entirely within the medulla, neither directly involving the auditory pathways nor affecting them by compression or deformation. Abnormalities in the I-III or III-V interpeak interval, or a combination of both, can be present, depending on the location of the tumor and the extent to which it affects surrounding brainstem tissue. Serial recordings may show deterioration of the BAEPs due to tumor growth. When a brainstem tumor shrinks in response to treatment, the BAEPs may demonstrate an improvement corresponding with an improvement in conduction within the brainstem auditory pathways.

Cerebrovascular Disease

Abnormalities in the I-III or III-V interpeak interval, or a combination of both, can be seen in patients with brainstem strokes. Posterior circulation vascular disease can also interfere with the blood supply to the cochlea via the internal auditory artery. If a cochlear stroke accompanies the brainstem stroke, all BAEP components will be absent following stimulation of the ear.

BAEP abnormalities are found in most patients with vertebrobasilar transient ischemic attacks, if they are recorded acutely.[35] These findings tend to resolve over time,[35,36] and the yield of abnormalities was lower in studies in which the BAEPs were recorded more than a week after the last transient ischemic attack. Persistent BAEP changes may represent small infarcts that are clinically silent.

Demyelinating Disease

One of the major clinical applications of evoked potential testing is in patients suspected of having a demyelinating disease such as multiple sclerosis. Evoked potentials can detect conduction slowing and temporal dispersion due to subclinical demyelination and thus help demonstrate the involvement of areas besides those accounting for the patient's clinical signs. In a meta-analysis by Chiappa[30] covering 1,000 patients with MS (in various categories) reported in the literature, abnormal BAEPs were found in 46 percent. When subdivided by categories of disease the rate of abnormal BAEPs was 67 percent in patients with definite MS, 41 percent in probable MS, and 30 percent in possible MS. BAEPs can detect silent lesions in 40%. However, BAEPs are less sensitive and specific than SSEP in detection of silent lesions.

BAEPs may display various patterns of abnormality in MS, depending on the areas that are involved by the disease process. Abnormalities in the I-III or I-V interpeak interval, or a combination of both, may be seen. Another pattern seen in MS is an abnormally small IV/V:I amplitude ratio in the presence of normal component latencies and interpeak intervals.

Coma and Brain Death

Coma can be caused by bilateral cerebral hemispheric dysfunction, brainstem dysfunction, or metabolic abnormalities that cause diffuse brain dysfunction. The BAEP findings depend on the cause of the coma and for structural lesions, on the location of the pathology. BAEPs are typically normal in patients with coma due to supratentorial disease, although they may subsequently deteriorate due to transtentorial herniation. The finding of normal-appearing BAEPs in a patient with brainstem dysfunction should prompt suspicion of a metabolic etiology such as a drug overdose, as BAEPs are highly resistant to central nervous system depressant drugs.

In patients on barbiturate anesthesia, BAEPs can persist with only minor changes despite high doses of barbiturates in both human patients[28,37,38] and animals.[39,40] High doses of intravenous lidocaine can transiently abolish BAEPs.[41]

Wave I attenuation is seen with metabolic and toxic encephalopathies, e.g., uremia.

Absence of waves III to V in a patient with anoxic-ischemic cardiac arrest or traumatic brain injury is invariably associated with death or persistent vegetative state. While patients with I-V interpeak interval greater than 4.48 m. sec invariably die or remain in a vegetative state.

Typically, the BAEP recording in patients with brain death contains no identifiable components except wave I. The presence of wave III is not compatible with total cessation of brainstem functions.

PRACTICAL PEARLS

Criteria for BAEP Abnormalities

- Absence of all BAEP waves I through V.
- Absence of all waves following wave I, II or III.
- Interpeak interval prolongation; I-III, III-V, I-V.
- Abnormal diminution of V/I amplitude ratio.
- Interaural differences; I-III, III-V, I-V interpeak intervals.

Clinical Tips

- Absence of wave I with normal wave V probably reflects technical problems in recording [Use external auditory meatus electrode referred to vertex to reveal normal wave I].
- Absence of wave III is significant only when wave V is also missing or delayed.
- A delayed wave V, with normal latency of wave I signifies delay after wave I.
- Wave I, II, III may be preserved while waves IV and V either are absent or prolonged are suggestive of brainstem lesion.
- Presence of wave I, with absence of all other waves indicates total functional destruction of brainstem.
- Absence of all waves suggest a deficit involving cochlea or eighth nerve.
- I-V interpeak interval prolongation suggest brainstem pathology.
- III-V interpeak interval prolongation indicates a deficit at or after superior olivary complex in either the high pons or the low midbrain.

References

1. Halliday AM, McDonald, WI and Mushin J. Delayed Pattern Evoked Responses in Optic Neuritis in Relation to Visual Acuity. Lancet 1972;1:982-85.
2. Celesia GG. Steady State and Transient Visual Evoked Potentials in Clinical Practice. Ann N Y Acad. Sci 1982;388:290-305.
3. Celesia GG. Evoked Potential Techniques in the Evaluation of Visual Function. J Clin Neurophysiol 1984;1:55-76.
4. Minckler DS. The Organization of Nerve Fiber Bundles in the Primate Optic Nerve Head. Arch Ophthalmol 1980;98:1630-36.
5. Hoyt WF and Luis O. Visual Fiber Anatomy in the Infrageniculate Pathway of the Primate: Uncrossed and Crossed Retinal Quadrant Fibers Projections Studied with Nauta Silver Stain. Arch Ophthalmol 1962;68:94-106.
6. Oppel O. Mikroskopische Untersuchungen Uber Die Anzahl und Kaliber der Markhaltigen Nervenfasern im Fasciculus Opticus des Menschen. Graefes Arch Ophthalmo 1963;166:19-27.
7. Ogden TE and Miller RF. Studies of the Optic Nerve of the Rhesus Monkey: Nerve Fiber Spectrum and Physiological Properties. Vision Res 1966;6:485-506.
8. Phelps ME, Mazziotta JC, Kuhl DE, Nuwer M, Packwood J, Metter J, Engel J. Topographic Mapping of Human Cerebral Metabolism: Visual Stimulation and Deprivation. Neurology 1981;31:519.
9. Fox PT, Rachile ME. Stimulus Rate Determines Regional Brain Blood Flow in Striate Cortex. Ann Neurol 1985;17:303.
10. Coupland SG and Kirkham TH. The Orientation Specific Visual Evoked Potential Deficits in Multiple Sclerosis. J Neurol Sci 1982;9:331-37.
11. Celesia GG and Tobimatsu S. Electroretinograms to Flash and to Patterned Visual Stimuli in Retinal and Optic Nerve Disorders. In Visual Evoked Potentials, Ed. and JE Desmedt 1990:45-55, Amsterdam: Elsevier.
12. Neima D and Regan D. Pattern Visual Evoked Potentials and Spatial Vision in Retro Bulbar Neuritis and Multiple Sclerosis. Arch Neurol 1984;41:198-201.
13. Celesia GG, Meredith JT and Pluff K. Perimetry. Visual Evoked Potentials and Visual Spectrum Array in Homonymous Hemianopsia. Electroencephalogr Clin Neurophysiol 1983;56:16-30.
14. Abe Y and Kuroiwa Y. Amplitude Asymmetry of Hemi Field Patterns Reversal VEPs in Healthy Subjects. Electroencephalogr Clin Neurophysiol 1990:77:81-85.
15. American Electroencephalographic Society. Guidelines for Clinical Evoked Potential Study. J Clin Neurophysiol 1984;1:3-53.
16. Barrett G, Blumhardt LD, Halliday AM, Halliday E and Kriss A. A Paradox in the Lateralization of the Visual Evoked Response. Nature 1976;261:253-55.
17. Blumhardt LD, Barrett G, Kriss A and Halliday AM. The Pattern Evoked Potential in Lesions of the Posterior Visual Pathways. Ann N Y Acad Sci 1982:388:264-89.
18. Cracco JB, Cracco RQ, Stolove R. Spinal Evoked Potential in Man: A Maturational Study. Electroencephalogr Clin Neurophysiol 1979;46:58.
19. Desmedt JE, Cheron G. Non-Cephalic Reference Recording of Early Somatosensory Potentials to Finger Stimulation in Adult or Aging Normal Man: Differentiation or Wadespread

N18 and Contralateral N20 from the Prerolandic P22 and N30 Components. Electroencephalogr Clin Neurophysiol 1981: 52:553.

20. Kakigi R. The Effect of Aging on Somatosensory Evoked Potentials Following Stimulation of the Posterior Tibial Nerve in Man. Electroencephalogr Clin Neurophysiol 1987:68:277.
21. Walsh JC. Yiannikas C. McLeod JG. Abnormalities of Proximal Conduction in Acute Idiopathic Polyneuritis: Comparison of Short Latency Evoked Potentials and F-waves. J Neurol Neurosurg Psychiatry 1984:47:197.
22. Aminoff MJ. Eisen AA. Somatosensory Evoked Potentials. Muscle Nerve 1998:21:277-90.
23. Shibasaki H. Electrophysiological Studies of Myoclonus. Muscle Nerve 2000:23:321-35.
24. Sedgwick EM. El-Negamy E. Frankel H. Spinal-cord Potentials in Traumatic Paraplegia and Quadriplegia. J Neurol Neurosurg Psychiatry 1980:43:823.
25. Rowed DW. McLean JAG. Tator CH. Somatosensory Evoked Potentials in Acute Spinal Cord Injury: Prognostic Value. Surg Neurol 1978:9:203.
26. Dorfman LJ. Perkash I. Bosley TM. Cummins KL. Use of Cerebral Evoked Potentials to Evaluate Spinal Somatosensory Function Patients with Traumatic and Surgical Myelopathies. J Neurosurg 1980:52:654.
27. American Electroencephalographic Society: Guideline nine: Guidelines on Evoked Potentials. J Clin Neurophysiol 1994; 11:40.
28. Stockard JJ. Stockard JE. Sharbrough FW. Nonpathologic Factors Influencing Brainstem Auditory Evoked Potentials. Am J EEG Technol 1978:18:177.
29. Rowe MJ. Normal Variability of the Brainstem Auditory Evoked Response in Young and Old Adult Subjects. Electroencephalogr Clin Neurophysiol 1978:44:459.
30. Chiappa K. Gladstone KJ. Young RR. Brainstem Auditory Evoked Responses Studies of Waveform Variations in 50 Normal Human Subjects. Arch Neuro 1979:36:81.
31. Legatt AD. Pedley TA. Emerson RG *et al.* Normal Brainstem Auditory Evoked Potentials with Abnormal Latency-Intensity Studies in Patients with Acoustic Neuromas. Arch Neurol 1988:45:1326.
32. Eggermont JJ. Don M. Mechanisms of Central Conduction Time Prolongation in Brainstem Auditory Evoked Potentials. Arch Neurol 1986:43:116.
33. De Moura LFP. Inner Ear Pathology in Acoustic Neurinoma. Arch Otolaryngol 1967.85:125.
34. Ferbert A. Buchner H. Bruckmann H *et al.* Evoked Potentials in Basilar Artery Thrombosis: Correlation with Clinical and Angiographic Findings. Electroencephalogr Clin Neurophysiol 1988:69:136.
35. Factor SA. Dentinger MP. Early Brainstem Auditory Evoked Responses in Vetebrobasilar Transient Ischemic Attacks. Arch Neurol 1987:44:544.
36. Rossi L. Amantini A. Bindi A *et al.* Electrophysiological Investigations of the Brainstem in the Vertebrobasilar Reversible Attacks. Eur Neurol 1983:22:371.
37. Drummond JC. Todd MM. U HS. The Effect of High Dose Sodium Thiopental on Brainstem Auditory Median Nerve Somatosensory Evoked Responses in Man. Anesthesiology 1985:63:249.
38. Newlon PG. Greenberg RP. Enas GG. Becker DP. Effects of Therapeutic Pentobarbital Coma on Multimodality Evoked Potentials Recorded from Severely Head Injury Patients. Neurosurgery 1983:13:613.
39. Bobbin RP. May JG. Lemonie RL. Effects of Pentobarbital and Ketamine on Brainstem Auditory Potentials: Latency and Amplitude Intensity Functions after Intraperitoneal Administration. Arch Otolaryngol 1979:105:467.
40. Sutton LN. Frewen T. Marsh R *et al.* The Affects of Deep Barbiturate Coma on Multimodality Evoked Potentials. J Neurosurg 1982:57:178.
41. Garcia-Larrea L. Artu F. Bertrand O *et al.* Transient Drug-Induced Abolition of BAEPs in Coma. Neurology 1988; 38:1487.

7 Chapter

ELECTROPHYSIOLOGY: SELECTED ADDITIONS

Bibek Talukdar

NEONATAL EEG

EEG in the neonate has been an area of great interest and constant exploration. Clinical detection of seizure in a neonate is often problematic due to its diverse manifestation. Recording and interpreting seizures in the neonate is also beset with problems. Certain technical difficulties are also there in recording neonatal EEG because of small head size. The placement and derivations of electrodes is often changed. With improved machines and techniques, the usual electrode placement (10-20 system) as used in older children can be used well.

In the NICU setting amplitude integrated EEG (aEEG) has been found to be useful in detecting seizure activity; however, it is technically difficult regarding establishing it in the environment where there are lot of mechanical noise. Also there are limitations in the recording as is only partial. One has to rely heavily in standard EEG.

Neonatal EEG has certain special characteristics of its own, specially in the premature babies. Some characteristic activities are shown below. The striking features are the changes related to maturation of the nervous system. It is important to be well versed with these maturation related changes; these can be confounders as they may mimic structural pathology or seizure. These changes are extremely useful in diagnosis of gestational age.

EEG activities have been recorded as early as 22-23 weeks of gestation. Early EEGs are characterized by prolonged period of inactivity (flat recording) intervened by periods of sharp activity; these records have been termed 'trace discontinua'. After about 32-36 weeks of gestation, it is replaced by 'trace alternans', where the EEG shows more or less regular activity with intermittent bursts.

Some other selected age-related patterns that may be seen are: Temporal saw tooth (27-29 weeks), Rhythmic theta (27-29 weeks), Delta brush (30-32 weeks), Sharp transients (Rolandic and temporal) (38-42 weeks), Frontal sharp transients (38-42 weeks) and Anterior slow dysrhythmia (38-42 weeks).

Some other states of the baby while recording needs careful notation as these needs to be considered while reporting. Some of these are wakefulness (sleep and awake), movements like chewing, sucking, swallowing etc. Active sleep is associated with rapid eye movement (REM sleep), irregular respiration and irregular theta-delta mix low voltage background activity and quite sleep shows no rapid eye movement (NREM sleep), regular respiration and continuous slow wave background activity. Active sleep starts appearing by 32 weeks and quite sleep by 34 weeks. Movements like chewing, sucking, swallowing often produces spiky activities mimicking seizure.

EEG pattern shows evolution with maturation of the nervous system. EEG findings correlates best with conceptional age (CA) that is gestational age (GA) + chronological age after birth on the date of EEG, the gestational age being counted from the first day of last menstruation period till the date of birth. Thus while reading neonatal EEG, findings are correlated to the CA.

Neonatal EEG however is extremely useful in diagnosis of seizure in newborn as detecting seizure in the newborn clinically is often difficult, especially the subtle seizures. Interpreting seizure in newborn is also not always easy mainly because of certain maturation related (age related) activities that mimics seizure as already mentioned may be confounding. Seizure is usually diagnosed only when the discharges are frequent/excessive. Seizures in the newborn can be focal, multifocal and generalized. Some traces of neonatal seizures done in our laboratory in cases admitted in our neonatal unit with seizures, are shown in the figures below.

Neonatal EEG is also extremely useful in diagnosis of depressed cerebral function like birth anoxia and hypoxic ischemic encephalopathy HIE. Depressed cerebral function is usually shows low voltage EEG.

Neonatal EEG has another usefulness regarding future neurodevelopment of the child. Several studies and observations have shown abnormal neonatal EEG is associated with later neurodevelopmental deviations.

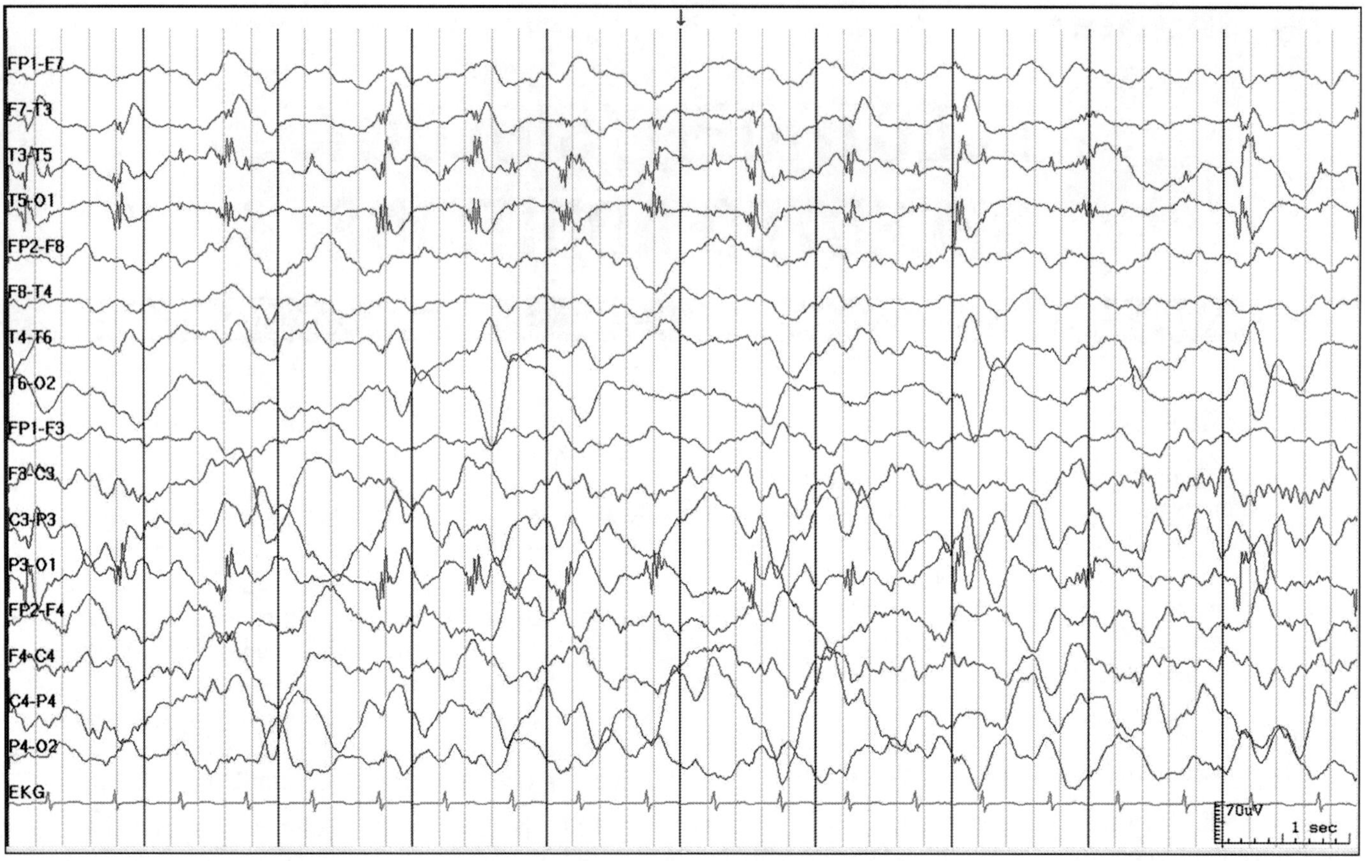

FP1-F7
F7-T3
T3-T5
T5-O1
FP2-F8
F8-T4
T4-T6
T6-O2
FP1-F3
F3-C3
C3-P3
P3-O1
FP2-F4
F4-C4
C4-P4
P4-O2
EKG
70uV
1 sec

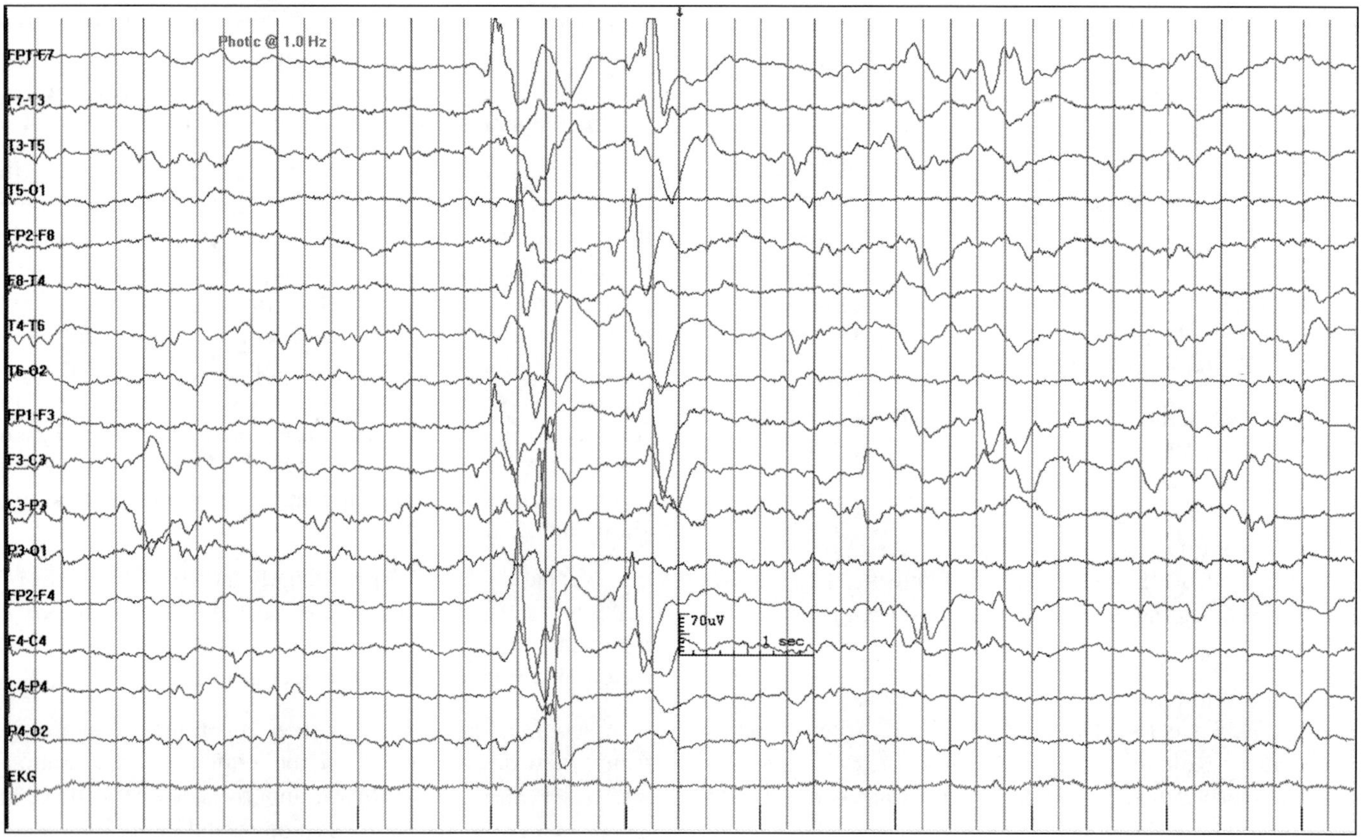

Photic @ 1.0 Hz
FP1-F7
F7-T3
T3-T5
T5-O1
FP2-F8
F8-T4
T4-T6
T6-O2
FP1-F3
F3-C3
C3-P3
P3-O1
FP2-F4
F4-C4
C4-P4
P4-O2
EKG
70uV
1 sec

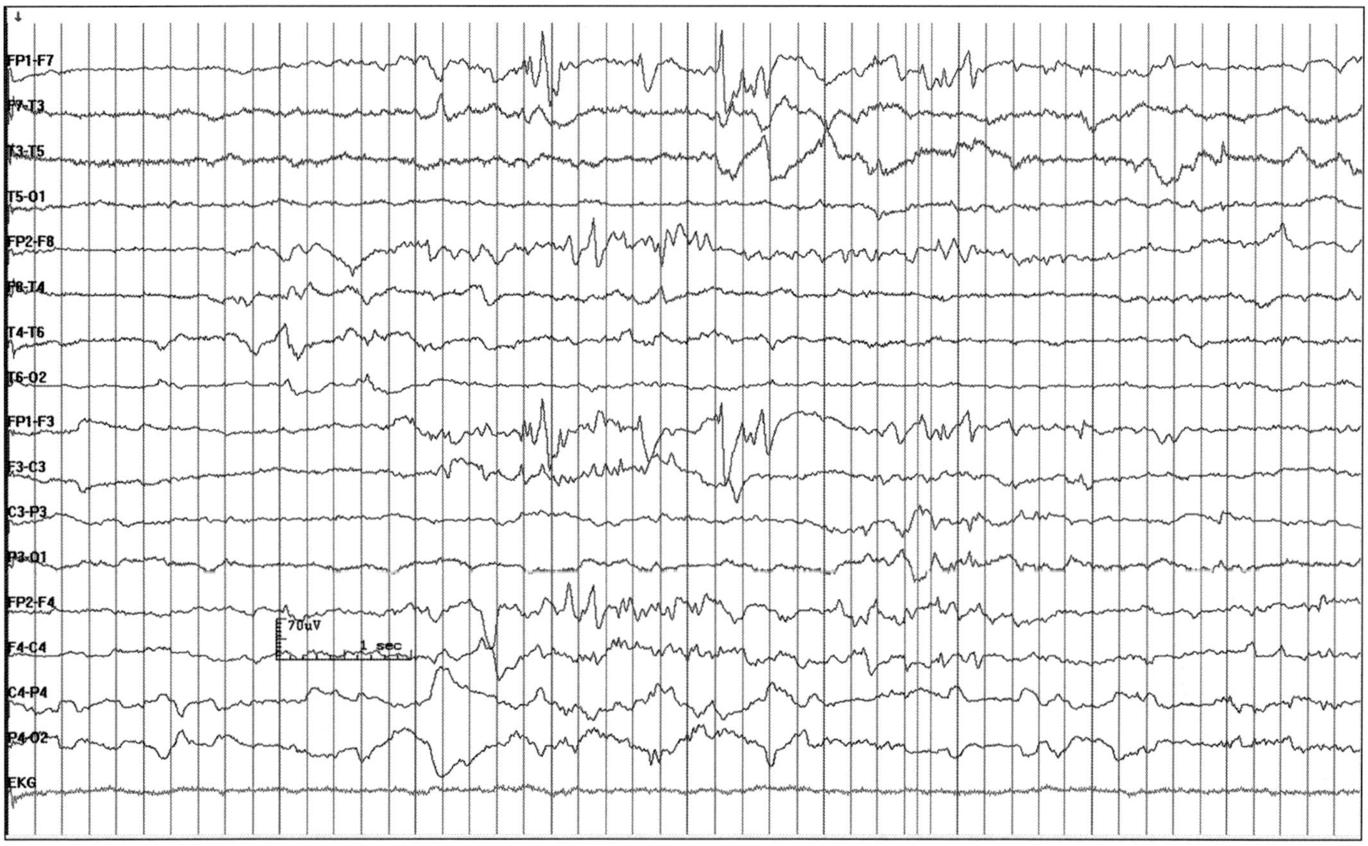

FP1-F7
F7-T3
T3-T5
T5-O1
FP2-F8
F8-T4
T4-T6
T6-O2
FP1-F3
F3-C3
C3-P3
P3-O1
FP2-F4
F4-C4
C4-P4
P4-O2
EKG

70uV
1 sec

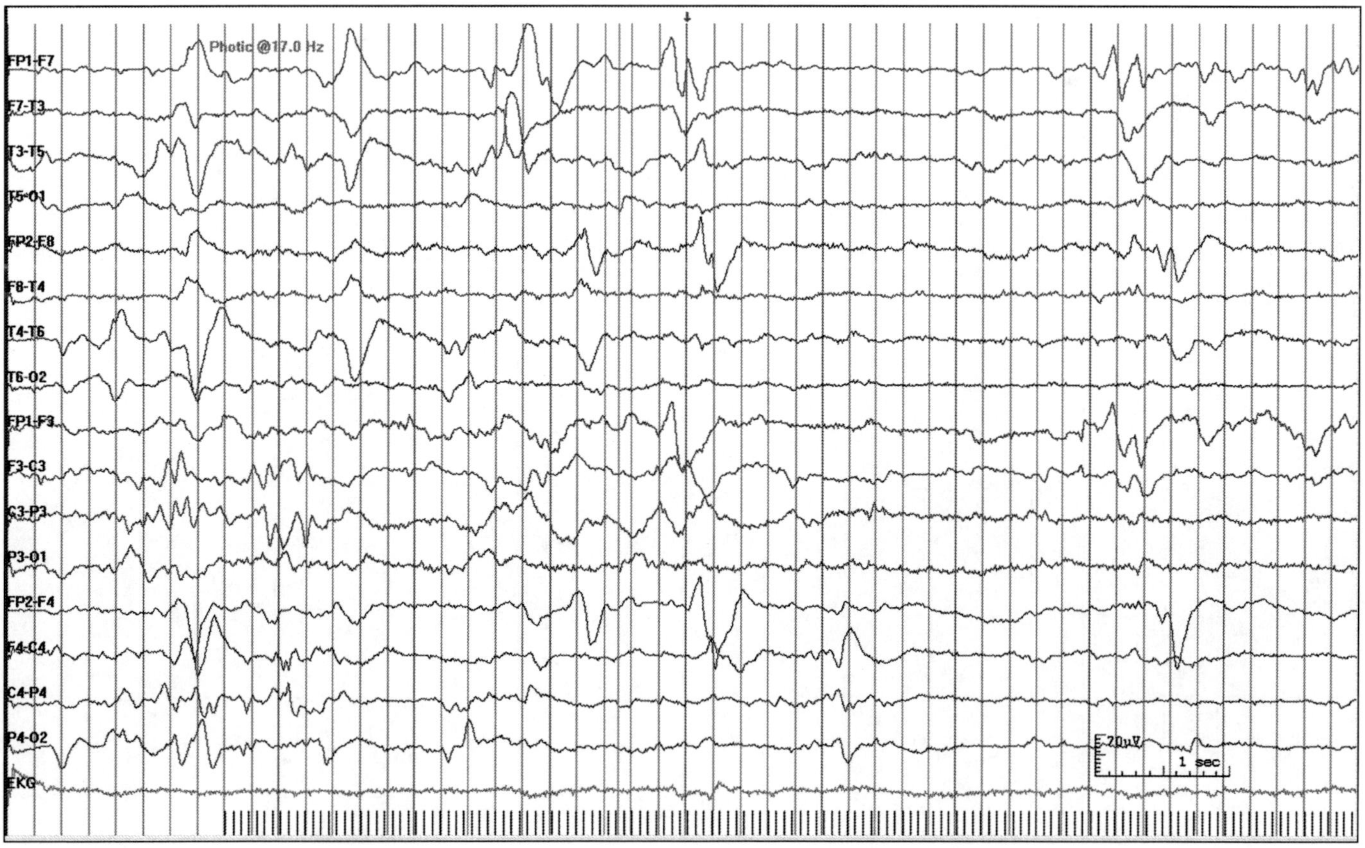

Photic @17.0 Hz

FP1-F7
F7-T3
T3-T5
T5-O1
FP2-F8
F8-T4
T4-T6
T6-O2
FP1-F3
F3-C3
C3-P3
P3-O1
FP2-F4
F4-C4
C4-P4
P4-O2
EKG

70uV
1 sec

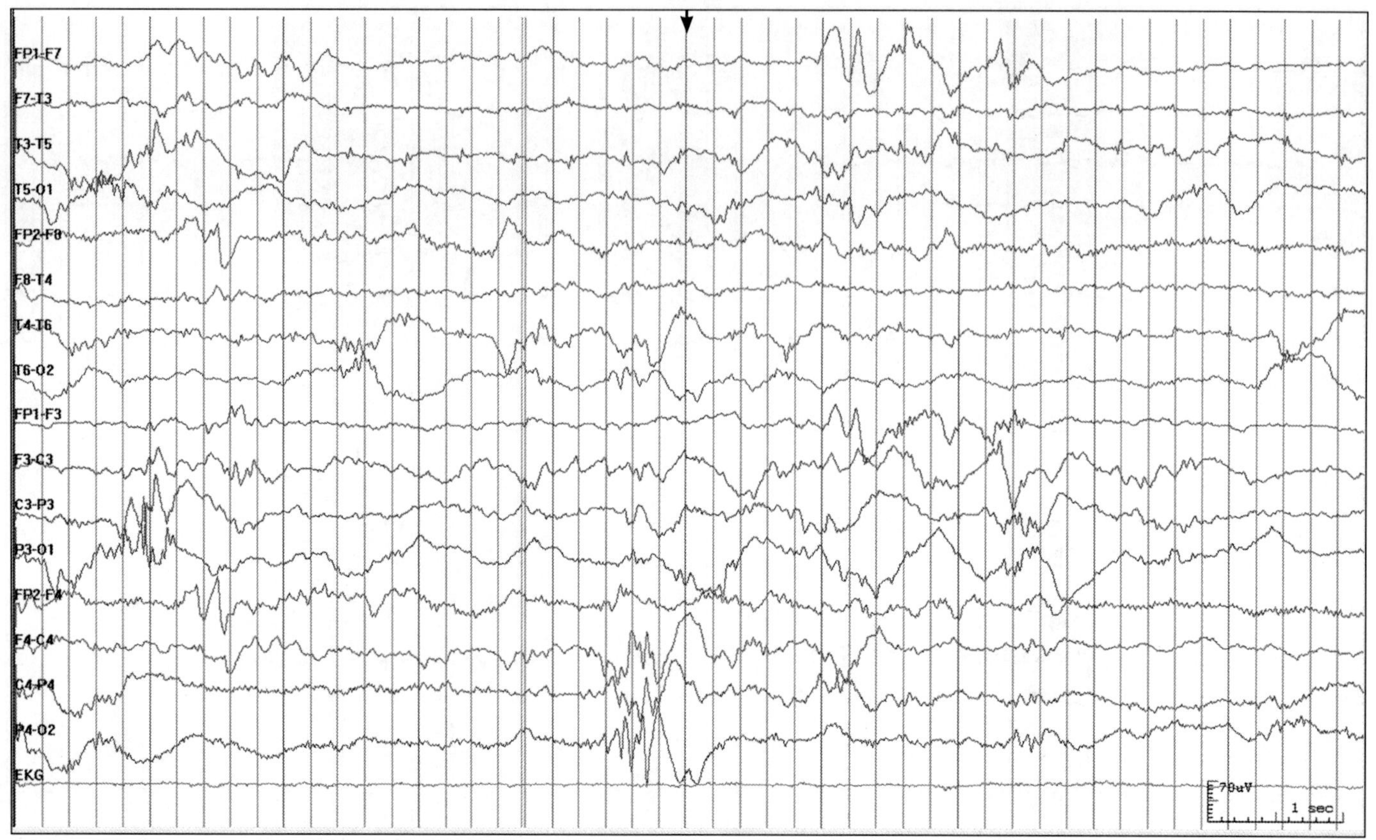

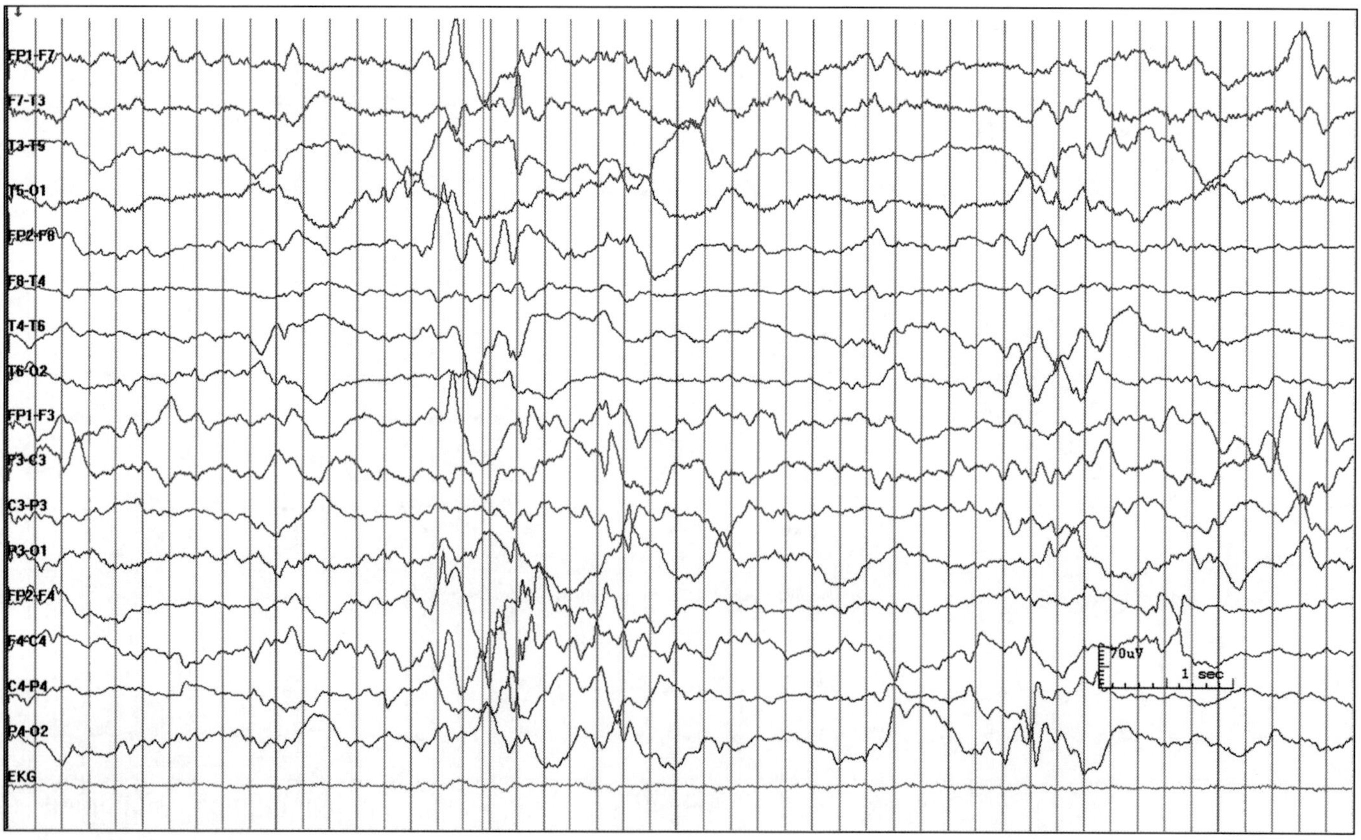

FP1-F7
F7-T3
T3-T5
T5-O1
FP2-F8
F8-T4
T4-T6
T6-O2
FP1-F3
F3-C3
C3-P3
P3-O1
FP2-F4
F4-C4
C4-P4
P4-O2
EKG
70uV
1 sec

FP1-F7
F7-T3
T3-T5
T5-O1
FP2-F8
F8-T4
T4-T6
T6-O2
FP1-F3
F3-C3
C3-P3
P3-O1
FP2-F4
F4-C4
C4-P4
P4-O2
EKG
70uV
1 sec

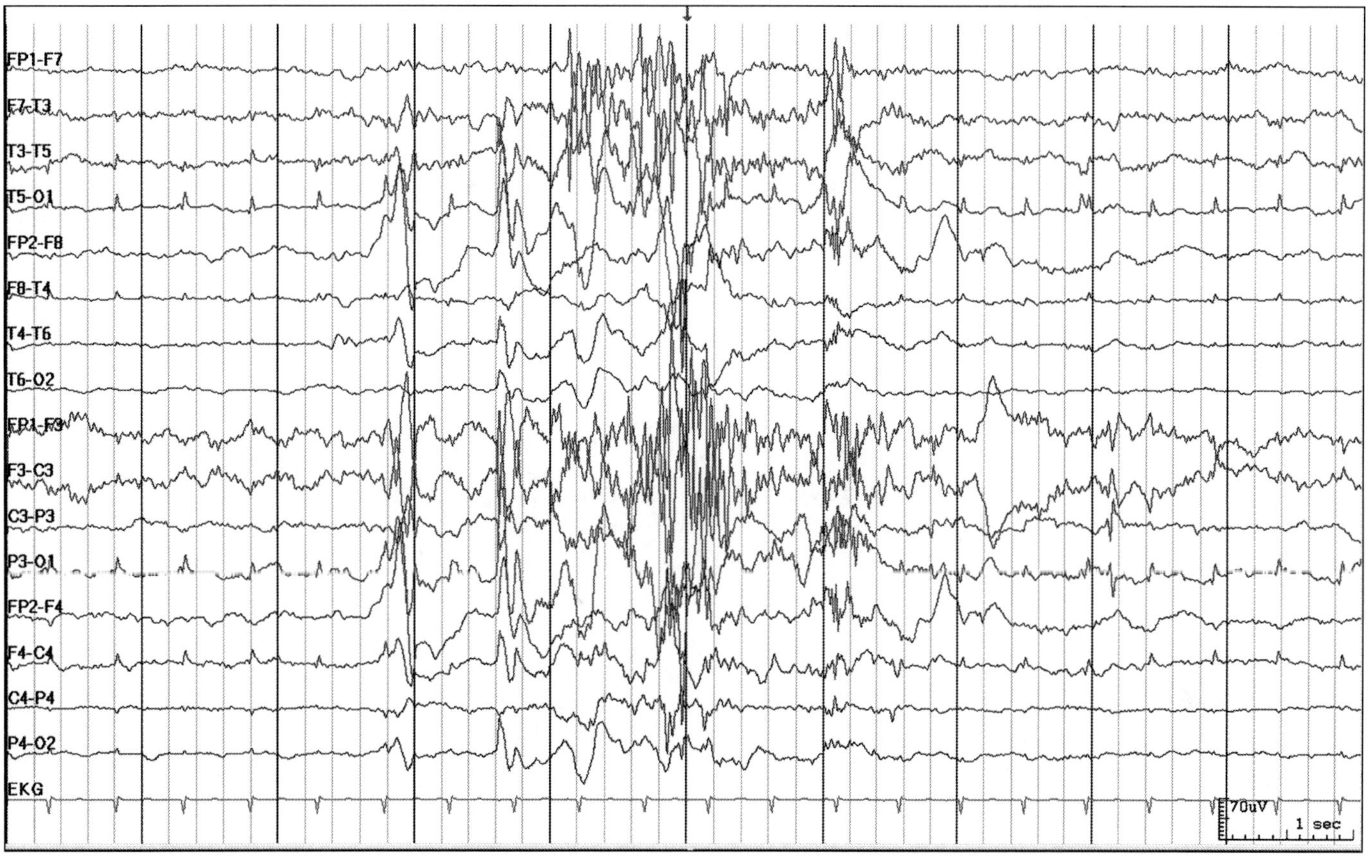

FP1-F7
F7-T3
T3-T5
T5-O1
FP2-F8
F8-T4
T4-T6
T6-O2
FP1-F3
F3-C3
C3-P3
P3-O1
FP2-F4
F4-C4
C4-P4
P4-O2
EKG
70uV
1 sec

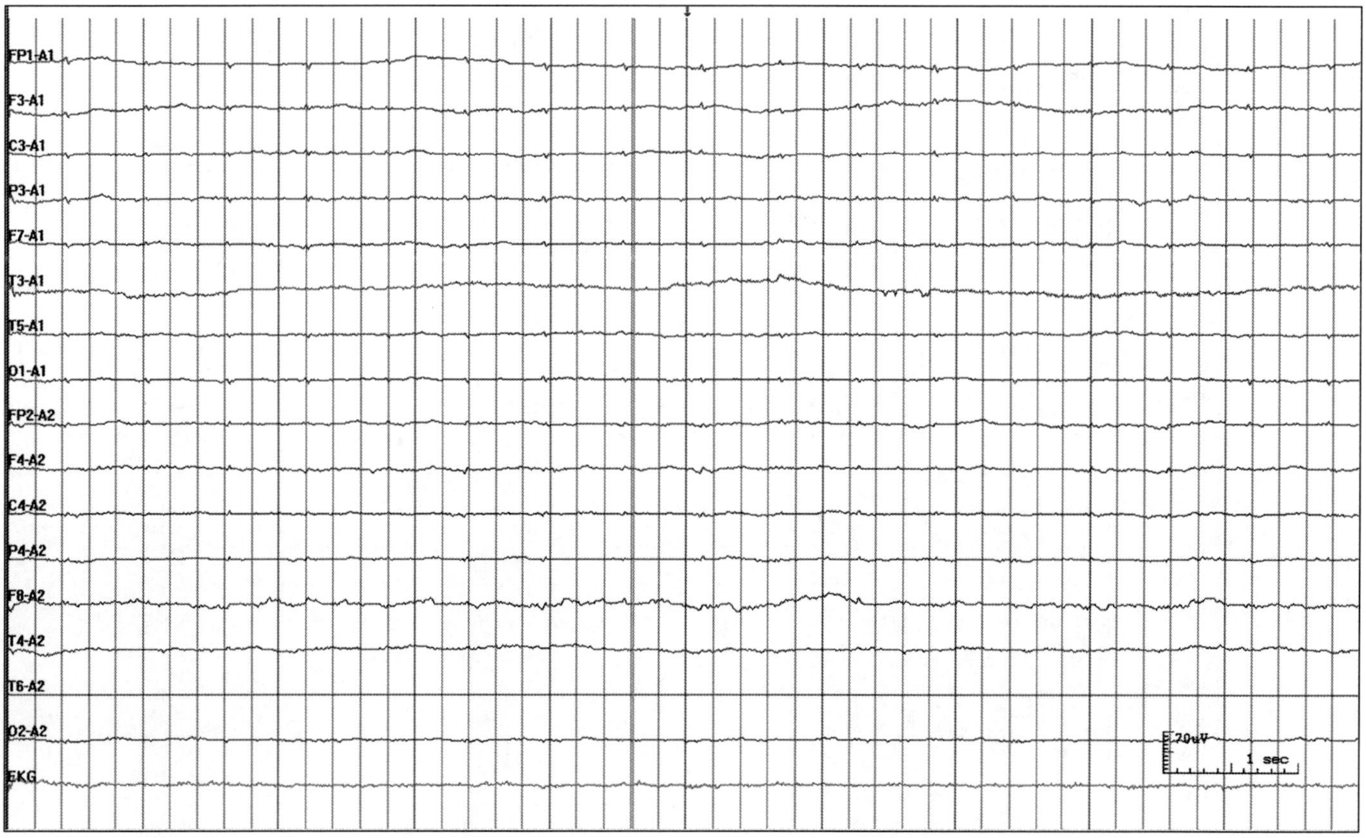

FP1-A1
F3-A1
C3-A1
P3-A1
F7-A1
T3-A1
T5-A1
O1-A1
FP2-A2
F4-A2
C4-A2
P4-A2
F8-A2
T4-A2
T6-A2
O2-A2
EKG
70uV
1 sec

EEG IN INFANTS AND OLDER CHILDREN

EEG is the most important tool for diagnosis of seizures in children. It is necessary for classifying seizures according to ILAE. It confirms the abnormal neuronal activity confirming the diagnosis of seizures, it shows the type of seizure and it is also essential for diagnosis of various epilepsy syndromes. EEG shows seizure activity in the form of spikes, spike and waves, sharp and slow waves and polyspikes/multispikes. Seizure activities can be focal, multifocal or generalized usually occurring in paroxysms simultaneously in both the cerebral hemispheres. Shown below are some of EEG tracings done in our laboratory of cases with seizures admitted / who attending our institution.

Focal Seizure

The seizure activities occur in one hemisphere and remain localized to the same area throughout the recording. Occasionally the focal activity becomes generalized involving the other hemisphere as well when it is classified as focal seizure evolving into generalized seizure. Some EEG traces of children who presented with focal seizure are shown below.

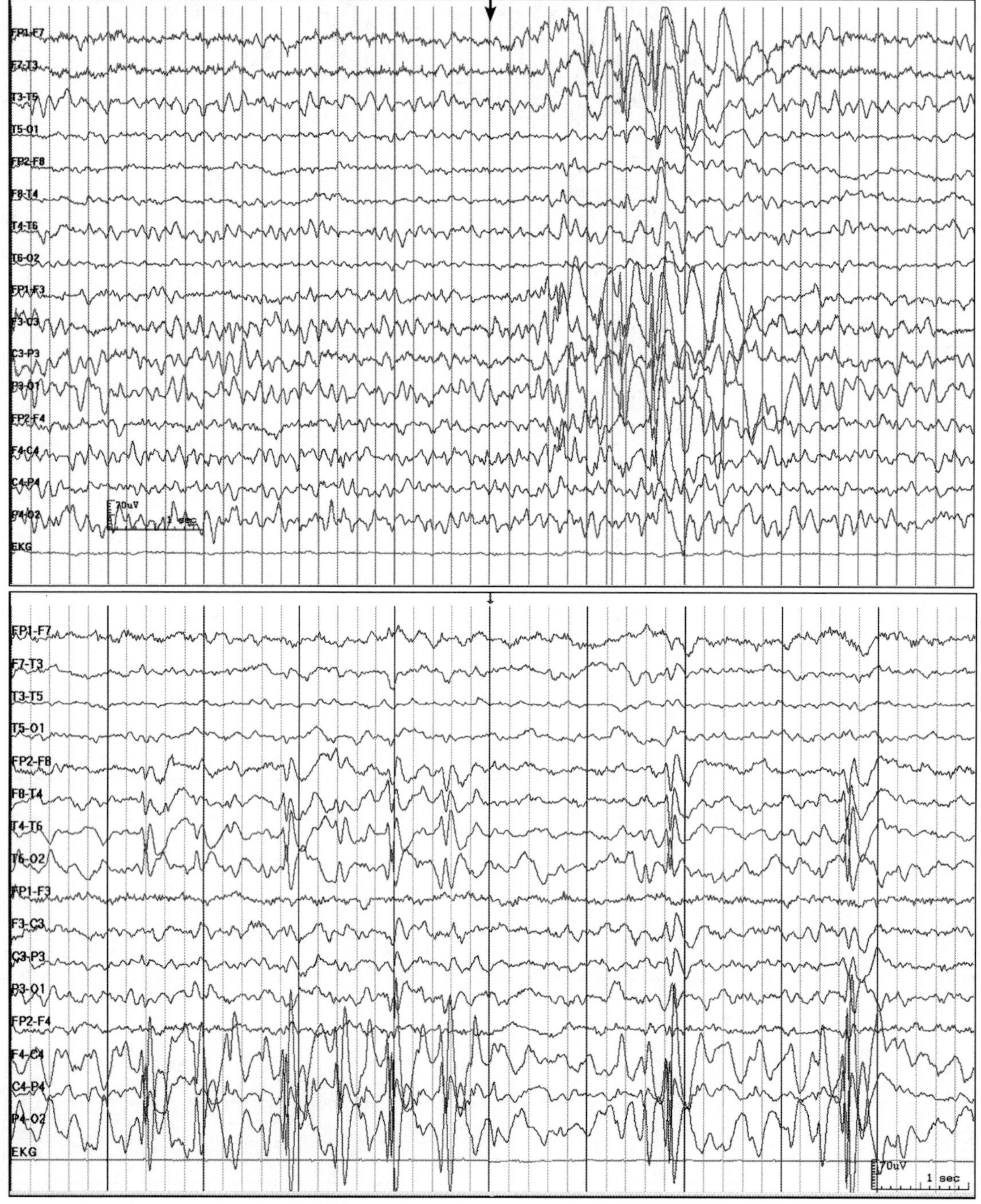

Generalized Tonic-Clonic Seizure

The seizure activities occur in both the cerebral hemispheres simultaneously. It may involve all the areas at a time or some particular areas in both the hemisphere. Frequently, however, the seizure activities occur in multifocal distribution in both the cerebral hemispheres. The discharges may be of varying amplitude and duration. Some traces of children done in our laboratory who had come to us with generalized seizure are shown below.

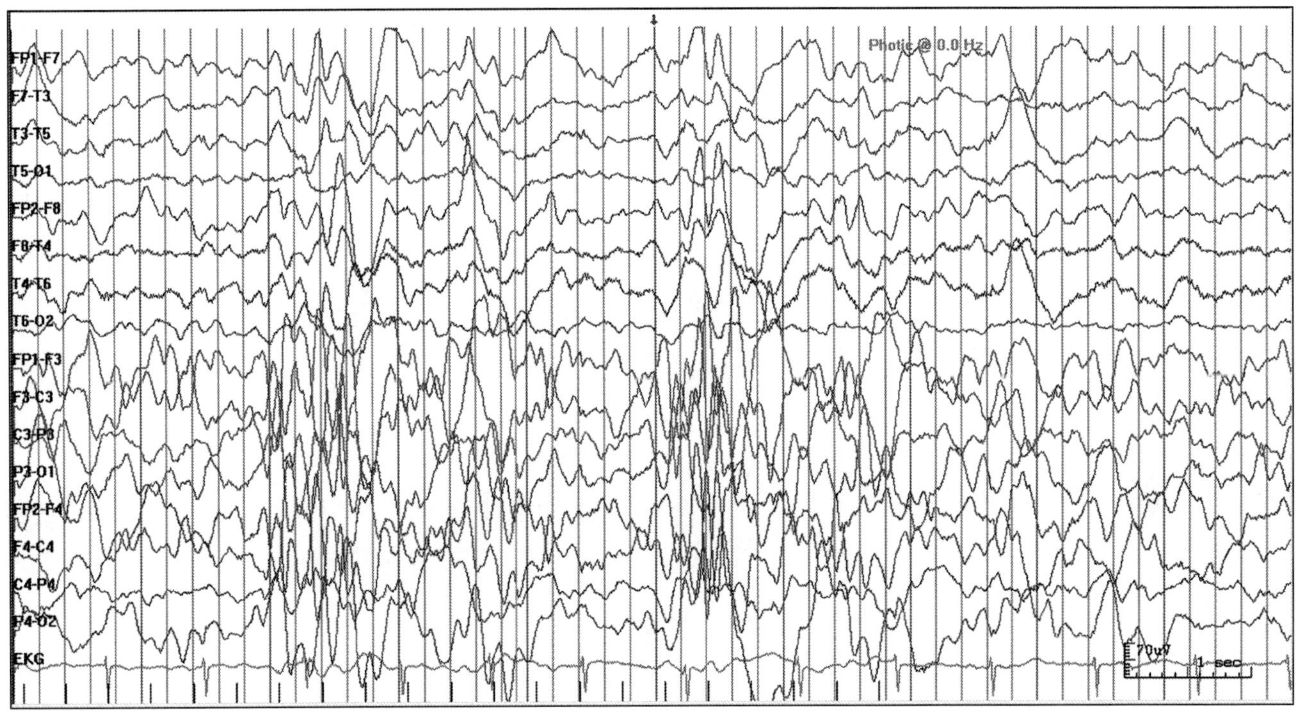

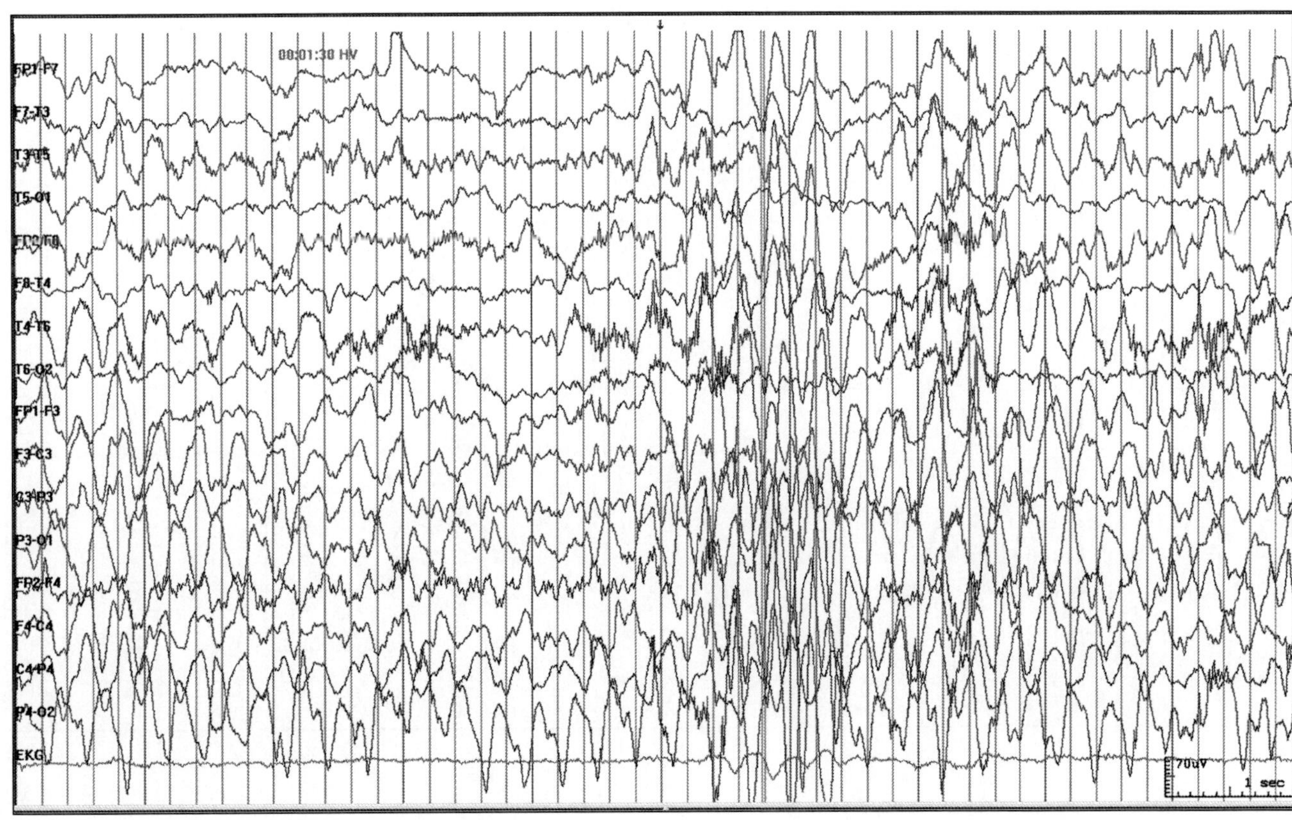

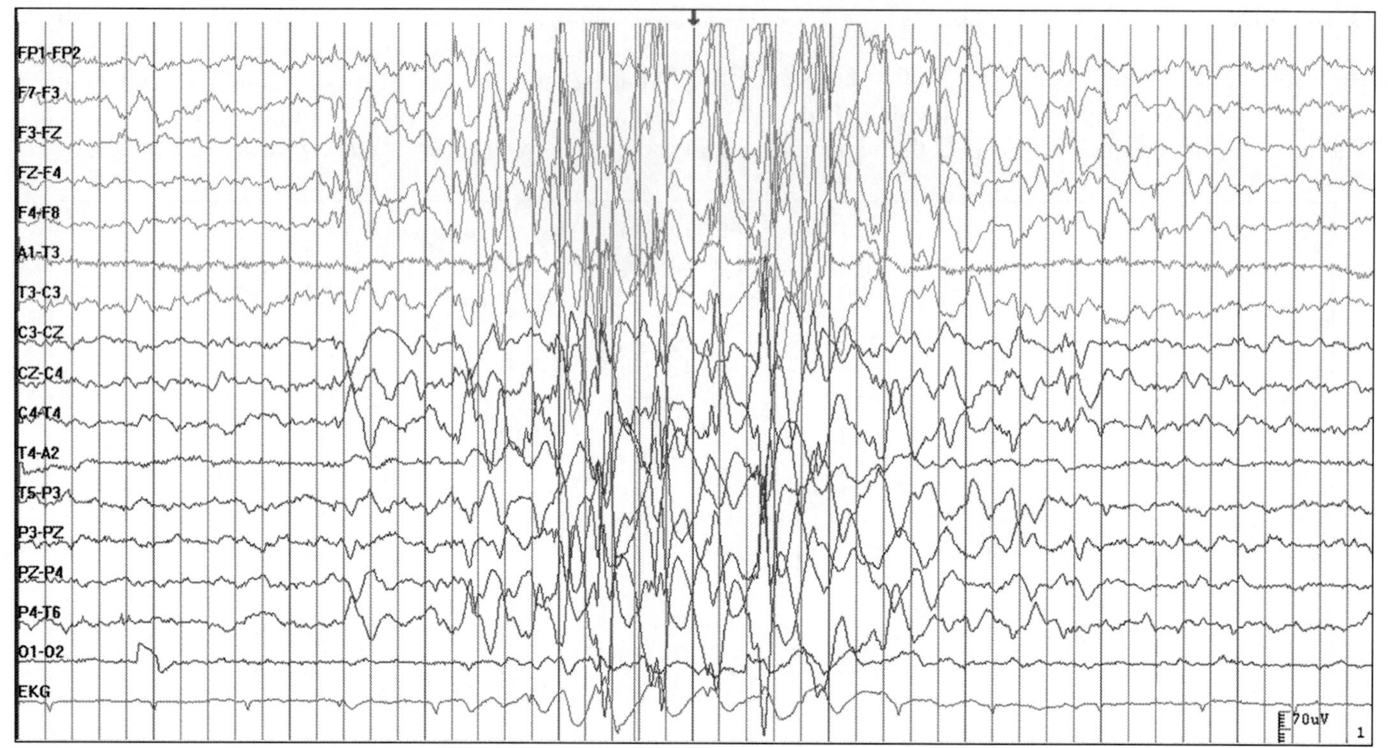
FP1-FP2
F7-F3
F3-FZ
FZ-F4
F4-F8
A1-T3
T3-C3
C3-CZ
CZ-C4
C4-T4
T4-A2
T5-P3
P3-PZ
PZ-P4
P4-T6
O1-O2
EKG
70uV
1

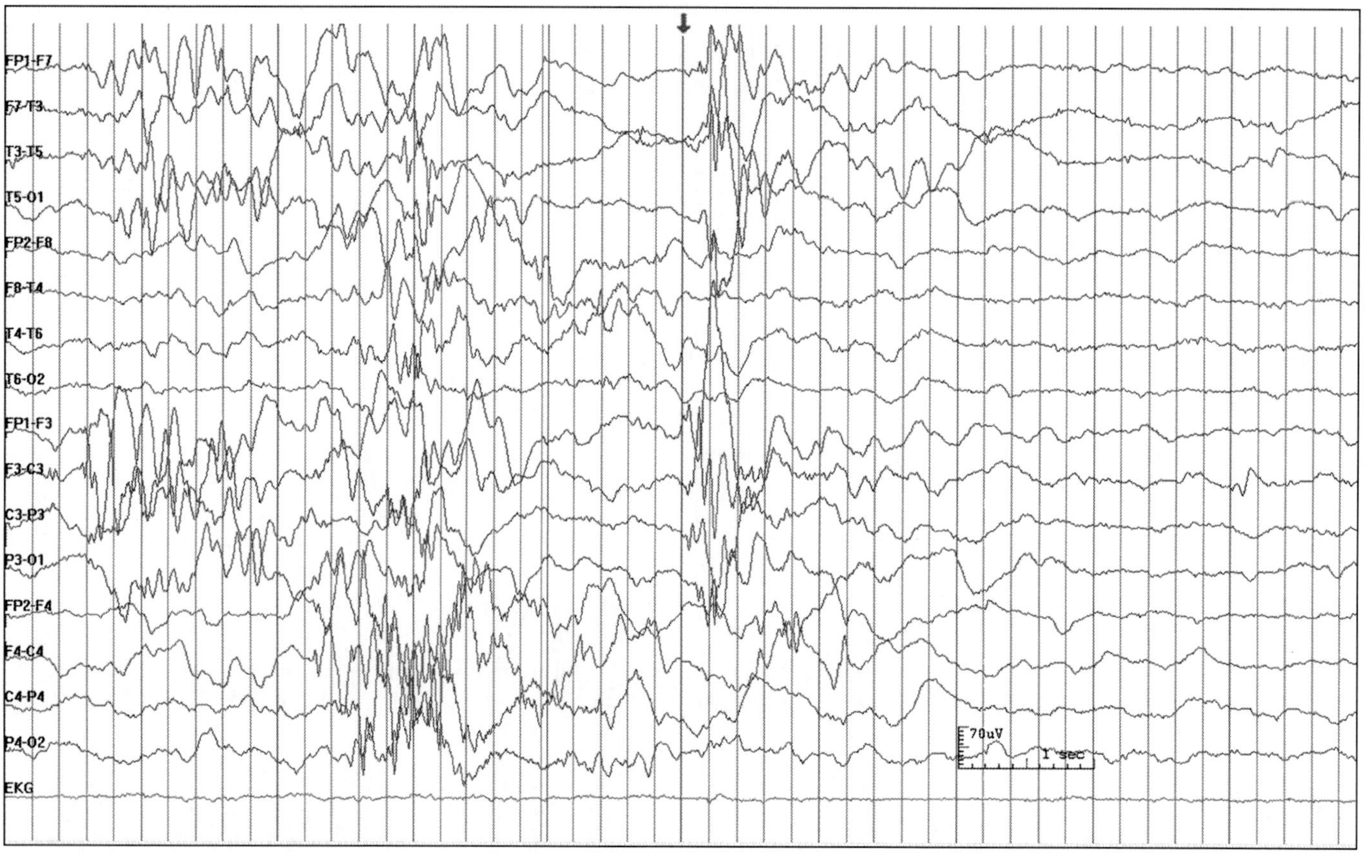

FP1-F7
F7-T3
T3-T5
T5-O1
FP2-F8
F8-T4
T4-T6
T6-O2
FP1-F3
F3-C3
C3-P3
P3-O1
FP2-F4
F4-C4
C4-P4
P4-O2
EKG
70uV
1 sec

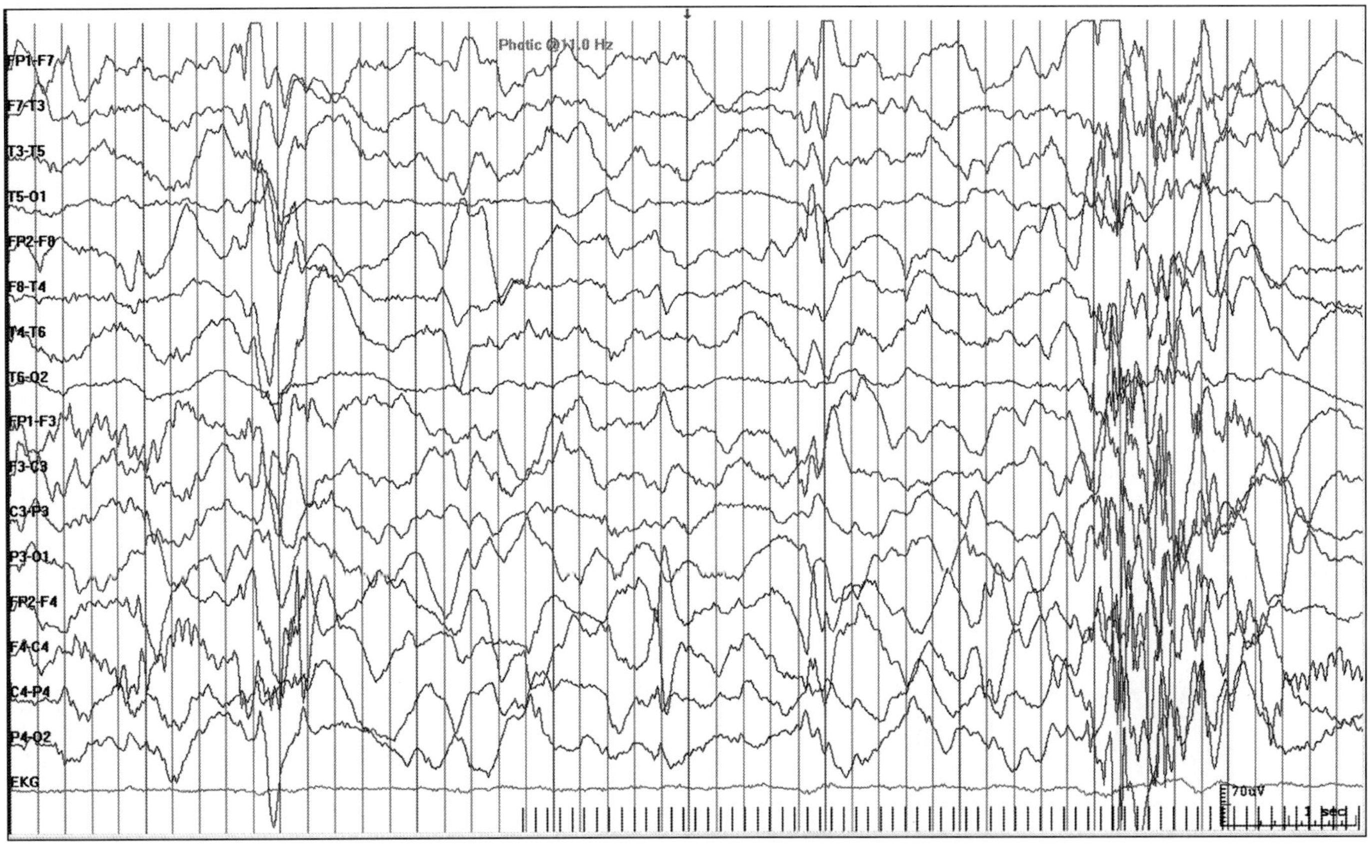

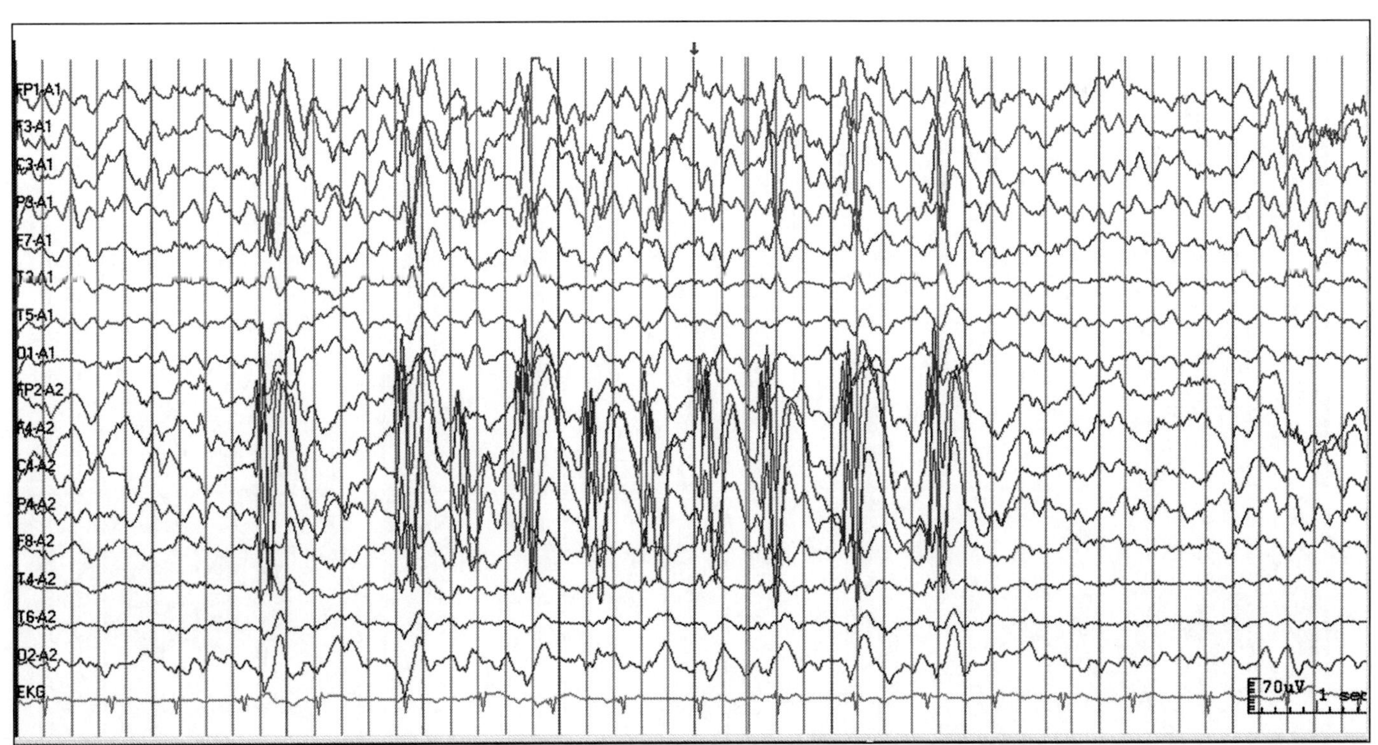
FP1-A1
F3-A1
C3-A1
P3-A1
F7-A1
T3-A1
T5-A1
O1-A1
FP2-A2
F4-A2
C4-A2
P4-A2
F8-A2
T4-A2
T6-A2
O2-A2
EKG
70uV
1 sec

Myoclonic Seizures

Myoclonic seizures are characterized by discharges with polyspikes/multispikes. These are usually generalized, but can be focal also. Show below are EEG traces of some children who presented to us with myoclonic jerks. The traces usually shows independent discharges as well.

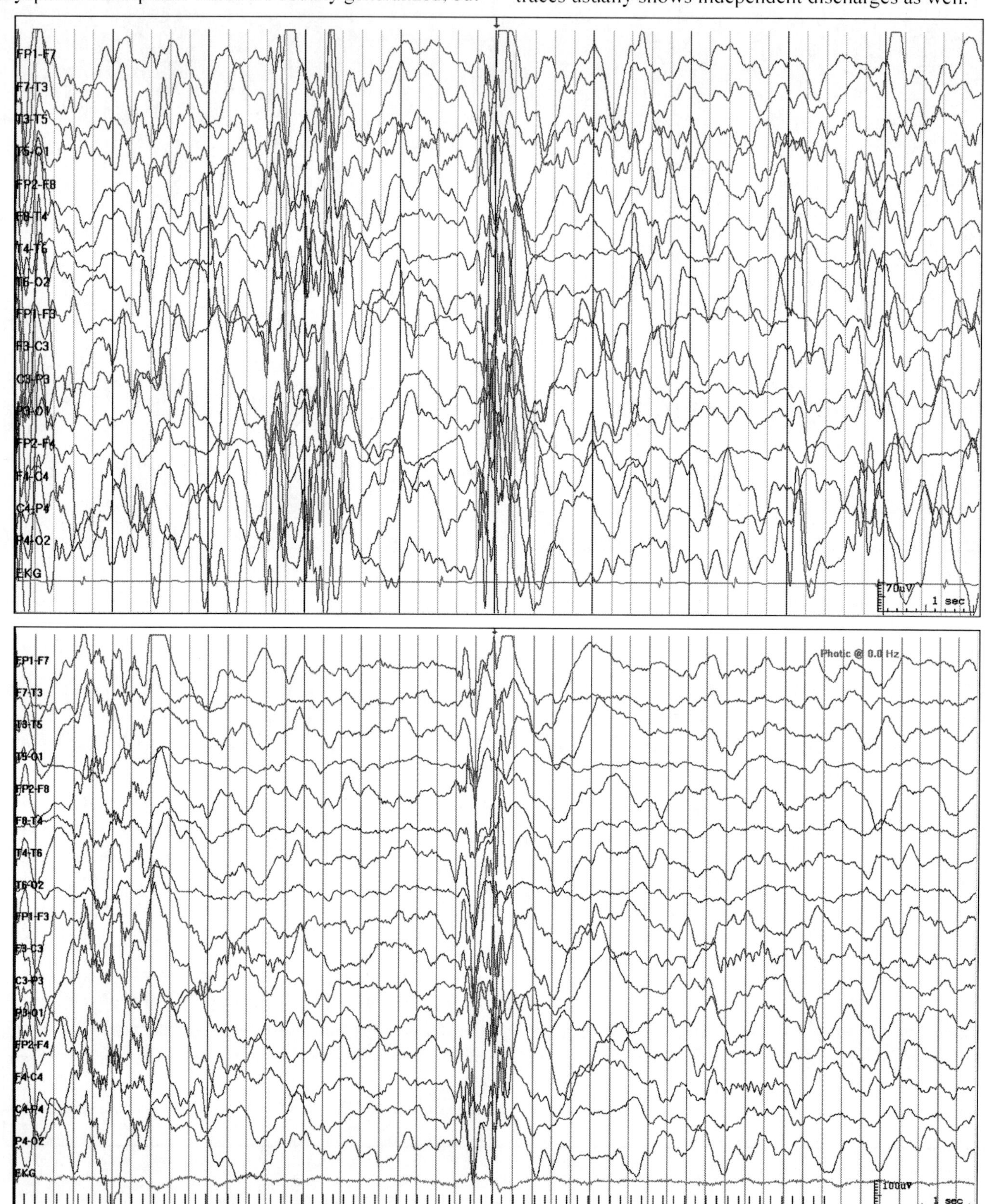

Atonic Seizure

Atonic seizures are clinically characterized by sudden loss of postural tone the child usually slumping to the ground. Atonic seizures are often confused with Lennox-Gastaut syndrome and myoclonic epilepsy. Below are traces of children who presented to us with typical atonic seizure.

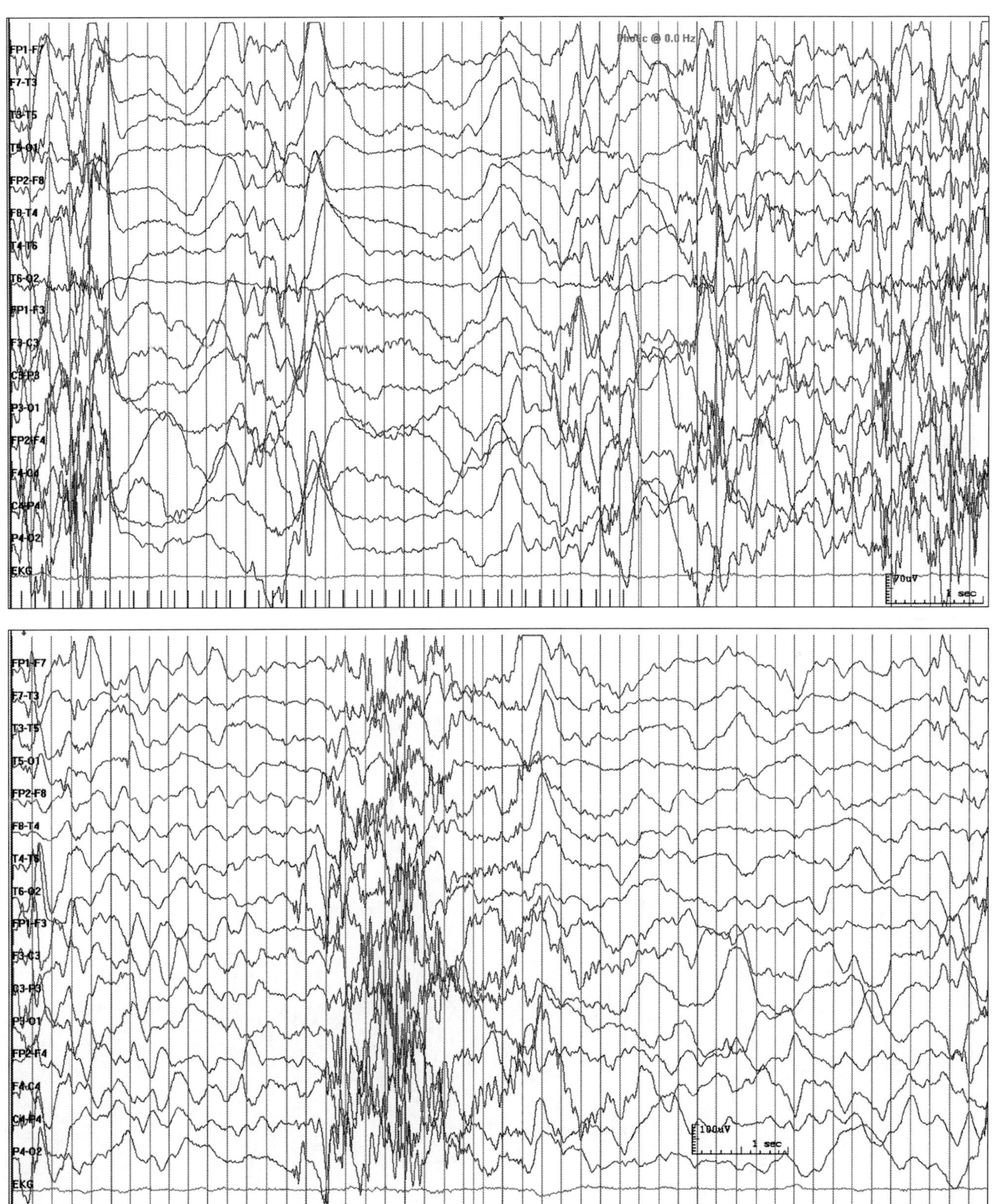

Absence Seizure

Absence seizures are characterized by presence of 3 Hz spike and waves in the record. A characteristic feature is abrupt onset and abrupt termination of the seizure activity. Below are some traces of children who presented to us with absence seizure.

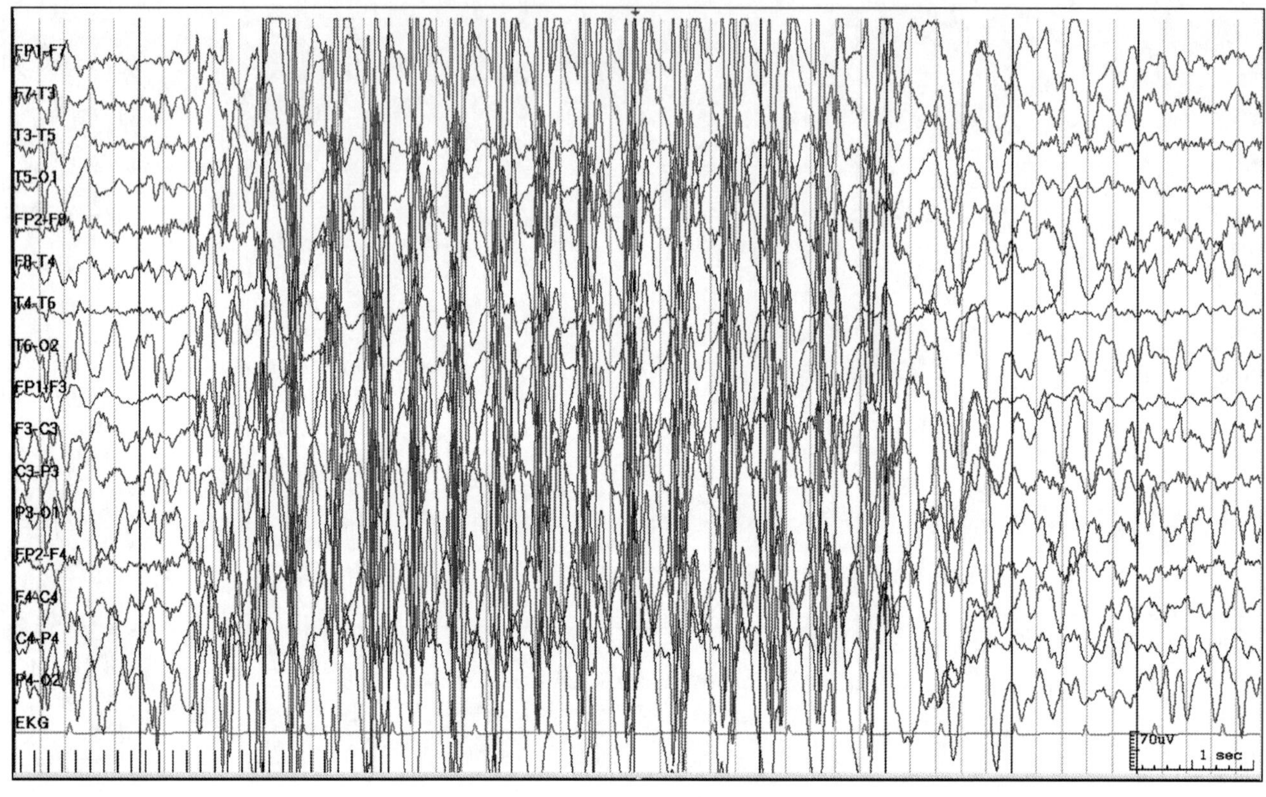

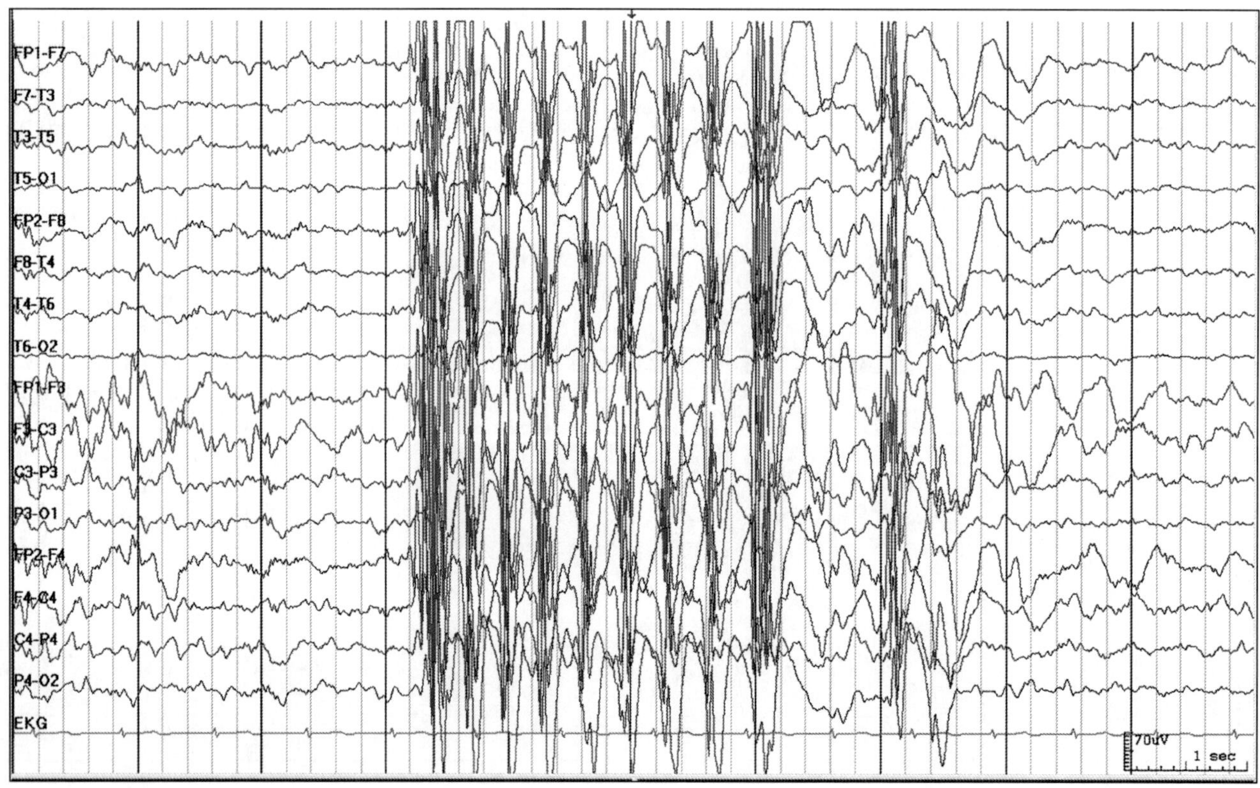

Epilepsy Syndromes

Epilepsy syndromes are characterized by seizures and certain features that age-related. EEG is useful and practically essential for diagnosis of syndromes, i.e., like West syndrome / Infantile spasm, Lennox-Gastaut syndrome, Rolandic epilepsy, JME etc.

Infantile Spasm

Infantile spasm / West syndrome is characterized by spasms / jerks occurring in cluster, with onset around 4-5 months of age, regression of milestones and EEG showing hypsarrhythmia. Hypsarrhythmia is characterized by bizarre background activity, high voltage slow waves, shifting spikes, often electrodecremental response in EEG. Some traces of cases of infantile spasms who had presented to us are shown below.

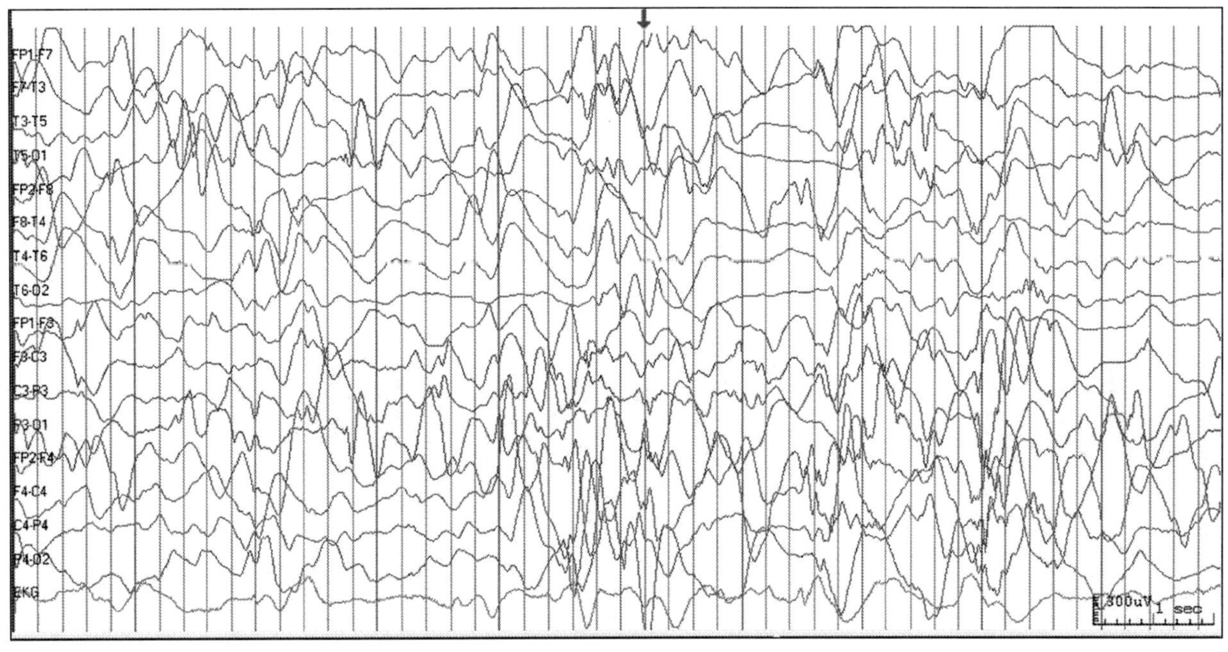

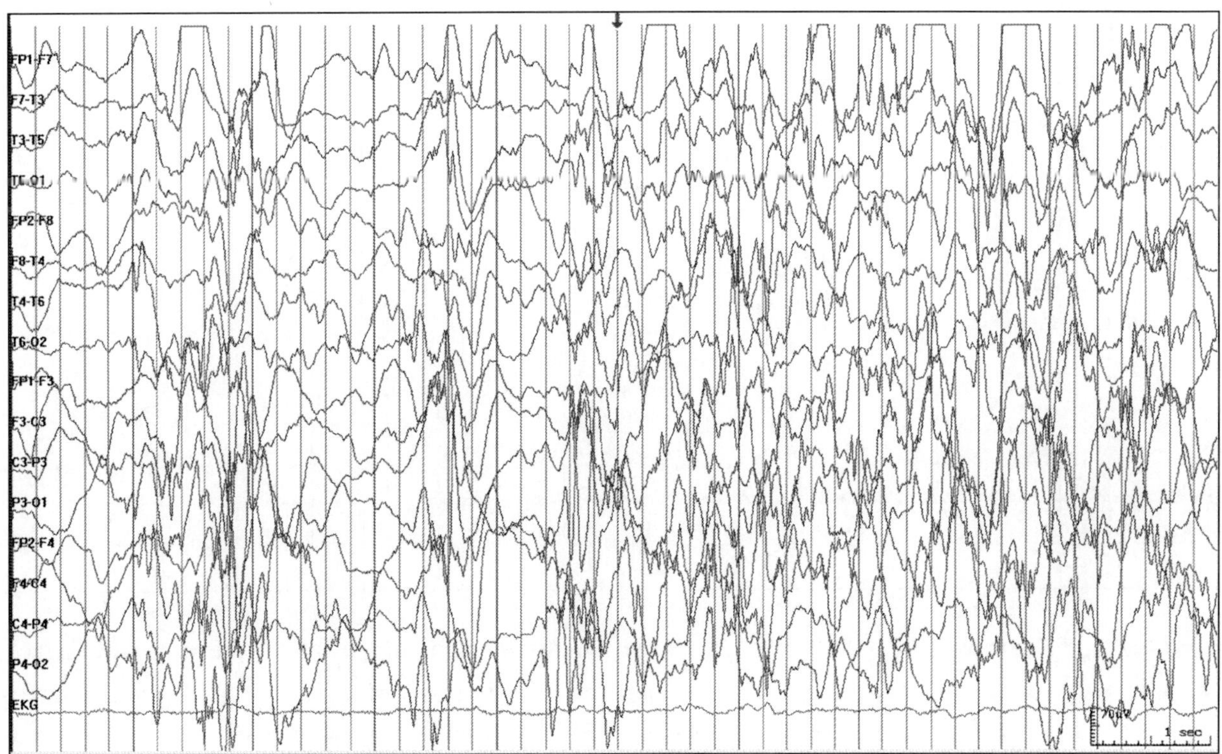

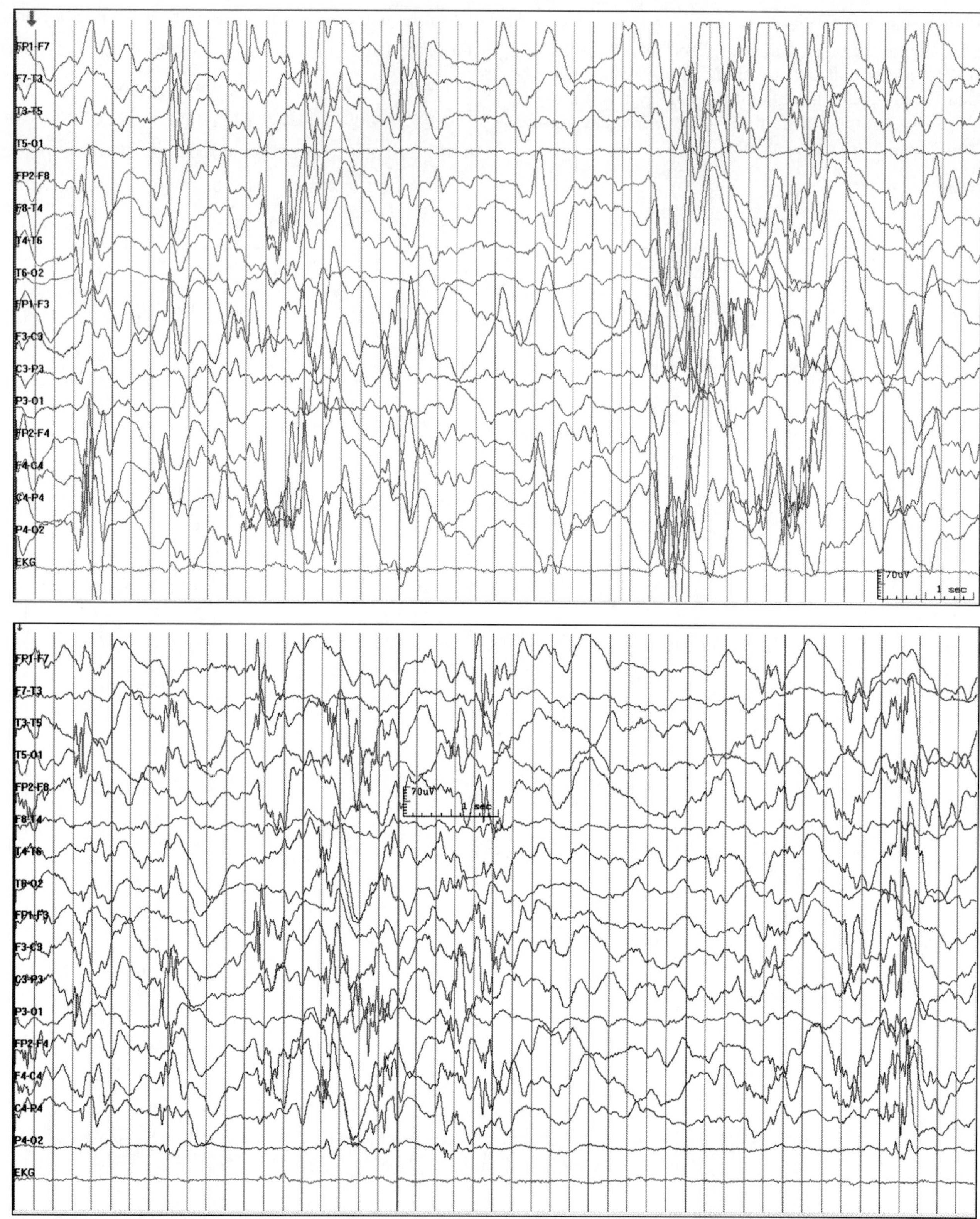

Lennox-Gastaut Syndrome

It is characterized by frequent myclonic jerks, often associated with falls. The falls are often so sharp that injury is common, specially to the forehead and face, often needing head-gear for protection. EEG is characterized by sharp and slow wave complexes. It is usually seen in 2-3 years of age, subsequently with some change in character of the seizure. Besides jerks some cases have associated tonic and tonic clonic seizures. Below are traces of cases of LGS presented to us.

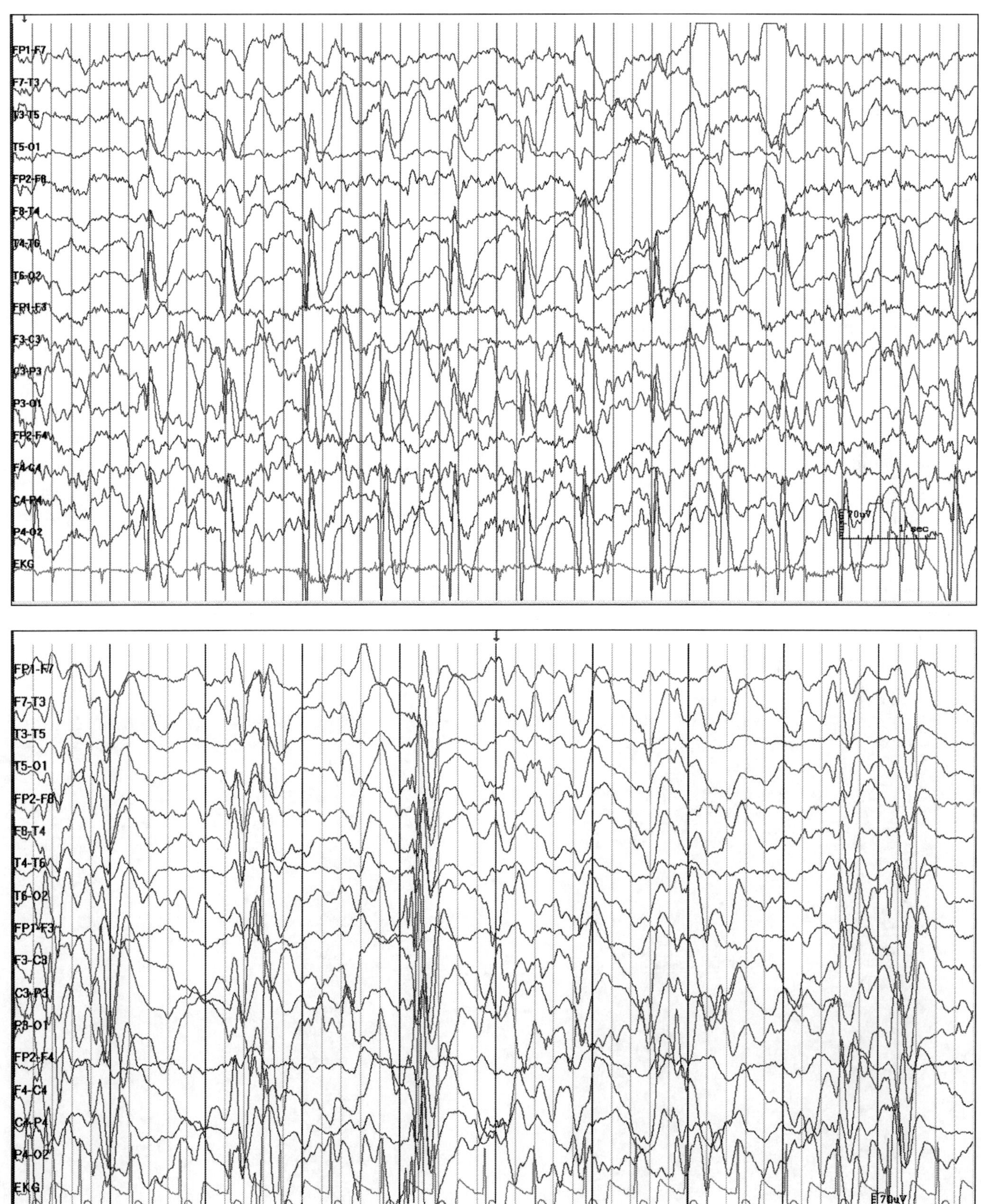

Usefulness of EEG in Miscellaneous Disorders

Besides detecting seizure activity, EEG is useful in some conditions/disorders involving the brain. Some such conditions are – various encephalopathies, focal pathology, diagnosis and monitoring coma, monitoring progress while on treatment.

When there is a pathology involving the brain as a whole, EEG usually shows suppression of background activity, usually generalized or diffuse. This occurs due to diffuse involvement of the brain parenchyma by the pathological process. Such findings are commonly seen in conditions like viral and even bacterial meningoencephalitis, diffuse cerebral edema from any cause, neurocysticercosis (encephalitic form), brain trauma, deep coma from any cause.

Focal pathology is usually shown in EEG as focal attenuation/suppression of the background activity and is due to focal involvement of the brain parenchyma. We commonly get such findings in conditions like stroke, mass lesion like brain abscess, neurocysticercosis, tuberculoma, brain tumour, cysts etc. Focal involvement can also be seen herpes encephalitis.

In deeply comatose patients also cerebral activity is suppressed and EEG shows generalize lowing. With improvement the EEG gradually returns to normal. EEG is also useful and is essential for diagnosis of brain death. The recording does not show any activity (flat tracing) in brain dead patients.

EEG shows certain characteristic/specific patterns in certain conditions and lend helpful clue to diagnosis. In SSPE the record often shows periodic discharges recurring at intervals of 3-11 sec. In stroke EEG frequently shows periodic lateralized epileptiform discharges (PLED).

AUDITORY EVOKED POTENTIAL (AEP)

Auditory Evoked Potential (AEP), also known as Brainstem Evoked Response Audiometry (BERA) and also known as Brainstem Auditory Evoked Potential (BAEP) is a useful objective tool for assessing the function of the auditory pathway. The fundamental principle of the technique is stimulation of the cochlea and subsequently the auditory nerve and the hearing pathway till the auditory cortex and examining the response produced by the stimulus. The response is detected/recorded in the form of waves that has been shown to correspond to different areas of the auditory pathway right, i.e., cochlea, auditory nerve and supranuclear auditory pathway. The waves produced are I, II, III, IV, V, VI and VII. Waves I - V are most consistent and are most useful clinically. The configuration, amplitude and latency between different waves give valuable information regarding the function of the different areas of the auditory pathways. The reader is referred to chapter 6 for details. Some examples of AEP done in cases in our laboratory are shown below.

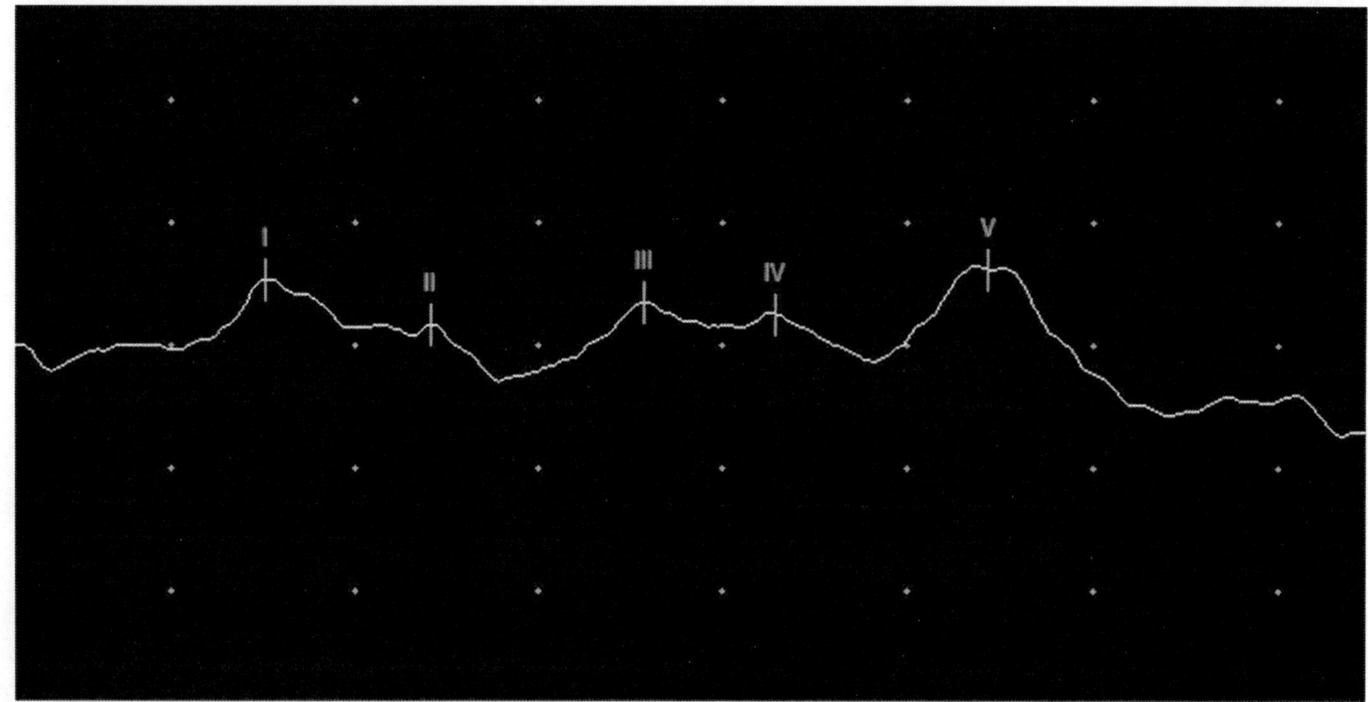

Fig. 7.1: Normal AEP waves in a 7-year-old boy

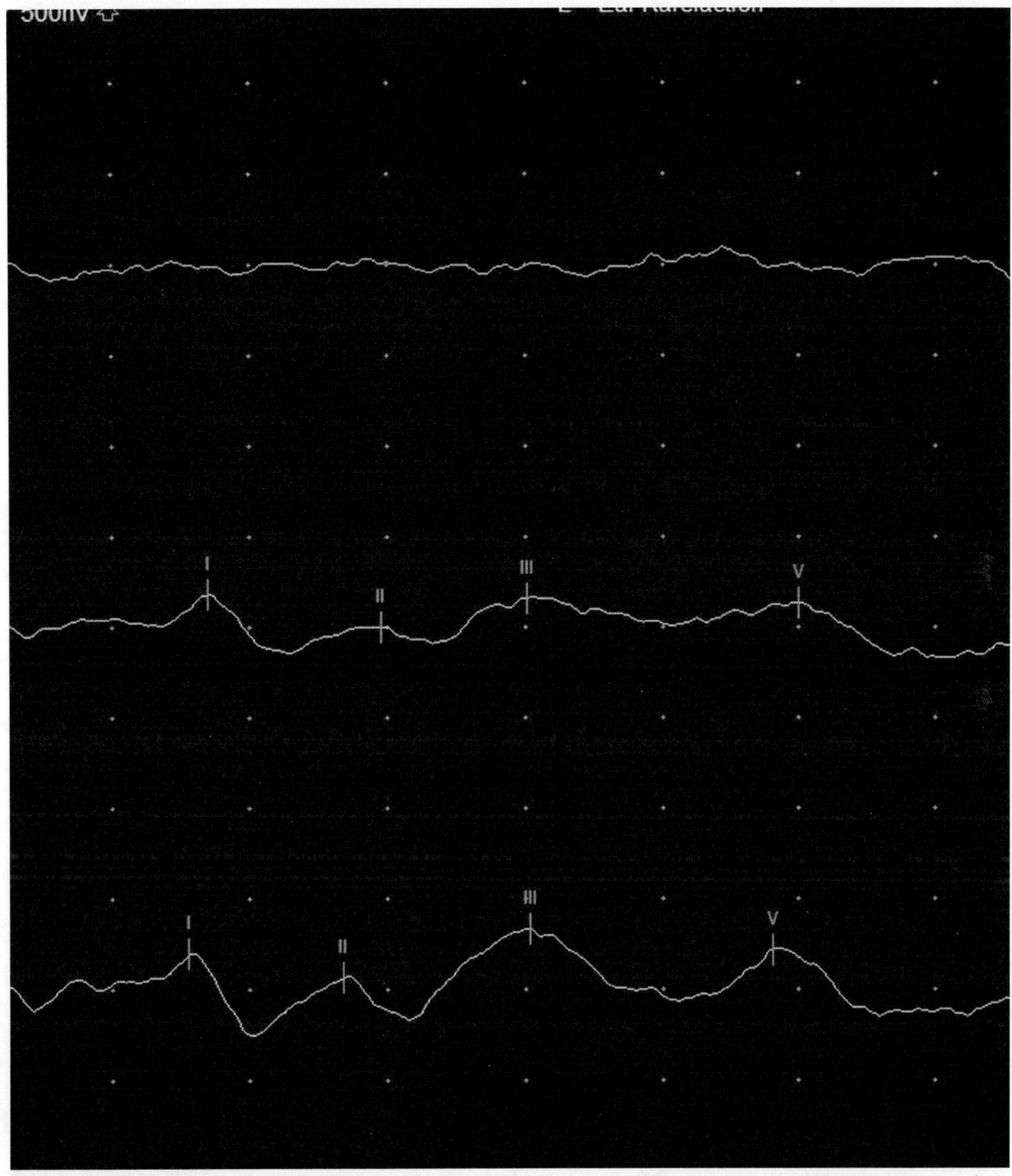

Fig. 7.2: Impaired response in a 1.10 years old boy, none at 40 dB, response seen at 75 and 90 dB with prolonged latency of wV

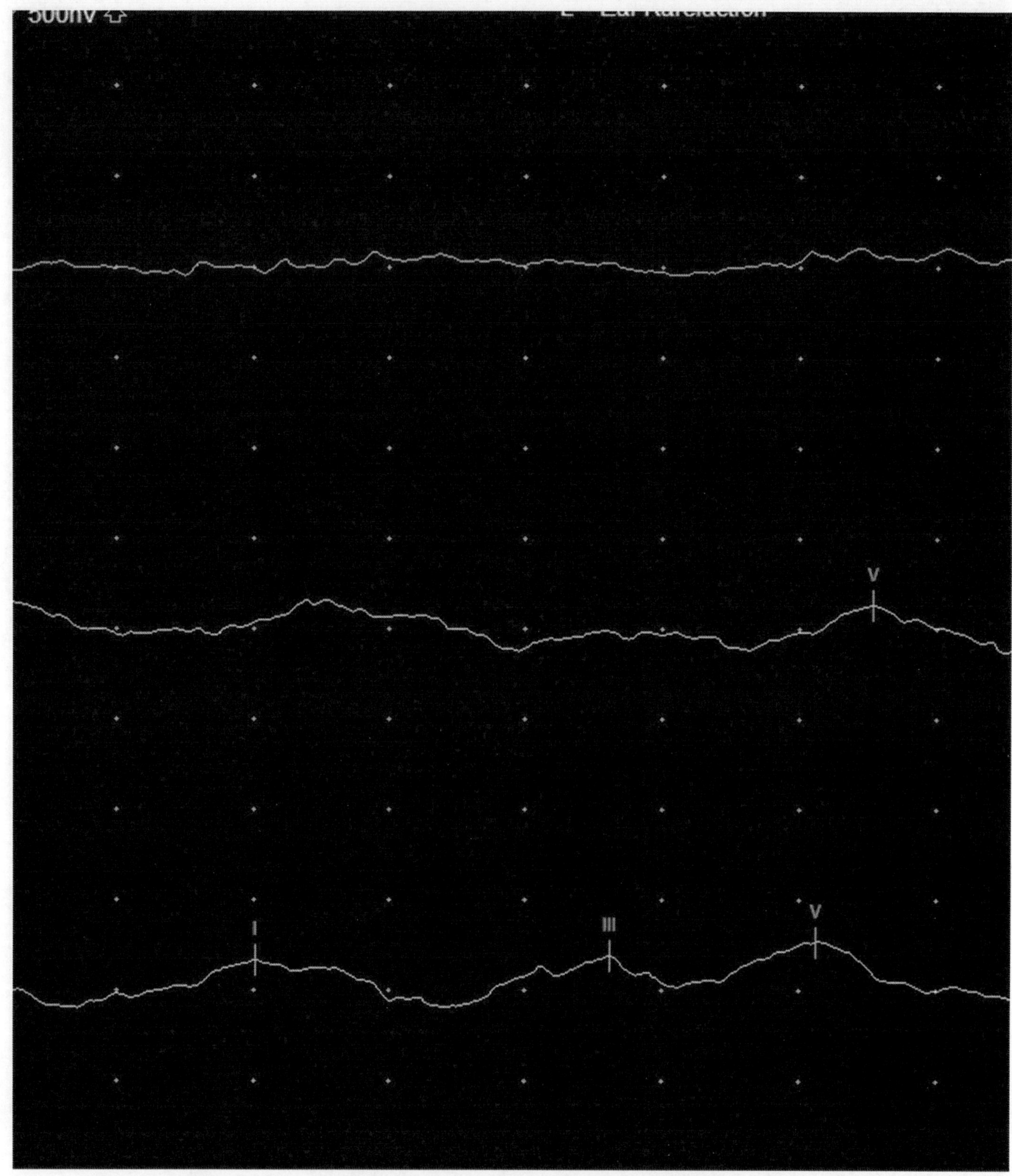

Fig. 7.3: Impaired response in a 3.7 years old girl, none at 75 dB and 90 dB prolonged wV and others seen

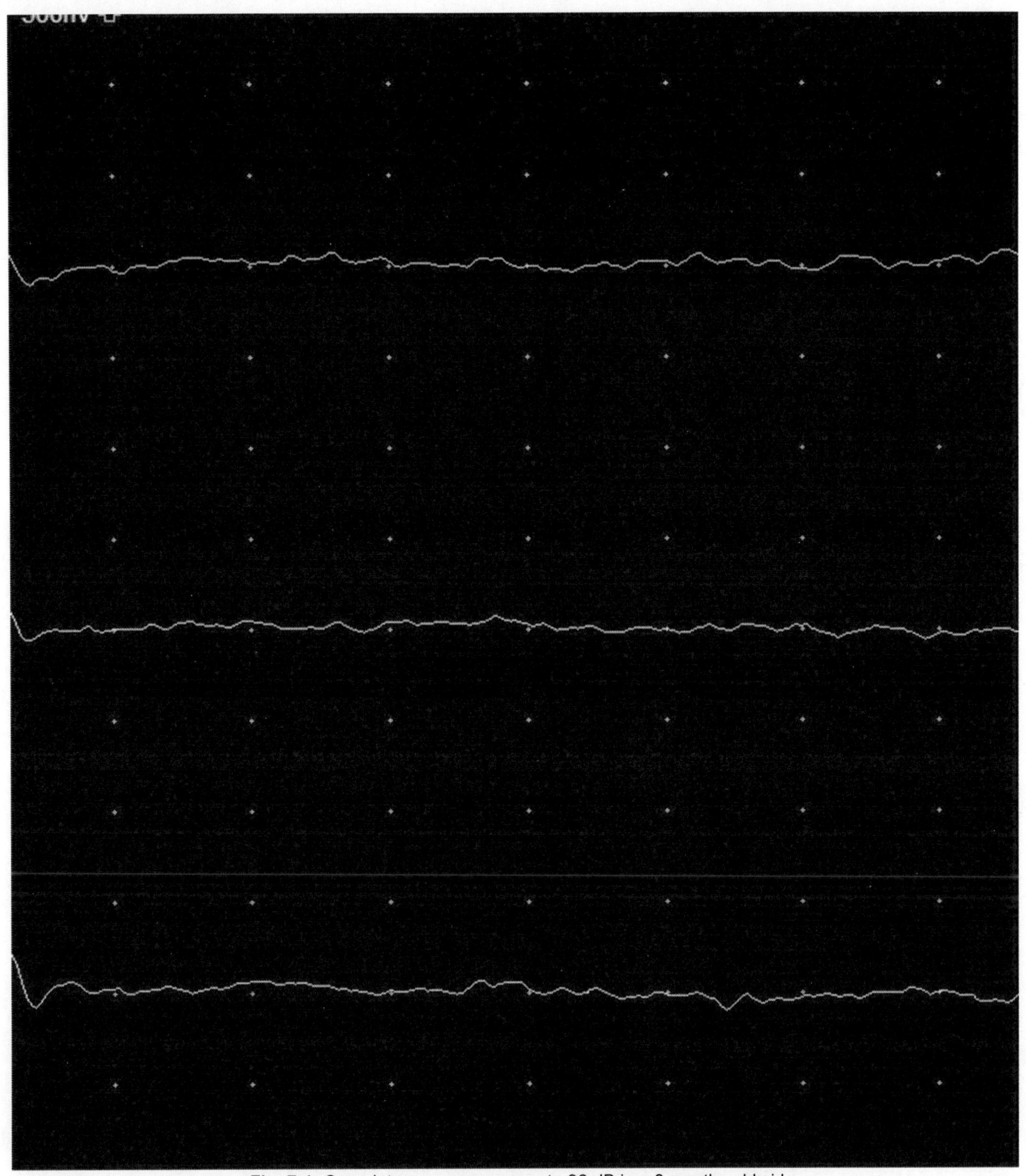

Fig. 7.4: Complete non-response up to 90 dB in a 3 months old girl

VISUAL EVOKED POTENTIAL (VEP)

Visual evoked potential (VEP) is a useful objective tool for assessing the function of the visual pathway. The basic principle of the technique is stimulation of the retina and recording the response that arises from the visual pathway from retina to visual cortex. The response is detected/recorded in the form of waves namely N75, P100 and N145. The reader is referred to chapter 6 for details. The most important clinically useful response is the P100 latency. Some examples of VEP done in cases in our laboratory are shown below.

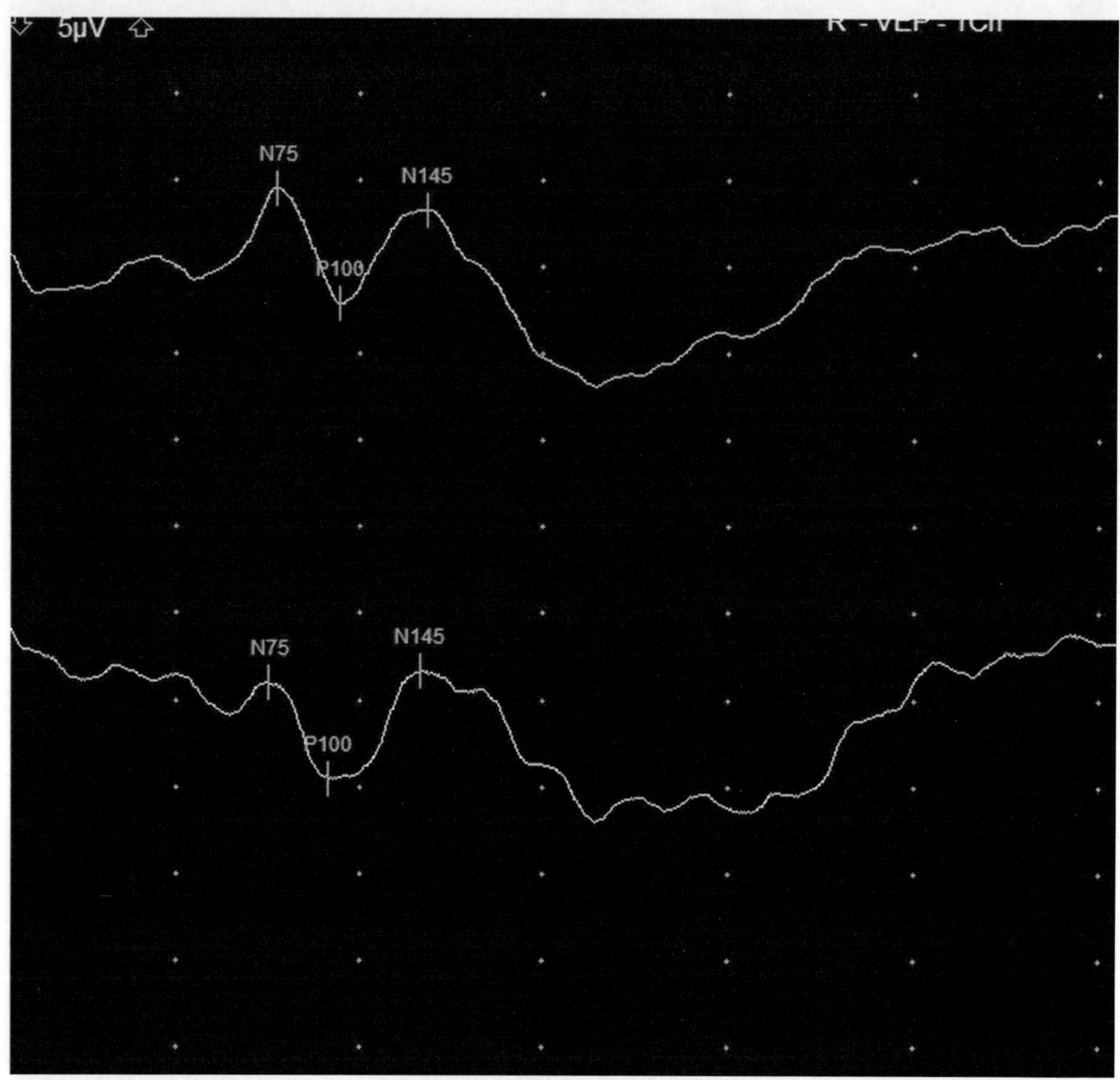

Fig. 7.5: Normal VEPs in a 6 years old girl

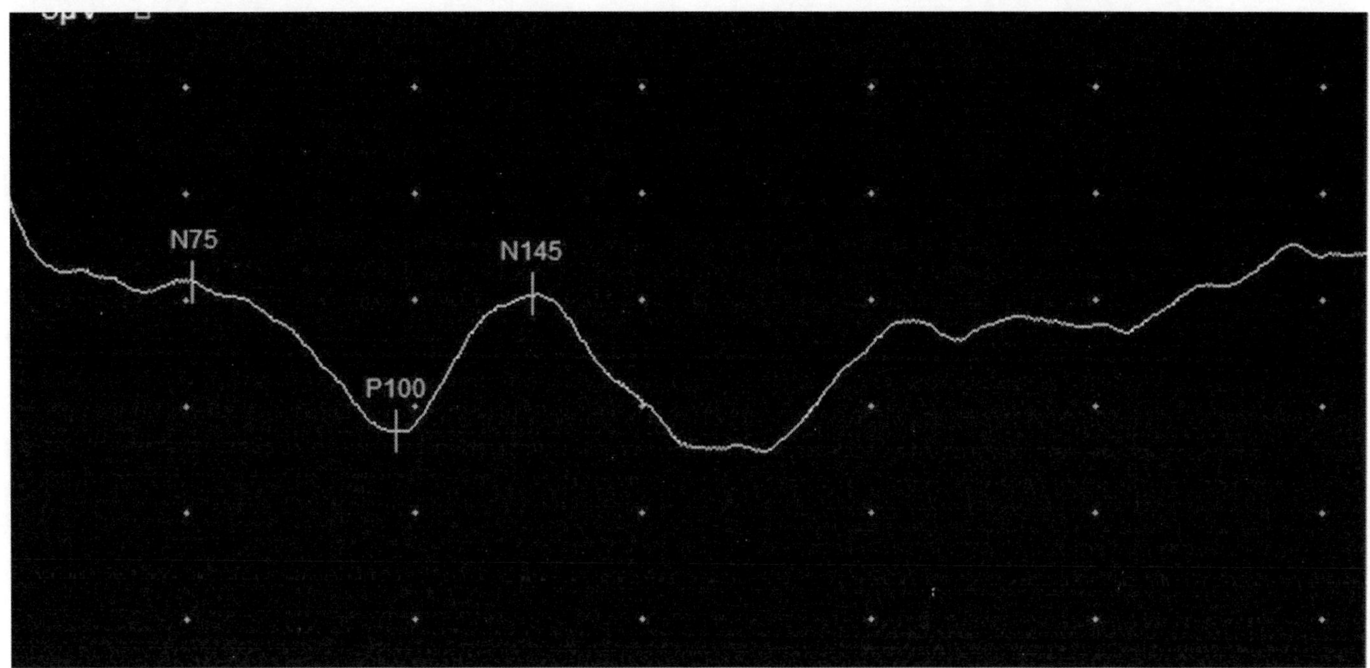

Fig. 7.6: Normal VEPs in a 9 months old boy

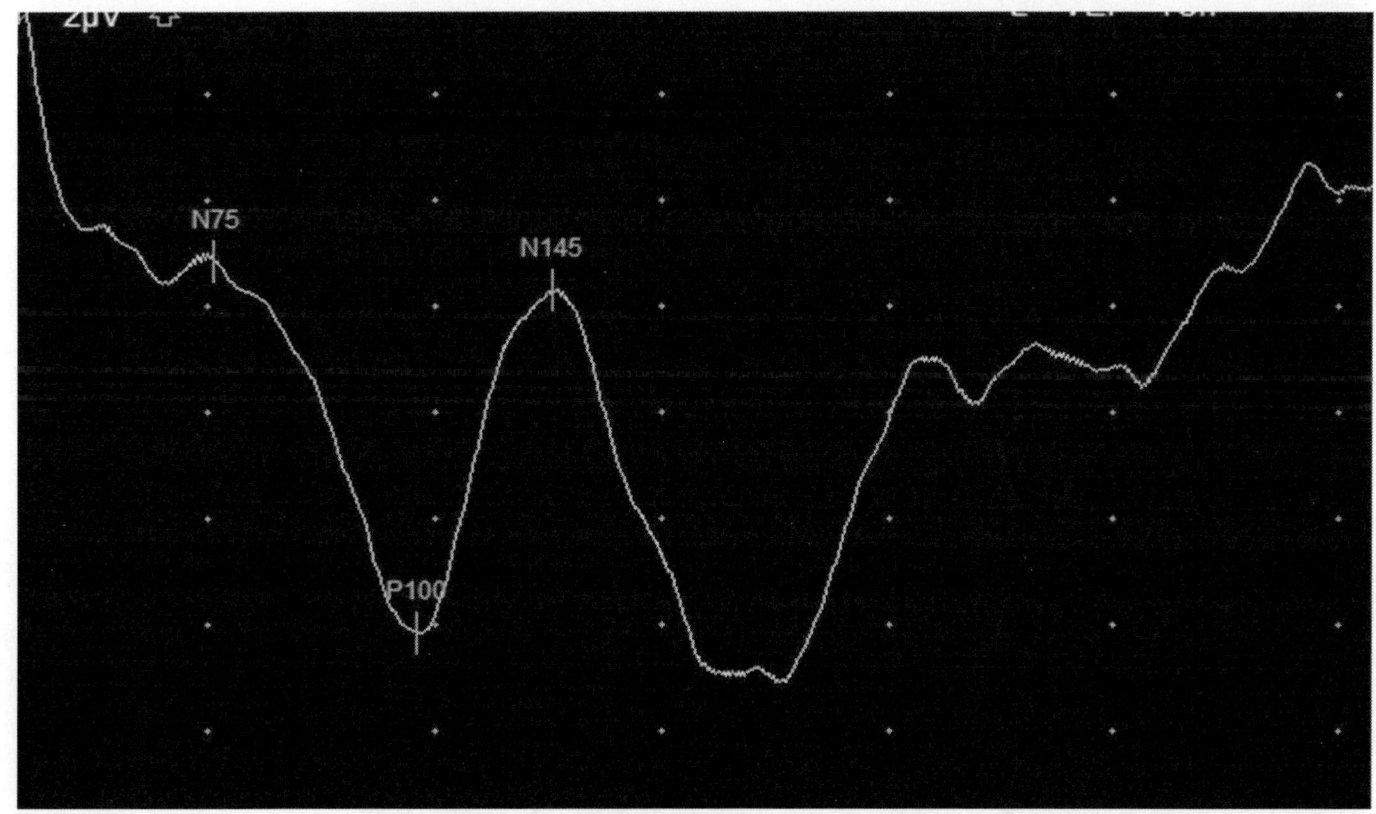

Fig. 7.7: Normal VEPs in a 1.6 years old girl

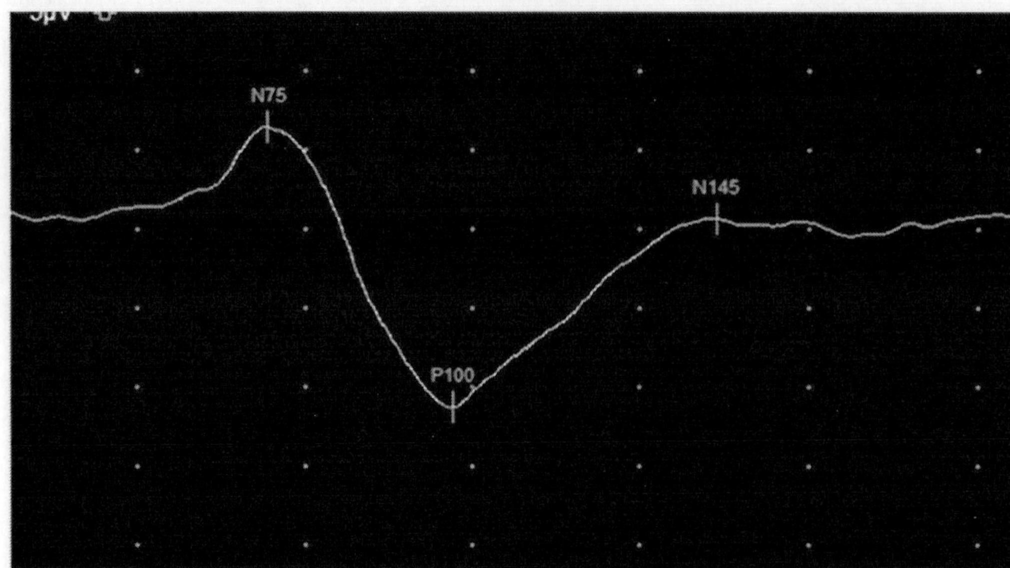

Fig. 7.8: Abnormal responses showing prolonged P100 latency in a 3.7 years old girl

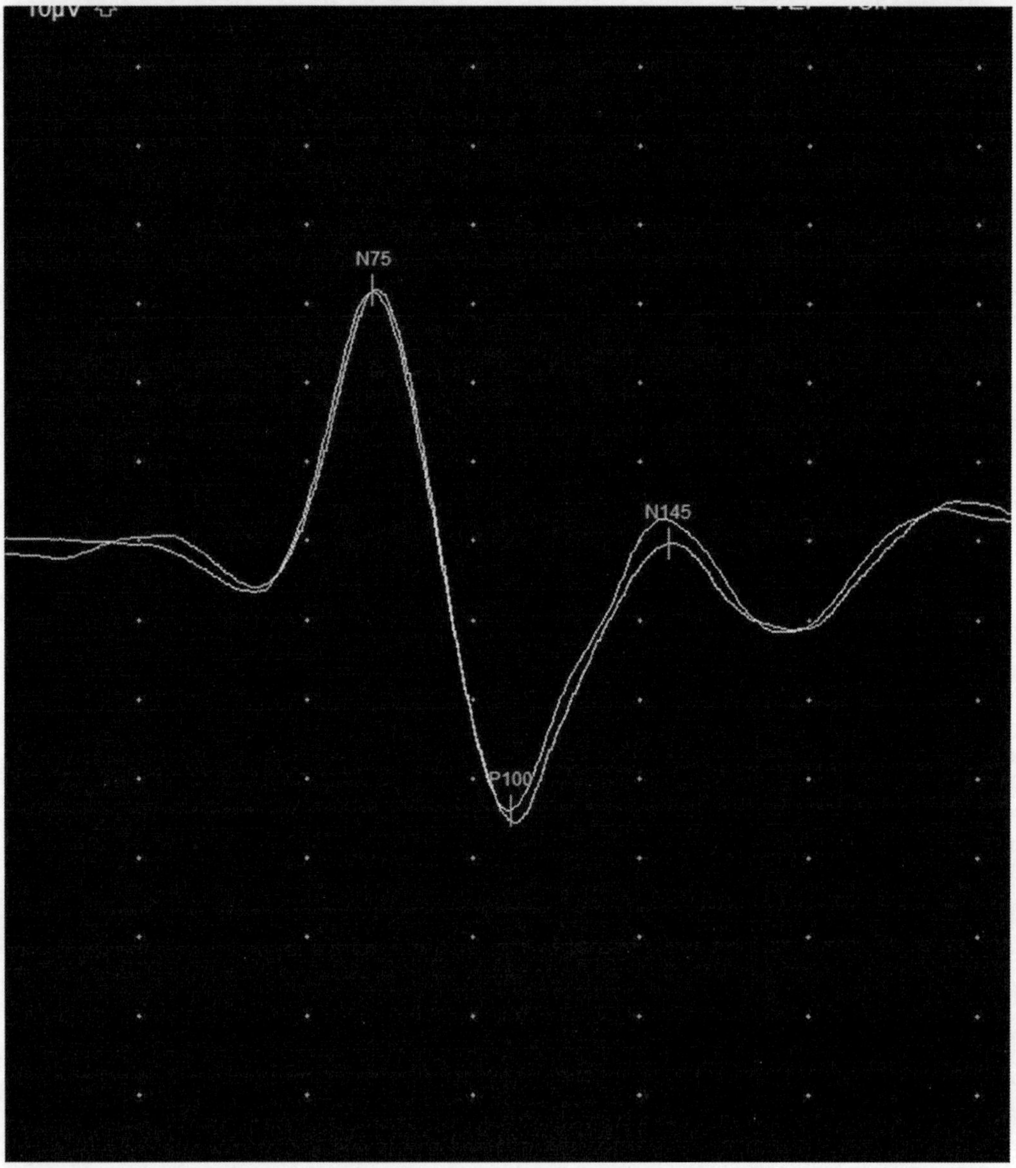

Fig. 7.9: Abnormal responses showing prolonged P100 latency in a 2 years old boy

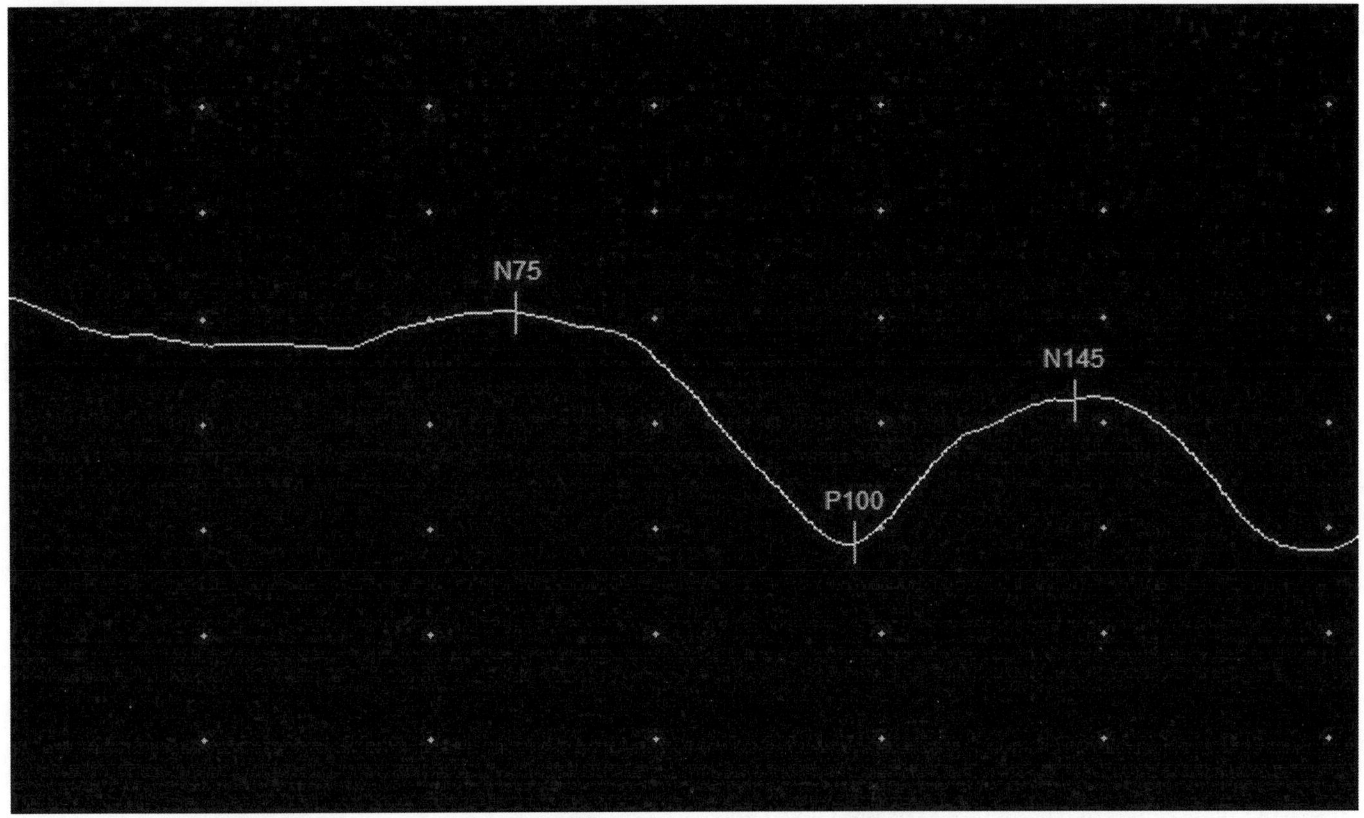

Fig. 7.10: Abnormal responses showing prolonged P100 latency in a 10 months old girl

Suggested Reading

- American Electroencephalographic Society. Guidelines in EEG, 1-7 (Revised 1985). J Clin Neurophysiol 1986:3:131-68.
- Dreyfus-Brisac C. Monod N. The Electroencephalogram of Full-term Newborn and Premature Infants. In: Lary CG (ed), Handbook of Electroencephalography and Clinical Neurophysiology, Amsterdam, Elsevier 1975:6:6-24.
- Flink R, Pedersen B, Guekht AB, *et al.* Guidelines for the Use of EEG Methodology in the Diagnosis of Epilepsy. International League Against Epilepsy: Commission Report. Commission on European Affairs: Subcommission on European Guidelines, Acta Neurol. Scand 2002:106:1-7.
- Gibbs FA, Gibbs EL. Atlas of Electroencephalography. Vol 1. IV. Normal and Abnormal Infants from Birth to 11 Months of Age. Reading, Mass: Addison-Wesley 1978:373.
- Hughes JR, Fino J, Gagnon L. Periods of Activity and Quiescence in the Premature EEG. Neuropediatric 1983:14: 66-72.
- Hughes JR. EEG in Clinical Practice, 2nd Edition, Butterworth-Heinmann, Boston, 1994.
- Kumar A, Gupta A, Talukdar B. Clinico-Etiological and EEG Profile of Neonatal Seizures, Indian J Pediatr 2007;74:33-37.
- Menache CC, Bourgeois BF, Volpe JJ. Prognostic Value of Neonatal Discontinuous EEG, Pediatr Neurol 2002 August; 27(2):93-101.
- Niedermeyer E, Lopes da Silva F. Electroencephalography, Basic Principles, Clinical Applications and Related Fields, Baltimore: Williams and Wilkins:1999.
- Stockard-Pope JE, Werner SS, Bickford RG, Curran JS. Atlas of Neonatal Electroencephalography, Second Edition, Raven Press, New York 1992.

8 Chapter

CONGENITAL MALFORMATIONS OF THE CENTRAL NERVOUS SYSTEM

Kausik Mandal

INTRODUCTION

Congenital malformations involving the central nervous system are one of the most common major malformations found in a fetus or a neonate.

Various environmental factors including folic acid deficiency and teratogens are implicated in the genesis of malformations of the central nervous system. Environmental causes form the major group, causing the maximum number of malformations, necessitating their prevention by prior knowledge and simple interventions. On the other hand, there are various chromosomal and single gene disorders which give rise to specific patterns of malformations; recognition of such genetic disorders is necessary for management, prognostication, diagnostic genetic testing and prenatal diagnosis to prevent recurrences.

CLASSIFICATION OF CONGENITAL MALFORMATIONS OF THE CENTRAL NERVOUS SYSTEM

Classification of malformations of brain and spinal cord is difficult; an exhaustive list will overlap with disorders of other systems and a precise list will miss out on many important disorders.

Various authors have tried to classify the disorders according to their embryological stages; however, as not all processes are discrete and time bound, such classification has not been universally used. Other methods are classifications according to the anatomical location of lesions and according to the underlying etiology; none were complete. For a better and complete understanding of brain malformations, a multi-disciplinary approach has been found to be more helpful. It involves various fields like neuro-embryology, neurogenetics, neurochemistry, pediatric neurology and pediatric neuroradiology. With the steady growth in facilities for neuroimaging, mutation detection by molecular methods like Sanger sequencing and multiplex ligation-dependent probe amplification (MLPA),[1] and identification of new genes by Next-Generation Sequencing (NGS) techniques; classifications involving pattern-recognition and underlying etiology have been helpful to understand the various CNS malformations. We will discuss the various disorders under the following headings:

(I) Neural tube defects (NTD).

(II) Midline malformations of the forebrain.

(III) Disorders of cerebral cortical development.

(IV) Agenesis or hypoplasia of corpus callosum.

(V) Agenesis of cranial nerves.

(VI) Disorders involving cerebellum and posterior fossa.

(VII) Phakomatosis.

(VIII) Anomalies associated with craniosynostosis.

(IX) Hydrocephalus and hydranencephaly.

(X) Specific malformations due to teratogens.

(XI) Other malformations like intracranial cysts, hamar-tomas and vascular malformations.

(I) NEURAL TUBE DEFECTS (NTD)

Neural tube defects can result from alterations in any of the processes that are involved in the formation of the primary neural tube. Though the molecular basis of neural tube closure defects is likely to be quite heterogeneous, periconceptional folic acid supplementation has been found to reduce the risk by around 70%.[2, 3] The process of neurulation occurs at the fourth week of human gestation. This gives the idea about the requirement of folic acid much early in the development; even before the woman has learned that she is pregnant as she misses a period. It is recommended that a woman should start taking folic acid as soon as she plans a pregnancy (at least three months prior to pregnancy) to prevent neural tube defects in the fetus. The common practice of starting folic acid after a positive pregnancy test; offers limited protection.

Embryology: During the process of neurulation, the neural plate is converted into the neural tube, which is covered by ectoderm. The neural tube later on differentiates into the brain and the spinal cord. Regulation of the neural tube formation is a complicated process involving multiple genes and multitude of processes involving cell migration and alterations in the cellular morphology. At a very early stage, signalling molecules induce the epithelia of the two-layered embryo to get thickened and form the neural plate. At this stage the neural plate lies over the notochord. It subsequently bends so that the lateral margins of the neural plate elevate to form the neural folds with the neural groove lying in between. In the rostral end neural folds bend inward at the dorsolateral hinge points. In addition to the bending motions, the movement of the neural folds is aided by the narrowing and lengthening of the cells of the neural plate. Two additional processes are fundamental to the creation and fusion of the neural tube. The first is apical constriction, whereby columnar epithelial cells are converted into wedge-shaped cells by cytoskeletal elements. The second is convergent extension, whereby the flat sheet of epithelial cells is remodelled, via intercalation, into a longer, narrower configuration. The neural tube, under the control of a multitude of genes working at a timely fashion, ultimately fuses at several discrete points, unlike the oversimplified model of a hollow tube that closes continuously in a "zipperlike" manner.[4,5,6] That the neural tube actually closes at multiple points can be exemplified by the occurrence of more than one defect in the neural tube in the same fetus (Fig. 8.1).

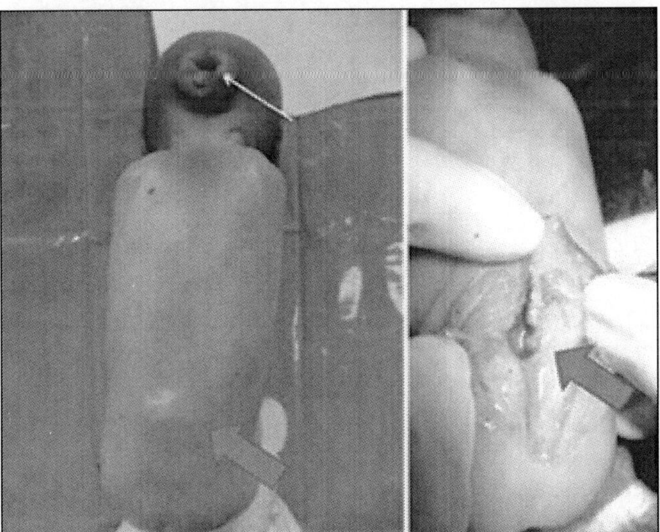

Fig. 8.1: More than one defect in the neural tube in the same fetus; occipital encephalocele (arrow) and lumbar meningomyelocele (broad arrow)

Classification: Though the processes for normal neural tube closure is quite complex, the gross phenotypic consequences are relatively homogeneous. The failure of neural tube closure is associated with defects in the overlying bony structures (i.e., cranial vault and neural arches) resulting in exposure of the underlying neural tissue. As a result, defects of primary neural tube closure are often referred to as "open" NTDs. Further classifications of the NTDs are based on the location and extent of the defect.

Anencephaly: In this condition there is absence of the cranial vault along with markedly diminished cerebral hemispheres (Fig. 8.2). The cerebellum might also be absent and the brainstem hypoplastic. As per severity anencephaly is classified as holocrania and mesocrania:

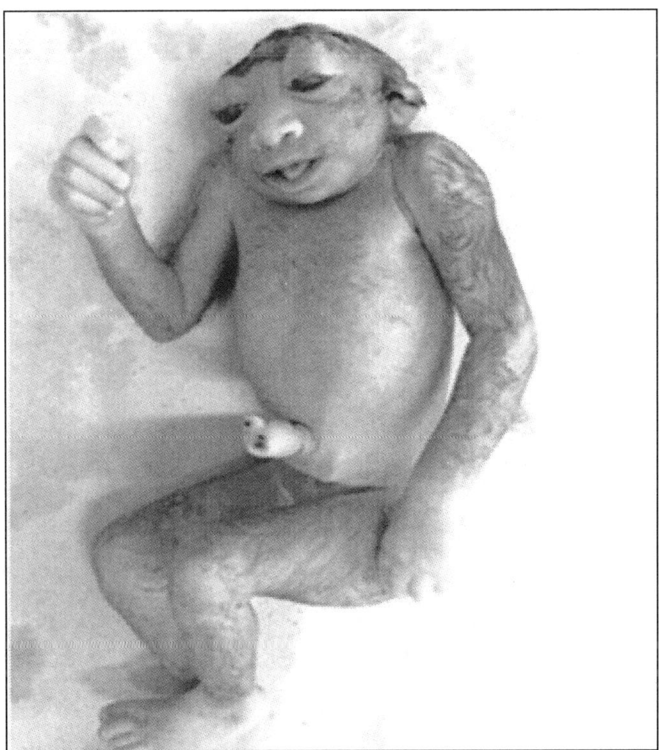

Fig. 8.2: Anencephaly

1. Holocrania – when the defect involves the foramen magnum.
2. Merocrania – when the foramen magnum is not involved.

Folic acid deficiency in mother is still considered to be the most common cause of anencephaly. Sometimes genetic or chromosomal disorders are also implicated. Rarely anencephaly is seen as a disruption sequence following amniotic band entanglement of the fetus in utero.

Most fetuses with anencephaly are either aborted spontaneously or undergo medical termination following detection of the defect by prenatal ultrasonography. On rare occasions, anencephalic infants are live born and can survive for short periods without significant medical support. This disorder is considered universally as a lethal disorder.

Acalvaria: Acalvaria is a condition often diagnosed as anencephaly. Unlike in anencephaly, there is not much diminution of brain size. The cranial contents in acalvaria are generally complete, though there can be associated pathologies in the brain. It consists of absence of the calvarial bones, dura mater and associated muscles in the presence of a normal skull base and normal facial bones. It is considered to be a postneurulation defect. The likely pathogenesis of acalvaria is faulty migration of the membranous neurocranium. The normal placement of the embryonic ectoderm, results in an intact layer of skin over the brain parenchyma. Some children are reported to live for some time in case studies.

Encephaloceles: They are characterized by protrusion of intracranial contents through a congenital defect in the dura and skull. They are usually midline defects and based on the anatomical locations they are named as:

- Occipital.
- Parietal.
- Temporal.
- Frontal or Frontoethmoidal (Sincipital).
- Transsphenoidal.
- Nasal.

As per the contents, pathologically they are sometimes classified as meningocele (leptomeninges and CSF), meningoencephalocele (leptomeninges, CSF and brain), meningoencephalocystocele (leptomeninges, CSF, brain and ventricles), atretic cephalocele (small nodule of fibrous fatty tissue) or gliocele (CSF lined by glial tissue).

Sometimes occipital encephaloceles are associated with known single gene defects, e.g., Meckel-Gruber syndrome, where there is occipital encephalocele associated with enlarged polycystic kidneys with or without polydactyly (Fig. 8.3).

Anencephaly: It is a rare neural tube defect that combines extreme retroflexion (backward bending) of the head associated with occipital bone defects and defects in the cervico-thoracic spine (Fig. 8.4).

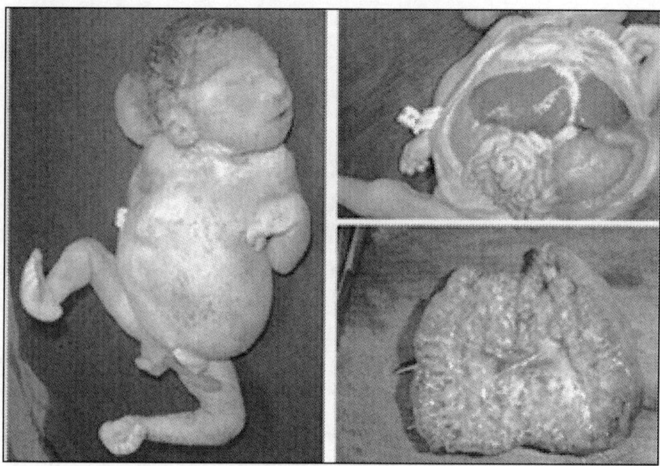

Fig. 8.3: Meckel-Gruber syndrome: Large occipital encephalocoele, protuberant abdomen, deformation effect on upper and lower limbs due to oligohydramnios. Large kidneys with cystic changes on cut section

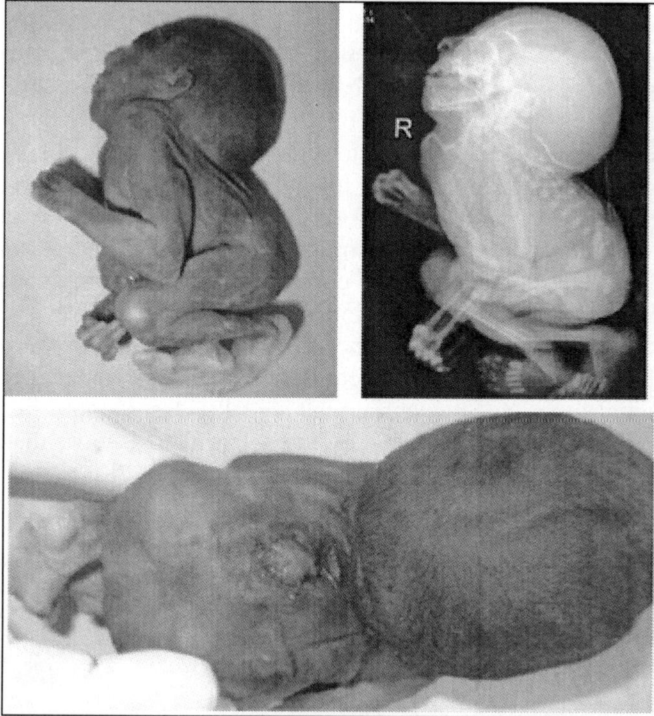

Fig. 8.4: Fetus with anencephaly showing extreme retroflexion (backward bending) of the head and an open spina bifida

Craniorachischisis: Craniorachischisis, also called craniospinal-rachischisis is failure of neural tube closure over the entire body axis (Fig. 8.5). It is a lethal condition.

Spina bifida: Neural tube closure defects that are restricted to the caudal portion of the neural tube are referred to generally as spina bifida or sometimes as meningomyeloceles. This condition is associated with bony defects in the overlying neural arches, through which the meninges and spinal cord tissue are exposed to the body surface.

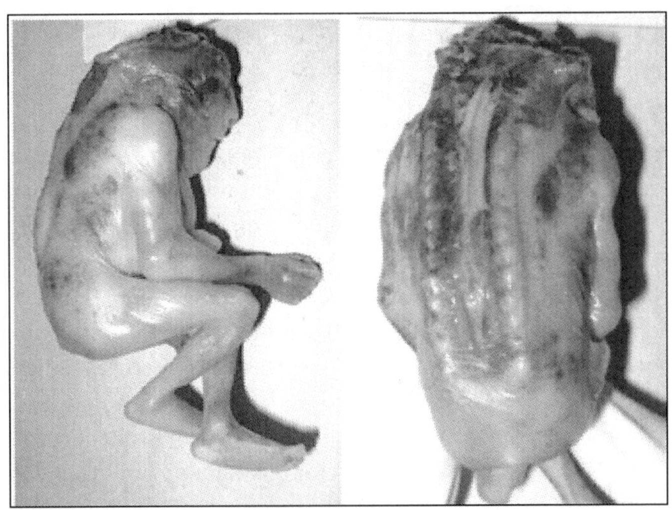

Fig. 8.5: Fetus with craniorachischisis showing failure of neural tube closure over the entire body axis

Most lumbosacral meningomyeloceles are associated with Chiari II (Arnold Chiari) malformation and ventricular dilatation (Fig. 8.6).

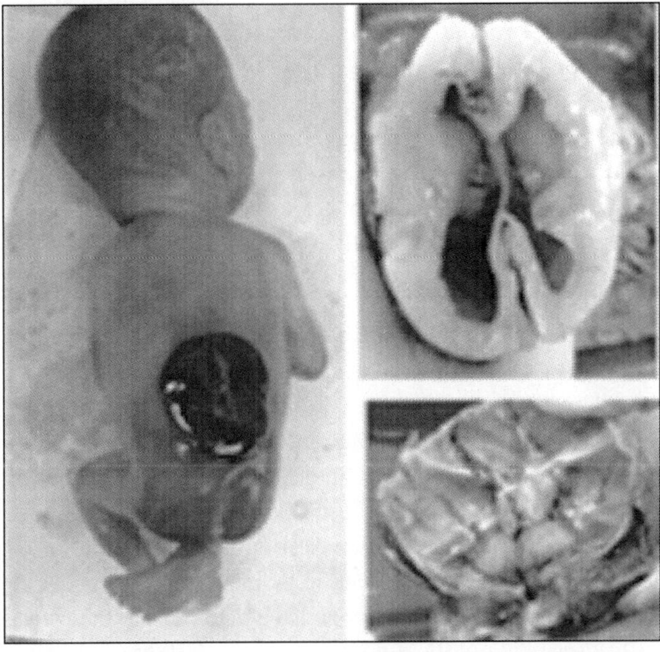

Fig. 8.6: Typical lumbosacral meningomyelocele with Arnold-Chiari malformation (caudally displaced cerebellar vermis) with lateral ventricular dilatation in brain. Such displaced and compressed cerebellum is described as "banana sign" in antenatal ultrasonography

The majority of babies with meningomyeloceles are live born. These babies need to be evaluated for associated ventricular dilatation and other neurological functioning like lower limb movements soon after birth. With proper neurosurgical intervention and medical treatment, survival into the adulthood is common. Neurosurgical interventions mainly comprise repair of the defect and ventriculoperitoneal shunt for associated hydrocephalus. However, many such babies might have residual neurodeficit like bladder incontinence and lower limb weakness even after successful surgical correction.

Occult spinal dysraphisms: Occult spinal dysraphisms (Fig. 8.7) includes meningocele (that may be partially skin covered), spinal lipomas (lipomyelomeningocele or lipomeningocele), myelocystocele, split cord malformations and various forms of sacral agenesis. A number of closed or skin-covered conditions like encephalocele, iniencephaly along with occult spinal dysraphisms are sometimes referred to as closed NTDs as opposed to the open NTDs (anencephaly, meningomyelocele or spina bifida and craniorachischisis). In general, the occult spinal dysraphisms are conditions, thought not to result from defects in primary neural tube closure but may arise due to defects in secondary neural tube development.

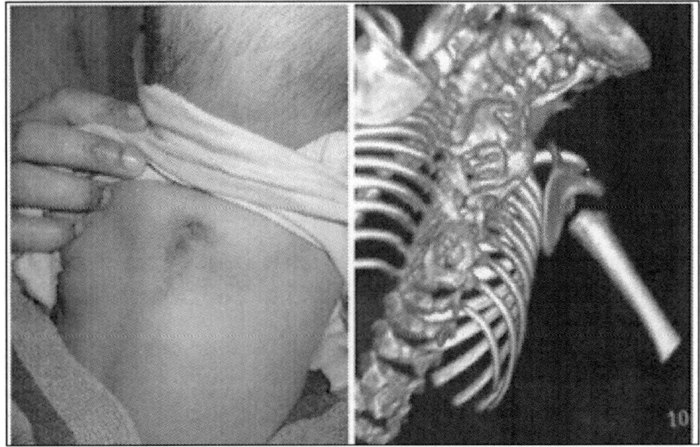

Fig. 8.7: Occult spinal dysraphism with overlying hairy skin cover. The spinal defect is visualised by CT (computerised tomography) with 3 D reconstruction

Risk factors for NTDs: The open NTDs, which are relatively common, are recognized as being etiologically heterogeneous.[7,8]

Folic acid deficiency: Folic acid deficiency in mother has been implicated as the single most important risk factor for NTDs. It has been shown that the incidence decreases by 50 to 70% by folic acid supplementation in women in child bearing age, in various studies.

Though found in small number of individuals, the following are other risk factors for NTDs:

- Maternal use of medications – Valproic acid, carbamazepine (CBZ) etc or other antifolate drugs.
- Family history – Risk in siblings of affected individuals is 3% to 8%.

- Maternal insulin-dependent diabetes.
- Obesity – The risk of having a child with an NTD increases with increasing maternal body mass index (BMI).
- Hyperthermia – There is an increased risk for NTDs, in particular anencephaly, in infants whose mothers were exposed to hyperthermia during the first trimester of pregnancy.
- Reproductive technologies – There is an association between assisted reproductive technologies and the risk of congenital malformations, including NTDs.
- Autoantibodies to folate receptors.
- Environmental occupational hazards.
- Chromosomal and genetic disorders – Though rare, some chromosomal and Mendelian disorders have been associated with NTD.

Prevention strategies: NTDs as a group is amenable to prevention at different stages.

Primary prevention: Use of periconceptional folic acid (starting 3 months prior to conception as a common practice) is being universally accepted as the best prevention strategy. The recommended dose is 0.5 mg daily; however, the preparation available in the market contains 5 mg of folic acid per tablet. Folic acid is a water soluble vitamin and the extra is supposed to be excreted in urine without any side effects.

Fortification of food with folic acid has been tried by some countries.

Secondary prevention: Screening to identify pregnant women who are at an increased risk of carrying an NTD-affected fetus can be achieved by the evaluation of maternal serum alphafetoprotein levels[9] as a part of biochemical screening for aneuploidies (like triple test). However, a more practical approach is a careful ultrasonography, as a part of anomaly scan. It is likely to pick up a high percentage of all NTDs before 20 weeks of gestation (legal gestational age for termination of the affected pregnancy). When a diagnosis of spina bifida is confirmed by ultrasound before 20 weeks of gestation, the couple need to be counselled about the advantages of detection of the anomaly before the legal gestational age of termination of pregnancy.[10] Ultrasonography and sometimes fetal MRI is used to identify spontaneous leg movements, spine deformities and the presence of associated Chiari II malformation. The couple can take decisions of termination of pregnancy or continuation of the same according to the associated complications, probable outcome after surgery and social and religious beliefs.

Management and outcome: Although anencephaly and craniorachischisis are lethal conditions, individuals with spina bifida can survive with appropriate medical and surgical treatment. Those babies who are live born with a spina bifina, is likely to get their spinal lesion closed postnatally early in the neonatal period, usually within 3 days after birth. In advanced centres, a small proportion of fetuses undergo surgeries in utero. Literature depicts better outcome in babies who undergo surgeries in utero; however, the expertise required for such procedures is high. Whether treated in utero or postnatally, children with spina bifida are at risk of hydrocephalus, complications of Chiari II malformations, lower limb paralysis, sensory loss, bowel and bladder dysfunction, spinal deformities and club foot. Though most children treated adequately have normal intelligence, some cognitive and learning problems are common in such children. The most important determinant of neurological outcome is the level of the lesion, the more proximal the lesion, the poorer the outcome. Post surgery, one year survival among individuals with spina bifida is around 85 to 90%, however, many of these individuals have significant comorbidities and increased mortality, sometimes presenting as sudden death.

Genetic counselling: Apart from the above mentioned issues for counselling, the couple must be counselled about the chance of chromosomal abnormality, single gene disorder, or teratogenic exposure in a small percentage of such babies. Prenatal testing for chromosomes and probable single gene disorders should be offered to all couples. Those who opt for termination with or without prenatal testing should be offered post-mortem examination. Such testing and examination is essential for effective genetic counselling which helps couples to take future reproductive decisions. Recurrence risk depends on the underlying cause, if any. When a chromosomal and single gene disorder is not identified, the empiric recurrence risk is around 3-5%. Special care should be taken during counseling of women, where there is a probable teratogenic cause. Women on anti-epileptic drugs need to be counselled about possible tertogenic effects including NTD. As a rule, possible monotherapy at possible lowest dose for effective control of seizures need to be adjusted pre-pregnancy. Valproate use should be preferably avoided in pregnant women by all possible means.

(II) MIDLINE MALFORMATIONS OF THE FOREBRAIN

Failed or incomplete separation of the forebrain early in gestation results in holoprosencephaly (HPE).

Classification of holoprosencephaly (HPE): Classic HPE includes a continuum of brain malformations and can be classified in order of decreasing severity as below:

- **Alobar HPE**, the most severe, in which there is a single monoventricle and no separation of the cerebral hemispheres.
- **Semilobar HPE**, in which the left and right frontal and parietal lobes are fused and the interhemispheric fissure is only present posteriorly.
- **Lobar HPE**, in which most of the right and left cerebral hemispheres and lateral ventricles are separated but the frontal lobes, most rostral aspect of the telencephalon, are fused, especially ventrally.
- **Middle interhemispheric** fusion variant (MIHF/ MIHV or syntelencephaly), in which the posterior frontal and parietal lobes fail to separate, with varying lack of cleavage of the basal ganglia and thalami and absence of the body of the corpus callosum but presence of the genu and splenium of the corpus callosum.[11]
- A **septopreoptic** type, in which non-separation is restricted to the septal and/or preoptic regions; described in small case series.
- **Microforms of HPE** with mild craniofacial anomalies without obvious neurologic findings on conventional neuroimaging.
- **Other structural CNS findings with HPE:** There are some other structural CNS findings that may occur with but are not specific to HPE:
- **Anomalies of midline structures:** Undivided thalami, absent corpus callosum, callosal dysgenesis, absent septum pellucidum, absent or hypoplastic olfactory bulbs and tracts (arrhinencephaly) and optic bulbs and tracts.
- Macrocephaly secondary to hydrocephalus.
- Dandy-Walker malformation.
- Neuronal migration anomalies.
- Abnormal circle of Willis.
- Caudal dysgenesis.

Craniofacial anomalies associated with HPE: HPE is accompanied by a spectrum of craniofacial anomalies in around 80%.[12] The facial changes help in recognition of the underlying anomalies of the brain (Fig. 8.8). Though it is generally believed that more severe facial anomalies are associated with severe brain anomaly, the facial anomalies may be subtle in severe forms of HPE as well. The spectrum of facial anomalies is as follows:

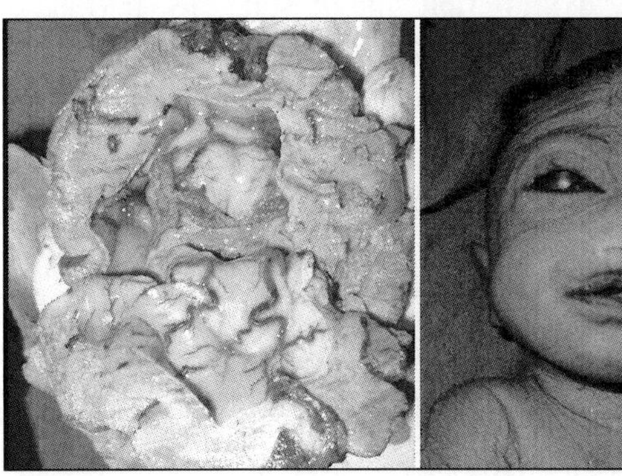

Fig. 8.8: Semilobar holoprosencephaly (HPE), in brain: The left and right frontal and parietal lobes are fused and the interhemispheric fissure is only present posteriorly. Note the closely spaced eyes with single-nostril in nose (cebocephaly) in the fetus

- **Cyclopia:** Single eye or partially divided eye in single orbit with a proboscis above the eye.
- Cyclopia without proboscis.
- **Ethmocephaly:** Extremely closely spaced eyes but separate orbits with proboscis between the eyes.
- **Cebocephaly:** Closely spaced eyes with single-nostril in nose.
- Closely spaced eyes (hypotelorism).
- Anophthalmia or microophthalmia.
- Premaxillary agenesis with median cleft lip, closely spaced eyes, depressed nasal bridge.
- Bilateral cleft lip.
- Palatal abnormalities like clefts, ridge, high arched palate, bifid uvula etc.
- Single maxillary central incisor.

Clinical Manifestations of HPE

- **Developmental delay** in variable degree is present in almost all individuals with the HPE, associated with CNS anomalies.
- **Microcephaly** is common in HPE.
- **Seizures** are common, many a times, difficult to control.
- **Hydrocephalus** can occur and may result in macrocephaly, instead of the more commonly observed microcephaly.

- **Neural tube defects** in a small proportion of individuals.
- **Hypothalamic and brainstem dysfunction** may lead to swallowing difficulties and instability of temperature, heart rate and respiration.
- **Pituitary dysfunction** manifesting as partial or complete panhypopituitarism.
- **Short stature** and **failure to thrive.**
- **Feeding difficulties** and choking episodes.
- **Excessive intestinal gas/colic**, irritability and constipation.
- **Altered sleep patterns.**

Prevalence of HPE: HPE is the most common forebrain defect in humans, with a prevalence of 1:250 in embryos and approximately 1:10,000 among live-born infants.

Etiology of HPE

Environmental Causes:

Maternal diabetes mellitus: Infants of diabetic mothers have a 1% risk (a 200-fold increase) for HPE.

Maternal use of cholesterol-lowering agents: Use of statins by mother has been associated with HPE.

Chromosomal anomalies: Around 25%-50% babies with HPE have a chromosomal abnormality.[13,14] Trisomy 13, trisomy 18 and triploidy (total 69 chromosomes) are the most common numerical chromosomal anomalies associated with HPE. Structural chromosomal abnormalities associated with HPE have been commonly reported with deletions and duplications involving chromosomes 13q (Fig. 8.9), 18p, 7q, 3p, 2p, 21q etc. probably denoting the areas of genome harbouring the various genes associated with HPE.

Single gene disorders: Mutation in single genes can cause syndromic and non-syndromic forms of HPE.

(a) Syndromic HPE (approximately 18%-25% of individuals with HPE):

- ***Autosomal dominant***
  - Pallister-Hall syndrome.
  - Rubinstein-Taybi syndrome.
  - Kallmann syndrome.
  - Martin syndrome (clubfoot, spinal anomalies).
  - Steinfeld syndrome (congenital heart disease, absent gallbladder, renal dysplasia, radial defects).
  - Hartsfield syndrome (ectrodactyly).
  - Otocephaly-agnathia spectrum disorder.
- ***Autosomal recessive***
  - Pseudotrisomy 13 syndrome.
  - Smith-Lemli-Opitz syndrome.

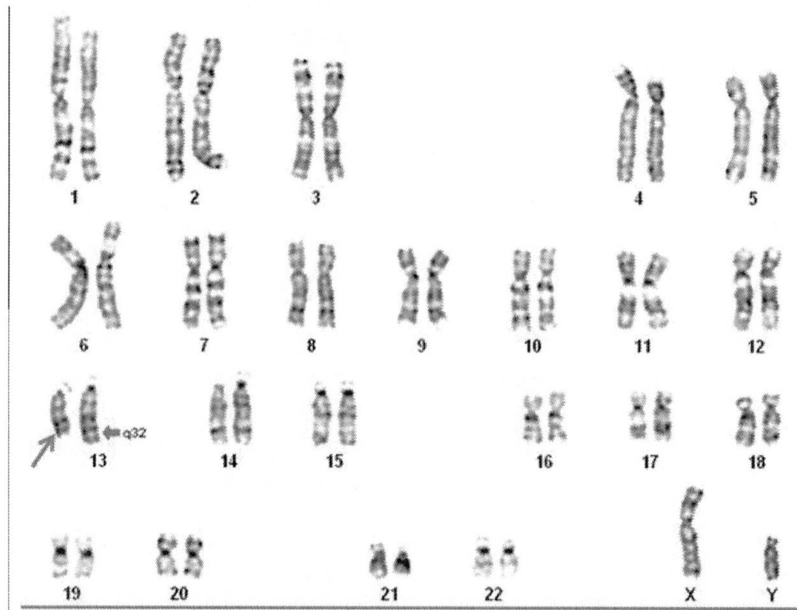

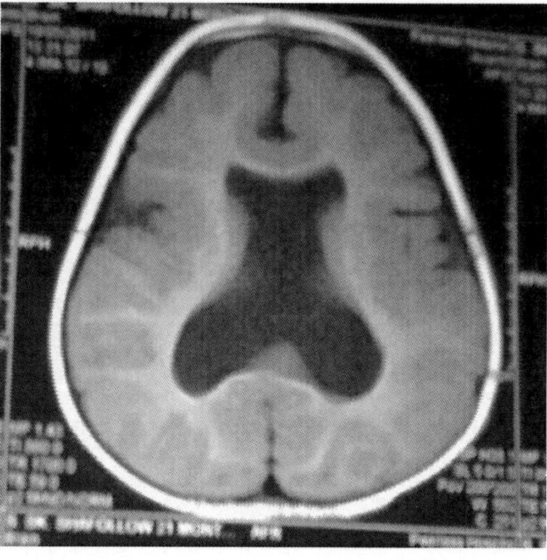

Fig. 8.9: Karyotype showing 13q deletion (arrow); deletion is noted from band q32 (shown in normal chromosome 13 with broad arrow). MRI brain of the child is showing dilated lateral ventricles, lack of interventricular septum – forming a single ventricle, and pachygyria. The child presented with developmental delay and limb anomalies

- Meckel syndrome.
- Genoa syndrome (craniosynostosis).
- Lambotte syndrome (microcephaly, prenatal growth retardation, widely spaced eyes).
- Hydrolethalus syndrome (hydrocephalus, polydactyly and other anomalies).
- Facial clefts and brachial amelia.

(b) **Nonsyndromic HPE:** The nonsyndromic forms of HPE are single gene disorders with HPE and facial features.[15,16] They are generally not associated with other obvious malformations and are not a part of a known syndrome with HPE. The clinical manifestations of individuals with nonsyndromic HPE is extremely variable, even within the same family. Most forms are autosomal dominant at the molecular level. The various common genes associated with nonsyndromic HPE are as below:

Genes associated with autosomal dominant non-syndromic HPE

Gene Symbol	Chromosomal Locus	Percentage of individuals with HPE and mutations in the mentioned gene	
		With family history	Simplex/ sporadic cases
SHH	7q36	30%-40%	< 5%
ZIC2	13q32	5%	2%
SIX3	2p21	1.3%	Rare

Other known genes are *GIF1, GLI2, PTCH1, DISP1, FGF8, FOXH1, NODAL, TDGF1 (CRIPTO), GAS1, DLL1* and *CDON*.

Outcome of HPE: Most fetuses affected with HPE do not survive, and mostly die in utero. Severely affected children do not survive beyond early infancy, whereas a significant proportion of mildly affected children survive past their infancy. Mildly manifesting individuals with "microform" HPE survive till adulthood and produce children.[17,18]

Diagnosis of HPE

- Imaging of the brain by CT or MRI confirms the diagnosis of HPE and may define the anatomic subtype. It also identifies associated CNS anomalies.
- Approximately 25%-50% of individuals with HPE have a numeric or structural chromosomal abnormality detectable by routine karyotype or chromosomal microarray.
- Approximately 18%-25% of individuals with monogenic HPE have a recognizable syndrome and the remainder nonsyndromic HPE. Around 10% of individuals with HPE have defects in cholesterol biosynthesis. Molecular genetic testing of putative genes is indicated either by Sanger sequencing or Next-generation sequencing (NGS) techniques is indicated in all monogenic forms of HPE. Deletion duplication analysis by multiplex ligation-dependent probe amplification (MLPA) or chromosomal microarray in case sequence variation is not identified.

Management: Treatment should be preferably by a multidisciplinary team. The various components of treatment are:

- Hormone replacement therapy for pituitary dysfunction.
- Antiepileptic drugs for seizures.
- Surgical treatments for feeding difficulties and gastroesophageal reflux - like gastrostomy tube and Nissen fundoplication.
- Special feeding devices and surgical repair of cleft lip and/or palate.
- Ventriculo-peritoneal shunt placement for hydrocephalus.
- Physiotherapy, occupational therapy and special education for developmental disabilities.
- Surveillance.
- Parental support and counseling.

Genetic counseling: Genetic counseling and recurrence risk assessment depend on determination of the specific cause of HPE in an individual. Mutation testing can be offered for prenatal testing if mutation is detected in the affected child. Prenatal ultrasonography is likely to detect most major brain anomalies and aid in prenatal diagnosis of HPE.

(III) DISORDERS OF CEREBRAL CORTICAL DEVELOPMENT

Embryology: Malformations of the cerebral cortex have their origins during the process of cortical development. Understanding normal cortical development is essential when considering these disorders.

The neurons of the human brain are formed in a pseudostratified columnar neuroepithelium of the ventricular zone. They gradually migrate radially and tangentially over considerable distances of several millimetres to reach their final destination. The neural progenitor cells give rise to postmitotic neurons and also to a secondary population of progenitor cells in the subventricular zone. The subventricular zone contains two major types of progenitors, the basal progenitors and the multipotent progenitors. The basal progenitors are short-lived, and produce individual cell types such as neuron or glia. The multipotential progenitors are only found in humans and mammals with a large cerebral cortex. The first group of cells, the postmitotic neurons produces a layer called the primordial plexiform layer or preplate. The preplate later on get slit into an outer layer ("marginal zone") and a deeper layer ("subplate") by a group of neurons that form the cortical plate. Neurons add to the cortical plate in an inside-out manner, with the newer-arriving neurons migrating past the older cortical plate neurons until they get arrested next to the marginal zone. The marginal zone, which contains specialized neurons called Cajal-Retzius cells, seems to be instrumental in establishing the inside-out laminar gradient of the cortical plate.[19,20] The migration of cortical plate neurons is guided by long radially aligned fibers of radial glial cells. Nonradial (tangential) neuronal migration is also common in the developing cortex. Tangential migration is seen particularly in inhibitory interneurons, originating outside of the cortex. A vast diversity of molecules has been implicated in the development of the cortex and the genetic basis is known for many developmental anomalies of the cortex.[21]

In the human cortex, postmitotic neurons start migrating out of the ventricular zone by the sixth and seventh week of gestation and form the primordial plexiform layer. Migration of neurons peaks between the 11th and 15th week of gestation. Although it is not clear when migration is finally completed in the cerebral cortex, the majority of neurons are found to have entered the cortex by the 24th week of gestation.

Classification: Although a universally applicable classification for malformations of cortical development is difficult to find, a system proposed by Barkovich *et al.* is helpful and is described below:

I. Malformations Due to Abnormal Neuronal and Glial Proliferation or Apoptosis

A. Decreased proliferation/increased apoptosis (microcephaly)

1. Microcephaly with normal or mildly simplified gyri.
   a. Microcephaly vera (primary autosomal recessive microcephaly).
   b. Microcephaly, seizures and developmental delay.
   c. Microcephaly with proportionate short stature.
   d. Others.
2. Microlissencephaly (severe microcephaly with significant simplification of gyri).
3. Microcephaly with other brain malformations (e.g., polymicrogyria, pontocerebellar hypoplasia).

B. Increased proliferation/decreased apoptosis (megalencephaly).

C. Abnormal proliferation and differentiation (non-neoplastic).

1. Cortical tubers of tuberous sclerosis.
2. Focal cortical dysplasia.
3. Hemimegalencephaly.

II. Malformations Due to Abnormal Neuronal Migration

A. Classical lissencephaly/subcortical band heterotopia

1. LIS1-associated lissencephaly.
2. X-linked lissencephaly 1.
3. X-linked lissencephaly 2.
4. TUBA1A-associated lissencephaly.

B. Cobblestone dysplasia

C. Gray matter heterotopia

1. X-linked periventricular heterotopia.
2. Autosomal recessive periventricular heterotopia with microcephaly.
3. Heterotopia due to chromosomal aberration.

III. Malformations Due to Abnormal Cortical Organization (Includes Later Stages of Neuronal Migration)

A. Polymicrogyria

1. Bilateral frontoparietal polymicrogyria.
2. Bilateral perisylvian polymicrogyria.

3. Bilateral occipital polymicrogyria.
4. Bilateral generalized polymicrogyria.
5. Other localized polymicrogyria syndromes.
6. Tubulin-associated polymicrogyria.
7. Polymicrogyria due to chromosomal aberration.

B. Schizencephaly.

IV. Malformations of Cortical Development, Not Otherwise Classified

A. Malformations secondary to inborn errors of metabolism.

B. Others.

Overview of Different Malformations of Cortical Development

Description of all above mentioned disorders is beyond the scope of this chapter. We will only be describing a few important terms and cover few important topics:

Classical Lissencephaly: Lissencephaly signifies a smooth brain with a lack or overt paucity of normal gyri (Fig. 8.10). Classical (or Type I) lissencephaly is characterized by a severely thickened cerebral cortex with three or four abnormal layers instead of the normal six layers of the cortex. On the other hand, "cobblestone" (or Type II) lissencephaly is a completely different entity histologically. Several clinical entities are associated with classical lissencephaly, including isolated lissencephaly sequence (ILS), Miller-Dieker syndrome (MDS), X-linked lissencephaly 1 and X-linked lissencephaly 2. The most common cause of classical lissencephaly is a mutation of a gene on chromosome 17p13 known as *LIS1*. Deletion or mutation in the *LIS1* gene is the cause of lissencephaly both in MDS and in ILS.[22, 23, 24] Additional clinical findings in MDS include dysmorphism in form an abnormal facies with microcephaly, bitemporal hollowing with narrowing at the temples, tall and prominent forehead with vertical furrowing, hypertelorism with upward slanting palpebral fissures and ptosis, short nose with upturned nares, low-set ears with minor flattening of the helices, prominent philtrum with thin vermilion border of the upper lip, and small mandible. Digital abnormalities, such as syndactyly, congenital heart disease, and other visceral abnormalities may be seen in patients with MDS. Almost all children with classical lissencephaly have profound developmental delay and intellectual disability; many of them die during infancy or childhood. The majority of the patients have seizures, typically starting during the first 6 months of life.

On imaging studies, the cerebral hemispheres show agyria (lack of gyri) or pachygyria (broadening of

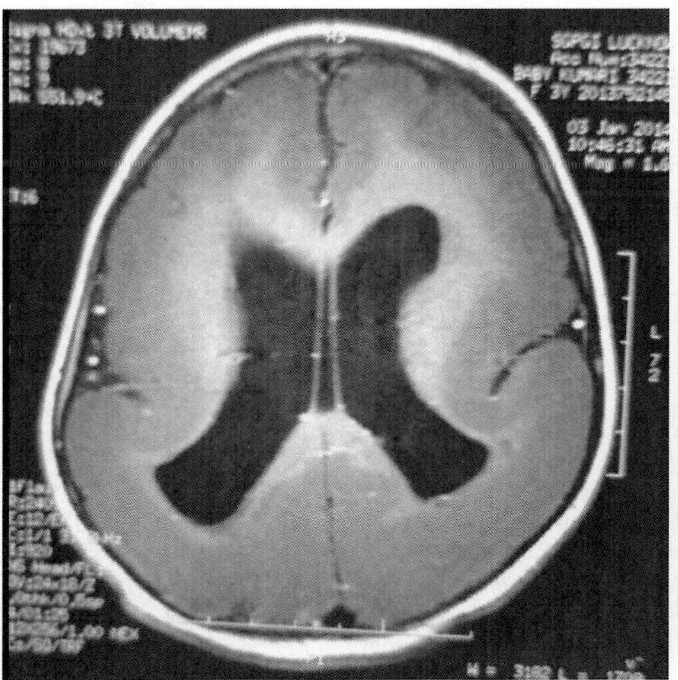

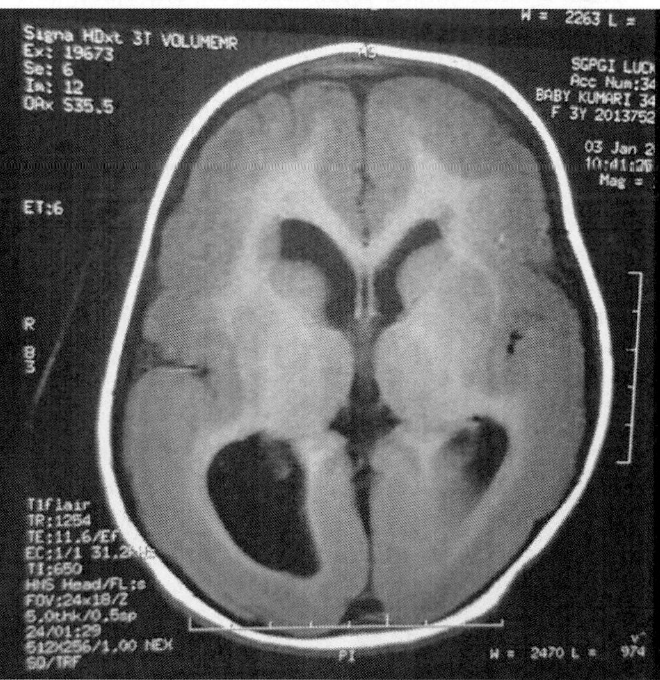

Fig. 8.10: Lissencephaly with agyria (lack of gyri) and pachygyria (broadening of gyri)

gyri): often these two features coexist. The frontal and temporal opercula (the parts of the brain that cover insular cortices) are not developed, leading to a characteristic "figure-of-eight" shape appearance of the brain on axial images with bitemporal hollowing. Agenesis or hypogenesis of the corpus callosum may be seen, and small midline calcifications in the region of the septum pellucidum may be observed in patients with MDS.

X-Linked Lissencephaly 1/Subcortical Band Heterotopia: A familial, X-linked form of lissencephaly (LISX1) has also been identified and is associated with a higher recurrence risk than classical lissencephaly due to LIS1 mutations. LISX1 manifests in affected males with severe intellectual disability, intractable seizures, lissencephaly with pachygyria/agyria, agenesis of corpus callosum, and death during infancy. Carrier females, typically mildly affected with intellectual disability and epilepsy, has subcortical band heterotopia (SBH), also known as double cortex syndrome. SBH is characterized by symmetric stretches of gray matter found in the central white matter between the cortex and the ventricular surface. The gene responsible for LISX1/ SBH is named doublecortin (DCX).[25, 26]

X-Linked Lissencephaly 2 (X-Linked Lissencephaly with Abnormal Genitalia): This is another form of X-linked lissencephaly, LISX2, associated with agenesis of the corpus callosum and ambiguous or underdeveloped genitalia. The causative gene for this syndrome was identified as the Aristaless-related homeobox transcription factor gene, ARX. ARX has been shown to regulate tangential migration of interneurons and neuronal proliferation.

Cobblestone Dysplasia: Cobblestone dysplasia is characterized by disorganized cortical layers. There is over migration of neurons onto the outside of the brain through breaches in the pial surface, and gliovascular proliferation giving a bumpy cobblestone-like appearance. The gyral pattern seen on imaging studies varies widely, including polymicrogyria, pachygyria and agyria. Cobblestone dysplasia is the characteristic brain malformation observed in a group of disorders, sometimes referred to as "dystroglycanopathies", which includes three characteristic autosomal recessive disorders: Fukuyama congenital muscular dystrophy (FCMD), Walker-Warburg syndrome (WWS), and muscle-eye-brain disease (MEB). All the three syndromes are associated with cobblestone dysplasia and affect the muscle and eye along with the brain. As the genetic studies of these disorders progressed, it became clear that there is significant clinical and genetic overlap among these conditions. In typical FCMD, the frontal lobes show polymicrogyria, and cobblestone dysplasia is limited to the temporo-occipital area. WWS presents more dramatically, with diffuse agyric or pachygyric areas, enlarged ventricles, hypoplasia of the pons and cerebellar vermis, fusion of the superior and inferior colliculi, and a diffuse abnormality of the cerebral white matter. Imaging findings of MEB are similar to that of WWS, but abnormalities are usually less extensive. Cerebellar polymicrogyria with or without small cysts can be seen in any of these disorders. The various genes implicated are FKTN (fukutin), FKRP (fukutin-related protein), POMGNT1 (protein O-mannose beta-1, 2-N-acetylglucosaminyl transferase), POMT1 (protein O-mannosyltransferases), POMT2, LARGE etc.

X-Linked Periventricular Heterotopia: Gray matter heterotopias are masses of well-differentiated neurons in abnormal locations, reflecting arrested radial neuronal migration. Periventricular heterotopia (PH) can be encountered as a sporadic condition, but there are several genetic syndromes in which heterotopias are a cardinal feature. One such syndrome is X-linked PH, for which many familial cases are known. In these pedigrees, typically only females were affected and there was a high rate of miscarriages among the affected females. These observations led to the suggestion that the condition was an X-linked disorder with prenatal lethality in males. Females affected with X-linked PH typically present with epilepsy, commonly generalized tonic-clonic or complex partial seizures. Typical age of onset is before the mid-twenties, and the average age is around 15 years. Intelligence is usually normal, although some patients have borderline intellectual disability, and dyslexia is remarkably common. An increased incidence of patent ductus arteriosus and stroke at young ages has been noted. Abnormalities in cardiac valve development have also been reported in some cases. An increasing number of affected patients have vascular manifestations of Ehlers-Danlos syndrome. Brain MRI of affected females typically shows bilateral PH nodules, which show the typical signal characteristics of normal gray matter. Pathologically, brains of females with X-linked PH show continuous bands or discontinuous nodules of gray matter along the periventricular region, consisting of well-differentiated cortical neurons. The heterotopic subependymal nodules of X-linked PH may initially be misdiagnosed as TSC nodules, but classical lesions of X-linked PH appear as roughly symmetric nodules as opposed to the less confluent and not necessarily symmetric nodules of TSC.

X-linked PH was mapped to distal Xq28, and subsequently mutations in the FLNA (filamin A) gene were identified to be the cause. Mutations in FLNA have been identified in almost 100% of familial cases of X-linked PH and 26% of sporadic patients with classical bilateral nodular PH. In rare instances, male patients with PH have FLNA mutations, but the majority of male patients are negative for FLNA mutations. FLNA mutations have also been identified in patients with various other disorders like otopalatodigital syndrome types 1 and 2, frontometaphysial dysplasia, Melnick-Needles syndrome, FG syndrome-2, terminal osseous dysplasia and cardiac valvular dysplasia. FLNA is expressed by the cortical neurons during migration, and possibly regulates the actin cytoskeleton in response to the extracellular signals during neuronal migration.

Other Genetic Heterotopia Syndromes: Heterotopias have been seen in association with various chromosomal anomalies like 5p anomalies, 5q deletion, 7q11.23 deletion and 1p36 deletion. An autosomal recessive syndrome with heterotopia associated with microcephaly was found to be caused by mutation in the ADP-ribosylation factor guanine nucleotide-exchange factor-2 gene (ARFGEF2).

Polymicrogyria: Polymicrogyria refers to a cortical malformation characterized by numerous small gyri. Clinical presentations of polymicrogyria depend on the extent and location of the abnormal cortex. When the abnormality is diffuse, severe developmental delay is the rule, but when it is focal, developmental delay is less severe. Some individuals with small regions of focal polymicrogyria have normal intelligence. Seizures are common in both groups. On MRI, small meandering gyri of polymicrogyric cortex may appear as thickened cortex, and it may be difficult to distinguish from "pachygyria" (thickened cortex). Irregularity of the junction between the cortex and white matter is usually evident with high-resolution imaging. In recent years, several distinctive syndromes of polymicrogyria have emerged. These syndromes, which are mainly distinguished by characteristic distributions of polymicrogyric cortex, include:

- Bilateral frontoparietal polymicrogyria (BFPP).
- Congenital bilateral perisylvian syndrome (CBPS) also known as bilateral perisylvian polymicrogyria (BPP).
- Bilateral generalized polymicrogyria (BGP).
- Bilateral occipital polymicrogyria (BOP).

BFPP is associated with moderate to severe developmental delay, seizures (usual onset after 4–5 years), bilateral pyramidal and cerebellar signs, and dysconjugate gaze. CBPS is characterized by diplegia of the facial, pharyngea, and masticatory muscles (pseudobulbar palsy). BGP is characterized by motor and cognitive delay and seizures.

Polymicrogyria is usually encountered as a sporadic condition; however, it has become evident that there are distinct genetic syndromes with polymicrogyria. It is associated with chromosome 22q11 deletions and recurrent copy number variations at 1p36.3, 2p16.1-p23.1, 4q21.21-q22.1, 6q26-q27 and 21q2. The gene mutated in BFPP was found to be GPR56, which encodes a G-protein coupled receptor. Recently, mutations in LAMC3, encoding a laminin protein that is characteristic of the pial basement membrane, has also been discovered in association with polymicrogyria in the occipital region. Intrauterine insults (e.g., cytomegalovirus infection) and metabolic disorders have been associated with polymicrogyria as well, but genetic forms of polymicrogyria always need to be considered. Bandlike calcification of the brain with simplified gyral pattern and polymicrogyria (OMIM 251290), which resembles TORCH (Toxoplasmosis, Other, Rubella, Cytomegalovirus, Herpes simplex virus) infection and sometimes referred to as pseudo-TORCH syndrome, is associated with mutations in a tight-junction protein gene, OCLN.

Tubulinopathies and Polymicrogyria: TUBA1A is a gene encoding a microtubule-related protein that is associated with brain malformations, typically lissencephaly with other features. Mutations in TUBA1A are also responsible for some cases of BPP. Mutations in the gene encoding β-tubulin, TUBB2B, have been reported in some cases of asymmetrical polymicrogyria. Mutations in TUBA8 have been implicated in a form of polymicrogyria associated with optic nerve hypoplasia and mutations in the gene TUBB3 have been seen in cases of frontally predominant polymicrogyria associated with basal ganglia dysmorphism, corpus callosum abnormalities and mild brainstem hypoplasia.

Schizencephaly: The term "schizencephaly" refers to a brain malformation characterized by full-thickness cleft of the cerebral mantle. The walls of the clefts are usually lined by polymicrogyric cortex. Schizencephaly can be divided into two subtypes, namely closed-lip schizencephaly and open-lip schizencephaly. In closed-lip schizencephaly, two walls are in apposition and form a so-called "pial-ependymal seam". On the other hand, in open-lip schizencephaly the two walls are apart and the space between the two walls is filled with cerebrospinal fluid (CSF). The clinical presentation varies depending on the extent and location of anatomical abnormalities. Closed-lip schizencephaly often presents with hemiparesis or motor delay, and open-lip schizencephaly may present with the same features as well as seizures.

Mutation in the EMX2 gene, in heterozygous state, has been reported in sporadic and familial cases of schizencephaly; however, subsequent effort failed to identify any pathogenic EMX2 mutation in more than 100 patients with schizencephaly. Recently, a few patients with WDR62 mutations were found to have schizencephaly as well as microcephaly. Schizencephaly can also definitely be caused by nongenetic aetiology such as death of monozygotic co-twin, in utero exposure to warfarin, alcohol and cocaine.

Malformations Secondary to Inborn Errors of Metabolism: Typically, inborn errors of metabolism cause degenerative cerebral lesions; however, several metabolic disorders are associated with developmental malformations of the cerebral cortex. For example, neuronal migration abnormalities, particularly perisylvian pachygyria and polymicrogyria, are a prominent feature of Zellweger syndrome. Other inborn errors of metabolism associated with developmental disorders of the cerebral cortex include multiple acyl-CoA dehydrogenase deficiency (glutaric aciduria type II) as well as mitochondrial disorders and disorders of pyruvate metabolism. Amish lethal Microcephaly, maternal phenylketonuria and phosphoglycerate dehydrogenase deficiency are metabolic causes of congenital microcephaly.

(IV) AGENESIS OR HYPOPLASIA OF CORPUS CALLOSUM

Dysgenesis of the corpus callosum, complete (agenesis) or partial (hypoplasia) represents an *in utero* developmental anomaly.

It can be divided into:

- **Primary agenesis:** The corpus callosum never forms.
- **Secondary dysgenesis:** The corpus callosum forms normally and is subsequently destroyed.

A true estimate of incidence is difficult to establish as many isolated cases are asymptomatic. It may be as common as 1:20,000 according to an autopsy series. There appears to be a male predilection (M:F ~2:1).

Embryology: The development of the corpus callosum occurs between the 12th and 16th weeks of gestation. It begins with the genu and then continues posteriorly along the body to the splenium. The rostrum is the last part to be formed.

Pathogenesis: Agenesis is a result of an insult occurring at approximately 8-12 weeks gestation resulting in failure to form the corpus callosum. The white matter tracts, which usually cross the midline horizontally, are instead oriented vertically. These bundles of white matter, known as Probst bundles, separate the lateral ventricles widely. The anterior commissure is usually present and often enlarged. The hippocampal formations are usually hypoplastic, with resultant dilatation of the temporal horns of the lateral ventricles. Dysgenesis (which may be complete or partial) is a result of encephalomalacia secondary to toxic, ischemic or traumatic events.

Associations: Most cases of corpus callosum agenesis are sporadic and may be isolated; however, an association with the following are being noted:

- **Chromosomal aneuploidy**
  - Trisomy 18.
  - Trisomy 13.
  - Trisomy 8.
- **Single gene and other syndromic conditions**
  - Aicardi syndrome.
  - Apert syndrome.
  - Coffin-Siris syndrome.
  - Fryns syndrome.
  - Gorlin syndrome.
  - Hydrolethalus syndrome.
  - Lowe syndrome.

- Zellweger syndrome.

- **Other CNS malformations**
  - Chiari II malformation.
  - Dandy-Walker spectrum.
  - Grey matter heterotopia.
  - Holoprosencephaly.
  - Interhemispheric cysts.
  - Intracranial lipoma.
  - Polymicrogyria.
  - Porencephaly.
- **Teratogenic condition**
  - Fetal alcohol syndrome.
- **Inborn errors of metabolism**
  - Non-ketotic hyperglycemia.
  - Pyruvate metabolism disorders.
  - Congenital lactic acidosis (due to mitochondrial respiratory chain defects).
  - Mucopolysaccharidoses.
  - Mucolipidoses.

Clinical Presentation: Isolated partial dysgenesis of the corpus callosum is often asymptomatic. The clinical picture in other cases is dictated by the associated abnormalities that are frequently found, especially in agenesis.

Radiographic Features: Though MRI is the modality of choice in evaluating both the corpus callosum and the frequently associated anomalies, an antenatal ultrasound often picks up the following signs:

- Lateral ventricles are widely spaced parallel bodies (racing car sign) with small frontal horns and colpocephaly: which can give a "tear drop" configuration on axial scans.
- Third ventricle is dilated, can be elevated or dorsally displaced, may communicate with the interhemispheric cistern, may project superiorly as a dorsal cyst and choroid may be seen as echogenic structure in the roof of the cyst.
- **Septum pellucidum:** Absent.

Aicardi Syndrome: Amongst all disorders with corpus callosum agenesis, Aicardi syndrome warrants special mention. It is characterized by a triad of callosal agenesis, infantile spasms, and chorioretinal lacunae ('holes'). Occurrence of flexion spasms in a normal looking female infant is the usual mode of clinical presentation. These spasms develop into epilepsy, which are difficult to treat. Children with Aicardi syndrome often have additional brain abnormalities, including asymmetry between the two sides of the brain, hydrocephalus and porencephalic cysts (Fig. 8.11).

In addition to chorioretinal lacunae, children with Aicardi syndrome may have other eye abnormalities such as microphthalmia or a coloboma in the optic nerve, causing blindness. These children often have gastrointestinal problems such as constipation or diarrhea, gastroesophageal reflux and difficulty in feeding.

The severity of Aicardi syndrome varies. Some children with this disorder have very severe epilepsy and may not survive past childhood. Less severely affected individuals may live into adulthood with milder signs and symptoms. Most affected children have moderate to severe developmental delay and intellectual disability.

The inheritance of Aicardi syndrome is X-linked dominant, with probable locus at Xp22. All cases are probably due to new mutations. Affected males die in utero.

(V) AGENESIS OF CRANIAL NERVES

Agenesis of cranial nerves is rare. They are sporadic in occurrence in most situations. Well described group of disorders are Moebius syndrome and bilateral optic nerve hypoplasia.

Moebius Syndrome: The most basic description of Moebius syndrome is a congenital facial palsy with impairment of ocular abduction. The facial nerve (cranial nerve VII) and abducens nerve (CN VI) are most frequently involved, but other cranial nerves may be involved as well. Other variable features include orofacial dysmorphism and limb malformations. Mental retardation has been reported in a subset of patients. Most cases of Moebius syndrome are sporadic, but familial occurrence has been reported. In MRI studies of patients with Moebius syndrome, features described are: straightening of the floor of the fourth ventricle and absence of the medial colliculus at the level of the pons, suggesting hypoplasia of the VIth (abducens) and VIIth (facial) nuclei, absence of the hypoglossal eminence at the medulla, consistent

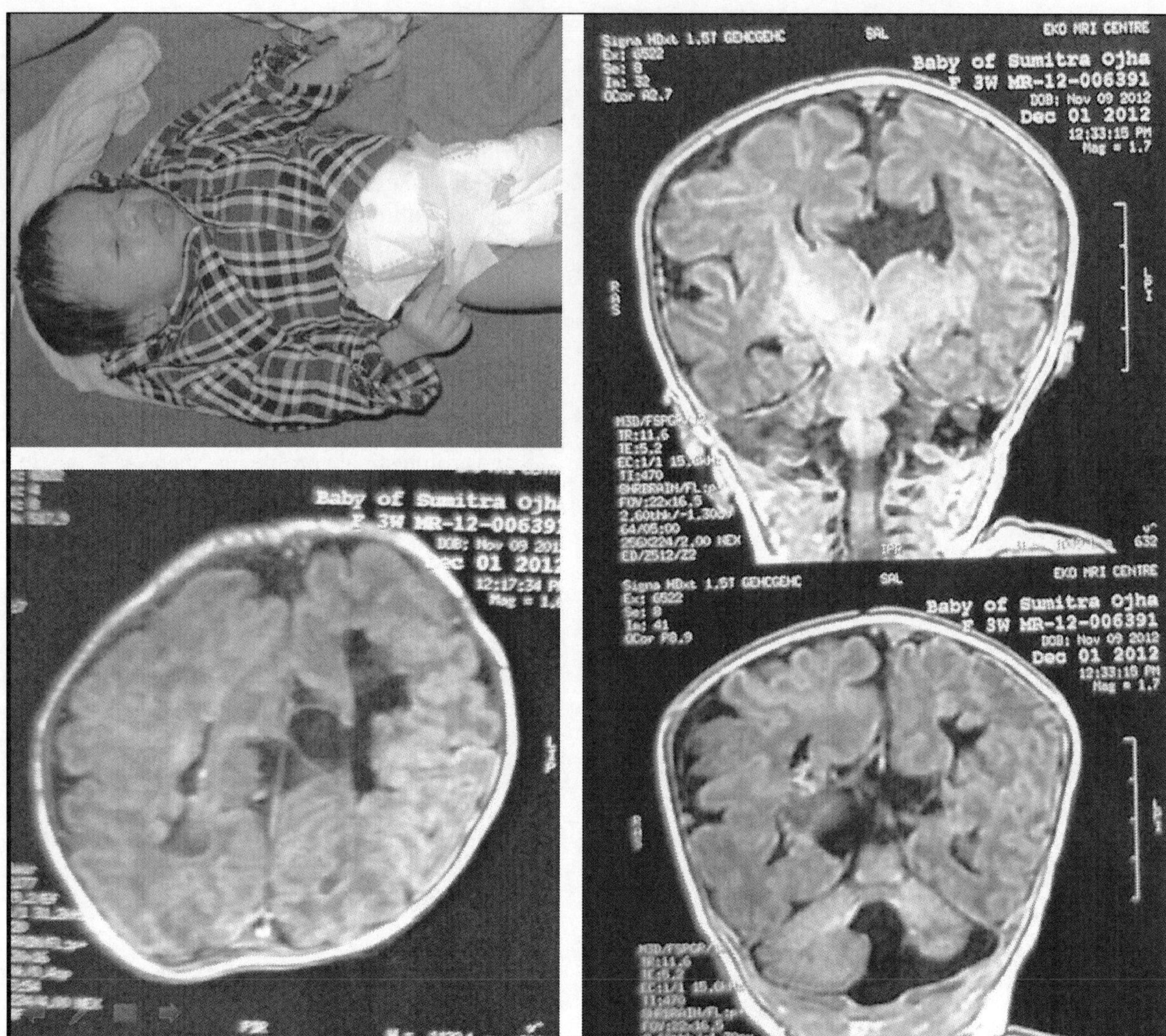

Fig. 8.11: Aicardi syndrome: Occurrence of flexion spasms in a normal looking female infant is the usual mode of clinical presentation. MRI brain is showing corpus callosum agenesis, asymmetry between the two sides of the brain and cysts

with hypoplasia of the hypoglossal nuclei and other associated structural anomalies of brain mostly involving the posterior fossa.

The definition and diagnostic criteria for Moebius syndrome have been controversial and problematic. The syndrome has most frequently been confused with hereditary congenital facial paresis. Hereditary congenital facial paresis (HCFP) is the isolated dysfunction of the facial nerve (CN VII). HCFP is considered to be distinct from Moebius syndrome, which shares some of the same clinical features. The condition is genetically heterogeneous. One locus for HCFP (HCFP1) has been mapped to chromosome 3q. Another locus (HCFP2) has been mapped to chromosome 10q. HCFP3 is caused by mutation in the HOXB1 gene chromosome 17q21.

Optic Nerve Hypoplasia: Optic nerve hypoplasia is the most common congenital anomaly of the optic disc. It may be an isolated finding or part of a spectrum of anatomic and functional abnormalities that includes partial or complete agenesis of the septum pellucidum, other midline brain defects, cerebral anomalies, pituitary dysfunction, and structural abnormalities of the pituitary. Hypopituitarism is a serious problem, and failure to recognize it carries a risk of adrenal crisis, hypoglycemia and death. The association of optic nerve hypoplasia with absent septum pellucidum, with or without pituitary dysfunction, has also been described. Mutations in the PAX6 gene have been identified in patients with bilateral optic nerve hypoplasia or aplasia.

(VI) DISORDERS INVOLVING CEREBELLUM AND POSTERIOR FOSSA

Cerebellar Agenesis: Isolated agenesis of cerebellum is uncommon and often asymptomatic. It has been associated with trisomy 13 and 18. Unilateral agenesis is common and usually asymptomatic. Agenesis of vermis may be partial, involving posterior vermis or occasionally complete when insult has occurred earlier. It may be asymptomatic. When symptomatic, patients show hypotonia, incoordination, tremors and truncal ataxia. Delayed motor milestones, nystagmus and decreased deep tendon reflexes may occur. Joubert's syndrome, as autosomal recessive form of agenesis of vermis, consists of episodic hyperpnea and apnea, rotatory nystagmus and mental retardation. The respiratory abnormality improves with maturation. Neuroimaging shows enlarged fourth ventricle and dilated cisterna magna.

Global Cerebellar Hypoplasia: The causes of global cerebellar hypoplasia are chromosomal and genetically determined diseases, Tay-Sachs disease, Menkes' kinky hair disease, spinal muscular atrophy and sporadic. Histologically, there is selective depletion of granule cells or a loss of Purkinje cells. Clinical features are developmental delay and generalized muscular hypotonia, truncal titubation and ataxia become evident after several months, and nystagmus and intention tremor in severe cases.

Focal Cerebellar Dysplasia: They are often clinically asymptomatic. Extensive lesions can present with cerebellar findings. They are a disorder of neuronal migration due to genetic defects or due to focal ischemic insults and exposure to cytotoxic drugs or viruses.

Dandy-Walker Malformation: It consists of malformation of the fourth ventricle and the cerebellum. It occurs in approximately one in 30,000 live births. The malformation most likely originates at around 32 days when fourth ventricle is formed. The fourth ventricle is misshaped into a large cyst extending into the spinal canal. Cerebellar hemispheres are rudimentary and displaced superiorly and posterior vermis is hypoplastic or absent. The aqueduct of Sylvius, third ventricle and lateral ventricles are grossly dilated. Posterior fossa is enlarged with upward displacement of lateral sinuses, tentorium and torcula. Many abnormalities like pachygyria, heterotopias, aqueductal stenosis, agenesis of corpus callosum, Klippel Feil syndrome etc. and non neural abnormalities like polydactyly, syndactyly, cleft palate, polycystic kidneys, abnormal lumbar vertebrae are also associated with Dandy-Walker syndrome.

Clinical Features: Usually presents in infancy with delayed motor milestones, hydrocephalus, nystagmus, spasticity, titubation, apnea etc. The posterior portion of the head is enlarged. If it presents in adolescence, then symptoms of raised intracranial pressure and ataxia dominate. Diagnosis can be achieved by cranial ultrasound, CT and MRI which shows cystic enlargement of fourth ventricle with hypoplasia of cerebellar vermis and hydrocephalus which should not be mistaken with arachnoid cyst. Familial forms with autosomal recessive inheritance are associated with polycystic kidneys, cataracts, retinal dysgenesis and choroidal coloboma.

Management: A shunt from the ventricles or cyst or both is the mainstay of treatment. Surgery is indicated when occipital bossing, distortion of CSF cisterns or compression of brain surrounding the cyst occurs in non-communicating cyst. A cystoperitoneal shunt may suffice when there is communicating cyst.

Chiari Malformations: In 1891 Hans Chiari, an Austrian pathologist, described types of anomalies affecting the cerebellum and the brainstem in association with hydrocephalus. In 1894 Arnold described a similar malformation of hindbrain in a case of meningomyelocele but without hydrocephalus. Arnold's pupils Schwalbe and Gredig (1907) termed the Type II abnormality of Chiari as Arnold Chiari malformation.

Type I: Cerebellar tonsils herniated into foramen magnum (no caudal displacement of medulla).

Type II : Cerebellar vermis displaced caudally (caudal displacement of medulla and pons).

Type III: Cerebellar herniation into high cervical meningocele (caudal displacement of medulla).

Type IV: Cerebellar hypoplasia.

Chiari type I malformation is the most common and the least severe of the spectrum, often diagnosed in adulthood. Its hallmark is caudal displacement of peglike cerebellar tonsils below the level of the foramen magnum, a phenomenon variably referred to as congenital tonsillar herniation, tonsillar ectopia, or tonsillar descent. The resultant impaction of the foramen magnum, compression of the cervicomedullary junction by the ectopic tonsils, and interruption of normal flow of cerebrospinal fluid (CSF) through the region produce the clinical syndrome.

Chiari type II malformation is less common and more severe, almost invariably associated with myelomeningocele. Because of its greater severity, it becomes symptomatic in infancy or early childhood. Its hallmark is caudal displacement of lower brainstem (medulla, pons, 4th ventricle) through the foramen magnum. Symptoms arise from dysfunction of brainstem and lower cranial nerves.

Chiari type III and IV malformations are exceedingly rare and generally incompatible with life and are, therefore, of scant clinical significance. The type III malformation refers to herniation of cerebellum into a high cervical myelomeningocele, whereas type IV refers to cerebellar agenesis.

Importantly, it is not at all clear that the 4 types of Chiari malformation represent a disease continuum corresponding to a single disorder. The 4 types (particularly types III and IV) are increasingly believed to have different pathogenesis and share little in common other than their names.

Joubert Syndrome and Related Disorders

Classic Joubert syndrome is characterized by three primary findings:

- A distinctive cerebellar and brainstem malformation called the molar tooth sign.
- Hypotonia.
- Developmental delays.[27]

Episodic tachypnea or apnea and atypical eye movements, though characteristic, are not always found. The breathing abnormalities improve with age and cerebellar signs like truncal ataxia develop over time. Cognitive abilities are variable. Additional findings in Joubert syndrome and related disorders (JSRD) are retinal dystrophy, renal disease, ocular colobomas, occipital encephalocele, hepatic fibrosis, polydactyly, oral hamartomas and endocrine abnormalities.

Diagnosis: The diagnosis is based on the presence of characteristic clinical features and magnetic resonance images (MRI) through the junction of the midbrain and pons (isthmus region) that resemble a "molar tooth". Biallelic mutations in around 20 genes are identified in about 50% of individuals. Some of the important genes are *NPHP1, CEP290, AHI1, TMEM67 (MKS3), RPGRIP1L, CC2D2A, ARL13B, INPP5E, OFD1* etc.

Management: Infants and children with abnormal breathing may require stimulatory medications (e.g., caffeine); supplemental oxygen; mechanical support; or tracheostomy in rare cases. Other interventions may include speech therapy for oromotor dysfunction; occupational and physical therapy; educational support, including special programs for the visually impaired; and feedings by gastrostomy tube. Surgery may be required for polydactyly and symptomatic ptosis and/or strabismus. Nephronophthisis, end-stage renal disease, liver failure and/or fibrosis are treated with standard approaches.

Surveillance: Annual evaluations of growth, vision, liver and kidney function; periodic neuropsychologic and developmental testing.

Agents/Circumstances to Avoid: Nephrotoxic medi-cations such as nonsteroidal anti-inflammatory drugs in those with renal impairment; hepatotoxic drugs in those with liver impairment.

Genetic Counseling: JSRDs are predominantly inherited in an autosomal recessive manner. JSRD caused by mutation of OFD1 is inherited in an X-linked manner. Digenic inheritance (mutations in two different genes giving rise to disease in an individual) has been reported.

(VII) PHAKOMATOSIS

Neurocutaneous syndromes (phakomatosis) represent a group of central nervous system disorders with associated lesions in the skin, eye, and possibly other organs. The neurocutaneous manifestations are related to the common ectodermal origin of these organs. The "phakomatosis" concept was formulated early in the twentieth century by the ophthalmologist van der Hoeve. He included 3 disorders in the group–neurofibromatosis, tuberous sclerosis complex, and von Hippel-Lindau syndrome, on the basis of the occurrence of patchy ophthalmologic manifestations in each disorder. The definition can be expanded to include other entities such as Sturge-Weber syndrome, incontinentia pigmenti, ataxia telangiectasia, nevoid basal cell carcinoma syndrome etc. The detailed description of each disorder is beyond the scope of this chapter and is being described in a separate chapter in the book.

(VIII) ANOMALIES ASSOCIATED WITH CRANIOSYNOSTOSIS

The genetic cause underlying most craniosynostosis syndromes involves the fibroblast growth factor receptor 3 (FGFR3) and TWIST genes. Such disorders are associated with abnormalities in the skull base along with some other associated CNS malformations. Impaired venous outflow is often caused by a hypoplastic jugular foramen. This causes an increase in the intracranial blood volume, thereby causing an increase in intracranial pressure. This can be further complicated with a possible Arnold-Chiari malformation, which can partially obstruct the flow of cerebrospinal fluid from the neurocranium to the spinal cord. The Chiari malformation may be asymptomatic or present with ataxia, spasticity or abnormalities in breathing, swallowing or sleeping. Due to the impaired venous outflow, which may be further complicated with an Arnold-Chiari malformation, there is often a clinical image of hydrocephalus present. Hydrocephalus is seen in 6.5 to 8% of patients with Apert's syndrome, 25.6% in patients with Crouzon's syndrome and 27.8% of those with Pfeiffer's syndrome. Ventriculomegaly is a usual finding in children with the Apert syndrome, sometimes detected in antenatal ultrasonography associated with hypolplastic corpus callosum.[28]

(IX) HYDROCEPHALUS AND HYDRANENCEPHALY

Though apart of CNS malformation the above entities are described separately.

(X) SPECIFIC MALFORMATIONS DUE TO TERATOGENS

During the first two weeks of gestation, teratogenic agents usually will either kill the embryo or cause no effects, popularly called the "all or none phenomenon". Major malformations are more common when exposure is during the period of organogenesis, between day 15 to day 60 of fetal life. Major congenital malformations are generally widespread; however, the following can be listed to be associated with CNS malformations:

- **Maternal diabetes:** Apart from various anomalies, it is associated with NTD.
- **Maternal phenylketonuria:** Severe mental retar-dation, if uncontrolled.
- **Fetal alcohol syndrome:** Microcephaly and low IQ along with craniofacial anomaly.
- **Maternal use of valproate:** NTD, develop-mental delay.
- **Maternal use of carbamazepine:** NTD.
- **Maternal use of retinoic acid (Vitamin A):** NTD.
- **Congenital rubella or German measles:** Triad of cataracts, cardiac malformation and deafness. May also cause mental retardation.
- Congenital cytomegalovirus infection is the most common viral infection of the fetus. Exposure later in the pregnancy results in intrauterine growth retardation, micromelia, chorioretinitis, blindness, microcephaly, cerebral calcifications, mental retardation and hepatosplenomegaly.
- Ionizing radiation can injure the developing embryo due to cell death or chromosome injury. The severity of damage to the embryo depends on the dose absorbed and the stage of development at which the exposure occurs. Study of survivors of the Japanese atomic bombing demonstrated that exposure at 10 to 18 weeks of pregnancy is a period of greatest sensitivity for the developing brain. Most X-ray exposure do not cause harm to the fetus. X-rays can cause injury to the brain only in very high dose.

(XI) OTHER MALFORMATIONS LIKE INTRACRANIAL CYSTS, HAMARTOMAS AND VASCULAR MALFORMATIONS

Some hamartomas and vascular malformations have already been discussed. Some of the important cystic lesions re-described below:

Choroid plexus cysts (CPCs) are non-neoplastic epithelial-lined cysts of the choroid plexus. They are the most common of all intracranial neuroepithelial cysts. Most are bilateral and located in the lateral ventricular atria. Most CPCs are asymptomatic and are found incidentally, typically during antenatal ultrasonography and in neonates. Symptomatic lesions are rare. Previously thought to be marker of chromosomal anomalies, once detected in antenatal ultrasonography, it is no longer considered an indication for amniocentesis if found isolated without any other malformation. Microscopic analysis of CPCs reveals neuroepithelial microcysts containing nests of foamy lipid-laden histiocytes.

Ependymal cysts are rare, benign, ependymal-lined cysts of the lateral ventricle or juxtaventricular region of the temporoparietal region and frontal lobe. Most are incidental, but symptomatic cysts may manifest with headache, seizure, and/or obstructive hydrocephalus. Ependymal cysts are thought to arise from sequestration of developing neuroectoderm during embryogenesis.

Neuroglial (also called glioependymal) cysts are benign epithelial-lined lesions that occur anywhere in the neuraxis. They are uncommon, representing fewer than 1% of intracranial cysts.

Arachnoid cysts are benign, congenital, intra-arach-noidal space-occupying lesions that are filled with clear CSF. They do not communicate with the ventricular system. The cysts tend to be unilocular, smoothly marginated expansile lesions that are molded by the surrounding structures. They are common, representing 1% of all intracranial masses. Most arachnoid cysts are supratentorial. Fifty to 60% are found in the middle cranial fossa, anterior to the temporal lobes. Other locations include the suprasellar cistern and posterior fossa (10%), where they occur most commonly in the cerebellopontine angle cistern. Arachnoid cysts are generally stable over time, although cases of sudden or progressive enlargement, as well as spontaneous resolution, have been reported. Once detected in a neonate, head circumference monitoring at regular intervals is recommended, and surgical correction is warranted in case of rapid growth or complications.

Intracranial epidermoid cysts are congenital inclusion cysts. Epidermoid cysts comprise 0.2%–1.8% of primary intracranial tumors and are four to nine times as common as dermoid cysts. The most common location for epidermoid cysts is the cerebellopontine angle cistern (40%–50%), where they are the third most common overall cerebellopontine angle cistern–internal auditory canal mass (after acoustic schwannoma and meningioma). Epidermoid cysts also occur in the fourth ventricle (17%) and the sellar and/or parasellar regions (10%–15%). Less common locations include the cerebral hemispheres or brainstem. Ten percent of epidermoid cysts are extradural, located in the skull or spine. All are located off the midline. Most are asymptomatic but may occasionally result in mass effect, cranial neuropathy, or seizure. Occasionally, epidermoid cysts rupture and may excite a granulomatous meningitis. To the surgeon or pathologist, the irregular lobulated surface of the epidermoid glistens with the sheen of mother-of-pearl. This so-called "beautiful tumor" has an irregular cauliflower-like outer surface that grows to encase vessels and nerves.

Dermoid cyst is another congenital ectodermal inclusion cyst. They are extremely rare, constituting fewer than 0.5% of primary intracranial tumors. These cysts increase in size by means of glandular secretion and epithelial desquamation. Growth can lead to rupture of the cyst contents, causing a chemical meningitis that may lead to vasospasm, infarction, and even death. Malignant transformation into squamous cell carcinoma has also been described.

Dermoid cysts arise from the inclusion of ectodermally committed cells at the time of neural tube closure (3rd–5th week of embryogenesis). The dermoid cyst is a well-defined, lobulated, "pearly" mass of variable size. The capsule is thicker than that of the epidermoid cyst and often contains plaques of calcification. Characteristically, the cyst contains thick, disagreeable, foul-smelling, yellow material due to the secretion of sebaceous glands and desquamated epithelium. The cysts may also contain hair and/or teeth.

Neurenteric cysts are congenital, benign, malformative endodermal lesions in the central nervous system. They are approximately three times as common in the spine, compared with the brain. Most intracranial neurenteric cysts are found in the posterior fossa. They are typically in the midline, anterior to the brainstem.

Porencephalic cysts are congenital or acquired cavities within the cerebral hemisphere that usually–although not invariably–communicate directly with the ventricular system. They can be cortical or subcortical, unilateral or bilateral.The location often corresponds to territories supplied by the cerebral arteries. Congenital porencephalic cysts originate from a fetal or perinatal encephaloclastic process that results from intrauterine vascular or infectious injury. Acquired cysts are secondary to injury later in life and are usually secondary to trauma, surgery, ischemia, or infection. Porencephalic cysts vary greatly in size. They are typically CSF-filled cavities with a smooth wall and are lined with gliotic or spongiotic white matter. The adjacent skull may demonstrate remodeling due to chronic CSF pulsations.

Acknowledgement: I acknowledge the contributions of my teacher Professor Shubha R Phadke for teaching me the pearls of human malformations.

References

1. Mandal K, Boggula VR, Borkar M, Agarwal S, Phadke SR. Use of Multiplex Ligation-Dependent Probe Amplification (MLPA) in Screening of Subtelomeric Regions in Children with Idiopathic Mental Retardation. Indian J Pediatr 2009 October;76(10):1027-31.
2. Blom HJ, Shaw GM, den Heijer M, Finnell RH. Neural Tube Defects and Folate: Case Far From Closed. Nat. Rev. Neurosci 2006;7(9):724-31.
3. Castilla EE, Orioli IM, Lopez-Camelo JS, Dutra Mda G, Nazer-Herrera J. Latin American Collaborative Study of Congenital Malformations (ECLAMC) Preliminary Data on Changes in Neural Tube Defect Prevalence Rates After Folic Acid Fortification in South America. Am. J. Med. Genet 2003: 123A:123-28.
4. Shum AS, Copp AJ. Regional Differences in Morphogenesis of the Neuroepithelium Suggest Multiple Mechanisms of Spinal Neurulation in the Mouse. Anat. Embryol (Berl.) 1996: 194:65-73.
5. Wallingford JB. Neural Tube Closure and Neural Tube Defects: Studies in Animal Models Reveal Known Knowns and Known Unknowns. Am. J. Med. Genet. C. Semin. Med Genet 2005;135:59-68.
6. Rifat Y, Parekh V, Wilanowski T, Hislop NR, Auden A, Ting SB, Cunningham JM, Jane SM. Regional Neural Tube Closure Defined by the Grainy Head-Like Transcription Factors. Dev. Biol 2010;345(2):237-45.
7. Kappen C, Kruger C, MacGowan J, Salbaum JM. Maternal Diet Modulates the Risk for Neural Tube Defects in a Mouse Model of Diabetic Pregnancy. Reprod. Toxicol 2011;31(1): 41-49.
8. Wagner C, Nau H. Alteration of Embryonic Folate Metabolism by Valproic Acid During Organogenesis: Implications for Mechanism of Teratogenesis. Neurology 1992;42 (4 Suppl. 5):17-24.
9. Wald NJ, Cuckle H, Brock JH, Peto R, Polani PE, Woodford FP. Maternal Serum-Alpha-Fetoprotein Measurement in Antenatal Screening for Anencephaly and Spina Bifida in Early Pregnancy. Report of U.K. Collaborative Study on Alpha-Fetoprotein in Relation to Neural Tube Defects. Lancet 1977;1(8026):1323-32.
10. Forrester MB, Merz RD. Prenatal Diagnosis and Elective Termination of Neural Tube Defects in Hawaii, 1986-1997. Fetal Diagnosis Ther 2000;15:146-51.
11. Barkovich AJ, Quint DJ. Middle Interhemispheric Fusion: An Unusual Variant of Holoprosencephaly. AJNR Am J Neuroradiol 1993;14:431-40.
12. Demyer W, Zeman W, Palmer CG. The Face Predicts The Brain: Diagnostic Significance of Median Facial Anomalies for Holoprosencephaly (Arhinencephaly). Pediatrics 1964;34: 256-63.
13. Bendavid C, Dubourg C, Pasquier L, Gicquel I, Le Gallou S, Mottier S, Durou MR, Henry C, Odent S, David V. MLPA Screening Reveals Novel Subtelomeric Rearrangements in Holoprosencephaly. Hum Mutat 2007;28:1189-97.
14. Bendavid C, Rochard L, Dubourg C, Seguin J, Gicquel I, Pasquier L, Vigneron J, Laquerrière A, Marcorelles P, Jeanne-Pasquier C, Rouleau C, Jaillard S, Mosser J, Odent S, David V. Array-CGH Analysis Indicates a High Prevalence of Genomic Rearrangements in Holoprosencephaly: An Updated Map of Candidate Loci. Hum Mutat 2009;30:1175-82.
15. Brown SA, Warburton D, Brown LY, Yu CY, Roeder ER, Stengel-Rutkowski S, Hennekam RC, Muenke M. Holoprosencephaly Due to Mutations in ZIC2, a Homologue of Drosophila Odd-paired. Nat Genet 1998;20:180-83.
16. Domené S, Roessler E, El-Jaick KB, Snir M, Brown JL, Vélez JI, Bale S, Lacbawan F, Muenke M, Feldman B. Mutations in the Human SIX3 Gene in Holoprosencephaly are Loss of Function. Hum Mol Genet 2008;17:3919-28.
17. Barr M Jr, Cohen MM Jr. Holoprosencephaly Survival and Performance. Am J Med Genet 1999;89:116-20.
18. Berry SA, Pierpont ME, Gorlin RJ. Single Central Incisor in Familial Holoprosencephaly. J Pediatr 1984;104:877-80.
19. Noctor SC, Martinez-Cerdeno V, Ivic L, Kriegstein AR. Cortical Neurons Arise in Symmetric and Asymmetric Division Zones and Migrate through Specific Phases. Nat. Neurosci 2004;7(2):136-44.
20. Haubensak W, Attardo A, Denk W, Huttner WB. Neurons Arise in the Basal Neuroepithelium of the Early Mammalian Telencephalon: A Major Site of Neurogenesis. Proc. Natl. Acad. Sci. USA 2004;101(9):3196-201.
21. Mochida GH, Walsh CA. Molecular Genetics of Human Microcephaly. Curr. Opin. Neurol 2001;14(2):151-56.
22. Miller JQ. Lissencephaly in 2 Siblings. Neurology 1963:158: 13:841-50.
23. Dieker H, Edwards RH, ZuRhein G, Chou S, Opitz JM. The Lissencephaly Syndrome. Birth Defects Orig., Artic. Ser 1969; 5,53-64.
24. Pollin TI, Dobyns WB, Crowe CA, Ledbetter DH, Bailey-Wilson JE, Smith AC. Risk of Abnormal Pregnancy Outcome in Carriers of Balanced Reciprocal Translocations Involving the Miller-Dieker Syndrome (MDS) Critical Region in Chromosome 17p13.3. Am. J. Med. Genet 1999;157:85(4): 369-75.

25. des Portes V. Pinard JM. Billuart P. Vinet MC. Koulakoff A. Carrie A. Gelot A. Dupuis E. Motte J. Berwald-Netter Y. *et al.* A Novel CNS Gene Required for Neuronal Migration and Involved in X-Linked Subcortical Laminar Heterotopia and Lissencephaly Syndrome. Cell 1998:171:92(1):51-61.

26. Gleeson JG. Allen KM. Fox JW. Lamperti ED. Berkovic S. Scheffer I. Cooper EC. Dobyns WB. Minnerath SR. Ross ME. *et al.* Doublecortin, a Brain-Specific Gene Mutated in Human X-Linked Lissencephaly and Double Cortex Syndrome. Encodes a Putative Signaling Protein. Cell 1998:172:92(1): 63-72.

27. Boltshauser E. Isler W. Joubert Syndrome: Episodic Hyperpnea. Abnormal Eye Movements. Retardation and Ataxia. Associated with Dysplasia of the Cerebellar Vermis. Neuropadiatrie 1977: 8:57-66.

28. Phadke SR. Mandal K. Ranganath P. Prenatal Diagnosis of Apert Syndrome in Second Trimester–A Case Report. Perinatology 2012:12:4:159-62.

9 Chapter

COMMON BEHAVIOR PROBLEMS

Monica Juneja, Ridhima Jain

Behavior is the way in which one acts, or conducts, or reacts to a situation. According to the 'transactional model of development', the individual's inherent characteristics ('nature') and environmental factors ('nurture') influence each other and together mold the child's development and behavior. During growing up majority of children have emotional and behavioral issues that are due to the stresses of development and adaptation to family and social expectations. These are usually transient in nature. A child is said to be manifesting a behavioral problem when the child demonstrates a behavior that is different from what is expected at home or in school, or community and is having serious negative consequences for a child's academic achievement and social development. Even though, behavioral problems are not serious enough to warrant an official Diagnostic and Statistical Manual of Mental Disorders (DSM)/International Classification of Diseases (ICD) diagnosis, they do need early identification, management and referral, especially if development of more serious behavior disorder is to be prevented.

The spectrum of behavior problems changes with age as along with increase in cognitive, motor and communication abilities of children, their social and emotional needs also change.

Common behavioral problems seen at various ages are listed in Table 9.1.

Table 9.1: Examples of Common Behavioral Problems at Different Ages

Age	Influencing factors	Common behavior problems
Infants (0 – 1 year)	Attachment, separation	Colic Breath-holding spells Repetitive behaviors (thumb sucking, head banging)
Toddlers (1 – 3 years)	More mobile and vocal, seeking autonomy/mastery	Breath-holding spells Temper tantrums Feeding problems (food fussiness, pica) Repetitive behaviors (thumb sucking, body rocking, bruxism, nail biting)
Preschoolers (3 – 6 years)	Rapid advancement of language, increased cognitive and social skills, more self-regulation, exposure to structured learning environment	Temper tantrums Sibling rivalry Oppositional behavior Power struggles around feeding and sleeping routines and toilet training Aggression, hyperactivity Anxiety
School age children (6 – 12 years)	Intellectual and social demands of school environment, peer pressure	Eating problems (pica, obesity) Elimination disorders (enuresis, encopresis) Bullying Repetitive behaviors (bruxism, nail-biting, body rocking) Hyperactivity, inattention Socialization problems

Contd.

Contd.

Adolescents (12–18 years)		Eating disorders (pica, anorexia nervosa, bulimia nervosa, cyclic vomiting syndrome) Bullying Elimination disorders (enuresis, encopresis) Recurrent pains Repetitive behaviors (trichotillomania, masturbation, habit cough, nail-biting)

Breath-holding Spells: Breath-holding spells (BHS) are dramatic, reflexic, nonepileptic, involuntary episodes that occur in otherwise healthy children. They have a prevalence of 0.1–4.6% in the age group of 6 months – 5 years. The typical breath-holding episode begins when a child becomes upset, is startled, or suffers a minor injury, and begins to cry. This is followed by a phase in which the child becomes silent, apneic and cyanosed or pallid. In simple BHS, the event resolves with no associated syncope or postural change while in severe BHS there is subsequent loss of consciousness and a brief period of limpness followed by increase in muscle tone or opisthotonos. Occasionally this may end in a seizure; which may be myoclonic, clonic or tonic-clonic. The entire episode lasts from several seconds to more than a minute and ends with a sudden, deep inspiration or return of normal breathing. The child may be lethargic for a brief period before complete recovery. Simple Breath-Holding Spells occur in 27% children and severe episodes may be seen in as many as 4.6%. Onset of breath-holding spells is nearly always before 18 months of age. Cyanotic breath-holding spells are triggered by anger or frustration whereas pallid spells are more frequently incited by a painful or frightful experience. Sometimes features of both pallor and cyanosis may be present and these are known as mixed BHS. Frequency varies from multiple episodes a day to once a year, with peaking of frequency and severity during the second and third years of life. By the time patients are 4 years old, about half of breath-holding cases have spontaneously resolved; by age 6, about 90% have done so; and by age 7 or 8, virtually all have resolved. A positive family history is found in 20% to 35% of all patients that is consistent with an autosomal dominant inheritance with reduced penetrance.

For many years, BHS were thought to derive from emotional or behavior problems since they occurred in the setting of anger, agitation, or frustration. Recent studies have shown that these episodes are the result of an involuntary reflex and are not intentional. Generalized autonomic dysfunction has been found in children with both types of BHS. In the pallid type, noxious stimuli may lead to centrally mediated cardiac inhibition through the vagus nerve, thus inducing bradycardia or brief asystole. Similarly, cyanotic episodes may be caused by central inhibition of respiratory movements, mediated through the vagus nerve. Clinical experience has shown a reduction in frequency of BHS with behavioral training of parents; indicating that though BHS is mediated by an involuntary reflex, the crying episode triggering the reflex is amenable to behavioral management. Breath-holding spells have also been associated with iron deficiency with or without anemia (IDA) and several studies have reported abatement of BHS with iron treatment. Although the underlying mechanism is still unknown, it has been proposed that iron may be involved in catecholamine metabolism and the functioning of neurotransmitters in the central nervous system. BHS is also seen with increased frequency in children suffering from familial dysautonomia, and transient erythroblastopenia of childhood.

Some potentially life-threatening conditions like seizures or cardiac rhythm disturbances may resemble BHS and need to be distinguished (Table 9.2). The

Table 9.2: Differential Diagnosis of Severe Breath-Holding Spells

Feature	Severe BHS	Seizures	Cardiac rhythm disturbances
Age at onset	Infancy - toddler	Any age	Variable
Family history	Frequently positive	Variable	
Inciting event	Always (anger, frustration, surprise, pain, fright)	Usually absent	Usually absent
State	Always awake	Asleep or awake	Awake, often with stressor

Contd.

Contd.

Pallor or cyanosis	Always occurs: Sequence is **before** loss of consciousness	May or may not occur: When occurs it is **after** loss of consciousness	May or may not occur
Crying	Always: precedes change in color and loss of consciousness	A single shrill cry may occur in tonic phase of a seizure: occurring after loss of consciousness	
Heart rate	Bradycardia in pallid	Usually tachycardia	Variable. May be irregular
Any type of jerks (myoclonic, clonic, tonic clonic)	Variable: few beats	Usually	Absent
Incontinence	Uncommon	Common	Absent
Post ictal confusion	Absent	Common	Absent
Duration of episode	Usually less than a minute	Usually more than a minute.	

differentiation between BHS and seizures is clinical and a thorough history is often enough to make a diagnosis. The sequence in which the events (crying, pallor/cyanosis, loss of consciousness) take place during the episode is the most helpful differentiating feature. Videos of the episodes recorded by parents can further help in establishing the diagnosis. A physical examination including neurological and cardiac examination should be carried out. As iron deficiency is prevalent in children with BHS, a complete hemogram as well as iron studies should be done. Electrocardiogram is usually done to rule out rare but potentially life-threatening Long QT syndrome or other arrhythmias. More extensive investigations (e.g., Holter monitoring, EEG etc.) are indicated only if history or examination are suggestive of a cardiac disorder or epilepsy rather than BHS.

The most important aspect of management is to reassure parents that although BHS are frightening to observe, they are not life threatening and do not affect the subsequent neurological development or increase the risk of epilepsy. Due to these fears, parents become overindulgent while trying to avoid crying episodes in their child, inadvertently reinforcing these crying episodes, which usually end in BHS. Parents are best advised to ignore the behavior. In cases in which a child loses consciousness, the child should be placed in a lateral supine position to help avoid injury and possible aspiration. In cases with iron deficiency, treatment with iron supplements has been found to significantly reduce the number of spells. In cases with bradycardia or asystole or in patients with multiple daily episodes, a 0.1 mg dose of oral atropine three times daily may be helpful. Individual case studies have used drugs, that act through autonomic system, like glycopyrrolate, oral theophylline, fluoxetine, melatonin with some success, but larger robust studies are required to confirm or refute their role. Anticonvulsants have no role even in those cases which have seizure-like manifestation. There have been some reports of implantation of permanent pacemakers in severe and frequent spells that are unresponsive to medication and are associated with seizures, life-threatening bradycardia, or asystole.

Colic: Colic refers to excessive crying in a young infant who is otherwise healthy and also not hungry. It occurs in 16-26% of all infants across all socioeconomic, racial and ethnic groups with no sex predilection. Mechanisms causing it are poorly understood. Even though the word colic has a gastrointestinal connotation, both gastrointestinal and non-gastrointestinal theories have been proposed. Interplay between multiple factors like biological, behavioral, social and neurodevelopmental, are likely to be causative. The suggested gastrointestinal mechanisms causing colic include lactase enzyme deficiency, food allergens/hypersensitivity, immaturity of enteric nervous system or intestinal dysmotility. There is growing evidence that gut microbiota of colicky infants differs from that of healthy infants. Implications of this difference in microbiota or of mode of delivery, as well as breastfeeding; on the severity or frequency and treatment of colic is still a subject of research. Gas, aerophagia or colonic fermentation does not however, cause colic. Non-gastrointestinal mechanisms implicated are altered parent-child interaction, improper feeding, immaturity of nervous system and maternal smoking. Recent case control studies examining the frequency of infantile colic history in children with migraine found strong association between the two (OR 5.6, p 0.004) suggesting colic could be an early form of migraine.

Colicky infants cry for more than 3 hours a day, more than 3 days a week and for more than 3 weeks. Excessive crying usually starts at 2 weeks of age, peaks at 6 weeks, starts decreasing after 8 weeks and usually subsides by 16 weeks of age. Crying episodes are unrelated to feeding and show a diurnal variation with increase in evening and night. Babies flex legs arch their backs and may pass a lot of flatus during the crying episodes. The diagnosis is made by detailed history, usually a normal examination in a baby who is gaining weight well. If failure to thrive is present, the diagnosis of colic should be questioned, and alternative diagnosis should be considered. Differential diagnosis includes otitis media, incarcerated hernia, gastroesophageal reflux (GER), lactose intolerance or milk allergy. These are easy to exclude by history and examination. Management is usually supportive. Reassuring the parents about the benign and self-limited nature of the problem, clarifying their queries and making them aware of what to expect goes a long way in minimizing parental anxiety. Dietary changes are not effective and drugs like simethicone or dicyclomine are not indicated. Recent studies have explored the role of probiotics in prevention and management of colic, but their results are inconclusive.

Temper Tantrums: Temper tantrums are brief episodes of disruptive, undesirable behavior or emotional outbursts that are extreme and severe in nature and are usually disproportionate to the situation. These are commonly seen between 18 months to 4 years, when the child starts developing autonomy while simultaneously seeking parental attention. They occur in 70-75% of toddlers and preschoolers. They are more common in boys (boy: girl ratio of 3.1:1). Temper tantrums are related to the individual personality trait of the child and the triggering situation. The underlying precipitating factor needs to be understood for successful management of the tantrum and prevention of a recurrence. Underlying precipitants include unfulfilled demands, frustration or attention seeking behavior. Fear, fatigue, an overstimulating environment, hunger and physical discomfort often evoke temper tantrums in younger children. Psychosocial factors associated with increased incidence are inconsistent parenting, failure to set limits or excessive disciplining, the use of corporal punishment, maternal depression, low social class.

Children may throw tantrums in the form of shouting, screaming, crying, falling to floor, flailing extremities, banging head, kicking and throwing items. Tantrums usually occur once a day in a toddler, lasting for 1–3 minutes, after which the child typically returns to his/her usual mood and behavior. As they get older, children learn to identify and communicate feelings to others and act appropriately rather than throwing tantrums. Thus, the severity, frequency and duration of tantrums decrease as child ages. Tantrums which are severe or atypical (See Table 9.3), usually indicate the presence of a serious underlying medical, neurodevelopmental or psychiatric disorder like language delays, autism spectrum disorder, intellectual disability, hearing deficit, major depressive disorder, etc. Frequent temper tantrums may be predictive of future anti-social behavior in older children. When associated with frequent defiance, breaking rules, aggression, physical injury to others, it becomes a part of *Disruptive, Impulse control and Conduct Disorders.*

Table 9.3: Severe Temper Tantrums	
1.	Continuing beyond 5 years age
2.	Causing injury to themselves or others during the tantrum
3.	Lasting longer than 15 min
4.	More than five times a day
5.	Persistent negative mood between tantrums

The evaluation of a child with temper tantrums begins with a complete history and physical examination. A thorough history will help in identifying atypical temper tantrums, which would warrant referral to a Developmental specialist for identification and management of underlying medical, behavioral or developmental disorder. It also provides information about family dynamics that may affect intervention. Physical examination is usually unremarkable; presence of neurocutaneous stigmata or dysmorphism indicate the need for further evaluation. Visual and hearing screening are also essential as undiagnosed vision or hearing impairment can cause frustration leading to or exacerbating tantrums. Effective management should be directed towards the cause as well as modification of parental responses to the temper tantrum. If the underlying cause is identified as fatigue or hunger, situations, which lead to such a state, should be pre-empted. When tantrums are due to a feeling of frustration, positive remarks and an understanding attitude may often decrease the outburst. In case, the tantrums are due to failure to fulfill some demand, ignoring the behavior is the most effective means of tackling it. In such a scenario, fulfilling the child's demands even sometimes, reinforces the tantrum throwing behavior. When the outburst is occurring, time and opportunity should be provided to the child to regain composure. If this fails it may be necessary to physically hold the child, but without emotion. This is usually done using "time-out" technique, especially if the nature of tantrum is disruptive and out of control. This involves removing the child from the reinforcing environment, calmly explaining what the offense is, escorting him/her to a designated time-out area where there are no reinforcers available, for a short duration (suggested one minute per year of age). Caregivers who respond with punitive anger run the risk of reinforcing the anger and teaching the child that out-of-control emotions are a reasonable response to frustration. It is of prime importance that parents model the anger control which they want their children to exhibit. Offering simple choices to the child before the tantrum has started or after the tantrum has aborted may make him feel more in control and develop a sense of autonomy.

Bullying

Bullying is defined as repetitive and negative (unpleasant or hurtful) behavior by an individual or a group directed against another with an intent to cause fear and/or harm to the victim in situations where there exists some sort of power differential between them. The power difference may be in terms of physical size, social status, or other factors. The prevalence of bullying and victimization across countries, ranges from 15-40%. The few studies available from India have reported a higher prevalence ranging from 50-61% in school going children.

Bullying can manifest in many forms:

(i) **Physical:** Any type of physical assault, hitting, kicking, choking, and forcefully taking something from the victim.

(ii) **Verbal:** Harassment or intimidation in the form of name calling, threatening, taunting, making faces or obscene gestures.

(iii) **Indirect:** Social exclusion of victims through the manipulation of social relationships by bullies, injuring the reputation of victims, gossiping sabotage, convincing peers to exclude victims.

(iv) **Cyberbullying:** Harm inflicted through threatening, harassing, taunting, and/or intimidating a peer using an electronic medium, such as computers, cellphones and other electronic medium. This is particularly insidious form of bullying as it is difficult to detect and verify, quickly reaches wide audience and easily assessable to adolescents. Most authors divide children experiencing bullying into bullies only, victims only and both bullies and victims. Persons witnessing bullying may be classified as bystanders, defenders, reinforcers and assistors.

Victims of bullying may experience anxiety, depression, poor school performance, psychosomatic complaints, difficulty sleeping, headaches, stomach upsets, and nightmares. Long-term consequences include lower self-esteem, poor academic achievement, poor psychosocial adjustments as adults, anxiety, depression and psychosis. Bullying is significantly associated with suicidal ideation and suicide attempts in victims. Bullies themselves often show poor school adjustment and academic performance, high rate of substance abuse, fighting and weapon carrying. Long-term consequences include anti-social development, intimate partner violence perpetration, unemployment, delinquency and criminality.

The first step in management of bullying is identification of bullying and victimization. Often victims present with psychosomatic complaints, symptoms of depression, phobia, inattention or poor school performance, rather than reporting being bullied. When bullying is suspected on the basis of these symptoms, especially in a child perceived as anxious or weaker; further enquiry is necessary. Probing should be gentle, with open-ended questions and without judgement or direct confrontation. Intervention starts with a sympathetic listening of the child's ordeal. An assurance (verbal as well as facial expressions and body language) that the child did not deserve to be treated negatively and such behaviours are hurtful can help counteract the negative consequences of bullying and building the child's self-esteem. Other interventions include counseling children and their families, coaching victims how to respond to bullying, screening, and managing comorbidities. School authorities or law enforcement agencies may need to be involved if bullying is severe, extreme or violent. School or community-based programs approach bullying as an adverse social phenomenon needing change in cultural attitudes and hence direct interventions involving schools, teachers or communities instead of only bullies or victims. The essential elements of a bullying prevention program consist of training of teachers and parents, strict consistent classroom rules for handling bullying and implementation of whole school anti-bullying policy. Interventions include awareness programs about negative consequences of bullying, social and behavioral skills training, playground supervision, etc. The Olweus Bullying Prevention Program is one of the first and also the most adopted, researched and accepted multidisciplinary school-based intervention program. It is based on an authoritative adult–child interaction wherein the adult (parent/teacher) sets firm limits to unacceptable behaviors, and consistently applies non-physical and non-hostile sanctions if those limits are violated. Expulsion or physical punishment of bullies have been ineffective in reducing bullying. Mediation sessions between bully and victim have failed to decrease bullying and have rather shown to increase victimization and are hence not recommended.

Pica: Pica is classified under *Feeding and Eating Disorders* in DSM-5. The word pica comes from the Latin word for magpie, a bird known for its large and indiscriminate appetite. It is typically defined as the persistent eating of non-nutritive and non-food substances for a period of at least 1 month duration, at an age in which this behavior is developmentally inappropriate and not part of a culturally sanctioned practice. This is usually beyond 24 months, since prior to this age young children ingest and mouth a variety of substances in the process of learning to distinguish between edible and non-edible substances. If it occurs in the context of another mental disorder for example Autism Spectrum Disorder, additional diagnosis of pica is given only if it is sufficiently severe to warrant clinical attention. Prevalence of pica is reported between 2% and 10% in the general population.

Pica is associated with a wide array of medical, physiological and psychiatric conditions. A recent meta-analysis has shown that pica was associated with lower zinc levels and 2.4 times greater odds of anemia. Thus, it may be seen commonly in children with iron efficiency anemia as well as sickle cell disease, children undergoing dialysis and those suffering from celiac disease. It has also been linked to many micronutrient deficiencies (thiamine, vitamin C, vitamin D). Increased incidence of pica is also seen in children with global developmental delay/intellectual disability, autistic spectrum disorder, pregnant women, schizophrenics and patients of Kleine-Levin syndrome. Several psychological factors have been implicated in exacerbating pica including parental neglect, parental separation, lack of communication between families and environmental deprivation. Traumatic events in one's life such as abuse, neglect, social isolation amongst others often have harmful and long lasting impact on an individual's psyche, which may predispose them towards developing pica like habits as a means of satisfying oral needs.

Individuals presenting with pica have been reported to mouth and/or ingest an exhaustive list of non-food substances, which include mud (geophagia) dirt, sand, stones (lithophagia), pebbles, hair (tricophagia), feces (coprophagia), lead (plumbophagia), laundry starch (amylophagia), vinyl gloves, plastic, pencil erasers, ice (pagophagia), fingernails, paper, paint chips, coal, chalk, wood, plaster, light bulbs, needles, string, cigarette butts, wire, and burnt matches (cautopyreiophagia). Although pica is considered a benign behavior, it may have life threatening consequences and can result in significant complications like anemia, hyperkalemia, metabolic alkalosis, hypercalcemia, hyper/hypophosphatemia, poisonings (lead/mercury/naphthalene), parasitic infestation, bowel obstruction/perforation and dental injury. Investigations, which need to be undertaken, may include a complete blood count, peripheral smear, serum electrolytes, liver function tests, iron, ferritin, lead and zinc levels. A plain abdominal radiograph, ultrasound/barium study may be necessary to distinguish obstruction from parasites or bezoars.

There is no specific medical treatment. Pica often remits spontaneously. When it persists, a multidisciplinary approach (psychologists, social workers, and developmental pediatricians) may be warranted. Development of the treatment plan must take into account the symptoms, contributory factors, as well as possible complications. When pica is for provision of environmental or sensory stimulation, addressing these issues and managing deprivation and social isolation may prove to be beneficial. Behavioral strategies which are employed are 'discrimination training' between edible and non-edible items; sensory contingent aversion using taste (lemon), smell (ammonia), physical sensation (water mist, brief physical restraint); and overcorrection. Occasionally self-protection devices that prohibit placement of objects in the mouth may be needed. Medical management incudes iron therapy in children diagnosed with anemia, multivitamin supplementation and treatment of co-existent disorders such as schizophrenia.

Enuresis: Enuresis is a common behavioral problem in children and adolescents, distressing for not only the children themselves but also their parents. It is classified under *Elimination disorders* in DSM-5. Enuresis is defined as the repeated voiding of urine into bed or clothes, whether involuntary or intentional after the developmental age when bladder control should have been established. A chronological age or equivalent development age of minimum 5 years is required for diagnosis, since more than 85% children achieve complete diurnal and nocturnal bladder control by this age. The remaining 15% gain continence at a rate of 15% per year. This behavior is clinically significant if frequency is at least twice a week for three consecutive months or is causing significant distress/impairment in social, academic or other important areas of functioning. It should not be exclusively due to direct physiological effect of a substance (e.g., diuretic) or another medical condition (e.g., diabetes). The prevalence of enuresis at age 5 years is 7% for males and 3% for females. By adolescence 0.5%-1% children continue to have enuresis.

Bed-wetting is categorized into primary and secondary enuresis. Primary enuresis means enuresis in a child more than 5 years of age, who has never been dry at night. This represents approximately 90% of all cases. Secondary enuresis means, a child who has been continent for at least 6 months begins to wet the bed again. This is usually seen between the ages of 5 to 8 years, is more transitory, usually due to psychosocial stressors, and has a better prognosis. Enuresis may also be classified according to the time of enuresis. Nocturnal enuresis is the passage of urine during sleep. It may be monosymptomatic with no day time urinary symptoms or non-monosymptomatic that is accompanied by day time urinary symptoms. Day time symptoms include increased (> 8 times) or decreased (< 3 times) voiding frequency, urgency, day time incontinence, hesitancy, straining, intermittency, weak stream, holding maneuver, feeling of incomplete emptying, postmicturition dribble, lower urinary tract pain, constipation or encopresis. Enuresis may negatively impact the child's self-esteem, emotional state and social development. Child may experience a feeling of failure, constant fear of being detected by peers, hesitancy in participating in social activities along with being at an increased risk of physical or emotional abuse from family members. Persistence of bed-wetting into older ages is associated with poorer performance in school and poorer quality of life among parents.

The pathogenesis of enuresis is multifactorial. Nocturnal enuresis involves three major pathogenic mechanisms: increased arousal threshold possibly due to immaturity of central nervous system, nocturnal polyuria associated with low overnight vasopressin levels and nocturnal detrusor over activity resulting in low functional bladder capacity during sleep. The most common cause of day time enuresis in preschool children is waiting until the last minute to void urine (micturition deferral). There is strong genetic predisposition, with the child having a 70% likelihood of having enuresis, if both parents have a positive history. Twin studies show that there is a marked familial pattern. Linkage studies have also implicated multiple chromosomes, particularly chromosome 22. Certain studies have also suggested the role of physiological factors like under secretion of arginine-vasopressin (AVP) in children who are less responsive to low plasma osmolality with fluid overload and alterations in the AVP receptors in the renal tubule. Psychosocial factors and stressful environmental events have also been implicated, more so in secondary enuresis. These include marital or domestic conflicts, birth of a sibling, death in the family and poor socioeconomic status. Attention deficit hyperactivity disorder is associated with increased incidence of primary nocturnal enuresis and its persistence beyond 10 years of age. Enuresis is more common in children who are obese and those who have an obstructive airway disease.

Management of the child with enuresis depends on an understanding of the possible specific causative factors. A detailed history is imperative to distinguish monosymptomatic from non-monosymptomatic nocturnal enuresis, identify associated or underlying constipation/ renal disease/diabetes/spinal or neurological disease and determine frequency and impact of enuresis. The presence of day time symptoms should alert the clinician to the probability of a urinary or neurological disorder. Psychosocial factors including emotional stress, parent-child maladjustments, immature toilet training must be evaluated. Physical examination must include examination of urogenitals, abdominal palpation for palpable bladder or fecoliths, perianal tears or fissures, spinal cord deformity and a neurological examination. Underlying medical conditions may be found rarely. A urinalysis should be performed in all cases to identify renal disease or urinary tract infection. Invasive procedures like urography and cystoscopy are indicated only when there is a suspected organic lesion. Parents should be asked to maintain a frequency volume chart or bladder diary. The diary should contain the timing and volume of urine and stool voids, documentation of any urine or stool leakage as well as fluid intake.

Prevention of this problem is crucial and can be achieved by stress-free proper bladder training at the appropriate developmental age (usually by the middle of the second year). Table 9.4 enumerates some strategies, which may be used by parents to ameliorate the problem. If these do not work behavior modification, using simple and inexpensive conditioning devices can be employed. Among these, the bell and alarm system has been found to be most effective and with fewer relapses. It consists of an alarm bell with the sensor placed in the underwear that activates the bell when there is initial wetting. The child can then be taken for complete evacuation. Success and relapse rates are around 70% and 30% respectively. A combination of strategies (alarm, night waking, and cleanliness training) has been found to have a success rate of 85%-100%.

Table 9.4: Guidelines for Behavioral Management of Enuresis	
1.	Parental counseling to avoid power and autonomy struggles, stress, punishment or humiliation
2.	The child should void before retiring
3.	Minimize fluid intake at least 2 hours before bedtime
4.	Avoid substances which cause diuresis (tea, coffee, soft drinks)

Contd.

Contd.

5.	Maintain an enuresis frequency chart with small rewards to be given for being dry
6.	Older children to be asked to launder soiled bed clothes and pajamas
7.	Wake the child by using an alarm clock for voiding 2–3 hours after falling asleep

Pharmacological agents should be used in those children in whom behavioral modification is unsuccessful. Imipramine (2.5 mg/kg/24 hours before bedtime) has shown a success rate of approximately 50%, with a relapse rate of 30%. Side effects are conduction defects and lethal overdoses. Desmopressin acetate nasal spray (DDAVP) has fast results and is used when rapid control of enuresis is desired. It is also administered at bedtime. However, the limiting factors are its cost, the relapse rate upon discontinuation, and side effects (hyponatremia and water intoxication).

Encopresis: Encopresis is also classified under *Elimination disorders* in DSM-5. It refers to the repeated passage of feces into inappropriate places (e.g., clothes, floor), whether involuntary or intentional after 4 years of age or equivalent developmental level. One such event should occur each month for at least 3 months to make a diagnosis and this behavior should not be due to the physiological effects of a substance (e.g., laxative) or another medical condition (except for constipation). It must be specified whether it occurs with or without constipation and overflow incontinence. Prevalence is approximately 1% of school-aged children. Encopresis may be retentive (associated with constipation) or non-retentive (without constipation). Many children may have abnormal anal sphincter physiology. In about two thirds of cases it is associated with chronic constipation, fecal impaction, and overflow incontinence. This may progress to psychogenic mega colon. Primary encopresis has a higher association with global developmental delay and enuresis, whereas secondary encopresis is seen more in children with high psychosocial stress levels and conduct disorders. In some children, encopresis may represent unconscious anger and defiance by the child. In addition, improper parental responses lead to loss of self-esteem.

Apart from a detailed history, rectal examination is warranted to evaluate for fecal retention, which is suggestive of chronic constipation and can be managed accordingly. Wherever indicated, the anal sphincter physiological function can be assessed by electromyography or by assessing the ability to defecate a rectal balloon. Management includes proper parental education regarding supportive reestablishment of proper toilet training. Coercive toilet training should be avoided. Attempts at toilet training should be temporarily stopped in children less than 2.5 years of age who are resistant to toilet training. Power and autonomy struggles should be avoided. Records of the child's elimination should be kept, with rewards being provided for compliance. In older children, relieving constipation and removing impactions can lead to significant improvement in about three fourths of cases. This can be achieved by initial short term use of enemas and laxatives and dietary interventions (mineral oil usage and increased quantities of fiber). Failure to respond to supportive measures may require psychotherapeutic intervention with the child and family. Other methods which are currently under investigation are biofeedback (a technique in which the anal sphincter muscle is trained) and the use of tricyclic anti-depressants. The addition of an intensive behavioral program to conventional medical therapy can be of substantial therapeutic benefit for most children. These include educating patients and families; giving specific toileting instruction about appropriate positioning and straining; designing a program of regular, timed, and uninterrupted toileting; maintaining a symptom and toileting diary; defining of specific achievable target behaviors; establishing age-appropriate rewards and consequences; and strongly emphasizing consistency.

Repetitive Behaviors: All children show repetitive patterns of movement at some developmental phase or the other. These include head banging, body rocking, thumb sucking, nail biting, hair pulling, teeth grinding (bruxism), nose picking, self-injurious behavior and body manipulations which the child is not able to control, are apparently purposeless but may be means of tension release. As children become older, they may learn to inhibit these habits, particularly in social situations. They are considered significant if they persist and start interfering with the child's physical, emotional, academic or social functioning or result in self-injury. The DSM-5 defines repetitive behaviors under stereotypic movement disorder. Apart from being repetitive, these movements are seemingly driven, and apparently purposeless. They also interfere with social, academic or other activities and may be self-injurious and are not attributable to direct effects of a neurological disorder. Fortunately, most repetitive behaviors in childhood do not match the criteria for a stereotypic movement disorder, are part of normal developmental trajectory and remit spontaneously without treatment, as the child grows older. Comorbid conditions frequently associated with repetitive behaviors include developmental disorders like global developmental delay, intellectual disability, autism spectrum disorder, learning disabilities, ADHD, anxiety disorders, tics and OCD, visual impairment or hearing deficit.

Head banging is the compulsive, repetitive, rhythmic movement of the head against a solid object. The exact etiology is unknown. Various suggested hypotheses include: It being an integral part of normal development, a kinesthetic drive, a tension releasing or attention-seeking maneuver, a consequence of emotional deprivation, and a response to various acute illnesses. The reported incidence in childhood varies from 5 to 15%. It is more common in boys (male : female ratio 3 or 4:1). The onset is usually in the latter half of the first year of life and generally ends spontaneously by four years of age. Head banging generally occurs before normal sleep. The duration may vary from a few minutes to an hour. The frontal-parietal region of the head is the most frequently struck site. Although head banging appears alarming, the child seldom inflicts significant damage to the head and physical examination is usually normal. Laboratory investigations are generally not indicated. Appropriate management is to offer the parents a supportive and reassuring explanation that brain damage is unlikely, and that the child will outgrow the problem.

Thumb sucking occurs in 23% to 46% of children aged 1 to 4 years. This behavior is generally not of concern, and most children cease sucking their thumb or fingers without intervention before they enter school. However, if finger sucking continues past 4 years of age certain health problems can develop, like dental malocclusion, digital deformities, speech difficulties and emotional problems. The best strategy is to ignore the symptom and provide lots of praise and encouragement for efforts to restrain thumb sucking.

CONCLUSION

Behavior problems if not appropriately managed may adversely impact the child's academic and social functioning as well as his/her family's psychosocial health. Since the pediatrician is usually the first professional who comes in contact with a child with behavioral problems, it is important to screen the child at every outpatient visit in accordance with the developmental phase of the child. On one hand one may encounter parents who are very anxious regarding their child's behaviors, many of which may be part of normal development. On the other hand, some parents may be unable to recognize certain behavior patterns in their child as problems. Pediatricians must identify children who have adverse symptoms that do not meet the criteria for a specific mental disorder yet do require intervention and distinguish them from those who require more sophisticated mental health care and referral to a specialist. Most behavior problems can be tackled by providing explanations about why they are occurring and guiding parents about appropriate responses to adverse behaviors.

Suggested Reading

- American Psychiatric Association, DSM-5 Task Force (2013). Diagnostic and Statistical Manual of Mental Disorders: DSM-5™ (5th Edition). Arlington, VA, US: American Psychiatric Publishing, Inc.
- Azab SF, Siam AG, Saleh SH, *et al.* Novel Findings in Breath-Holding Spells: A Cross-sectional Study. Medicine (Baltimore) 2015;94(28):e1150.
- Brazzelli M, Griffiths P. Behavioural and Cognitive Interventions With or Without Other Treatments for Defecation Disorders in Children. Cochrane Database Syst Rev 2001: CD002240.
- Daoud AS, Batieha A, Al-Sheyyab M, Ebuekteish F, Hijazi S. Effectiveness of Iron Therapy on Breath-Holding Spells. J Pediatr 1997;130:547-50.
- DiMario FJ Jr, Burleson JA. Autonomic Nervous System Function in Severe Breath-Holding Spells. Pediatr Neurol 1993;9:268-74.
- DiMario FJ. Prospective Study of Children with Cyanotic and Pallid Breath-Holding Spells. Pediatrics 2001 February;107(2): 265-69.
- Evans JHC. Evidence Based Management of Nocturnal Enuresis. BMJ 2001;17:323(7322):1167-69.
- Gleason MM, Goldson E, Yogman MW. AAP Council On Early Childhood. Addressing Early Childhood Emotional and Behavioral Problems. Pediatrics 2016;138(6):e20163025.
- Gupta SK. Is Colic a Gastrointestinal Disorder? Curr Opin Pediatrics 2002;14:588-92.
- Har AF, Croffie JM. Encopresis. Pediatr Rev 2010;(9):368-74.
- Kelly AM, Porter CJ, McGoon MD, Espinosa RE, Osborn MJ, Hayes DL. Breath-Holding Spells Associated With Significant Bradycardia: Successful Treatment With Permanent Pacemaker Implantation. Pediatrics 2001;108(3):698-702.
- Miao D, Sera L, Young CD, Golden A. Meta-Analysis of Pica and Micronutrient Status. Am J Hum Biol 2015;27:84-93.
- Neece CL, Green SA, Baker BL. Parenting Stress and Child Behavior Problems: A Transactional Relationship across time. Am J Intellect Dev Disabil 2012;117(1):48-66, doi:10.1352/1944-7558-117.1.48.
- Olweus D. Bullying at School: What It Is and What We Can Do. Cambridge (United Kingdom): Blackwell; 1993.
- Potegal M, Davidson RJ. Temper Tantrums in Young Children: Behavioural Composition. Journal of Developmental and Behavioural Pediatrics 2003;24:140-48.
- Prakash Jyoti, Mitra AK, Prabhu HRA. Child and Behaviour: A School Based Study, Delhi Psychiatr J 2008;11(1):79-82.

- Romanello S, Spiri D, Marcuzzi E, *et al.* Association between Childhood Migraine and History of Infantile Colic. JAMA 2013;309:1607-12.
- Savino F, Juncker A, Opramolla A, Tarasco V, Ceratto S, Bonde I, *et al.* Metagenomic Analysis of Fecal Samples from Healthy and Colicky Infants. Journal of Pediatric Gastroenterology and Nutrition 2013;56(2):154.
- Srinath S, Girimaji SC, Gururaj G, Seshadri S, Subbakrishna DK, Bhola P, *et al.* Epidemiological Study of Child and Adolescent Psychiatric Disorders in Urban and Rural Areas of Bangalore, India. Indian J Med Res 2005;122:7-79 [PubMed: 16106093].
- Vurucu S, Karaoglu A, Paksu SM, Oz O, Yaman H, Gulgun M, Babacan O, Unay B, Akin R. Breath-Holding Spells May be Associated with Maturational Delay in Myelination of Brain Stem. J Clin Neurophysiol 2014 February;31(1):99-101.
- Wessel MA, Cobb Jc, Jackson EB, Harris G Sjr, Detwiler AC. Paroxysmal Fussing in Infancy, Sometimes Called 'Colic'. Pediatrics 1954;14:421-35.

10 Chapter

ATTENTION DEFICIT HYPERACTIVITY DISORDER

MS Bhatia, Anubhav Rathi, Shruti Srivastava

Attention deficit hyperactivity disorder (ADHD) is the most common mental disorder in childhood (Olfson 1992). Although widely researched in children and having the distinction of being one of the most researched disorders in medicine (Goldman *et al.*, 1998), till recently it was thought of only in the context of children and was considered a childhood condition which remits with age. The Diagnostic and Statistical Manual has been relatively slow to acknowledge the disorder's persistence into adulthood, although this hesitation is consistent with the psychiatric community's and the general public's knowledge of adult ADHD. A growing literature supports the persistence of the disorder and/or associated impairment into adulthood in a majority of cases. Hyperactive and impulsive symptoms decrease more rapidly than inattentive symptoms with age (Faraone *et al.* 2000).

DEFINITIONS OF ADHD IN VARIOUS DSM EDITIONS

The Diagnostic and Statistical Manual, Second Edition (DSM-II) definition, hyperkinetic syndrome, emphasized motoric over activity as a core symptom in children with this disorder. In 1980, the Diagnostic and Statistical Manual of Mental Disorders, Third Edition DSM-III emphasized for the first time inattention (with and without hyperactivity) and designated an attention deficit disorder (ADD) diagnostic category. This allowed the diagnosis of non-hyperactive individuals with simple inattention, an important issue for adolescents and adults. DSM-III briefly mentions that it is possible for ADHD to persist into adolescence or adulthood, but it provides no description of symptoms (APA, DSM-III, 1980). In this edition, inattentiveness was central to the diagnosis; the disorder could be diagnosed without evidence of hyperactivity, and there was a heavier emphasis placed on impulsiveness than exists today as it listed six symptoms of impulsivity and five symptoms of inattention and hyperactivity.

The Diagnostic and Statistical Manual of Mental Disorders, Revised Third Edition (APA, DSM-III-R, 1987) stated that "approximately one-third of children with ADHD continue to show some signs of the disorder in adulthood". Though this edition still did not code adult ADHD as a separate category, it was the first edition that seriously recognized the possibility of ADHD in adolescents and adults. The other changes in the revised third edition included changing the name of the disorder to attention deficit/hyperactivity disorder from attention deficit disorder and placing more emphasis on overactivity than DSM-III did.

The Diagnostic and Statistical Manual of Mental Disorders, Fourth Edition (DSM-IV) is the first to acknowledge that full-fledged ADHD can persist into adolescence and adulthood. This edition states that "symptoms attenuate during late adolescence and adulthood, although a minority experience the full complement of symptoms of ADHD into mid-adulthood" (APA, DSM-IV, 1994). By DSM-IV and DSM-IV-TR (APA, DSM-IV-TR, 2000) definition, ADHD must begin in childhood, and evidence of the condition must be demonstrated by age 7. Another change in the fourth edition was placing impulsive and hyperactive symptoms in the same list but keeping them separately identified. A distinction was also drawn between inattention symptoms and other symptom clusters. Although both DSM-III-R and DSM-IV acknowledge that symptoms persist into adolescence and adulthood for many people who are diagnosed as children, both editions describe symptoms much more in terms of the phenomenon in a child than that in an adult.

This further changed in the latest edition of DSM-5, according to which (APA, DSM-5, 2013) there are five main diagnostic criteria:

(1) An onset before age 12 years.

(2) Duration greater than 6 months.

(3) An 18-item symptom list of which 6 of 9 inattention or 6 of 9 hyperactive/impulsive symptoms have persisted for at least 6 months to a degree that is maladaptive and inconsistent with developmental level.

(4) Some impairment in two or more settings; and

(5) Symptoms that do not occur exclusively during the course of a pervasive developmental disorder, schizophrenia, or other psychotic disorder and are not better accounted for by another mental disorder, such as depression.

Epidemiology

The prevalence of ADHD is estimated at 5% in children and 2.5% in adults (APA, DSM-5, 2013). It has been estimated that persistence of ADHD into adolescence and adulthood is there in approximately 66% to 85% of cases (Weiss *et al.*, 1985; Barkley *et al.*, 1990 and 2002; Biederman *et al.*, 1996). In a recent study from India, the prevalence of ADHD in primary school children is 11.3% (Venkata and Panicker, 2013).

Boys are two to four times more likely to be diagnosed with ADHD than girls (Cornejo *et al.*, 2005; Neuman *et al.*, 2005; Fontana *et al.*, 2007). The male/female ratio ranges from 2:1 in population based studies to 9:1 in clinical studies (Bhatia *et al.*, 1991 and 1999; Venkata and Panicker, 2013). This difference in prevalence rates may be probably due to the fact that girls have ADHD with a higher predominance of inattention and fewer comorbid symptoms of conduct disorder, causing less trouble to the family and at school, resulting therefore in fewer referrals to treatment (Luis *et al.*, 2004). Thus, as in childhood, ADHD continues to be one of the most common neuro-psychiatric disorders in adolescence also.

PREDISPOSING AND PROGNOSTIC FACTORS

Although the exact etiology of ADHD is yet to be determined, both nature (Genetics) and Nurture (Environment) appear to have a role in its etiopathogenesis. There is a growing consensus that the pathophysiology of ADHD involves functional and structural dysfunction of Pre-Frontal Cortex (PFC) and cortico-basal ganglia-thalamo-cortical circuitry. A lot of research has taken place in the field of genetics, animal studies, neurobiology, structural and functional imaging in the past 20 to 30 years which have led to the greater understanding of the etiology and management of ADHD. A highly integrated story is emerging regarding the etiology and pathophysiology of ADHD which in turn informs its management. ADHD still remains underdiagnosed, misdiagnosed and undertreated (Hamed *et al.*, 2015).

Genetics of ADHD

Genetic studies (family, twin and adoption studies) implicate a robust genetic contribution to ADHD with heritability estimates ranging from 60-90% among studies (Sharp *et al.*, 2009; Gizer *et al.*, 2009). Genome-wide association studies have failed to come up with any associations that are significant after correction for multiple testing (Franke *et al.*, 2009) though multiple candidate genes have been identified.

Studies have reported alterations in the genes encoding for molecules involved in catecholamine signaling, e.g., the dopamine (DA) receptors (D1 and D5 receptors (Daly *et al.*, 1999; Tahir *et al.*, 2000; Kustanovich *et al.*, 2004; Bobb *et al.*, 2005), D4 receptor) (Sunohara *et al.*, 2009), Norepinephrine (NE) receptors (the alpha 2A receptor) (Comings *et al.*, 2001; Xu *et al.*, 2001; Roman *et al.*, 2003), the DA and NE transporters (Daly *et al.*, 1999; Bobb *et al.*, 2005; Durston *et al.*, 2005; Mill *et al.*, 2006) and dopamine beta hydroxylase (the enzyme needed for the synthesis of NE) (Daly *et al.*, 1999; Roman *et al.*, 2002 and 2003). There are also associations with the catabolic enzyme, monoamine oxidase, and some serotonergic genes (Faraone *et al.*, 2005). Associations with DISC 1 Gene (Implicated with Schizophrenia) have also been reported (Jacobsen *et al.*, 2013). ADHD symptoms are also found in well-defined genetic mutations like Tuberous Sclerosis Complex, Fragile X syndrome and Turner Syndrome. The role of cytokine gene polymorphism has also been reported (Anand *et al.*, 2017).

The Neurochemical Correlates of ADHD– The Central Role of Catecholamines Norepinephrine (NE) and Dopamine (DA)

Catecholamines constitute the mainstay of the neuro-chemical environment of Pre-Frontal Cortex, with too much (stress) or too little (drowsy) both conditions being detrimental to its optimal functioning. Thus this region of brain is very sensitive to genetic and environmental insults affecting these neurotransmitters (Rathi *et al.*, 2013). While NE stimulation of alpha-2A receptors enhances PFC function by strengthening appropriate network connections (increasing "signals"), DA stimulation of D1 receptors exerts its beneficial effects by weakening inappropriate connections (decreasing "noise") (Arnsten, 2007). Medications effective in ADHD normalize catecholamine transmission in their therapeutic doses thus optimizing the neurochemical environment of PFC in patients with genetic abnormalities of these pathways (Rathi *et al.*, 2013).

Environmental Factors

High lead exposure and maternal smoking have been associated with higher incidence of ADHD (Greenhill *et al.*, Kaplan Comprehensive Textbook of Psychiatry, 9th Edition). Children coming from a lower social class is another factor considered important by many (Chawla *et al.*, 1981; Sacachar *et al.*, 1989) in causation of ADHD. Many authors have found increase incidence of broken homes, persistent parental discord of spontaneous complaints of aggressive behavior by parents etc. as compared with control group (Cohen *et al.*, 1983; Singhal *et al.*, 1987).

Clinical Features

ADHD is characterized by three core Behaviors–Inattentiveness, impulsiveness and hyperactivity. As per DSM-5, for a diagnosis of ADHD, following criteria need to be fulfilled: Either (1) and/or (2):

1. Inattention

Six (or more) of the following symptoms of inattention have persisted for at least 6 months to a degree that is inconsistent with developmental level and that negatively impacts directly on social and academic/occupational activities:

Note: The symptoms are not solely a manifestation of Oppositional Behavior, defiance, hostility, or failure to understand tasks or instructions. For older adolescents and adults (age 17 years and older), at least five symptoms are required.

(a) Often fails to give close attention to details or makes careless mistakes in schoolwork, work, or during other activities (e.g., overlooks or misses details, work is inaccurate).

(b) Often has difficulty sustaining attention in tasks or play activities (e.g., has difficulty remaining focused during lectures, conversations, or lengthy reading).

(c) Often does not seem to listen when spoken to directly (e.g., mind seems elsewhere, even in the absence of any obvious distraction).

(d) Often does not follow through on instructions and fails to finish schoolwork, chores, or duties in the workplace (e.g., starts tasks but quickly loses focus and is easily side-tracked).

(e) Often has difficulty organizing tasks and activities (e.g., difficulty managing sequential tasks; difficulty keeping materials and belongings in order; messy, disorganized work; has poor time management; fails to meet deadlines).

(f) Often avoids, dislikes, or is reluctant to engage in tasks that require sustained mental effort (e.g., schoolwork or homework; for older adolescents and adults, preparing reports, completing forms, reviewing lengthy papers).

(g) Often loses things necessary for tasks or activities (e.g., school materials, pencils, books, tools, wallets, keys, paperwork, eyeglasses, mobile telephones).

(h) Is often easily distracted by extraneous stimuli (for older adolescents and adults, may include unrelated thoughts).

(i) Is often forgetful in daily activities (e.g., doing chores, running errands; for older adolescents and adults, returning calls, paying bills, keeping appointments) six (or more) of the following symptoms of hyperactivity impulsivity have persisted for at least 6 months to a degree that is inconsistent with developmental level and that negatively impacts directly on social and academic/occupational activities.

Note: The symptoms are not solely a manifestation of Oppositional Behavior, defiance, hostility, or failure to understand tasks or instructions. For older adolescents and adults (age 17 years and older), at least five symptoms are required.

2. Hyperactivity/Impulsivity

- Often fidgets with hands or feet or squirms in seat.
- Often leaves seat in classroom or in other situations in which remaining seated is expected (e.g., leaves his or her place in the classroom, in the office or other workplace, or in other situations that require remaining in place).
- Often runs about or climbs excessively in situations in which it is inappropriate (in adolescents or adults, may be limited to feeling restlessness).
- Often unable to play or engage in leisure activities quietly.
- Is often "on the go" or acting as if "driven by a motor" (e.g., is unable to be or uncomfortable being still for extended time, as in restaurants, meetings; may be experienced by others as being restless or difficult to keep up).
- Often talks excessively.

Impulsivity

- Often blurts out answers before questions have been completed (e.g., completes other people's sentences; cannot wait for turn in conversation).
- Often has difficulty awaiting turn (e.g., while waiting in line).
- Often interrupts or intrudes on others (e.g., butts into conversations, games, or activities; may start using other people's things without asking or receiving permission; for adolescents and adults, may intrude into or take over what others are doing).
- Some hyperactive impulsive or inattentive symptoms that caused impairment were present prior to the age of 12 years.
- Some impairment from the symptoms is present in two or more settings (e.g., at home, school or work; with friends or relatives; in other activities).
- There must be clear evidence that symptoms interfere with, or reduce the quality of social, academic, or occupational functioning.
- The symptoms do not occur exclusively during the course of a pervasive developmental disorder, schizophrenia, or other psychotic disorder and are not better accounted for by another mental disorder (e.g., mood disorder, anxiety disorder, dissociative disorder, or a personality disorder).

Code Based on Type

- 314.01 (F90.2) Attention Deficit/Hyperactivity Disorder, Combined Type: If both Criteria A1 and A2 are met for the past 6 months.
- 314.00 (F90.0) Attention Deficit/Hyperactivity Disorder, Predominantly Inattentive Type: If Criterion A1 is met but Criterion A2 is not met for the past 6 months.
- 314.01 (F90.1) Attention Deficit/Hyperactivity Disorder, Predominantly Hyperactive-Impulsive Type: If Criterion A2 is met but Criterion A1 is not met for the past 6 months.
- **Coding note:** For individuals (especially adolescents and adults) who currently have symptoms that no longer meet full criteria, "In Partial Remission" should be specified.

The neuroimaging studies have shown ADHD (Combined type) is distinct from ADHD (Inattentive type) i.e., former shows distributed atypical connectivity with predominant findings in default network whereas latter shows predominant findings in control systems (ADHD-200-Consorium 2012, Fair *et al.*, 2013).

Children and adolescents with ADHD often seem emotionally immature, compared with their same-age peers (Hoy *et al.*, 1978). They often do best when interacting with younger children or in the environment of adults who tolerate their immature behaviors. Adolescents and children with ADHD often display affect, both negative and positive, that is excessive for the situation (Barkley *et al.*, 1992). Other symptoms can be "becoming frustrated easily" and having a "short fuse", with sudden outbursts of anger. These impairments may have widespread effects that often seem like behavioral problems and are not recognized as part of the ADHD (Wolraich *et al.*, 2005).

Adolescents diagnosed with ADHD and comorbid disruptive behavior disorders during childhood report high levels of aggression associated with increased emotionality in the form of anger, but not hostile cognitions. These findings suggest that in addition to inattention and hyperactivity/impulsivity, emotional dysregulation may be an important component of ADHD, particularly as it presents in adolescence (Harty *et al.*, 2009). The clinical picture is further complicated by features of associated comorbidities like oppositional defiant disorder, conduct, anxiety, substance abuse and mood disorders.

Comorbidity

Comorbidity is very common with ADHD patients, with estimates as ranging from 50-80% (Pliszka, 1998; Waxmonsky, 2003; Kunwar *et al.*, 2007; Biederman *et al.*, 1993; Barkley, 1998). A review done in 2004 by Klassen showed that a significant minority of children and adolescents with ADHD have more than one comorbidity, whereas a 2008 review by Elia J *et al.*, found that the mean number of concurrent comorbid diagnosis among ADHD adolescents were 2.1 inclusive of ADHD. Thus, assessing the absence or presence of symptoms of other disorders is a key part of ADHD diagnosis. Various comorbidities associated with ADHD are:

I. **Disruptive Behavioral Disorders (Oppositional Defiant Disorder (ODD) and Conduct Disorder (CD)):** Studies show a high prevalence of comorbidity between ADHD and disruptive behavioral disorders (conduct disorder and oppositional defiant disorder), which ranges from 30% to 50% (Biederman, 1991; AACAP practice parameters, 1997; Berenson, 1998; Goldman *et al.*, 1998; Elia, 2008; Spencer *et al.*, 2007; Rathi *et al.*, 2012).

Adolescents with ODD are chronically much more argumentative, negativistic and defiant than most other adolescents (APA, DSM-IV, 1994). CD is considered more severe, and involves habitual rule breaking defined by aggression, destruction and lying. It is correlated with a more severe course of ADHD.

II. Anxiety Disorders: Anxiety disorders occur in up to 25% to one third of patients with ADHD against an average of 3-5% in general population (Biederman *et al.*, 1991; AACAP practice parameters, 1997; MTA cooperative group, 1999; Pliszka *et al.*, 1999; Tannock, 2000, Waxmonsky, 2003; Kunwar *et al.*, 2007; Rathi *et al.*, 2012). In a review by Souza *et al.*, in 2005 Generalized anxiety disorder was the most prevalent disorder (12.8%), followed by social phobia (3.84%) and separation anxiety disorder (3.8%).

Adolescents with comorbid ADHD and anxiety may present a complicated clinical picture, because these disorders are characterized by thinking too little (ADHD) and thinking too much (anxiety). Careful assessment is important when attempting to diagnose these comorbid conditions (Wolraich *et al.*, 2005).

III. Mood Disorders: The prevalence of mood disorder in patients with ADHD is more controversial, with studies showing 0% to 33% of patients with ADHD meeting criteria for a depressive disorder (Pliszka *et al.*, 1999). Prior systematic studies of children and adolescents found rates of ADHD ranging from 57% to 98% in bipolar children and rates of bipolar disorder of 22% in ADHD inpatients (Faraone *et al.*, 1997). The mood disorders, including major depression, bipolar disorder, and dysrhythmia, have a comorbidity rate with ADHD ranging from 19% to 37% (Waxmonsky, 2003; Kunwar *et al.*, 2007 Rathi *et al.*, 2012).

Both mania and depression can both complicate an ADHD diagnosis, due to shared developmental and clinical features. Thus, they require careful and more often than not, multiple assessments to make a definitive diagnosis.

IV. Substance Use and Abuse: The range for comorbid alcohol abuse is 32% to 53%, and for other types of substance abuse, including marijuana and cocaine abuse, the comorbidity rate is 8% to 32% (Barkley *et al.*, 1998). Individuals with ADHD start smoking at a younger age (Hartsough *et al.*, 1987) and have higher rates of smoking than do individuals without ADHD (Lambert *et al.*, 1998). Fifteen percent to 19% of patients with ADHD will start to smoke (Milberger *et al.*, 1997) or develop other substance abuse disorders (Biederman *et al.*, 1997; Rathi *et al.*, 2012).

Clinicians should therefore be cautious in making an ADHD diagnosis during adolescence when substance use is present and childhood symptoms are absent. It may be best to reassess an adolescent suspected of having ADHD after at least a 1 month period of abstinence from all psychoactive drugs (Wolraich *et al.*, 2005). Individuals with ADHD, independent of comorbidity, tend to maintain their addiction longer than do their non-ADHD peers (Wilens *et al.*, 1998). The presence of ADHD is also associated with greater severity of substance use disorders, including higher rates of substance-related motor vehicle accidents and treatment episodes (Carroll *et al.*, 1993; Biederman *et al.*, 1997; Schubiner *et al.*, 2000). Although adolescents with ADHD are at greater risk of substance use, the evidence suggests that appropriate treatment of ADHD, including the use of psychostimulant medication, does not increase that risk (Faraone *et al.*, 2003).

V. Learning Disorders: Various studies and reviews have estimated the comorbidity of learning disabilities from 10 to 60% with some estimates as high as 92% depending on the psychometric definitions used as against 5-15% in general adolescent population (Silver, 1981; Barkley, 1988; Biederman *et al.*, 1991; Shapiro *et al.*, 1993; AACAP practice parameters, 1997; Shaywitz, 1998; Pliszka, 1998, 2000; AAP, Clinical Practice Guidelines, 2000; Waxmonsky, 2003; Kunwar *et al.*, 2007).

It is known that children with Specific learning disorder/ADHD have 'more severe' learning problems than children who have Specific learning disorder but no ADHD, and also 'more severe' attention problems than children who have ADHD but no Specific learning disorder (Mayes *et al.*, 2000; Singh 2012, Tosto 2015). They also tend to have more behavioral problems such as aggressive and withdrawn behaviors because of a lack of self-esteem and frustrations due to their poor school performance (Pisecco *et al.*, 1996).

VI. Tic Disorders: Association has been found between ADHD and TS (Tourette's Syndrome). In a study 250 consecutive cases of TS were taken; 62% were found to have ADD and 48.8% were having ADD with hyperactivity (Comings *et al.*, 1985). Most of these patients began with history of ADD. 2-3 years prior to the development of tics, OCD was also a common finding in this group. Various other studies (Comings *et al.*, 1987) have reported ADHD in 21-90% of GTS (Giles de la Tourette's Syndrome) patients. But the relationship between these two disorders is still not clear.

Rating Scales

Several Rating Scales are useful for assessing the severity and presence of ADHD. The most commonly used are the Conners (1985), and the Achenbach scales, which are available in parents and teacher version. For rating the severity of ADHD, ADHD-RS (DuPaul *et al.*,1998) is used. The Child Behavior Check List (CBCL) is a 138 item parent report questionnaire and is useful with children from ages 4 to 16 years. This instrument assesses a broad range of behavior problems and impotencies. The family members report more commonly than school teachers (Visser *et al.*, 2015).

DIAGNOSIS AND INVESTIGATIONS

Recently FDA has approved the first brain wave test for aiding in the diagnosis of ADHD in children and adolescents between the age group of 6 and 17 years. This test is based on electroencephalogram technology. It computes the ratio of theta and beta brain waves in 15 to 20 minutes. Children and adolescents with ADHD have a higher theta-beta ratio than those who do not have the disorder (http://www.medscape.com/viewarticle/807869). However, for the most part, ADHD remains a clinical diagnosis with careful history taking from multiple reliable informants, ruling out differential diagnosis and systematic observations playing an invaluable role. Differential diagnosis of ADHD include General Medical Conditions (e.g., lead toxicity, thyroid disorders etc.); Neurological and Developmental issues (e.g., PANDAS, intellectual disabilities, learning disorders, static encephalopathy etc.); Psychiatric Disorders (anxiety disorders, disruptive behavior disorders, OCD, PTSD, mood disorders, substance abuse etc.) and Environmental problems (ineffectual parental practices or classroom management, child maltreatment and bullying, socioeconomic dis-advantage etc.) (French 2015). Untreated ADHD can lead to many complications such as impaired relationships and quality of life, reduced employment, proneness to addiction, depression and anxiety, accident proneness and suicide (Gaffen and Forster 2018).

Management

Multidisciplinary approach is needed to provide an adequate care to these children. Medications, behavioral approaches and various educational programs are required together to bring about better outcomes.

Psychopharmacological Approach–Stimulants

Stimulant medication has already been proved to be effective in controlling various hyperactive symptoms in particular and also improve the attention span as well as information processing in these children. All these medicines are equally effective and one particular medicine may be more useful in specific group according to the situation. Methylphenidate, dextroamphetamine and pemoline; all these are first line drugs. Out of these Amphetamines and Pemolines are not available in India. Pemoline has also been banned from various countries on account of its toxicity.

Methylphenidate still remains the first choice in most of these cases as it has the most robust effect size among all the drugs available for treatment of ADHD (Bachman *et al.*, 2017). It is given in 0.5-1 mg/day divided in morning and mid day doses. It is available in immediate release, sustained release and osmotic release preparations. *The common side effects reported with this drug are decreased appetite, weight loss and abdominal pain. Type, dose or duration of drug makes no changes as evident from a recent meta-analysis (Holmskov et al., 2017).* Starting the treatment with stimulants results in a better interpersonal relationship between parents and the child and its lead to an enhanced effectiveness of behavioral approaches (Schachar *et al.*, 1987). A few characteristics like young age of patient, clearly disturbed attention span, an average IQ and low level of associated anxiety predict a better response to the stimulants. Besides having an abuse potential these drugs also cause a reversible growth retardation, depression, tachycardia and hypertension rarely (Dulkan *et al.*, 1988).

Non-Stimulant Medications

Atomoxetine

Atomoxetine is a norepinephrine reuptake inhibitor (NRI). Its putative mechanism of action is thought to involve selective inhibition of the presynaptic norepinephrine transporter (Spencer *et al.*, 1998). It is prescribed in the dose of 1.4 mg/kg/day. It has less abuse potential as compared to other stimulants like methylphenidate. Common side effects of this drug are decreased appetite, dyspepsia, dizziness, fatigue, sedation, nausea, vomiting, mood swings and growth delay.

Tricyclic Antidepressants

Imipramine, Desipramine and Nortriptyline in a dose of 3 mg/kg/day have been found useful in reducing the symptoms of ADHD. They are useful for selected nonresponders to stimulants and patients with comorbid tics or mood disorder. Regular ECG and blood estimation are to be done especially in patients receiving more than 50 mg/day. If at all it is to be combined with methylphenidate all precautions to be taken regarding repeated tests as the chances of toxicity are high in combination.

Bupropion

It is a norepinephrine and dopamine reuptake inhibitor (NDRI) that has shown efficacy in ADHD but is less effective than TCAs or stimulants. It is available in extended release preparation (SR and XL) and the recommended doses are up to 200-300 mg/day. Higher doses (above 400 mg/day) are not recommended due to seizure risk.

Alpha-Adrenergic Agents

Although not FDA approved but these are frequently used by clinicians along with clinicians in ADHD which is comorbid with tics. Total daily doses greater than 0.3 mg are not recommended (Greenhill *et al.*, Kaplan Comprehensive Textbook of Psychiatry, 9th Edition). The other agent that is sometimes used is Guanfacine.

Non-Pharmacological Treatments

The short-term benefits of stimulant intake are clear, long term ones are not. Behavioral interventions play a key role for long-term improvement of executive functioning and organizational skills (Rajeh *et al.*, 2017).

These include different modalities, such as psycho-education, academic organization, skill teaching and remediation, parent training, behavior modification, cognitive–behavioral therapy (CBT) (Schachar *et al.*, 2004, Danielsen *et al.*, 2017), social skills training, neurobiofeedback and individual therapy.

Of these modalities, parent training (Cunningham *et al.*, 1993), intensive behavior modification, and social skills training (MTA Cooperative Group 1999b) have shown efficacy for children with ADHD in controlled trials. Parental satisfaction has been found to be more in ADHD patients without conduct symptoms (Goyal *et al.*, 2013).

The role of diet needs further research (Pelsser *et al.*, 2017).

Suggested Reading

- ADHD-200-Consortium (2012). The ADHD-200 Consortium: A Model to Advance the Translational Potential of Neuro-imaging in Clinical Neuroscience. Front. Syst. Neurosci., 6:62. doi: 10.3389/fnsys. 2012.00062.
- Anand D, Colpo GD, Zeni G, Geni CL,Teixeira AL. Attention Deficit/Hyperactivity Disorder and Inflammation: What Does Current Knowledge Tell Us? A Systematic Review. Front Psychiatry, 09 November 2017 Accessed from https://doi .org/10.3389/fpsyt.2017.00228.
- American Academy of Child and Adolescent Psychiatry (AACAP). Practice Parameters for the Assessment and Treatment of Children, Adolescents and Adults with Attention. Deficit/Hyperactivity Disorder. J Am Acad Adolesc Psychiatry 1997:36S10:85-121.
- American Academy of Pediatrics. Clinical Practice Guideline: Diagnosis and Evaluation of the Child with Attention-Deficit/ Hyperactivity Disorder, Pediatrics 2000;105:1158-70.
- American Psychiatric Association Diagnostic and Statistical Manual of Mental Disorders. 3rd Edition. Washington (DC): American Psychiatric Press 1980.
- American Psychiatric Association, Diagnostic and Statistical Manual of Mental Disorders, 3rd Edition, Revised. Washington (DC): American Psychiatric Press 1987.
- American Psychiatric Association. Diagnostic and Statistical Manual of Mental Disorders. 4th Edition. Washington (DC): American Psychiatric Press 1994.
- American Psychiatric Association. Diagnostic and Statistical Manual of Mental Disorders. 4th Edition. Text Revision. Washington (DC): American Psychiatric Press 2000.
- American Psychiatric Association. Diagnostic and Statistical Manual of Mental Disorders. 5th Edition. Text Revision. Washington (DC): American Psychiatric Press 2013.
- Arnsten AF. Catecholamine and Second Messenger Influences on Prefrontal Cortical Networks of "Representational Knowledge": A Rational Bridge Between Genetics and the Symptoms of Mental Illness. Cerebral Cortex 2007;17(S 1): i6-i15.
- Bachman CJ, Philipsen A, Hoffman F. ADHD in Germany: Trends in Diagnosis and Pharmacotherapy. ODifsch Arzlebl Int 2017:114(9):141-48.
- Barkley RA. Attention-Deficit/Hyperactivity Disorder: A Handbook for Diagnosis and Treatment. New York, NY: Guilford Press.1988.
- Barkley RA. Attention Deficit Hyperactivity Disorder: A Handbook for Diagnosis and Treatment, 2nd Edition. New York: Guilford 1990.
- Barkley RA, Murphy KR. Attention Deficit/Hyperactivity Disorder: A Clinical Workbook, 2nd Edition, Guilford Publications, Incorporated 1998.
- Barkley RA, Fischer M, Smallish L, Fletcher K. The Persistence of Attention Deficit/Hyperactivity Disorder Into Young Adulthood as a Function of Reporting Source and Definition of Disorder. J Abnorm Psychol 2002;111(2):279-89.
- Berenson CK. Frequently Missed Diagnosis in Adolescent Psychiatry. Psychiatr Clin North Am 1998;21:917-26.

- Bhatia MS. Nigam VR. Bohra N. Malik SC. Attention Deficit Disorder with Hyperactivity Among Pediatric Outpatients. J Child Psychol Psychiatry 1991:32:297-306.
- Bhatia MS. Choudhary S. Sidana A. Attention Deficit Hyperactivity Disorder Among Psychiatric Outpatients. Indian Pediatr 1999:36:583-87.
- Biederman J. Newcom J. Sprich S. Comorbidity of Attention Deficit Hyperactivity Disorder with Conduct. Depressive. Anxiety and Other Disorders. Am J Psychiatry 1991:148: 564-77.
- Biederman J. Faraone SV. Spencer T. Wilens T. Norman D. Lapey KA. *et al.* Patterns of Psychiatric Comorbidity. Cognition and Psychosocial Functioning in Adults with Attention Deficit/ Hyperactivity Disorder. Am J Psychiatry 1993: 150(12):1792-98.
- Biederman J. Farone S. Milberger S. *et al.* A Prospective 4-Year Follow-up Study of Attention Deficit Hyperactivity and Related Disorders. Arch Gen Psychiatry 1996:53:437-46.
- Biederman J. Wilens T. Mick E *et al.* Is ADHD a Risk Factor for Psychoactive Substance Use Disorders? Findings from a Four-year Prospective Follow-up Study. J Am Acad Child Adolesc Psychiatry 1997:36:21-29.
- Bobb AJ. Addington AM. Sidransky E. Gornick MC. Lerch JP. Greenstein DK. *et al.* Support for Association Between ADHD and Two Candidate Genes: NET1 and DRD1. Am J Med Genet B Neuropsychiatr Genet 2005:134:67-72.
- Carroll K. Rounsaville BJ. History and Significance of Childhood Attention Deficit Disorder in Treatment-Seeking Cocaine Abusers. Compr Psychiatry 1993:34:75-82.
- Chawla PL. Shashi G. Sunderam KR. Mehta M. A Study of Prevalence Pattern of Hyperactive Syndrome in Primary School Children. Ind J Psychiatry 1981:23:313-23.
- Cohen NJ. Minde K. The Hyperactive Syndrome in Kindergarten Children Comparison of Children with Pervasive and Situational Symptoms. J Child Psychol Psychiatr 1983:24: 443-55.
- Comings DE. Comings BG. Tourette-Syndrome: Clinical and Psychological Aspects of 250 Cases. Am J Hum Genet 1985:37:435-50.
- Comings DE. Comings BG. A Controlled Study of Tourette Syndrome I-VII. Am J Hum Gen 1987:41:701866.
- Comings DE. Clinical and Molecular Genetics of ADHD and Tourette Syndrome. Two Related Polygenic Disorders. Ann N Y Acad Sci 2001:931:50-83.
- Conners CK. Barkley RA. Rating Scales and Checklists for Child Psychopharmacology. Psychopharmacol Bull 1985: 21(4):809-43.
- Cornejo JW. Osio O. Sanchez Y. *et al.* Prevalence of Attention Deficit Hyperactivity Disorder in Colombian Children and Teenagers. Rev Neurol 2005:40:716-22.
- Cunningham CE. Davis JR. Dunn KN and Rzasa T. Coping Modeling Problem Solving Versus Mastery Modeling: Effects on Adherence. in-session Process. and Skill Acquisition in a Residential Parent Training Program. J Consult Clin Psychol 1993:61:871-77.
- Daly G. Hawi Z. Fitzgerald M. Gill M. Mapping Susceptibility Loci in Attention Deficit Hyperactivity Disorder: Preferential Transmission of Parental Alleles at DAT1. DBH and DRD5 to Affected Children. Mol Psychiatry 1999:4(2):192-96.
- Danielsen ML. Visser SN. Chronis-Tuscano A. DuPaul GJ. A National Description of Treatment Among US Children and Adolescents with Attention Deficit/Hyperactivity Disorder. J Peds 2018:192:240-46.
- Dulkan MK. Treatment of Children and Adolescents. In: Textbook of Psychiatry Eds. Talbott JA. Hales RE. Yudofsky SC. Washington DC. American Psychiatric Press Inc 1988: 985-1020.
- Dupaul GJ. Power TJ. Anastopoulos AD. Reid R. The ADHD Rating Scale-IV: Checklists. Norms and Clinical Interpretation. New York:Guilford. 1998.
- Durston S. Fossella JA. Casey BJ. Hulshoff Pol HE. Galvan A. Schnack HG. *et al.* Differential Effects of DRD4 and DAT1 Genotype on Frontostriatal Gray Matter Volumes in a Sample of Subjects with Attention Deficit Hyperactivity Disorder. Their Unaffected Siblings and Controls. Mol Psychiatry 2005:10:678-85.
- Elia J. ADHD Characteristics: I. Concurrent Comorbidity Patterns in Children and Adolescents. Child Adolesc Psychiatr Ment Health 2008:2:15.
- Fair DA. Nigg JT. Iyer S. *et al.* Distinct Neural Signatures Detected for ADHD Subtypes After Controlling for Micro-Movements in Resting State Functional Connectivity MRI Data. Front Syst. Neurosci 04 February 2013: Accessed from https://doi.org/10.3389/fnsys.2012.00080.
- Faraone S. Biederman J. Wozniak J. *et al.* Is Comorbidity with ADHD a Marker for Juvenile-Onset Mania? J Am Acad Child Adolesc Psychiatry 1997:36:1046-55.
- Faraone SV. Biederman J. Spencer T. Wilens T. Seidman LJ. Mick E. *et al.* Attention Deficit/Hyperactivity Disorder in Adults: An Overview. Soc Biol Psychiatry 2000:48:9-20.
- Faraone SV. Wilens T. Does Stimulant Treatment Lead to Substance Use Disorders? J Clin Psychiatry 2003:11(s 64): 9-13.
- Faraone SV. Perlis RH. Doyle AE. Smoller JW. Goralnick JJ. Holmgren MA. *et al.* Molecular Genetics of Attention Deficit/ Hyperactivity Disorder. Biol Psychiatry 2005:57:1313-23.
- Fontana Rda S. Vasconcelos MM. Werner J Jr. Góes FV. Liberal EF. ADHD Prevalence in Four Brazilian Public Schools. Arg Neuropsiquiatr 2007:65:134-37.
- Franke B. Vasquez AA. Johansson S. Hoogman M. Romanos J. Boreatti-Hummer A. *et al.* Multicenter Analysis of the SLC6A3/DAT1 VNTR Haplotype in Persistent ADHD Suggests Differential Involvement of the Gene in Childhood and Persistent ADHD. Neuropsychopharmacology 2009: 35(3):656-64.
- French WP. Assessment and Treatment of Attention Deficit/ Hyperactivity Disorder: Part 1. Pediatr Ann 2015:44(3): 114-20.
- Gaffen J. Forster KT. Treatment of ADHD: A Clinical Perspective. Ther Adv. Psychopharmacol 2015:6:168.

- Gizer IR. Ficks C. Waldman ID. Candidate Gene Studies of ADHD: A Meta-Analytic Review. Hum Genet 2009:126: 51-90.
- Goldman S. Genel M. Bezman R. Slanetz P. Diagnosis and Treatment of Attention Deficit/Hyperactivity Disorder in Children and Adolescents. JAMA 1998: 279:1100-07.
- Goyal S. Sagar R. Mehta M. Parental Satisfaction Assessment for Treatment in ADHD Patient With and Without Conduct Symptoms. Delhi Psychiatry J 2013:16(1):80-82.
- Greenhill LL. Hechtman LI. Attention Deficit/Hyperactivity Disorder. In. Sadock. Benjamin J: Sadock. Virginia A: Ruiz. Pedro (ed). Comprehensive Textbook of Psychiatry. 9th Edition. Philadelphia. Lippincott Williams and Wilkins 2009: 3561-72.
- Hamed AM. Kauer AJ. Stevens HE. Why the Diagnosis of Attention Deficit Hyperactivity Matters? Front Psychiatry 2015:6:168.
- Hartsough C. Lambert NM. Pattern and Progression of Drug Use Among Hyperactives and Controls: A Prospective Short-term Longitudinal Study. J Child Psychol Psychiatry 1987:28: 543-53.
- Harty SC, Miller CJ. Newcorn JH, Halperi JM. Adolescents with Childhood ADHD and Comorbid Disruptive Behavior Disorders: Aggression, Anger and Hostility. Child Psychiatry Hum Dev 2009;40(1):85-97.
- Holmskov M. Storebo OJ. Moreira-Maia CR. *et al.* Gastro-intestinal Adverse Events During Methylphenidate Treatment of Children and Adolescents with Attention Deficit Hyperactivity Disorder: A Systematic Review with Meta-Analysis and Trial Sequential Analysis of Randomized Clinical Trials. Hills RK. ed. PLoS ONE 2017;12(6):e0178187.
- Hoy E. Weiss G. Minde K. Cohen N. The Hyperactive Child at Adolescence: Emotional. Social and Cognitive Functioning. J Abnorm Child Psychol 1978:6:311-24. http://www.medscape.com/viewarticle/807869.
- Jacobsen KK *et al.* DISC1 in Adult ADHD Patients: An Association Study in Two European Samples. Am J Med Genet Part B 2013.162B.227-34.
- Klassen AF. Health-Related Quality of Life in Children and Adolescents Who Have a Diagnosis of Attention Deficit/ Hyperactivity Disorder. Pediatrics 2004;114(5).
- Kunwar A. Dewan M. Faraone SV. Treating Common Psychiatric Disorders Associated with Attention Deficit/Hyper-activity Disorder. Expert Opin Pharmacother 2007:8:555-62.
- Kustanovich V. Ishii J. Crawford L. *et al.* Transmission Disequilibrium Testing of Dopamine Related Candidate Gene Polymorphisms in ADHD: Confirmation of Association of ADHD with DRD4 and DRD5. Mol Psychiatry 2004;9: 711-17.
- Lambert N. Hartsough C. Prospective Study of Tobacco Smoking and Substance Dependence Among Samples of ADHD and Non-ADHD Subjects. J Learn Disabil 1998;31: 533-54.
- Luis A Rohde. Recent Advances on Attention Deficit/Hyper-activity Disorder J Pediatr (Rio J) 2004; 80(S 2):S61-S70.
- Mayes SD. Calhoun SL. Crowell EW. Learning Disabilities and ADHD: Overlapping Spectrum Disorders. J Learn Disabil 2000:33:417-24.
- Milberger S. Biederman J. Faraone SV. Chen L. Jones J. ADHD is Associated with Early Initiation of Cigarette Smoking in Children and Adolescents. J Am Acad Child Adolesc Psychiatry 1997:36:37-44.
- Mill J. Caspi A. Williams BS. Craig I. *et al.* Prediction of Heterogeneity in Intelligence and Adult Prognosis by Genetic Polymorphisms in the Dopamine System Among Children with Attention Deficit/Hyperactivity Disorder: Evidence from 2 Birth Cohorts. Arch Gen Psychiatry 2006:63:462-69.
- MTA Cooperative Group. Moderators and Mediators of Treatment Response for Children with Attention Deficit Hyperactivity Disorder: The MTA Study. Arch Gen Psychiatry 1999b:56:1088-96.
- Neuman RJ. Sitdhiraksa N. Reich W. Ji TH. Joyner CA. Sun LW. *et al.* Estimation of Prevalence of DSM-IV and Latent Class Defined ADHD Subtypes in a Population-Based Sample of Child and Adolescent Twins. Twin Res Hum Genet 2005; 8:392-401.
- Olfson M. Diagnosing Mental Disorders in Office-Based Pediatric Practice. J Dev Behav Pediatr 1992:13:363-65.
- Pelsser LM. Frankena K. Toorman J. Rodrigues PR. Diet and ADHD. Reviewing the Evidence: A Systemic Review of Meta-Analyses of Double Blind Placebo Controlled Trials Evaluating the Efficacy of Diet Interventions on the Behavior of Children with ADHD. PLoS One 2017;12(1):e0169277.
- Pisecco S. Baker DB. Silva PA. Brooke M. Behavioral Distinctions in Children with Reading Disabilities and/ or ADHD. J Am Acad Child Adolesc Psychiatry 1996;35: 1477-84.
- Pliszka SR. Comorbidity of Attention Deficit/Hyperactivity Disorder with Psychiatric Disorder: An Overview. J Clin Psychiatry 1998;59(S7):50-55.
- Rajeh A. Amanullah S. Shivakumar K. Cole J. Interventions in ADHD: A Comparative Review of Stimulant Medications and Behavioral Therapies. Asian J Psychiatry 2017:25:131-35.
- Rathi A. Sitholey P. Agrawal V. Sivakumar T. Bhatia MS. Sharma S. A Comparative Study of Phenomenology. Psychiatric Comorbidities and Global Functioning of People with ADHD from Childhood to Adulthood. Delhi Psychiatry J 2012;15(1):14-21.
- Rathi A. Bhatia MS. Neurobiology of ADHD. Indian J Biol Psychiatry 2013;1(1):20-27.
- Roman T. Schmitz M. Polanczyk GV. Eizirik M. Rohde LA. Hutz MH. Further Evidence for the Association Between Attention Deficit/Hyperactivity Disorder and the Dopamine-Betahydroxylase Gene. Am J Med Genet 2002:114(2):154-58.
- Roman T. Schmitz M. Polanczyk GV. Eizirik M. Rohde LA. Hutz MH. Is the Alpha-2A Adrenergic Receptor Gene (ADRA2A) Associated with Attention-Deficit/Hyperactivity Disorder? Am J Med Genet B Neuropsychiatr Genet 2003; 120:116-20.

- Safren SA. Psychosocial Treatments for Attention Deficit/ Hyperactivity Disorder Psychiatr Clin N Am 2004:27:349-60.
- Schachar R, Rutter M, Smith A. The Characteristics of Situationally and Pervasively Hyperactive Children: Implications for Syndrome Definition. J Child Psychol Psychiatry 1989b: 30:691-709.
- Schachar RJ, Taylor E, Wieselberg M. Changes to Family Function and Relationship in Children Who Respond to Methylphenidate. J Am Acad Child Adolesc Psychiatry 1987; 26:728-32.
- Schubiner H, Tzelepis A, Milberger S. Prevalence of Attention Deficit Hyperactivity Disorder and Conduct Disorder Among Substance Abusers. J Clin Psychiatry 2000:61:244-51.
- Shapiro BK, Gallico RP. Learning Disabilities. Pediatr Clin North Am 1993:40:491-505.
- Sharp SI, McQuillin A, Gurling HM. Genetics of Attention Deficit Hyperactivity Disorder (ADHD). Neuropharmacology 2009;57:590-600.
- Shaywitz SE. Dyslexia. N Engl J Med 1998;338:307-12.
- Silver LB. The Relationship between Learning Disabilities, Hyperactivty, Distractibility and Behavioral Problems. J Am Acad Child Psychiatry 1981:20:385-97.
- Singhal R, Taylor E, Wieselberg M, Thorley G, Rutter M. Changes in Family Function and Relationships in Children Who Respond to Methylphenidate. J Am Acad Child Adolesc Psychiatry 1987;26:728-32.
- Singh AP. Cognitive Functions Among Children with ADHD and Emotional Disorders. Delhi Psychiatry J 2012:15(1): 148-59.
- Souza I, Pinheirol MA, Mattos P. Anxiety Disorders in An Attention Deficit/Hyperactivity Disorder Clinical Sample. Arqu Neuropsiquiatr 2005;63:407-09.
- Spencer T. Effectiveness and Tolerability of Atomoxetine in Adults with Attention Deficit Hyperachivity Disorder. Am J Psychiatry 1998;155:693-95.
- Spencer J, Biederman J, Mick E. Attention Deficit/Hyperactivity Disorder: Diagnosis, Lifespan, Comorbidities and Neurobiology. Ambul Pediatr 2007;7:73-81.
- Sunohara GA, Roberts W, Malone M, Schachar RJ, Tannock R, Basile VS. *et al.* Linkage of the Dopamine D4 Receptor Gene and Attention Deficit/Hyperactivity Disorder. J Am Acad Child Adolesc Psychiatry 2000;39(12):1537-42.
- Tahir E, Yazgan Y, Cirakoglu B, Ozbay F, Waldman I, Asherson PJ. Association and Linkage of DRD4 and DRD5 with Attention Deficit Hyperactivity Disorder (ADHD) in a Sample of Turkish Children. Mol Psychiatry 2000:5(4):396-404.
- Tannock R. Attention Deficit Disorders with Anxiety Disorders. In: Attention Deficit Disorders and Comorbidities in Children, Adolescents and Adults, Brown TE, Edition, New York: American Psychiatric Press 2000:125-75.
- Tosto MG, Momi SK, Asherson P, Malki K. A Systemic Review of Attention Deficit Hyperactivity Disorder (ADHD) and Mathematical Ability: Current Findings and Future Implications. BMC Med 2015;13:204.
- Venkata JA, Panicker AS. Prevalence of Attention Deficit Disorder in Primary School Children, Indian J Psychiatry 2013;55(4):338-42.
- Visser SN, Zablotsky B, Halbrook JR, Danielsen ML, Bitsko RH. Diagnostic Experiences of Children with Attention Deficit/Hyperactivity Disorder. Natl Health Stat Report 3rd September, 2015;81:1-8.
- Waxmonsky J. Assessment and Treatment of Attention Deficit Hyperactivity Disorder in Children with Comorbid Psychiatric Illness. Curr Opin Pediatr 2003;15:476-82.
- Weiss G, Hechtman L, Milroy T, Perlman T. Psychiatric Status of Hyperactives as Adults: A Controlled Prospective 15-Year Follow-up of 63 Hyperactive Children. J Am Acad Child Psychiatry1985;24(2):211-20.
- Wilens T, Biederman J, Mick E. Does ADHD Affect the Course of Substance Abuse? Findings From A Sample of Adults With and Without ADHD. Am. J. Addict 1998;7:156-63.
- Wolraich ML, Wibbelsman CJ, Brown TE, *et al.* Attention Deficit/Hyperactivity Disorder Among Adolescents: A Review of the Diagnosis, Treatment and Clinical Implications. Pediatrics 2005;115(6).
- Xu C, Schachar R, Tannock R, Roberts W, Malone M, Kennedy JL, *et al.* Linkage study of the alpha 2A Adrenergic Receptor in Attention Deficit Hyperactivity Disorder Families. Am J Med Genet 2001;105:159-62.

11 Chapter

AUTISM SPECTRUM DISORDERS

MS Bhatia, Anubhav Rathi, Shruti Srivastava

Autism Spectrum Disorders (ASDs) are a group of disorders that affect cognitive, motor, linguistic and developmental domains of the suffering children. Autism was first described by Kanner (1943) after studying 11 children who had in common behavioral abnormalities, e.g., delayed echolalia, pronoun reversal, communication deficits in speech as well as non-verbal modes, apathy, and repetitive behavior. These children had difficulty in relating people but appeared of normal intelligence. At the same time Asperger (Asperger, 1944) described a group of children whose behavior was closely similar with above mentioned symptoms. It was initially thought to be an early onset form of schizophrenia but later was distinguished from Schizophrenia in 1970s. More recently in DSM-5, subgroup of these related disorders, i.e., Autistic Disorder, Asperger's Disorder and Pervasive Developmental Disorder–Not Otherwise Specified (PDD-NOS), have been referred to as Autism Spectrum Disorders (ASDs) and are classified under Neurodevelopmental Disorders. Of these Autistic Disorder is the prototype of these disorders (ASDs) and most extensively studied.

EPIDEMIOLOGY

The prevalence estimates of ASDs have increased over time and the latest Epidemiological studies estimate the median global prevalence rate of ASDs to be 62 per 10,000. The existing evidence does not support differences in their prevalence by geographic region nor of a strong impact of ethnic/cultural or socioeconomic factors (Elsabbagh *et al.*, 2012). Autism is more common in males, in a ratio of about 3-4 to 1, although a wide variation has been reported (Fombonne, 2005; Autism and Developmental Disabilities Monitoring Network Principal Investigators, 2007; Autism and Developmental Disabilities Monitoring Network 2006; Principal Investigators, 2009; Christensen *et al.*, 2016). The male excess appears to be greater in case of those with an IQ in the normal range (~6:1) and least in those who are profoundly retarded (~1.5:1). This gender bias is even more profound in Asperger's Disorder (~9:1) (Fombonne and Tidmarsh, 2003; van Wijngaarden-Cremers *et al.*, 2014)). In India, ASDs has been reported to be more common in rural areas (Raina *et al.*, 2015).

ETIOPATHOGENESIS

Psychosocial Theories

Kanner speculated that emotional factors might play a role in the pathogenesis of autism led early researchers to prematurely conclude that this condition was always caused by the presence of a 'refrigerator' mother who was not responsive to the child's needs. Subsequent research has unequivocally ruled out that this is not the case.

Contemporary Thinking

Emerging genetic and epidemiological research clearly indicate that autism is a complex disorder which results from a combination of genetic and environmental interactions. While important advances have been made in genetic research, the research of the environmental factors has lagged behind along with the research on gene-environment interactions.

BIOLOGICAL

Neuropathology

The literature on microscopic neuropathology of autism has rapidly been accruing. Specific brain areas of the cerebellum, limbic system, and cortex appear to be more affected. For example, the forebrain (both limbic-hippocampus, entorhinal cortex, amygdala, anterior and posterior cingulate cortex, and neocortex as well as the face processing area in the fusiform gyrus of the temporal lobe) and the hindbrain (cerebellum and inferior olivary complex) are affected (Blatt, 2012).

Microscopically, altered cortical organization characterized by more frequent and narrower mini columns and early overgrowth of the frontal portion of the brain, which affects connectivity have been found. Abnormalities include cytoarchitectonic laminar differences, excess white matter neurons, decreased numbers of GABAergic cerebellar Purkinje cells, and other events that can be traced developmentally and cause anomalies in circuitry. Problems with neurotransmission are evident especially in the inhibitory GABA system thus likely contributing to an imbalance of excitatory/inhibitory neurotransmission (Blatt, 2012).

Neuroimaging

A meta-analysis by Stanfield *et al.* (2008) of 43 structural imaging studies of over 800 subjects revealed enlarged total brain volume, hemispheres, cerebellum and caudate in ASD, and decreased volumes in other brain regions including midbrain regions, regions of the cerebellar vermis, and area of the corpus callosum.

Meta-analysis of Voxel Based Morphometric (VBM) studies on gray matter (Via *et al.*, 2011) revealed differences in amygdala-hippocampus complex and medial parietal regions. White matter volume (Radua *et al.*, 2011) studies revealed differences in areas relevant to language and social cognition.

Meta-analyses of functional magnetic resonance imaging (fMRI) studies by Philip *et al.*, 2012 revealed a tendency for decreased activation in ASD across several prefrontal and subcortical brain regions during tasks tapping executive function. Activation patterns in the superior temporal gyri were significantly different between ASD and controls across several domains, although the direction varied: ASD had decreased activation during tasks related to auditory and language processing, but increased during tasks of simple social processing, and mixed findings as demands became increasingly complex.

Meta-analyses of Diffusion Tensor Imaging (DTI) studies by Travers *et al.*, in 2012 revealed that persons suffering from ASDs have decreased fractional anisotropy and increased mean diffusivity in white matter tracts spanning many regions of the brain but most consistently in regions such as the corpus callosum, cingulum, and aspects of the temporal lobe. The review also raised a possibility of atypical lateralization in some white matter tracts of the brain and atypical developmental trajectory of white matter microstructure in persons with ASD.

Neurophysiology

A higher incidence of EEG abnormalities and seizures in these children indicates that this is an organic disorder rather than a psychogenic one. Seizures are common in early childhood with a second peak at adolescence. Generalized tonic-clonic seizures are most frequent. Diffuse spike and slow waves and paroxysmal spike and wave activity are most common abnormalities (Lord *et al.*, 1994).

Nocturnal production of melatonin has been found to be reduced in autism and has been postulated to be the probable reason of sleep disturbances found in these children (Tordjman *et al.*, 2005;2015).

Evoked Potentials

Researchers using Evoked Response Potentials have demonstrated abnormalities in the early stages of face processing in autism. McPartland and colleagues (2004) found slower than normal peak N 170 responses but normal latency. Similarly Dawson and colleagues (2002) showed that P400 and Nc components of autistic children did not differentiate between familiar and unfamiliar faces unlike typically developing controls. These findings show that these children have abnormality in face processing circuitry and is believed to be a functional trait marker for genetic risk of autism.

Neurochemistry

Although abnormalities in the CSF serotonin, norepinephrine, dopamine, 5-HIAA levels have been found but most of the findings are inconclusive. The opioid theory proposes that autism appears due to early, long-term overload of CNS with opioids which are probably exogenous and derived from incompletely digested dietary gluten and/or casein. This may be secondary to deficient barrier at intestinal mucosa or at brain level, which may be inherited or acquired (Berney, 2000). Few studies have emphasized the role of GABAergic neurotransmission and synaptic vesicle proteins in the pathogenesis of ASD indicating ASD as a "synaptic neuropathology" (Cellot and Cherubini, 2014; Giovedi *et al.*, 2014).

GENETIC FACTORS

Association of autism has been shown with fragile X syndrome, Phenylketonuria (PKU), neurofibromatosis and tuberous sclerosis. Of these tuberous sclerosis and fragile X syndrome has been found most consistently with autism. Studies have been conducted to find out the involved chromosomes and linkage with 7q, 10q, 15q, 16p, 16q and 17p have been reported (Lauristen *et al.*, 1999).

The recurrence rate of autism in siblings of affected children is approximately 2% to 8%, much higher than the prevalence rate in the general population but much lower than in single-gene diseases. Twin studies reported 60% concordance for classic autism in monozygotic (MZ) twins versus 0% in dizygotic (DZ) twins, the higher MZ concordance attesting to genetic inheritance as the predominant causative agent. Re-evaluation for a broader autistic phenotype that included communication and social disorders increase concordance remarkably from 60% to 92% in MZ twins and from 0% to 10% in DZ pairs. Though exact identity and number of genes involved remain unknown, the wide phenotypic variability of the autistic spectrum disorders likely reflects the interaction of multiple genes within an individual's genome and the existence of distinct genes and gene combinations among those affected (Muhle *et al.*, 2004).

The first mutations identified in idiopathic autism involve synaptic genes like NLGN3 and NLGN4X (Jamain *et al.*, 2003; Laumonnier *et al.*, 2004) or SHANK3 (Durand *et al.*, 2007; Gauthier *et al.*, 2009; Moessner *et al.*, 2007). In ASD associated with specific genetic syndromes like Fragile X Syndrome, the most common cytogenetic abnormality found is 15q11–q13 duplication of the maternal allele which affects synaptic plasticity. The candidate genes at this loci are FOXP2, RAY1/ST7, IMMP2L and RELN genes at 7q22-q33 and the GABA (A) receptor subunit and UBE3A genes. Subsequently structural genetic variations in other synaptic genes such as SynGAP and DLGAP2 (Marshall *et al.*, 2008; Berkel *et al.*, 2010; Pinto *et al.*, 2010) were found. The detection of Copy Number Variants (CNVs) in these genes have consistently confirmed the importance of synaptic function in autism (Szatmari *et al.*, 2007). The analysis of CNVs have revealed other pathways which are affected in the etiopathogenesis of autism like cellular proliferation and motility, GTPase/Ras signaling, and neurogenesis (Pinto *et al.*, 2010; Gilman *et al.*, 2011, Ben-David *et al.*, 2012) like SLC25A12 gene found on chromosome 2 (Ramoz *et al.*, 2004).

ENVIRONMENTAL

Epigenetic and Transcriptome Abnormalities

Several lines of evidence indicate epigenetic and transcriptome abnormalities in persons with ASDs. Several syndromes associated with autism like Rett syndrome [MeCP2 gene mutation (Chahrour *et al.*, 2008) are caused by mutations in genes involved in epigenetic and transcription regulation. Several chromosomal regions subject to parental imprinting (transcriptional regulation of either the maternal allele or the paternal allele inducing monoallelic expression] were associated with autism (Vorstman *et al.*, 2006; Bremer *et al.*, 2010). Studies have shown association of ASD with single nucleotide polymorphisms in a gene directly involved in DNA methylation (Mohammad *et al.*, 2009; Liu *et al.*, 2011). Lastly, comprehensive gene-expression analysis of brains of patients with ASD have reported differences in transcriptome organization as compared to non-autistic individuals (Voineagu *et al.*, 2011).

Prenatal and Perinatal Factors

Generally higher incidence of prenatal problems is found in these children compared to normal population. These include gestation diabetes, maternal bleeding during pregnancy and maternal medication (like valproate (Kolozi *et al.*, 2009), anti-depressant exposure (Croen *et al.*, 2011), organophosphate insecticides (Landrigan, 2010)) in first trimester (Gardener *et al.*, 2009), advanced maternal age, meconium staining, prematurity, post maturity of early or midtrimester bleeding. It is usually not associated with perinatal problems. Epidemiologic studies indicate that environmental factors such as perinatal insults, and prenatal infections such as rubella and cytomegalovirus account for few cases. However, finding of its association with MMR has not always been replicated (Fombonne *et al.*, 2001).

Findings from a large number of studies have been summarized in two comprehensive books (Bauman *et al.*, 1994; Gillberg *et al.*, 2000). This area of study is problematic because we know relatively little about the function of normal brain and even less about the acquisition of skills during development.

Metabolic Factors

Autism may also occur in the context of abnormal cellular metabolism, such as mitochondrial disease or dysfunction. Untreated phenylketonuria is a well-documented metabolic cause of autism, however, the exact mechanism is uncertain. Some clinic-based studies report high levels of uric acid secretion in up to one quarter of patients with autism and amelioration of certain symptoms with anti-hyperuricosuric metabolic therapy. However, the genes that are responsible for this type of "purine autism" are yet to be identified (Muhle, 2004).

Immune Dysfunction

Several studies have shown abnormalities in the peripheral immune system such as T-cell dysfunction, autoantibody production, increase in the number of activated B cells and NK cells, and increase in proinflammatory cytokines in persons with ASDs (Gupta *et al.*, 1998; Singh *et al.*, 1997; Ashwood *et al.*, 2011). Studies have provided evidence for microglial and astroglial activation in the cerebellum and cerebral white matter (Vargas *et al.*, 2005) and also in Dorsolateral Prefrontal Cortex (DLPFC) (Morgan *et al.*, 2010).

DIAGNOSIS

At present we have two diagnostic guidelines–ICD and DSM. Both the systems have overlapping criterion and require the onset of symptoms before 36 months and disruption in three domains namely–social, communication and restricted and stereotyped behavior and interests. A variety of symptoms in these domains appear.

DSM-5 Diagnostic Criteria for Autism Spectrum Disorder (ASD) 299.0 (F84.0)

Must meet criteria A, B, C and D:

A. Persistent deficits in social communication and social interaction across contexts, not accounted for by general developmental delays, and manifest by all 3 of the following:

1. Deficits in social-emotional reciprocity; ranging from abnormal social approach and failure of normal back and forth conversation through reduced sharing of interests, emotions and affect and response to total lack of initiation of social interaction.
2. Deficits in nonverbal communicative behaviors used for social interaction; ranging from poorly integrated–verbal and nonverbal communication, through abnormalities in eye contact and body-language, or deficits in understanding and use of nonverbal communication, to total lack of facial expression or gestures.
3. Deficits in developing and maintaining relationships, appropriate to developmental level (beyond those with caregivers); ranging from difficulties adjusting behavior to suit different social contexts through difficulties in sharing imaginative play and in making friends to an apparent absence of interest in people.

B. Restricted, repetitive patterns of behavior, interests, or activities as manifested by at least two of the following:

1. Stereotyped or repetitive speech, motor movements, or use of objects (such as simple motor stereotypes, echolalia, repetitive use of objects, or idiosyncratic phrases).
2. Excessive adherence to routines, ritualized patterns of verbal or nonverbal behavior, or excessive resistance to change (such as motoric rituals, insistence on same route or food, repetitive questioning or extreme distress at small changes).
3. Highly restricted, fixated interests that are abnormal in intensity or focus (such as strong attachment to or preoccupation with unusual objects, excessively circumscribed or perseverative interests).
4. Hyper- or hypo-reactivity to sensory input or unusual interest in sensory aspects of environment (such as apparent indifference to pain/heat/cold, adverse response to specific sounds or textures, excessive smelling or touching of objects, fascination with lights or spinning objects).

C. Symptoms must be present in early childhood (but may not become fully manifest until social demands exceed limited capacities).

D. Symptoms together limit and impair everyday functioning.

There are also 3 new "Severity Levels" for ASD:

Level 3: 'Requiring Very Substantial Support'

- Severe deficits in verbal and nonverbal social communication skills cause severe impairments in functioning; very limited initiation of social interactions and minimal response to social overtures from others.
- Preoccupations, fixated rituals and/or repetitive behaviors markedly interfere with functioning in all spheres. Marked distress when rituals or routines are interrupted; very difficult to redirect from fixated interest or returns to it quickly.

Level 2: 'Requiring Substantial Support'

- Marked deficits in verbal and nonverbal social communication skills; social impairments apparent even with supports in place; limited initiation of social interactions and reduced or abnormal response to social overtures from others.
- RRBs and/or preoccupations or fixated interests appear frequently enough to be obvious to the casual observer and interfere with functioning in a variety of contexts. Distress or frustration is apparent when RRB's are interrupted; difficult to redirect from fixated interest.

Level 1:'Requiring Support'

- Without supports in place, deficits in social communication cause noticeable impairments. Has difficulty initiating social interactions and demonstrates clear examples of atypical or unsuccessful responses to social overtures of others.
- May appear to have decreased interest in social interactions.
- Rituals and repetitive behaviors (RRB's) cause significant interference with functioning in one or more contexts. Resists attempts by others to interrupt RRB's or to be redirected from fixated interest.

One important point to remember while diagnosing patients with autism is that it is a 'dynamic disorder' that means a nuanced interpretation is required according to age as its expression changes according to age.

This disorder can be diagnosed as early as 18 months using the CHAT (Checklist for autism in toddlers). Consistent failure on three key items, i.e., proto-declarative pointing, gaze-monitoring and pretend play diagnose children with risk of autism at the age of 18 months (Baron-Cohen *et al.,* 1992 and 1996). However, case reports are there where diagnosis was made as early as 15 months (Klin *et al.,* 2004).

Social Deficits

This is probably the most specific and most handicapping of all. The most characteristic abnormality is lack of social reciprocity and impaired ability to develop loving relationship on the basis of personal relationships. There is a poor integration of social, communicative and emotional features–as for example, expected in greeting behavior (Bailey *et al.,* 1996). These infants do not hold their arms up when an attempt is made to lift them up, do not adjust their body while being held while others may be very clingy. They do not pay attention to family members. Human faces are usually attractive stimulus for normal infants, but not to children with autism. They do not imitate gestures.

In preschool years they do not take interest in making friends, have limited facial expressions and abnormal eye contact. They are less likely to use their parents as a secure base or to provide comforts to youngsters in need (Lord *et al.,* 1994).

Child with autism has difficulty in either starting or continuing relations. They may walk past people or bump into them as they do not see them. Gaze avoidance may persist until adulthood, although it is most susceptible to improvement with training. They are unable to understand the other person's feelings. However, a lot of variation in terms of severity and frequency is common. Depending upon the social skills they can be divided into three groups:

(1) Aloof children who are essentially cut off socially.

(2) Passive children that are more reachable but tend to gravitate away from social interaction unless actively engaged.

(3) Active-but-odd children who can initiate interaction but do so in an awkward, stilted, inappropriate manner.

Communication

Children with autism show a delay in language development but it is basically the deviant pattern of language use that is more specific of autism. This includes a lack of social chit-chat even when language is fully developed (Bailey *et al.,* 1996).

Use of gestures in these infants is delayed and they often babble less frequently. They sometimes do not respond to sounds appearing deaf, and at other times respond consistently to a particular music or a peculiar sound, e.g., as one generated by candy wrapper.

In contrast to non-autistic dysphasic children, virtually all preschool autistic children have impaired comprehension of language. When speech develops, they do not carry to and fro conversation, even at the level of toddler.

Autistic children often do not enquire about other persons state of mind, they are rather interested in upcoming events (When will we go outside?) or something that holds their interest. If the child is talkative speech is usually stereotyped or a monologue. They usually talk to themselves and do not need a partner. These individuals find it difficult to maintain an ongoing topic of conversation, are poor at building a conversational interchange on what the other person has said, and are impaired in adapting their communication to different social contexts.

They may produce fluent unintelligent jargon with little communicative meaning. On closer scrutiny, it may found containing bits and pieces of memorized television commercials or part phrases (Delayed echolalia). Other peculiarity is pronoun reversal, i.e., they refer themselves as 'you' or 'he'. Recent echolalia, repetition, neologisms, aprosodia are also common. They may perseverate and ask the same question repeatedly even when they know the answer fully. Nonverbal communication and language use (pragmatics) are also deficient. When unable to communicate verbally they rarely use gestures to get their point (Lord *et al.*, 1994).

Restricted Interests and Stereotypy

These children often do not use toys in the intended fashion. They are rather preoccupied with a part of it, e.g., spinning wheel of a car or repeatedly opening or closing the door of a house.

Imaginative play, e.g., dressing or feeding up a doll or pretending to talk on a phone is also absent. Less retarded children may engage themselves in complex routine with objects that they act over and over again. Many autistic children are interested in sensory parts of the objects, e.g., smell or taste of the objects. Peering at object using peripheral vision is also common.

Autistic children regularly display repetitive movements such as flapping of hands when excited, twirling, humming, running around in circles, rocking, head banging, twisting of fingers and so on. They resist change in routine or environment and have unusual tolerance for monotony, e.g., they spend hours playing with water, shaking a string, flipping a light switch, tearing a paper etc.

Verbally autistic children may spend weeks and months studying some narrow topic viz., dinosaurs, or time table to the point where they know all about it, and talk about them, unaware of the boredom of those in vicinity.

OTHER ASSOCIATED FEATURES

Disturbances of Developmental Rate

Autistic children show deviations from normal sequential motor, language and social milestones. In particular even the course of normal development is disrupted. For example, they may precociously sit without support but delayed in pulling themselves in standing position. Sequences of spurts and plateaus are common. Some researchers believe that this history can be used in differentiating them from severe retardation (Ornitz *et al.*, 1976).

Mood and Affect

They have been described as having flat affect due to lesser responsiveness, or they may be happy or irritable. Some children are unable to understand the consoling behavior of their parents and often cry for hours, disrupting the family life. Some are aggressive and may pinch or hit without provocation. Strong fears and anxiety are usually present (Rapin, 1991).

Intelligence

Numerous studies have shown that mental retardation is present in about three quarters of cases of autism but most investigators now agree that autistic children have a wide range of intelligence ranging from profound mental deficiency to superior intelligence. However, the mean IQ of autistic population is low. Some autistic children have exceptionally superior skills for a narrow range of abilities (savants), for example, calculation, puzzles or rote verbal memory, in the face of overall cognitive deficits (Rapin, 1991). In a study, the significant intellectual disabilities at 19 years age are predicted by age 2 in 85% of the time (Anderson, Liang and Lord, 2014).

Attention and Arousal

Few are inattentive and some are hyperactive. Without intending to be disruptive they may create chaos. On the other hand few remain engaged for hours in activities that please them (Rapin, 1991). They also have disrupted sleep pattern. Recently it has been found that sleep parameters such as time in bed, sleep period time, and total sleep time are significantly lower in subjects with autistic disorder than in normal controls; moreover, patients with autistic disorder had lower REM latency and decreased Stage 1 sleep. Density of muscle twitches was significantly higher in patients with autistic disorder than in normal controls (Elia *et al.*, 2000).

Sensorimotor Skills

Toe walking and hypotonia is common. Some children walk late, drool, are clumsy and have difficulty imitating movements and learning how to use tools. A striking abnormality is insensitivity to pain. Some of them do not cry even when severely hurt (Rapin, 1991).

Epilepsy

Epilepsy occurs in 30% cases of autism (Berney, 2000). More than one third of all cases with infantile spasms show autistic behavior. Few authors report higher frequency of GTCS while others say that complex partial seizures are more common in this population. The most peculiar feature of epilepsy in autistic individuals is its onset in adolescence.

Sensory Deficits

Moderate to severe hearing loss (> 25 dB) occur in at least 20% of these cases. In one in five children of autism show reduced visual acuity (Steffenberg, 1991). Some blind children particularly those with retinopathy of prematurity have a very high rate of autism (Ek *et al.*, 1998).

COMORBIDITY

Autism has familial links with other disorders like Depression, OCD, epilepsy (30%) and motor tics. It has also association with learning disorders, mental retardation (70% cases), ADHD (Berney, 2000).

COURSE

Most of the children with autism are identified by parents in second year of life. Parents usually identify difficulties that are not specific to autism, e.g., language delay, difficulty in settling, eating or sleeping. One third of parents report loss of speech in first year. Two strongest predictors for adult outcome are IQ (An IQ below 50 is strongest predictor of poor social outcome) and language function at age 5 (useful level of spoken language associated with good outcome). Variations in symptomatology and prognosis depend on both severity and the extent of underlying brain dysfunction. Small proportions (17%) of individuals in adolescence develop catatonia thus adding to the burden of care (Wing *et al.*, 2000).

ASSESSMENT OF AUTISTIC CHILDREN

Information about child's history, behavior and cognitive skills can only be acquired through reports of parents and teacher, direct observation and standardized assessment.

It is always better to ask a chronological history starting from the present complaints, duration, age of onset, developmental milestones before the onset of symptoms and then going back to perinatal and prenatal history. Then information regarding specific symptoms of autism must be considered (Lord *et al.*, 1994). Since the symptoms are more conspicuous in preschool years, behavior of this duration is of great importance.

Interview/Observation of Child

Observation of child's spontaneous social behavior is of utmost importance. However, if clinician is creating an environment so well where every child has to respond, it becomes difficult to assess. On the other hand if these children are left in completely unstructured environment they do not do anything and very little information is gained. So clinician must be very careful in creating the environment when they want to assess child's social interactions. Unusual motor behavior, rituals and repetitive actions are apparent directly on examination.

Cognitive Assessment

It is better to employ a test that separates verbal from performance skills (Wechsler scales) or to compare scores on non-verbal test (Raven's matrix test) with verbal scores. It is important to use the tests that hold the child's attention. Communication and language must be assessed for articulation, comprehension, and expressive language. However, measurement of intelligence in these children needs experience as these children are often not interested in performing the test.

Medical Examination

Main goal of examination is to assess the physical comorbidities, their treatment and to consider them during therapy. Among people with ASD, 10%-25% have an associated medical disorder (Kielinen *et al.*, 2004).

Diagnostic Checklists and Interviews

At presently no single instrument is sufficient to serve as an objective tool for sound diagnosis. However, following instruments can be used as adjunctive measures:

1. **Childhood Autism Rating Scale (CARS):** It is most widely used diagnostic instrument. Its scoring is done immediately after a child is observed in classroom or home. For each subscale there are instructions on how to create opportunities to observe behavior of interest (Schopler *et al.*, 1980, 1986).

2. **Diagnostic Checklist for Behavior Disturbed Children (DBCL):** The most frequently studied version of Rimlands diagnostic checklist Form E-2, contains 80 items regarding development and behavior from birth to age 5 to be completed by parent (Rimland, 1964).

3. **Autism Diagnostic Interview:** It is structured interview protocol used with child's principal caregiver. Its items cover recent concepts of autism. It is time consuming and primarily intended for research (Le Couteur *et al.*, 1989).

4. **Checklist for Autism in Toddlers (CHAT):** It is a very brief screening instrument designed specially for the early detection of autism at about 18 months of age. It is perhaps too brief to be consistently accurate (Baron-Cohen *et al.*, 1992).

5. **Other batteries:** The two most comprehensive batteries of psychological tests used for the diagnosis of autism, especially in research, are the autism diagnostic observation schedule (ADOS) (Lord *et al.*, 1989) and autism diagnostic interview (ADI). Together,

they represent a complete structured interview and an observation method for the objective assessment of social skills, communication skills, and behavior of autistic individuals, ranging from speechless children to adults who are able to communicate relatively well.

Disability Certification

Ministry of Social Justice and Empowerment issued an extraordinary Gazette notification in the year 2016 for certifying disability in persons suffering from Autism. Indian Scale of Assessment of Autism for Assessment of Disability is used for children more than 6 years of age. Both the State and Central government can carry out the certification which can provide benefits under this category. A medical board comprising the following members need to be constituted:

A. Clinical Psychologist/Rehabilitation Psychologist.

B. Psychiatrist.

C. Pediatrician or General Physician.

The certificate can be both temporary (valid for 5 years) or permanent depending on the severity of disability.

DIFFERENTIAL DIAGNOSIS

Severe Psychosocial Deprivation

These children often lack language comprehension difficulties, social interaction is normal and reciprocity is also good unlike autistic child. Moreover, a history of deprivation is also an important clue to diagnosis.

Elective Mutism

These are socially unresponsive but they usually do not show the language difficulties associated with autism. They carry on conversation, creative, playful and normal attachment with family members.

Receptive Expressive Language Disorder

Only verbal language delay is present, other symptoms of autism viz., poor nonverbal communication, poor social interactions and repetitive motor movements are absent.

Rett's Syndrome

This has different course from autism and found almost exclusively in the girls. Development is normal in first year but in second year head growth begins to decelerate, there is a loss of purposeful hand movements and verbal skills. There is social impairment and stereotyped hand movements, e.g., hand wringing and clapping near the midline. Gait and truncal ataxia is common at the age of 3 years.

Disintegrative Disorder

Heller's disease occurs when child show deterioration after normal development for approximately 2 years, often in association with loss of coordination of bowel and bladder functions. Social withdrawal, reduced response to sounds, complete loss of communication is common thus mimicking autism. But it differs in the loss of self help skills also.

Asperger's Disorder

This disorder simulates autism except that symptoms develop in persons with normal intelligence and without language delay. It is now considered under the rubric of ASDs.

Epilepsy

It occurs in up to 30% of autistic children. Behavior change similar to autism occur in Landau-Kleffner syndrome in which clinical seizures are absent in 30% patients, and diagnosis of epilepsy rests upon EEG. Similarly paroxysmal EEG is present in autistic children, particularly at later stage of regression. This highlights the importance of EEG in diagnosis of autism as a routine investigation (Berney, 2000). Yet the data are far from conclusion as only 5% of autism sufferers respond to anticonvulsant.

Schizophrenia

Confusion mainly occurs due to wide variety of phenotypes in both diseases. Quite often, Shizotypal and Schizoid personality disorders create diagnostic difficulties especially in adolescence.

GENETIC COUNSELING

Genetic counseling justifies testing, but until autism genes are identified and their functions are understood, prenatal diagnosis will exist only for the rare cases ascribable to single-gene defects or overt chromosomal abnormalities. Parents who wish to have more children must be told of their increased statistical risk. Parents need to understand that they and their affected children are the only available sources for identifying and studying the elusive genes responsible for autism.

TREATMENT AND INTERVENTION

Early intervention programs can make an enormous difference and result in significant and long-lasting gains.

It has been supposed that individuals with autism and other associated diseases, such as tuberous sclerosis, will have a different prognosis from those without severe disorders associated, but this has not been clearly demonstrated. It is common knowledge that better and more widely available educational and community services will be able to change the long-term prognosis of autistic patients. The dramatic increase in recognition of ASD is producing high demands on health care systems for timely and accurate diagnosis (Anagnostou *et al.*, 2014).

Goals of treatment are:

1. Fostering Social and Communicative Developments.
2. Enhancing Learning and Problem Solving.
3. Decreasing Behaviors That Interfere With Learning and Access To Opportunities For Normal Experiences.
4. Helping Families Cope With Autism.

Modes of Treatments

Education

Education has been the most powerful source of improvement for children with autistic spectrum disorder for last 50 years (National Research Council, 2001). Appropriate education has been consistently shown to improve the learning of autistic children and they have shown use of better academic achievements provided they have been given opportunity. They show better results if kept in special classes with structured programs. Increasingly emphasis has been placed on children proactive behaviors, e.g., learning to communicate using objects and pictures, being able to respond to teachers direction in a group, rather than eliminating negative behaviors, with the assumption that many problem behaviors decrease with the child's understanding and acquisition of skills (Carr *et al.*, 1999).

Family Support

It is important to recognize that different families function differently. Families must be helped in accepting the disappointment and fear and they should be made to feel that the clinician is with them in the treatment.

Specific Therapies

Speech therapy, occupational therapy, physical therapy, facilitated communication and auditory training are integral part of program. Social skills training and social groups may be beneficial. A functional analysis that identifies the contingencies in the environment that sustain a child's problem behavior is a crucial part of this approach (Lord *et al.*, 2004).

Pharmacological Therapies

Antipsychotics

The use of drugs to treat autism is still recent. Neuroleptics, especially haloperidol, have been widely used to treat behavioral disorders in autistic patients. However, possible side effects restrict their use in chronic disorders, such as autism. Haloperidol has proved to remarkably reduce aggressiveness, stereotypies and self-injurious behaviors in autistic individuals.

Atypical antipsychotics seem to have positive effects on target symptoms, such as irritability, aggressiveness, and hyperactivity in autistic disorder spectrum patients. Risperidone in dose of 0.5 to 3 mg/day is effective. It is also effective in reducing stereotypies. Side effects, sedation and weight gain were relatively mild. Uncontrolled studies have demonstrated similar benefits with other atypical antipsychotics also. However, the risk of metabolic syndrome (olanzapine, quetiapine, risperidone), prolactin elevation (risperidone, amisulpiride and quetiapine). Possibly significant side effects, such as elevation of prolactin and long QT syndrome (Ziprasidone) should be carefully monitored (Gadia *et al.*, 2004). However, a recent study reported that risk of weight gain with Risperidone gradually slow over time and weight gain at 1 month may be predictor of final weight at 6 months.

This means that those patients who significantly develop weight with this drug can be made drug free at the earlier stage (Martin *et al.*, 2004).

Antidepressants

Clomipramine (tricyclic antidepressant and nonselective serotonin reuptake blocker) has shown to be efficient in the treatment of obsessive-compulsive behavior, in the minimization of stereotypies and self-injurious behavior in autistic patients. However, the risk of cardiac arrhythmias and its side effect profile has restricted its use (Gadia *et al.*, 2004).

Selective serotonin reuptake inhibitors, such as fluoxetine (DeLong *et al.*, 1998), fluvoxamine, paroxetine, sertraline and escitalopram have been used in autistic individuals in an attempt to reduce obsessive behaviors, rituals and stereotypies with variable efficacy. They are usually well tolerated. Akathisia or "excessive activation" seems to be a relatively frequent dose dependent side effect.

Naltrexone

There has been some interest in opioid antagonism, particularly to promote social engagement and decrease self injurious behavior (Tsai, 1999). Naltrexone may be helpful in reducing over activity (Campbell *et al.*, 1993) but other researchers have concluded no positive effect (Gillberg, 1995).

D-Cycloserine

Recently D-cycloserine has been tried in autistic children and it has been found to improve the social withdrawal after 4 weeks therapy. Its effect has been hypothesized to act through NMDA receptors (Posey *et al.*, 2004).

Buspirone

Buspirone, 5 HT receptor agonist, may have a positive effect by reducing anxiety and has shown efficacy in reducing stereotyped or self-injurious behaviors.

Alpha-Agonists

Clonidine seems to be useful in the treatment of hyperactivity, impulsivity, and aggressive behavior, although very few studies have been conducted to confirm this clinical impression. It has been reported that pyridoxine (vitamin B_6) and magnesium may increase the state of alertness and minimize self-injurious behaviors. Most of these studies had methodological problems and their results have not been confirmed by controlled studies (Gadia *et al.*, 2004).

Others

Behavioral interventions that emphasize synchrony of circadian rhythm have shown substantial improvement in ASD, when combined with melatonin (Tordjman *et al.*, 2015).

CONCLUSIONS

Thus it can be concluded that autism is a childhood disorder with lesser frequency but with grave prognosis. Major advances have been made over years in our understanding of its etiopathogenesis and management, however, many important questions still remain unanswered. Early diagnosis and multi-modal intervention is important to reduce the social burden as no specific therapy is available till date.

Suggested Reading

- American Psychiatric Association. Diagnostic and Statistical Manual of Mental Disorders. 5th Edition. Text Revision. Washington (DC): American Psychiatric Press, 2013.
- Anagnostou E, Znaigenbaum L, Szatmari P, *et al.* Autism Spectrum Disorders: Advances in Evidence-Based Practice. CMAJ 2014:186(7):509-19.
- Anderson DK, Liang JW, Lord C. Predicting Young Adult Outcome Among More or Less Cognitively Able Individuals with Autism Spectrum Disorders. J Child Psychol Psychiatry 2014:55:485-94.
- Ashwood P, Corbett BA, Kantor A, Schulman H, Van de Water J, Amaral DG. In Search of Cellular Immunophenotypes in the Blood of Children with Autism. PLoS One 2011:6:e19299.
- Asperger Hans. Die "Autistichen Psychopathen" im Kindersalter. Archive fur Psychiatrie und Nervenkrankheiten, 1944:117:76-136.
- Autism and Developmental Disabilities Monitoring Network Principal Investigators. Prevalence of Autism Spectrum Disorders, 14 Sites, United States, 2002. MMWR, Surveill Summ 2007:56(1):12-28.
- Autism and Developmental Disabilities Monitoring Network 2006 Principal Investigators. Prevalence of Autism Spectrum Disorders, United States, 2006, MMWR, Surveill Summ 2009;58(SS-10):1-20.
- Bailey A, Phillip W, Rutter M. Autism: Toward an Integration of Clinical, Genetic, Neuropsychological and Neurobiological Perspectives. J Child Psychol Psychiaty 1996;37(1):89-126.
- Baron-Cohen S, Allen J, Gillberg C. Can Autism be Detected at 18 months? The needle, The Haystack and The CHAT. Br. J. Psychiatry 1992;161:839-43.
- Baron-Cohen S, Cox A, Baird G, *et al.* Psychological Markers in Detection of Autism in Infancy in a Large Population. Br. J. Psychiatr 1996:168:158-63.
- Bauman ML, Kemper TL. Neurobiology of Autism 1994. Johns Hopkins University Press, Baltimore.
- Ben-David E, Shifman S. Networks of Neuronal Genes Affected by Common and Rare Variants in Autism Spectrum Disorders. PLoS Genet 2012:8:e1002556.
- Berkel S, Marshall CR, Weiss B, *et al.* Mutations in the SHANK2 Synaptic Scaffolding Gene in Autism Spectrum Disorder and Mental Retardation. Nat Genet 2010;42:489-91.
- Berney TP. Autism–An Evolving Concept. Br J Psychiatry 2000:176:20-25.
- Blatt GJ. The Neuropathology of Autism. Scientifica (Cairo). 2012:2012:16 pages.
- Bremer A, Giacobini M, Nordenskjold M, *et al.* Screening for Copy Number Alterations in Loci Associated with Autism Spectrum Disorders by Twocolor Multiplex Ligation-Dependent Probe Amplification. Am J Med. Genet B Neuropsychiatr Genet 2010:153B:280-85.
- Campbell M, Anderson LT, Small AM, *et al.* Naltrexone in Autistic Children: Behavioral Symptoms and Attentional Learning. J Am Acad Child Adolesc Psychiatry 1993;32: 1283-91.

- Carr EG. Horner RH. Turnball AP. *et al.* Positive Behavior Support for People with Developmental Disabilities. American Association with Mental Retardation Monograph Series. Washington DC. 1999.
- Cellot G. Chrubini E. GABAergic Signaling as Therapeutic Target for Autism Spectrum Disorders. Front Pediatr 2014:2:70.10.3389/fped.2014.00070.
- Chahrour M. Jung SY. Shaw C. *et al.* MeCP2. A Key Contributor to Neurological Disease. Activates and Represses Transcription. Science 2008:320:1224-29.
- Christensen DL. Baio J. Braun KVN. *et al.* Prevalence and Characteristics of Autism Spectrum Disorder Among Children Aged 8 Years–Autism and Developmental Disabilities Monitoring Network. 11 sites. United States. 2012 MMWR. Suveill Summ 2016:65(3):1-23.
- Croen LA. Grether JK. Yoshida CK. Odouli R. Hendrick V. Antidepressant Use During Pregnancy and Childhood Autism Spectrum Disorders. Arch Gen Psychiatry 2011:68:1104-12.
- Dawson G. Carver L. Meltzoff AN. *et al.* Neural Correlates of Face and Object Recognition in Young Children with Autism Spectrum Disorder. Developmental Delay and Typical Development. Child Dev 2002;73(3):700-17.
- DeLong GR. Teague LA. Kamran MM. Effects of Fluoxetine Treatment in Young Children with Idiopathic Autism. Develop Med. Child Neurol 1998;40:551-62.
- Durand CM. Betancur C. Boeckers TM. *et al.* Mutations in the Gene Encoding the Synaptic Scaffolding Protein SHANK3 are Associated with Autism Spectrum Disorders. Nat Genet 2007: 39:25-27.
- Ek U. Fernell E. Jacobsson L. *et al.* Relationship Between Blindness Due to Retinopathy of Prematurity and Autistic Spectrum Disorders. A Population Study. Dev. Med. Child Neurol 1998;40:297-301.
- Elia M. Ferri R. Musumeci SA. *et al.* Sleep in Subjects with Autistic Disorder: A Neurophysiological and Psychological Study. Brain Dev 2000:22(2):88-92.
- Elsabbagh M. Divan G. Koh Y. *et al.* Global Prevalence of Autism and Other Pervasive Developmental Disorders. Autism Res 2012:5:160-79.
- Fombonne E. Chakrabarti S. No Evidence for A New Variant of Measles-Mumps-Rubella-Induced Autism. Pediatrics 2001; 108(4):E58.
- Fombonne E. Epidemiology of Autistic Disorder and Other Pervasive Developmental Disorders. J Clin Psychiatry 2005: 66(S 10):3-8.
- Fombonne E. Tidmarsh L. Epidemiologic Data on Asperger Disorder. Child and Adolescent Psychiatric Clinics of North America 2003:12(1):15-21.
- Gadia CA. Tuchman R. Rotta NT. Autism and Pervasive Developmental Disorders. J Pediatr 2004;80(Suppl 2):S83-94.
- Gardener H. Spiegelman D. Buka SL. Prenatal Risk Factors for Autism: Comprehensive Meta-analysis. Br J Psychiatry 2009;195:7-14.
- Gauthier J. Spiegelman D. Piton A. *et al.* Novel de Novo SHANK3 Mutation in Autistic Patients. Am J Med Genet B Neuropsychiatr Genet 2009:150B:421-24.
- Giovedi S. Corradi A. Fassio A. Benfenati F. Involvement of Synaptic Genes in the Pathogenesis of Autism Spectrum Disorders: The Case of Synapins. Front Pediatr 2014:2:94.10. 3389/fped.2014.00094.
- Gillberg C and Coleman M. The Biology of Autistic Syndrome. 3rd Edition. MacKeith Press. London. 2000.
- Gillberg C. Endogenous Opioids and Opiate Antagonists in Autism: Brief Review of Empirical Findings and Implications for Clinicians. Dev Med Child Neurol 1995:37:239-45.
- Gilman SR. Iossifov I. Levy D. Ronemus M. Wigler M. Vitkup D. Rare de novo Variants Associated with Autism Implicate A Large Functional Network of Genes Involved In Formation and Function of Synapses. Neuron 2011:70:898-907.
- Gupta S. Aggarwal S. Rashanravan B. Lee T. Th1- and Th2-like cytokines in CD4+ and CD8+ T Cells in Autism. J Neuroimmunol 1998:85:106-09.
- Jamain S. Quach H. Betancur C. *et al.* Mutations of the X-linked Genes Encoding Neuroligins NLGN3 and NLGN4 are Associated with Autism. Nat Genet 2003;34:27-29.
- Kanner L. Autistic Disturbance of Affective Contact. Nerv Child 1943:2:217-50.
- Kielinen M. Rantala H. Timonen E. *et al.* Associated Medical Disorders and Disabilities in Children with Autistic Disorder: A Population-Based Study. Autism 2004;8:49-60.
- Klin A. Chawarska K. Paul R. Autism in a 15-Month Old Child. Am J Psychiatry 2004;161(11):1981-88.
- Kolozsi E. Mackenzie RN. Roullet FI. deCatanzaro D. Foster JA. Prenatal Exposure to Valproic Acid Leads to Reduced Expression of Synaptic Adhesion Molecule Neuroligin 3 in Mice. Neuroscience 2009;163:1201-10.
- Landrigan PJ. What Causes Autism? Exploring the Environmental Contribution. Curr Opin Pediatr 2010;22:219-25.
- Laumonnier F. Bonnet-Brilhault F. Gomot M. *et al.* X-linked Mental Retardation and Autism are Associated with a Mutation in the NLGN4 Gene, a Member of the Neuroligin Family. Am J Hum Genet 2004;74:552-55.
- Lauristen M. Mors O. Mortensen PB *et al.* Infantile Autism and Associated Autosomal Chromosome Abnormalities: A Register Based Study and Literature Survey. J Child Psychol Psychiatry 1999:40(3):335-45.
- Le Couteur A. Rutter M. Lord C. *et al.* Autism Diagnostic Interview: A Standardized Investigator Based Instrument. J Autism Dev Disord 1989;19:363-87.
- Liu X. Solehdin F. Cohen IL. *et al.* Population- and Family-Based Studies Associate the MTHFR Gene with Idiopathic Autism in Simplex Families. J Autism Dev Disord 2011;41: 938-44.
- Lord C and Bailey A. Autism Spectrum Disorders. In Child and Adolescent Psychiatry. Eds. Rutter M. Taylor E. Blackwell Science Ltd, London 2004:636-63.
- Lord C, Rutter M. Autism and Pervasive Developmental Disorders. In: Child and Adolescent Psychiatry Modern Approaches. Eds. Rutter M. Taylor E. Blackwell Science Ltd. London 1994:569-93.

- Lord C, Rutter M, Goode S, *et al.* Autism Diagnostic Observation Schedule: A Standardized Observation of Communicative and Social Behavior. J Autism Dev. Disorder 1989;19:185-212.
- Marshall CR, Noor A, Vincent JB, *et al.* Structural Variation of Chromosomes in Autism Spectrum Disorder. Am J Hum Genet 2008;82:477-88.
- Martin A, Scahill L, Anderson GM and *et al.* Weight Gain and Leptin Changes Among Risperidone Treated Youth with Autism: 6 Months Prospective Data. Am J Psychiatry 2004;161:1125-27.
- McPartland J, Dawson G, Webb SJ, Panagiotides H, Carver LJ. Event-related Brain Potentials Reveal Anomalies in Temporal Processing of Faces in Autism Spectrum Disorder. J Child Psychol Psychiatry 2004;45(7):1235-45.
- Moessner R, Marshall CR, Sutcliffe JS, *et al.* Contribution of SHANK3 Mutations to Autism Spectrum Disorder. Am J Hum Genet 2007;81:1289-97.
- Mohammad NS, Jain JM, Chintakindi KP, Singh RP, Naik U, Akella RR. Aberrations in Folate Metabolic Pathway and Altered Susceptibility to Autism. Psychiatr Genet 2009;19:171-76.
- Morgan JT, Chana G, Pardo CA, *et al.* Microglial Activation and Increased Microglial Density Observed in the Dorsolateral Prefrontal Cortex in Autism. Biol Psychiatry 2010:68:368-76.
- Muhle R, Trentacoste SV, Rapin I. The Genetics of Autism. Pediatrics 2004;113(5):e472-86.
- National Research Council. Educating Children with Autism. Committee on Educational Intervention for Children with Autism. Division of Behavioral and Social Science Education, National Acadamy Press, Washington DC, 2001.
- Ornitz EM, Ritvo ER. The Syndrome of Autism: A Critical Review. Am J Psychiatry 1976;133:609-21.
- Philip RCM, Dauvermann MR, Whalley HC, Baynham K, Lawrie SM, Stanfield AC. A Systematic Review and Meta-analysis of the fMRI investigation of Autism Spectrum Disorders. Neurosci Biobehav Rev 2012:36:901-42.
- Pinto D, Pagnamenta AT, Klei L, *et al.* Functional Impact of Global Rare Copy Number Variation in Autism Spectrum Disorders, Nature 2010;466:368-72.
- Posey DJ, Kem DL, Sweizy NB, *et al.* A Pilot Study of D-cycloseriene in Subjects with Autistic Disorders. Am J Psychiatry 2004;161(11):2115-17.
- Radua J,Via E, Catani M, Mataix-Cols D. Voxel-Based Meta-Analysis of Regional White-Matter Volume Differences in Autism Spectrum Disorder Versus Healthy Controls, Psychol Med 2011:41:1539-50.
- Raina SK, Kashyap V, Bhardwaj AK, *et al.* Prevalence of Autism Spectrum Disorders Among Children (1-10 years of age)–Findings of a Midterm Report from Northeast India. J Postgrad Med 2015:61(4):243-46.
- Ramoz N, Reichert JG, Smith CJ, *et al.* Linkage and Association of Mitochondrial aspartate/glutamate carrier SLC25A12 Gene with Autism. Am J Psychiatry 2004;161(4):662-69.
- Rapin I. Autistic Children: Diagnosis and Clinical Features. Paediatrics 1991;S:751-60.
- Rimland B. Infantile Autism, NewYork: Appleton-Century-Crofts,1964.
- Schopler E, Reichler RJ, Renner BR. The Childhood Autism Rating Scale. Los Angeles: Western Psychological Services, 1988.
- Schopler E, Reichler RJ, de Vellis RF, *et al.* Towards Objective Classification of Childhood Autism: Childhood Autism Rating Scale (CARS). J Autism Dev Disord 1980;10:91-103.
- Singh VK, Warren R, Averett R, Ghaziuddin M. Circulating Autoantibodies to Neuronal and Glial Filament Proteins in Autism. Pediatr Neurol 1997;17:88-90.
- Stanfield AC, McIntosh AM, Spencer MD, Philip R, Gaur S, Lawrie SM. Towards a Neuroanatomy of Autism: A Systematic Review and Meta-Analysis of Structural Magnetic Resonance Imaging Studies. Eur. Psychiatry 2008;23:289-99.
- Steffenburg S. Neuropsychiatric Assessment of Children With Autism: A Population Based Study. Dev Med Child Neurol 1991;33:495-11.
- Szatmari P, Paterson AD, Zwaigenbaum L, *et al.* Mapping Autism Risk Loci Using Genetic Linkage and Chromosomal Rearrangements. Nat Genet 2007;39:319-28.
- Tordjman S, Anderson GM, Pichard N, *et al.* Nocturnal Excretion of 6-sulphatoxymelatonin in Children and Adolescents with Autistic Disorder. Biol Psychiatry 2005;57(2): 134-38.
- Tordjman S, Davlantis K, Georgieff N, *et al.* Autism as a Disorder of Biological and Behavioral Rhythms: Towards New Therapeutic Perspectives. Front Pediatr 2015:3:1.10.3389/fpeed.2015.00001.
- Travers BG, Adluru N, Ennis C, Tromp DPM, Destiche D, Doran S, *et al.* Diffusion Tensor Imaging in Autism Spectrum Disorder: A Review. Autism Res 2012:5(5):289-13.
- Tsai LY. Psychopharmacology in Autism. Psychosomatic Med 1999:61:651-65.
- van Wijngaarden-Cremers PJM, van Eeten E, Groen WB, *et al.* Gender and Age Differences in the Core Triad of Impairments in Autism Spectrum Disorders: A Systematic Review and Meta-Analysis. J Autism Dev Disord 2014;44:627-35.
- Vargas DL, Nascimbene C, Krishnan C, Zimmerman AW, Pardo CA. Neuroglial Activation and Neuroinflammation in the Brain of Patients with Autism. Ann Neurol 2005:57:67-81.
- Via E, Radua J, Cardoner N, Happe F, Mataix-Cols D. Meta-Analysis of Gray Matter Abnormalities in Autism Spectrum Disorder: Should Asperger Disorder be Subsumed Under a Broader Umbrella of Autistic Spectrum Disorder? Arch Gen Psychiatry 2011;68:409-18.
- Voineagu I, Wang X, Johnston P, *et al.* Transcriptomic Analysis of Autistic Brain Reveals Convergent Molecular Pathology. Nature 2011;474:380-84.
- Vorstman JA, Staal WG, van Daalen E, van Engeland H, Hochstenbach PF, Franke L. Identification of Novel Autism Candidate Regions Through Analysis of Reported Cytogenetic Abnormalities Associated with Autism. Mol Psychiatry 2006; 11:18-28.
- Wing L, Shah A. Catatonia in Autism Spectrum Disorders. Br. J Psychiatry 2000;176:357-62.
- http://disabilityaffairs.gov.in/upload/uploadfiles/files/Autism%20Guidelines-%20Notification_compressed.pdflast accessed on 3/09/2018.

12 Chapter

LEARNING DISORDERS

Shahzadi Malhotra

INTRODUCTION

Learning is acquisition of new knowledge, skills or attitude. Children during their early years of development learn to understand the spoken language first and then learn to speak. Subsequently during their school years they learn to read, write and do arithmetic, according to their age and intellectual capacity. But some children may not be able to learn one or more of these skills as per their age and intellectual capacity. For example, an 8-year-old child, studying in third standard having average intellectual capacity may be reading and writing like a child in the first standard or a student in ninth class may not be able to do the arithmetic sums like his classmates in spite of having above average intellectual ability. Thus, it seems that there are some children, who, in spite of having average or above average intellectual ability and unimpaired visual, hearing or physical abilities are unable to acquire one or more age appropriate language and/or arithmetic skills, even when adequate opportunities for learning are provided. These children have specific learning disorder (SLD). Interestingly, inability to learn certain skills is not restricted to only reading, writing and arithmetic. Children may have difficulty in understanding and expressing age appropriate communication due to which they may not be able to understand jokes or the abstract meanings of phrases or tell a story in an organized manner. Similarly, some children may not develop age appropriate motor coordination as a result of which they may not be able to learn certain skills like skating or dancing requiring high level of coordination.[1]

The National Joint Commission of Learning Disabilities[2] states that learning disabilities is a general term that refers to a heterogeneous group of disorders manifested by significant difficulties in the acquisition and use of listening, speaking, reading, writing and mathematical abilities. These disorders are intrinsic to the individual, presumed to be due to central nervous system dysfunction and occur across life span. Lyon *et al.*[3] point out that this definition addresses the issues of heterogeneity, persistence, intrinsic etiology and comorbidity. However, this definition according to Lyton *et al.* is vague and overly broad. At the current time, there is an increasing consensus that a single definition is not the best approach to address learning disorders, and that separate definitions for each of the areas that can be affected is more acceptable approach.[4] Problems in self-regulatory behavior, social perception and social interaction may exist with learning disabilities but do not by themselves constitute a learning disorder.[5]

Conceptualization

The field of learning disorders emerged on two fronts. First was the desire by researchers to gain a scientific and clinical knowledge of individual differences in learning among children and adults, who although intellectually average displayed specific deficits in spoken or written language. The other was the practical need to provide services to youngsters exhibiting these patterns.[3] Beginning in the later part of the 19th century, neurological basis of the observed difficulties were postulated.[6,7] In the 20th century, it was initially hypothesized that a lack of left hemispheric dominance for the processing of linguistic symbols underlay the disorder.[8] While neither his theory nor the centrality of reversals to the disorder has stood the test of time,[9] his influence on the time has been tremendous.

Since the 1970s, the field of learning disorders has gradually responded to research involving the specific deficits involved in reading, written expression and mathematics. Increasingly, assessment and remediation have targeted the specific academic areas of need via direct instruction, as opposed to focusing on the remediation of underlying processes, and the field now stresses optimally delivered academic instruction rather than instruction tailored to a particular student's pattern of processing strengths and weaknesses.

The aforesaid changes in the conceptualization of learning disorders have been reflected in the successive versions of the DSM.

The current literature and the DSM–V[10] have come up with the term learning disorders in place of learning disabilities. Specific learning disorders (SLD) in place of learning disability is considered to be more appropriate term for various reasons.

(1) The term–'Learning disability' is used in some countries like UK for mentally retarded individuals. Though, in some children the problem in reading and writing may be very severe almost like a disability, in most of the children it may not be very severe and disabling. So instead of 'disability' it is better to use 'disorder'.

(2) Frequently, the disability in learning, in these children, may not be generalized and may be explicit, restricted to only one area. For example, the child may have difficulty only in arithmetic and not in reading or writing. So it is more appropriate to have a prefix 'specific' as in 'specific learning disorder'.

(3) The term used in ICD-10[11] 'Specific developmental disorders of scholastic skills' does not clearly bring out the issue of difficulty in learning these skills which the children having this disorder have.

(4) Reading, writing and arithmetic are the language skills and not necessarily only 'scholastic skills'. The adjective 'developmental' has now being considered to be less acceptable as the diagnosis is based on the clinical features and not on the presumed contributory etiological factors.

Over the past twenty years, much research in the field of LD has taken place, and with that research, the community of professionals has gained new knowledge. This knowledge is reflected not only in the way that LD is assessed and diagnosed, but also in the way teachers and specialists' work with students who have LD. The DSM IV had placed an individual's learning disorder into one of three categories – Specific Reading Disorder, Specific Math Disorder and Disorders of Written Expression. It is now well understood that these three classifications frequently overlap; research has substantiated that the three disorders are highly inter-related and should not be considered separate.[12] Therefore, the DSM V (APA, 2013) has revised the diagnosis into a single category, Specific Learning Disorder, which captures the overall difficulty experienced in the academic domain; allowing the diagnostician to specify the details of the areas of academic impairment as well as the severity of the disorder: mild, moderate or severe.

Types of Learning Disorders

The most common types of specific learning disorders are those that impact the areas of reading, math and written expression. They may co-occur with other disorders of attention, language and behavior, but are distinct in how they impact learning. Following are the main types of learning disorders (Fig. 12.1).

Dyslexia is defined as difficulty in reading. When children are learning to read and write in kindergarten and first grade, it is not uncommon for them to misinterpret "b" as "d", "6" as "9", the word "on" as "no", "god" as "dog" and so forth. An important consideration in such cases is that this is not a vision problem; rather, the brain is reversing, inverting or mis-sequencing the information it receives from the eyes. Most children outgrow this condition by age seven or so. For dyslexic youngsters, however, the reading problems persist.

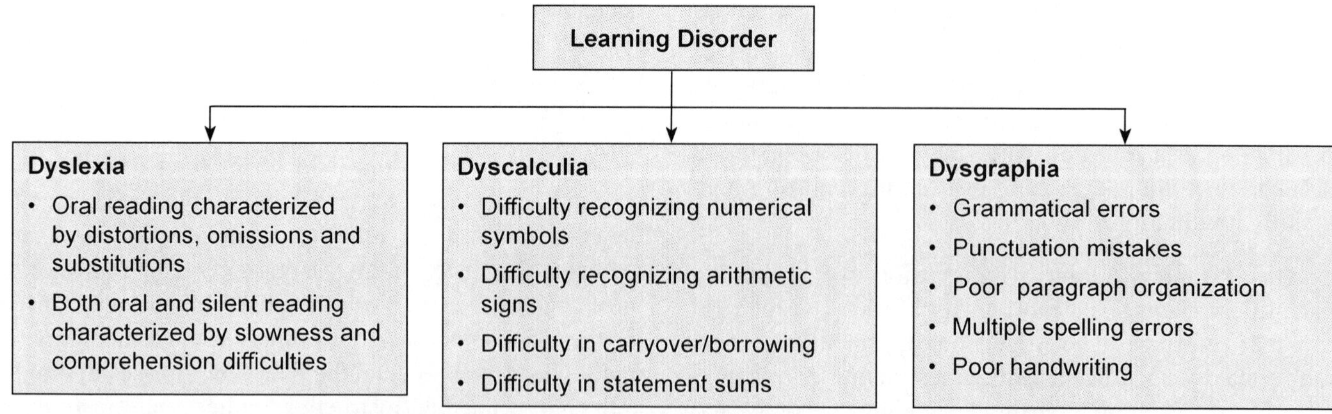

Fig. 12.1 Common types of learning disorders with their presenting symptoms

Dyslexia is the term associated with specific learning disorder in reading. Although features of LD in reading vary from person to person, common characteristics include difficulty with phonemic awareness (the ability to notice, think about and work with individual sounds in words), phonological processing (detecting and discriminating differences in phonemes or speech sounds), difficulties with word decoding, fluency, rate of reading, rhyming, spelling, vocabulary, comprehension and written expression. Dyslexia is the most prevalent and well-recognized of the subtypes of specific learning disorders.

Dyslexia may occur in one of the three ways.[13] First, the ability to decode might be impaired but comprehension is intact. Second, decoding may be intact but comprehension impaired. This is called hyperlexia wherein the child can read almost anything but does not understand what he read. Thirdly, both decoding as well as comprehension could be impaired. This third kind of impairment results from a general cognitive impairment and is called reading backwardness.

Most of the students who have reading disorder have difficulty acquiring the knowledge and skills essential for rapid automatic decoding. Reading comprehension is thus limited by weak decoding skills. Further, since spelling also use the same decoding skills as are required for word recognition, spelling is also frequently impaired in these children.

Dyscalculia is the term associated with specific learning disorder in math. Although features of learning disorder in mathematics vary from person to person, common characteristics include difficulty with counting, learning number facts and doing math calculations, difficulty with measurement, telling time, counting money and estimating number quantities, trouble with mental math and problem-solving strategies.

Children and adolescents with mathemetics disorder may exhibit a wide range of symptoms including delays in the basic number and spatial concepts.

Dysgraphia is the term associated with specific learning disorder in writing. Dysgraphia could be a result of either one or more of the following: A result of dyslexia, poor motor coordination or problems understanding space. Common characteristics of dysgraphia include: tight, awkward pencil grip and body position, getting tired quickly while writing, and avoiding writing or drawing tasks, trouble forming letter shapes as well as inconsistent spacing between letters or words, difficulty writing or drawing on a line or within margins, trouble organizing thoughts on paper, trouble keeping track of thoughts already written down, difficulty with syntax structure and grammar, large gap between written ideas and understanding demonstrated through speech.

The specific manifestation of dysgraphia depends upon the cause. The written work of a child with dysgraphia due to dyslexia will contain many illegible and/or misspelled words, whereas motor clumsiness or defective visual-spatial perception affects only handwriting, not spelling. It is used to capture both the physical act of writing and the quality of written expression. Features of learning disorder in writing are often seen in individuals who struggle with dyslexia and dyscalculia, and will vary from person to person and at different ages and stages of development.

It is essential to distinguish between a fine motor problem that results in difficulty with the mechanics of writing and a language based learning disorder that results in problems with the writing of language.[13] Individuals with a disorder of written expression might have a fine motor problem but always have a language based disorder, resulting in difficulty with capitalization, spelling, punctuation, grammar and / or composition.

Poor spelling might be the first observed sign of learning disorder in writing. By third or fourth grade, additional writing problems are apparent. Children with a writing disorder exhibit grammatical and punctuation errors at sentence level. Their paragraphs show poor organization.

Prevalence

The prevalence of LD among school-age children of various cultures ranges from 5-15%, demonstrating that this disorder afflicts a great number of individuals world wide.[10] Although Specific Learning Disorders (SLDs) are one of the most common neurodevelopmental disorders affecting children, there is still high variability in SLD prevalence estimates, due to a lack of univocal diagnostic criteria. Differences in prevalence data might be due to varying definitions of SLD, to the different methods used for diagnosis, as well as to the different age ranges that are considered in the various studies.

Bhat and Shah[1] have reported that in each class of about 40 to 50 students, right from nursery and kindergarten to 10 standard, it seem that on an average 2 students have learning disorder. It means that in India, where there are about 250 million school going children, there are about 12.5 million (1.25 crore) children suffering from learning disorder.[1]

Indian studies have reported the prevalence of various types of specific learning disorders to be between 3 and 13% among student population.[14-18] In a study from northern region, one per cent of children attending an outpatient clinic of a tertiary hospital were found to be having specific learning disorder.[19] The issue of identification of specific learning disorder cases in Indian context is perhaps more complex as still in most places, classroom conditions are far from ideal, along with problems of socio-economic factors, bilingualism and multilingualism, limited proficiency in medium of instructions may play a significant role in Indian educational system.[20-21] The class sizes are big, and there is no screening tool available for teachers to identify SLD. The issue of assessment of Specific Learning Disorders is further complicated by the fact that various Education Boards (Central and State Boards) have differing level of academic difficulty.

Gender Differences

SLD are reported to be more frequent in males than females.[14,22-23] In India also, similar findings have been reported. Barring arithmetic disorder which may be more common in girls, all other learning disorders seems to be 3 to 4 times more common in boys.[1]

Effects of Mother-Tongue and Medium of Instruction

Different languages have different writing systems and variations in prevalence depend on factors like the spelling opacity of each language. Shah and Bhat[1] have reported that learning disorders are seen worldwide and occurs in students irrespective of their mother-tongue and medium of instruction in the school which may be English or any other vernacular language such as Hindi, Gujarati, Urdu, Tamil, Telugu, Bengali, etc. It has been further reported that the difficulty faced by children having learning disorders may be more obvious in non-phonetic languages like English than in phonetic vernacular languages. However, it has been documented that changing medium of instruction does not help. Children who learn in Chinese or Japanese language in which there are only symbols may also have learning disorder. The Italian language has a shallow orthographical system, for this reason, it may be expected that there would be a lower prevalence of SLD in Italy. However, the prevalence rate of SLD in Italy is very large–between 0.88% and 10%.[24-29]

Bhat and Shah have also reported that learning disorder may also be detected even in students who are blind or deaf; they may not be able to learn "brail language" or "sign language" respectively as per their age, in spite of having good intellectual capacity and adequate opportunities to learn these languages.

Thus, SLD occurs in all languages although the prevalence and severity may differ depending on the opacity of spelling in any given language.

Comorbidity

Comorbidities are very common in Neuropsychiatric diseases, including LD, during developmental age. Understanding comorbidity is important because the presence of an additional disorder may affect the expression and severity of the clinical picture, requiring specific treatments and interventions. Children with comorbidity compared to those without comorbidity usually exhibit more severe neurocognitive impairment, negative academic experience and social outcomes and lower treatment response.

The most common comorbidity associated with specific learning disorder is Attention Deficit Hyperactivity Disorder (ADHD). Almost 20-25% of the children with Specific Learning Disorder may have comorbid ADHD. As suggested earlier both these disorders may have common etiological factor–brain insult. It is very important to detect this comorbidity and treat it simultaneously with appropriate medications and behavior therapy. Dyslexia is the most extensively investigated learning disorder in the national and international studies regarding its features and also its comorbidity. Some old and less replicated studies have suggested that reading disorder might be the primary deficit, which causes secondary symptoms of ADHD.[30-33] Recent data have shown that there are common cognitive deficits between the two disorders[34] according to a possible similar genetic etiology, as demonstrated by families studies in twins.[35-36] It is reported that approximately 60% of patients with dyslexia also meet the criteria for at least one neuropsychiatric disorder.[37-38] Comorbidity with ADHD is present from 10% to 50% of LD children, while comorbidity with dyslexia is present from 25 to 40% of ADHD patients.[37,39-41]

The other disorder, which may be found frequently, though not as frequently as ADHD, is Oppositional Defiant Disorder (ODD). Children with specific learning disorders may make various unreasonable demands and throw temper-tantrums if their demands are not met with. Initially when the parents are not aware about SLD, they may promise various incentives to their child for completing the books or the home-work. After sometimes this may become a habit and child may start demanding unreasonable things for any study related activities which if not met would result in temper-tantrum. Some children due to fear of poor performance and subsequent punishment or humiliation may develop severe anxiety related to their performance in exams. Few days before the exams they may not be able to fall asleep, develop headache, vomiting or other somatic complaints and may seek repeated reassurance about their performance from the parents.[1]

Recently, a bi-directional relationship between anxiety, depression and academic achievement has been hypothesized.[42] Anxiety and depressed mood could negatively impact learning process, alternatively children with LD may develop anxiety and mood problems, because they often reported adverse academic experiences. Although, comorbidity with anxiety and mood disorders has been also reported in some studies but in others no difference was reported in the symptoms of anxiety and depressed mood among children with and without LD.[39,43-49]

Language disorders may precede or be associated with dyslexia. International studies have estimated that 30-40% of children with Specific Language Disorder receive a diagnosis of reading disorder later on[50-52] and a percentage between 55%[53] and 77%[54] of dyslexics meets the diagnostic criteria for Specific Language Disorder. In Italy, comorbidity with Specific Language Disorder has been found from 15% to 20% of dyslexic children.[43,55]

In addition, children with LD often have motor, sensory, perceptual abnormalities.[56-60] Chabrolle *et al.*[61] in a review found that the impairment of motor development is a feature of nearly 50% of patients with dyslexia and that dyslexia is common among dyspraxic patients. Motor coordination disorder was reported in a percentage from 10.3% to 26% of dyslexics.[43,55] These data support the "cerebellar theory" of dyslexia[62] according to which, the cerebellum, that is responsible for motor control and automate over learned tasks (i.e., reading), in LD may exert an insufficient motor control influencing articulation, phonological representation and ability to form appropriate connections between graphemes and phonemes.

The classification system DSM-5 does emphasize that SLD can co-occurs with neurodevelopmental disorders (e.g., ADHD, communication disorders, developmental coordination disorder, autistic spectrum disorder) or other mental disorders (e.g., anxiety disorders, depressive and bipolar disorders). Further investigations, in accordance to new classification criteria, are needed to better define comorbidities and prognostic profiles of specific learning disorders to implement appropriate intervention strategies.

Diagnostic Criteria

The DSM -V and ICD 10 classification systems distinguish specific learning disorders from intellectual disability (or mental retardation), specific language delays, and acquired learning problems associated with traumatic brain injury. Both systems then offer a sub-classification of specific scholastic disabilities through reference to the specific skill in which the deficits are exhibited, for example, reading, spelling or arithmetic.

As per the diagnostic criteria laid down by DSM-V, one essential feature of specific learning disorder is persistent difficulties in learning keystone academic skills (Criterion A), with onset during the years of formal schooling (i.e., the developmental period). A second key feature is that the individual's performance of the affected academic skills is well below average for age (Criterion B). One robust clinical indicator of difficulties in learning academic skills is low academic achievement for age or average achievement that is sustainable only be extraordinarily high levels of effort or support. A third core feature is that the learning difficulties are readily apparent in the early school years in most individuals (Criterion C). However, in others, the learning difficulties may not manifest fully until later school years, by which time learning demands have increased and exceed the individual's limited capacities. Low achievement scores on one or more standardized tests or subtests within an academic domain (i.e., at least 1.5 standard deviations [SD] below the population mean for age, which translates to a standard score of 78 or less, which is below the 7th percentile) are needed for the greatest diagnostic certainty. However, precise scores will vary according to the particular standardized tests that are used. On the basis of clinical judgment, a more lenient threshold may be used (e.g., 1.0-2.5 SD below the population mean for age), when learning difficulties are supported by converging evidence from clinical assessment, academic history, school reports, or test scores. Moreover, since standardized tests are not available in all languages, the diagnosis may then be based in part on clinical judgment of scores on available test measures. It is noteworthy that the criteria are rather statistically prescriptive. DSM-5 considers "low achievement scores" to be at least 1.5 standard deviations below the population mean for age. As a caution, individual variability and clinical judgment need to be highlighted in determining a diagnosis of learning disabilities. There is a concern that there could be too much reliance on actual numbers, just as there was too much reliance on a statistical calculation in the IQ-Achievement Discrepancy model. Potentially this could be disadvantageous to individuals with learning disabilities. The importance of analyzing the pattern of reading skills, written expression skills or mathematical skills is undervalued, in that such an analysis can provide information that is highly relevant in understanding the reasons why given interventions may or may not be successful, and where compensatory, rather than remedial options need to be considered. The emphasis with the DSM-5 is on the score and the more qualitative aspect of diagnosis is overlooked. Cognitive Processing DSM-5 does not require impairments in cognitive processes related to learning for diagnosis. The diagnostic criteria for a Specific Learning Disorder (SLD) requires the presence of "symptoms… difficulties learning and using academic skills... One essential feature of specific learning disorder is persistent difficulties learning keystone academic skills".

The DSM-V defines specific learning disorder as a neurodevelopmental disorder of biological origin manifested in learning difficulties and problems in acquiring academic skills markedly below age level and manifested in the early school years, lasting for atleast six months; not attributed to intellectual disabilities, developmental disorders, or neurological or motor disorders. The DSM-V further gives specifiers as – with impairment in reading (315.00), with impairment in written expression (315.2) and impairment in mathematics (315.1). It also provides for specifying the current severity as mild, moderate or severe.

The four diagnostic criteria are: (Adapted from APA, DSM V, 2013)[10]

A. A persistent difficulty learning academic skills for at least 6 months despite intervention targeting the area(s) of difficulty. Many schools use a RTI model of academic skill assessment and progress monitoring to determine the effectiveness of interventions. The areas of documented academic skill difficulties include:
   1. Word decoding and word reading fluency.
   2. Reading comprehension.
   3. Spelling.
   4. Writing difficulties such as grammar, punctuation, organization and clarity.
   5. Number sense, fact and calculation.
   6. Mathematical reasoning.

B. The affected academic skills are substantially below expectations given the individual's age and result in impaired functioning in school, at work and in activities of daily living.

C. LD is readily apparent in the early years, however, it is not to be diagnosed until the onset of school years; in some individuals the disorder is not apparent until the onset of a demand for higher-level skills.

D. The academic and learning difficulties occur in the absence of:
   1. Intellectual disabilities.
   2. Visual or hearing impairments.
   3. Mental disorders (e.g., depression, anxiety, etc.).
   4. Neurological disorders.
   5. Psycho-social difficulty.
   6. Language differences.
   7. Lack of access to adequate instruction.

Specific learning disorder is distinguished from the academic and cognitive-processing difficulties associated with schizophrenia or psychosis, because with these disorders there is a decline (often rapid) in these functional domains. If there is an indication that another diagnosis could account for the difficulties in learning keystone academic skills described in Criterion A, specific learning disorder should not be diagnosed.

Signs of Learning Disorders

Teachers, parents and clinicians may look out for the following signs of specific learning disorders:

Specific Reading Disorders

- Slow rate of oral or silent reading.
- Inability to answer questions about what is being read.
- Lack of skill in using skills to locate information such as index or table of contents.
- Reading word by word rather than in groups of words.
- Lack of expression in oral reading.
- No regard for punctuation.
- Mispronunciation of words.
- Omission of words and/or letters.
- Insertion of words and/or letters.
- Substitution of words.
- Repetitions.

Specific Learning Disorder of Writing

- Difficulty in copying.
- Difficulty in aligning letters properly.
- Use of squibbles that are not really letters.
- Difficulty in writing from left to right.
- Poor spacing of words and letters.
- Irregular letter size.
- Poor letter formation.
- Written work shows fatigue.
- Very slow.
- Reversals for example writing "b" for "d"; or "pat" in place of "tap".

Specific Learning Disorder of Arithmetic

- Rotation of numbers.
- Reversal of digits For example 12 is written as 21.
- Inadequate concept of place value for example 1008 is read as one, zero, zero, eight.
- Writing the number as we say them. For example Four hundred and fifty as 40050.
- Difficulty doing basic mathematical operations (addition, subtraction, multiplication and division).
- Difficulty in carryover.
- Difficulty in borrowing.
- Difficulty solving application based problem sums.

Etiology

Learning disorders are proposed to be due to genetic and/or neurobiological factors or injury that alters brain functioning in a manner, which affects one or more processes related to learning. Specific learning disorder is a neurodevelopmental disorder with a biological origin that is the basis for abnormalities at a cognitive level that are associated with the behavioral signs of the disorder. The biological origin includes an interaction of genetic, epigenetic, and environmental factors, which affect the brain's ability to perceive or process verbal or nonverbal information efficiently and accurately. These disorders are not due primarily to hearing and/or vision problems, socio-economic factors, cultural or linguistic differences, lack of motivation or ineffective teaching, although these factors may further complicate the challenges faced by individuals with learning disorder. The learning difficulties are not better accounted for by intellectual disabilities, uncorrected visual or auditory acuity, other mental or neurological disorders, psychosocial adversity, lack of proficiency in the language of academic instruction, or inadequate educational instruction.

The etiology of specific learning disorder in reading may be understood within the context of theories about development of reading skills. The phonic theory argues that in order to read, children must first learn the sounds associated with letters, and then use these phonic building blocks to read and spell whole words.[63] The argument is that children build up the word rat from the three sounds associated with the letters "r", "a" and "t".

In contrast to the phonic theory, the whole language theory proposes that children learn to recognize whole words rather than piecing together individual letters and/or sounds. According to the whole language theory, the sound of unfamiliar words is learned by guessing from the meaning of the context within which they occur and obtaining feedback from teachers and parents.[64] In line with this theory, one may assume that a child learns that the word "rat" sounds like "rat" because it is written under the picture of rat or in sentence that says "the cat chased the rat".

None of the theories have received complete support and day-to-day practical experience points towards role of both the theories. And therefore, any deficits in either of the above two pathways may lead to specific learning disorders. A large body of evidence suggests that children who develop the skills of recognizing phonological and orthographic similarities at an early age become good readers, and those who do not do so develop reading problems.

Assessment

Assessment in the present context refers to the global mapping of the strengths and weaknesses in reading, writing, spelling and comprehension. Diagnostic assessment refers to the fine grained delineation of the condition and the profile of the child for effective instruction. Both generalized assessment and specific diagnostic assessment are required for effective intervention. John *et al.*[5] have laid down Indian guidelines for assessment of specific learning disability. According to the guidelines laid by them: the assessment of specific learning disability by a Clinical Psychologist allows the clinician to:

- Make diagnosis of specific learning disability.
- Understand the severity of disability.
- Construct a learning profile of the child.
- Make recommendations for specialized instructions and accommodations for the child.

The child must be assessed in all areas related to the suspected disability such as health, vision, hearing, social and emotional status, general intelligence, academic performance, communicative status and motor abilities.[65]

An ideal assessment for LD is a long process requiring several sessions with a qualified clinical psychologist. Apart from administering a battery of tests, the psychologist also gathers relevant information about the child from the teachers and school records.

The assessment procedure for LD involves the following steps:

1. **Parent Interview:** The academic, developmental and medical history along with the linguistic usage and

communications patterns of the child must be obtained from the parents. The parent must be involved in the planning of the intervention program such as attending a resource room, provision of accommodation and modifications to the child. Gathering Information from the Teachers/School. The psychologist must also observe the child in his/her school setting to know about the child's performance and behavior in the class, and gain insights from the teacher. Review of previous grades will show the pattern of academic progress. These may throw light into the problem areas of the child. A student's current classroom performance can be compared to Test scores. Looking at Student Workbooks Regrettably, in the present educational setup, very often the notebooks don't reflect the learning difficulties faced by the child due to rote learning especially when the child can easily copy from the blackboard. The examination papers may give a clearer picture of the specific nature of difficulty. Only through collecting data through a variety of approaches (observations, interviews, tests, curriculum-based assessment, etc.) and from various sources such as parents, teachers, peers, adequate picture be obtained of the child's strengths and weaknesses. Synthesized, this information can be used to determine the specific nature of the child's special needs, whether the child needs special services and if so, to design an appropriate program.[65] A number of approaches being used recently include curriculum-based assessment, task analysis, dynamic assessment, and assessment of learning style. These approaches yield rich information about students and are especially important when assessing students from culturally or linguistically diverse backgrounds, and therefore, are critical methods in the overall approach to assessment.[65]

2. **Interview with the Child:** Along with parents and teachers, detailed interview with the child is important to assess child's viewpoint regarding his problems. Interview with the child also serves to know what other factors might be contributing to child's poor academic performance. For example, a child may be undergoing severe emotional disturbances owing to bullying at school due to which he might not be able to perform well at school. Furthermore, it is also important to interview the child so to get an in-depth knowledge and understanding the psychological impact of poor school performance due to learning disorder. Useful insights regarding child's psychosocial support can also be obtained from interviewing the child.

3. **Formal Testing:** Essentially, the tests for LD have two major components:

   1. **Testing for Potential:** Performance Discrepancy.

   2. **Testing Processing Abilities:** A two-year discrepancy between potential and performance is an indicator of a possible LD. Validity of a significant discrepancy will be evaluated on a case by case basis (Hirisave U, *et al.*, 2002).

The recommended psycho-educational tests are discussed below under various heads:

1. **Intellectual Assessment:** To begin with the psychologist must carry out assessment of intellectual abilities of the child/adolescent. This would help in ascertaining the discrepancy between his potential and his performance. For example, MAlin's Intelligence Scale for Indian Children or the Woodcock Johnson Tests of Cognitive Ability may be administered to assess child's intellectual functioning.

2. **Achievement:** After assessing child's intellectual abilities, it is important to assess his academic performance and achievement. This can be done using various psychoeducational tests. For example, Grade Level Assessment Devise,Woodcock Johnson Psycho-Educational Battery-Revised.

3. **Cognitive Processing Abilities:** In addition to assessing intellectual abilities and academic performance, it is of utmost importance to assess various cognitive functions. For this, the following tests may be used–Woodcock Johnson Psycho-Educational Battery Revised (Part 1 – Tests of Cognitive Ability), Weschler Memory Scales Revised, Benton Visual Retention Test, Berry Visuo-Motor Integration Test, Raven Colored Progressive Matrices, Rex Auditory-Verbal Learning Test, Bender Visual Motor Gestalt Test, Halstead-Reitan Neuropsychological Test Battery, Memory-For-Designs Test, Nimhans Index.[66]

Some frequently used psychological tests are listed in Table 12.1. Depending on the age at the time of assessment, a battery of the following tests is used, ensuring that all the relevant areas are evaluated to arrive at a diagnosis.

Table 12.1: Frequently Used Psychological Tests		
Test Name	**What it Measures**	**Age Ranges**
Malin's Intelligence Scale for Indian Children	Verbal intelligence, Performance intelligence, IQ	6 to 15 years
Wechsler Intelligence Scale for Children – Fourth Edition (Indian Adaptation) (WISC-IV)	Verbal Comprehension, Perceptual Reasoning, Working Memory, Processing Speed)	6-16 years 11 months
Binet Kamat Test of Intelligence	IQ	Mental age 3 years to 23 years
Wechsler Adult Performance Intelligence Scale-PR Indian Adaptation (WAPIS-PR)	Performance IQ	15-44 years
Verbal Adult Intelligence Scale (VAIS) Indian Adaptation of Wechsler Adult Intelligence Verbal Scale	Verbal IQ	20-69 years
Bender Visual Motor Gestalt Test	Visuo perceptual abilities	
Wide Range Achievement Test – Expanded (WRAT–Expanded)	Reading comprehension	5 years and above
Wide Range Achievement Test - 4 (WRAT-4)	Basic academic skills	5 years and above
Woodcock Johnson III – Tests of Achievement	Writing fluency, math fluency, calculation, applied problems, quantitative reasoning	2 years and above
Woodcock Johnson III – Tests of Cognitive Abilities	Short-term memory, cognitive fluency, processing speed, working memory	2 years and above
Screening of Early Reading Process Test	Reading	KG to 2nd Grade
Individual/Informal Reading Inventory	Basic academic skills	1st-12th Grade
Grade Level Assessment Device	Basic academic skills	1st-4th grade
NIMHANS SLD Battery	Cognitive functions, academic skills	5-12 years
Dyslexia Screening Test–Junior, Indian Adaptation	Reading	6 years 6 months-11 years 5 months
Diagnostic Test of Reading Disorder	Reading	6-13 years
Diagnostic Test of Learning Disabilities	Cognitive functions	6-13 years

Curriculum based assessments (CBA) may also be used. "Tests" of performance in this case come directly from the curriculum. For example, a child may be asked to read from his or her reading book for one minute. Information on the accuracy and the speed of reading can then be compared with other students in the class. CBA is quick and offers specific information about how a student may differ from his peers.[65] Because the assessment is tied to curriculum content, it allows the teacher to match instruction to a student's current abilities and pinpoints areas where curriculum adaptations or modifications are needed. CBA provides information that is immediately relevant to instructional 167 programming (National Information Centre for Children and Youth with Disabilities, 2000). The merits of a CBA are lost in a system with a rigid curriculum based mainly on memorization as is true in India where CBA may not be the right option.

Neurocognitive Aspects in Learning Disability

Cognitive processes go beyond what is measured in standardized IQ tests, although the clusters of abilities assessed by IQ tests can provide valuable information about cognitive abilities and suggest areas of difficulty that warrant further exploration. Academic learning difficulties are logically related to observed deficits in cognitive processes. Examples of cognitive processes under consideration include phonological processing, language processing, attention and memory (working memory, long-term memory and short-term memory), processing speed, visual perception, visual-motor processing and executive functions. This information, together with a growing body of evidence linking cognitive processing deficits to academic achievement, is important for describing an individual learner's profile of strengths and needs. It is this profile that is critical for designing intervention for a student with learning disorder. In clinical practice, there are a wide range of profiles which describe strengths and needs in cognitive and academic areas. Recommendations for intervention are individualized based on the individual's profile and typically include ideas for teaching approaches, remediation strategies, skills, content, compensatory strategies, accommodations and assistive technology. At a clinical level, the understanding of underlying cognitive processes is important for both classroom and individualized programming.[67] It has been reported that there are deficits in phonological processing, processing speed, and verbal working memory in children with reading disorders.[68] Impairments in executive functioning, processing speed, and short-term memory were linked to math disorders.[68]

Children with learning disorders are often seen to have Auditory Processing Deficit (or Auditory Processing Disorder) which creates difficulties/weakness in the ability to understand and use auditory information. Related to this deficit children may have difficulties in one or more of the following abilities–auditory discrimination (the ability to notice, compare and distinguish the distinct and separate sounds in words–a skill that is vital for reading), auditory figure-ground discrimination (the ability to pick out important sounds from a noisy background), auditory memory (short-term and long-term abilities to recall information presented orally), auditory sequencing (the ability to understand and recall the order of sounds and words), spelling, reading and written expression.

Visual Processing Deficit (or Visual Processing Disorder) is the term used to describe a weakness in the ability to understand and use visual information. Individuals with these types of difficulties often have trouble with, visual discrimination (the ability to notice and compare the features of different items and to distinguish one item from another), visual figure-ground discrimination (the ability to distinguish a shape or printed character from its background), visual sequencing (the ability to see and distinguish the order of symbols, words or images), visual motor processing (using visual feedback to coordinate body movement), visual memory (the ability to engage in short-term and long-term recall of visual information), visual closure (the ability to know what an object is when only parts of it are visible), spatial relationships (the ability to understand how objects are positioned in space).

Children with learning disorders have been reported to have deficits in their attention, verbal and visual memory, and visuospatial functioning.[69-73]

Although children with Specific Learning Disorder typically (but not invariably) exhibit poor performance on psychological tests of cognitive processing. However, it remains unclear whether these cognitive abnormalities are the cause, correlate, or consequence of the learning difficulties. Thus, assessment of cognitive processing deficits is not required for diagnostic assessment. There are no known biological markers of specific learning disorder. As a group, individuals with the disorder show circumscribed alterations in cognitive processing and brain structure and function. Genetic differences are also evident at the group level. But cognitive testing, neuroimaging, or genetic testing are not useful for diagnosis at this time.

While not designated as specific subtypes of LD, there are a number of areas of information processing that are commonly associated with LD. Weaknesses in the ability to receive, process, associate, retrieve and express information can often help explain why a person has trouble with learning and performance. The inability to process information efficiently can lead to frustration, low self-esteem and social withdrawal, and understanding how these areas of weakness impact individuals with LD and can be beneficial in planning for effective instruction and support. Ongoing research is uncovering the specific nature and impact of these problems.

Lobe	Impaired Neuropsychological Function
Frontal Lobe	Motor Speed
	Selective Attention
	Sustained Attention
	Focussed Attention
	Executive Functions • Design Fluency • Verbal Working Memory • Visuospatial Working Memory • Planning • Set shifting
Parietal Lobe	Visuo Perceptual Ability
	Visuo Conceptual Ability
	Visuoconstructive Abilities
Temporal Lobe	Verbal Comprehension
	Verbal Learning and Memory
	Visual Learning and Memory

Differential Diagnosis

It is important to keep following differential diagnoses in mind while evaluating these children and rule them in or out by taking meticulous history, physical, neurological, vision and auditory examination and appropriate psychological and education test before confirming the diagnosis of specific learning disorder. The child with borderline intellectual capacity is usually confused with the child having specific learning disability.

1. **Intellectual disability:** The child with mild mental retardation may also present with poor scholastic performance and repeated failures in school. When clinically it is difficult to differentiate, the performance on tests of intelligence, i.e., child's IQ, may resolve

the problem. The mentally retarded child would have an IQ below 70.

2. **Borderline intellectual functioning:** The child with borderline intellectual capacity may present with difficulty in reading and writing, and poor scholastic performance. His difficulties are more general and are due to his borderline intellectual capacity. These children are also called "slow learners".

3. **Hearing or visual impairment:** Rarely, it may happen that a child is slow in writing and unable to complete his books due to hearing or visual impairment. This can be easily corrected by appropriate glasses or hearing aids.

4. **Neurological deficits such as myopathy:** The difficulty in writing may be secondary to neurological problem such as myopathy. In this kind of situation parents may be asked to take a certificate of physical disability to take advantage of concessions.

5. **Writer's cramp:** In writer's cramp the student starts getting pain and spasms in hands after writing for sometimes. Students having writer's cramp are also entitled for a writer in exams.

6. **Pervasive developmental disorders:** Pervasive developmental disorders are relatively rare and with the other associated features it is usually not difficult to differentiate them from receptive and expressive language disorders.

7. **Receptive and expressive language disorder:** One of the most striking clinical features of children having pervasive developmental disorder is very poor language development. It may have to be differentiated from receptive and expressive language disorders.

8. **Language problems/Discrepancy between mother-tongue and language of schooling:** Sometimes one may get an impression that the child is not able to do well in his studies as his mother-tongue may not be English or nobody in the home speaks or understands English. In this kind of situation generally the child would not able to speak English fluently and may make more grammatical mistakes but he would able to write fast and complete his books.

9. **Inadequate facilities for schooling:** Once in a while, when a student who has studied in a less sophisticated village school and then gets an admission in a more sophisticated city school, he may show poor performance in city school in spite of being intelligent. This may be due to lack of adequate facilities in the village school. This may also be noticed when the child is shifted from one board to other board, i.e., from SSC-board to ICSC or CBSE board. Most of the time, this kind of difficulty is only during the first couple of months and most of the intelligent children are able to overcome this problem over next few months.

Intervention

Treatment of SLD is directed at the underlying academic difficulties by use of educational interventions. Psychological interventions are also directed at any existing emotional, social, or family difficilties. In addition, social skills training may be helpful. Counseling and psycho-education of students, parents and teachers. Rarely, it may happen that a child is slow in writing and unable to complete his books due to hearing or visual impairment. This can be easily corrected by appropriate glasses or hearing aids. It is essential that remediation programmes for children with specific learning disorders be based on a thorough assessment of the child's abilities and the potential resources within the family, the school and the wider social and professional network for remediating the child's learning difficulties. Till now no medication has been found to be effective in treatment of SLD. However, if there is any comorbid condition that may require pharmacotherapy, it is important to start with pharmacotherapy. For example, for a child having comorbid ADHD along with SLD, it is important that medication be used to minimize the hyperactivity, distractability or impulsivity that may be aggravating child's learning problems.

All programmes for children with specific learning disorder should be structured, with graded difficulty level as the child progresses. Direct instruction in reading as well as writing and spelling is considered is essential for treatment for a child with specific learning disorder. These techniques used by trained professionals emphazise explicit instruction in letter sound associations. Instructions are usually given in multisensory modalities. Children see a letter, say its name and sound, and write the letter. Sounds and letters are then blended to form words. Reading, writing and spelling are taught simultaneously. Instruction involves extended practice and is supplemented by speech segmentation training and study skills instructions.

The treatment for writing disorder might involve a skills approach or a holistic approach. Skills programmes are often used with younger children and focus on letter-sound associations, with emphasis on reading and spelling. Children may be asked to listen carefully for the sounds in words and then to represent these sounds with written letters, saying each letter aloud as it is written. The holistic approach to writing begins with the students' ideas. It involves a series of highly structured steps to narrowing ideas to one topic, writing a first draft, reading it aloud to an audience of peers, and then refining organization and language. Most interventions for writing combine both these approaches. Children with a SLD in writing need direct sequential instruction in letter sound associations and spelling rules as well as in sentence structures and the connections between sentences and paragraphs that make text cohesive and meaningful.

Course and Prognosis

Learning disorders are lifelong. The way in which they are expressed may vary over an individual's lifetime, depending on the interaction between the demands of the environment and the individual's strengths and needs. The learning difficulties begin during school-age years but may not become fully manifest until the demands for those affected academic skills exceed the individual's limited capacities (e.g., as in timed tests, reading or writing lengthy complex reports for a tight deadline, excessively heavy academic loads). Changes in manifestation of symptoms occur with age, so that an individual may have a persistent or shifting array of learning difficulties across the lifespan. Learning disabilities are suggested by unexpected academic under-achievement or achievement, which is maintained only by unusually high levels of effort and support. The affected academic skills are substantially and quantifiably below those expected for the individual's chronological age, and cause significant interference with academic or occupational performance, or with activities of daily living, as confirmed by individually administered standardized achievement measures and comprehensive clinical assessment. For individuals age 17 years and older, a documented history of impairing learning difficulties may be substituted for the standardized assessment.

References

1. Shah N, Bhat T. Clinical Practice Guidelines for the Specific Learning Disorders. Ind J Psychiatry 2009:51:68-95.
2. National Joint Committee on Learning Disability. Operationalising on NJCLD Definition of Learning Disabilities for Ongoing Assessment in Schools. Learning Disabilities Quarterly 1998:21:186-93.
3. Lyon G Reid, Shaywitz Sally E, Shaywitz, Bennett A. A Definition of Dyslexia. Annals of Dyslexia 2003:53:1-14.
4. Abramowitz A. Developmental Disabilities: Learning Disorders. In Sexson SB (Eds). Child and Adolescent Psychiatry (2nd Edition), Blackwell Publishing 2006:79-90.
5. John A, Sadasivan A, Bhola P, David NJ, Manickam LSS. Indian Association of Clinical Psychologists: Practice Guidelines for Learning Disabilities. Ind J Clin Psychologists 2013:40(1): 65-88.
6. Wernicke C. Grundriss der Psychiatrie: Psycholphysiologische Eindeitung, 1894, Wiesbaden, Germany.
7. Broca PP. Localization des Functions Cerebrales: Siege du Langage Aricule. Bulletin de la Societe d Anthropologie de Paris 1863:4:200-03.
8. Orton S. Reading, Writing and Speech Problems in Children: A Presentation of Certain Types of Disorders in the Development of the Language Faculty 1937: NY: WW Norton.
9. Torgesen JK, Wagner RK, Rashotte CA, Burgess SR, Hecht SA. The contributions of Phonological Awareness and Rapid Automatic Naming Ability to the Growth of Word Reading Skills in Second to Fifth Grade Children, Scientific Studies of Reading 1997;1:161-85.
10. American Psychiatric Association: Diagnostic and Statistical Manual of Mental Disorders, Fifth Edition (DSM-5), Washington DC: American Psychiatric Publishing; 2013.
11. World Health Organization (1994). ICD-10 DCR Classification of Mental and Behavioural Disorders: Diagnostic Criteria for Research. Oxford University Press, Oxford.
12. Tannock R (2013, May 1). Rethinking Learning Disorders. Retrieved from: http://blogs.scientificamerican.com/mind-guest-blog/2013/05/01/rethinking-learning-disorders, 2013.
13. Shepherd MJ, Uhry J. Segmentation/Spelling Instruction as Part of a First-Grade Reading Program: Effects on Several Measures of Reading, Reading Research Quarterly 1993; 28(3):21.
14. Arun P, Singh BC, Bhargava R , Sharma A, Kaur J. Prevalence of Specific Developmental Disorder of Scholastic Skill in School Students in Chandigarh, India, Indian J Med Res 2013 July;138,89-98.
15. Altarac M, Saroha E. Lifetime Prevalence of Learning Disability Among US Children. Pediatrics 2007;119(Suppl 1): S77-S83.
16. Ramaa S. Two Decades of Research on Learning Disabilities in India, Dyslexia 2000;6:268-83.
17. Agarwal KN, Agarwal DK, Upadhyay SK, Singh M. Learning Disability in Rural Primary School Children. Indian J Med Res 1991;94:89-95.
18. Singh S, Sawani V, Deokate M, Panchal S, Subramanyam AA, Shah HR. Specific Learning Disability: 5 Years Study from India. Int J Contemp Pediatr 2017;4:863-68.
19. Kohli A, Malhotra S, Mohanty M, Khehra N, Kaur M. Specific Learning Disabilities in Children: Deficits and Neuropsychological Profile. Int J Rehabil Res 2005;28:165-69.
20. Karanth P. Introduction. In: Karanth P, Rozario J, Editors. Learning Disabilities in India: Willing the Mind to Learn, New Delhi, Sage Publications 2003;17-29.
21. Snow CE, Burns MS, Griffin P. Preventing Reading Difficulties in Young Children, Washington, DC: US National Research Council Report, 2000.

22. Rutter M, Caspi A, Fergusson D, Horwood LJ, Goodman R, Maughan B, Moffitt TE, Meltzer H, Carroll J. Sex Differences in Developmental Reading Disability: New Findings from 4 Epidemiological Studies. JAMA 2004;291 (Suppl 16):2007-12.

23. Hawke JL, Olson RK, Willcut EG, Wadsworth SJ, DeFries JC. Gender Ratios for Reading Difficulties. Dyslexia 2009;15 (Suppl 3):239-42.

24. Bishop DVM, Snowling MJ. Developmental Dyslexia and Specific Language Impairment: Same or Different? Psychol Bull 2004;130:858-86.

25. Catts HW, Adlof SM, Hogan TP, Weismer SE. Are Specific Language Impairment and Dyslexia Distinct Disorders? J Speech Lang Hear Res 2005;48:1378-96.

26. Pennington BF, Bishop DV. Relations Among Speech, Language and Reading Disorders. Annu Rev Psychol 2009; 60:283-306.

27. Newbury DF, Paracchini S, Scerri TS, Winchester L, Addis L, Richardson AJ, Walter J, Stein JF, Talcott JB, Monaco AP. Investigation of Dyslexia and SLI Risk Variants in Reading- and Language-Impaired Subjects. Behav Genet 2011;41 (Suppl 1):90-104.

28. Capellini SA, Coppede AC, Valle TR. Fine Motor Function of School-aged Children with Dyslexia, Learning Disability and Learning Difficulties. Prò-Fono Revista de Atualizacao Cientìfica 2010;22:3.

29. Lingam R, Golding J, Jongmans MJ, Hunt LP, Ellis M, Emond A. The Association Between Developmental Coordination Disorder and Other Developmental Traits. Pediatrics 2010;126(Suppl 5):1109-18.

30. Cunningham CE, Barkley RA. The Role of Academic Failure in Hyperactive Behaviour. J Learn Disabil 1978;11:15-21.

31. Rabiner D, Coie JD, the Conduct Problems Prevention Research Group: Early Attention Problems and Children's Reading Achievement: A Longitudinal Investigation. J Am Acad Child Adolesc Psychiatry 2000;39:859-67.

32. McGee R, Prior M, Williams S, Smart D, Sanson A. The Long-Term Significance of Teacher-Rated Hyperactivity and Reading Ability in Childhood: Findings from Two Longitudinal Studies. J Child Psychol Psychiatr 2002;43:1004-17.

33. Dally K. The Influence of Phonological Processing and Inattentive Behaviour on Reading Acquisition. J Educ Psychol 2006;98:420-37.

34. Willcutt EG, Betjemann RS, McGrath LM, Chhabildas NA, Olson RK, DeFries JC, Pennington BF. Etiology and Neuropsychology of Comorbidity between RD and ADHD: The Case for Multiple-Deficit Models. Cortex 2010;46(Suppl 10):1345-61.

35. Ebejer JL, Coventry WL, Byrne B, Willcutt EG, Olson RK, Corely R, Sammuelson S. Genetic and Environmental Influences on Inattention, Hyperactivity-Impulsivity and Reading: Kindergarten to Grade 2. Sci. Stud Read 2010;14: 293-316.

36. Greven CU, Rijsdijk FV, Asherson P, Plomin R. A Longitudinal Twin Study on the Association between ADHD Symptoms and Reading. J Child Psychol Psychiatry 2012;53(Suppl 3):234-42.

37. Dally K. The Influence of Phonological Processing and Inattentive Behaviour on Reading Acquisition. J Educ Psychol 2006;98:420-37.

38. Willcutt EG, Betjemann RS, McGrath LM, Chhabildas NA, Olson RK, DeFries JC, Pennington BF. Etiology and Neuropsychology of Comorbidity between RD and ADHD: The Case for Multiple-Deficit Models. Cortex 2010;46(Suppl 10):1345-61.

39. Ebejer JL, Coventry WL, Byrne B, Willcutt EG, Olson RK, Corely R, Sammuelson S. Genetic and Environmental Influences on Inattention, Hyperactivity-Impulsivity and Reading: Kindergarten to Grade 2. Sci. Stud Read 2010;14: 293-316.

40. Greven CU, Rijsdijk FV, Asherson P, Plomin R. A Longitudinal Twin Study on the Association Between ADHD Symptoms and Reading. J Child Psychol Psychiatry 2012;53(Suppl 3):234-42.

41. Grills-Tacquerel AE, Fletcher JM, Vaughn SR, Stuebing KK. Anxiety and Reading Difficulties in Early Elementary School: Evidence for Unidirectional or Bidirectional Relations? Child Psychiatr Hum. Dev. 2012;43(Suppl 1):35-47.

42. Grills-Tacquerel AE, Fletcher JM, Vaughn SR, Stuebing KK. Anxiety and Reading Difficulties in Early Elementary School: Evidence for Unidirectional or Bidirectional Relations? Child Psychiatr Hum. Dev 2012;43(Suppl 1):35-47.

43. Carroll JM, Maughan B, Goodman R, Meltzer H. Literacy Difficulties and Psychiatric Disorders: Evidence for Comorbidity. J Child Psychol Psychiatr 2005;46(Suppl 5): 524-32.

44. Li H, Morris RJ. Assessing Fears and Related Anxieties in Children and Adolescents with Learning Disabilities or Mild Mental Retardation. Res Dev Disabil 2007;28(Suppl 5): 445-57.

45. Li H, Morris RJ. Assessing Fears and Related Anxieties in Children and Adolescents with Learning Disabilities or Mild Mental Retardation. Res Dev. Disabil 2007;28(Suppl 5): 445-57.

46. Terras MM, Thompson LC, Minnis H. Dyslexia and Psychosocial Functioning: An Exploratory Study of the Role of Self-Esteem and Understanding. Dyslexia 2009;15(Suppl 4): 304-27.

47. Kempe C, Gustafson S, Samuelsson S. A Longitudinal Study of Early Reading Difficulties and Subsequent Problem Behaviors. Scand J Psychol 2011;52 (Suppl 3):242-50.

48. Nelson JM, Gregg N. Depression and Anxiety Among Transitioning Adolescents and College Students with ADHD, Dyslexia, or Comorbid ADHD/dyslexia. J Atten Disord 2012;16(Suppl 3):244-54.

49. Rietz CS, Hasselhorn M, Labuhn AS. Are Externalizing and Internalizing Difficulties of Young Children with Spelling Impairment Related to Their ADHD Symptoms? Dyslexia 2012;18(Suppl 3):174-85.

50. Pieters S, Desoete A, Van Waelvelde H, Vanderswalmen R, Roeyers H. Mathematical Problems in Children with Developmental Coordination Disorder. Res Dev Disabil 2012; 33(Suppl 4):1128-35.

51. Westendorp M. Hartman E. Houwen S. Smith J. Visscher C. The Relationship Between Gross Motor Skills and Academic Achievement in Children with Learning Disabilities. Res. Dev. Disabil 2011:32(Suppl 6):2773-79.

52. Fawcett AJ. Nicolson RI. From Dyslexia: The Role of the Cerebellum. In Dyslexia in Context: Research. Policy and Practice. Chapter 2. Edited by: Reid G. Fawcett AJ. London: Whurr Publishers: 2004.

53. Willcutt E. Pennington B. DeFries JC. Twin Study of the Aetiology of Comorbidity Between Reading Disability and Attention-deficit/Hyperactivity Disorder. Am J Med Genet 2000:96:293-301.

54. Trzienewski K. Moffitt T. Caspi A. Taylor A. Maughan B. Revisiting the Association Between Reading Achievement and Antisocial Behavior: New Evidence of An Environmental Explanation from A Twin Study. Child Dev 2006:77:72-88.

55. Kain W. Landerl K. Kaufmann L: Comorbidity of ADHD. Monatsschr Kinderheilkd 2008:8:757-67.

56. Kempe C. Gustafson S. Samuelsson S. A Longitudinal Study of Early Reading Difficulties and Subsequent Problem Behaviors. Scand J Psychol 2011:52(Suppl 3):242-50.

57. Nelson JM. Gregg N. Depression and Anxiety Among Transitioning Adolescents and College Students with ADHD. Dyslexia. or Comorbid ADHD/Dyslexia. J Atten Disord 2012:16(Suppl 3):244-54.

58. Rietz CS. Hasselhorn M. Labuhn AS. Are Externalizing and Internalizing Difficulties of Young Children with Spelling Impairment Related to Their ADHD Symptoms? Dyslexia 2012:18(Suppl 3):174-85.

59. Cunningham CE. Barkley RA. The Role of Academic Failure in Hyperactive Behaviour. J Learn Disabil 1978:11:15-21.

60. Rabiner D. Coie JD. The Conduct Problems Prevention Research Group: Early Attention Problems and Children's Reading Achievement: A Longitudinal Investigation. J Am Acad Child Adolesc Psychiatry 2000:39:859-67.

61. Achenbach MT. Child Behavior Checklist for Ages 6-18. ASEBA: University of Vermont: 2001.

62. McGee R. Prior M. Williams S. Smart D. Sanson A. The Long-term Significance of Teacher-rated Hyperactivity and Reading Ability in Childhood: Findings from Two Longitudinal Studies. J Child Psychol Psychiatr 2002:43:1004-17.

63. Perfetti CA 1985. Reading Ability. Oxford University Press. New York.

64. Goodman KS Reading: A Psycholinguistic Guessing Game. In Singer H. and Ruddell RB (Eds.). Theoretical Models and Processes of Reading. 1976: 2nd Edition. 497-508.

65. National Information Centre for Children and Youth with Disabilities. Assessing Children for the Presence of a Disability: Methods of Gathering Information. [Online]. 2000.

66. Kapur M. John A. Rozario J. Oomen A. NIMHANS Index of Specific Learning Disabilities. In Hirisave U. Oommen A. Kapur M. (Eds). Psychological Assessment of Children in Clinical setting. Bangalore. Department of Clinical Psychology National Institute of Mental Health and Neurosciences 2002: 88-126.

67. Fuchs D. Hale JB and Kearns DM. On the Importance of A Processing-Deficit Perspective: An Introduction. Journal of Learning Disabilities 2011:44:99-104.

68. Cortiella C and Horowitz SH. The State of Learning Disabilities: Facts. Trends and Emerging Issues. New York: National Center for Learning Disabilities. 2014.

69. Kohli A. Malhotra S. Mohanty M. Khehra N. Kaur M. Specific Learning Disabilities in Children: Deficits and Neuropsychological Profile. Intern J Rehab Res 2005:28(2): 165-69.

70. Snow JH. Mental Flexibility and Planning Skills in Children and Adolescents with Learning Disabilities. J Learning Disab 1992:25(4):265-70.

71. Reiter A. Tucha O. Lange KW. Executive Functions in Children with Dyslexia. Dyslexia 2005:11(2):116-31.

72. Malhotra S. Rajender G. Sharma V. Singh TB. Bhatia MS. Neurocognitive Functioning in Children with Learning Difficulties. Delhi Psychiatry Journal 2009:12(2):276-81.

73. Krishna R. Oomen A. Rao SL. Neuropsychological Profile of Learning Disability in the Indian Population–Preliminary results. Ind J Cl Psych 2007:34(1):69-75.

13 Chapter

INTELLECTUAL DISABILITY DISORDERS: CLINICAL APPROACH

Bibek Talukdar

Intellectual Disability Disorder (IDD), earlier known as mental retardation (MR), is an important problem in pediatric neurology primarily because it impairs the process of learning that is vital for a meaningful life. Impaired learning is often associated with a variety of behavioral abnormalities that limits normal social functioning. This disorder adds to our handicapped population and is an important socio-economic burden. Prevalence of IDD seems to be around 1-3% as reported in some population based studies and observations.[1,2] The prevalence in India is not well-known; however, observations based on limited population suggests that this could be around 4.4/1000 population in semi-urban areas[3] (Satapathy *et al.*). The incidence, however, is likely to be different now due to change in diagnostic criteria; in earlier studies diagnosis of IDD (MR) was based solely on IQ without taking into consideration the adaptive behaviour. The incidence and prevalence of IDD also may change in times to come due to socio-cultural changes, specially the mild category.

There is practically no cure of established IDD although many conditions are potentially preventable. The management of children with IDD is beset with variety of problem especially in developing countries with limited resources. In large number of cases it is difficult to pinpoint the cause and the unsatisfied parents keep shopping doctors in the hope of getting a cause and a cure. A good clinical work-up is needed for every child with IDD aimed at knowing its severity and finding the cause; these will put the management of these in right perspective.

Definition of Intellectual Disability (ID)

Intellectual disability basically implies impaired mental development from early in life and continuing to persist in later life. Defining intellectual disability satisfactorily is problematic and different definitions has been suggested by different groups. The diagnostic criteria for IDD formulated by the American Psychiatric Association (APA) and published in DSM V[4] is commonly accepted. The approach of the American Association on Intellectual and Developmental Disability (AAIDD)[5] is also similar. As envisaged in DSM V, diagnosis of IDD requires both intellectual deficit and deficit in adaptive functioning to be considered. Deficit in adaptive functioning results in failure to meet the standards for personal independence. In the current approach more emphasis has been given on linking intellectual deficits to adaptive deficit, IQ is not the sole criteria for determining IDD. ICD 11 has proposed this disorder to be termed as intellectual developmental disorder.[6] The essence of all these definitions are that the problem is to be projected as a general disability than a mental disability alone. Less emphasis is to be placed on IQ sore and greater emphasis on adaptive functioning.

As projected by APA and AAIDD, IDD currently is defined as significant impairment in general intellectual function and adaptive behavior acquired before the age of 18 years.

Similar approach has also been proposed in ICD 11. The diagnosis ID thus has to be based on the following criteria:

1. Significant impairment in *intellectual functioning* with IQ score below 70 obtained after an individually administered test of intelligence (this is 2 SD below the mean).

2. Significant impairment in *adaptive behaviour* judged by impairment in day-to-day functioning or daily living skills resulting from cognitive dysfunction; this is to be based on significant delay in 1 of 3 sets of skills, i.e., conceptual, social and practical.

3. Onset before the *age of 18 years*.

For assessment of impairment in *intellectual functioning* various mental abilities are considered like reasoning, problem solving, planning, abstract thinking, judgment, academic learning (ability to learn in school via traditional teaching methods) and experiential learning (the ability to learn through experience, trial and error, and observation). These mental abilities are measured by IQ tests. A score of approximately two standard deviations below the mean represents a significant cognitive deficit. The tests used to measure IQ must be standardized and culturally appropriate.

Adaptive behavior assessment involves 3 broad sets of skills, i.e., conceptual, social and practical. Conceptual skills include language, reading, writing, money concept and self direction. Social skills include interpersonal skills, personal responsibility, self-esteem, gullibility, nativite and ability to follow rules, obey laws and avoid victimization. Practical skills include activities of daily living like dressing, feeding, toilet, bathing and mobility. All the skills have to be age appropriate. These skills are needed to live in an independent and responsible manner, without which a person needs additional help and support in different areas like schooling, daily living. Deficits in adaptive functioning are measured using standardized, culturally appropriate tests.

The accurate diagnosis of IDD in infants and young children below 5 years of age continues to be difficult as the standard tests for intelligence and adaptive behavior are not easily applicable in this age group. Developmental quotient (DQ) still remains the best tool in this age group more so till about 3 years of age.

The *degree of the disability* continues to be categorized as mild, moderate and severe according to the IQ score; mild 50-69 moderate 35-49, severe < 35. The term profound is often applied when IQ is < 25. Frequency of cases in these different grades of severity is variable due to variability in characteristics of study population and also methodology. In a multicentric ICMR study[7] that included 1314 children (tests based on primarily IQ and where only apparently idiopathic cases were included), the proportion of children in these different groups were found to be as follows–mild 42.3%, moderate 25.3%, severe 19.2% and profound 13.1%. In another recent hospital based study (sample size 101) these were found to be as follows – mild in 11.7%, moderate in 21.7%, severe in 30.6% and profound in 35.6%.[8]

Mild ID: They usually have poor school perfor-mance (academic failure) and thus they are detected when they reach school age. Ability to learn depends on the degree of severity majority reaching mid school level. These usually do not have much clinical abnormality. Most of them learn self care and skills needed in day-to- day life, although may be little slow in acquiring them.

Moderate ID: These cases usually are apparent in the first year of life. Speech delay is common in them. They need considerable support in study usually have limited ability to learn. They usually lag behind in skills needed for day-to-day life (feeding, dressing, bathing, communication and other social skills) and need considerable support in these areas.

Severe ID: They need intensive support and supervision practically in every field of day-to-day life. Many need whole time care giver.

The term global developmental delay (GDD) is often used in young children who has delay acquiring developmental milestones in two or more domains.

ID occurs as co-morbidity in several other neuro-psychiatric disorders like ADHD, anxiety disorders, autism spectrum disorders, stereotypic movement disorder, self-injurious behavior, aggression and disruptive behaviour, bipolar disorder and depression.[9]

Pathogenesis and Causes of IDD

Normal mental development is considered to depend on genetic endowment, structural and functional integrity of the brain and external environmental stimuli. Abnormalities in any of these areas can be associated with IDD. There may often be an interplay of these factors. The etiopathology of IDD is diverse and in many situations it remains unclear despite extensive investigations. Genetic and developmental disorders are common causes. In cases with mild IDD the brain is often normal or shows minor changes that are difficult to correlate with the development of IDD. Advancements in investigative techniques suggest that a complex interplay of molecular, genetic, metabolic and other factors is likely to be operative in development of IDD.

Many systemic disorders are known to be associated with IDD. It is still not clear whether these disorders are causes or associations, although considered as causes for all practical purpose. Some of the relatively common and important conditions associated with IDD grouped into certain categories from clinical point of view, based on some reports in Indian literature,[3,10-13] are shown in Table 13.1. The exact incidence of different disorders associated with or causing IDD are difficult to know because of variable methods of case selection, investigation and different ways of categorization of the cases in the reported studies and also due to difference in type of studies whether hospital based or epidemiologic. Extent of investigation is another important factor, specially in terms of genetic and metabolic aspect.

Table 13.1: Aetiology of Intellectual Disability

The common and important disorders associated with Intellectual Disability can be grouped into categories as follows:

Genetic-Chromosomal

Chromosomal disorders, genetic syndromes

Congenital Malformations

Hydrocephalus, microcephaly, megalencephaly, lissencephaly, spinal dysruphysm

Metabolic Disorders

Many inborn errors of metabolism

Systemic Disease

Endocrinal–Hypothyroidism

CNS–Neurodegenerative disorders, neuroectodermosis, cerebral palsy

Prenatal-Intranatal-Neonatal (PIN) Insult

Congenital infections TORCH

Birth anoxia, birth trauma

Prematurity and LBW

Neonatal sepsis, neonatal hyperbilirubinemia, neonatal sepsis

Environmental

Sequelae of CNS insult– Meningitis, encephalitis, drowning, poisoning, stroke, severe dehydration

Sequelae of malnutrition occurring in early age

Familial

Idiopathic

Disorders reported in a few relatively larger earlier studies from India.[3,10-13] The frequency of the etiology observed in these studies appear to be as follow– *chromosomal anomalies*, 2.6-19.3%,[3,10,11,13] *prenatal, intranatal and neonatal (PIN) factors*, 9-31.7%,[3,10-13] *environmental factors* in 2.6-42%[3,10-13] and metabolic factors 0.6-1.3% of cases. *Multifactorial* aetiology have been reported in 4.7-26.1% cases.[3,10,11] *No cause* could be found in about 24.5-35.5% cases in these studies.[3,10,12,13] In a multicentric study by ICMR done earlier,[5] among 1314 patients, chromosomal anomalies were found in 23.7%, metabolic defects in 5.0% and identifiable genetic syndromes in 11.6% of the patients; in the remaining 59.7 per cent patients, no known genetic cause could be identified. In an well investigated hospital based study reported recently[6] where the etiology could be established in 82.1% of the cases, the frequency of different etiologies were as follows–genetic 61.4%, perinatal acquired 20.4%, CNS malformations 12%, external prenatal 3.6%, and postnatal acquired 2.4%; no etiology could be established in 17.9% cases.

Genetic-Chromosomal Factors are responsible for significant proportion of cases, probably majority of the cases of IDD.[16] These disorders can be familial or sporadic. Some of examples of genetic disorders associated with IDD are shown in Inset 13.1. Down syndrome, seems to top the list of IDD worldwide and is a classic example of IDD. High prevalence, of about 1 in 1150 births, has made it the most common chromosomal abnormality associated with IDD in India.[17-20] It is also the most common chromosomal anomaly reported from India in studies on ID, i.e., 2.6-14.7% of the cases.[3,10,11,13] Subtelometric deletions seems to follow trisomy 21 in frequency of occurrence of IDD/MR.

Inset 13.1: Some Genetic-Chromosomal Disorders Associated with Well-Documented IDD

Trisomies–Trisomy 18 (Edwarde Syndrome), Trisomy 21 (Down Syndrome), Mosaicism, *Deletions*–4p- (Wolf-Hirschhorn syndrome), 5p- (Cri-du-chat syndrome), 9p-, 13q-, 18p-,18q-, 21q-, *Microdeletions*–7q11.23 (Williams), 8q24.1- (Langer-Giedion), 11p13- (WAGR), 15q11-13 (pat) (Prader Willi), 15q11-13 (mat) (Angelman), 16p13- (Rubinstein-Taybi), 17p11.2 (Smith-Magenis), 17p13.3 (Miller-Diecker), 20p12- (Alagille Syndrome), 22q11.2 (Valocardiofacial Di George Syndrome), *Ring chromosome, Subtelometric deletions, Sex chromosome anomalies*–Turner's syndrome, Klinefelter's syndrome, Fragile X syndrome, Mosaicisms–isochromosome 12p (Pallister-Killian Syndrome)

Many congenital malformations are associated with IDD. Most common are those with developmental malformations involving the brain. Many other disorders and syndromes often displaying dysmorphology are associated with IDD[21] (Inset 13.2). Many cases have genetic basis. However, genetic defects are not seen consistently. Some cases display clear familial transmission even if there is no clear genetic-chromosomal abnormality.

Inset 13.2: Some Syndromes with Dysmorphology and IDD

With chromosomal abnormality – Cornelia de Lange Syndrome, Carpenter syndrome, Beckwith-Widemann syndrome, Smith-Lemli-Opitz Syndrome, X-linked hydrocephalus, meningo-myelocele, Velocardiofacial Syndrome, *Without clear/consistent chromosomal abnormality but often showing familial transmission*–Ellis Van Crevald syndrome, Joubert syndrome, Menkes syndrome, Laurence-Moon-Biedl syndrome, Penna-Shokier syndrome, Russel-Silver syndrome, Aicardi syndrome, Seckel syndrome, Noonan syndrome, Soto syndrome, Larsen-Sjogren syndrome, Pfeiffer syndrome, Apert syndrome, *Without chromosomal abnormality and at times showing familial transmission*–Dubowitz syndrome, Johanson syndrome, Kabuki syndrome, Weaver syndrome, Marshal-Smith syndrome, X-linked hydrocephalus syndrome, Schinzel-Giedon syndrome, Marden-Walker syndrome, Fraser syndrome, Branchio-oculo-facial syndrome, Carpenter syndrome.

Metabolic factors are important causes of IDD. Many inborn errors of metabolisms are well-known to be associated with IDD (Inset 13.3).[30] In Indian studies IDD has been reported in relatively smaller number of cases probably due to technical difficulties; there have been occasional reports of phenylketonuria (PKU), homocystinuria, tyrosinosis and cystinosis and mucopolysacharidosis.[3,10,11]

Inset 13.3: IEMs associated with documented MR
Aminoacidopathies–Phenylketonuria, Tyrosinemia type II and type III, Homocystinuria, *Organic academias*–Maple syrup urine disease, Multiple carboxylase deficiency, Biotinidase deficiency, 3-Methylglutaconic acidurias, Cytosolic acetoacetyl CoA thiolase deficiency, Mevalonic aciduria, Propionic acidemia, *Aminoacid metabolism defects*, Non ketotic hyperglycinemia, Creatine deficiency, 3–Phosphoglycerate dehydrogenase deficiency, Prolidase deficiency, Glutathione synthetase deficiency, Gamma glutamyl transpeptidase deficiency (glutationemia), GABA transaminase deficiency, Gama-hydroxybutyric aciduria, *Hyperammonemias* Orotic aciduria, Argininosuccinic acid synthetase deficiency (citrulinemia), Argininosuccinic aciduria, Arginase deficiency, Hyperammonemia–hyperornithinemia–hypercitrulinemia (HHH syndrome), *Others* Lysine protein intolerance (familial protein intolerance), Canavan disease, *Lipids* Adrenoleukodystrophy, GM 1 Gangliosidosis, GM 2 Gangliosidosis (Tay-Sachs disease, Sanhoff disease), Gaucher Disease type 2, Niemann-Pick type A and type C, Metachromatic Leucodystrophy, Krabbe Disease, *Carbohydrate* Leigh Disease, Sialidosis, Galactosemia, *Mucopolysaccharide* MPS I (Hurler), MPS II (Hunter), MPS IIIA (Sanfilippo A), MPS VII (Sly).

Many **systemic disorders** are associated with IDD (Inset 13.4). CNS disorders, commonly static, developmental, degenerative and metabolic ones seem to be the most common of the systemic disorders. Hypothyroidism is the most well-known endocrine disorder associated with IDD/MR. It has been reported to occur in 0.6-3% cases in studies on IDD in Indian children.[3,10-13] Many neuromuscular disorders are associated with IDD.

Inset 13.4: Systemic disorders associated with ID
CNS disorders – Congenital-developmental malformations, some encephalopathies, neurodegenerative disorders, neurometabolic disorders, some neuromuscular disorders.
Endocrine disorders – Hypothyroidism.

Prenatal, Intranatal and Neonatal (PIN) factors like prenatal maternal infections, birth trauma and anoxia, prematurity and low birth weight are well established causes of IDD. The most common factors reported in Indian literature are birth trauma and anoxia in about 7.9-18.6% of cases[3,10-14] and low birth weight and prematurity in about 0.9-13.2% of cases.[10-13]

Environmental factors are mostly of sequelae of CNS infections, head trauma, dehydration, malnutrition and toxicity like lead poisoning.[15] The most common factor reported in the Indian studies are sequelae of CNS infections and encephalopathies like viral encephalitis, meningitis, bacterial and tuberculous, with an incidence of 2.6-21.1%.[3,10-13] Malnutrition, occurring in early life, can cause retarded cell division and reduction in number of cerebral neurons and subsequent retardation in brain growth and thus can cause of IDD in developing countries.[23-29]

Familial ID

Cases of IDD without clear genetic basis or any known disorder associated with IDD, at times is found to run in families. Proportion of such cases has been reported to be 8.2-10.8% in some Indian studies.[10,12] In some instances parents are also of deficient intelligence. It is likely that these cases of familial IDD have some pathology underneath yet to be detected and defined; most of them could be genetic or metabolic. Better availability of genetic and metabolic studies is likely to reduce the incidence of such cases. *Consanguinity*, a factor well-known for its contribution to propagation of genetic disorders, is also common in India, reported in 8.8%-70% of cases, especially in cases of familial IDD;[10,11] the wide variability in incidence of consanguinity is due to different culture influencing marriage practices.[10,11]

IDD is **idiopathic** in varying proportion of cases no cause being found despite extensive work up. The incidence of such cases in the studies on IDD reported from India varies from 26.2-35.5%.[3,11,13] It is likely, however, that these cases have some underlying causes yet to be identified. With advances in diagnostic techniques, the proportion of idiopathic cases is likely to go down. Therefore, one should always keep an open mind; a case thought to be idiopathic today may turn out to be due to some cause tomorrow.

Many idiopathic cases may be genetic. Some of these cases may due to more than one etiological factor operative at different times, i.e., meningitis in a child who had severe malnutrition and also history of birth anoxia. The incidence of such cases of IDD having more than one causative factor have been reported to be 4.7-26.1% in Indian studies.[3,10] In such cases with multifactorial aetiology it is possible that one factor is primary while others contribute to aggravation of IDD to variable extent or all may be of equal significance that is however not easy to establish. Complex interplay between organic and genetic factors with socio-cultural and environmental factors is recognized.[31]

Many case of IDD could be due to socio-cultural factors, often referred to as *psychosocial*, sometimes as *socio-cultural*, due to lack of inadequate cognitive stimulation, i.e., inadequate and inappropriate learning stimuli.[2,23-28] The problems can be further compounded by malnutrition, inadequate health care and variety of diseases and other environmental factors. The attitude of the family and the society also probably can play important role in causation or aggravation of it.[13] Psychosocial IDD is more likely to be prevalent in developing countries. Most of these cases belong to mild to moderate category. It is however possible that some such cases that appear to be psychosocial do have some underlying pathology, including genetic or metabolic, and the diagnosis should be made after careful evaluation and exclusion of any pathology.

Clinical Presentation

The children with intellectual disability are usually brought by parents with complaints of *neurodevelopmental lag* in case of infants and young ones and *inferior mental functions and academic failures* in the case of older ones. The common complaints of the parents in case of young children are – 'the child is dull and lethargic', 'he is still not walking or speaking well', 'his activities are behind that of others of his age', 'he does not understand things', 'he appears to be immature', and 'his behaviour is abnormal', The common complaints of the parents, in case of older children are–'he does not give attention to studies', 'he is not doing well in studies', 'he has failed several times', 'teachers frequently complain that he is unable to cope up with studies', 'his memory is weak', 'his brain is weak', and 'he does not understand things'.

A variety of *abnormal behaviour* is frequently complained of by parents. Hyperactivity, inattentiveness, undue lethargy, inappropriate and undesirable activities are common complaints. Emotional disorders like too shy and withdrawn too talkative, emotional lability are also common. Sometimes parents come with complaints that are due to disorders often associated with IDD like motor handicaps, seizures and speech, hearing and visual problems.

Some children are brought for some other disease and IDD is suspected by the physician during examination. Children with congenital malformations, seizures and metabolic disorders and hepatosplenomegaly are common examples of it.

Evaluation of a Case of IDD

A suspected case of IDD should be worked up with the following aims:

(a) Establishing that there is really intellectual disability.

(b) Establishing the degree of the disability.

(c) Establishing the cause.

(d) Diagnosing any associated problems like behavior disorder, seizure, hearing and visual problems.

The clinical tools for establishing IDD are history, physical examination and developmental assessment. The clinical diagnosis of IDD however has to be confirmed and its degree established through formal psychometric evaluation. Therefore all cases of clinically suspected IDD should be subjected to psychometric evaluation by a clinical psychologist, preferably one skilled in assessing children (clinical child psychologist).

Establishing the cause of IDD involves history, examination and investigations. It is to be realized that IDD is not a physical disease per say but a symptom in true sense and a host of disorders and factors discussed already can be associations or causes of it. Clinical evaluation and investigation of IDD actually centers round establishing the cause. If a cause is found the management of a case of IDD definitely gets a clear direction. The cause may be treatable or amenable to preventive approach besides appropriate counseling. Many a times even if nothing much can be done, finding of a cause itself give satisfaction to the parents as well as the caring physician that some cause has been found in the child.

History

Keeping the various causes of mental retardation in mind, it is important to explore any parental *consanguinity, bad obstetrical history, PIN problems, history of feeding, past history, family history and socio-economic and cultural history,* abnormal findings in these areas can give clue to the aetiologic diagnosis.

Detailed *prenatal history* is important. It should include history of maternal infections specially those suggestive of TORCH infections, maternal medication and addictions, maternal exposure to radiation, maternal malnutrition and systemic diseases like toxemia, hypertension, heart disease and renal failure. These adverse events specially occurring in the first trimester coinciding with the period of organogenesis, are well known causes of fetal brain damage and subsequent development of

IDD (16 R). Pregnancy complications like hydramnios, oligohydramnios, malposition, twinning and breech pregnancy should be noted. *Bad obstretical history* specially previous miscarriages and stillbirths, congenital anomalies at birth should be looked for; this may be a pointer to the diagnosis of chromosomal disorders as these problems are frequently associated with chromosomal; disorders.[21,22] Parental *consanguinity* that facilitates transmission hereditary disorders, specially autosomal recessive ones, should be looked for carefully that will help the diagnosis of genetically transmitted disorders as the cause.

Intranatal events like ante partum hemorrhage, obstructed labour and prolonged labour. These events are often associated with intrapartum and neonatal anoxia. Mode of delivery should be recorded; forceps delivery is sometimes associated with various birth trauma and LSCS is known for its association with neonatal respiratory distress. Aided delivery of any kind is often indirect evidence of intrapartum anoxia as these modes of delivery are often resorted to under emergency circumstances.

All the important events in the immediate *neonatal period* should be noted. Special enquiry should be made about birth trauma, birth asphyxia, prematurity, low birth weight, seizures, sepsis, meningitis, hyperbilirubinemia and feeding problems. Parents sometimes may not remember the exact events but they often say that the perinatal and neonatal periods were stormy. History of active medical help to the newborn, admission of the baby into an intensive care unit and/or keeping the baby in hospital for prolonged period suggest the possibility of the baby suffering from adverse neonatal/perinatal stress.

History of *feeding behaviour,* specially in infancy and early years of life is important. Retarded children often show lack of interest in feeding usually interpreted by parents as lack of appetite. Subsequently the child may not learn self-feeding properly or at all, specially the severely retarded ones. Feeding problems often lead to malnutrition in these children.

Detailed study of *postnatal physical growth and development* are extremely important. Retarded physical growth of varying degree is common in cases with IDD as many of them suffer from chronic disorders known to cause growth failure.

Neurodevelopmental history is the most valuable tool for the clinician for making a clinical diagnosis of IDD.Knowledge of developmental milestones and parameters are essential. Lag in normal development is strongly suggestive of IDD[33] (Gassel, Illingworth). In infants developmental assessment remains the most important tool for diagnosis of IDD. In older children also, developmental history remains the most useful tool for suspecting early developmental delay and hence IDD.

While assessing neurovevelopment, *behaviour disorders* should also be inquired about. Abnormal behaviour that we frequently come across in cases in children with IDD are hyperactivity, quarrelsome, destructiveness, inattentiveness, undue lethargy, inappropriate and undesirable activities, biting self and even others, casting, throwing, pica and urinary and fecal soiling. Other behavior problems reported in Indian literature are beating others, snatching away food from passersby, speaking obscene languages, unsocial behaviour and activity, excessive dependency, speech difficulty, bed wetting, obstinancy, aggressiveness, inattentiveness, disobedience, irritability, excessive fear, have been reported in Indian literature.[13] Some *established behaviour disorders reported in Indian literature are hyperactivity, temper tantrum, enuresis, pica,* stammering, nail biting and thumb sucking. IDD can be associated with ADHD, autism and even other psychiatric disorders. Common emotional disorders that are seen in cases of IDD are emotional lability, unusual shyness, withdrawn behaviour and stubbornness.[13]

While assessing development and behaviour, it is important to look for any *regression or loss of milestones* that is suggestive of neurodegenerative disorders.

In the school-going children, it is important to enquire about the child's *school performance* including failures. Poor school performance or academic failure is the most important pointer towards the diagnosis of IDD in school-going children.

Past history of head trauma, CNS infections, episodes of severe dehydration, poisoning, seizure disorders and other chronic CNS disorders should be looked for. History of prolonged hospitalization should be asked for in every case as this may lead to some clue regarding serious illness affecting the nervous system.

Family history of IDD and other neuropsychiatric illness can throw light on genetically linked causes of IDD. Family tree should be studied in all cases of IDD that is helpful in establishing a disorder as genetically linked and also the mode of inheritance. It is extremely important to know the pattern of inheritance in genetically linked IDD for management. History of goiter and thyroid disorders in family members should also be sought.

In the *socio-economic and cultural history*, the home environment and the educational and cultural background should be studied in detail, besides income and living condition. It may give clue to quality of child care, quality of cognitive stimulation, nutritional disorders and environmental insult to the CNS like lead poisoning. Socio-economic and cultural history is important for the diagnosis of IDD due to PIN insult, environmental factors and also psychosocial factors.

Physical Examination

Detail physical examination, both general physical and systematic, should be carried out in every case aimed at finding clues to the pathological causes of IDD. Many abnormal clinical findings on general physical examination are well-known to be associated with IDD that can be found in any textbook of pediatrics. Such findings should be specially looked for in each case some of which are shown in Inset 13.5. While examining a case of IDD it is always useful to keep in mind the established causes (see Table 13.1) this should reduce the chances of missing diagnoses.

Inset 13.5: Useful Findings in Etiologic Diagnosis of IDD
Short stature–Down syndrome, congenital malformation, Tall stature–Marfan syndrome, *Small head*–Microcephaly, craniostenosis, prenatal infection, LBW, *Large head*–Hydrocephalus, meagalencephaly, *Blonde hair*–Phenylketonuria, *White forelock*–Waardenburg syndrome, *Fractured, kinky hair*–Menke's syndrome, *Facial Dysmorhism*–Chromosomal disorders, MPS, *Flat bridge of nose*–Down, cretinism, MPS *Mongoloid slant*–Down syndrome, *Brushfield's spot in cornea*–Down syndrome, *Corneal opacity*–MPS (Hurler's syndrome), *Cataract*–Galactosemia, congenital rubella, *Lenticular dislocation*–Marfan syndrome, *Telangiectasia in face and eyes*–Ataxia telangiectasia, Sturge-Weber syndrome, *Blue sclera/iris*–PKU, *Nystegmus*–Cerebellar disorders, *Chorioretinitis in fundus*–Congenital infection specially toxoplasmosis *Pigmentations in fundus*–Laurence-Moon-Biedl syndrome, Refsum's disease, *Cherry red spot*–Gangliosidosis commonly Tay-Sach's disease, *Optic atrophy*–Neurodegenerative disorders like Leber's optic atrophy, neuronal ceroid lipofuschinosis, leucodystrophy, *Dry, rough, coarse skin*–Hurler's syndrome, hypothyroidism, *Skin cold to touch*–Hypothyroidism, *Adenoma sebaceum*–Tuberous sclerosis, *Eczema*–PKU, *Dermatoses*–Inborn errors of metabolism like Hartnup disease, biotinidase deficiency, *system related-hepatosplenomegaly*–Storage disorders, Abnormal dermatoglyphic specially altered triradii Down syndrome, Bradycardia–Hypothyroidism *Polydactily* – Laurence-Moon-Biedl syndrome, multiple congenital malformations–Chrosomal anomalies.

Anthropometry specially weight, height and head circumference should be recorded in each case. *Microcephaly* is often associated with IDD. Most cases of *hydrocephaly* are also associated with IDD. Underweightness in many cases of IDD is due to secondary malnutrition resulting from feeding problems. Occasional case may be obese due to forced feeding by parents, unusual eating habits developed by the child and or lack of activity. *Short stature* is commonly found in conditions like hypothyroidism, chromosomal disorders and many other conditions associated with IDD. Growth failure in varying parameters and to varying extent is however common in most of the cases of IDD as the disorders they suffer from are basically chronic ones.

The **appearance and behaviour** should be noted carefully. The *dull look* of many mentally retarded children is often characteristic. Abnormal look, frequently associated with drooling of saliva is common in severely retarded children. The *facies* in Down syndrome, hypothyroidism, Hurler's syndrome are characteristic. Dysmorphologic features (Inset 13.6) should be looked for carefully in every child with IDD as they are important pointers to genetic and familial disorders. Many *abnormal behaviour* noted during history taking may be confirmed during observation.

Inset 13.6: Common and Important Dysmorphologic Features Suggestive of Genetic Defects
Brachycephaly, Plagiocepgaly, Scaphocephaly, Posterior parietal whorle, Brachydactyly, Polydactyly, Syndactyly, Camptodactyly, Clinodactyly, Hypoplastic nail, Low-set ears, Hypertelorism, depressed bridge of the nose, Mongoloid slant, Anti-mongoloid slant, Short palpebral fissures, Telecanthus, short limbs, other congenital anomalies.

The blond *hair* suggests PKU and the white forelock Waardenberg syndrome. The *eyes* may have blue sclera suggestive of PKU, corneal opacities in Hurler's syndrome, cataract in galactosemia and congenital rubella. The eye findings of Down syndrome are characteristic, most important being the mongoloid slant. The *skin* should be thoroughly examined by proper exposure of the body for evidence of neurocutaneous stigmata like adenoma sebaceum, cutaneous fibromas, hypopigmented macules, café-au-spots and cutaneous angiomata, eczema suggestive of PKU, and dermatoses suggestive of inborn errors of metabolism. *Smell* of body and body and body fluids like urine sweat should also be noted that can give clue to inborn errors of metabolisms like musty or mousy (PKU), burnt sugar, sweet odour (MSUD), boiled cabbage (tyrosenemia, hypermethionenemia), sweaty feet (isovaleric academia), smell of swimming pool (Hawakinsinuria), tomcat urine (multiple carboxylase deficiency), rotten fish (trimethylaminuria).[30]

Special attention should be given to features of well-known chromosomal abnormalities. Congenital *malformation* and *skeletal abnormalities* also should be looked for carefully as many such abnormalities are associated with genetic/chromosomal disorders. A mixture of facial dysmorphism, congenital malformations and skeletal and other systemic abnormalities are seen in a large number of syndromes associated with IDD (Inset 13.4).[21,22]

Systemic examination can be useful clues to the cause. *Nervous system* should be examined thoroughly with particular attention to intelligence, memory, hearing, vision, speech, emotional state, muscle tone power, focal deficit and fundus. Focal deficits and evidences of pyramidal and extra pyramidal abnormalities are often seen in intracranial structural lesions and many metabolic and neurodegenerative disorders. Chorioretinitis in the *fundus* is often seen in cases of prenatal infection with TORCH group of organisms.

Hearing and *vision* should be examined carefully in all cases and investigated appropriately specially in infant and young ones as abnormalities in these areas may give clue to diagnosis like congenital infections and meningoencephalitis. *Cardiac defects* are common in some chromosomal disorders like Down syndrome (commonly endocardial cushion defect, VSD), congenital infections like rubella (commonly PDA) and some syndromes like Marfan syndrome (aortic regurgitation). *Hepatosplenomegaly* is common in some metabolic and endocrinal disorders like storage disorders (commonly Gaucher, Niemann-Pick) and hypothyroidism.

In cases with no clear abnormality, one should keep in mind that some of these could be due to inborn errors of metabolisms, even chromosomal anomalies and hence the important features of these disorders should be looked for again as subtle abnormalities may be missed at the initial examination. Some pointers to these disorders are shown in Inset 13.7.

Inset 13.7: Suspecting Genetic and Metabolic Disorders Causing IDD
Clues to genetic/chromosomal anomalies–Dysmorphology, congenital anomalies, classic features of established disorders family history.
Clues to inborn errors of metabolism–Acidosis, seizures, vomiting, failure to thrive, CNS deficits, family history of similar problems, seizures and ID and features of well established metabolic disorders.

Finally a thorough *developmental examination* has to be done in every case of IDD. From the history it is usually possible to have a fair idea about the child's level of development. However, parent's recollection of the time of appearance of the milestones may not always accurate. Therefore, it is important to examine the neurodevelopment in every child as appropriate. Developmental examination helps in judging the neurologic maturation and finally determining how much a child, suspected to have IDD, is lagging behind normal and this will give an idea of the degree of retardation. Development assessment is the best way by which a clinician can suspect/diagnose IDD in the infant and young children. To establish developmental problem, developmental status of the child has to be compared with standard norms.

Every effort should be made to find out whether the IDD is *genetic or non-genetic* since this has tremendous bearing on management, i.e., genetic counseling is the most important step in management of genetic IDD. That IDD is genetic can be suspected from positive family history, pedigree charting showing affected individual, and specific clinical signs of genetic/chromosomal disorders as mentioned already. Chromosomal anomalies should be suspected in presence of congenital anomalies and dysmorphology and the classic features of established syndromes and disorders. IEM should be suspected in presence of features of these like acidosis, seizures, vomiting, failure to thrive, diverse CNS deficits, family history and seizures, and also features of well established disorders.

Psychometric Evaluation

All cases of suspected or clinically diagnosed to have IDD should be subjected to psychometric evaluation. Final diagnosis of IDD ultimately rests on the level of intelligence (IQ) and adaptive behaviour as already stated under definition. This is necessary to confirm IDD and to know the severity of it. Knowing the severity is useful in management. Only after confirmation, categorical diagnosis of IDD should be conveyed to the parents since declaring IDD in a child may have a devastating effect on the family. Cases where the diagnosis is yet to be confirmed through appropriate psychological assessment, should be kept as 'IDD suspects' and the parents be conveyed the message as such. Specific learning disorders like dyslexia should also be looked for. Associated behavior disorders should also be looked for defined.

Investigations

Once IDD is confirmed by appropriate clinical and psychometric evaluation, cases should be investigated appropriately to find the cause/associations that help in appropriate management. The extent of investigations will vary according to the suspected etiology. Investigations are more likely to be positive in severe and moderate IDD that is well established.

In cases suspected to be due to genetic/chromosomal disorders, appropriate *genetic* studies has to be done. It is always advised to have a discussion with genetic experts for tests. Karyotyping and hybridizations are commonly done in such cases. Some cases will need other studies for associated malformations that are common in these cases. In cases where the cause is suspected to be due to *metabolic* disorder, commonly IEM, appropriate tests has to be done to establish the diagnosis.

In cases of IDD due to *systemic* disorders appropriate investigations should be done to establish the clinical suspicion. In cases of IDD due to PIN factors, investigations may be needed only in selected cases to establish any continuing or established pathology, i.e., serologic studies and imaging for suspected TORCH infection in an infant. In cases of IDD due to environmental factors investigation may be to establish any suspected pathology like lead poisoning. In cases of IDD suspected to be multifactorial, investigations may have to be done to establish any suspected organic pathology.

Imaging studies are of immense value in confirming pathologies like hypoxic ischemic encephalopathies, congenital infections and malformations, structural lesions, developmental or acquired and disorders. Although most of the time these findings do not have much curative or therapeutic implication, they tell about a pathology in the brain that is usually reassuring to the parents and also the clinician who is looking for a cause.

Every case should be looked for associated problems and investigate as necessary. Common associated abnormalities in cases of IDD that we commonly see are hearing abnormalities, visual abnormalities, speech delay and seizures. These abnormalities may be detrimental for cognitive functions and need initiation of remedial measures as early as possible. Behaviour disorders should be looked for and assessed appropriately, is to be remembered that it may be difficult to be definite whether the behavior abnormalities are due to IDD alone or due to the underlying pathology or due to both.

Idiopathic ID: A common and still not resolved problem is investigation of cases of IDD where there are no abnormal findings on clinical evaluation and no cause could be found. Whether these cases should be investigated at all or if investigated, what should be the direction and extent of investigation remains unclear. Such cases are often subjected to radiological, metabolic and even chromosomal studies, which are frequently non-contributory. However, it has been observed that imaging studies (CT/MRI) often show changes like atrophy and other findings that may be a clue to some developmental problems and even problems having genetic implications, of the CNS. Therefore routine imaging studies specially MRI because of better resolution are, indicated in such cases.[30,32] Chromosomal analysis/genetic studies have been shown to give diagnostic clue in 3-12% of cases of otherwise unexplained IDD and hence the American College of Medical Genetics recommends a minimum band level of 500 on a g-banded karyotype in otherwise unexplained IDD.[33] Routine cytogenetic studies and molecular testing for fragile X mutation have been advocated by certain research groups because of higher yield of 3.5-10% even in the absence of dysmorphic features or features suggestive of a specific syndrome.[32]

The proportion of cases due to IEM in such cases also remains unclear; the yield of IDD in most non targeted metabolic screening is extremely low, about 1%, and hence routine metabolic screening is not indicated in the initial evaluation of a child with mental retardation.[32] However, if there is strong suspicion screening for relatively common disorders may be sought.

While evaluating and investigating the cases of IDD, care should be taken *not to miss the preventable causes of IDD* for which there is specific treatment early institution of which can successfully prevent the development of IDD or reasonably halt further progression of it. The classic examples are hypothyroidism and PKU. These disorders must be picked up as early as possible.

Steps of Clinical Work-up of a Case of IDD

After confirming ID through history, examination and psychometric evaluation, search should be made for the cause. Searching the cause usually involves investigations many of which are costly and difficult to get and a judicious approach is necessary. For this, categorizing the cases after history and examination as shown in Table 13.1 should be useful. This should be helpful in giving an idea about type and extent investigations to be carried out in different cases. A plan of work up of a case of IDD is shown in the Figure 13.1.

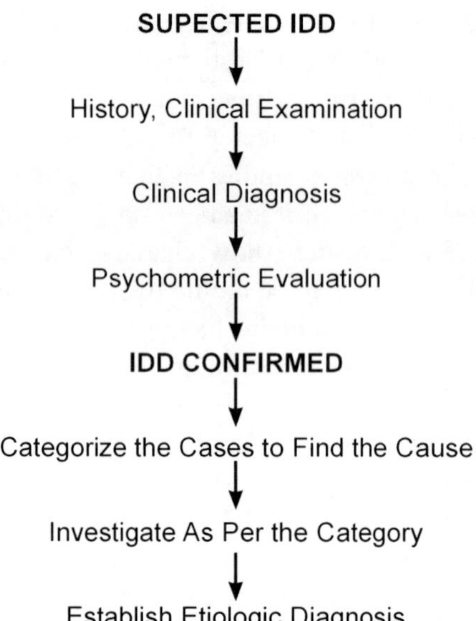

Fig. 13.1: Steps of clinical work-up and evaluation of IDD

Differential Diagnosis

Some conditions may give an impression of IDD and need to be excluded carefully. We come across children with rickets, talepes, dislocation of hip, chronic arthropathies like TB hip, being brought by parents for developmental delay specially in walking. Primary disorders of hearing and vision can make the child appear retarded, although these may be associated with IDD as such. Specific learning disorders like dyslexias also can give an impression of IDD in the school going children. Similarly children with attention deficit hyperactive disorders (AHDH), autism and certain emotional and behavioural disorders like too shy and withdrawn, may appear to be cases of IDD at the initial contact although these disorders can be associated with IDD.

PRINCIPLES OF TREATMENT

Goals of Management

IDD does not have a cure at present and treatment is basically supportive that will vary from patient to patient depending upon the severity IDD and also the primary disorder the child is suffering from. Every child with IDD has to be assessed carefully for the degree of IDD, the cause and the associated problems and appropriate/possible remedial measure instituted. The most important long-term issues in management of cases of IDD are education and vocational guidance. The mildly retarded ones can be managed reasonably well with acceptable educational and vocational achievement. Others will need a variety of support depending on severity, cause and associated problems.

IDD is a disability than a disease. There is no cure of established IDD. However with appropriate support many can learn and make up deficits to certain extent. They basically need support in appropriate area, stimulation, teaching as needed (academic, daily living and social) and upto the capability of the child, and managing associated problems, behavior and emotional issues. Rehabilitation is aimed at supporting developmental disability, improving daily living skills, job oriented programmes in school upto capability. Specific programmes are needed to make them learn basic life skills. Family oriented strategies are needed like empowering the family with skills needed to support and encourage the child with IDD. Audio-visual techniques are quite useful in many areas. Other useful areas of intervention are psychosocial treatments, cognitive and behavioural treatment including language and social skill acquisition. Ultimate goal for all intervention technique is giving the child a sense of self-independence using the acquired skills he/she has.

Treatment of Associated Problems and Disorders

Associated problems like *seizures, visual defects and hearing defects*, should be treated appropriately. These problems are known for their detrimental effect cognitive development and also create problems in proper management. Any *primary disorder* the child is suffering from, i.e., cerebral palsy, should be managed appropriately. *Psychological and psychiatric problems* should also be taken care of as needed.

Treatment of Behaviour Problems and Emotional Disorders

The child with IDD often shows a variety of behaviour and emotional disorders as detailed already and these should be managed appropriately. Behavior and emotional problems are at times much more problematic issues than even the IDD. Certain problems in the environment in which the child with IDD lives are common, like:

(a) Improper attitude of parents, i.e., disgust, handing over the care of the child to others, indifference, over protection, rejection.

(b) Improper attitude of other members of the family, i.e., indifference.

(c) Improper attitude of other people in the environment, i.e., teasing, beating, making fun.[3,13] Such environmental problems can be conductive to aggravation of behaviour problems in these children that in turn might aggravate IDD. Correction of these environmental problems might help in halting further deterioration of IDD. Managing these problems in a retarded child, however, is not easy and needs helping hand from psychiatrist, child psychologist, medical social worker. Parental counseling and guidance, talking to neighbours, talking to teachers, special schooling etc are needed. Efforts should be made to change the attitude of the parents to the child.

Taking Care of General Health

Normal *nutrition* should be advised. Prompt treatment of acquired illnesses like *infections* should be done. Appropriate *immunization* should also be ensured. Under-nutrition/malnutrition is common in retarded children because of multiple factors like primary disorders they suffer from, feeding difficulties and often parental neglect.

Parental Guidance and Support

Parents of mentally retarded children are usually victims of variety of misconceptions about the child's problems, physical stress, emotional strain, anxiety about the future of the child and also financial burden. Doctor shopping is common expecting some miracle. They need help. At the same time management of this chronic problem is impossible without co-operation of parents. Much of the problems of the parents can be resolved through removing misconceptions, if any, proper explanation of the disease and providing appropriate guidance how to go about. It is extremely important to adopt a sympathetic approach to the child as well as the parents. Such an approach will ensure parental cooperation that is vital in management of a child with IDD.

Educational and Vocational Guidance

A vital issue in management of IDD is taking care of the educational and vocational aspect. It depends largely on the severity of IDD and associated problems. Educable ones may be sent to normal school as far as possible with special help like extra classes for the slow learners. Special schools are helpful, if available. Appropriate vocational guidance, should be provided depending upon severity of IDD, age, scope and availability.

Providing Learning Stimulus

Psychosocial IDD, supposed to be common in developing countries, should improve with provision of better learning and other cognitive stimuli that however needs to be studied. Observations in rural Indian setting showing positive effect on psychosocial development of factors like parents spending time with the child, telling stories and taking the child for outing[34] suggest that there is scope for early institution of learning stimulus in IDD associated with environmental factors specially psychosocial.

Prevention of IDD

IDD results from a wide variety of disorders some of which can be prevented to certain extent and this may help in reducing the incidence of IDD. Early diagnosis and early institution of treatment may help in preventing the progression of IDD in certain situation. Established MR is not curable and therefore any chance for possible prevention of IDD should not be missed. Current research also should be directed more to prevention.

Preventing worsening of IDD through early institution of treatment: It has been established that further progression of IDD and even probably development of IDD can be halted by early instituting specific treatment available for a few conditions like *hypothyroidism*, *PKU* and *galactosemia*. It is, therefore, extremely important to diagnose and/or not to miss these few conditions. These few conditions should always be kept in mind while working up a case of IDD. Routine screening for PKU soon after birth is done many countries for this purpose.

Reducing the incidence of IDD: Successful genetic counseling should lead to reduction of the incidence of genetically linked IDD. Genetic counseling involves prenatal diagnosis and appropriate counseling for putting a halt to further transmission of the abnormal gene. Advent in molecular and cytogenetic diagnosis of genetic disorders has made it possible to make accurate diagnosis of many such disorders prenatally and institution of appropriate therapeutic measures.

It should be possible to reduce the incidence of IDD due to PIN factors (like birth anoxia, neonatal seizures, neonatal hypoglycemia and neonatal infections) and environmental factors (like CNS infections, head trauma, dehydration and metabolic and toxic disorders of the CNS with well established therapy) to some extent through quick and effective treatment and also possible preventive measures, i.e., good care during birth and delivery, measures to prevent infections in community (like safe drinking water, personal hygiene). Development of malnutrition can be prevented through measures to improve knowledge of good nutrition in the community. Improvement in socio-cultural and educational status of a community also should help to a great extent. Such measures should be conductive to reduction in incidence of IDD associated with PIN and environmental factors.

OUTCOME

Outcome of IDD depends on the severity of IDD and also the etiology. Many severe cases of IDD perish in early life. More or less normal life can be expected in mild cases without gross pathology.

References

1. World Health Organization. Mental Health Around the World. World Health Day 2001, Geneva:WHO:2001.
2. Hageberg B, Kyllermann M. Epidemiology of Mental Retardation: A Swedish Survey. Brain Dev1993:5:441.
3. Satapathy RK, Ghose JM, Sarangi B. Survey of Mentally Retarded Persons. Indian Pediatr 1985:22:825-28.
4. American Psychiatric Association. Diagnostic and Statistical Manual of Mental Disorders, 5th Edition, Washington, DC: American Psychiatric Association, 2013.
5. Schalock RL, Borthwick-Duffy S, Bradley VJ, *et al.* Intellectual Disability: Definition, Classification and Systems of Supports, 11th Edition, Washington, DC: American Association on Intellectual and Developmental Disabilities; 2010.
6. Salvador-Carulla L, Reed GM, Vaez-Azizi LM, *et al.* Intellectual Developmental Disorders: Towards A New Name, Definition and Framework for 'Mental Retardation/Intellectual Disability' in ICD-11. World Psychiatry 2011; 10:175-80.
7. Multicentric Study on Genetic Causes of Mental Retardation in India. ICMR Collaborating Centres and Central Co-ordinating Unit. Indian J Med Res 1991; 94:161-69.
8. Jain S, Chowdhury V, Juneja M, Kabra M, Pandey S, Singh A, Bhattacharya M, Kapoor S. Intellectual Disability in Indian Children: Experience with A Stratified Approach for Etiological Diagnosis. Indian Pediatr 2013 December:50(12):1125-30. Epub. 2013:June 5.
9. Haris JC, Curr Opin Psychiatry 2013;26(3):260-62.
10. Sincliar S. Etiological Factors in Mental Retardation: A Study of 470 Cases. Indian Pediatr 1972;9:391-96.
11. Joshua GE. Mental Retardation in Children-1-An Etilogical Study of 303 Cases 1974;11:47-51.
12. Subramanyam G, Agarwal KN, Agarwal SP, Jaiswal A. Clinical and Etiological Study of Childhood Mental Retardation. Indian Pediatr 1974;11:723-27.
13. Mudgil A, Singh SB, Srivastava JR. An Etiological and Psychological Study of Mentally Retarded Children. Indian Pediatr 1982;19:689-93.
14. Volkman FR, Dykens E. Mental Retardation. In: Child and Adolescent Psychiatry, Lewis M (Ed), 3rd Edition, Lippincott, Williams and Wilkins, Philadelphia 2002:603-11.
15. Shapiro BK, O'Neill ME. Developmental Delay and Intellectual Disability. In: Kliegman RM, St Geme III JW, Blum NJ, *et al.* editors. Nelson Textbook of Pediatrics, 21st edition. Philadelphia, PA: Elsevier 2020:283-93.
16. Chromosomal Aberrations in Pediatric Patients with Developmental Delay/Intellectual Disability: A Single-Center Clinical Investigation. Hu Ting, Zhang Zhu, Wang Jiamin, Li Qinqin, Zhu Hongmei, Lai Yi, Wang He and Liu Shanling.
17. Verma IC. Genetic Causes of Mental Retardation. In: Niermeijer M, Hicks E (eds); Mental Retardation, Genetics and Ethical Considerations, Amsterdam, Reidel 99-106.
18. Verma IC, Anand NK, Modi UJ, Bharucha BA. Study of Malformations and Down Syndrome in India–A Multi-Centric Study, 1998, Bhabha Atomic Research Centre, Trombay, Department of Atomic Energy, India. (Verma IC. In: Kumar D (ed). Genetic Disorders of the Indian Subcontinent, Kluwer Academic Publishers, Dordrecht 2004:81-87).
19. Verma IC. Cytogenetic Studies in Down Syndrome. Indian Pediatr 1991:28:991-96.
20. Thomas IM, Rajangam S, Hedge S. Cytogenetic Investi-gation in Down Syndrome Patients and Their Parents. Indian J Med Res 1992:96:366-71.
21. Wynshaw-Boris A and Biesecker LG. Dysmorphology. In: Nelson Textbook of Pediatrics, Kleigman RM, Behrman RE, Jenson HB, Stanton BF (Eds), 18th Edition, Saunders, Philadelphia 2007:786-93.
22. Jones KL. Smith's Recognizable Pattern of Human Malformation, 6th Edition, Elsevier Saunders, Philadelphia 2006.
23. Dobbing J, Smart JL Vulnerability of Developing Brain and Behaviour. Br Med Bull 1974:30:164-68.
24. PS, Dorsey J, McKhann GM. The Effect of Malnutrition on the Synthesis of Myelin Lipid, Pediatrics 1967:40: 551-59.
25. Benítez-Bribiesca L, Rosa-Alvarez IDL, Mansilla-Olivares A. Dendritic Spine Pathology in Infants With Severe Protein-Calorie Malnutrition. Pediatrics 1999;104:21.
26. Birch HG. Malnutrition, Learning an Intelligence. Am J Public Health 1972:62:773-84.
27. Srikantia SG, Sastri CY. Observations on Malnutrition and Mental Development. Indian J Med Res 1971:59 (6 Suppl): 216-20.
28. Champakam S, Srikantia SG, Gopalan C. Kwashiorkor and Mental Development. Am J Clin Nutr 1968:21:844-52.
29. Martin H. Nutrition: Its Relationship to Children's Physical, Mental and Emotional Development. Am J Clin Nutr 1973 July:26(7):766-75.
30. Barkovich AJ. Pediatric Neuroimaging. Raven Press, New York, 1990.
31. Rutter M, Simonoff E, Plamin R. Genetic Influence on Mild Mental Retardation: Concepts, Findings and Research Implications. L Biosos Sc 1996:28:509-26.
32. Shevell M, Ashwal S, Donley D, Flint J, Gingold M, Hirtz D, Majnemer A, Noetzel M, Sheth RD. Practice Parameter: Evaluation of The Child with Global Developmental Delay: Report of the Quality Standards Subcommittee of the American Academy of Neurology and The Practice Committee of the Child Neurology Society, Neurology, 2003 February11:60(3): 367-80.
33. Curry CJ, Stevension RF, Aughton D *et al.* Evaluation of Mental Retardation: Recommendations of A Consensus Conference. Am J Med Genet 1997:72:468.
34. Vazir S, Naidu AN, Vidaysagar P. Role of Early Intervention–Early Detection and Intervention. Nutritional Status and Home Environment are Important in Psychomotor Development (WHO Report of the Workshop of Investigators the Collaborative Study on Physical Growth and Psychosocial Development. Maternal and Child Health and Family Planning Division. World Health Organization, Geneva 1991; MCH/91.8).

14 Chapter

PSYCHOLOGICAL APPROACH TO A CHILD WITH NEURODEVELOPMENTAL DELAY

Shahzadi Malhotra, Shweta Tandon

The importance of early diagnosis and treatment of children with developmental delay and intellectual disability has emerged in recent years as a matter of growing concern among pediatricians. Early identification of children with delayed development has important implications for their treatment and in preventing risks of future disabilities and secondary problems related to family dysfunction, peer difficulties and school failure. Psychological assessment is needed to confirm diagnosis of intellectual disability. This is extremely important for management planning of the child concerned and bad dressing parental concerns.

Developmental Screening

Developmental screening is a brief testing procedure designed to identify children who should receive more intensive diagnosis or assessment. Screening refers to the detection of unsuspected deviations from normal development that would not otherwise be identified in routine pediatric practice. The goal of screening is to identify, as early as possible, developmental disabilities in children at high risk so that a treatment or remediation can be initiated at an early age when it is most effective. Early screening does not merely mean the administration of a single test at one point of time, rather it is a set of processes and procedures used over a period of time.

There is a need to distinguish developmental screening from developmental assessment. Developmental assessment refers to a more detailed investigation of developmental delay and is diagnostic in scope. On the other hand, developmental surveillance is a continuous, flexible and comprehensive process, which includes all activities related to the detection of developmental problems and the promotion of development during primary child health care visits.

Screening is the brief cross-sectional process of evaluating children by screening tools with good psychometric qualities (sensitivity and specificity >70-80%), that have been norm-referenced and standardized on populations representative of the target population. Lack of screening means delay in detection, initiation of intervention, increased morbidity and parental anguish, more health service utilization and poorer prognosis.

However, in India, there are multiple challenges to practice of universal developmental surveillance and screening. Parents are unaware of the existence and need of these services. Health care seeking is prioritized for acute illnesses, which are not appropriate opportunities for screening. A heterogeneous population of doctors with variable proficiency caters to the health needs of Indian children. Well-child visits are primarily for immunization with a few perfunctory questions asked about development, if at all. Further, informal evaluation has been proved unreliable in detecting developmental delay. Recognition is difficult in early childhood unless specifically looked for in a structured way, since changes in development are rapid, there is intra-domain overlap, and early indicators are often subtle.

THE ASSESSMENT PROCESS

Detailed Child Birth and Developmental History

A child referred to clinical psychologist for psychometric evaluation is initially assessed through detailed birth and developmental history from a reliable informant, preferably the mother. However, if the mother is not available then some other reliable caregiver may be involved in assessment process. It involves eliciting information about prenatal, perinatal and post-natal events; any significant post-natal issues. Along with these history also involves details about developmental milestones and current level of functioning. Direct observations of child's abilities and behaviours are also done during this session.

These interview and observation sessions are important to know the nature of the problem and the apparent psychopathology. These also give insights to the type of tests that need to be used and are most suitable for a particular child. Also, the test results have to be interpreted in relation to other behavioural observations and history, never in isolation. The initial interview and observation sessions also help in rapport formation, which is vital for optimum test performance and results.

Standardised Tests of Development and Intellectual Functioning

After the interview and clinical observation, the psychometric assessments are to be done. The psychometric tests are aimed primarily at evaluating the development level/intellectual functioning level and adaptive functioning. Tests are selected based on the age of the child, suspected degree of delay/retardation and also socio-cultural as well as educational background. Tests that are chosen must have high reliability and validity and preference should be given to those tests that have been standardised on the population under evaluation. While conducting assessments, the clinician must ensure that the child is not fatigued, anxious or stressed as these physical and emotional states are bound to have adverse effects on the test results. Personality issues, organicity will also have effects on test results. When using and interpreting test results, due consideration must be given to child's socio-cultural background as well as any associated handicaps.

Some of the widely used psychometric tests for assessment of development and intelligence are discussed in this section. These are:

For developmental assessment, the frequently used test include:

- Gessel Developmental Schedule.
- Developmental Screening Test (DST).
- The Denver Development Screening Test (DDST).
- Yale Developmental Schedules.
- The Trivandrum Developmental Screening Chart.
- Bayley Scale of Infant Development.

Tests that are frequently used for Adaptive Functioning assessment are:

- Vineland Social Maturity Scale.

For assessment of intellectual functioning, the following tests are frequently used:

- Seguin Form Board Test.
- Binet Kamat Test of Intelligence (BKT).
- Malin Intelligence Scale for Indian Children (MISIC).
- Wechsler Intelligence Scale for Children (WISC-IV).
- Wechsler Preschool and Primary Scale of Intelligence (WPPSI).
- Colored Progressive Matrices.

All the above listed tests for assessment of development, adaptive functioning and intelligence are discussed below.

Gessel Developmental Schedule[1]: Arnold Gessel was the first to develop the norms of development, describing the development of infants and children from newborn period to the age of five years. Based on the developmental norms, a large number of developmental scales and screening tests were developed. The first developmental assessment tool was Gessel schedules, published in 1925. It consists of eleven schedules of development corresponding to the eleven age levels from 15 months to 6 years.

Developmental Screening Test (DST) which was designed by Bharath Raj[2] is a reliable and valid test to screen the mental development of children in the Indian context. The Developmental Screening Test measures mental development of children from birth to 15 years of age. Developmental schedule consists of a simple chart with items on it. These items are descriptions of behavior that may be observed in an infant or elicited in a child. The items are arranged age-wise from 3 months to 15 years. First group of items describe the type of behavior that a baby from birth to 3 months may show for example, birth cry present, rolling over. Items are arranged at 3, 6, 9 months; 1, 1½, 2 years. And then onwards at every one year level till 15 years. The items progressively depict greater level of physical and social maturity and independence. The tester starts with the item closest to chronological age of the child to establish a 'Basal Age'. This is the age at which all items are likely to be passed or the behavior described is likely to be present. Gradually tester moves through upper age levels. Each item could be evaluated either by observing the child (e.g., Steadiness of head) or by asking the parent (e.g., combing hair by self) or by asking the child (e.g., repeat 3 digits). Larger number of items at the early age levels permits assessment of very young children. The test provides a brief and fairly dependable assessment without requiring the use of performance tests. The DQ was calculated by the concepts of DA and CA. Final version of DST consist of 88 items.

DST has a correlation of +.75 with Columbia Mental Maturity Scale. Inter scorer reliability (+.928) and test retest reliability (.98) were also found to be high and satisfactory.

The Denver Development Screening Test (DDST)[3] is the most widely used test all over the world. It has been translated in 7 languages. This was first described by Frankenburg and Dodd in 1967 and has had several revisions. The DDST was primarily designed by doctors to be used in a medical setting. The test is mainly concerned with attainment of various skills and many of these items are passed by the parents' report.

Developmental Assessment Scale for Indian Infants (DASII)[4]: DASII is a revision of 1970 Baroda norms from one month to 30 months. It is based on Bayley scales of infant development. The scale consists of 67 items for motor development and 163 items for mental development, with a total of 230 items. Based on the performance of the child, his motor age, mental age and corresponding motor development quotient and mental developmental quotient are calculated.

The Trivandrum Developmental Screening Chart[5]: The TDSC was developed in 1991 in Child Development Center, Kerala, India for target age group–0-2 years. It consists of seventeen test items that include mental and motor developmental milestones over the first 2 years of age. Items included in the tool have been taken from the Baroda norms for the Bayley. The range for each test items was taken from the norms given in the Bayley Scales of Infant Development (Baroda norms). A vertical line is drawn, or a pencil kept vertically, at the level of the chronological age of the child being tested. If the child fails to achieve any item on the left side of the line they are considered to have developmental delay. It assesses functional skills rather than non-functional outcomes. It has a sensitivity of 66.8% and specificity of 78.8%. It has been validated against the Denver Developmental Screening Test in a two-stage study.

Bayley Scale of Infant Development[6]: The Bayley scales of infant development, first developed in 1969, had been the most commonly used development assessment schedules used in clinical and research settings. The first edition of the scale could be used from birth to 15 months of age. These scales can be used with infants between 3 and 30 months of age. The scales included a mental scale, motor scale, and behaviour rating scale, and the performance was evaluated in the form of mental developmental index (MDI) and the psychomotor developmental index (PDI). The mental scales assess receptive and expressive language skills, visual motor coordination, visual spatial skills and social responsiveness. The physical (motor) skills evaluate fine and gross motor coordination. Bayley Scale of Infant Development II was developed and released in 1993 using re-standardised norms. It consisted of three subscales but the age range was extended from 1 month to 42 months with new items from expanded age range. The time taken to administer the scale is 30-90 minutes depending on the age of the child. BSID II was used as a primary diagnostic tool when determining eligibility for early intervention services in United States. The third revision of Bayley Scale of Infant Development (BSID III) was done in 2006 and is currently in use. It consists of social emotional and adaptive behaviour questionnaire in addition to motor, cognitive and language scale, which can be completed by caregiver or parent. It also consists of growth charts for cognitive, motor and social emotional scales.

Vineland Social Maturity Scale (VSMS)[7]: The Vineland Social Maturity Scale (VSMS) was designed and standardized for Indian children by A.J. Malin (1965), which measures the differential social capacities of an individual. It provides an estimate of Social Age (SA) and Social Quotient (SQ), and shows high correlation (0.80) with intelligence. It is designed to measure social maturation in eight social areas: Self-help general (SHG), Self-help eating (SHE), Self-help dressing (SHD), Self direction (SD), Occupation (OCC), Communication (COM), Locomotion (LOM) and Socialization (SOC). The scale consists of 89 test items grouped into year levels, i.e., from birth to 15 years. The information on VSMS test items regarding child's abilities through direct observation and supplement is collected by interviewing the mother of the child. The item will be recorded as pass if the child is able to perform correctly and fail if otherwise. Half credits may be given if it can be presumed that the child could have passed the item if the opportunity was present. These half credits receive full credit if they lie between two passed items. By adding up passed scores (full and half) the Social Age (SA) of the child will be known. The Social Quotient (SQ) is obtained by dividing SA by CA and multiplying by 100. The maturity levels is assessed both in terms of SA and SQ for each of the eight social areas by referring VSMS norms and social maturity constellation is recorded.

Seguin Form Board Test[8]: In 1856 Seguin developed a simple performance-based intelligence test using form boards to evaluate eye-hand coordination, shape concept, visual perception, and cognitive ability through nonverbal means. It is used to assess the participants' motor dexterity, visuomotor coordination, spatial organization, and speed and accuracy of performance, and can be used in children as young as 3 years. The form board consists of 10 differently shaped wooden blocks, and the participants are required to fit the differently shaped blocks into their respective slots on the form board. This culture-fair test, which can be easily administered in 10 minutes is used for preliminary assessment of mental age in a normal population. The task administration involved three consecutive trials with an instruction to start placement of blocks at the command "Start". Speed is stressed at the start of the test, with no further between cues or assistance being provided to the child. The best time from three trials was used to determine a mental age from the standard chart, which was subsequently used in determination of the intelligence quotient (IQ).

Binet Kamat Test of Intelligence (BKT)[9]: Binet-Kamat (B-K) test is a modified version of Stanford Binet Scale measuring intelligence of Indian children. It is an age scale where in the tests are grouped into age levels extending from 3 years to superior adult level. Each age level consists of six tests. There is no test for ages 11, 13, 15, 17, 18, 20, 21 years, due to declaration of mental development at these ages. Alternative tests are also provided at each age level, which can be substituted for regular test. B-K test include both verbal and performance tests. It is both power and speed test since some of the test items are timed. The test provides an estimate of MA and IQ (Indian adaptation by Dr. V. V. Kamat, 1958) from 3-22 years. Pattern analysis of the test items provide estimate of specific cognitive functions as, comprehension, memory, reasoning and other abilities. The reliability of the Binet - Kamat test of intelligence is reportedly above 0.7 and the validity of this test for normal children against estimation of intelligence quotient by teachers is 0.5 (Kamat, 1967).

Wechsler Intelligence Scale for Children (WISC)[10] developed by David Wechsler, is an individually administered intelligence test for children between the ages of 6 and 16. Currently, in India the 4th edition of WISC (WISC-IV-India) that has Indian norms and has been standardized on Indian population is in use. The WISC-IV takes 45-65 minutes to administer. It generates a Full Scale IQ (formerly known as an intelligence quotient or IQ score) that represents a child's general intellectual ability. It also provides five primary index scores: Verbal Comprehension Index, Visual Spatial Index, Fluid Reasoning Index, Working Memory Index, and Processing Speed Index. These indices represent a child's abilities in discrete cognitive domains. Five ancillary composite scores can be derived from various combinations of primary or primary and secondary subtests.

Wechsler Preschool and Primary Scale of Intelligence (WPPSI)[11] is an intelligence test designed for children ages 2 years 6 months to 7 years 7 months developed by David Wechsler in 1967. It is a descendent of the earlier Wechsler Adult Intelligence Scale and the Wechsler Intelligence Scale for Children tests. Since its original publication the WPPSI has been revised three times in 1989, 2002 (followed by the UK version in 2003) and 2012. The current version is WPPSI-IV. It provides subtest and composite scores that represent intellectual functioning in verbal and performance cognitive domains, as well as providing a composite score that represents a child's general intellectual ability (i.e., Full Scale IQ).

Malin's Intelligence Scale for Indian Children or MISIC[12]: The Indian adaptation of the Wechsler Intelligence Scale for Children, measures verbal and performance abilities, and can be administered to children to assess intelligence from 6 years to 15 years. The intelligence scale measures the full IQ which is obtained from six verbal subscales and five performance subscales. The verbal scale measures verbal information and language development and comprehension, using the following subtests: Information, similarities, arithmetic, vocabulary, comprehension, and digit span. The performance scale has the following subtests: picture completion, coding, picture arrangement, block design, and object assembly. The raw scores obtained from the verbal subscales are converted into standardized scores to derive the verbal IQ. Similarly, the performance subscales yield the performance IQ, and the cumulative score of the verbal and performance subscales gives the full-scale IQ. The test has a reliability coefficient of about 0.9, and the concurrent and congruent validity scores are both around 0.6.

Woodcock-Johnson Tests of Cognitive Abilities[13] is a set of intelligence tests first developed in 1977 by Richard Woodcock and Mary E. Bonner Johnson. It was revised in 1989, again in 2001, and most recently in 2014; this last version is commonly referred to as the **WJ IV**. They may be administered to children from age two right up to the oldest adults (with norms utilizing individuals in their 90s). The abilities measured are Comprehension-Knowledge, Long-Term Retrieval, Visual-Spatial Thinking, Auditory Processing, Fluid Reasoning, Processing Speed, Short-Term Memory, Quantitative Knowledge and Reading-Writing. A General Intellectual Ability (GIA) or Brief Intellectual Ability (BIA) may be obtained.

Raven's Progressive Matrices[14] (often referred to simply as **Raven's Matrices**) or **RPM** is a nonverbal group test typically used in educational settings. It is usually a 60-item test used in measuring abstract reasoning and regarded as a nonverbal estimate of fluid intelligence. It is the most common and popular test administered to groups ranging from 5-year-olds to the elderly. It is made of 60 multiple choice questions, listed in order of difficulty. This format is designed to measure the test taker's reasoning ability, the educative ("meaning-making") component of Spearman's **g** (g is often referred to as general intelligence). The tests were originally developed by John C. Raven in 1936. In each test item, the subject is asked to identify the missing element that completes a pattern. All of the questions on the Raven's progressives consist of visual geometric design with a missing piece. The test taker is given six to eight choices to pick from and fill in the missing piece.

Colored Progressive Matrices[14]: Designed for children aged 5 through 11 years of age, the elderly, and mentally and physically impaired individuals. This test contains sets A and B from the standard matrices, with a further set of 12 items inserted between the two, as set Ab. Most items are presented on a coloured background to make the test visually stimulating for participants. However, the very last few items in set B are presented as black-on-white; in this way, if a subject exceeds the tester's expectations, transition to sets C, D and E of the standard matrices is eased.

CONCLUSION

After thorough assessment of the child's developmental; adaptive and intellectual level, intervention needs to be planned. A thorough assessment is vital in providing a detailed understanding of child's strengths and weaknesses so as to enable the service providers to plan individualized early intervention and at later stages individualized education programmes for adequate education, training and rehabilitation. Thus, a thorough psychological assessment done by a trained Clinical Psychologist using standardised tests in the first step in rehabilitation of children with intellectual disabilities.

References

1. Gessel A. The First Five Years of Life: A Guide to the Study of the Preschool Child. London, Metheun and Company, 1950: 1-20.
2. Bharath Raj J (1983). DST Manual + Know Your Child's Intelligence and How to Improve It. Sri Meera Printers: Mysore.
3. Frankenburg WK. Dodds JB. The Denver Developmental Screenig Test. J Pediatr 1967:71(2):181-91.
4. Phatak P. Mental and Motor Growth of Indian Babies (1-30 months). Final Report. Department of Child Development MSUB. Baroda 1970:1-85.
5. Nair MK. George B. Philip E. Lekshmi S. Haran J and Sathy N. Trivandrum Developmental Screening Chart. Indian Pediatrics 1991:28:869-72.
6. Bayley N. Bayley Scales of Infant Development Manual. New York. The Psychological Corporation. 1969.
7. Malin AJ. Indian Adaptation of Vineland Social Maturity Scale. Lucknow. Indian Psychological Corporation. 1971.
8. Basavarajappa S. Venkatesan D. Vidya M. Normative Data on Seguin Form Board Test. Indian J Clin Psychol 2009:35(2): 93-97.
9. Kamat VV. 4th Edition. London: Oxford University Press: 1983: neuropsychological Assessment.
10. Wechsler D (2003). The Wechsler Intelligence Scale for Children. Fourth Edition. London: Pearson.
11. Wechsler D (1989). Wechsler Preschool and Primary Scale of Intelligence–Revised. San Antonio. TX: The Psychological Corporation.
12. Malin AJ. Malin's Intelligence Scale for Children–Manual. Lucknow: Indian Psychological Corporation;1969.
13. Woodcock-Johnson III Normative Update (NU) Tests of Cognitive Abilities, 2014; Riverside Publishing.
14. Raven J, Raven JC and Court, JH (2003, updated 2004) Manual for Raven's Progressive Matrices and Vocabulary Scales. San Antonio. TX: Harcourt Assessment.

15 Chapter

EPILEPTOGENESIS

Vinod Puri, Neera Chaudhry, Shruti Jain

INTRODUCTION

Epilepsy is one of the world's oldest recognised disorders, first described by Hippocrates in the 5th century BC.[1] At present, around 50 million people worldwide have active epilepsy with continuing seizures that need treatment, and 30% of patients are drug refractory. Nearly 90% of epilepsy cases are in low income countries, and in India, for example, the total cost for an estimated 5 million cases of epilepsy has been shown to be equivalent to 0.5% of the gross national product.[2] Epilepsy, one of the most common disorders of the brain, is characterized by recurrent, usually unprovoked, epileptic seizures, and by the cognitive, psychosocial, and social consequences of this condition.[3] Epilepsies can be divided into three major categories on the basis of etiology: idiopathic, symptomatic, and presumed symptomatic (also called "cryptogenic"). Idiopathic epilepsies are generally thought to arise from genetic abnormalities that lead to alteration of basic neuronal regulation. Symptomatic (acquired) epilepsies arise from the effects of an epileptic lesion, whether that lesion is focal, such as a tumor, or a defect in metabolism causing widespread injury to the brain. Cryptogenic epilepsies involve a presumptive lesion that is otherwise difficult or impossible to uncover during evaluation.[4] In approximately 40% of all epilepsy cases, the etiology is known, including brain insults such as traumatic brain injury (TBI), ischemic stroke, intracerebral hemorrhage, infections, tumors, cortical dysplasia, several neurodegenerative diseases, and prolonged acute symptomatic seizures such as complex febrile seizures or status epilepticus (SE).[5,6] Thus, epilepsy is one of the only brain diseases known to man in which people at risk can be identified, but there is no prophylactic treatment to prevent the development of epilepsy in those at risk.

CONCEPT OF EPILEPTOGENESIS

Currently, the terms epileptogenesis or latency period are used synonymously as operational terms to refer to a period that begins after the occurrence of insult (e.g., traumatic brain injury [TBI] or stroke), or even during the insult (prolonged febrile seizure, status epilepticus [SE], or encephalitis), and ends at the time of the appearance of the first spontaneous seizure. Epileptogenesis refers to a dynamic process that progressively alters neuronal excitability, establishes critical interconnections, and perhaps requires intricate structural changes before the first spontaneous seizure occurs. These changes can include neurodegeneration, neurogenesis, gliosis, axonal damage or sprouting, dendritic plasticity, blood-brain barrier (BBB) damage, recruitment of inflammatory cells into brain tissue, reorganisation of the extracellular matrix, and reorganisation of the molecular architecture of individual neuronal cells. In addition to symptomatic or acquired epilepsy, epileptogenesis also operates in cryptogenic causes of epilepsy, which are far more common than the acute symptomatic forms with identifiable disease processes or injuries. Furthermore, the latent period between gene mutations and first onset of spontaneous seizures in idiopathic epilepsies indicates that an epileptogenic process is induced by the mutation, which is substantiated by experimental data suggesting that early pharmacological intervention can prevent or modify the development of genetic epilepsies.[7]

EXPERIMENTAL MODELS FOR EPILEPTOGENESIS

Experimental models can be divided into whole animal (in vivo) versus in vitro studies. Whole animal models of acquired epilepsies typically involve single or multiple treatments to the animal that produce some form of injury or stimulation that results in later development of spontaneous seizures. Examples of these induced injuries include Status Epilepticus (chemoconvulsant and electrical), kindling, hypoxia and head trauma. In genetic models, a spontaneous or induced genetic mutation or deletion results in seizures that happen spontaneously. Seizure activity must be carefully defined for several reasons. Typically, rhythmic, stereotyped, altered behaviour is observed and characterized as seizure activity. As in the clinical literature, EEG has become the gold standard for correlating altered behaviour with seizures. In vitro studies involve removal and subsequent manipulations of whole brain structures, slices of brain structures or isolation, and culture of separated brain cells (neurons and glia). These studies allow detailed manipulations and measurements but are limited in a key way. While it is tempting to designate repetitive electrical discharges as a seizure, seizures defined in the whole animal are associated with a change in behaviour or sensation, which cannot be appreciated in these in vitro models and thus must be referred to as "seizure-like" events or an ictus to avoid confusion.

ANIMAL MODELS FOR EPILEPTOGENESIS

In recent decades, animal models of epileptogenesis have greatly enhanced the understanding of the processes leading to epilepsy and thus of potential targets for antiepileptogenic therapies. However, not all models are suitable for testing antiepileptogenic or disease-modifying therapies. Reasons include a long latency period and low incidence of spontaneous seizures, which complicates drug studies. On the basis of such logistical considerations, a models workshop organized by the National Institutes of Health/National Institute of Neurological Disorders and Stroke (NIH/NINDS) in 2002 thus recommended only two groups of models as potentially useful tools for antiepileptogenic treatment discovery: kindling and post-SE models of TLE.[8]

A. The Kindling Model of Temporal Lobe Epilepsy

Kindling, which was described in 1969 by Graham Goddard and colleagues is a model in which repeated excitatory stimuli initially induce subconvulsive or partial seizures.[9] The stimuli usually consist of electrical stimulation of a specific brain region, such as amygdala or hippocampus, via chronically implanted depth electrodes. Repetition of the same stimuli results in a progressive increase in the severity and duration of the seizures (i.e., acquisition of kindling). Fully kindled seizures resemble complex partial seizures with secondary generalization, so that amygdale or hippocampal kindling is considered a model of TLE. Once an animal has been kindled, the heightened response to the stimulus seems to be permanent, indicating the development of chronic brain alterations. If daily kindling is repeated over many weeks and months ("overkindling"), spontaneous convulsive seizures develop in approximately half of the rats, indicating a very prolonged latent period.[10,11] Some indication of kindling in humans stems from anecdotal reports of seizures occurring in the setting of thalamic stimulation for treatment of chronic pain and of development of spontaneous seizures some time after repeated sessions of electroconvulsive therapy.[12] One important drawback of this model is that electrical kindling needs long-term implantation of an electrode into a region of temporal lobe such as amygdala or hippocampus, the brain injury caused by electrode implantation may play a role in the kindling process.[13]

B. Post Status Epilepticus Models of Temporal Lobe Epilepsy

SE is a common, serious, potentially life-threatening, neurologic emergency characterized by prolonged seizure activity. Epidemiologic studies indicate that epilepsy develops in up to 43% of patients with SE.[14] For post-SE rodent models of TLE, a variety of different chemoconvulsants and intracerebral electrical stimulation patterns have been used to induce SE, which is followed, after a latent period of days to weeks, by spontaneous recurrent seizures. Chemically induced SE models–Bicuculline model, Cobalt-Homocysteine model, Kainic acid model, Lithium/Pilocarpine model, Soman (nerve agent model).

BICUCULLINE MODEL

Bicuculline is a highly potent alkaloid inhibitor of GABA-mediated neuronal inhibition that has been used to induce experimental status epilepticus in baboons and rats when injected intraperitoneally or intravenously.[15]

COBALT-HOMOCYSTEINE MODEL

This is a model of secondarily generalised convulsive SE that closely approximates human GCSE in the natural history and characteristics of induced seizures, the EEG changes and the response to anti status drugs. Cobalt has been known to induce focal onset seizures but the mechanism remains unknown. Homocysteine appears to be a NMDA agonist and it induces seizures by activation of EAA receptors. In this model, an epileptic lesion is created over the motor cortex by placing powdered cobalt on to the dura when epidural screw electrodes are implanted. When the lesion becomes electrographically active, SE is induced by intraperitoneal administration of homocysteine.[16]

CHOLINESTERASE INHIBITOR MODEL

Soman (pinacolyl methylphosphonofluoridate) is an organophosphorus cholinesterase inhibitor nerve agent that causes peripheral signs of cholinergic poisoning, convulsions, respiratory arrest and death. Almost all studies of these agents have been done with rats, guinea pigs and rhesus monkeys and most have been conducted by military investigators. Administration is subcutaneous. Initiation and early expression of seizures are cholinergic phenomenon reversible with anti-cholinergic agents. With prolonged epileptiform activity, the seizures enter a predominantly non cholinergic phase and becomes progressively refractory to pharmacologic therapy.[17,18]

PILOCARPINE MODEL

The first evidence that rats with brain damage induced by cholinergic agent pilocarpine develop spontaneous recurrent seizures after a silent period of 14-15 days was provided by Turski *et al.* This natural history is reminiscent of that of human TLE, which often begins with prolonged status epilepticus in infancy and develops with recurrent seizures in later life. Epileptogenic effects of pilocarpine depends on the facilitation of burst discharges in hippocampal pyramidal neurons by means of a block of the potassium transmembrane current which leads to cell death, axonal sprouting, and a synaptic reorganisation of hippocampal circuitry.[19]

KAINIC ACID MODEL

Kainic acid is a highly potent glutamate agonist that is obtained from the seaweed Digenea simplex and used as an ascaricide. Kainic acid was found to be excitatory when applied iontophoretically to the rat cortex and to induce seizures when injected intracranially or systemically. Kainic acid induced cell injury is attributed to an excitotoxic mechanism triggered by the activation of excitatory amino acid (EAA) receptors and is particularly prominent in the hippocampus. The earliest seizures characterising the acute phase consist of behavioral arrest that progress to a more complex phenomenology, including facial automatisms, forelimb clonus and generalised tonic clonic seizures. The seizures disappear during the latent phase but relapse during the chronic phase with characteristics similar to those of acute phase. The permanent changes in hippocampus underlying chronic seizures is ascribed to neuronal damage of the vulnerable hilar mossy cells due to kainic acid excitotoxicity or the ensuing sprouting of mossy fibres.[20]

Of the various systemic chemoconvulsants, kainate and pilocarpine have been the best characterized with regard to seizure phenomenology, electroencephalographic (EEG) features, cognitive outcome, and neuropathology. In both models, rats develop spontaneous recurrent partial and secondarily generalized seizures, hippocampal and extra hippocampal damage, and behavioral and cognitive alterations resembling the clinical characteristics of TLE. Typically, in models with systemic administration of kainate or pilocarpine, SE is terminated after 60 to 90 min by AEDs (such as diazepam) or general anesthetics (such as pentobarbital) to reduce the otherwise high mortality associated with chemically induced SE. In addition, lithium can be used to potentiate the convulsant activity of pilocarpine.[21] An alternative to systemic administration of kainate or pilocarpine is unilateral focal injection into amygdala or hippocampus, which avoids the widespread brain damage associated with systemic administration, thus creating more realistic models of human TLE.[22] Most of the SE models have the advantage of a latent period of days to weeks during which spontaneous seizures do not occur. The duration of the latent period depends on the severity of the initial SE. After the latent period, spontaneous recurrent seizures typically escalate in frequency over time. The latent period offers an opportunity to introduce therapy and measure its effect on prevention. Post-SE models of TLE are frequently associated with cognitive impairment and behavioral psychopathology. Another appealing feature of these models is their similarity to human TLE with partial seizures with or without secondary generalization. The consequences of chemically and electrically induced SE differ in a number of important factors. First, although a SE duration of 60 to 90 min is sufficient to induce epilepsy in the majority of rats or mice with systemic administration of pilocarpine or kainate, 3 to 4 hours of SE are needed in this respect in models in which SE is induced by focal electrical stimulation of amygdale or hippocampus.[23] Chemically induced SE is more severe than SE induced by electrical stimulation and more difficult to terminate by AEDs such as diazepam. An additional difference from electrical models is that the neurotoxic effects of chemoconvulsant may add to the effects of SE.

TOXIN MODEL

Tetanus Toxin Model

Tetanus toxin is a protein with a molecular weight of 150 kDa released by Clostridium tetani. Animals that are injected with the toxin in either the hippocampus or neocortex develop seizures 3-7 days after the injection. Hippocampal injections induce limbic seizures that eventually develop into tonic clonic seizures whereas neocortical injections induce early focal motor seizures that later on generalise. The tetanus toxin dependent epileptogenic process has various phases. At the very beginning, the toxin induces epileptiform discharges in the injection site as a result of a block of GABA release leading to the impairment of local inhibitory circuits established by the GABA interneurons in both the hippocampus and the neocortex. In a second phase, the toxin is transported through the axons to even remote sites, where it can move transsynaptically inside local GABAergic neurons and generate a mirror foci. The epileptic activity persisting in the chronic phase is attributed to seizure induced plastic changes in the hippocampal or neocortical circuits, leading to the functional disconnection of the GABAergic neurons or the sprouting of new excitatory neurons.[24]

BRIEF SEIZURE MODELS

Pentylenetetrazole and flurothyl are GABAergic antagonists that are administered systemically or inhaled, respectively. They both induce relatively short seizures, with flurothyl being very brief and limited nearly to the length of exposure to the vapors. As a result, both agents are used to mimic conditions involving single or multiple brief, generalized seizures. The major limitations of these models are that the mechanism of seizure induction does not clearly parallel any human condition, and the animals never develop spontaneous seizures. Both agents are thought to act on all susceptible brain regions, including cortex and hippocampus.[25]

MECHANISMS OF EPILEPTOGENESIS

1. Neurodegeneration

Classic hippocampal sclerosis involves a characteristic pattern of selective neuron loss in the CA1 and CA3 regions and the dentate hilus, whereas the CA2 and dentate granule cell layers of the hippocampal formation are relatively spared. Dentate hilar neurons are presumed to govern dentate granule cell excitability, so that hilar neuron loss has been suggested as the common pathological denominator and primary network defect underlying development of a hippocampal seizure "focus". In addition to neuronal damage, gliosis and mossy fiber sprouting, the growth of aberrant collaterals of granule cell axons, are also common and have been implicated in epileptogenesis.[26,27]

2. Neurogenesis

Occurrence of neurogenesis in human brain was demonstrated by Eriksson and co-workers 10 years ago.[28] Neural precursor cells can be isolated from surgical specimens obtained from patients with intractable TLE and propagated or differentiated into neuronal and glial lineages. It is still, however, unclear whether epileptogenic insults or epileptic seizures have an effect on hippocampal neurogenesis in humans. In animals, it has been shown that even brief induced or spontaneous seizures, in addition to SE, can trigger neurogenesis. After SE, increased neurogenesis can be detected within a few days and remains elevated for several weeks. In epileptic rodent brain, seizure activity can disturb the migration of newly born neurons, resulting in their ectopic location in the hilus, aberrant connectivity, and, consequently, enhanced excitability.[29] Another line of evidence suggests that newly born cells in an "epileptogenic environment" could actually adapt to the situation and become less sensitive to glutamate and more sensitive to GABA than in the normal hippocampus. It is important to realize that other clinically relevant epileptogenic brain insults such as stroke and TBI can also induce neurogenesis. Further, altered neurogenesis has been linked to, for example, learning and memory impairment, as well as depression, which are not uncommon comorbid conditions in patients with epilepsy.[30]

3. Gliosis

Glial cells can contribute to the epileptogenic process in several ways, including structural support, water and ionic homeostasis (aquaporins), regulation of neuro-transmission, inflammatory responses, and neuro-genic potential. Most of the data available on glial cells in the epileptogenic process come from astrocytes and microglia. Astrocytes are presumed to regulate the levels of extracellular potassium, as well as glutamate uptake and synaptic glutamate concentrations, to be active participants in metabolism, and to synthesize various molecules (e.g., proteases) that are needed for the recovery process. Data also point to their role in regulation of synaptic transmission and seizure activity. Importantly they also synthesize and release inflammatory mediators during the early post injury phase, as well as in animals and patients with chronic epilepsy. They can also form a "barrier" that isolates, for example, the cortical lesion from ingrowing axons and blood vessels compromising the self-repair process. Microglia commonly undergo activation in response to the brain insult. Activated microglia become secretory and release a number of compounds with harmful effects on neurons, such as pro-inflammatory cytokines (interleukin-1, interleukin-6, tumor necrosis factor a) and their receptors, proteases, and nitric oxide. On the other hand, activated microglia can secrete transforming growth factor b, brain-derived neurotrophic factor (BDNF), neurotrophin-3, or nerve growth factor, which have a neuroprotective effect and can promote regeneration. Another beneficial function of microglia is clearing the dying neurons and glia from the tissue. The net effect of the harmful and protective actions of microglia is controversial.[31,32]

4. Axonal Growth

Sprouting of glutamatergic granule cell axons or mossy fibers is the most widely studied form of axonal plasticity in epilepsy. Excitotoxic loss of mossy cells in the dentate gyrus (which may occur following status epilepticus or other insults) may lead to sprouting of dentate axons, known as mossy fibers (MFs). The sprouted MFs make aberrant excitatory connections locally in the dentate gyrus and distantly in CA3 creating an abnormal excitatory feedback circuit. These abnormal connections are further dysfunctional, with a higher probability of activation, a larger NR (noradrenergic receptor) stimulation component, and recruitment of kainate receptors. These disturbances, coupled with permanent altera-tions in GABARs, are thought to result in a circuit prone to trigger seizures in other regions, such as CA3.[23]

5. Dendritic Plasticity

Loss of dendritic spines, changes in spine morphology, and reduced dendritic branching have been described both in experimental TLE models and in persons with TLE. It is likely that these alterations could affect the availability of various receptor types as well as their stoichiometry and, thus, compromise the information flow from afferent inputs.[33]

6. Angiogenesis

Damage to the blood-brain barrier (BBB) and consequent expression of angiogenic factors, proliferation of endothelial cells, and angiogenesis are features common to various epileptogenic insults such as SE, TBI, and stroke, as well as human TLE, and are most active during the first month after injury. Molecular profiling data indicate activation of expression of angiogenic factors after electroconvulsive seizures as well as following status epilepticus.[34]

7. Changes in Extracellular Matrix

Post injury epileptogenesis involves a remarkable remodelling of neuronal circuits which is accompanied by changes in extracellular matrix. Recent molecular profiling studies have pinpointed the regulation of expression of a large number of enzymes contributing to ECM degradation and remodeling. In particular, the plasminogen system including tissue-type plasminogen activator (tPA), urokinase plasminogen activator (uPA), and their inhibitors TIMP-1 and -2, as well as metalloproteinases, appear to be involved in tissue remodeling following insult.[35]

8. Acquired Channelopathies

Molecular analysis of ion channels after epileptogenic insults, particularly SE, has revealed that brain injury can result in changes in both ligand-gated and receptor-gated ion channels that are associated with altered function when investigated using single-cell electrophysiology. This phenomenon, called acquired channelopathy, has been described in the dendritic, somatic, and axonal channels. Some of the subunit and functional changes can last even weeks and, thus, can contribute to the establishment of lowered seizure threshold in parallel with other plastic alterations. Early studies of in vitro brain slice models indicated that alterations in NMDA Receptors (NRs) with the successive prolongation of seizure-like discharges correlated with epileptogenesis.[36] The mechanism of non-NR-mediated calcium influx via calcium permeable Glutamate receptors (GluRs) is also thought to underlie cell death in adult models of seizures and hypoxia. GluR1 upregulation and downregulation of GluR2 can lead to seizures and hippocampal injury in animal models of kainite induced SE.[37] Transient alteration in the properties of synaptically activated GluRs consistent with calcium permeable GluRs following hypoxic seizures in developing animals has been postulated to mediate the cascade resulting in later-life alterations in this model. Seizures induced by kainate in infant rats results in altered LTP (long-term potentiation), kindling and learning associated with enhanced inhibition in the dentate gyrus and mechanistically linked to reduced NR2A and altered trafficking of GluR1.[38] In adult, epileptic animals following pilocarpine SE, GABAergic signaling is altered by specific reduction of GABA A receptor $\alpha 1$ subunits and an increase in $\alpha 4$ subunits in the dentate gyrus, resulting in a reduction in benzodiazepine sensitivity and enhanced inhibition by zinc.[39] Altered function of VGSCs (voltage gated sodium channels),

T-type calcium channels and potassium channels have been described in epileptic animals and are thought to contribute to the epileptic state. In the hyperthermia model of febrile seizures, a single prolonged seizure results in permanent susceptibility to convulsants, enhanced in vitro kindling, mechanistically linked to enhancement of the voltage-gated potassium channel HCN.[40] The signaling pathways that regulate the plasticity in ion channel expression during epileptogenesis are just beginning to be elucidated. For example, recent studies have demonstrated that the mechanisms that regulate differential expression of GABAR α-subunits in hippocampus after SE include the CREB/ICER, JAK/STAT, BDNF, and Egr3 signaling pathways.[41] Targeting signaling pathways that alter the expression of genes involved in epileptogenesis may provide novel therapeutic approaches for preventing or inhibiting the development of epilepsy after a precipitating insult.

9. Epigenetic Mechanisms

The term epigenetic refers to changes in genes that occur without directly affecting DNA sequence. This can be achieved by chemical modification of DNA or chromatin, such as DNA methylation and alterations in the methylation or acetylation status of histones. Such modifications strongly influence gene expression and, therefore, are of importance for cell function. Seizure-induced or SE-induced histone modifications have been reported for promoters of a number of genes, including those involved in neuronal plasticity, such as transcription factors c-fos, c-jun, and CREB, the neurotrophin BDNF, and the glutamate receptor GluR2. By influencing the level of growth factor production, the epigenetic mechanism may control the formation of aberrant neuronal connections. At the same time, deacetylation of histones at the GluR2 promoter leads to its decreased expression, which can result in enhanced epileptogenesis. Another clue to the involvement of the epigenetic mechanism in epilepsy was provided by the discovery that the potent antiepileptic drug valproate can act as an inhibitor of histone deacetylases (HDACs) and also can influence gene expression.[42,43]

ROLE OF GENETICS IN EPILEPTOGENESIS

Advances in genetics have allowed for several human epilepsy syndromes associated with single gene defects to be further characterized. Following determination of the analogous gene in mice, similar defects can be introduced through cloning techniques in order to better understand how epilepsy develops in these syndromes as well as determine which treatments might be more efficacious. Often, the nature of the genetic defect, whether it represents a gain or loss of function, is not clear until the altered resulting protein is expressed in an intact, cloned animal model. In the animal model of Dravet syndrome, genetic knock-in of human mutations in VGSCs (NaV1.1) results in a phenotype very similar to that seen in humans. Importantly, these studies have highlighted how the balance between excitation and inhibition is a critical modifier in this disorder.[44] Similarly, genetic knock-in of human mutations in KCNQ2 and KCNQ3 has many similarities to the human phenotype of benign familial neonatal convulsions.[45] Enhanced function of T-type calcium channels in thalamocortical circuits has been postulated to mediate childhood absence epilepsy. While specific mutations in T-type calcium channels have not been determined in the human condition; specific genetic targeting of enhanced expression of T-type calcium channels in this circuit have been found to mimic the human condition.[46]

SUMMARY

Epileptogenesis results from a temporal progression of cascading molecular and cellular changes that lead to network reorganization, most of which occur during the latent phase. Animal models, despite their limitations, have advanced our understanding of the mechanisms of seizures and epileptogenesis. Specifically, substantial gains have been made in understanding the ability of the hippocampus and cortex to rewire themselves following insults to result in circuits capable of spontaneous seizures. The increasing comprehension of these epileptogenic processes might aid in the development of targeted antiepileptogenic drugs to complement the currently available antiepileptic agents.

References

1. Adams F. On The Sacred Disease. In: The Genuine Works of Hippocrates, Vol II. London: Sydenham Society 1849:831-58.
2. WHO. Epilepsy. http://www.who.int/mediacentre/factsheets/fs999/en/index.html (accessed November 19,2010).
3. Engel JJ and Pedley TA (2008) Epilepsy: A Comprehensive Textbook.. Lippincott Williams and Wilkins, Philadelphia.
4. Banerjee PN, Filippi D, Allen Hauser W. The Descriptive Epidemiology of Epilepsy–A Review, Epilepsy Res 2009;85: 31-45.
5. Dichter MA. Posttraumatic Epilepsy: The Challenge of Translating Discoveries in the Laboratory to Pathways to a Cure. Epilepsia 2009a; 50 (Suppl 2):41-45.

6. Dichter MA. Emerging Concepts in The Pathogenesis of Epilepsy and Epileptogenesis. Arch Neurol 2009b;66:443-47.

7. Lukasiuk K. Pitkanen A. Seizure-induced Gene Expression. In: Encyclopedia of Basic Epilepsy Research. Oxford: Academic Press 2009;1302-09.

8. Stables JP. Bertram EH. White HS. Coulter DA. Dichter MA. Jacobs MP. *et al.* Models for Epilepsy and Epileptogenesis: Report from the NIH Workshop. Bethesda. Maryland. Epilepsia 2002;43:1410-20.

9. Goddard GV. McIntyre DC. Leech CK. A Permanent Change in Brain Function Resulting from Daily Electrical Stimulation. Exp Neurol1969:25:295-330.

10. Morimoto K. Fahnestock M. Racine RJ. Kindling and Status Epilepticus Models of Epilepsy: Rewiring the Brain. Prog Neurobiol 2004;73:1-60.

11. McIntyre DC, Poulter MO, Gilby K. Kindling: Some Old and Some New. Epilepsy Res 2002;50:79-92.

12. Reisner AD. The Electroconvulsive Therapy Controversy: Evidence and Ethics. Neuropsychol Rev 2003;13:199-219.

13. Loscher W. Wahnschaffe U. Ho¨Nack D Rundfeldt C. Does Prolonged Implantation of Depth Electrodes Predispose the Brain to Kindling? Brain Res 1995;697:197-204.

14. Hesdorffer DC, Logroscino G, Cascino G, Annegers JF, Hauser WA. Risk of Unprovoked Seizure After Acute Symptomatic Seizure: Effect of Status Epilepticus. Ann Neurol 1998; 44:908-12.

15. Meldrum BS, Horton RW, Convulsive Effects of 4 - Deoxy-pyridoxine and of Bicuculline in Photosensitive Baboons (Papiopapio) and in Rhesus Monkeys (Macacamulatta). Brain Res 1971;35:419-36.

16. Walton NY, Treiman DM. Experimental Secondarily Generalized Convulsive Status Epilepticus Induced by D, L-Homocysteine Thiolactone. Epilepsy Res 1988:2:79-86.

17. McDonough JH Jr. Shih TM. Pharmacological Modulation of Soman-Induced Seizures. Neurosci Biobehav Rev. 1993; 17:203-215.

18. McDonough JH Jr; Shih TM. Neuropharmacological Mechanisms of Nerve Agent-induced Seizure and Neuro-pathology. Neurosci. Biobehav. Rev 1997;21,559-79.

19. Curia G. Longo D. Biagini G. *et al.* The Pilocarpine Model of Temporal Lobe Epilepsy. J Neurosci Methods 2008;172: 143-57.

20. Ben-Ari Y. Cossart R. Kainate. A Double-agent That Generates Seizures: Two Decades of Progress. Trends Neurosci 2000: 23(11):580-87.

21. Cavalheiro EA, Naffah-Mazacoratti MG, Mello LE, Leite JP. The Pilocarpine Model of Seizures. Models of Seizures and Epilepsy 2006;433-48. Elsevier. Amsterdam.

22. Dudek FE. Clark S. Williams PA and Grabenstatter HL. Kainate-induced Status Epilepticus: A Chronic Model of Acquired Epilepsy. Models of Seizures And Epilepsy 2006: 415-32. Elsevier. Amsterdam.

23. Pitkanen A. Kharatishvili I. Narkilahti S. Lukasiuk K. Nissinen J. Administration of Diazepam During Status Epilepticus Reduces Development and Severity of Epilepsy in Rat. Epilepsy Re 2005;s 63:27-42.

24. Benke TA. Swann J. The Tetanus Toxin Model of Chronic Epilepsy. Recent Advances in Epilepsy Research. 16th Edition. New York: Kluwer Academic. 2003.

25. Velisek L. Veliskova J. Ptachewich Y. *et al.* Age-Dependent Effects of Gamma-Aminobutyric Acid Agents of Flurothyl Seizures. Epilepsia 1995;36(7):636-43.

26. Cavazos JE. Jones SM. Cross DJ. Sprouting and Synaptic Reorganization in the Subiculum and CA1 Region of the Hippocampus in Acute and Chronic Models of Partial-onset Epilepsy. Neuroscience 2004;126:677-88.

27. Jutila L. Immonen A. Partanen K. *et al.* Neurobiology of Epileptogenesis in the Temporal Lobe. Adv. Tech Stand Neurosurg 2002:27:3-22.

28. Eriksson PS. Perfilieva E. Björk-Eriksson T. *et al.* Neurogenesis in the Adult Human Hippocampus. Nat Med 1998;4:1313-17.

29. Parent JM. Yu TW. Leibowitz RT. Geschwind DH. Sloviter RS. Lowenstein DH. Dentate Granule Cell Neurogenesis is Increased by Seizuress and Contributes to Aberrant Network Reorganization in The Adult Rat Hippocampus. J Neurosci 1997:17:3727-38.

30. Siebzehnrubl FA. Blumcke I. Neurogenesis in the Human Hippocampus and Its Relevance to Temporal Lobe Epilepsies. Epilepsia 2008;49(Suppl 5):55-65.

31. Wetherington J. Serrano G. Dingledine R. Astrocytes in The Epileptic Brain. Neuron 2008;58:168-78.

32. Jorgensen MB. Finsen BR. Jensen MB. Castellano B. Diemer NH. Zimmer J. Microglial and Astroglial Reactions to Ischemic and Kainic Acid-Induced Lesions of the Adult Rat Hippocampus. Exp Neurol 1993;120:70-88.

33. Isokawa M. Remodeling Dendritic Spines of Dentate Granule Cells in Temporal Lobe Epilepsy Patients and the Rat Pilocarpine Model. Epilepsia 2000;41(Suppl. 6):S14-17.

34. Rigau V. Morin M. Rousset MC. *et al.* Angiogenesis is Associated with Blood-Brain Barrier Permeability in Temporal Lobe Epilepsy. Brain 2007;130 (Pt.7):1942-56.

35. Lukasiuk K. Kontula L. Pitkänen A. CDNA Profiling of Epileptogenesis in the Rat Brain. Eur J Neurosci 2003;17: 271-79.

36. Stasheff SF. Anderson WW. Clark S. *et al.* NMDA Antagonists Differentiate Epileptogenesis from Seizure Expression in an in Vitro Model. Science 1989;245:648-51.

37. Sommer C. Roth SU. Kiessling M. Kainate-Induced Epilepsy Alters Protein Expression of AMPA Receptor Subunits GluR1, GluR2 and AMPA Receptor Binding Protein in the Rat Hippo-campus. Acta Neuropathologica 2001:101:460-68.

38. Lynch M, Sayin U, Bownds J, *et al.* Long-Term Consequences of Early Postnatal Seizures on Hippocampal Learning and Plasticity. Eur J Neurosci 2000;12:2252-64.

39. GABAergic System Contribute to Development of Spontaneous Recurrent Seizures in the Rat Lithium-pilocarpine Model of Temporal Lobe Epilepsy. Hippocampus 2001;11:452-68.

40. Ellerkmann RK, Remy S, Chen J, *et al.* Molecular and Functional Changes in Voltage-Dependent Na(+) Channels following Pilocarpine-induced Status Epilepticus in Rat Dentate Granule Cells. Neuroscience 2003;119:323-33.

41. Lund IV, Hu Y, Raol YH, *et al.* BDNF Selectively Regulates GABAA Receptor Transcription by Activation of the JAK/STAT Pathway. Sci Signal 2008;1:ra9.

42. Graff J, Mansuy IM. Epigenetic Codes in Cognition and Behaviour. Behav Brain Res 2008;192:70-87.

43. Huang Y, Doherty J, Dingledine R. Altered Histone Acetylation at Glutamate Receptor 2 and Brain-Derived Neurotrophic Factor Genes is An Early Event Triggered by Status Epilepticus. J Neurosci 2002;22:8422-28.

44. Kalume F, Yu FH, Westenbroek RE, *et al.* Reduced Sodium Current in Purkinje Neurons from Nav1.1 Mutant Mice: Implications for Ataxia in Severe Myoclonic Epilepsy in Infancy. J Neurosci 2007;27:11065-74.

45. Singh NA, Otto JF, Dahle EJ, *et al.* Mouse Models of Human KCNQ2 and KCNQ3 Mutations for Benign Familial Neonatal Convulsions Show Seizures and Neuronal Plasticity Without Synaptic Reorganization. J Physiol 2008;586:3405-23.

46. Ernst WL, Zhang Y, Yoo JW, *et al.* Genetic Enhancement of Thalamocortical Network Activity by Elevating Alpha 1g-Mediated Low-voltage-activated Calcium Current Induces Pure Absence Epilepsy. J Neurosci 2009;29:1615-25.

16 Chapter

FEBRILE SEIZURES

Mahesh Kamate

Febrile seizures (FS) are the most common seizures of childhood, occurring in children. Although they are benign, they can be extremely frightening, emotionally traumatic and anxiety provoking when witnessed by parents.

Definition: National Institute of Health (NIH) consensus statement defines febrile seizures as 'an event in infancy or childhood usually occurring between 3 months and 5 years of age, associated with fever but without evidence of intracranial infection or defined cause for the seizure'. The definition excludes children with previous afebrile seizures. The International League Against Epilepsy ILAE defines febrile seizures as 'a seizure occurring in childhood after one month of age, associated with a febrile illness not caused by an infection of the central nervous system, without previous neonatal seizures or a previous unprovoked seizures, and not meeting criteria for other acute symptomatic seizures'.

Careful review of the two definitions reveals that both are very similar, except for lower age limit; they do not exclude children with prior neurological impairment; do not provide a specific temperature criterion or defines a seizure. Febrile seizures are to be distinguished from epilepsy that is characterized by recurrent non-febrile seizure.

Three criteria that are critical in definition are age, fever and seizure:

1. **Age:** Most of the episodes of febrile seizures occur in children between 6 months and 3 years with the peak incidence at 18 months. Only 6-15% of febrile seizures occur after 4 years and onset after 6 years is very unusual. This unique age predisposition suggests the specificity of the maturing brain's sensitivity to fever, enhanced neuronal excitability during the normal brain maturation.
2. **Fever:** Occurrence of fever is a must for febrile seizure. Many febrile seizures occur early in the illness and may be the presenting feature. There is no data to support the significance of rate of rise of temperature versus peak temperature in the occurrence of febrile seizures. However, the peak of temperature is related to recurrent febrile seizure. Febrile seizure at fever less than 38.9 degrees Celsius usually has focal features or repeats within same febrile episode.
3. **Seizure:** The term seizure has not been defined in definition. But, definitely the definition excludes events like rigors, syncope, reflex anoxic seizures, breath-holding spell and apnea which may also be associated with fever. The seizures usually occur in the first few hours of the febrile illness and within 24 hours in the vast majority of cases although it can occur during the later part of the illness as well. Seizures occurring after 24 hours of fever onset are uncommon even if the temperature remains high.

Epidemiology

Febrile seizure is the most common type of seizure disorder in childhood and occurs in about 2-4% of all children. The prevalence appears to be little higher in Asian countries (8-10%) probably due to higher incidence of infection and social practice like children sleeping with parents, that is conductive to spread of infection and also prompt detection of seizure. This is likely to hold good for Indian subcontinent as well, although data is limited.

Type of Seizure

Febrile seizures are usually generalized and tonic, clonic or tonic-clinic in nature. Often it is only tonic, the child becoming stiff and rigid with up-rolling of the eyeballs. In some cases it may be only clonic from the beginning. Occasionally the child becomes limp. Pallor is a frequent accompaniment. Focal seizure is seen in about 4% of cases. Recently, febrile myoclonic seizures also have been recognized.

Febrile seizures are generally brief lasting for a minute or two (87% of children: Duration is less than 10 minutes). Prolonged seizures lasting for more than 15 minutes are seen in about 9% of cases. Majority of children have only one seizure during one episode of febrile illness, in about 16.2% of cases more than one seizure occur within 24 hours.

Classification: Febrile seizures are classified into simple or complex depending on the characteristics of the seizures. Simple or typical febrile seizures are single, brief and generalized type. They are termed as complex if the seizures are of focal type, if it lasts for more than 10-15 minutes and if the seizures recur within 24 hours or in the same febrile episode. Instead of the term complex or atypical febrile seizures it is preferable to use precise terms "prolonged", "focal" and "multiple". The significance of recognition of complex febrile seizures is that it is associated with increased risk of developing unprovoked seizure. Complex febrile seizure at first attack has been reported to occur in about 9-35% of cases. Febrile seizure, even the first episode, can present as status epilepticus. Febrile seizure is one of the most common cause of status epilepticus in children and accounts for about 25% of all episodes of status epilepticus in children.

Basic Mechanisms: The pathogenesis of febrile seizure is not well understood. Lower seizure threshold of the developing brain, the child's susceptibility to infections and propensity to have high fever and a genetic factor affecting the seizure threshold; all probably combine to precipitate febrile seizures in young children.

Fever and Febrile Seizures: Activation of the cytokine network in presence of infection/immunization may have a role in the pathogenesis of febrile seizure as suggested by a few preliminary works. Fever is associated with inflammation and release of pro-inflammatory cytokines, tumor necrosis factor-alpha (TNF-alpha), interleukin-1 alpha, interleukin-1 beta and interleukin 1Ra (IL-1). IL-1 influences neuronal excitability and causes seizures. Thus, fever itself not the cause of FS, but IL-1 links fever and seizures. But interleukins are released in older children and adults also but they do not develop febrile seizures. IL-1 probably acts as a modulator and in young children with immature brain it results in seizure. Elevated concentration of these CSF pro-inflammatory cytokines TNF-alpha, IL-1 beta, interleukin-1 alpha are seen in CSF. Recently, an association between a regulatory polymorphism in the genes encoding interleukin-1beta and interleukin-1Ra and febrile seizures was reported; however this has been contradicted by others.

Immunologic Derangements: Some studies have found zinc deprivation and iron deficiency and immunoglobulin deficiency to be common in febrile seizure and these have been speculated to have some role in etiopathogenesis of febrile seizure. There is a possibility of immunological derangements in the cytokine and interferon axis in FS that may play a part in causation of febrile seizure.

Age Selectivity: Certain highly reactive mechanisms specific for the immature age. Fever results in compensatory hyperventilation that causes alkaline shift in pH (due to CO_2 wash out). Elevated brain pH is thought to enhances neuronal excitability. Experiments in young rats have proven that hyperthermia results in greater increase in brain pH as compared to adult rats.

Familial Occurrence and Genetics of Febrile Seizures

The presence of positive family history in 25-40% of patients with febrile seizures, higher concordance in monozygotic twins, doubling of risk for developing febrile seizure when both parents have had febrile seizure (40-80% risk) suggests a genetic basis for occurrence of febrile seizures. About 8-14% of parents and 9-22% of sibs are found to have such history. But the mode of inheritance is unclear. An autosomal dominant pattern with incomplete penetrance has been suggested as the most common mode of inheritance but polygenic mechanism may also be involved and the mode of inheritance may vary from family to family. Linkage studies have given links to genes located on 2q, 5q, 5, 8q, 19p and 19q chromosomes. Work in this direction suggests that genetic abnormalities primarily mutations in several genes may be responsible for susceptibility to FS. Six susceptibility FS loci have been identified on chromosomes 8q13-q21 (FEB1), 19p (FEB2), 2q23-q24 (FEB3), 5q14-q15 (FEB4), 6q22-q24 (FEB5), and 18p11 (FEB6). Furthermore, mutations in the voltage-gated sodium channel alpha-1, alpha-2 and beta-1 subunit genes (SCN1A, SCN2A and SCN1B) and the GABA(A) receptor gamma-2 subunit gene (GABRG2) have been identified in cases of febrile seizure. Possibility of febrile seizure being primarily a channelopathy has been postulated in view of the mutations in the genes encoding ion channels in brain neurons like SCN1B.

The strongest linkage is to chromosome 2q, which codes for a protein in sodium channel receptors (SCN1A). The same locus is also associated with genetic epilepsy with febrile seizures plus (GEFS+) syndromes.

Genetic Epilepsy with Febrile Seizure Plus (GEFS+)

An interesting finding of genetic abnormalities found in cases of FS continuing beyond the usual age of occurrence has led to the development of the concept of GEFS+, a genetic epilepsy syndrome. GEFS has a spectrum of phenotypes including febrile seizure and febrile seizure plus. The syndrome comprised a childhood onset (median 1 year) of multiple FC, but unlike the typical FC syndrome, attacks with fever, at times without fever, continue beyond 6 years of age. Mutations in the voltage-gated sodium channel alpha-1, alpha-2 and beta-1 subunit genes (SCN1A, SCN2A and SCN1B) and the GABA(A) receptor gamma-2 subunit gene (GABRG2) have been identified in cases of GEFS+.

Risk Factors for Developing First Febrile Seizure: Fever is a common problem in children, but all children who have fever do not convulse. Majority of children (almost 50%) with febrile seizures do not have any risk factors. However, it has been observed that febrile seizures commonly occur in the following situations:

1. Family history of febrile seizure especially in first degree relative. Risk of febrile seizure for siblings is 10-45%. There is doubling of risk when both parents have febrile seizure.
2. Underlying brain disorder (Premature birth, delayed discharge from neonatal intensive care unit and developmental delay are potential markers for sub-optimal brain dysfunction).
3. Infection with human herpes virus-6 (HHV-6), influenza, metapneumovirus.
4. Attendance at day care centre has also been shown to be a risk factor.

Recurrent Febrile Seizure: One third of patients with febrile seizure will have recurrence and there is 50% risk if a child has more than 2 recurrences and age of the child at presentation is less than 12 months. About 9% of children with the first febrile seizure have more than 3 recurrences. The following are the risk factors for recurrent febrile seizures:

1. **Age:** Single, strongest, most consistent risk factor. There is 50% risk of recurrence in the first year, and over 90% recur within two years.
2. Family history of febrile seizure (but not epilepsy) in a first degree relative.
3. Initial febrile seizure with a relatively low fever.
4. Neurodevelopmental abnormality.
5. Shorter duration of fever before the initial febrile seizure.
6. Multiple initial seizures during the same febrile episode.

It is important to note that recurrent febrile seizure will be prolonged if the initial febrile seizure is also prolonged and febrile status epilepticus however does not appear to be associated with increased a risk recurrence.

Future Epilepsy: The most important event of which the parents are worried is the risk of future epilepsy. After first febrile seizure, 2-4% of children develop at least one unprovoked seizure (4 times higher risk when compared to the risk of epilepsy in general population). The risk is 1-1.5% in simple febrile seizures and 4-15% in complex febrile seizures. In other words, between 13-19% of children with afebrile seizure will have had one or more previous febrile seizures. Epilepsies to which febrile seizures predisposes include:

1. Idiopathic generalized epilepsy like GEFS+ (Genetic epilepsy with febrile seizures plus syndrome).
2. Severe myoclonic epilepsy of infancy (SMEI).
3. Mesial temporal lobe epilepsy (MTLE).

Risk Factors for the Occurrence of Future Epilepsy in a Child include:

1. Family history of epilepsy.
2. Complex features during the first episode of febrile seizure.
3. Early onset neurodevelopmental abnormalities.

Probability of epilepsy before 7 years of age is 1% if there are no risk factors (60% of febrile seizure population), 2% with only one risk factor (34% of febrile seizure population) and 10% with 2-3 risk factors (6% of febrile seizure population).

Febrile Seizure and Temporal Lobe Epilepsy (TLE)

This is the most controversial issue in epilepsy. Many retrospective studies have revealed that up to 40% of adults with intractable TLE had complex especially prolonged febrile seizure. While some studies have shown that prolonged and focal febrile seizure in childhood lead to hippocampal sclerosis on MRI of brain and they later developed TLE, other studies that performed MRI of brain within 48 hours of prolonged febrile seizure showed only hippocampal edema that on subsequent follow-up (MRI within 12 months) did not show mesial temporal sclerosis (MTS). Based on the available literature, the current opinion is:

1. Association between prolonged febrile seizure and pre-existing lesions within the temporal lobe and this may subsequently facilitate the development of hippocampal atrophy.
2. Complex interactions with genetic or environmental factors or both facilitate the development of TLE in patients with complex febrile seizure and hippocampal atrophy.

Outcome of Febrile Seizure: Febrile seizures are benign with risk of epilepsy of just 2-4%. There is no association between simple or complex febrile seizure (including SE) and later development of neurological deficits like hemiplegia, mental retardation, cerebral palsy, overall cognitive functioning, or specific memory impairment. It is important to emphasize that there is no increased risk or incidence of mortality in children with febrile seizure. This needs to be emphasized to parents while counseling. Most parents are reluctant to enquire about this but they expect this reassurance from the treating physician.

Clinical Presentation

The disease is characterized by sudden onset of seizure preceded by a brief febrile illness. Sometimes the initial manifestation is only a seizure, the fever going unnoticed by the parents initially, but detected later by the physician or by the parents themselves. The seizure generally is simple, sometimes complex and occasionally can take the form of a status. The termination of the seizure is usually abrupt. In the majority of cases there is hardly any post-ictal phase except a few where there can be drowsiness to deep sleep for varying duration. After the attack is over, the child appears well.

History may reveal features related to the cause of the fever like cold, cough, skin rash and diarrhea. Fever is the most important examination finding. Occasional child, usually the one having a focal seizure, can have Todd's palsy. Other findings are related to the cause of the fever like nasopharyngitis (in cases of upper respiratory infection), crepitations in chest (in cases of pneumonia) and splenomegaly (in cases of malaria) and any other preexisting morbidity.

Evaluation of a Child with Febrile Seizure

A detailed history of the fever onset, peak of temperature, site of infection, the type of seizure and family history of febrile seizure, epilepsy and sudden deaths should be elicited. Seizures need to be differentiated from rigors/ reflex anoxic seizure or other non-epileptic event which can occur with fever. A detailed examination for evidence of meningitis, underlying neurological deficits, asymmetry or stigmata of a neurocutaneous syndrome, microcephaly or metabolic disorder should be undertaken. Routine blood tests are not indicated unless clinically indicated.

Diagnosis

The diagnosis of febrile seizure is made solely by clinical features. Occasionally it may be differentiated from meningitis, encephalitis, brain abscess, toxic encephalopathy, Reye's syndrome, cerebral malaria and even cerebrovascular accidents. The most important condition is however bacterial meningitis which may mimic febrile seizure very closely in infants and young children. A thorough clinical examination is mandatory in every case.

Role of Lumbar Puncture: Excluding bacterial meningitis and doing a lumbar puncture in febrile seizure continues to be an important issue. The signs and symptoms of bacterial meningitis are often non-specific in infants and young ones and may even be absent specially in infants less than one year of age. Lumbar puncture is frequently done in infants and young children for the scare of missing bacterial meningitis. The tap however is normal, almost always. Studies on CSF examinations in febrile seizure have shown that extremely low yield as regards bacterial meningitis and the estimated incidence of meningitis in children who present with an apparent febrile seizure is 2-5%. Thus most of the taps that are done in febrile seizure were really unwarranted. On the other hand lumbar tap in a child immediately after a seizure is not without danger.

Yield of lumbar puncture is generally low in the absence of risk factors like focal seizures, and suspicious clinical findings. Definitive signs of meningitis like meningism and photophobia are more reliable in children more than 2 years and should not be dependable in younger children. Literature reveals that in approximately 13%-16% of children with meningitis, seizures are the presenting sign of disease and in approximately 30%-35% of these children (especially less than 18 months), meningeal signs and symptoms may be lacking *(Practice Parameter American Academy of Pediatrics 1996)*.

Lumbar puncture should be considered in children less than 2 years in the following situations:

1. History of irritability, decreased feeding and lethargy before or after seizure.
2. Seizure prolonged, focal or multiple febrile seizure occurring as a part of same febrile illness.
3. Physical signs of meningitis/encephalitis.
4. Prolonged post-ictal altered sensorium or neurological deficit.
5. Pretreatment with oral antibiotics.

American Academy of Pediatrics (1996) has issued guidelines for the management of febrile seizures and they recommend that in all infants of less than 12 months with febrile seizures, lumbar puncture to be strongly considered and in children between 12-18 months, lumbar puncture needs to be considered as signs and symptoms are subtle. With improvement in the immunization coverage of children, the incidence of meningitis is coming down. Hence, the updated AAP guideline (2011) no longer supports the routine lumbar puncture in infants with simple febrile seizures who are fully immunized against both H influenza B and S. pneumoniae. Lumbar puncture is optional in any infants with a simple febrile seizures who are missing immunizations or have an indeterminate immunization status.

Electroencephalography (EEG) in Febrile Seizure: EEG is not indicated in a normal child, irrespective of whether febrile seizure is simple or complex. Even in recurrent or complex febrile seizure also EEG is not justified, as it is of no use in identifying a structural abnormality or predicting recurrent febrile seizure or the development of epilepsy. At the same time EEG should be considered in children with complex febrile seizure who recur with afebrile convulsions and in children who recur with febrile seizures and exhibit developmental delays or abnormal neurological signs and symptoms.

Neuroimaging: Not indicated in a child with simple febrile seizure. It is indicated when there is:

1. Micro/macrocephaly, a neurocutaneous syndrome or preexisting neurological deficit.
2. Post-ictal neurological deficit persisting for more than a few hours following the febrile seizure.
3. Recurrent complex febrile seizure and particularly where there was any doubt whether the seizures were febrile in origin.

Magnetic resonance imaging (MRI) is always preferred to computed tomography (CT) of head when indicated.

Blood Studies: In evaluation of child with first febrile seizure, the biochemical investigations (serum electrolytes, calcium, phosphorous, magnesium, complete blood counts, blood glucose) should not be routinely performed *(AAP Practice Parameter 1996)*. However, estimation of random blood glucose can be considered if there is prolonged post-ictal obtundation. Further investigations will depend upon the nature of any comorbidity like rickets, neurodevelopmental anomaly and inborn errors of metabolism.

Treatment

The treatment of an attack of febrile seizure consists of terminating the seizure and lowering the body temperature. Acute treatment is indicated for prolonged seizures in the form of with intravenous diazepam in a dose of 0.3 mg/kg body weight or rectal diazepam (0.5 mg/kg) or buccal (0.4-0.5 mg/kg) or intranasal (0.2-0.5 mg/kg) midazolam. This can be administered at home for a seizure lasting for more than 5 min. Randomized controlled trials have shown that midazolam has superior efficacy to diazepam.

Occasionally a child does not respond to diazepam. Such cases usually respond to loading doses of intravenous valproate, 15-20 mg/kg/dose, or phenobarbitone 15-20 mg/kg/dose as loading dose. We should be careful about the risk of respiratory depression while using phenobarbitone after initial doses of benzodiazepines. Because of a possible potential role of sodium channel mutations in the causation of febrile seizures, sodium channel blockers like phenytoin are not as effective in management of febrile status epilepticus.

Subsequently the cause of fever should be treated appropriately. Lowering the body temperature is achieved by the use of antipyretic like paracetamol and tepid sponging. Cooling down the environment through fan, air coolers, air conditioners should be useful in hot weather. It is important to note and convey to parents in clear terms that antipyretics per se do not reduce risk of febrile seizures. As discussed earlier, fever itself not the cause of FS, but the inflammatory mediators like IL-1 by influencing neuronal excitability links fever and seizures. Antipyretics only reduce the fever and reduce the discomfort but cannot block the effects of the inflammatory mediators in the causation of seizures.

But most children present to hospital after the occurrence of seizure. In these children, we should assess the risk of recurrence and counsel accordingly. Based on detailed history taking if there are no risk factors for either recurrent FS or epilepsy and if the number of febrile seizures is less than 2, then follow 'wait and see' principle.

Prevention of Recurrence of Febrile Seizure

An intricately involved issue in this relatively benign disorder characterized by flurry of recurrences that subsides with age is prevention of recurrences. Recurrence of febrile seizures, that gives immense worries and anxieties to the parents, is a vexed problem. Counseling of parents about the benign nature of the disease, absence of any long-term morbidity in terms of memory disturbances or poor school performance and no risk of mortality is what is required in most of the cases.

Use of antiepileptic drugs like phenobarbitone, promidone, sodium valproate, to prevent recurrences are no longer advocated because of their unwanted side effects like behaviour disturbance and cognitive dysfunction with phenobarbitone and fatal hepatotoxicity with valproate that outweighs any benefit in a relatively benign disorder like febrile seizure. Recurrences also have virtually no serious consequences. Further, use of these drugs cannot prevent the development of later epilepsy.

Intermittent Febrile Seizure Prophylaxis: The seizures occur occasionally and the use of a drug to prevent occurrence of an attack during a febrile episode is more reasonable than continuous drug prophylaxis with its side effects. Benzodiazepines (oral or rectal diazepam or clobazam) are best suited for this purpose. They are used whenever the child is febrile and before the child starts seizing. Evidence shows that it is effective (decreases the febrile seizure recurrence rate by 1/3; 12% vs. 40%), but results in drowsiness, ataxia and interferes in assessment of patient.

Because the risk of recurrence of febrile seizures is low after a first febrile seizure, there is no need of prophylaxis after the first seizure.

Indications for intermittent prophylaxis:

1. History of prolonged FS (> 15-20 min).
2. Two or more risk factors and those with > 2 FS.
3. Frequent FS occurring over a short period of time, i.e., twice in half a day; ≥ 3 in 6 months; ≥ 4 in a year.
4. Remote place, away from medical facilities.

Dosage: Oral diazepam in a dose of 0.6 to 0.8 mg/kg/day in three divided doses starting from the first sign of febrile illness until the second day after recovery has also been found to be effective in preventing recurrences, although less effective than rectal diazepam, due to erratic absorption. Diazepam rectal or oral, used as above has the disadvantage of making the child little drowsy and even ataxic with the possibility missing an occasional case of bacterial meningitis; parents therefore should be asked to report immediately if it so happens. Parents must be made to understand the importance of anticipating the febrile episode.

The other option is use of oral clobazam at a dose of 0.75-1.0 mg/kg in two divided doses for three days with the occurrence of fever. This well tolerated as compared to diazepam.

Final decision on the use of benzodiazepines depends on the potential benefits (reduced recurrence, sense of satisfaction) vs. risks of its use, parental wishes and concerns and lastly the child's frequency and pattern of febrile illnesses and type of febrile seizure.

Long-Term Prophylaxis: Either phenobarbitone or valproate when administered continuously and maintained in therapeutic range, febrile seizure recurrence can be reduced in up to 90% of patients. Both phenytoin and carbamazepine not effective in preventing febrile seizure recurrence. There is no evidence that prophylactic AED significantly reduces the risk of late epilepsy. Hence both the American Academy of Pediatrics (AAP) and United Kingdom (UK) guidelines do not recommend prophylactic AED in children with either simple or complex febrile seizure. Despite the benign nature of febrile seizures and risk associated with long-term use of anti-epileptic drugs, there are some clinical situations where we have to use long-term prophylaxis.

Indications for daily or continuous use of anti-epileptic drugs:

1. Two or more seizures with a low fever (< 38.0 c) especially those from rural areas with poor access to medical facilities.
2. Prolonged FS where intermittent BDZ may not be given in time, as parents may fail to notice fever before the onset of seizures.
3. Prolonged FS where there is history of failed prevention using timely administration of diazepam.

Antihistaminics and Febrile Seizures: Because of associated rhinitis commonly antihistaminic and antipyretic combinations are commonly used. Due to their central nervous system effects (anticonvulsive central histaminergic system), H1 antagonists should be avoided in children with febrile seizures and epilepsy. It has been found that the time from fever detection to seizure onset was significantly shorter and the duration of seizures was significantly longer in the antihistamine group.

Vaccination and Febrile Seizures: None of the current standard vaccinations are contraindicated. They need to be given under doctor's supervision and measures for coping with fever and seizures should be explained. With measles vaccine, the risk of fever and hence febrile seizure occurence is around one week after vaccination. This needs to be emphasized to parents.

Information to Parents

Observing a seizure is probably one of the most frightening experiences for the parents. Parents of children with febrile seizure are a terribly worried lot regarding the future of the child. They are haunted by fears of accident during the attack and fears about the future of the child specially development of mental retardation, epilepsy. They often go round shopping doctors' clinics and hospitals in search of a permanent cure. To avoid these, the families should be provided with proper information about the disease and reassurance about the consequences and outcome of febrile seizure. They should be told in clear language that the disease is benign and self limiting, the children usually outgrowing it with age and the outcome including subsequent neurodevelopment is good although a small number of cases can develop epilepsy. Neurodevelopmental abnormalities, manifested by some of these children later, are likely to be due to preexisting disorders and not as a consequence of febrile seizures. What the parents need in mostly is reassurance.

Parental Advice: To allay anxiety in parents of febrile seizure children appropriate scientific information to parents need to be given, which should be both verbal and written. The following points needs to be emphasized:

1. Febrile seizure are common, recurrences are likely.
2. Risk of brain damage and later epilepsy are very rare.
3. Reassure that no evidence that any child has ever died as a result of febrile seizure.
4. They should be advised to keep a close watch on the temperature of the child whenever he is not looking well and/or is having cold, cough or diarrhea etc. Whenever they feel or find rise in body temperature, antipyretic and/or tepid sponging should be started in order to keep the temperature low. They may start diazepam orally or rectally.
5. What to do during febrile illness, and when child has a febrile seizure?
6. To seek doctor's help when seizure last > 5-10 min and shows no sign of stopping, frequently repeating short-term seizures with continued disturbance of consciousness in between, partial seizures, seizures in infants < 6 months age and in the presence of neurological symptoms such as prolonged disturbance of consciousness, post-ictal paralysis are present in addition to fever and seizures.
7. Advice as to what to do when a child has a febrile seizure?

   Not to panic, remain calm; to loosen the child's clothing particularly around the neck; if unconscious, place the child in supine position, keeping the head lower than the body, and turn the head so as to face side ways while tilted upwards; to record temperature, observe and record the duration and features of seizure; not to give any drugs or fluids orally and to stay near the patient until the seizure is subsided.

Suggested Reading

- AAP Practice Parameter: The Neurodiagnostic Evaluation of The Child with a First Simple Febrile Seizure. American Academy of Pediatrics. Provisional Committee on Quality Improvement Subcommittee on Febrile Seizures. Pediatrics 1996;97:769-75.
- Ad Hoc Task Force of LICE Guidelines Commission. Recommendations for The Management of "Febrile Seizures". Epilepsia 2009;50(Suppl.1):2-6.
- Expert Committee on Pediatric Epilepsy, Indian Academy of Pediatrics. Guidelines for Diagnosis and Management of Childhood Epilepsy, Indian Pediatrics 2009;46:681-98.
- Sadleir LG, Scheffer IE. Febrile Seizures, BMJ 2007;334:307-11.
- Steering Committee on Quality Improvement and Management. Subcommittee on Febrile Seizures. Febrile Seizures: Clinical Practice Guideline for the Long-term Management of the Child With Simple Febrile Seizures. Pediatrics 2008;121:1281-86.
- Subcommittee on Febrile Seizures American Academy of Pediatrics. Febrile Seizures: Clinical Practice Guideline for the Long-term Management of the Child with Simple Febrile Seizures. Pediatrics 2008;121:1281-86.
- Subcommittee on Febrile Seizures. Febrile Seizures: Clinical Practice Guideline for the Neurodiagnostic Evaluation of the Child With a Simple Febrile Seizure. Pediatrics 2011;127:389-94.
- Virta M, Hurme M, Helmmen M. Increased Plasma Levels of Pro and Anti Inflammatory Cytokines in Patients with Febrile Seizures. Epilepsia 2002;43:920-23.
- Waruiru C, Appleton R. Febrile Seizure: An Update. Arch Dis Child 2004;89:751-56.

17 Chapter

SEIZURE DISORDERS IN INFANCY AND EARLY CHILDHOOD

Suvasini Sharma

INTRODUCTION

Seizures are a common neurological problem in infancy and childhood. Seizures are the most common neurological problem encountered in children and are often a frightening experience for the parents. Seizure is a symptom of central nervous system dysfunction due to any cause. Epilepsy is a condition characterized by the occurrence of recurrent unprovoked seizures. For epidemiological purposes, epilepsy is defined as the occurrence of two or more unprovoked seizures more than 24 hours apart.

Approach to An Infant or A Young Child With Seizures

When faced with an infant or a young child who presents with a seizure, certain questions need to be answered.[1]

Is It a Seizure or a Seizure Mimic?

Many paroxysmal conditions in infants and young children mimic seizures. Examples include breath-holding spells, benign sleep myoclonus, gratification disorders, shuddering attacks and Sandifer syndrome. The parents should be asked what the child was doing at the time of the attack. They should be asked to describe or enact the movement. With the common availability of smart phones, home videos are a very good way to see the episodes when the episodes are frequent.

What is the Type of Seizure(s)?

Many seizure types can occur in infants and young children including focal, tonic, myoclonic, atonic, generalized tonic clonic and epileptic spasms. Generalized tonic clonic seizures are rare in children. One child may have more than one seizure type. Recognition of the precise seizure type is important for syndromic diagnosis (as described below) and for appropriate treatment.

Is It a Provoked or An Acute Symptomatic Seizure?

Has the seizure occurred as a result of an acute illness such as bacterial meningitis? Is there a metabolic or an electrolyte imbalance such as hypoglycemia, hyponatremia or hypocalcemia which has resulted in the seizure. Such seizures which occur as a result of acute illnesses are called acute symptomatic seizures. These do not constitute epilepsy. Hypocalcemic seizures are very common in infants especially in infants who are fed with cow's milk.

Another special category in young children is febrile seizures. A febrile seizure is a seizure accompanied by fever, without CNS infection or dyselectrolytemia that occurs in infants and children between 6 and 60 months of age and without prior history of afebrile seizures. Febrile seizures are the most common cause of seizures in infants and young children and do not constitute epilepsy. The evaluation and management of a child with febrile seizures is discussed in another chapter.

What is the Developmental Status of the Child?

Is the child developmentally normal or delayed? How was the child prior to the onset of seizures? Has there been a developmental delay, arrest or regression after the onset of seizures? This will help to formulate the syndromic diagnosis as well as give clues to the underlying etiology.

Does It Constitute An "Epilepsy Syndrome"?

Epilepsy syndromes are "electro-clinical" syndromes which are identifiable on the basis of a typical age of onset, specific EEG characteristics, seizure types, and often other features (such as the developmental status of the child and family history) which, when taken together, permit a specific diagnosis. The diagnosis in turn often has implications for treatment, management and prognosis. Not all children with epilepsy will be classifiable into an epilepsy syndrome. But recognition of these syndromes aids in planning the investigations, management and for prognostication. The common epilepsy syndromes in infancy and childhood are discussed below.

Epilepsy syndromes in infants and young children are often categorized into "benign" and "catastrophic". Benign epilepsy syndromes are characterized by epileptic seizures that are easily treated or require no treatment and remit without sequelae. Catastrophic epilepsy syndromes are characterized by refractory and difficult-to-treat seizures and associated comorbid developmental delay/regression and poor neurodevelopmental outcome. Another term that is used for such conditions is epileptic encephalopathy. Epileptic encephalopathies refer to a group of disorders in which the unremitting epileptic activity contributes to severe cognitive and behavioral impairments above and beyond what might be expected from the underlying pathology alone.

BENIGN EPILEPSY SYNDROMES

Benign Myoclonic Epilepsy of Infancy

This is a rare condition that is commoner in boys. Myoclonic seizures occur in a neurologically normal infant between 6 months and 2 years of age. The myoclonic seizures have EEG correlates of spike-wave or polyspike-wave discharges which distinguishes this from benign myoclonus of early infancy but the interictal EEG is normal.[1] The myoclonus tends to occur in the awake state but not during sleep. A family history of epilepsy is present in 25-30% of the patients. The treatment of choice is sodium valproate.

Benign Infantile Seizures (Familial and Non-Familial)

This constitutes an age-related idiopathic syndrome of infancy. The seizures are focal and the infants are otherwise normal. The age of onset is from 3-20 months. Seizures characteristically occur in clusters of 5-10 per day for 1-3 days and may recur after 1-3 months.[2] The interictal EEG is normal. Prognosis is good and the seizures remit within 1-2 years of onset. Carbamazepine or sodium valproate may be used for treatment.

Panayiotopoulos Syndrome

This is also known as early onset benign childhood occipital epilepsy. The age of onset is between 3 and 6 years. It is a predominantly "autonomic" epilepsy as the seizure features are predominantly autonomic. The seizures typically occur in sleep. Ictal emesis and retching is a predominant symptom. The child may have gaze deviation and limb jerking. Other autonomic features which may occur include pallor and mydriasis. The children often have a prolonged loss of consciousness after the seizure but are completely well when awake. EEG shows multifocal spikes with occipital predominance (Fig. 17.1). The prognosis is remarkably benign. 50% of

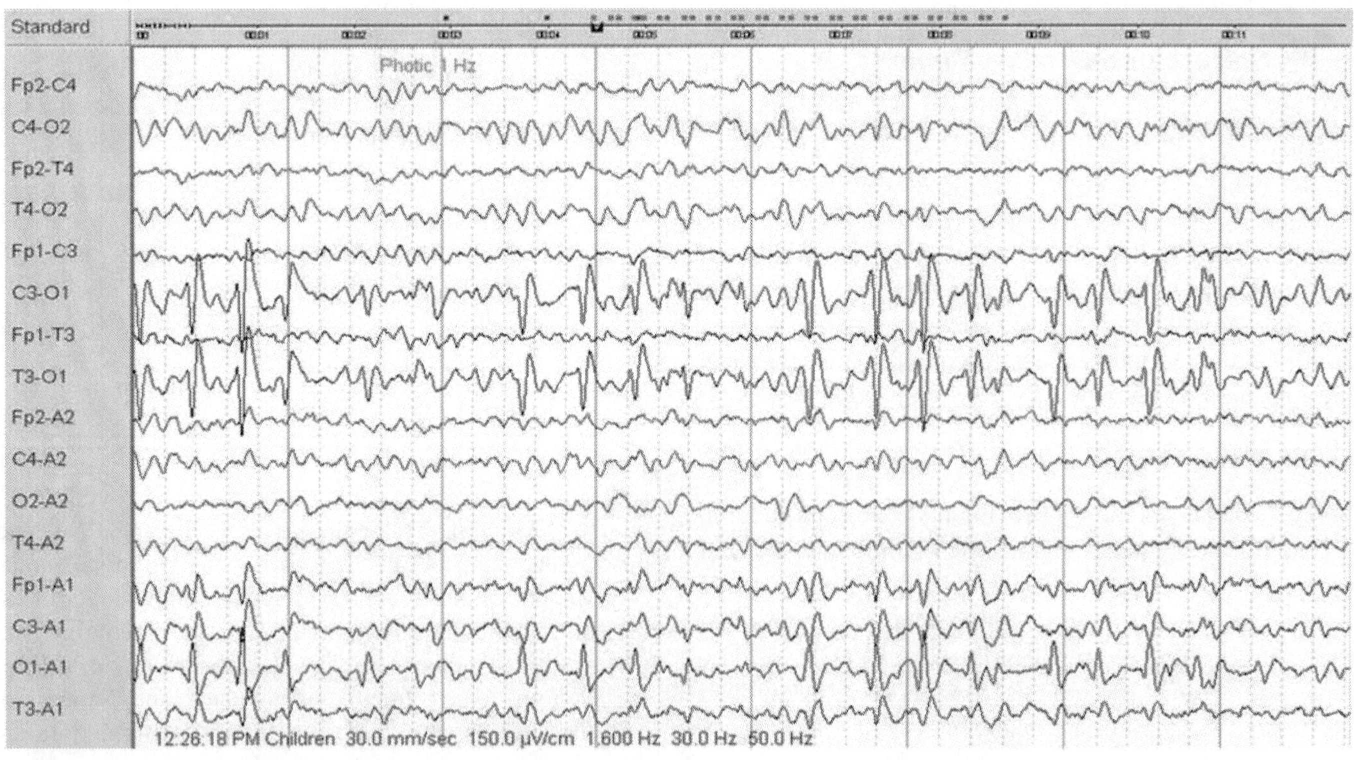

Fig. 17.1: EEG showing left sided occipital spike wave discharges in a child with Panayiotopoulos syndrome

the children have 1-5 seizures. 90% of patients go into complete remission within 1-2 years of onset.[2] Treatment is not indicated for few seizures. For frequent seizures, carbamazepine or sodium valproate may be used.

Catastrophic Epilepsy Syndromes/Epileptic Encephalopathies

Ohtahara Syndrome

Ohtahara syndrome occurs with onset ranging from intra-uterine period to 3 months of age. Tonic seizures are the defining seizure type, which are very frequent and occur in both sleep and wakeful states. The interictal EEG shows burst suppression pattern with no sleep-wake differentiation. The majority of cases are attributable to static structural brain lesions such as focal cortical dysplasia, hemimegalencephaly, and Aicardi syndrome.[3] Few genetic mutations have been described. The medical management of seizures is not rewarding. The prognosis is uniformly poor with survivors left with severe psychomotor retardation.[4] There may be age-dependent evolution to West syndrome and then subsequently to Lennox-Gastaut syndrome.

Early Myoclonic Encephalopathy

This presents within first 3 months of age and mostly within the neonatal period. Fragmentary, erratic myoclonia, partial seizures and less frequently tonic spasms are seen. The interictal EEG shows burst suppression pattern more prominent during the sleep. Inherited metabolic disorders such as non-ketotic hyperglycinemia, organic acidemias, Menke's disease, Zellweger syndrome, molybdenum cofactor deficiency and pyridoxine dependency and genetic factors are the most important etiologies.[3] These seizures are often refractory to conventional anti-epileptic drugs. The prognosis is dismal.

West Syndrome

West syndrome was first described by W.J. West in 1841 and is characterized by epileptic spasms or '*salaam attacks*', hypsarrhythmia on EEG and developmental delay or regression.[4] The typical onset is between 3 and 12 months of age. Epileptic spasms are clusters of sudden, brief (0.2-2 seconds), diffuse or fragmented, tonic contractions of axial and limb muscles. This may be accompanied by cry, laughter or autonomic changes.[2] They may be flexor (most common), extensor, mixed or subtle. Spasms usually occur on awakening. Hypsarrhythmia is the classical interictal EEG finding and is characterized by chaotic background with nearly continuous random asynchronous high voltage slow waves and spikes arising from multiple foci (Fig. 17.2).[5]

The etiology is diverse. West syndrome has been classically classified into symptomatic (identifiable neuro-

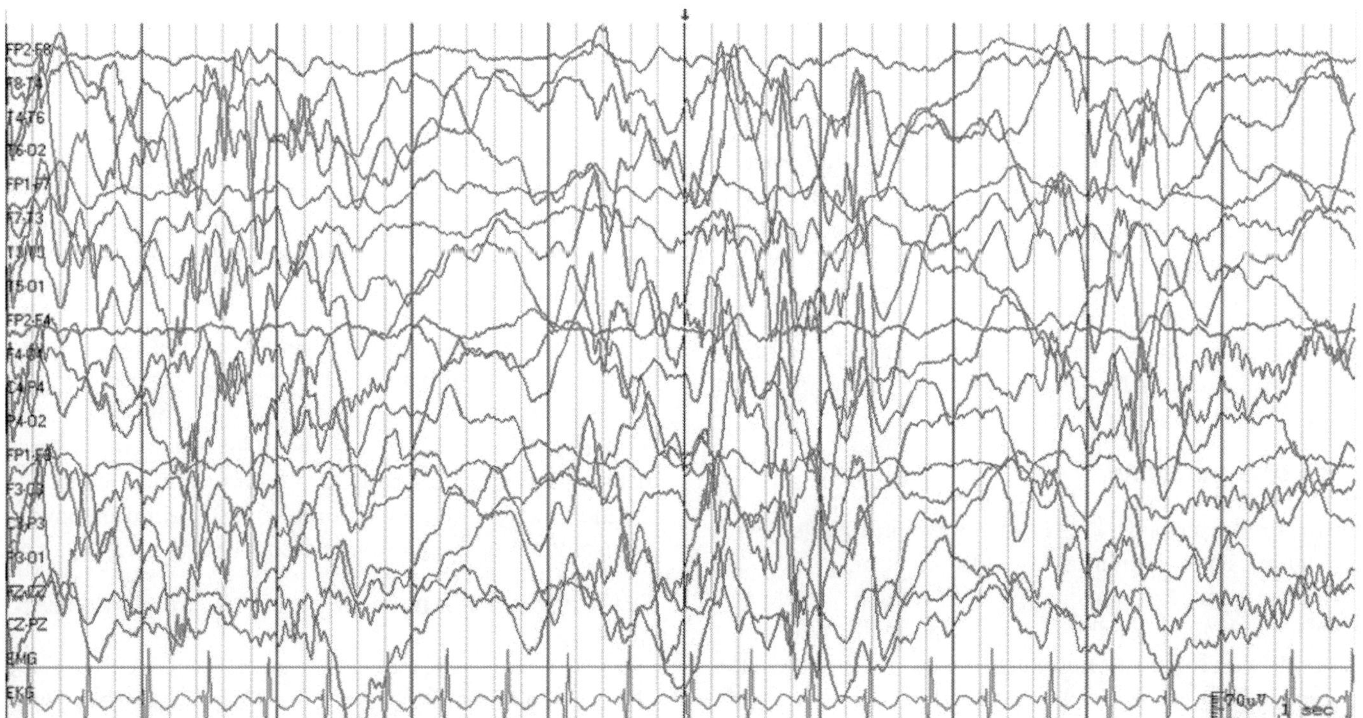

Fig. 17.2: EEG showing chaotic high voltage slow waves with intermixed spike wave discharges suggestive of hypsarrhythmia

logical insult), cryptogenic (probably symptomatic but with no known etiology) and idiopathic (normal premorbid development and unknown etiology) forms (see Table 17.1). Thus, a thorough clinical evaluation followed by appropriate neuroimaging and genetic and metabolic work-up is warranted in a child with West syndrome.

Table 17.1: Classification of West Syndrome
Symptomatic
Pre-, peri- and post-natal cerebral ischemia
Cerebral malformations
Neuro-infections sequelae
Neurocutaneous syndromes: Tuberous sclerosis, incontinentia pigmenti
Genetic: CDKL-5, MeCP 2, ARX, STXBP-1, SPTAN1, PLC-β1
Chromosomal disorders: Down syndrome, 1p36 deletion, Pallister-Killian syndrome
Inborn errors of metabolism: Biotinidase deficiency and other organic acidurias, phenylketonuria, mitochondrial disorders, Menkes disease, non-ketotic hyperglycinemia, antiquitin deficiency
Hypothalamic hamartoma
Cryptogenic
Idiopathic

Adrenocorticotrophin hormone (ACTH) is the drug of choice for short-term treatment of epileptic spasms. High dose oral steroids may also be an alternative, especially in resource-constrained settings.[6] Vigabatrin is a second-line drug except in children with Tuberous Sclerosis Complex where it is the preferred drug over ACTH. Pyridoxine and biotin trial should always be considered in refractory spasms. Ketogenic diet has also shown to be beneficial. Resective neurosurgery may be warranted in refractory cases with structural lesions.

The prognosis is guarded and is governed by the underlying etiology and the treatment. The affected children are left with variable psychomotor retardation, epilepsy or psychiatric disorders.

Dravet Syndrome

It was first described by Charlotte Dravet in 1978 as severe myoclonic epilepsy of infancy (SMEI). The onset is usually between 5 and 8 months of age with frequent, prolonged febrile unilateral clonic convulsions with alternating pattern in a previously normal child. Non-febrile seizures may also be present. This stage is followed by emergence of multiple seizure types (myoclonic, atypical absences and complex focal seizures) which frequently progress to status epilepticus and associated severe psychomotor deterioration. The relentless progression stops at around 10-12 years of age with decrease in seizure frequency and persisting neurologic sequelae.[7]

The interictal EEG is normal initially. Soon, the EEG deteriorates with background slowing, asymmetric paroxysms of generalized polyspike/spike-slow-wave discharges and multifocal epileptiform abnormalities.[4] Mutations in the SCN1A gene encoding the alpha-1 subunit of the sodium channel are detectable in 70-80% of patients with Dravet syndrome.[8] Seizures are usually refractory. Drugs like carbamazepine, phenytoin and lamotrigine are contraindicated. Early initiation of ketogenic diet has been advocated.

Lennox-Gastaut Syndrome

Lennox-Gastaut syndrome (LGS) is a severe form of epileptic encephalopathy with onset between 1 and 8 years of age, mainly between 2 and 5 years of age. It is characterized by intractable mixed types of seizures including tonic, atypical absence, atonic and myoclonic seizures. "Drop attacks", tonic or atonic, seen in 50% children frequently causes injuries.[9] Twenty percent children have history of epileptic spasms.[10] Cognitive impairment is common and fluctuates with the seizure frequency.

The pathognomonic interictal EEG finding is bilateral, synchronous, slow-spike-and-wave discharges (1.5 - 2.5 Hz) with fronto-central voltage dominance with abnormal background. Paroxysmal fast activity of bilateral synchronized bursts of 10-20 Hz frontally-dominant activity lasting for few seconds is also seen (Fig. 17.3).

The etiology of Lennox-Gastaut syndrome is heterogenous and similar to epileptic spasms. One-third of children have no antecedent history or evidence of cerebral pathology.

Valproate and clobazam are the preferred drugs. Levetiracetam, rufinamide, lamotrigine, topiramate and zonisamide are the second line drugs. Steroids and intravenous immunoglobulins may be indicated during periods of increased seizure frequency or status epilepticus.[2] The prognosis is guarded with more than 80% children having persistent epilepsy and severe neurocognitive sequelae.

Evaluation of An Infant or Young Child with Seizures

The evaluation begins with a detailed history, which should include details of the pregnancy, delivery and postnatal factors. A detailed family history and a three-generation pedigree should be made. The presence of other

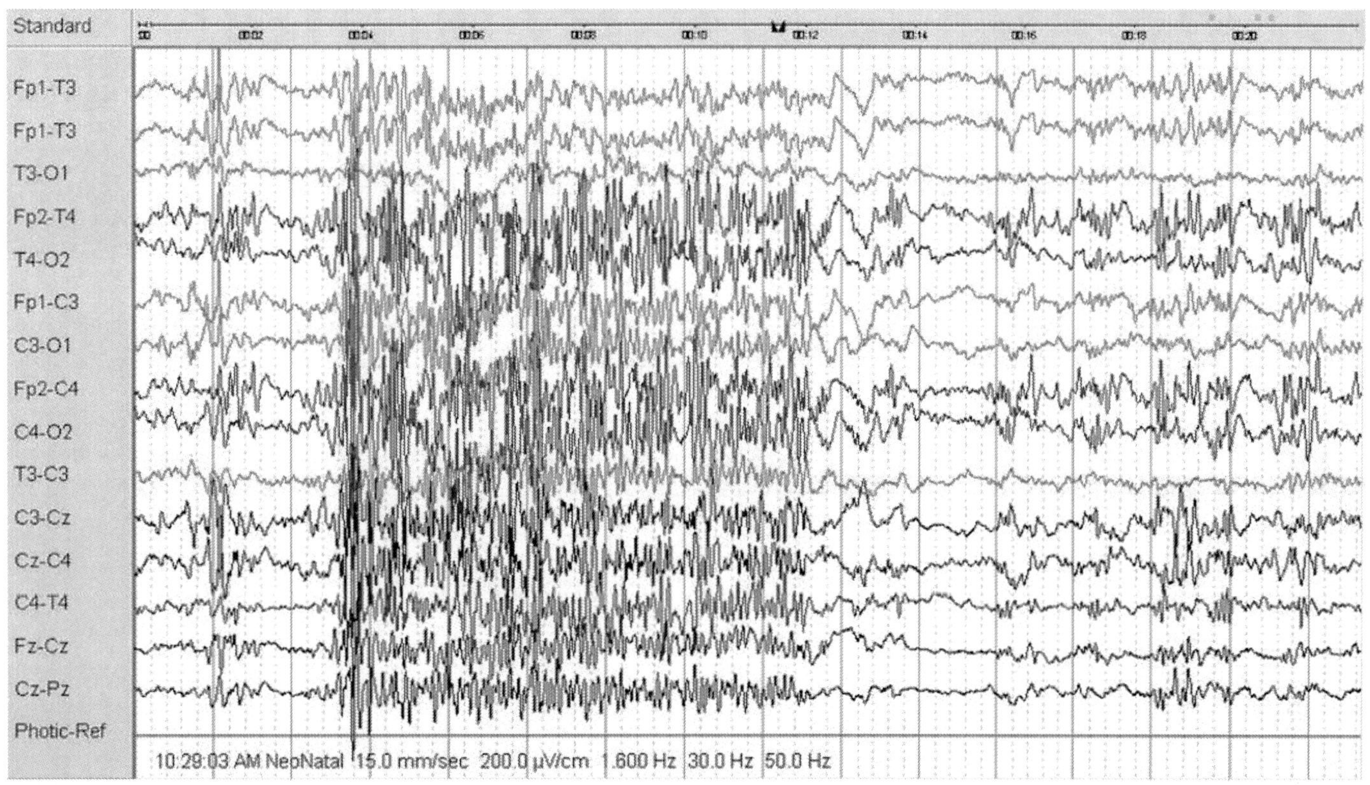

Fig. 17.3: EEG showing generalized paroxysmal fast activity in a child with Lennox Gastaut syndrome

neurological problems such as autistic features, stiffness, vision and hearing problems must be screened for.

A general physical examination must be performed to look for craniofacial dysmorphic features (chromosomal abnormalities, peroxisomal disorders, abnormal fat pads in congenital disorders of glycosylation), and neurocutaneous markers such as ash leaf macules, which are characteristic of tuberous sclerosis. Alopecia and seborrheic dermatitis is characteristic of biotinidase deficiency.

Neurological examination must be performed to assess tone abnormalities, and associated movement disorders such as dystonia, choreoathetosis and stereotypies. The ocular fundi must be examined for the presence of chorioretinitis and/or changes of a pigmenetary retinopathy, optic atrophy, which may point towards the presence of infantile neuronal ceroid lipofucscinosis, and mitochondriopathies.[11]

All infants and young children with epilepsy should undergo an EEG. A video-EEG is preferable over a routine EEG, especially if there are very frequent seizures. A neuroimaging study, preferably an MRI of brain, must be performed in all infants and young children with epilepsy. MRI is diagnostic for brain malformations, tuberous sclerosis, perinatal insult sequelae such as asphyxia, while an MR spectroscopy performed simultaneously can be of diagnostic value in patients with inborn errors of metabolism (glycine encephalopathy, creatine deficiency syndromes), and mitochondriopathies (elevated lactate).[11]

Chromosomal karyotyping must be performed if dysmorphic features are present. If no clue has been found by clinical evaluation, and neuroimaging, metabolic etiology must be looked for, especially keeping in mind treatable conditions. If the initial metabolic investigations exclude hypoglycemia, hypocalcemia, hypomagnesemia, elevations of lactate and ammonia, the focus of investigation and management should continue to vigorously search for treatable epileptic encephalopathies. A CSF examination must be performed to look for low glucose levels and low CSF to serum glucose ratio (glucose transporter defect), elevated lactate (mitochondriopathies), elevated glycine (non-ketotic hyperglycinemia), serine (serine biosynthesis defects), or pipecolic acid (pyridoxine dependency), and neurotransmitters (abnormalities seen in Pyridoxal phosphate dependency).[11]

Treatment

Treatment depends on the types of seizures and epilepsy syndrome, if identified. If an epilepsy syndrome has been identified, appropriate treatment should be given as mentioned above. If no syndrome has been identified, treatment is as per the seizure type. For focal seizures, carbamazepine, oxcarbazepine or levetiracetam are used. For generalized seizures (generalized tonic clonic, myoclonic, atonic, absence etc), sodium valproate is preferred as it is a broad spectrum agent. Sodium valproate should be avoided in children with suspected inherited metabolic disorders, mitochondrial disorders and comorbid liver disease.

A sequential therapeutic trial with vitamin B_6, folinic acid and pyridoxal phosphate should be considered early in all infants with epileptic encephalopathy and poor response to antiepileptic treatment. Biotin should be administered if there is alopecia with/without seborrheic dermatitis.

CONCLUSION

Seizures in infants and young children are a common neurological problem. The approach should be to first confirm if the event is epileptic, then see the seizure type, and see if an epilepsy syndrome diagnosis can be made. Genetic and metabolic etiologies should be considered in these children.

References

1. Alam S, Lux AL. Epilepsies in Infancy. Arch Dis Child 2012 November;97(11):985-92.
2. Panayiotopoulos CP. A Clinical Guide to Epileptic Syndromes and Their Treatment. Springer Publications 2010.
3. Ohtahara S, Yamatogi Y. Epileptic Encephalopathies in Early Infancy with Suppression-burst. J Clin Neurophysiol 2003: December:20(6):398-407.
4. Jain P, Sharma S, Tripathi M. Diagnosis and Management of Epileptic Encephalopathies in Children. Epilepsy Res Treat 2013:2013:501981. doi: 10.1155/2013/501981. Epub 2013 July 22.
5. Gibbs F, Gibbs E. Atlas of Encephalography. Cambridge, MA: Addison-Wesley: 1952.
6. Chellamuthu P(1), Sharma S(2), Jain P(3), Kaushik JS(4), Seth A(5), Aneja S(2). High Dose (4 mg/kg/day) Versus Usual Dose (2 mg/kg/day) Oral Prednisolone for Treatment of Infantile Spasms: An Open-Label, Randomized Controlled Trial. Epilepsy Res 2014 October:108(8):1378-84.
7. Dravet C. The Core Dravet Syndrome Phenotype. Epilepsia 2011April:52 Suppl.2:3-9.
8. Marini C, Scheffer IE, Nabbout R, *et al.* The Genetics of Dravet Syndrome. Epilepsia 2011April;52 Suppl 2:24-29.
9. Camfield PR. Definition and Natural History of Lennox-Gastaut Syndrome. Epilepsia 2011August:52 Suppl5:3-9.
10. Markand ON. Lennox-Gastaut Syndrome (Childhood Epileptic Encephalopathy). J Clin Neurophysiol 2003December:20(6): 426-41.
11. Sharma S, Prasad AN. Genetic Testing of Epileptic Encephalopathies of Infancy: An Approach. Can J Neurol Sci 2013 January;40(1):10-16.

18 Chapter

ABSENCE SEIZURES

Vinod Puri, Neera Chaudhry, Ashish Kumar Duggal

Absence seizure is a subgroup of the primary generalized epilepsies with absence (loss of consciousness) as its fundamental and may be the sole manifestation. It account for 5% to 10% of all seizures in childhood and occurs in children with a strong familial propensity for seizures. Characteristically bilateral synchronous spike and wave or multiple-spike-wave electroencephalographic changes are seen during ictal and interictal period. Absence seizure responds poorly to barbiturates and hydantoins while ethosuximide, valproate and lamotrigine are medications of choice.

Historical Aspects

Poupart (1705) gave the vivid description of absence, "at the approach of an attack the patient would sit in a chair, her eyes open, and would remain there immobile and would not afterwards remember falling into this state. If she had begun to talk and the attack interrupted her, she took it up again at precisely the point at which she had stopped and she believed she had talked continuously."[1] Tissot in 1770 used the term petit while Esquirol (1805) introduced the term petit mal. It was left to Calmeil who coined the present nomenclature of absence to such attacks. Huglings Jackson[2] was the first to clearly distinguish between non-convulsive seizures of temporal lobe origin and petit mal. Of course he relied more upon the presence of automatism that suggested a temporal lobe origin. He did recognize that partial complex seizures could very closely resemble petit mal. It was left to the era of electroencephalography to adequately separate these two types of seizures.

In 1935 Gibbs *et al.*[3] described the typical EEG picture of 3 Hz spike-wave pattern that accompanies these seizures. The international league against epilepsy[4,5] discarded the term petit mal for absence to these types of seizures.

Two major types of absence seizures are recognized:

- **Typical Absence Seizures:** These are characteristically seen with the idiopathic (primary) generalized epilepsies of following types:
  1. Childhood absence epilepsy (CAE).
  2. Juvenile absence epilepsy (JAE).
  3. Juvenile myoclonic epilepsy (JME).
- **Atypical Absence Seizures:** These are seen in patients with symptomatic or cryptogenic generalized epilepsies, especially Lennox-Gastaut syndrome.

Typical absence seizures (Classic absence) are of various types:

a. Simple absence

b. Complex absence

   i. Absence with mild clonic component.

   ii. Absence with increase in postural tone.

   iii. Absence with decrease in postural tone.

   iv. Absence with automatism.

   v. Absence with autonomic components.

   vi. Mixed forms (combination of i to v).

Incidence

Hauser and Kurland[6] estimated an annual incidence of 1/10,000 in the population of Rochester, Minnesota. Among children with epilepsy Cavazutti[7] found 8% to have absence seizures while Viani *et al.*[8] could not find a single case of myoclonic absence out of 645 patients. However, juvenile absence was found in 16%. Penry *et al.*[9] observed simple absence in 9.4% while 90.6% had complex absence.

CLASSIC ABSENCE

Clinical Features

Classic Absence

Typically, seizures commence between the ages of 4-8 years in a child without a prior history of unprovoked or non-febrile seizures. The description of seizure is mostly given by a parent or teacher as brief lapses in awareness where the child stares and becomes unresponsive or ceases an ongoing activity and afterwards he resumes prior activity. At times only deterioration in school performance is noted. Many such attacks may occur each day. Normal intelligence and normal neurological examination is the rule, however, mental retardation and/or abnormal neurological examination has been reported in 5.1 to 24%.[10,11] In some cases, a period of retrograde amnesia has also been observed.[12] Although majority of patients with absence seizures have its onset between 4-8 years, in a few it may begin between 1-4 or after 8 years of age and rarely there is adult onset.[13]

Simple Absence

Absence with impairment of consciousness only, is the simple absence seizure. The manifestation of these is cessation of ongoing activities and a loss of responsiveness. There may be a brief upward movement of the eyes. The attack usually last for less than 10 seconds.

Complex Absence

Absence with additional phenomena like mild clonic component, atonic component, tonic component, automatism and autonomic component either singly or in varying combination is called complex absence.

1. **Absence with Mild Clonic Component:** The clonic activity may occur as blinking, twitching of corner of mouth, fingers, arms, shoulder or neck flexors. These movements usually do not impair posture although they may cause the patient to lose control of objects in his hand. Contraction of the neck flexors may jerk the head forwards, leading to some difficulty in distinguishing this attack from the one associated with loss of muscle tone.

2. **Absence with Increase in Postural Tone:** Increased tone may affect flexors or extensors and may be symmetric or asymmetric. If standing, increased tone may lead to retropulsion. An asymmetric increase in tone may pull the head and trunk to one side. Occasionally slight clonic activity may interrupt the tonic contraction resulting in intermittent postural deviation.

3. **Absence with Decrease in Postural Tone**: Tone may be diminished in postural as well as limb musculature. Loss of postural tone may be symmetric or asymmetric. The head or trunk may slump forward, dropping of the arms, relaxation of grip or buckling at the knees may result. Rarely, tone may be sufficiently diminished to cause the patient to fall.

4. **Absence with Automatism:** Automatisms are apparently purposeful movements occurring without awareness during the absence attack. Automatisms may be perseverative or de novo type. Perseverative automatisms represent persistence of activity engaged in before the onset of the seizures such as walking or handling of objects, although these activities are distorted during the seizures. De novo automatisms are movements initiated after the onset of the seizure. Lip smacking, chewing and fumbling with fingers are the most common de novo automatisms. Others include swallowing, lip licking, grimacing, yawning, scratching, shuffling the legs, walking and stepping in place. Some de novo automatisms may appear responsive to environmental stimuli.

5. **Absence with Autonomic Components:** The most commonly observed autonomic phenomena are circumoral pallor and pupillary dilatation. Others include flushing, tachycardia, piloerection, salivation, urinary incontinence, respiratory arrest, decreased gastric and esophageal motility.

6. **Mixed Form:** Seizures may be combination of two or more of previous categories. Penry *et al.*[9] analyzed 374 absence seizures in 48 patients. Mild clonic component occurred in 45% of all seizures. 87% of these movements were of eyelids. Decreased postural tone occurred in 22.5% while increased tone was rare 4.5%, 88% experienced automatism with absence seizure. The probability of an automatism occurring during an absence seizure increases as seizure duration increases and in a seizure lasting 3 seconds or less was 22.5%, while for those lasting 18 seconds or more the probability was 95%.

EEG FEATURES

EEG Pattern During Ictal Phase

The classic ictal EEG abnormality is 3 Hz spike and wave pattern. The discharges begin and end abruptly. Usually they are bilaterally symmetrical but may show a shifting emphasis between the two hemispheres. With maximal expression at the superior frontal electrodes. Often the discharges commence at a frequency of 3.5 to 4 Hz, gradually slowing to 2.5-3 Hz. As a burst progresses the spike discharges may become smaller. The National Institute of Health group examined over 600 absence seizures recorded on split screen videotape with simultaneous recording of the clinical seizure and EEG and observed all absence seizures were accompanied by bilateral spike wave or multiple spike wave discharges of 2-4 Hz. Careful analysis of the morphology of the waveforms shows them to be quiet complex.[14] Some complexes may show two negative spikes, a positive transient and a negative slow wave. In any one pattern the morphology may vary from one region to another.

Interictal Pattern

The background activity is usually normal, although paroxysmal activity may occur as spikes or spike-slow wave complexes.[13] Rhythmic delta activity of 3 Hz may occur posteriorly in about 15% of cases. Cobb *et al.*[15] described it as being more common in children who had an early age of seizures. Presence of this slow activity has a prognostic significance of cessation of absence attacks by the age of 10-12 years and a lesser tendency to develop grand mal seizures. Lugaresi[16] and Gastaut[17] felt this activity was enhanced in contrast to 3 Hz spike wave pattern, which disappeared while under effective treatment with Ethosuximide.

Effect of Precipitation Procedures on EEG Pattern

1. **Hyperventilation**: Spike and wave paroxysms can almost always be precipitated by hyperventilation in untreated patients with absence seizures.[10] As a patient responds to treatment, discharges may only be seen during hyperventilation and in majority of cases not even then. Adams and Lueders[19] claimed that 5 minutes of hyperventilation was more reliable than a 6 hours recording as a guide to seizure frequency.
2. **Photic Stimulation:** Spike wave paroxysms can be provoked by photic stimulation in 10-13% of absence seizures.[20] Majority of cases with photo paroxysmal response on EEG later on develop tonic clonic seizures, in addition.
3. **Hypoglycemia:** Like hyperventilation hypoglycemia is also a potent stimulator of spike wave paroxysms.
4. **Sleep:** During sleep the character of the spike slow wave paroxysms changes. Sato *et al.*[21] described increasing irregularities of the paroxysms during stage I and II of sleep with a somewhat periodic character especially in stage II while in stage III and IV the number of spikes increases and the waves become longer in duration and more distorted.

   REM sleep shortens the duration of paroxysms however the basic morphology remained similar to that during wakefulness. These changes were most apparent during the first sleep cycle.[21]

Clinical Significance of Spike Wave Discharges

All absence seizures are accompanied by spike wave paroxysms. Studies of spike wave paroxysms have revealed altered responsiveness during the paroxysms, which gradually improve before the pattern, has disappeared from EEG but never returns to normal until background is restored.[22] Mirsky and Van Buren[23] and Gallerand Galler[24] reported impaired visual attentiveness 0.5 seconds before the onset of 3 Hz seizure pattern. Orren[25] has shown decreased visual evoked potential amplitude 200 to 500 msec before the start and that persisted during the paroxysms. Brown *et al.* found normal auditory reaction time 1 second before the paroxysms but only 45% of them were normal at the start of paroxysms, which further dropped to 4% in the first second of the discharge. Several studies have suggested that spike wave paroxysms may have deleterious effect on memory. Retrograde memory deficits for verbal or visual material presented during a period several seconds prior to spike wave paroxysms, have been reported.[24,26] Erba and Cavazzuti[27] observed impairment of the ability to perform complex tasks without any significant impairment of motor control, vigilance or memory during the paroxysms. The 3 Hz spike wave paroxysms can be single or fragmentary or may repeat for several seconds at a time. Those lasting longer than 3 seconds have a readily recognized clinical accompaniment.

The conclusion from these studies is that significant impairment in performance occurs during short spike wave bursts even in the absence of clinical evidence for seizures and therefore, the aim of treatment should be the abolition of the discharges. Counting spike wave bursts on prolonged EEG recording is a valid method of evaluating the effectiveness of anti-absence drugs.

Etiology

The evidence suggests absence seizure is an expression of genetic factors triggered by an additional abnormally possibly biochemical.

Typical cases of absence seizures have been described in patients with mesial frontal lesion,[28,29] diencephalic lesion,[30,31] diffuse neuronal disease[32] and even withdrawal from sedatives.[33] However, most of these do not have precise 3 Hz spike wave discharge. Till now no biochemical abnormality has been implicated except the finding of increased thermolability of benzodiazepine receptors in a Papio Papio baboon who had spontaneous seizure.[34] The only child with absence seizures whose brain was studied at postmortem showed no abnormality.[35]

The preponderance of evidence favors a genetic etiology of absence seizures but the mode of inheritance is debatable. Lennox and Lennox[36] reported: (i) 34% of patients with 3 Hz spike wave pattern had family history of epilepsy (ii) 95% of monozygotic twins had absence seizures (iii) 85% of monozygotic twins had identical EEG abnormalities. Metrokos and Metrokos[37,38] claimed an autosomal dominant mode of inheritance for generalized spike and wave pattern with an age dependent maximal penetrance at 4-16 years, regardless of the presence of seizures. However, they included all types of spike wave abnormalities with only 81 of 211 probands having the 3 Hz spike wave pattern. Doose *et al.*[39] believed the inheritance to be polygenic. They suggested that epilepsies with spike wave absence were not inherited by a single autosomal dominant gene but by several genetic factors, some being independent and some either reinforcing or inhibiting the others. These findings are supported by animal studies.[40] The locus for absence seizures has been found to be chromosome 8q24, although the gene and the gene product have not yet been identified.

Pathophysiology

The unclear pathophysiological mechanisms of absence seizure are explained by following theories:

1. Centrencephalic theory.
2. Cortical theory.
3. Corticoreticular theory.

Centrencephalic Theory: Morison and Dempsey defined specific and non-specific thalamic activating system.[41] Penfield and Jasper[42] suggested the pathophysiologic mechanism must involve structures, which have widespread connections to the hemispheres. They explained the loss of consciousness, a fundamental feature of absence seizure resulted from a disturbance involving upper brainstem. Jasper and Droogleevar-Fortuyn[43] produced bisynchronous 3 Hz spike and wave discharge by electrical stimulation of the intralaminar nucleus of the thalamus in cats. Alumina implantations into the intralaminar nucleus of thalamus, reticular formation of midbrain also produced typical 3 Hz spike wave pattern with seizures.

Cortical Theory: Several clinical and experimental studies, suggested that cerebral cortex, played a primary role. Bancaud *et al.*[44] showed the electrical stimulation of human mesial frontal cortex produced clinical and EEG activity indistinguishable from spontaneous spike wave burst and absence seizure. Tucket and Jasper[45] suggested anterior parasagittal and mesial lesions being the originating areas. In experimental animals stimulation of premotor areas, produced typical EEG burst pattern of 3 Hz.[46,47] Thus there is evidence for both the cortical and centrencephalic theories.

Cortico-Reticular Theory: Gloor[48] concluded from his experimental work in animals, that there is a pre-existence of mild generalized cortical hyperexcitability and the epileptiform discharges and seizures are triggered by incoming thalamocortical volleys. The 3 Hz spike wave pattern represents an abnormal response pattern of cortical neurons to afferent thalamocortical volleys normally involved in elicitation of spindles. Such a response occurs under conditions of diffuse mild cortical hyper-excitability that causes cortical neurons to generate an increased number of action potentials per afferent volley. This secondarily leads to powerful activation of the intra-cortical recurrent inhibitory pathway. The result is an alteration of short periods of increased cortical excitation corresponding to the EEG spike with longer lasting periods of intense cortical inhibition, corresponding to the wave component of the spike and wave complex. The widespread fluctuations between increased excitation and increased inhibition disrupts the neuronal activity resulting in alteration of various components of higher mental functions like perception, memory, voluntary motor activity and cognition–the essential features of absence seizures.

Gloor and Testa[49] felt this cortical hyperexcitability was particularly prominent at the time when ascending reticular system was inactive. Clooland and Booker[50] observed that the seizure best developed during drowsiness and by partial sensory restrictions. Papini *et al.*[51] found 53.9% of absence seizures occurred during inactive wakefulness, 31.5% during drowsiness and only 8.1% during active wakefulness.

Gloor's hypothesis involves interaction of two anatomical areas:

(i) Diffusely hyperexcitable cortex.

(ii) Thalamus and mesencephalic reticular formation. The hyperexcitable state of cortex is due to inherited and/or biochemical trait and alteration of brainstem function is not a factor in the genesis of spike wave discharge. Although the Gloor's hypothesis is quite attractive and convincing, altered brainstem evoked potentials have been reported during absence seizures, a point at variance from Gloor's hypothesis.

Functional MRI Studies

So while cortex and thalamus are both involved in the generation of 3 Hz generalised spike-wave discharges, it is still unclear which structure initiates the cascade of processes underlying absence seizures. EEG-fMRI studies in patients with idiopathic generalized epilepsy (IGE) showed that thalamus, default mode areas, i.e., precuneus or parietal cortex,[52] and caudate nuclei are involved in short GSW paroxysms[53,54,55] (Aghakhani *et al.*, 2004; Gotman *et al.*, 2005; Hamandi *et al.*, 2006) and absence seizures. Moeller *et al.* found that, patient-specific BOLD signal changes were remarkably consistent in space and time across different absences like a fingerprint of one patient but were quite different from other patients, despite having similar EEG pattern and clinical semiology. They found that cortical activations and deactivation in default mode areas and caudate nucleus occurred earlier than the thalamus. So early frontal activation could support the cortical focus theory but this is patient specific.[56]

Differential Diagnosis

A number of non-epileptic conditions resemble absence seizures like inattentiveness due to lack of interest or fatigue, hypoglycemia, and various psychological factors. None of these have the characteristic EEG findings and with a careful history can be readily differentiated. Partial complex seizures have many superficial resembling features to absence seizures but have certain differentiating features as described in Table 18.1.

Table 18.1: Differentiating Features of Complex Partial and Absence Seizures

	Complex Partial	Absence
Onset	May have simple partial onset	Abrupt
Duration	Usually >30 s	Usually <30 s
Automatisms	Present	Duration dependent
Awareness	No	No
Ending	Gradual-postictal	Abrupt

Treatment

Aim should be a complete resolution of the seizures and elimination of all spike wave pattern from the EEG. Failure to activate epileptiform discharges during hyperventilation is a good indicator of optimum therapy. The treatment should be started with a single agent and only after an adequate trial and with compliance confirmed by therapeutic blood level, should a second agent be added. The refractory cases may need two agents.

Ethosuximide: It is the drug of choice. It has an elimination half-life of 20-60 hours. And reaches steady state concentration after 8-10 days of chronic administration. Treatment is started with 10 mgm/kg/day and gradually increased to 20-30 mgm/kg/day if seizures are not controlled with lesser dosage. The therapeutic blood level range 40-100 microgram/ml. Once daily dose provides adequate blood level but it may produce drowsiness or gastric irritation and so twice daily schedule is better. Ethosuximide is extremely effective in controlling both clinical absence seizure and 3 Hz spike wave discharge on EEG. Winstein and Allen[57] reported 70% of patients obtain 90% or better seizure control with ethosuximide. About 1-7% of patients with this drug develop leucopenia, which is reversible if detected early.

Valproic Acid: Valproic acid is extremely effective in controlling clinical absence seizures as well as 3 Hz spike-wave discharges on EEG but due to its cost and potential lethal hepatotoxicity it remains the drug of second choice. It has a half-life of 8-15 hours. Treatment is started with 10 mgm/kg/day and slowly increased until seizure control is achieved. Dose of upto 60 mgm/kg/day may be required. The therapeutic blood level range is 5-120 microgram/ml. Valproic acid interacts more often with other antiepileptic drugs decreasing serum level of hydration or carbamazepine while increasing of Phenobarbital. 15-30% of patients show a transient asymptomatic increase in SGOT level while several fatal cases of hepatotoxicity have been reported till date.[58,59] Valproate is the drug of choice where absence seizures are complicated by concurrent grand mal seizures. The side effects of the drug are sedation, transient alopecia, pancreatitis, stomatitis, tremors similar to essential tremors, thrombocytopenia, poor platelet aggregation and chronic use makes the hair then and lusterless.

Lamotrigine: Lamotrigine is now being used as a monotherapy particularly in absence seizures. It has a life of 29 hours as monotherapy, 15 hours if used with enzyme inducing drugs and 60 hours if used with valproate as comedication. Its mechanism of action is by stabilization of neural membrane by blocking voltage dependent sodium channel conductance. It is well absorbed orally with bioavailability about 100% with peak concentration in 1-3 hours. It is 55% bound to plasma protein. The dose in children depends on the co-medication for those co-medicated with valproate the schedule is for first two weeks 0.15 mgm/kg, for weeks 3 and 4; 0.3 mgm/kg and then 0.3 mgm/kg increments every one to two weeks to achieve a maintenance dose of 1-5 mgm/kg. Monotherapy dose for children is initially 0.5 mgm/kg/day raising to 1 mgm/kg after two weeks with a maintenance dose ranging between 2 and 8 mgm/kg. It is also effective for atypical absences.

Clonazepam: Clonazepam is as effective as ethosuximide[60] but its high rate of side effects particularly drowsiness, ataxia and development of tolerance limits its use. Treatment is started with 0.05 to 0.2 mgm/kg/day with a low increment of 0.25 to 0.5 mgm every 4-5 days to a maximum of 8 mgm/day.

Others: *Acetazolamide* may be of benefit in some patients but it is usually a transient effect. There is no role currently for agents as methosuximide, phensuximide or trimethadione.

Newer Anti-Epileptic Drugs like Levetiracetam and Zonisamide have been found to be promising in the management of absence seizures in small case series, however their efficacy needs to be substantiated by larger randomized trials.

Tiagabine, vigabatrin and possibly gabapentin has been associated with exacerbation of absence seizures. The use of carbamazepine also has been associated with exacerbation of absence seizures in some patients.

Duration of Treatment

After a seizure free interval of 2-3 years, the drug should be carefully withdrawn.

Prognosis

50-70% of patients with absence seizure cease to have seizures spontaneously in teenage years. Sato *et al.*[61] found that following prognostic factors were useful for predicting cessation of absence seizures:

(i) Normal or above normal intelligence.

(ii) Normal EEG background.

(iii) Negative history of tonic clonic seizure.

(iv) Negative family history of seizure disorders.

About 90% of patients with all of these prognostic factors cease having seizures of any type. Most authorities agree that:

(a) Absence of any seizure before onset of absence[61]

(b) Onset between 4 and 8 years.[62]

(c) A shorter duration of seizures.[57]

(d) Prompt response to treatment;[61, 62] and

(e) Normal intelligence and neurological examination are good prognostic indicators.[63]

25-30% of patients with absence seizure also develop tonic clonic seizures. Livingstone[64] suggested that children with absence seizure should also be treated with an agent effective against tonic clonic seizures. Most authorities do not agree on prophylactic treatment for tonic clonic seizure. Tonic clonic seizures when develop do so after 8 years of age.

Majority of patients with absence seizures have normal intelligence, however, 20-30% of patients have IQs of less than 90. This may occur due to social factors as falling behind at school, attitude to the disease, or adverse effect of the antiepileptic drugs.

ATYPICAL ABSENCE

Lennox and Davis[65] was the first to describe subtle motor manifestation and/or absence with atypical spike wave activity in the EEG. Gastaut *et al.*[66] distinguished the types of atypical absence seizure depending upon whether alteration of consciousness is complete or incomplete. Most authorities believe the former to be a variant of tonic seizures. The latter, referred as atypical absence seizure has decreased responsiveness and the onset and cessation are more gradual than in typical absence seizures. Erba and Cavazzuti[67] reported that during slow spike wave activity certain patients have selective and variable impairment of high cortical function while they are still responsive and able to attend to the assigned task. This variety of incomplete absence seizure may also be accompanied by automatisms, an increase or decrease of postural tone (more marked than in typical absence seizures or autonomic phenomena).

Etiology and Pathophysiology

Only a minority of patients with atypical absence seizures have primarily generalized epilepsy and these suggest genetic predisposition. While the majority are symptomatic of an underlying acquired encephalopathy of a fixed or progressive nature.

The mechanisms responsible for the production of atypical absence seizure are similar to those responsible for the production of absence seizures.

EEG

The ictal EEG shows diffuse often asymmetrical slow spike wave bursts of 1-2.5 Hz usually 5 to 15 seconds in duration. The interictal EEG of atypical absence of idiopathic type is normal. However, if there is an underlying encephalopathy the EEG background is usually abnormal and show slow spike wave discharges or other forms of slowing, spikes or irregular spike wave activity. These abnormalities are often asymmetrical.

Treatment

Lamotrigine, Topiramate, Valproic acid and clonazepam are effective while ethosuximide is effective in only a minority of patients.

Juvenile Absence Epilepsy

The age of onset of this syndrome is around puberty, males and females being equally affected. The seizures are clinically similar to those in childhood absence epilepsy but with important differences: they occur infrequently and often sporadically, retropulsive eye movements are less common during the absences, and they are associated with a less complete impairment of cognition (although some impairment of consciousness is invariable). Generalized tonic clonic seizures nearly always occur, usually on awakening. Myoclonic seizures may also be present.

Spike-wave discharges on the EEG have a frequency greater than 3 Hz usually 3.5-4 Hz. Juvenile absence epilepsy does not remit, but absences may become less frequent after the age of 30 years.

Treatment

Lamotrigine, Topiramate, Valproic acid and clonazepam are effective. Levetiracetam and Zonisamide have been found to be promising, however, more studies are required to substantiate this.

Myoclonic Absence

It is characterized by brief unconsciousness with a staring, automatism and bilateral symmetric clonic jerks. The EEG shows spike wave discharge of 3 Hz. Myoclonus with absence differs from myoclonic absence in that the jerks are asymmetric, automatism reactive.

Myoclonic absences are rare. Only 0.5-1 per cent of a selected population of children with epilepsy had this seizure type.[68] The onset and offset of myoclonic absences are abrupt. Seizures occur frequently throughout the day and are of 10-60 seconds' duration. Consciousness may not be completely lost, though it is impaired in most instances. The motor component consists of a rhythmic jerking of the shoulders, head and arms, and staggering. Falls are unusual. An arrest or alteration in the respiratory pattern may be observed. Some patients are incontinent during the attacks. A tonic contraction may follow the initial myoclonia.

Generalized tonic clonic seizures are also seen in some patients. Hyperventilation will precipitate the attacks in about two thirds of the cases, and about half the children are photosensitive. Wakening from sleep may also precipitate attacks.

Males are affected more commonly than females. The attacks may begin at almost any age during childhood. In about half the cases, mental retardation precedes the onset of seizures.

Differential Diagnosis

- Myoclonic absences differ from other absences by the relative prominence of motor symptoms.
- Other syndromes with myoclonia tend to have 2 Hz spike wave discharges on EEG rather than the 3 Hz frequency seen in this syndrome.

Etiology

Epilepsy with myoclonic absences may be intermediary between idiopathic generalized and symptomatic generalized epilepsies. Genetic factors appear to be important. A family history of epilepsy is present in 25 per cent of cases; otherwise, nothing is known of the aetiology. Chromosomal abnormalities, for example 12p, may rarely be associated with this syndrome.[69]

Treatment

A combination of sodium valproate and ethosuximide is most likely to control the seizures. Lamotrigine was effective in a small number of patients who failed to respond to ethosuximide, valproate or clonazepam.[70]

Prognosis

- **Seizures:** The seizures remit in some cases. In others, they become complicated by the appearance of tonic attacks and atypical absences such as occur in the Lennox-Gastaut syndrome. The EEG then shows slow spike wave discharges rather than 3 Hz paroxysm.

- **Neurological handicaps:** Gross disturbances do not usually occur, but most affected children are mildly ataxic and some have moderate or severe dyspraxia.
- **Cognition:** Of the children who are intellectually normal at the onset of the myoclonic absences, about half later lose cognitive skills. About 75 per cent are finally intellectually impaired.
- **Behavior:** No specific behavior has been related to epilepsy with myoclonic absences.

Absence Status

Absence status can be best subdivided into at least two separate syndromes, with overlapping clinical and EEG features. Both should be distinguished from complex partial status, which can take a similar clinical form.

- **Typical absence status:** Non-convulsive status, occurring in the syndrome of idiopathic generalized epilepsy.
- **Atypical absence status:** Status that occurs largely in secondarily generalized epilepsy of the Lennox-Gastaut type, and also in other patients with compromised cerebral function.
- Whilst this is a tidy classification scheme, there are transitional cases which do not fit happily into either category.

Typical Absence Status

Absence status occurs in about 3-9% of patients with typical absence.[71] The attacks can recur, and can last for hours or occasionally days precipitating features are common and include menstruation, withdrawal of medication, hypoglycemia, hyperventilation, flashing or bright lights, sleep deprivation, fatigue and stress. The main clinical feature is clouding of consciousness. This can vary from slight clouding to profound stupor. At one extreme, patients have nothing more than slowed ideation and expression, and deficits in activities requiring sustained attention, sequential organization or spatial structuring. Amnesia may be slight or even absent. At the other extreme, there may be immobility, mutism, simple voluntary actions performed only after repeated requests, long delays in verbal responses, monosyllabic and hesitant speech. Typically, the patient is in an expressionless, trance-like state with slow responses and a stumbling gait. Motor features occur in about 50% of cases, including myoclonus, atonia, rhythmic eyelid blinking, quivering of the lips and face. Facial, especially eyelid, myoclonus is common in absence status, but rare in complex partial status. Episodes of absence status are often terminated by a tonic clonic seizure. The diagnostic electrographic pattern is continuous or almost continuous bilaterally synchronous and spike/wave activity.

Atypical Absence Status: This form of status is common in patients with diffuse cerebral damage and is typically seen as part of the Lennox-Gastaut syndrome. Although the clinical phenomenology of typical and atypical absence status overlap greatly, there are important differences. The clinical context is very different; typical absence status occurs in patients without intellectual deterioration, very unlike the clinical picture of the Lennox-Gastaut syndrome. The episodes of atypical absence status are usually longer and more frequent, with a gradual onset and offset. Atypical absence status is often preceded by changes in motor activity, mood or intellectual ability, for hours or days before the overt seizures develop. This prodromal stage might be caused by sub clinical status. Atypical absence status tends to fluctuate and minor motor, myoclonic or, more typically, tonic seizures interrupt, but do not terminate an episode. In some patients, the mental state fluctuates gradually in and out of this ill-defined epileptic state over long periods of time, some attacks last weeks or even months with little distinction possible between ictal and interictal phases. Unlike typical absence status, tonic clonic seizures seldom occur at the beginning or end of the status episode, and atypical absence status often responds poorly to injection of a benzodiazepine. Indeed antiepileptic drug therapy has little effect, and condition fluctuates apparently uninfluenced by external factors. Atypical absence status is more likely to occur if the patient is drowsy or understimulated, and it is thus important not to overmedicate these patients. The EEG during atypical absence status may show continuous irregular slow (2Hz) spike/wave, hypsarrhythmia or more discrete ital patterns.

De Novo Absence Status of Late Onset

This is a condition which presents in later life, usually without a history of recent epilepsy. It is commonly caused by drug withdrawal (especially psychotropic drugs or benzodiazepines).

Treatment

1. **Absence Status Epilepticus:** There is no evidence that absence status epilepticus induces neuronal damage, and thus aggressive treatment is not warranted. Typical absence status (petit mal status) can usually be terminated by intravenous benzodiazepine therapy, diazepam of 0.2-0.3 mg/kg, clonazepam 1 mg (0.25-0.5 mg in children) or lorazepam 0.07 mg/kg (0.1

mg/kg in children), repeated if required. If this is ineffective, intravenous phenytoin or valproate can be used. Once controlled maintenance therapy with valproate, Lamotrigine or ethosuximide is required.

2. **Atypical Absence Status Epilepticus:** This is usually poorly responsive to intravenous benzodiazepines, which should in any case be giving cautiously as they induce tonic status epilepticus in occasional cases. Oral rather than intravenous treatment is usually more appropriate, and the drugs of choice are valproate, lamotrigine, clonazepam and clobazam. Sedating medications like carbamazepine have been reported to worsen these seizures. Conversely, arousal or stimulation can terminate the status. Often the episodes are self-limiting and therapy is not required.

3. **De Novo Absence Status of Late Onset:** As it is commonly caused by drug withdrawal (especially psychotropic drugs or benzodiazepines), and can be safely treated by intravenous diazepam, lorazepam. Long-term maintenance therapy is not usually required.

References

1. Temkin O. The Falling Sickness. A History of Epilepsy from the Greeks to the Beginning of Modern Neurology. Baltimore: John Hopkins Press 1971:2nd Edition.
2. Jackson JH. On Temporary Mental Disorders After Epileptic Paroxysms In: Taylow J (Edition). Selected Writings of John Hughling Jackson, Vol. 1, London, Hodder and Stoughton 1981:119-34.
3. Gibbs FA, Davis H, Nennox WG. The EEG in Epilepsy and Conditions of Impaired Consciousness. Arch. Neurol Psychiat 1935:34:1134-48.
4. Dreifuss FE. Proposal for Revised Clinical and Electrophysiologic Classification of Epileptic Seizures. Epilepsia 1981:22:489-501.
5. Gastaut H. Clinical Electroencephalographical Classification of Epileptic Seizures. Epilepsia 1975:16:1-66.
6. Hauser WA, Kurland LT. Epidemiology of Epilepsy in Rochester. Minnesota 1935-1967. Epilepsia 1975:16:1-66.
7. Cavazutti GB. Epidemiology of Different Types of Epilepsy in School Age Children of Modena, Italy, Epilepsia 1980:21:57-62.
8. Viani F, Beghi EH, Atza G and Gulotta MP. Classification of Epileptic Syndrome. Advantages and Limitations for Evaluation of Childhood Epileptic Syndromes in Clinical Practice, Epilepsia 1988:29:440-45.
9. Penry JK, Proter RJ and Dreifuss FE. Simultaneous Recording of Absence Seizure with Video Tape and Electroencephalography. A Study of 374 Seizures in 45 Patients, Brain 1975:98:427-40.
10. Livingstone S, Torres L, Pauli LL. Petit Mal Epilepsy, Result of a Prolonged Follow-up Study of 117 Patients, JAMA 1965:194:113-18.
11. Holowwach J, Thurston DLO'Leary JL. Petit Mal Epilepsy. Pediatrics 1962:30:893-901.
12. Ounstead C, Hutt SJ, Lee D. The Retrograde Amnesia of Petit Mal. Lancet 1963:1:671.
13. Sto S, Dreifuss FE and Penry JK. Prognostic Factors in Absence Seizures. Neurology 1976:26:778-96.
14. Weir B. The Morphology of the Spike Wave Complex. Electroenceph. Clin. Neurophysiol 1965:19:284-90.
15. Cobb WA, Gordon N, Mathews C. The Occipital Delta Rhythm in Petit Mal. Electroenceph. Clin. Neurophysiol 1961:13:142-43.
16. Luqaresi E. Discussion Remarks in Gastaut H, Waltregny A, Poire R, Regis H Eds. Les Activities Electriques Cerebrals Spontaneous.
17. Gastaut H. Discussion Remarks in Gastaut H, Waltrogny A, Poire R, Regis H, eds. Les Activites Electriques Spontaneous et evoquees chez L'homme 1967:217-18.
18. Brown TR, Dreifuss FE, Penry JK *et al.* Clinical and EEG Estimates of Absence Seizure Frequency. Arch Neurol 1983:40:469-72.
19. Adams DJ, Lueders H. Hyperventilation and Six-hour EEG Recording in Evaluation for Absence Seizures, Neurology 1981:31:1175-77.
20. Newmark ME and Penry JK. Photosensitivity and Epilepsy. A Review, New York, Raven Press 1979.
21. Sato S, Dreifuss FE, Penry JK. The Effect of Sleep on Spike Wave Discharges in Absence Seizure, Neurology 1973:23:1335-45.
22. Browne TR, Penry JK, Porter RJ *et al.* Responsiveness Before, During and After Spike Wave Paroxysm, Neurology 1974:24:655-59.
23. Mirsky AF, Van Buren JM. On the Nature of the Absence of Centrencephalic Epilepsy. A Study of Some Behavioral, Electroencephalographic and Autonomic Factors, Electroenceph, Clini, Neurophysiol 1965:18:334-48.
24. Geller M, Geller A. Brief Ammestic Effects of Spike Wave Discharges. Neurology 1970:20:1089-95.
25. Orren MM. Evoked Potential, Studies in Petit Mal Epilepsy. In:cobb WA, Van Duyn H eds. Contemporary Clinical Neurophysiology (EEG Suppl. No. 34) Amsterdam: Elsevier 1978.
26. Mirsky AF and Van Buren JM. On the Nature of the Absence on Centrencephalic Epilepsy. A Study of Some Behavioral Electrencephalograpic and Autonomic Factors. Electroencephalogr. Clin. Neurophysiol 1965:18:334.
27. Erba G and Cavazzuti V. Incomplete Absence Selective and Variable Functional Loss During Spike Wave Activity. Electroencephalogr. Clin. Neurophysiol 1980:50:217.
28. Steward LF, Dreifusas FE. Centrencephalic Seizure Discharges in Focal Hemispheric Lesions. Arch. Neurol 1972:26:409-19.
29. Loissau P, Cohadon F, Cohadon S. Recordings of Absence of Petit Mal Type in a Man of 40 with Epileptic Attacks Since

the Age of 3. Who had A Frontal Glioma. Electroenceph. Clin. Neurophysiol 1971;30:251.

30. Neidermeyer E. The Generalized Epilepsies. Springfield. III: Charles C Thomas 1972.

31. Scherman R. Abraham K. Centrencephalic Electroencephalographic Patterns in Precocious Puberty. Electroencephl. Clin. Neurophysiol 1963:15:559-67.

32. Andermann F. Absence Attacks and Diffuse Neuronal Disease. Neurology 1967:17:205-21.

33. Wikler A. Essiq CF. Withdrawal Seizures following Chronic Intoxication with Barbiturates and Other Sedative Drugs. In: Neidermeyer E eds. Epilepsy. Recent Views on Theory. Diagnosis and Therapy of Epilepsy. 1970. Basel. Karper170-84.

34. Swquires R. Naquet R. Richo D *et al.* Increased Thermolability of Benzodiazepine Receptors in Cerebral Cortex of a Baboon with Spontaneous Seizures. A Case Report. Epilepsia 1979: 20:215-21.

35. Cohn R. A Neuropathological Study of a Case of Petit Mal Epilepsy. Electroencephl. Clin. Neurophysiol 1968;24:282.

36. Lennox WG and Lennox MA. Epilepsy and Related Disorders Vol. I Boston: Little Brown 1960.

37. Metrakos JD and Metrakos K. Genetics of Convulsive Disorders. Part I. Introduction. Problems. Methods and Baselines. Neurology 1960:10:228-40.

38. Metrakos JD and Metrakos K. Genetics of Convulsive Disorders. Part II. Genetic and Electroencephalographic Studies in Centrencephalic Epilepsy. Neurology 1961;11: 464-83.

39. Doose H. Gerken H. Horstmann T *et al.* Genetic Factors in Spike Wave Absences. Epilepsia 1973;14:57-75.

40. Seyfried TN. TuRK. Glaser GH. Genetic Analysis of Audiogenic Seizure Susceptibility C57BL/6JK DBA/2J Recombinant Inbred Strains of Mice. Genetics 1980;94: 197-210.

41. Morison RS. Dempsey EW. A Study of Thalamocortical Relations Am J Physiol 1942:135:281-92.

42. Penfield W and Jasper H. Epilepsy and the Functional Anatomy of the Human Brain. Boston Little. Brown 1954.

43. Jasper HH. Doorgleever. Fortuyn J. Experimental Studies on the Functional Anatomy of Petit Mal Epilepsy. Res Publ. Assoc. Res. Nerv. Ment. Dis 1946;26:272-98.

44. Bancand J. Talairach P. Morel M. *et al.* Generalized Epileptic Seizures Elicited by Electrical Stimulation of the Frontal Lobe in Man. Electroencephl. Clin. Neurophysiol 1974;37:275-82.

45. Tukel K. Jasper H. The Electroencephalogram in Parasagittal Lesions. Electroenceph. Clin. Neurophysiol 1952;4:481-94.

46. Pollon DA. Experimental Spike and Wave Responses in Petit Mal Epilepsy. Epilepsia 1968;9:221.

47. Marcus EM. Experimental Models of Petit Mal Epilepsy. In Purpura DP *et al.* eds. Experimental Models of Epilepsy. New York. Raven Press 1972.

48. Gloor P. Quesney LF. Zumstein H. Pathophysiology of Generalized Epilepsy in the Cat. The Role of Cortical and Subcortical Structures. II. Topical Application of Penicillin to the Cerebral Cortex and Subcortical Structures. Electroenceph. Clin. Neurophysiol 1977;43:79-94.

49. Gloor P. Testa G. Generalized Pencillin Epilepsy in the Cat. Effects of Intracarotid and Intravertebral Pentylenetetrazol and Amobarbital Injections. Electroenceph. Clin. Neurophysiol 1974;36:499-515.

50. Clooland CS. Booker HE. Petit Mal Evoked by Arousal During Sensory Restriction. Arch. Neurol 1967;17:324-30.

51. Papini M. Pasquinelli A. Armellin M *et al.* Alertness and Incidence of Seizures in Patients with Lennox-Gastaut Syndrome. Epilepsia 1984;25:161-67.

52. Raichle ME. Mintun MA. Brain Work and Brain Imaging. Annu Rev Neurosci 2006;29:449-76.

53. Aghakhani Y. Bagshaw AP. Benar CG. Hawco C. Andermann F. Dubeau F. Gotman J. fMRI Activation During Spike and Wave Discharges in Idiopathic Generalized Epilepsy. Brain 2004;127:1127-44.

54. Gotman J. Grova C. Bagshaw A. Kobayashi E. Aghakhani Y. Dubeau F. Generalized Epileptic Discharges Show Thalamocortical Activation and Suspension of the Default State of the Brain. Proc Natl Acad Sci USA 2005;102: 15236-40.

55. Hamandi K. Salek-Haddadi A. Laufs H. Liston A. Friston K. Fish DR. Duncan JS. Lemieux L. EEG fMRI of Idiopathic and Secondarily Generalized Epilepsies. Neuroimage 2006; 31:1700-10.

56. Moeller F. Maneshi M. Pittau F. Gholipour T. Bellec P. Dubeau F. Grova C and Gotman J (2011). Functional Connectivity in Patients with Idiopathic Generalized Epilepsy. Epilepsia 52:515-22.

57. Weinstein AW. Allen RJ. Ethosuximide Treatment of Petit Mal Seizures. Am J Dis Child 1966;111:63-67.

58. Willmore LJ. Wilder BJ. Bruni *et al.* Effect of Valproic Acid on Hepatic Function. Neurology 1978;28:961-64.

59. Sussman NM. Mclain LW. A Direct Hepatotoxic Effect of Valproic Acid. JAMA 1979;242:1173-74.

60. Sato S. Pensy JK. Dreifuss *et al.* Clonazepam in the Treatment of Absence Seizures. A Double Blind Clinical Trial. Neurology 1977;27:371.

61. Sato S. Dreifuss Fe. Penry JK. Prognostic Factors in Absence Seizures. Neurology 1976;26:788-96.

62. Roger J. Prognostic Features of Petit Mal Absence. Epilepsia 1974;15:433.

63. Loiseau P. Postro M. Darligues JF *et al.* Long Term Prognosis in Two Forms of Childhood Epilepsy. Typical Absence Seizures and Epilepsy with Rolandic (centre temporal) EEG Foci. Ann. Neurol 1983;13:642-48.

64. Livingstone S. Torres I. Pauli LL *et al.* Petit Mal Epilepsy. Result of a Prolonged Follow-up Study of 117 Patients. JAMA 1965;194:113-18.

65. Lennox WG and Davis JP. Clinical Correlates of the Fast and Slow Spike Wave Electroencephalog. Pediatrics 1950:5: 626-29.

66. Gastaut H. Generalized Non Convulsive Seizures Without Local Onset. In Vinken PJ and Bryun GW (eds.) Handbook of Clinical Neurology. Vol. 15. The Epilepsies. Amsterdam. Elsevier 1974.

67. Erba G and Cavazzuti V. Incomplete "Absence" Selective and Variable Functional Loss During Spike Wave Activity. Electroencephalogr. Clin. Neurophysiol 1980:50:217-22.

68. Tassinari CA. Bureau M. Thomas P. Epilepsy with Myoclonic Absences. In: Epileptic Syndromes in Infancy. Childhood and Adolescence. Eds. Roger J. Bureau M. Dravet CH. Dreifuss FE. Perret A. Wolf P. John Libbey. London 1992:151-60.

69. Elia M. Guerrini R. Musumeci SA *et al.*. Myoclonic Absence Like Seizures and Chromosome Abnormality Syndromes. Epilepsia 1998:39:660-63.

70. Manonnani V. Wallace SJ. Epilepsy with Myoclonic Absences. Archieves of Disease in Childhood 1994:70:288-90.

71. Shorvon SD. Emergency Treatment of Epilepsy: Acute Seizures. Serial Seizures. Seizures Clusters and Status Epilepticus. In: Handbook of Epilepsy Treatment. Blackwell Science Ltd. 2000:173-94.

19 Chapter

FOCAL SEIZURES

N Thilothammal

Focal seizures are disturbances that arise in more or less a well-defined area of the brain and the nature of seizures depends on the site of abnormal discharge. Although focal epileptic episode may confine to a part of the body at the onset, it may spread and become generalized, thus becoming a secondarily generalized seizure. The secondary generalization may be so fast that the initial features of focal nature may not be apparent to the observer. The patient may however experience specific motor, sensory or autonomic symptoms giving a clue to the epileptic focus.

The focal seizures are usually classified into focal aware seizure and focal impaired awareness seizures based on the conscious state of the patient. In focal aware seizure, consciousness is not lost during the attack and in focal impaired awareness seizure, consciousness is altered or lost. Earlier focal impaired awareness seizure was called complex partial seizure and it is also known as temporal lobe epilepsy or psychomotor seizure.

The ILAE recently reclassified seizures and epilepsies. The classification still depends primarily on clinical and electroencephalography (EEG) features but with modest changes in some of the terminology[1,2] (Table 19.1). The term focal onset replaces the term partial onset, and focal onset seizures are placed into two categories: aware and impaired awareness. Focal seizures that become generalized seizures are now referred to as "focal to bilateral tonic-clonic" instead of "partial with secondary generalization". Many of the descriptions of the motor and non-motor activity that occurs during the seizure remain the same.

Table 19.1: ILAE Seizure Classification, 2017

Focal onset	
Aware	**Impaired Awareness**
Motor onset	
Automatism	
Atonic	
Epileptic spasm	
Hyperkinetic	
Myoclonic	
Tonic	
Non-Motor onset	
Autonomic	
Behavioral arrest	
Cognitive	
Emotional	
Sensory	
Focal to bilateral tonic-clonic	

Old terms	New terms
Partial	Focal
Simple partial	Focal aware
Complex partial	Focal impaired awareness
Psychic	Cognitive
Secondary generalized tonic-clonic	Focal to bilateral tonic-clonic
Arrest, Freeze, Pause, Interruption	Behavior arrest
Dyscognitive	Focal impaired awareness
Astatic (Focal or generalized)	Atonic
Psychomotor	Focal impaired awareness

Focal aware seizures (Simple partial seizures) are not uncommon in children and seen in 5% and focal impaired awareness seizure (complex partial seizures) in about 30% of all seizures.[3] The focal seizures thus form a sizeable type of seizure disorder in children which merit detailed evaluation in order to help in treatment and prognostication.

PATHOPHYSIOLOGY OF FOCAL SEIZURES

Focal Aware Seizures (Simple Partial Seizures)

The spontaneous and repetitive abnormal discharges arise from a group of cortical neurons. They may spread through cerebral cortex to the corresponding site in the opposite hemisphere forming a mirror focus with no clinical change or spread through associate fibers and extend into wider areas of cortex or establish a thalamocortial circuit of impulses. When the epileptic discharges continue for hours or days, it is known as epilepsia partialis continua and is not common in children. If the discharge is in a regular march through motor or sensory area, it becomes Jacksonian epilepsy. When the impulses from a focus in one hemisphere spread through medial nuclei of thalamus bilaterally into reticular formation, consciousness is lost and thereafter the discharges spread upwards involving both hemispheres.[4,5]

Focal Impaired Awareness Seizure (Complex Partial Seizures)

Pathophysiology is exclusively confined to the temporal lobe and its connections with the limbic system. The limbic system is also known as visceral brain. It is a very intricate circuit comprising hippocampus, which fuses anteriorly with the tail end of caudate nucleus forming amygdale, posteriorly extends as fornix and finally ends in mamillary bodies of hypothalamus. The mamillothalamic tract connect the fornix and mamillary bodies with anterior thalamic nuclei which in turn project to cingulated gyrus and frontal cortex. There are also connections with insula and corresponding areas in the opposite hemisphere.[3] It is thus understandable that disturbances in such a complex and integrated system which is the seat of autonomic functions, emotional expression, olfaction, momory, regulation of cardiovascular, respiratory and alimentary systems are bound to produce complex symptomatology.[5,6]

Etiology

The causative factors of focal seizures are sometimes known, suspected or may remain unknown. Genetic predisposition is an important etiologic factor and is exemplified in bengin childhood focal epilepsies. It includes Rolandic epilepsy, Panayiotopoulos syndrome and idiopathic childhood occipital epilepsy of Gastaut.[5]

Hypoxic damage, post-traumatic insult to brain is common causes of focal seizures. Infection of brain, metabolic factors like hypernatremia or hyponatremia, dehydratiom and rarely hypoglycemia are known to cause focal seizures. Prolonged or clusters of febrile convulsion in childhood are found to cause damage to temporal lobes and focal seizures in later years. Space occupying lesions like tuberculoma, neurocysticercosis or Sturge-Weber Syndrome are common causes of recurrent focal seizures. Tuberculoma was found in 23% of cases with focal epilepsy.[7] Infarction was equally common etiologic factor in focal seizures. Children with hemiplegia, cerebral palsy, tuberous sclerosis and porencephalic cyst are invariably associated with focal seizures. Neurodegenerative disorders in children may give rise to focal seizures initially or rarely epilepsia partialis continua.

Symptomatology

Focal seizures are divided into three main categories:

- Focal aware seizures, in which there is no alternation of consciousness. It can be motor or non-motor seizure. In motor type, which is more common presentation in focal aware seizure, some type of movement occurs during the event. For example twitching, jerking or stiffening movements of a body part. In non-motor type, symptoms such as changes in sensation or autonomic functions occur.
- Focal impaired awareness seizures, in which consciousness is altered or lost. Non-motor symptoms are characteristic features that include changes in sensation, emotions, thinking or experiences. Focal awareness seizure can present with motor symptoms like automatism (automatic movements like licking lips, rubbing hands, walking or running).
- Focal to tonic-clonic seizures in which focal seizure develops into generalized seizure.

Auras: The term aura, which describes symptoms a person may feel in the beginning of a seizure, is not in the new classification. It's important to know that in most cases, these early symptoms may be the start of a seizure.

Focal seizures arising in different anatomical locations take different forms. About 60% of focal impaired awareness seizures have their origin in the temporal lobe and about 40% are extratemporal and focal aware seizures are more commonly extratemporal.[8] Both focal aware and focal impaired awareness seizures arising from any cortical area can spread to other regions.

Focal Aware Seizures

Most focal aware seizures are lasting a few seconds. Prolonged focal aware motor seizures tend to be confined to a limited anatomical region, and take the form of epilepsia partialis continua. The sub-classification of focal aware seizures with motor, sensory, autonomic and psychic symptoms is based on the distinct aura corresponding to the site of discharge. The cephalic aura (sense of discomfort, odd sensations and headache) is a common manifestation of an epileptic discharge in any cortical area.

Focal Aware Seizures with Motor Manifestation

The primary manifestations are jerking, dystonic spasm and posturing. They most commonly occur in epilepsies arising in frontal or central regions. The jerking can affect any muscle group, and the jerks may 'march' (the Jacksonian march) from one part of the body to another as the discharge spreads over the motor cortex. Head or eye turning can occur as an initial seizure manifestation (the adversive seizure).

If the seizure is initiated in or evolves to affect supplementary motor areas, posturing of the arms may develop, classically with adversial head, and eye deviation, abduction and external rotation of the contralateral arm and flexion at the elbows, often combined with posturing of the legs, and speech arrest or stereotyped vocalizations. Consciousness is usually maintained unless secondary generalization occurs. There is often an aura in these seizures, consisting of a very brief jolt, shock or emotional sensation. The classical posture is named by Penfield the 'fencing posture' (resembling as it does the en garde position).

Focal Aware Seizures with Somatosensory and/or Special Sensory Manifestation (Parietal Lobe Epilepsy)

Parietal lobe epilepsy generally causes focal aware seizures with somatosensory symptoms such as paresthesias (tingling or numbness, less commonly an electric-shock-like feeling, burning, pain or a feeling of heat), apraxia, and distortion of body image. These symptoms are most common in epileptic foci in central or parietal regions. Visual phenomena consisting of well-formed hallucinations have been reported and it consists of pictures of people, animals, or scenes. A receptive type of aphasia can occur if the epileptic activity is located on the dominant hemisphere.

Focal Aware Seizures with Visual Manifestations

Simple visual phenomena occur if the calcarine cortex is affected. Occipital lobe epilepsy is characterized by simple elementary visual symptoms, such as patterns or flashes of light or colors. Contralateral eye deviation and ictal blindness also are described.

Focal Aware Seizures with Autonomic Manifestations

Autonomic symptoms such as changes in skin colour, blood pressure, heart rate, pupil size and piloerection usually occur as a component of generalized or complex partial seizures of frontal or temporal origin. An epigastric sensation (often described as nausea, an empty or sick feeling), which may rise up to the throat, is the most common manifestation of a partial seizure arising in the temporal lobe and is frequently associated with psychic symptoms or alterations in consciousness:

Focal Aware Seizures with Psychic Manifestations

Psychic 'areas' can occur with very discrete discharges, and patients may retain normal awareness. Although there are recognized patterns, auras are not of reliable localizing value as discharges may activate widely distributed neuronal circuits. There are six principal categories:

- Dysphasic symptoms occur if cortical speech area (frontal or temporoparietal) are affected. Speech usually ceases or is several reduced. Repetitive vocalization with formed words may occur if a discharge originates in the non-dominant temporal lobe.
- Dysmnestic symptoms (disturbance of memory) may take the form of flashbacks, déjà vu, jamis vu or panoramic experiences (recollections of previous experiences, former life or childhood), and occur with temporal lobe seizure discharges.
- Cognitive symptoms include dreamy and sensations of unreality or depersonalization and occur primarily in temporal lobe seizures.
- Affective symptoms include fear (the most common symptom, which is sometimes very intense), depression, anger and irritability, and may be accompanied by autonomic effect. Elation, erotic thoughts, serenity or exhilaration may occur. Affective is most commonly seen with mesiobasal temporal lobe foci.
- Illusion of size (macropsia), shape, weight, distance, or sound occur, progressing as the seizure evolves. These symptoms are characteristic of temporal or parieto-occipital epileptic foci.

- Structured hallucination of visual, auditory, gustatory, or olfactory forms, which can be crude or elaborate, are usually due to epileptic discharges in the temporal or parieto-occipital association areas.

Epilepsia Partialis Continua (EPC)

This form of status epilepticus is defined as spontaneous regular or irregular clonic twitching of cerebral cortical origin, sometimes aggravated by action or sensory stimuli, confined to one part of the body, and continuing for hours, days or weeks.[9] This condition in children is most often due to chronic focal encephalitis (Rasmussen's chronic encephalitis). Other reported etiologies include cerebral infarction, harmorrphage, tumour, metabolic encephalopathy, mitochondrial disease non-ketotic hyperglycemia and Alper's disease.

Benign Childhood Focal Epilepsies

Benign childhood focal seizures and related idiopathic epileptic syndromes affect approximately 22% of children with non-febrile seizures. They comprise three identifiable electro-clinical syndromes recognized by International League Against Epilepsy (ILAE); Rolandic epilepsy, Panayiotopoulos syndrome and the Idiopathic childhood occipital epilepsy of Gastaut (ICOE-G).[10]

Rolandic Epilepsy (Benign Childhood Epilepsy with Centro-Temporal Spikes)

Rolandic epilepsy is the most common benign childhood focal epilepsy and it is genetically determined. The age of onset ranges from 1 to 14 years with 75% starting between 7 and 10 years. There is a 1.5 male predominance. The cardinal features of Rolandic epilepsy are focal seizures consisting of unilateral facial sensorimotor symptoms (30% of patients), oro-pharyngo-laryngeal symptoms (OPLS) (53%), speech arrest (40%) and hypersalivation (30%). Ictal manifestations indicative of temporal lobe involvement do not occur in Rolandic epilepsy, and the term 'centro-temporal' refers only to the spike topography where it is partly a misnomer.

Hemifacial sensorimotor seizures are mainly localized in the lower lip and may spread to the ipsilateral hand. Motor manifestations are clonic contractions sometimes concurrent with ipsilateral tonic deviation of the mouth, and sensory symptoms consist of numbness in the corner of the mouth. OPLSs are unilateral sensorimotor symptoms of numbness or paraesthesias (tingling, prickling or freezing) inside the mouth, associated with strange sounds, such as death rattle, gargling, grunting and guttural sounds.

Consciousness and recollection are fully retained in more than half (58%) of rolandic seizures. Progression to hemiconvulsions or generalized tonic-clonic seizures (GTCS) occurs in around half of children. Three-quarters of rolandic seizures occur during non-REM sleep, mainly at sleep onset or just before awakening. Rolandic seizures are usually brief lasting for 1-3 minutes.

Opercular status epilepticus usually occurs in children with atypical evolution or may be induced by carbamazepine or lamotrigine.This state lasts for hours to months and consists of ongoing unilateral or bilateral contractions of the mouth, tongue or eyelids, positive or negative subtle perioral or other myoclonus, dysarthria, speech arrest, difficulties in swallowing, buccofacial apraxia and hypersalivation.

EEG: By definition, centro-temporal spikes (CTS) are the hallmark of benign childhood epilepsy with CTS. However, although called centro-temporal, these spikes are mainly localized in the high central or low central (supra-sylvian) and not temporal electrodes (Fig. 19.1).

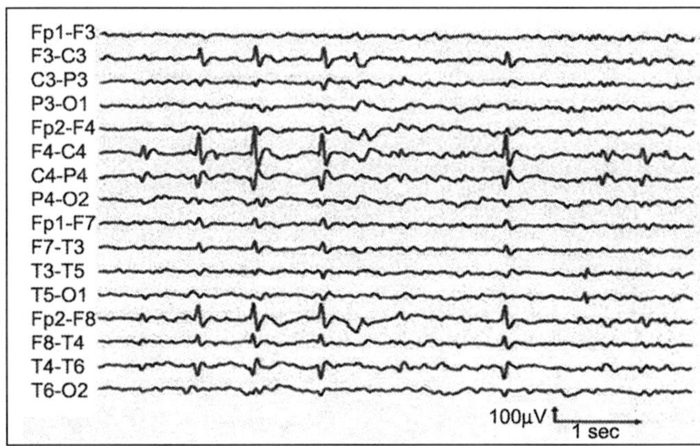

Fig. 19.1: Cento-temporal spikes in Rolandic epilepsy

Prognosis: For Rolandic seizures prognosis is almost invariably excellent, with probably < 2% risk of developing absence seizures and less often GTCS in adult life. Remission occurs within 2–4 years from onset and before the age of 16 years.

Panayiotopoulos Syndrome (PS)

PS is defined as benign age-related focal seizure disorder occurring in early and mid-childhood. It is characterized by seizures, often prolonged, with predominantly autonomic symptoms, and by an EEG that shows shifting and/or multiple foci, often with occipital predominance. Onset is from age 1 to 14 years with 76% starting between 3 and 6 years. PS, like Rolandic epilepsy, is probably genetically determined.

Ictal Autonomic Symptoms

Seizures commonly commence with autonomic manifestations (80-90%), while consciousness and speech, as a rule, are preserved. Ictus emeticus (nausea and retching) culminates in vomiting in 74–82% of seizures; Emesis is usually the first apparent ictal symptom, but it may also occur long after the onset of other manifestations. Other autonomic manifestations include pallor (28%), incontinence of urine (19%) and feces (3%), hypersalivation (10%), cyanosis (12%), mydriasis (7%) and less often miosis (2%), coughing and abnormalities of intestinal motility (3%). Breathing (7%) and cardiac irregularities may be more common than reported. Syncopal-like manifestations occur in at least one-fifth of seizures. The child becomes 'completely unresponsive and flaccid like a rag doll', which may precede, be concurrent with other seizure symptoms or be the sole manifestation of a seizure. They may occur while the patient is standing, sitting, lying down or asleep and last from 1-2 minutes to half an hour.[10]

Ictal Behavioural Changes

Restlessness, agitation, terror or quietness, may occur at the onset of seizures, often in combination with other autonomic manifestations.

Ictal Non-Autonomic Symptoms

In the majority of seizures, autonomic manifestations are followed by conventional seizure symptoms. Nearly always, the child gradually or suddenly becomes confused or unresponsive. Other non-autonomic manifestations include in order of prevalence, unilateral deviation of the eyes or eyes opening (60-83%), speech arrest (8-13%), hemifacial convulsions (6-13%), visual hallucinations (6-10%).The seizures may end with hemiconvulsions often with Jacksonian marching (19-30%), or generalized convulsions (21-36%).

The seizures are usually lengthy, last over 6 minutes and almost half of them last for >30 minutes to many hours, thus constituting autonomic status epilepticus. Even after the most severe seizures and status, the patient is normal after a few hours' sleep. There is no record of residual neurological abnormalities. Two-thirds of seizures start in sleep. The seizure type and duration are variable in a child.

EEG

In about 90% of cases, the EEG reveals mainly multifocal, high amplitude, sharp slow wave complexes that may appear in any area, often shifting from one region to another in the same or the contralateral hemisphere in sequential EEGs of the same child. Occipital spikes predominate but they do not occur in a third of patients (Fig. 19.2).

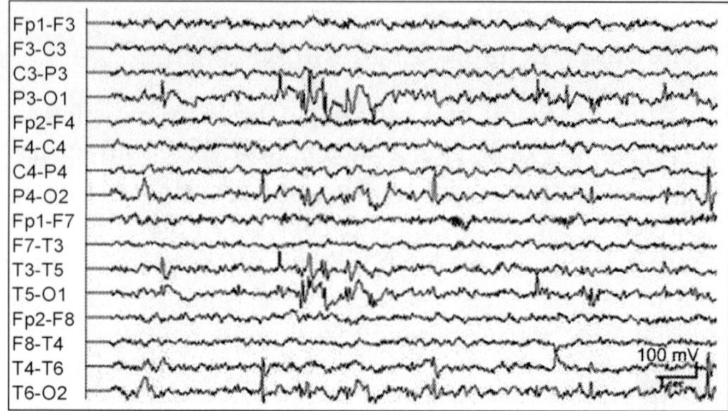

Fig.19.2: It shows normal background with high amplitude sharp and slow wave complexes similar to rolandic sharp waves. All brain regions are involved with posterior predominance

Prognosis

PS is remarkably benign. Remission often occurs within 1-2 years of onset but probably 10% may have more protracted active seizure periods. The risk of epilepsy in adult life appears to be no higher than in the general population and prognosis for cognitive function is good.

Idiopathic Childhood Occipital Epilepsy of Gastaut (ICOE-G)

The ICOE-G is a relatively rare form of pure occipital epilepsy accounting for about 2-7% of benign childhood focal seizures. Age at onset ranges from 3 to 15 years, but most start between 8 and 11 years. Both sexes are equally affected. Seizures are occipital and primarily manifest with elementary visual hallucinations, blindness or both. They are usually frequent, brief and diurnal.

Visual Ictal Symptoms

Elementary visual hallucinations are the most common and characteristic ictal symptom of ICOE-G. They are frequently the first and often the only seizure symptom consisting of small multicoloured circular patterns. Ictal blindness is probably the second most common symptom and is sudden, usually total. Complex visual hallucinations such as faces and figures occur in < 10% of patients.

Non-Visual Ictal Occipital Lobe Symptoms and Signs

Non-visual occipital symptoms usually appear after the elementary visual hallucinations and they are deviation of the eyes, eyelid fluttering or repetitive eye closures, pain and sensory hallucinations of ocular movements. Deviation of the eyes, often associated with ipsilateral turning of the head. Consciousness is intact during the visual symptoms (simple focal seizures), but may be disturbed or lost in the course of the seizure, usually before or at the time of eye deviation or convulsions. Elementary visual hallucinations or other ictal symptoms may progress to complex focal seizures (14%), hemiconvulsions (43%) or GTCS (13%). Postictal headache, mainly diffuse, but also severe, unilateral, pulsating and indistinguishable from migraine headache, occurs in half the patients.[10]

Seizure Stereotype

For any one patient, in every seizure, the elementary visual hallucinations have a fingerprint with a stereotypic appearance regarding morphology, colours, location, movement and other characteristics.

Visual seizures are usually brief, lasting from a few seconds to 1-3 minutes if they occur alone without other occipital or extraoccipital spreading. Visual seizures are predominantly diurnal and occur at any time of the day. If untreated, the majority of patients experience frequent brief visual seizures ranging from several every day to one per week or month.

Electroencephalography

The interictal EEG shows occipital paroxysms often demonstrating fixation off sensitivity (FOS).

Prognosis

The prognosis of ICOE-G is unclear, although available data indicate that remission occurs in 50 to 60% of patients within 2-4 years of onset. Rarely, atypical evolutions to epilepsy with CSWS (continuous spike and wave during sleep) and cognitive deterioration may occur. The performance scores for attention, memory and intellectual functioning are lower in patients with ICOE-G than control subjects.

Focal Impaired Awareness Seizure

Focal impaired awareness seizures arise from the temporal lobe in about 60% of cases and the frontal lobe in about 30%. Within the temporal lobe it may be (1) Mesio-basal origin or (2) Lateral neocortical origin. The typical focal impaired awareness seizure of temporal lobe has three components; aura, absence and automatisms.

Aura

An aura can occur in isolation as a focal aware seizure or the initial manifestation of a focal impaired awareness seizure.[11,12] It is typically comprises visceral, cephalic, gustatory, dysmnestic, or affective symptoms. The rising epigastric sensation is the most common aura, and other auras include perceptual or autonomic aura. Speech usually ceases or is severely reduced, but occasionally repetitive vocalization may occur. Simple auditory phenomena such as humming, buzzing, shissing and roaring may occur if the discharges occur in the superior temporal gyrus; and olfactory sensation, which are usually unpleasant and difficult to define, with seizure in the Sylvian region. More complex hallucinatory or illusionary states are produced with seizures discharges in association area (e.g., structural visual hallucination, complex visual patterns and musical sounds and speech).

Seizures frequently are preceded by an aura (epigastric discomfort, de´ja` vu ["already seen"], de´ja` entendu ["already heard"]), psychic symptoms such as fear, or automatisms (oroalimentary repetitive movements, vocalizations).

Absence/Altered Consciousness

This may follow the aura or evolve simultaneously. The altered consciousness takes the form of motor arrest, during which the patient is motionless and inaccessible. There is sometimes no outward sign; the patient's eyes may appear vacant or glazed, though sometimes minor motor sign, posturing or tone changes occur. Unilateral dystonic posturing of the limbs is common and is contralateral to the side of seizure onset.

Automatism

Automatism occur during or after the impairment of consciousness. An automatism is more or less coordinated involuntary motor activity usually followed by amnesia of the event.[11,12] Automatism (in distinction to aura) is of no localizing value and should be distinguished from simple postictal confusion, hysterical fugues, acute confusional states and somnambulism. Automatism are usually divided into:

- **Oro-Alimentary:** Orofacial movements such as chewing, lip smacking, swallowing, or drooling.
- **Mimicry:** With emotional expression, including displays or laughter or fear, anger or excitement.
- **Gestural:** Common movements include fiddling with the hands, tapping, patting, rubbing, ordering

and tidying movements; complex actions such as undressing; and genital directed actions.

- **Ambulatory Automatism:** Include walking, circling, running; sometimes the patient may wander around carrying out more or less purposeful, complex activity.
- **Verbal Automatism:** Sometimes these are meaningless sounds, humming, whistling, grunting and sometimes words which may be repeated, or formed sentences.
- **Responsive Automatism:** In which there is quasi-purposeful behavior, seemingly responsive to environmental stimuli.

Violent behavior sometimes occurs in an automatism, there is generally total amnesia for the events of the automatism, although a patient may not recognize that consciousness was fully lost.

Epilepsy Arising in the Frontal Lobe

Seizure of frontal lobe origin can take the form of focal impaired awareness seizures, focal aware seizures, and focal to bilateral tonic-clonic seizure.[13,14] Typically the seizures are frequent with a tendency to cluster. The attacks are brief, with a sudden onset and offset. Some types of frontal lobe seizure occur during sleep, and in some patients the epilepsy comprises frequent short nocturnal attacks (paroxysmal nocturnal dystonia). A brief, non-specific 'cephalic aura' may occur, which is a vague sensation of dizziness, strangeness, headache or the feeling that an attack is coming on. The absence (motor arrest) is usually short, and may be obscured by the prominent motor signs of the automatisms.

Frontal lobe automatism are typically gestural, especially comprising bilateral movements (e.g., cycling, stepping and kicking). The automatism are often highly excited, violent or bizarre and this leads, not frequently, to a misdiagnosis of non-epileptic attacks (pseudoseizures). Vocalization is common in frontal lobe automatisms. This can be a cry, sometimes very shrill and loud, other sounds or speech fragments. Postictal recovery is usually rapid, with a shorter period of postical confusion.[14]

Frontal lobe focal seizures have a more marked tendency to secondarily generalization than focal seizures of temporal lobe origin, and there is also commonly a history of status epilepticus, of both the tonic-clonic and non-convulsive types[15] (Table 19.2).

Diagnosis

A detailed history of evolution of the symptoms, aura if any, ictal and postictal events should be recorded. Behavioral data must also be noted.

Plain X-ray of Skull

Not generally informative. It may show calcification in a hamartoma or a depressed fracture of skull or constriction of middle cranial fossa.

Biochemical Assessment

Estimation of blood sugar, serum calcium, sodium, magnesium or lead, to eliminate metabolic triggering factors, when suspected.

Electroencephalography

Focal abnormality in the form of spike or spike and slow wave discharge is seen. The secondarily generalized seizures will be associated with high frequency and high amplitude waves during tonic phase followed by interrupted cortical spikes. Cessation of seizure is marked by isoelectric record followed by high amplitude irregular slow waves and appearance of original focal abnormality. Spikes are seen in central area unilaterally or bilaterally in benign epilepsy of childhood.

Table 19.2: Differentiation of Temporal and Frontal Focal Impaired Awareness Seizure

	Temporal	Frontal
Aura	More common, varied, at times suggesting	Nonspecific; vague cephalic sensations; forced thinking
Duration	1-2 minutes	10-60 seconds
Frequency	Several per week/month	Multiple per day, often in clusters
Onset	Arrest with stare or oroalimentary, automatism early	Vocalization; fearful facies
Automatism	Simple, oroalimentary. Picking at clothes	Bizarre, semipurposeful, complex; bimanual/bipedal; sexual
Vocalization	Simple, speech possible	Bizarre (screaming, cursing)
Generalization	Uncommon	Common
Postical	Confusion, lethargy, aphasia; up to 30 minutes	Minimal or absent

In focal impaired awareness seizures, routine recording of EEG may fail to reveal the epileptic focus as it lies deep in temporal lobe. Sleep record, natural or drug induced is better than routine EEG and is three times more rewarding.[12] Hyperventilation and photic stimulation are useful provocative techniques in detecting the focus. An EEG may show bilateral foci in children thus confusing the laterality of the epileptic activity. Moreover in children the coexisting generalised onset or other seizures may complicate the EEG findings. EEG with sphenoidal electrodes though useful are not applicable in children. Nasopharyngeal electrodes however is safe in children and will help to tap the discharge from the undersurface of temporal lobe. In view of the limitations of routine EEG recording, more accurate and sophisticated techniques like EEG monitoring with video recording, telemetry and ambulatory recording have been discovered to enable localization of epileptic focus. It is however too costly and requires an elaborate setup.

CT Scan: Abnormal CT scan has been reported in 30-50% of focal impaired awareness seizures[4,7] CT scan also helps in delineating vascular malformation in the brain.

MRI gives good resolution of the image and helps in accurate localization. The common pathologies identified with MRI are hippocampal sclerosis, focal cortical dysplasia, low grade tumors and vascular malformations. A successful postoperative outcome is less likely in imaging-negative patients with both temporal and frontal lobe epilepsy.[16]

Positron Emission Tomography is a costly metabolic scanner. It is helpful in precise localization of epileptic focus with quantification of underlying physiological process.

Medical Management

Drugs of choice are carbamazepine, sodium valproate, phenytoin sodium, phenobarbitone clonazepam and clobazam. When the focal seizure is due to tuberculoma or neurocysticerosis specific therapy for the underlying disease should be added. If the seizure control is poor with first ling drugs, newer antiepileptic drugs need to be considered. A small percentage of cases remain seizure free and successful in life. Another group may not respond to medical treatment and become intractable seizures. With newer anticonvulsants chances of better control seizure seems likely.[17,18,19]

In children with newly diagnosed or untreated focal-onset seizures, Oxcarbazepine (OXC) is the only medication with established efficacy and effectiveness (Class I evidence). Nine other AEDs Carbamazepine (CBZ), Clobazam (CLB), Lamotrigine (LTG), Phenobarbitone (PHB), Phenytoin (PHT), Topiramate (TPM), Valproate (VPA), Vigabatrin (VGB) and Zonisamide (ZNS) have Class III evidence for efficacy/effectiveness as initial monotherapy meaning they may be effective but the clinical trial data are weak. The situation is much better for adjunctive therapy of intractable focal onset seizures, where there is Class I efficacy/effectiveness evidence for Gabapentin (GBP), Lamotrigine (LTG), Levetiracetam (LEV), Oxcarbazepine (OXC) and Topiramate (TPM) in children.[20,21]

Oxcarbazepine: Initial starting dose 5-10 mg/kg/day and the maintenance dose is 30-40 mg/kg/day.

Valproate: Starting dose is 15 mg/kg/day and the maintenance dose is 20-40 mg/kg/day.

Lamotrigine: Starting dose as monotherapy 0.3 mg/kg/day; with enzyme inducers 0.6 mg/kg/day and with valproate 0.15 mg/kg/day. The maintenance dose as monotherapy 2-8 mg/kg/day; with enzyme inducers 5-8 mg/kg/day and with valproate 1-5 mg/kg/day.

Topiramate: It is a useful adjunctive therapy for focal and generalized seizure in children of 2 years of age and older. Therapy should be started at an initial dose of 0.5-1 mg/kg/day and increased by 0.5-1 mg/kg/day at 1 to 2 week intervals. With enzyme inducers, starting dose is 1-2 mg/kg/day and maintenance dose is 5-9 mg/kg/day is two-divided dose. When used as monotherapy the starting dose is 0.5-1.5 mg/kg/day and the maintenance dose is 3-5 mg/kg/day.

Tiagabine: It is indicated as an adjunctive drug for focal seizures in children over 12 years of age. Starting dose is 0.1 mg/kg/ day with subsequent increase of 0.1 mg/kg/day in 1-2 weeks. Target dose is 0.6 mg/kg/day in children who are not taking enzyme inducing antiepileptic drugs and 1 mg / kg/day in those who are taking these drugs.

Zonisamide: It has been approved for adjunctive treatment of focal seizure, GTCS, myoclonic epilepsy and refractory absence seizure both in adults and in children. Initial dose is 1-2 mg/kg/day and increased every 1-2 weeks upto a dose of 4-8 mg/kg/day as a single dose or divided twice daily.

Levetiracetam: It has been proved to be effective as adjunctive therapy in children with focal seizures. Starting dose is 20 mg/kg/day and the maintenance dose is 30-40 mg/kg/day.

Lacosamide: It is used in children with refractory epilepsy with 30-50% of children having more than 50% reduction in seizure frequency.[22]

Perampanel: It is a selective, non-competitive antagonist of AMPA-type glutamate receptors. Efficacy and tolerability of adjunctive perampanel in patients aged >12 years with refractory partial-onset seizures has been demonstrated in three phase III, randomized, double-blind, placebo-controlled trials.[23]

Management of Benign Childhood Focal Seizures

In the acute stage, control of the seizure is of paramount importance. Benzodiazepines are used to terminate long lasting seizures (>10 min) and status epilepticus. Continuous prophylaxis consists of daily monotherapy using any AED that has proven efficacy in focal seizures and minimal adverse effects in children. Carbamazepine and valproic acid have equivalent efficacy. Others AEDs like phenobarbital, phenytoin and clonazepam are also effective. Carbamazepine may exaggerate seizures in a minority of children. Recommended newer AED include levetiracetam, gabapentin and lamotrigine. Lamotrigine on rare occasions may cause seizure exacerbation and cognitive deterioration. Treatment is to be continued for 1-3 years of seizure free period.

Surgical Treatment

Surgical intervention is considered for those with intractable seizures. The emergence of surgery in treatment of intractable epileptic has been accepted as a logical and meaningful approach. Mental retardation, status epileptic and abnormalities in background rhythm in EEG, has unfavourable prognostic factors in a child with temporal lobe epilepsy.[24] It is believed that children with fulminant clinical course of focal impaired awareness seizures with progressive intellectual impairment, may benefit from surgery. If there is clear EEG and clinical evidence of localization related epilepsy, with rigorous exclusion of childhood absence epilepsy and benign childhood epilepsy with centrotemporal spikes, and if the seizures are truly intractable and disabling despite aggressive medication trials for two or three years, then it is appropriate to consider epilepsy surgery.

Various surgical techniques employed are resection of mesial temporal lobe structures or resection of anterior 4-5 cm of lateral temporal lobe plus 23 cm of hippocampus. Some advocate resection of amygdalo-hippocampus, preserving the lateral temporal cortex.[21] The preoperative evaluation requires a battery of tests that include EEG localization of lesion, neuroradiologic findings, neuropsycholigical rating and correlation with areas of cerebral dysfunction. Postoperative outcome is based on seizure control and improvement in behavioral changes. If emotional maladjustment persists then it is considered bad prognosis.[3,25] When operable space occupying lesions are responsible for simple partial seizure, they need to be excised.

References

1. Scheffer IE, Berkovic S, Capovilla G, Connolly MB, French J, Guilhoto L. *et al.* ILAE Classification of the Epilepsies: Position Paper of the ILAE Commission for Classification and Terminology. Epilepsia 2017;58:512-21.
2. Fisher RS, Cross JH, French JA, Higurashi N, Hirsch E, Jansen FE, *et al.* Operational Classification of Seizure Types by the International League Against Epilepsy: Position Paper of the ILAE Commission for Classification and Terminology. Epilepsia 2017;58:522-30.
3. Simon D Shorvon. Epilepsy – A General Practice Perspective. Published by Cibageigy 1988:10-15.
4. O' Donohoe NV. Epilepsies of Childhood, 2nd Edition, London, Butterworth 1985:83-105.
5. Aicardi J. Epileptic Syndromes in Childhood–Recent Advances in Childhood Epilepsy. Epilepsia Suppl 3 1988;29:S1-S5.
6. Fenwick P. Behavioural Therapy of Epilepsy: Recent Advances in Epilepsy. Pedley TA and Meldrum BS (eds.) Vol. 5 1992:223-35.
7. Kamala D. *et al.* Focal Convulsions in Children – Abstract of Paper Presented in 24th Ann. Conf. of IAP 1987.
8. Manford M, Hart YM, Sander JWAS, Shorvon SD National General Practice Study of Epilepsy (NGPSE):Partial Seizure Patterns in a General Population. Neurology 1992b;34: 1911-17.
9. Obeso JA, Rothwell JC Marsden CD. The Spectrum of Cortical Myoclonus, Brain 1985:108:193-224.
10. Chrysostomos P. Panayiotopoulos, Michael Michael, Sue Sanders, Thalia Valeta and Michael Koutroumanidis. Benign Childhood Focal Epilepsies: Assessment of Established and Newly Recognized Syndromes, Brain 2008;131:2264-86.
11. Delgado–Escueta AV, Bascal FE, Treiman DM. Complex Partial Seizures on Closed Circuit Television and EEG: A Study of 691 Attacks in 79 Patients, Ann Neurol 1982;11:292-300.
12. Kotagal P, Luders H, Williams G, Wyllie E, Nichols T, McPherson J. Temporal Lobe Complex Partial Seizures: Analysis of Symptom Clusters and Sequences, Epilepsia 1988:29:661.
13. Chauvel P, Delgado-Escueta A, Halgren E, Bancaud J 1992a. Frontal Lobe Seizures and Epilepsies, Advance in Neurology 57, Raven Press, New York.
14. Williamson PD, Spencer DD, Spencer SS, Noveelly RA, Mattson RH: Comples Partial Seizures of Frontal Lobe Origin. Ann Neurol 1985:18:497-504.

15. Daniel Luciano. Partial Seizures of Frontal and Temporal Origin. In H.I. Hurteg and MB Stern (eds): Neurologic Clinic. Epilepsy 1: Diagnosis and Treatment 1993:11:805-22.

16. Semah F. Picot MC, Adam C. *et al.* Is the Underlying Cause of Epilepsy A Major Prognostic Factor for Recurrence? Neurology 1998:51:1256-62.

17. Ilo E. Leppik. Nina Graves and Orrin Devinsky. New Antiepileptic Medications. In H.I.Hurtig and M.B.Stern (eds): Neurologic Clinics. Epilepsy I Diagnosis and Treatment 1993: 11:923-50.

18. JT Gilman. Drug Treatment Children. In J. Oxbury. C. Polkey and M. Duchowny (eds): Intractable Focal Epilepsy. London. WB Saundars 2000:491-504.

19. Trieiman DM. Gamma Vinyl Gaba–Current Role in Management of Drug Resistant Epilepsy. Epilepsia Vol. 30. Suppl. 3,1989:S31-S35.

20. Guerreiro MM. Vigonius U. Pohlmann H. de Manreza ML. Fejerman N. Antoniuk SA. *et al.* A Double-Blind Controlled Clinical Trial of Oxcarbazepine Versus Phenytoin in Children and Adolescents with Epilepsy. Epilepsy Res 1997:27(3): 205-13.

21. Glauser T. Ben-Menachem E. Bourgeois B. Cnaan A. Chadwick D. Guerreiro C. *et al.* ILAE Treatment Guidelines: Evidence-Based Analysis of Antiepileptic Drug Efficacy and Effectiveness as Initial Monotherapy for Epileptic Seizures and Syndromes. Epilepsia 2006:47(7):1094-120.

22. Buck ML. Goodkin HP. Use of Lacosamide in Children with Refractory Epilepsy. J Pediatr Pharmacol Ther 2012:17:211-19.

23. Buck ML. Goodkin HP. Use of Lacosamide in Children with Refractory Epilepsy. J Pediatr Pharmacol Ther 2012:17:211-19.

24. Roger J *et al.* Severe Partial Epilepsies in Childhood – Modern Perspectives of Child Neurology. Fukuyama *et al.* (Edition) 1990:223-30.

25. Rutecki PA and Grossman RG. Evaluation and Surgical Treatment of Patients with Complex Partial Seizures – Current Neurology. SH (ed.) Vol 10. 1990:293-313.

20 Chapter

GENERALISED TONIC CLONIC SEIZURE

Bibek Talukdar

Generalized tonic clonic seizure (GTCS) is the most common type of generalized seizure disorder childhood. The incidence of generalized tonic clonic seizures in epidemiologic studies (both adult and children inclusive) in earlier report is about 23/100000 population.

The seizure activity originates at some point within the brain rapidly spreading throughout the brain; the spread occurs through bilaterally distributed network that includes cortical and subcortical structures but not necessarily the entire cortex. Although individual seizure onsets can appear localized, the location and lateralization are not consistent from one seizure to another. GTCS can be asymmetric (Berg *et al.*, 2010).

Clinically GTCS is characterized by bilateral and symmetric convulsive movements. Some variation in symmetry including head and eye deviation can however be seen. Typically there is bilateral rhythmic jerking of the body.

The convulsive movements can be only clonic or tonic clonic. The tonic clonic seizure consists typically of a tonic phase followed by the clonic phase, however variations such as clonic tonic clonic are also seen. The tonic phase is characterized by bilateral increase in tone of the limbs lasting for seconds to a minute. In the clonic phase there occurs bilaterally rhythmic jerking that may occur alone or in combination with tonic activity. The jerking in clonic seizure is more sustained and rhythmic than that seen in myoclonc seizure.

Aetiopathogenesis

GTCS can result from/or associated with a wide variety of causes. The causes can be infective, structural, genetic, metabolic, immunologic and unknown as categorized in the recent IALE classifications (Scheffer *et al.*, 2017). The common conditions causing GTCS that we see in our practice are given in the chapter on 'approach to diagnosis and management of seizures and seizure disorder'.

GTCS can be sometimes be precipitated by certain physical, psychological and environmental factors that are not diseases. Some such well-known precipitating factors are fatigue, emotional stress, sleep deprivation, exercise, flickering light and fever.

Clinical Features: The Seizure

The onset is usually abrupt usually with loss of consciousness and fall that is often sharp. Injury sometimes occurs during the fall. Almost simultaneously, there is uprolling of the eyeballs frequently accompanied by deviation of the head to one side as well as stiffening of the trunk and extremities with fisting and clenching of teeth, striking features of the *tonic phase*. Breathing becomes slow because of diaphragmatic contraction and even cyanosis can occur. The tonic phase is followed by the *clonic phase* in which there is rhythmic jerking of the body, more marked in the extremities. The respiration becomes jerky, irregular, often with apnea, and noisy and at times expiratory grunt occurs due to forced expiration against a closed glottis. While the seizure activity is going on, frothing from mouth commonly occurs and occasionally involuntary passage of urine and stool. Tongue biting and tooth injury are also seen at times. The jerks become progressively slow diminishing infrequency but become more violent and finally come to a halt often with a 'sigh' indicating the termination of the seizure activity and the post-ictal stage ensues. In the *post-ictal stage*, the child usually goes to sleep, varying in depth and duration. On regaining consciousness, the child more or less appears well; some children may be little lethargic and may complain of headache. Uncommonly other symptoms like fatigue, irritability, headache, vomiting, confusion, abnormal behaviour, speech disturbance and ataxia may dominate the post-ictal state. Focal deficit in an extremity (Tod's palsy) is observed at times which usually improves within a day or two. Persistent weakness should make one suspect a focal pathology in the brain. After the child recovers fully, he does not remember what had happened.

Some **associated phenomena** occurring during an attack of GCS are quite characteristic. A host of *autonomic disturbances* occur, important ones being increase in heart rate and blood pressure, pupillary abnormalities like mydriasis, pallor, flushing of face, cyanosis, increased secretion of skin and salivary glands and increased urinary bladder pressure with contraction of the detrussors and tone of the gut. These occur most at the end of the tonic phase. '*Drooling*' or '*frothing*' from the mouth are common accompaniments of GTCS; these occur because of accumulation of pharyngeal secretion due to inability to swallow these as a result of dyscoordination of the pharyngeal muscles compounded by increased salivary secretions resulting from autonomic disturbance. Urinary incontinence is common and fecal incontinence is also seen at times; these are commonly seen during the tonic phase or at the end of clonic phase. Vomiting is also not infrequent. '*Tongue biting*' with or without bleeding occurs in some children, usually during the tonic phase, but can occur during the clonic phase as well. '*Injuries*' resulting from abrupt fall, commonly to the forehead, can occur and these are seen frequently in case with intractable epilepsies.

The duration of the seizure varies from patient to patient. Usually the tonic phase lasts 10-30 seconds, clonic phase 30-50 seconds and post-ictal phase 5-15 minutes. The tonic clonic phases lasts approximately about 1-2 minutes. Sometimes an episode of seizure becomes quite prolonged or continue to occur repeatedly without regaining consciousness in between resulting in 'status epilepticus'.

The attacks of GTCS however do not always conform to the classic description given above and *variations are common* in clinical practice. This is mostly seen in duration of different stages. Loss of consciousness may be very brief and at times may be incomplete and may go unnoticed. It may be predominantly tonic or predominantly clonic. Post-ictal phase may be quite variable–brief, negligible or even absent. In younger children, GTCS tend to be predominantly clonic. The associated phenomena like uprolling of eyeballs, head deviation, frothing, involuntary passage of urine and stool, tongue biting and other injuries may not always be present. In our experience uprolling of eyeballs and varying degree frothing are very common.

Some children speak of some '*premonitory symptoms*' (warning sign) like headache, giddiness, lethargy, loss of appetite and peculiar feeling before the attack. Some children with recurrent GTCS and even their parents become so familiar with such symptoms that they can accurately predict an attack. Uncommonly some older children may speak of 'aura' usually in cases of GTCS form a very quick focal attack.

The whole episode of seizure is extremely terrifying and emotionally traumatic to the parents. They feel that the child is going to die. They are also extremely worried about the future of the child. A skilled management is thus warranted.

DIAGNOSIS

GTCS is diagnosed on the basis of the typical history and clinical presentation/sequence of events. Diagnosis is aided to a great extent by EEG. Diagnostic work up should include thorough examination and appropriate investigation aimed at finding the etiology.

History

Physicians witness a small proportion of the attacks of GTCS right from the beginning since majority of these occur at home and are over or almost over by the time the child is with the doctor. Most of the cases come to the out patients department with history of an attack. The physician has to rely quite a lot on history.

A thorough and accurate history of the *sequence of evens is the most important tool in the diagnosis of GTCS*. If the attack is found to occur in sequence of loss of consciousness, fall, tonic stage, clonic stage, post-ictal stages followed by recovery and the child does not remember what had happened, it is a GTCS. Sometimes the attendants or the parents mix up the sequences but the clinician usually can make it out. Associated phenomena like aura, uprolling of eyeballs, head deviation, frothing, involuntary passage of urine and stool and injury if present, lend further support to the diagnosis and should be routinely asked for. History of GTCS should thus include a precise description of the sequence of events besides associated phenomena as stated above. While eliciting the history of the attack, the parents should be allowed to narrate freely at the beginning whatever they had observed, if necessary they may be asked to demonstrate the events; observant and intelligent parents often give a vivid description and demonstration of an attack.

Loss of consciousness, even if brief, is the most important event in GTCS and should be meticulously looked for. Brief loss of consciousness is often missed by the parents. Uprolling of eyeballs that is quite common and often prolonged, serves as an important diagnostic pointer. The associated phenomena like frothing or drooling of saliva, tongue biting and other injuries and bladder/bowel incontinence are extremely useful supportive evidence of

GTCS. These features are particularly helpful in diagnosis of doubtful cases where there was no witness to the seizure or the clinical picture of the attack is not typical or appears vague. Froth at the pillow or wet undergarment or bed sheet in a previously continent child are strong pointers to the occurrence of a nocturnal seizure.

After confirming that the event was a GTCS, attention should be paid to explore what could be the *cause of the seizure*. Questions relevant to a probable cause should be asked whenever felt necessary at any stage of the process of history taking. The prenatal, intranatal and neonatal history (PIN), past history, family history and developmental history need special attention besides other usual history. History of PIN insult to the developing brain, developmental delay, seizures in the family and seizures and other CNS disorder in the past are often associated with GTCS.

History of any *precipitating event* like fatigue, emotional stress, sleep deprivation, exercise, flickering light and fever as mentioned above should also be looked for that has therapeutic implications.

Examination

Thorough examination, general physical and systemic with special emphasis on neurologic examination, is mandatory in every child with GTCS primarily aimed at finding the cause. Head circumference should be measured in every child. Developmental examination should be done in infants and young children. One should look for evidence of facial dysmorphism, congenital malformations and neurocutaneous stigmata. Focal neurological deficit should be noted and also any evidence of head trauma. Abnormalities that we commonly encounter on examination in cases of GTCS are microcephaly, hydrocephalus, features of cerebral palsy, mental retardation, dysmorphology and congenital malformations, neurocutaneous stigmata and cranial nerve palsies and hemiplegia. In many cases of GTCS physical examination however is normal except occasional non-specific findings.

LABORATORY STUDIES

Electroencephalogram (EEG)

EEG is most useful tool in diagnosis of GTCS as it confirms the diagnosis by detecting the seizure activity in the brain and is indicated in all cases of GTCS. Besides confirming the clinical diagnosis of seizure by detecting seizure activity in brain, EEG helps in establishing the type of seizure that is essential for proper classification of the disease and in selecting the right AED therapy. EEG also has some value in prognostication of the outcome, more related to the type of seizure. EEG is also helpful in excluding seizure-mimickers.

The EEG findings are paroxysmal activities in the form of epileptiform discharges, i.e., spikes, spike and waves and sharp waves. These can be ictal (during an attack) or interictal (in between an attack). The *ictal EEG* in GTCS typically shows burst of generalized 10-25 Hz fast activities that progressively slows down and increases in amplitude and finally comes to a halt. Generalized fast rhythmic spikes are seen in the tonic stage. The frequency increases quickly after the onset that is often termed epileptic recruiting rhythm. These start becoming discontinuous as they progress into the clonic phase. The clonic phase is characterized by bursts of spikes and after-coming slow waves that are synchronous with the clonic jerks. The burst subsequently slows down further and finally stops usually with a single spike followed by slow wave or atypical spike and wave. In the post-ictal stage EEG usually shows irregular slow waves or flat tracings often followed by spikes and sharp waves that subsequently slow down. Recording an ictal EEG however is not possible routinely; it may be picked up when continuous monitoring is going on in ICU or if a child throws an attack during routine EEG recording. Ictal EEG is an excellent confirmation of GTCS.

The *interictal EEG* may show focal or multifocal or generalized discharges. Routine interictal EEG recorded over 20-30 minutes, usually has low sensitivity that shows abnormalities in about 20-40% cases of GTCS; this can however be increased about 60-80% with prolonged recording and using activation procedures other than routine, i.e., sleep deprivation. While interictal EEG may not always show abnormalities even in cases with typical history of GTCS, about 5-8% of normal children may show such abnormalities in EEG. EEG findings, therefore has to be correlated clinically. Abnormal inerictal EEG is thus highly corroborative but not always diagnostic of GTCS. For all practical purpose, abnormal interictal EEG in a case with history suggestive of GTCS confirms it. Normal interictal EEG in a clinically undoubted case of GTCS however does not rule out the diagnosis as picking up discharges is a matter of chance.

Following a first attack of GTCS, EEG is usually advised as it may be of help in confirming that the attack was epileptic in nature, knowing the type of seizure and also in predicting the outcome as it has been observed that chances of recurrence is less if the EEG is normal.

Video-EEG

Simultaneous video and EEG recordings allow visualization and study of both clinical and electrical seizures. This modality is extremely useful in diagnosis of pseudoseizures and also other seizure mimickers. Doubtful GTCS also can be confirmed. It is also useful prior to epilepsy surgery as it helps in accurate localization of the epileptogenic focus.

Continous/Ambulatory EEG Monitoring

Continous EEG monitoring with appropriately secured electrodes is useful in differentiating pseudoseizures from true seizures. It is also useful in some difficult to treat or intractable seizures by detecting the exact type of seizure that is helpful in selection of right AED. Ambulatory EEG, where recording is done in a cassette with the scalp electrodes appropriately secured, is useful in detecting the seizure type and the epileptogenic focus in intractable epilepsies.

Neuro-Imaging Studies

Many structural lesions of the brain that cause GTCS can be picked up by imaging techniques like CT and MRI scans and even ultrasound in the infant. It is indicated in all cases of GTCS.

Other Investigations

Whenever a lesion or a disease is suspected or found to be the cause of the seizure, appropriate investigations should be done to further confirm the diagnosis as necessary. In infants and young children with GTCS common metabolic causes should be ruled out. Hypocalcemia causing GTCS is quite common in cases with rickets and malnutrition. Ruling out metabolic causes, specially inborn errors of metabolism, is important in intractable GTCS specially in young children.

Except EEG and imaging studies, all other laboratory investigations in GTCS, including a first attack or a single seizure, should thus be selective based on clinical suspicion arrived at after history and examination. It is however important to find a cause and also remain vigilant for future; a case where no definite cause was found at initial contact may be found to have one later on.

Treatment

GTCS usually presents as acute attacks that may be brief or prolonged/severe (status epilepticus). It may be a one-time event or may continue to recur. Treatment of GTCS thus involves:

(a) Treatment of an acute attack; and

(b) Treatment of recurrent attacks/epilepsy.

Treatment of an Acute Attack of GTCS

The treatment of an acute attack primarily centers round:

(a) *Termination of seizure; and*

(b) *Simultaneous stabilization of the child.* Most of the acute attacks of GCS are usually brief lasting for about a minute or so and is over at home without any medication. Cases having relatively prolonged attacks/status epilepticus usually need hospitalization.

Immediate attention should be given to airway and vital signs and stabilization of the child as necessary. To keep the airway free from obstruction due to accumulation of froth and falling back of the tongue, the child should be placed in lateral decubitus and the throat should be suctioned. A plastic airway that helps in maintaining the patency of the airway by preventing the tongue from falling back, if available, is quite useful, specially when the seizure tends to be prolonged. Any tight clothing should be removed.

Suitable anticonvulsant is used to terminate an acute attack. Several anticonvulsants have been found to be effective for termination of seizure like benzodiazepines (commonly diazepam, lorazepam, midazolam), phenytoin/fosphenytoin, phenobarbitone, valproic acid and levitiracetum. Anyone can be used in order to control an acute attack depending on what is at hand. However cost, availability, and quickness of action are important consideration in choosing the agent to be used. Benzodiazepines like diazepam and lorazepam, midazolam are commonly used. (The reader is referred also to chapter on 'drugs and doses' and also 'approach to a child with seizures and epilepsy').

Diazepam, a short acting benzodiazepam, is commonly used as for initial therapy. It is administered intravenously in a dose of 0.3 mg/kg/dose (maximum 10 mg) slowly at a rate not exceeding 1 mg/minute. The drug has a quick onset of action and most of the cases are controlled with it within 1-2 minutes. While injecting diazepam, it is important to be watchful of the child's respiration (diazepam can cause sudden respiratory arrest specially if given rapidly) and see that there is no extravagation of the drug into the surrounding tissue as it can cause tissue necrosis and subsequent thrombophlebitis. If seizure recurs it can be repeated. *Lorazepam*, a longer acting benzodiazepam, can be used if available, in a dose of 0. 1 mg/kg (loading) over

2-5 minutes. Action of the drug is smiliar to diazepam, but is more sustained and subsequent recurrence is less because of its longer half life and many prefer to use this as the initial drug in status. If seizure recurs it can be repeated in a dose of 0.05 mg/kg/dose (bolus) over 10-15 minutes. *Phenytoin* is given in a dose of 15-20 mg/kg/dose loading dose) intravenously at a rate of 0.5-1.0 mg/kg/minute. *Fosphenytoin* can also be used if available in a dose of 20 mg/kg. *Phenobarbitone* can also be used intravenously in the same dose at a rate less than 50 mg minute. While administering these drugs it is important to keep a watch on their side effects, commonly respiratory depression, hypotension and cardiac arrhythmias. *Valproic acid* can be used in a dose of 20 mg/kg. *Levetiracetum* can also be used in a dose of 20 mg/ kg. In case of difficulty in getting IV access, buccal midazolam, intranasal midazolam and rectal diazepam can be used.

While measures to control the seizure is going on any specific cause found during examination and evaluation, that should go on simultaneously, should be treated promptly.

Genearalized tonic clonic seizures at times presents as convulsive *status epilepticus (SE), convulsive,* that is defined as five or more than five minutes of continuous seizures or one or more discrete seizures between which there is incomplete recovery of consciousness (Lowenstein *et al.*, 1999, Trinka *et al.*, 2015, American Epilepsy Society guideline, 2013). Any episode of GTCS can progress to SE. Status epilepticus is a medical emergency as it can result in significant morbidity, mortality and neurological sequele. These are resultant of neuronal damage secondary to probable multiple factors like hypoxia and biochemical derangements (like hypoglycemia, acidosis, electrolyte disturbances), respiratory depression, cerebral edema and intracranial hypertension. *The aim of treatment of status epilepticus should thus be termination of the seizure as quickly as possible and simultaneous systemic metabolic stabilization besides treating the treatable cause if found.* Treatment of status epilepticus needs special attention and use of defined protocols. The drugs used for controlling an acute attack are also used for SE, however in specific sequences, considering the emergency nature of the conditions so that the seizure can be aborted as quickly as possible (Chapter 24).

TREATMENT OF RECURRENT ATTACKS OF GTCS/EPILEPSY WITH GTCS

Antiepileptic Drug Prophylaxis

Recurrent attacks, the child becoming epileptic, occurs in about 70% of cases GTCS. Antiepileptic drug (AED) prophylaxis is the mainstays of treatment of these cases aimed at preventing such recurrences. *(Referred to chapters on drugs and doses and also approach to a child with seizures and epilepsy).* Many AEDs are available for this purpose. Current evidence as per on ILAE survey (based on trials in children) suggests that the following AEDs are useful for using as initial monotherapy in generalized onset tonic clonic seizures in children namely carbamazepine (CBZ), phenobarbitone (PB), phenytoin (PHT), topiramet (TPM), valproic acid (VPA) and oxcarbazepine (OXC). Level of evidence however are poor – CBZ, PB, PHT, TPM and VPA (possible level C) and OXC (level D) (Glauser *et al.*, 2013).

Decision on starting AED prophylaxis needs a very rational approach. Selection of suitable AED, Initiation and maintenance of the AED therapy, monitoring while AED therapy is going on need careful approach. Duration of AED prophylaxis needs to be properly planned. Withdrawal of AED needs extremely careful approach. Any treatable cause found has to be treated on a priority basis. Currently surgery has an important role in epilepsy especially in difficult cases. (The reader is referred also to chapters on ‘approach to a child with seizures and epilepsy’ and ‘drugs and doses’).

The important pharmacologic parameters of the commonly used AEDs useful in day-to-day management of the cases are shown in Table 20.1.

Table 20.1: Important Pharmacologic Parameters of Commonly used AEDs in GTCS for Chronic Prophylaxis

AED	Dose (mg/kg/d) and schedule of dosing	Therapeutic concentration (µg/ml)	Time to steady state (days)	Important side effects
Carbamazepine	10-30 q tid/bid	6-12	3-4	G.I. disturbance, drowsiness, rash, diplopia, ataxia, leukopenia
Oxcarbazepine	20-40 q bid	13-28 mg/l		G.I. headache, rash, somnolence, hypertrichosis, gingival hypertrophy
Lamotrigine	5-15 q tid/bid	1-15		G.I. headache, ataxia, Stevens-Johnson syndrome, liver toxicity

Contd.

Contd.

Phenytoin	5-8 OD/bid	10-20	7-10	Cosmetic (gingival hypertrophy, hirshuitism, acne) lymphadenopathy, rash, ataxia, nystagmus, anemia
Phenobarbitone	3-5 OD/bid	15-40	14-21	Behaviour disturbance (hyperactivity, lethargy, irritability), cognitive dysfunction, rash
Valproic Acid	10-60 bid/ tid	40-150	1-2	G.I. disturbance, sedation, rash, weight gain, tremor, alopecia, loss of appetite, stomatitis, thrombocytopenia, coma, hepatitis, pancreatitis
Levitiracetum	20-40 tid/bid	6-20 mg/l		Somnolence, dizziness, behavior problems
Topiramet	3-9 tid/bid	2-25 mg/l		Cognitive dysfunction, hypohydrosis, renal calculi, fever, glaucoma

OUTCOME

GTCS can be *non-recurrent* occurring as one time event in life (only a single episode or closely occurring few episodes, without subsequent recurrence) or can be *recurrent* becoming a chronic disorder the child becoming *epileptic*. Outcome of GTCS is ultimately determined by the primary brain pathology. The probability of being in remission of 20 years after diagnosis of GCS in general is about 85%. In children it is around 74.5% after withdrawal of antiepileptic therapy. The most significant factors predicting recurrence after withdrawal of therapy are symptomatic epilepsy with a known cause and presence of neurological abnormalities (focal neurologic signs) with or without mental retardation.

Suggested Reading

- American Academy of Neurology (1989b). Assessment: Intensive EEG Video Monitoring for Epilepsy. Neurology 1989b;39:1101-02.
- Annegers JF, Hauser WA, Elveback LR. Remission of Seizures and Relapse in Patients with Epilepsy. Epilepsia 1979;20: 729-37.
- Arts WFM, Visser LH, Loonen CB, Tjiam AT, Stroink H, Stuurman PM, Poortvliet DCJ. Follow-up of 146 Children with Epilepsy After Withdrawal of Antiepileptic Therapy. Epilepsia 1988;29:244-50.
- Berg AT, Berkovic SF, Brodie MJ, Buchhalter J, Cross JH, van Emde BW, Engel J, French J, Glauser TA, Mathern GW, Moshe SL, Nordli D, Plouin P, Scheffer IE (2010) Revised Terminology and Concepts for Organization of Seizures and Epilepsies: Report of the ILAE Commission on Classification and Terminology, 2005-2009. Epilepsia 2010:51:676-85.
- Bernd Pohlmann-Eden, Ettore Beghi, Carol Camfield, Peter Camfield. The First Seizure and Its Management in Adults and Children. BMJ 2006 (11th February):332(7537):339-42.
- Blom S, Heijbel J and Bergfors PG. Incidence of Epilepsy in Children: A Follow-up Study Three Years After The First Seizure. Epilepsia 1978;19:343-50.
- Dodson WE, Pellock JM. Pediatric Epilepsy. New York. Demos Publications, 1993.
- Ebersole JS, Leroy RF. An Evaluation of Ambulatory Cassette Monitoring, Detection of Interictal Abnormalities. Neurology 1983:33:8-18.
- Evidence-Based Guideline: Treatment of Convulsive Status Epilepticus in Children and Adults: Report of the Guideline Committee of the American Epilepsy Society. Epilepsy Currents, Vol. 16, No. 1 (January/February) 2016;48-61.
- Gastaut H, Broughton R. Epileptic Seizures. Springfield IL. Charles C Thomas, 1972.
- Gastaut H, Tissinary CA. Lack of Discharges in Different Types of Seizures. In Remond A (Ed). Handbook of Electro-encephalography and Clinical Neurolophysiology, Vol. 13A. Amsterdam, Elsevier 1975;13-45.
- Glauser T, Ben-Menachem E, Bourgeois B, Cnaan A, Guerreiro C, Kalviainen R, Mattson R, French JA, Perucca E, Toson T, for the ILAE Subcommission on AED Guidelines. Updated ILAE Evidence Review of Antiepileptic Drug Efficacy and Effectiveness as Initial Monotherapy for Epileptic Seizures and Syndromes. Epilepsia 2013:54(3):551-63. doi:10.1111/ epi.12074.
- Hirtz D, Ashwal S, Berg A, Bettis D, Camfield C, Camfield P *et al*. Practice Parameter: Evaluating a First Non Febrile Seizure in Children: Report of the Quality Standards Subcommittee of the American Academy of Neurology, The Child Neurology Society and the American Epilepsy Society. Neurology 2000; 55:616-23.
- Holmes GL. Diagnosis and Management of Seizures in Children. Philadelphia. WB Saunders Company 1987:163-71.

- Lowenstein DH, Blek T, Macdonald RL. It's Time to Revise the Definition of Status Epilepticus. Epilepsia 1999;40: 120-22.
- Scheffer IE, 1 Berkovic S, Capovilla G, Connolly MB, French J, Guilhoto L, Hirsch E, Jain S, Mathern GW, Moshe SL, Nordi DR, Perucca E, Tomson T, Wiebe S, Zhang YH, Zuberi SM. ILAE Classifications of Epilepsies: Position Paper of the ILAE Commission for Classification and Terminology. Epilepsia 2017;58(4):512-21. doi: 10.1111/epi.13709.
- Trinka E, Cock H, Hesdorffer D, Rosetti AO, Scheffer IE, Shinnar S, Shorvon S, Lowenstein DH. A Definition and Classification of Status Epilepticus – Report of the ILAE Task Force on Classification of Status Epilepticus. Epilepsia 2015;1-9. doi: 10.1111/epi.13121.

21 Chapter

MYOCLONIC SEIZURES AND EPILEPSY

Biswaroop Chakrabarty

Myoclonus is defined as sudden, jerky, irregular, shock like contractions of axial and appendicular musculature. Myoclonus can be of cortical or subcortical origin. Myoclonic epilepsies are of cortical origin, however there are entities where both cortical and subcortical myoclonus can co-exist. The characteristic electroencephalogram (EEG) correlate for epileptic myoclonus is a polyspike discharge.

This chapter describes benign and intractable myoclonic epilepsies of childhood in a chronological sequence starting from neonatal period to childhood and adolescence.

Myoclonic Epilepsy with Onset in Neonatal Period and Infancy

Early Myoclonic Encephalopathy (Aicardi Syndrome): This is characterised by neonatal onset of irregular, fragmentary myoclonic seizures. The EEG shows characteristic burst suppression pattern (Fig. 21.1). It may be associated with underlying metabolic disorders like non ketotic hyperglycinemia and cortical malformations. Unlike its mimicker Ohtahara syndrome, pure genetic causes have not been defined. Response to treatment is usually poor and neurodevelopmental outcome is grave. Levetiracetam and benzodiazepines like clonazepam have been tried without much effect.

However, one should be careful in differentiating benign neonatal sleep myoclonus from these entities, as it is present only during sleep, is not an epilepsy, does not require treatment and does not affect neuro-developmental outcome.

Benign Myoclonic Epilepsy of Infancy (BMEI): This entity is seen from 4 months to 3 years of age with characteristic myoclonic jerks, primarily of upper extremities. Associated febrile seizures and family history of epilepsy is present in upto one-third of cases. It may show photosensitivity and may be stimulus provoked. The characteristic EEG finding is ictal generalised spike and wave discharges, whereas the interictal EEG is usually normal. Neurodevelopmental outcome is usually good and seizures usually resolve within 1-2 years of diagnosis. The treatment of choice is Valproate, occasionally clonazepam or clobazam is added.

West Syndrome: This entity is characterised by the triad of spasm, hypsarrhythmia on EEG and psychomotor delay or regression. Usually the onset is between 4-8 months of age and it is always before 2 years of age.

A spasm is characterised by brief, symmetrical, bilateral contraction of the axial muscle groups, however unilateral variants have been described. It is longer than a myoclonus and shorter than a tonic seizure. Depending on the muscle group involved it can be flexor, extensor (least common) or mixed (most common). Typically, the spasms occur in clusters and in getting up from sleep. Associated findings include behavioural arrest, eye deviation and nystagmoid eye movements and alteration in respiratory pattern.

The classical EEG pattern is hypsarrhythmia, characterised by random, chaotic, high amplitude slow and polyspike-spike wave complexes (Fig. 21.2). Other types, called modified hypsarrhythmia or hypsarrhythmia variants have been described; hemispheric hypsarrhythmia, burst suppression, focal spikes, generalised slowing and increased interhemispheric synchrony.

Etiologically the cases are divided into prenatal, perinatal and postnatal categories. Prenatal includes cortical malformations, chromosomal anomalies, single gene disorders (ARX, CDKL5/STK9), neurocutaneous disorders, TORCH infections and neurometabolic disorders. Treatable neurometabolic disorders include phenylketonuria, GLUT-1 transporter defect and micronutrient responsive states (pyridoxine, biotin, folinic acid and

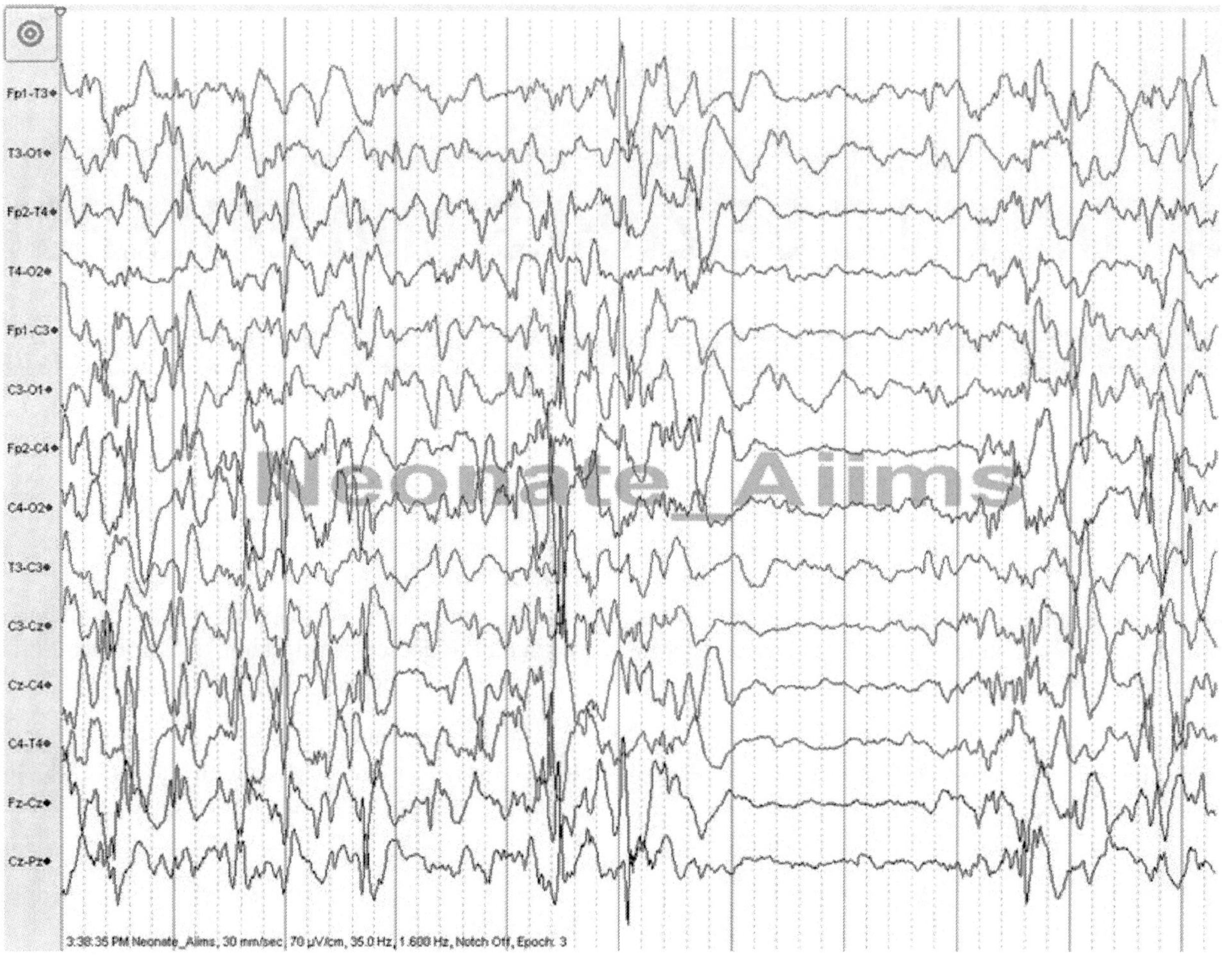

Fig. 21.1: Burst suppression pattern

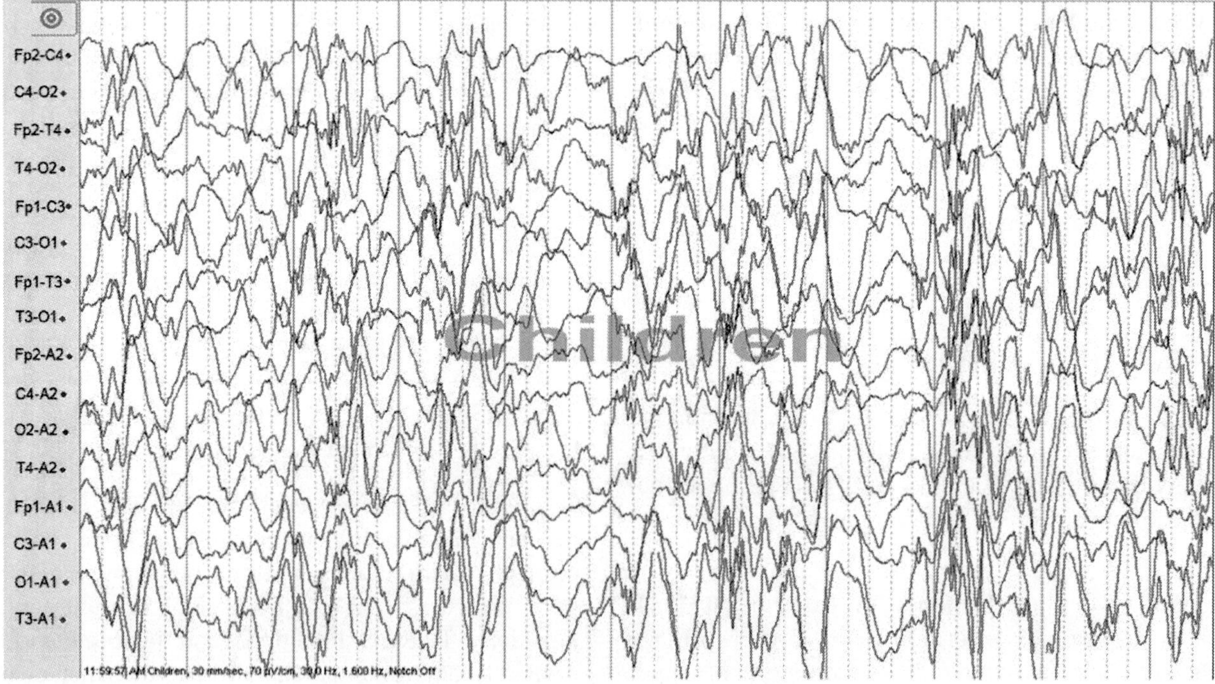

Fig. 21.2: Classical hypsarrhythmia pattern

pyridoxal phosphate). Metabolic disorders without definitive treatment include mitochondrial cytopathy, non-ketotic hyperglycinemia, sulphite oxidase deficiency and Menke's disease. Perinatal and postnatal causes include acquired structural brain injuries.

Multimodal neuroimaging reveals a diagnosis in 70% cases. In rest, depending on the clinical and etiological clues as mentioned above, investigations are planned.

Except for metabolic conditions described above with definitive treatment, the treatment of choice is parenteral steroid (ACTH). Studies have shown even oral steroids to be equally efficacious (prednisolone). Vigabatrin is the drug of choice in spasm associated with Tuberous Sclerosis. Upto 75% cases remit after drug of choice therapy, however, 20-30% may have a relapse. Antiepileptic drugs like valproate, levetirecetam, zonisamide, topiramate, lamotrigine and clonazepam may be effective. In pharmacoresistant cases, dietary therapy and epilepsy surgery may be useful.

Earlier the initiation of treatment of choice, better is the outcome. However, upto 50% may evolve into other epilepsies including Lennox-Gestaut syndrome and have psychomotor deficits.

Severe Myoclonic Epilepsy of Infancy: It is now preferably called as Dravet syndrome as presence of myoclonic epilepsy is not obligatory for diagnosis. It starts by second half of infancy usually with focal febrile and afebrile (upto 35%) seizures. This is usually followed by myoclonic, focal, atypical absence and generalised tonic clonic seizures. A specific clinical state, called 'obtundation status' has been described with this entity, in which the child continues to have segmental, fragmentary, erratic myoclonus with preserved consciousness; it may last for few days.

In upto 85% of patients with Dravet syndrome, an underlying SCN1A mutation is seen. The EEG is usually normal in the beginning, but later evolves into a nonspecific generalised or multifocal spike and wave discharges with or without background disturbances. MRI Brain is usually normal.

It is one of the potential drug refractory epilepsies. Variable response has been seen with valproate, topiramate, benzodiazepines, levetirecetam and zonisamide. Stiripentol can be added to refractory cases. Drug intractable cases may respond favourably to dietary therapy. Seizures are worsened by sodium channel blocking agents like carbamazepine, lamotrigine and phenytoin.

Long-term neurodevelopment, although variable, is usually poor. Premorbid development is generally normal and the clinical phenotype stabilises by 5 years of age.

Myoclonic Epilepsy with Onset in Early Childhood

Myoclonic Astatic Epilepsy: This entity is called Doose syndrome and is characterised by myolonic jerk usually followed by an atonic fall. The intensity of myoclonus can vary from a subtle head drop to a generalised axial myoclonic jerk. Atypical absences may be present with associated upper limb myolconus. Although association with SCN1A mutation has been described, the genotype phenotype correlation needs further evaluation. The onset is between 2-6 years of age.

The EEG shows generalised spike polyspike activity usually with a preserved background (Fig. 21.3).

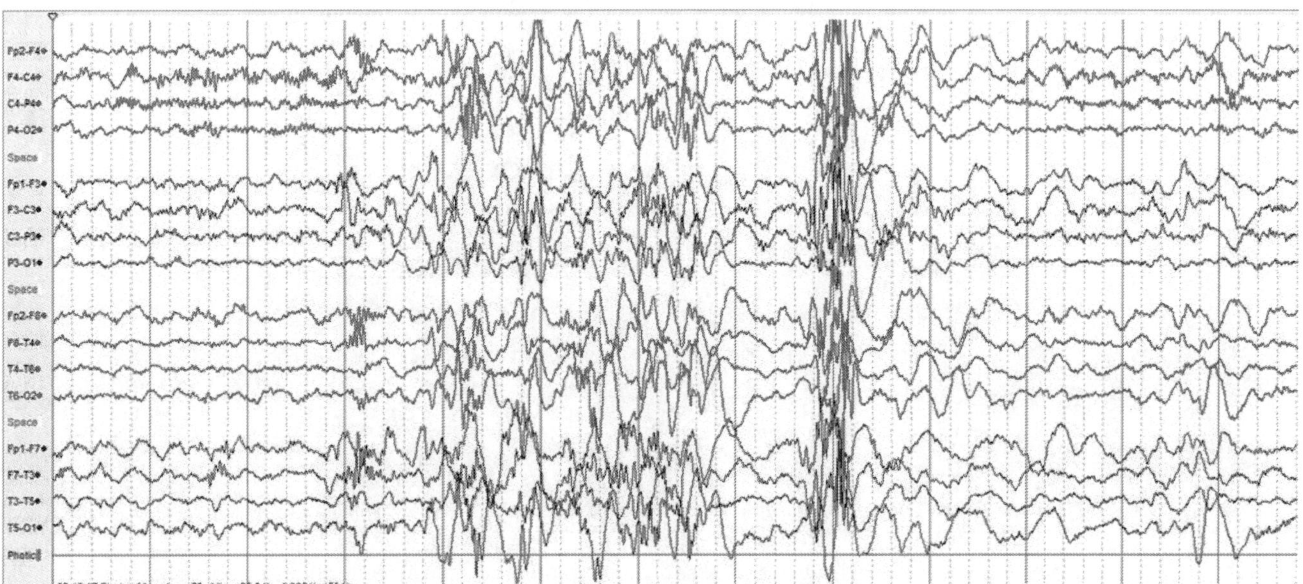

Fig. 21.3: Multifocal and generalised spike-polyspike wave discharges with preserved background

Occasionally 3 Hz spike and wave activity and occipital intermittent rhythmic delta activity (OIRDA) attenuating with eye opening is seen. MRI Brain is usually normal.

Antiepileptic drug therapy is usually effective. Valproate, topiramate, benzodiazepines, levetirecetam and zonisamide show favourable response. Drug intractable cases may respond favourably to dietary therapy.

Long-term neurodevelopment is dependent on epilepsy control. Seizure remission may occur in around 3 years from onset. Presence of tonic seizures is associated with poor prognosis and a small proportion of patients may evolve to Lennox-Gastaut Syndrome (LGS).

Lennox-Gastaut Syndrome: This entity is characterised by multiple seizure semiologies with onset at 3 to 5 years of age. The most common seizure type is generalised tonic seizure followed by myoclonic, atonic, generalised tonic clonic (GTC) and atypical absences. Isolated myoclonic variants are also described. It is characterised by multiple seizures, upto 100 per day.

Etiologically an underlying cause is identified in upto 65% cases. Upto one-third of west syndrome evolves into LGS. The underlying causes include hypoxic ischemic injuries, cortical malformations, neurocutaneous disorders like Tuberous sclerosis, posttraumatic brain injuries, stroke, hemorrhages, hypoglycemic brain injury, neuro-infection and congenital infections. Primary genetic causes have not yet been identified.

The EEG shows 1.5-2.5 Hz spike and slow wave activity, polyspikes and paroxysmal fast activity (Fig. 21.4). MRI Brain reveals findings of the underlying cause.

Usually it is a medically intractable epilepsy. Antiepileptic drug therapy, which may be effective, are valproate, lamotrigine, topiramate, benzodiazepines, levetiracetam and zonisamide. Drug intractable cases may respond favourably to dietary therapy. Palliative surgical options like subpial transaction and corpus callosotomy are available, particularly for those in whom neurodevelopmental potential is poor.

Long-term outcome in terms of seizure control and cognition is variable. Along with intellectual disability, behavioural problems like autism and hyperactivity are not rare.

Atonic Seizures: Semiologically this is characterised by sudden loss of tone, followed by fall and a brief period of unconsciousness. It rarely occurs in isolation and is usually seen with myoclonic epilepsy. In children, it has been described with LGS and Doose syndrome.

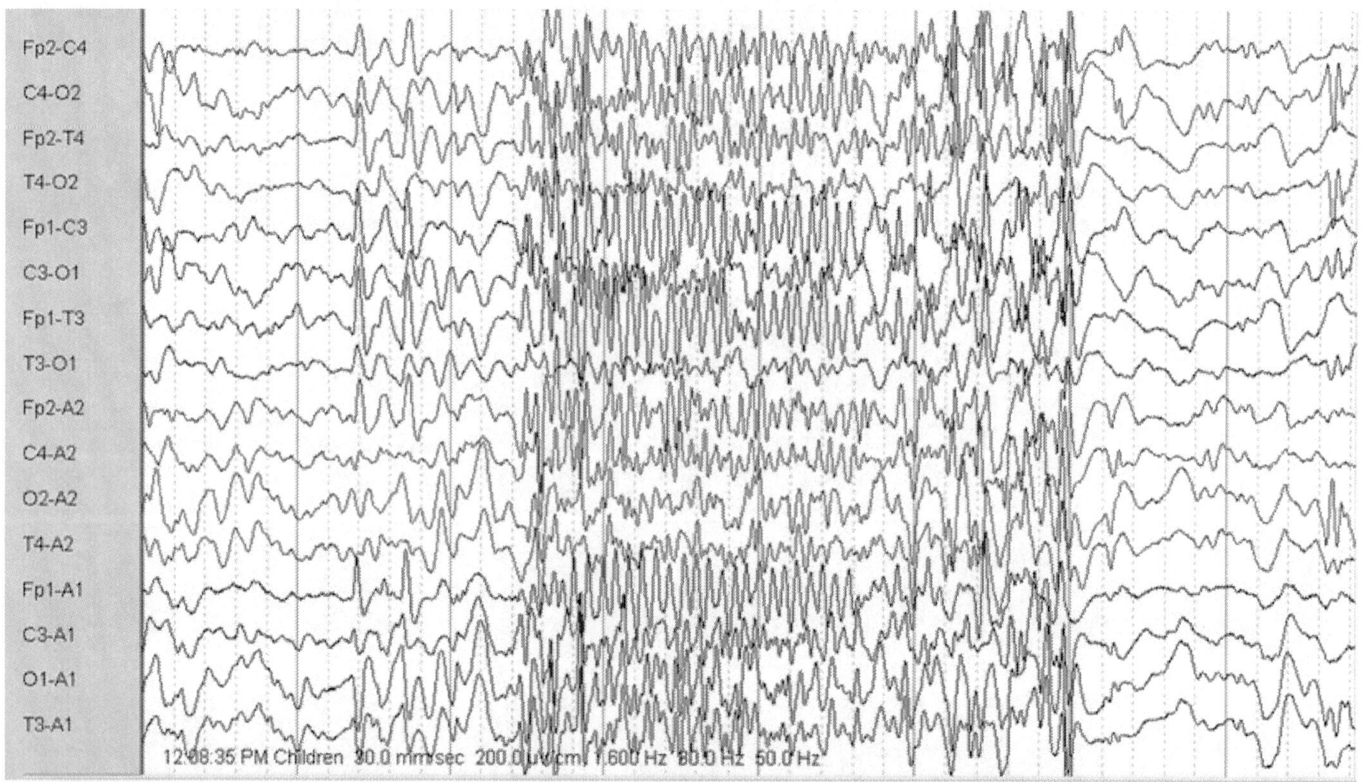

Fig. 21.4: 2-2.5 Hz spike and slow wave activity, generalised paroxysmal fast activity and generalised polyspike-spike wave discharges

Myoclonic Epilepsy with Onset in Late Childhood and Adolescence

Juvenile Myoclonic Epilepsy (JME): It is the most common form of primary generalised epilepsy (upto 1/4th) and constitutes 10% of all epilepsies. Onset is in late first decade or adolescence and is more common in females. Early morning myoclonic jerks precede development of GTCS and absences by 6-12 months. Underlying genetic defects have been identified in calcium, potassium and chloride channels.

The classical EEG findings are 4-6 Hz spike and polyspike activity (60%) accentuated by photic stimulation (Fig. 21.5) and 3 Hz spike and wave activity (15%).

The mainstay of therapy is valproate and benzodiazepines. However, levetiracetam, lamotrigine, zonisamide and topiramate have also been found to be effective.

Cognition is preserved but usually lifelong therapy is required.

Epilepsy with Myoclonic Absences: This entity is known as Tassinari syndrome. It is a rare entity with 0.5 to 1% incidence in tertiary centres. Usual age of onset is 3 to 12 years (peak 7 years) with male preponderance (70%). Etiologically, it can be secondary to cerebral palsy, or primarily due to chromosomal disorders (trisomy 14, 12, Angelman syndrome and INV-DUP 15) and genetic disorders (SYNGAP1, glutamate dehydrogenase and GLUT1).

Clinically, it is characterised by axial myoclonia followed by tonic contraction of bilateral upper limbs and behavioural arrest lasting upto 30 seconds. Rarely, GTCS, atonic and tonic seizures are seen. On EEG, generalised polyspike discharges and 3-4 Hz spike and wave discharges, accentuated by hyperventilation and photic stimulation are seen.

Drug of choice is valproate. In refractory cases, lamotrigine and benzodiazepine are helpful. Experience with levetiracetam, zonisamide and topiramate is limited. Upto one-third cases remit, whereas rest may evolve into long-term epilepsies. Those with tonic seizures may evolve into LGS. Cognitive impairment is seen in upto 70% cases.

Epilepsy with Eyelid Myoclonia and Absences (ELMA): Also known as Jeavons syndrome, it is

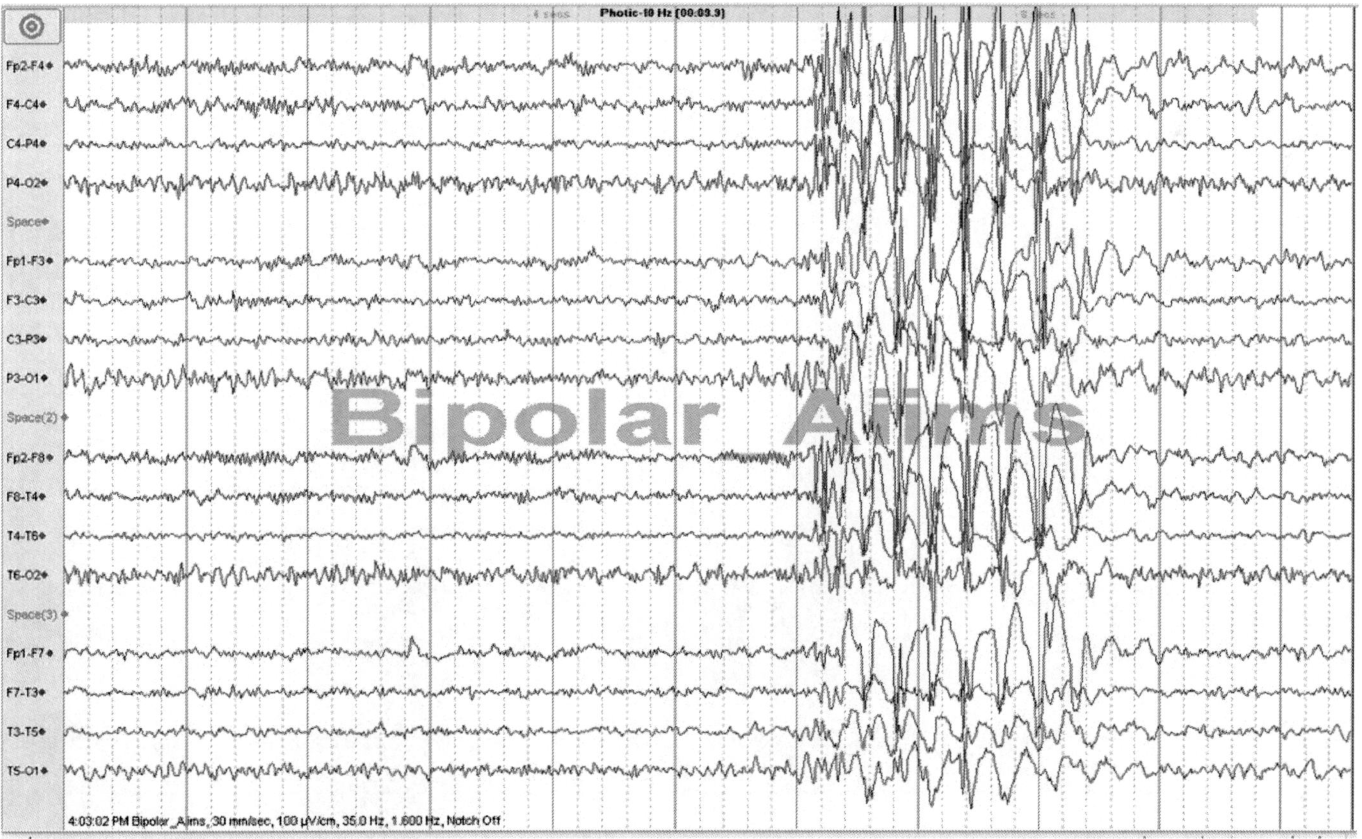

Fig. 21.5: Generalised 4-6 Hz spike-polyspike wave discharges precipitated by photic stimulation

characterised by triad of eyelid myoclonia, photosensitivity and eye closure sensitivity. It is important to recognise this triad as eyelid myoclonia is also associated with JME and BMEI. Overlap syndromes are described between JME and ELMA. It is a rare disorder with female preponderance and peak age of onset around 6-8 years (2-14 years range). It has a complex multigenic inheritance with *CHD2* linkage. Premorbid neurodevelopmental status is usually normal.

Other semiologies described are absences, GTCS and focal seizures mainly of occipital onset.

It is characterised on EEG by spike and polyspike wave discharges accentuated by eye closure (Fig. 21.6), photic stimulation, hyperventilation and sleep and 3Hz generalised discharges classically seen with absence epilepsy.

Rarely, an eyelid myoclonia status has been described, occasionally associated with arm myoclonus. A phenomenon of self-induction has been described, particularly in intellectually disabled.

Valproate and clonazepam are the most effective drugs. Levetiracetam is also helpful. Non-pharmacological treatment like wearing special glasses is also useful in photosensitive patients. Phenytoin, lamotrigine and oxcarbamazepine may worsen and precipitate status.

Usually response to drugs is unsatisfactory and patients may require lifelong therapy. Associated intellectual disability, learning difficulties and behavioural problems are not uncommon.

The salient features of all the above described epilepsies have been summarised in Table 21.1.

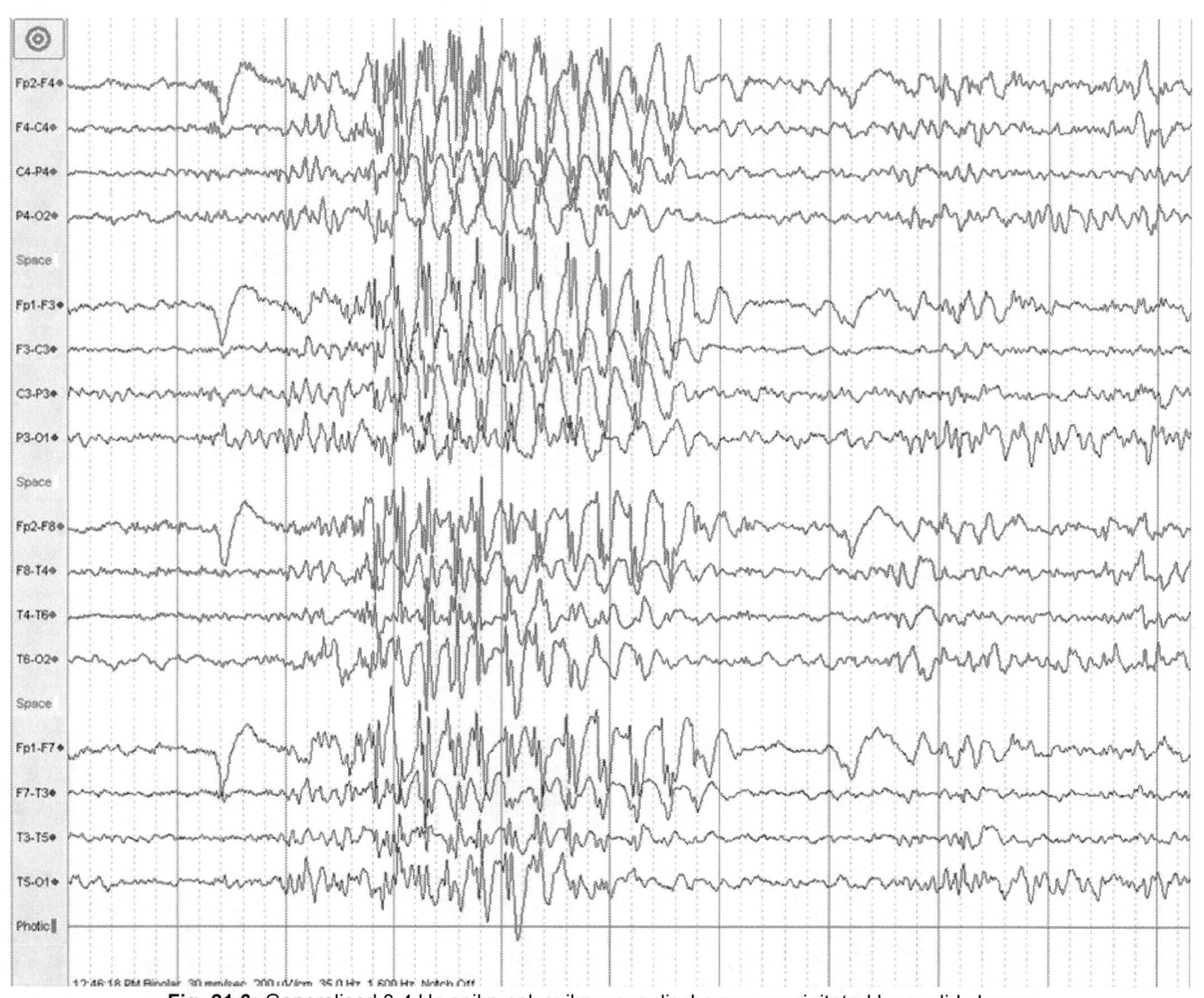

Fig. 21.6: Generalised 3-4 Hz spike-polyspike wave discharges precipitated by eyelid closure

Table 21.1: Salient Features of Childhood and Adolescent Onset Myoclonic Epilepsy

Disease	Age at onset	Seizure semiology	EEG finding	Response to therapy
Aicardi syndrome	Neonatal period	Irregular, fragmentary myoclonus	Burst suppression	Poor
Benign myoclonic epilepsy of infancy	4 months 3 years	Upper limb myoclonus	Ictal generalised discharges, interictal normal	Good
West syndrome	4-8 months	Spasm	Hypsarrhythmia	Variable
Dravet syndrome	6-12 months	Focal febrile and afebrile, myoclonus, atypical absence, GTCS	Multifocal or generalised discharges with normal or abnormal background	Variable
Doose syndrome	2-6 years	Myoclonic astatic, atypical absence, tonic	Generalised polyspike spike wave discharges with preserved background	Variable
LGS	3-5 years	Tonic, atypical absence, myoclonic, GTCS	1.5-2.5 Hz spike and slow wave, generalised PFAs and polyspike wave discharges	Usually poor
JME	Late first decade and adolescence	Early morning myoclonus, absence, GTCS	4-6 Hz polyspike and spike wave activity accentuated by photic stimulation	Good, lifelong therapy may be required
Tassinari syndrome	3-12 years	Axial myoclonus of bilateral upper limbs, GTCS, atonic, tonic	Generalised polyspike and 3 Hz spike and wave discharges accentuated by photic stimulation and hyperventilation	Variable
Jeavon syndrome	2-14 years	Eyelid myoclonia with photosensitivity and eyelid closure sensitivity, absences, GTCS, occipital seizures	Spike and polyspike wave discharges accentuated by eye closure, photic stimulation, hyperventilation and sleep and 3 Hz generalised discharges	Variable

(EEG: Electroencephalogram, GTCS: Generalised tonic clonic seizure, LGS: Lennox-Gestaut syndrome, PFA: Paroxysmal fast activity, JME: Juvenile myoclonic epilepsy)

Progressive Myoclonic Epilepsy (PME)

This heterogenous group of disorder is characterised by both cortical and subcortical myoclonus, developmental delay or regression, ataxia and tremors. The age at onset is usually late childhood and adolescence, with variable progression for different entities. Photosensitivity, particularly photo-paroxysmal responses on low frequency (0.5 Hz) photic stimulation, is demonstrable on EEG (Fig. 21.7).

The myoclonus is typically precipitated by posture, action, external stimuli like light, sound and touch and semiologically can be focal or segmental, asynchronous, arrhythmic, asymmetric and massive. Predominantly it is visible on the face and distal extremities. Other associated seizure types include GTCS, absences, tonic and focal seizures. The six predominant forms are being described below.

Unverricht Lundborg Disease (ULD)

The age at onset is 6-15 years with variable progression. The disease process usually stabilises beyond the age of 40. It is also called progressive myoclonic epilepsy type 1 (EPM 1) and has an autosomal recessive inheritance with underlying molecular defect in cystatin B gene. The EEG shows bursts of epileptiform discharges with background slowing and preserved sleep architecture.

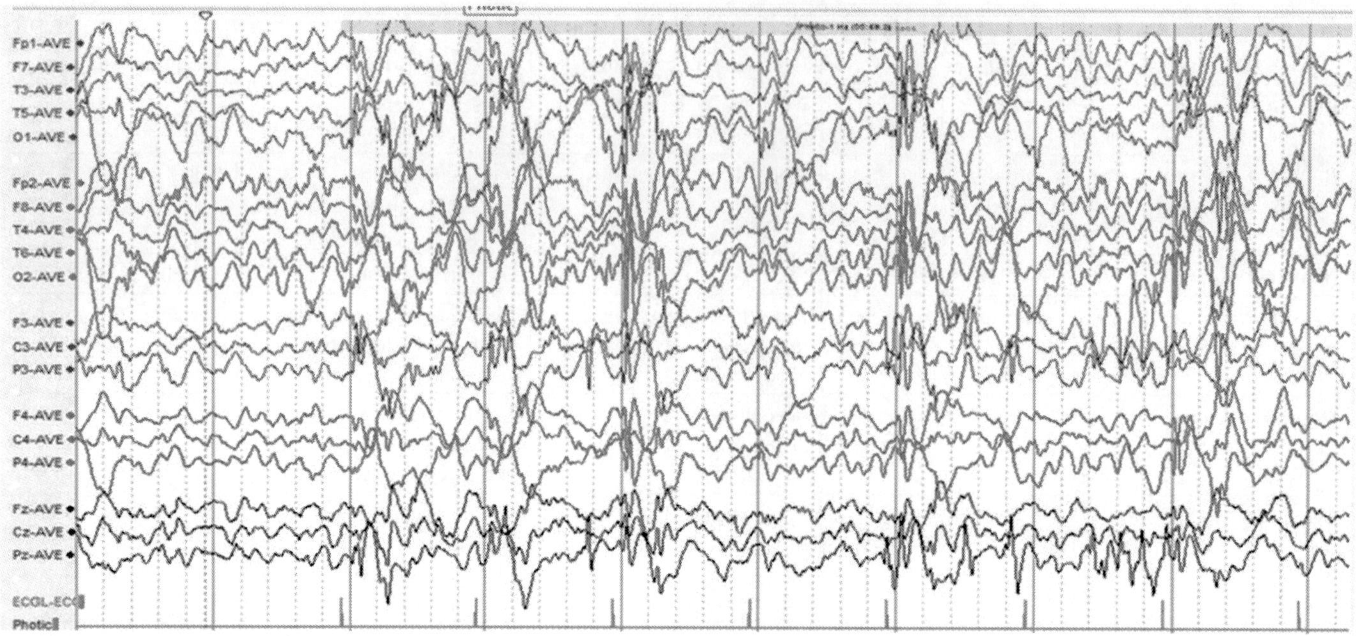

Fig. 21.7: Low frequency photic stimulation causing photo paroxysmal response in late infantile NCL

Lafora's Disease

This entity is characterised by onset at 12-15 years of age and occipital seizures in the form of visual hallucinations apart from the general features of PME phenotype. Neuroregression begins only after onset of seizures. Usually patients die within 10 years of onset. The EEG is characterised by multifocal discharges with progressive background and sleep abnormalities. The characteristic pathological finding is the presence of Lafora bodies which are periodic acid (PAS) positive polyglucosan inclusion bodies located predominantly in neurons, skin (sebaceous glands), liver and muscle. The underlying molecular defect is in the EPM2A (laforin) and EPM2B (several proteins including kinesin) gene.

Myoclonic Epilepsy with Ragged Red Fibres (MERRF)

This is a disorder of mitochondrial origin characterised by myoclonus and cerebellar ataxia with often associated myopathy, neuropathy, deafness, dementia, short stature, and optic atrophy and occasionally cardiomyopathy, retinitis pigmentosa, pyramidal signs, ophthalmoparesis, multiple lipomas and diabetes mellitus.

The EEG shows multifocal or generalised spike polyspike discharges with altered sleep and background architecture. The MRI brain is characterised by generalised atrophy with signal changes and calcification in deep grey matter nuclei. Muscle biopsy shows the characteristic ragged red fibres (muscle fibres interrupted by enlarged and distorted mitochondria) in modified Gomori trichrome stain (Fig. 21.8). Oxidative stains show reduced staining.

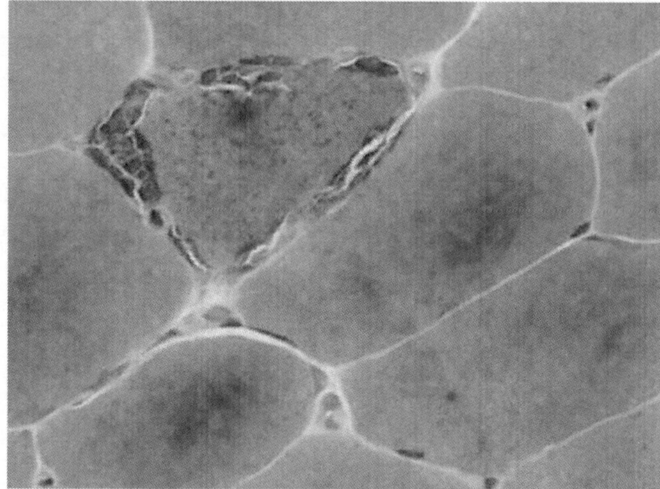

Fig. 21.8: Muscle biopsy showing ragged red fibres on modified Gomori trichrome stain (X 400) in a case of MERRF (*Courtesy:* Professor M.C.Sharma, Department of Pathology, AIIMS, New Delhi)

More than 80% patients show molecular defect (A8344G) in the t-RNA lysine gene. Rare molecular defects are T8356C and G8363A in the same gene.

Neuronal Ceroid Lipofuscinosis (NCL)

This is a group of disorder characterised by 5 subtypes which may manifest as PME, out of which 4 are autosomal recessive and 1 autosomal dominant. The presence of autofluorescent lysosomal storage material, ceroid lipofuscin is demonstrable in all the subtypes on electron microscope in one of the four or mixed forms; osmiophilic granular deposits (GROD), curvilinear (CV), fingerprint like (FP) and rectilinear (RL) inclusion bodies. The MRI brain shows generalised atrophy with deep white matter signal changes. Molecular testing is directed by presence of inclusion bodies in skin, conjunctiva or muscle biopsy. The various subtypes are briefly described below.

Classical Late Infantile: This is the most prevalent form of NCL that presents as PME. It has an onset between 2.5 to 4 years of age. The illness heralds with refractory epilepsy. Ophthalmoscopy reveals macular degeneration and vessel narrowing. The child succumbs within 5 years of disease onset.

Electron microscope characteristically shows curvilinear bodies and there is diminished activity of tripeptidyl peptidase enzyme in leukocyte or fibroblasts. The underlying molecular defect is in CLN2 gene.

Finnish Variant Late Infantile: This variant is restricted only in Finnish with underlying molecular abnormality in CLN5 gene. The age at onset is 5 years with slowly progressive loss of vision and myoclonus begins around 8 years of age. The characteristic inclusion bodies are fingerprint and rectilinear.

Egyptian/Indian Variant Late Infantile: This shows similar age at onset and slow progression with underlying molecular defect in CLN6 gene. Death occurs by third decade of life.

Juvenile NCL: The onset in this variant is between 4-10 years of age with vision loss. Death occurs around 8 years from onset. The underlying molecular defect is in CLN3 gene.

Adult Form: Also known as Kufs disease, this is characterised by adolescent or adult onset, preserved vision and mixed inclusion bodies.

Sialidosis

This entity is called myoclonic syndrome with cherry red spot. It has a juvenile or adult onset with slow progression and relatively preserved cognition. There is deficiency of α neuraminidase and urine chromatography reveals high levels of sialylated oligosaccharide.

Dentatorubral-Pallidoluysian Atrophy (DRPLA)

This is an autosomal dominant disorder of trinucloetide CAG repeat expansion. There are 3 forms; choreoathetoid, pseudo-Huntington and PME. Those with disease onset before 20 years of age always manifest with PME. Background EEG activity is usually preserved.

Treatment

Treatment is mainly supportive, rehabilitative and symptomatic. Drugs used for myoclonus are valproate, levetiracetam, zonisamide and clonazepam. Valproate should be avoided in suspected mitochondrial cytopathy. The only definitive treatment, recently approved by FDA is Cerliponase α (Brineura) for CLN2. Mitochondrial disorders may be empirically treated with antioxidant vitamins and cofactors like thiamine, riboflavin, coenzyme Q, carnitine and vitamin E.

The salient features of PME spectrum disorders is summarised in Table 21.2.

Table 21.2: Salient Features of Progressive Myoclonic Epilepsy Disorders

Disease	Age at onset	Specific clinical feature	Diagnostic clue
ULD	6-15 years	Slowly progressive with stabilisation beyond 40 years	Preserved EEG background
Lafora's disease	12-15 years	Occipital seizures	Lafora bodies on skin biopsy
MERRF	Variable	Multiorgan involvement	Ragged red fibres on muscle biopsy
NCL	Variable	Vision involvement may precede onset of myoclonus	Autofluoroscent lipofuscin inclusion bodies on skin biopsy
Sialidosis	Juvenile and adult onset	Cherry red spot	Urine chromatography showing sialylated oligosaccharide
DRPLA	Juvenile and adult onset	Inherited through principle of anticipation	Preserved EEG background

(ULD: Unverricht Lundborg disease, EEG: Electroencephalogram, MERRF: Myoclonic epilepsy with ragged red fibres, NCL: Neuronal Ceroid Lipofuscinosis, DRPLA: Dentatorubral-pallidoluysian atrophy)

Subacute Sclerosing Panencephalitis (SSPE)

This acquired neurodegenerative disorder is a PME mimicker. Ocular involvement can precede other features and is seen in a significant proportion with necrotising retinitis being the most characteristic lesion. It is a disease more prevalent in the developing world because of incomplete immunisation coverage.

The incidence of SSPE as per WHO estimates is 4-11/1,00,000 measles cases. The latency from a primary measles infection is usually 2-10 years and the age at onset is 5-15 years. Boys are affected twice more than girls. Occasional presence of multiple cases within a family points towards a genetic predisposition as well.

A mutant and aberrant measles virus is responsible for SSPE. The most commonly affected part of measles virus is the matrix protein, which in genetically predisposed immune dysregulated individuals, leads to persistent measles virus infection of the central nervous system affecting primarily oligodendroglia and neurons.

The progression of SSPE is described in the following clinical stages:

(a) Personality and behavioural changes, onset of cognitive decline.

(b) Myoclonic jerks, seizures.

(c) Extrapyramidal features; and

(d) Autonomic dysfunction, vegetative state progressing to coma.

The diagnosis of SSPE is based on clinical features supported by EEG, cerebrospinal fluid (CSF), neuroimaging and brain biopsy features.

The characteristic finding on EEG are generalised periodic or pseudoperiodic epileptiform discharges (GPEDs) (Fig. 21.9). A ratio of CSF to serum antimeasles antibody titre of 1:4 to 1:128 is characteristic of the disorder. The MRI brain findings are nonspecific with early involvement of posterior deep white matter and gradual involvement of rest of the brain. Only in atypical cases or cases with inconclusive findings on the above mentioned tests and strong clinical suspicion, brain biopsy and molecular testing of mutated measles virus genome is required.

There is no definitive cure and palliative measures like symptomatic and supportive therapy including antiepileptics are not much effective. The most effective therapy to start with is combination of oral isoprinosine and intrathecal interferon α. Isoprinosine is administered at a dose of 50-100 mg/kg/day. The starting dose of interferon α 2b is 1,00,000 units/m^2 which is escalated to 1,000,000 units/m^2 over 5 days, subsequently 1,000,000 units/m^2 twice a week is given. This combination is given

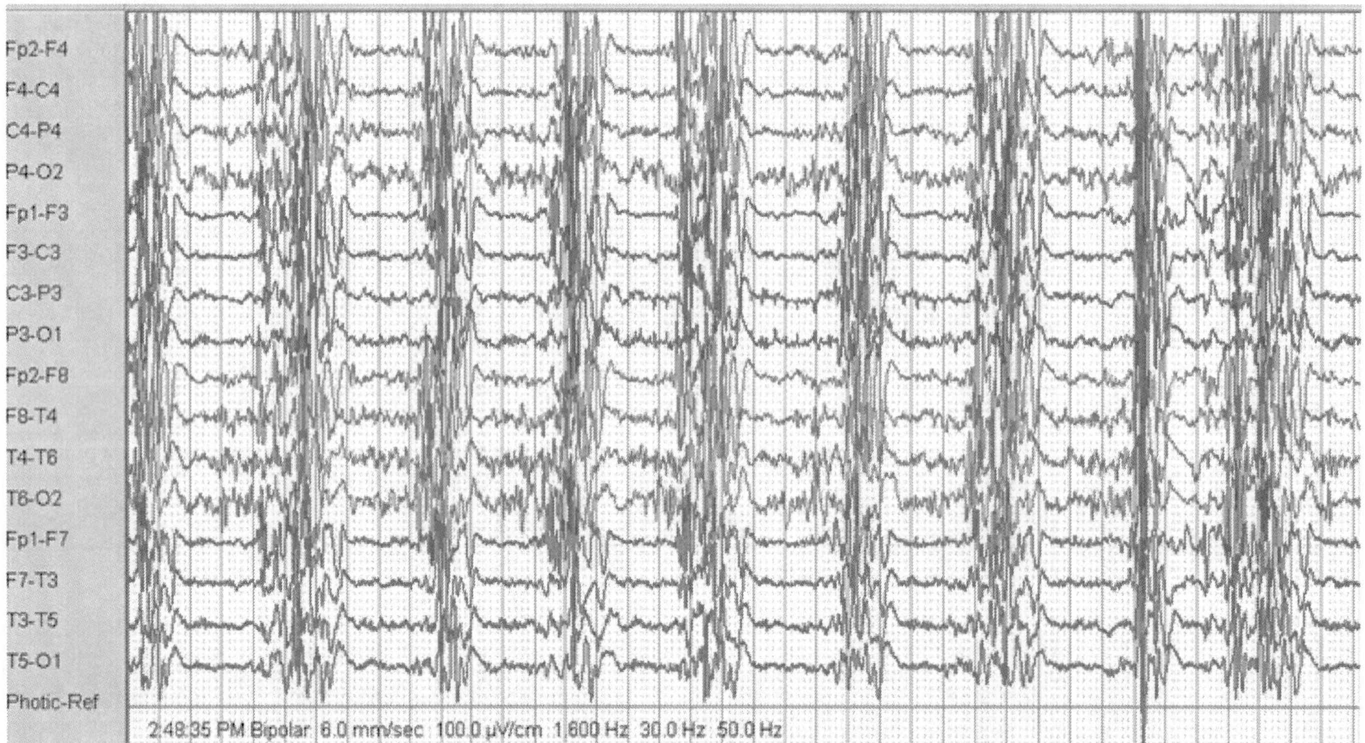

Fig. 21.9: Generalised periodic epileptiform discharges (GPEDs)

for 6 months and then need for further therapy is assessed. Other therapies that have been tried include interferon β, lamivudine and ribavarin.

Overall the prognosis is grim and death usually occurs in 1-3 years from onset. The only effective strategy against SSPE is vaccination against measles.

CONCLUSION

Myoclonic seizures encompass a wide variety of disease spectrum in the pediatric and adolescent age group. There are specific entities pertaining to different age groups. Early and appropriate diagnosis is important for proper treatment and prognostication.

Suggested Reading

- Cantalupo G, Tassinari CA, Bernardina BD. School Age Epilepsy with Myoclonic Absences and Epilepsy with Eyelid Myoclonia and Absences. In: Pellock's Pediatric Epilepsy: Diagnosis and Therapy. Pellock JM, Nordli DR, Sankar R, Wheless WJ. Fourth Edition. 2017. Demos Medical Publication 323-36.
- De Siqueira LFM. Progressive Myoclonic Epilepsies: Review of Clinical, Molecular and Therapeutic Aspects. J Neurol 2010;257:1612-19.
- Garg RK. Subacute Sclerosing Panencephalitis. J Neurol 2008;255:1861-71.
- Gutierrez J, Issacson RS, Koppel BS. Subacute Sclerosing Panencephalitis: An update. Dev. Med. Child Neurol 2010;52: 901-07.
- Singhal NS, Harini C, Sullivan J. Epileptic Spasms and myoclonic epilepsy. In: Swaiman's Pediatric Neurology: Principles and Practice, 6th Edition. Swaiman K, Ashwal S, Ferrlero D, Schor N. 2017. New York. Elsevier Publications. e1283-1301.

22 Chapter

METABOLIC SEIZURES AND EPILEPSY

Suvasini Sharma, Deepshikha Rani

INTRODUCTION

Metabolic disorders make up a special category of causes of neonatal and early infantile seizures. They are particularly important because many conditions are treatable, and the inborn errors of metabolism have a risk for recurrence in the same family.

Metabolic disorders cause seizures in the following ways:

- Alteration of intracellular osmolality.
- Depletion of substrates essential for cellular metabolism or membrane function.
- Intracellular accumulation of toxic substances.
- Primary or secondary disturbances in the neurotransmitter pathways.

Accumulation of compounds may cause direct neurotoxicity, and certain triggers, such as fever or intercurrent infections, may precipitate seizure onset and encephalopathy. It is believed that symptoms remain latent until the accumulation of toxic products is sufficient to interfere with cell functions, as in urea cycle disorders and organic acidurias. Primary or secondary disturbances in the neurotransmitter pathways with excess of excitation or lack of inhibition in the immature brain can also enhance seizure activity.

HYPOGLYCEMIA

Hypoglycemia is a frequent yet correctable metabolic cause for neonatal seizures. A blood glucose must be immediately measured in any infant with seizures. Some of the common causes being prematurity, infant of diabetic mothers, hypoxia, liver failure secondary to any cause.

The rare causes for hypoglycemia being hypopituitarism, congenital adrenal insufficiency pancreatic lesion and some inborn errors of metabolism. The symptoms and signs may be non-specific such as refusal to feed, lethargy, jitteriness, hypotonia, apnea and seizures. The hypoglycemia must be corrected immediately as the incidence of neurologic symptoms increases with increased duration of hypoglycemia.

HYPOCALCEMIA

There are 2 peaks. The early onset hypocalcemia commonly seen in the premature babies, low birth weight infants, infants of diabetic mothers and those who have sustained hypoxic injury is seen in the first 2-3 days of life. Late onset hypocalcemia manifests by the end of first week and is predominantly seen in full-term babies fed with formula feeds with inappropriate phosphorus to calcium or magnesium ratios. It may be accompanied by hypomagnesemia too. Late onset hypocalcemic seizures respond very well to calcium supplementation and have an excellent long-term prognosis. Other causes being maternal hyperparathyroidism or rarely a parathyroid agenesis as in Di George syndrome.

INBORN ERRORS OF METABOLISM

These disorders can present across all age groups with variable features such as encephalopathy, seizures, movement disorders, metabolic acidosis, developmental delay or regression, cyclical vomiting, organomegaly or multisystem involvement. In newborns and young infants, IEM may mimic or share overlapping features with common disorders such as sepsis and birth asphyxia. Timely and accurate diagnosis is essential for treatment and for genetic counseling purposes.

Though IEM are a relatively infrequent cause of epilepsy, epileptic seizures are a common feature in several IEM. IEM may present with epileptic encephalopathies when presenting in infancy and early childhood years, at other times the presentation may be that of a movement disorder which may be mistaken for epileptic seizures, e.g., in neurotransmitter disorders.

Classification of Epilepsies Associated With Inborn Errors of Metabolism

Epilepsy associated with IEM may be classified on the basis of a specific biochemical pathway or organelle involved, e.g., disorders of amino acid metabolism, carbohydrate metabolism, urea cycle defects, lysosomal storage disorders, neurotransmitter disorders, etc. Alternatively, they may also be classified by the age at presentation into disorders presenting in the (1) Neonatal period and early infancy (2) Late infancy and childhood; and (3) Adolescent and adult disorders. Mitochondrial disorders may present across the life span.

Clinical Presentations of Epilepsy in Inborn Errors of Metabolism

As stated earlier, inborn errors of metabolism are genetically transmitted enzyme deficiencies that block or interfere with cellular metabolic pathways.

Most inborn errors of metabolism present with progressive neurologic and systemic symptoms. Seizures may be one component of multiple neurological features at presentation or may be the dominant and/or the sole feature of the disease.

The clues to the presence of IEM in children with epilepsy include:

- Positive family history.
- Parental consanguinity.
- Neurodevelopmental delay/regression.
- Lethargy, feeding difficulties, vomiting.
- Failure to thrive.
- Presence of other neurological abnormalities (such as movement disorders, abnormal oculomotor movements, tone abnormalities or ataxia, coma).
- Dysmorphism.
- Hearing or ophthalmological problems (cataracts, retinitis pigmentosa etc.).
- Visceromegaly (hepatosplenomegaly, cardiomegaly etc).

Metabolic Epilepsies Presenting in the Neonatal Period and Early Infancy

The incidence of seizures is higher in the neonatal period given the vulnerability of the immature neonatal brain in terms of the excitation-inhibition imbalance. IEM may also be associated with seizures in the neonatal period with or without encephalopathy in the form of poor feeding, lethargy and vomitting. Excessive irritability, abnormal crying, abnormal sleep and hiccups are typical clinical markers.

Pyridoxine-Dependent Epilepsy

Pyridoxine-dependent epilepsy (PDE) is characterized by recurrent seizures in the prenatal, neonatal, and/or postnatal periods that are resistant to conventional anti-epileptic drugs but responsive to pharmacological dosages of pyridoxine. The underlying genetic defect is in ALDH7A1 gene resulting in the deficiency of α-aminoadipic semialdehyde dehydrogenase (antiquitin), which is involved in cerebral lysine catabolism.

PDE usually presents within hours or days of birth with seizures, gastrointestinal symptoms such as emesis and abdominal distension, or with features of hyperalertness, hyperacusis, irritability, paroxysmal facial grimacing and abnormal eye movements. The seizure types include multifocal and generalized myoclonic jerks, often intermixed with tonic seizures, and partial motor seizures.

Measurement of serum pipecolic acid and α aminoadipic acid semialdehyde (elevated) and serum pyridoxal-5-phosphate (decreased) needs to be performed before mutational analysis and initiation of trials. An initial dose 100 mg of pyridoxine can be given intravenously. This should be followed by oral pyridoxine supplementation (30 mg/kg/day in two divided doses) for 3-7 days. If the treatment is successful and/or the diagnosis confirmed by biochemical and/or molecular genetic testing, pyridoxine treatment must be continued indefinitely.

Pyridox(am)ine 5'-phosphate Oxidase (PNPO) Deficiency

Babies with PNPO deficiency are often born premature and present with encephalopathy, seizures, lactic acidosis and hypoglycemia. These infants present with pyridoxine resistant but pyridoxal phosphate responsive seizures. EEG may show a burst suppression pattern. However, a definitive diagnosis can only be established by molecular genetic testing for mutations in the PNPO gene. The treatment is enteral administration of pyridoxal phosphate (upto 60 mg/kg/day).

Folinic Acid Responsive Seizures

They also present similarly with epileptic encephalopathy and refractory seizures. They are considered similar to pyridoxine dependent epilepsy both biochemically and genetically. They respond to folinic acid supplementation in addition to pyridoxine supplementation. The dose of folinic acid is 3-5 mg/kg/day.

Biotinidase and Holocarboxylase Synthetase Deficiency

Biotinidase deficiency is an autosomal recessively inherited neurocutaneous disorder. In biotinidase deficiency, the endogenous recycling of biotin is impaired. Epilepsy usually starts after the first 3 or 4 months of life, and often as infantile spasms. Clinical manifestations include: hypotonia; seizures; eczematous skin rash; alopecia; respiratory problems, such as hyperventilation, laryngeal stridor, and apnea; conjunctivitis, candidiasis; ataxia; developmental delay; hearing loss; and vision problems, such as optic atrophy. It is often associated with intermittent metabolic acidosis, ketosis, lactic acidosis, organic aciduria, and mild hyperammonemia. The seizures and skin manifestations respond promptly to small doses of biotin, usually 5-20 mg/day while other features, such as developmental delay, optic atrophy, and hearing loss, are usually irreversible once they occur. In holocarboxylase synthase deficiency, symptoms start during the neonatal period. Seizures are less frequent, occurring in 25-50% of all children. Biotin is effective although a higher dose may be needed in some cases.

Glucose Transporter Defect (GLUT1 Deficiency Syndrome)

It occurs due to deficiency of cerebral glucose transporter (GLUT1) leading to impaired glucose transport to the brain. It classically presents with AED resistant infantile onset epilepsy, developmental delay, acquired microcephaly, hypotonia, spasticity, and movement disorders such as choreoathetosis, ataxia and dystonia. Patients usually appear normal at birth, and present with refractory focal motor seizures in early infancy. Beyond infancy, generalized seizures are common. Finding of a low CSF glucose in fasting (< 40) can help in diagnosis. However, genetic testing for pathogenic mutation in the SLC2A1 gene is considered the gold standard. The manifestations of the disease is usually responsive to ketogenic diet.

Nonketotic Hyperglycinemia

Nonketotic hyperglycinemia accumulation of glycine in the brain. Patients with the classic nonketotic hyperglycinemia phenotype present in the newborn period with hypotonia, feeding difficulties, encephalopathy, seizures and apneas. The presence of hiccups are an important clinical clue. Characteristically EEG recordings show a burst suppression pattern which later evolves to hypsarrhythmia and multifocal epilepsy.

Magnetic resonance spectroscopy demonstrates a glycine peak in the proton MRS spectra. The diagnosis is performed by testing glycine levels in the plasma and CSF. There is an increased ratio of CSF to plasma glycine > 0.04. The definitive diagnosis again is established by molecular genetic testing. Sodium benzoate and 1dextromethorphan (NMDA receptor antagonist) may be helpful in some milder forms of the disease, alongside AED and general supportive care.

Urea Cycle Defects, Organic Acidemias and Aminoacidopathies

Urea cycle disorders represent disorders in the pathway of ammonia detoxification into urea. Babies with urea cycle defects are normal at birth but soon develop lethargy, poor feeding, seizures, and tone abnormalities in the first 4-7 days of life. Diagnosis is suspected by the presence of high ammonia levels in the absence of metabolic acidosis or ketosis. Confirmation is done by testing for the deficient enzyme activity and molecular genetic testing.

Organic acidemias such as methylmalonic aciduria, propionic aciduria have similar presentation as urea cycle defects. The biochemical hallmark is the presence of significant metabolic acidosis with or without ketosis and hyperammonemia. The diagnosis is established by means of quantitative analysis of plasma amino acids and acylcarnitines, as well as urinary organic acids. Special dietary formulae, cofactor supplementation are essential for seizure management and prevent irreversible long-term sequelae.

The classic variant of maple syrup urine disease also presents in the neonatal period with encephalopathy, tone abnormalities and/or seizures usually at the end of the first week of life. There is no acidosis or hyperammonemia; the biochemical diagnostic clue is the presence of urine ketones.

Peroxisomal Disorders

Peroxisomes are intracellular organelles responsible for oxidation of branched-chain as well as very-long-chain fatty acids (VLCFAs). Peroxisomal disorders associated with early onset seizures include Zellweger syndrome, neonatal adrenoleukodystrophy, and infantile Refsum's disease. **Zellweger syndrome** is a multisystem disorder characterized by craniofacial abnormalities, eye abnormalities, neuronal migration defects, hepatomegaly, and chondrodysplasia punctata. Seizures occur in 70-90% of the patients and are difficult to control. Diagnosis is established by demonstration of elevated plasma VLCFA levels and relevant pathogenic mutation in one of the PEX genes. There is no definitive treatment.

EPILEPSIES ASSOCIATED WITH INBORN ERRORS OF METABOLISM PRESENTING IN LATE INFANCY AND CHILDHOOD

Disorders of Creatine Biosynthesis and Transport

Creatine deficiency syndromes present with developmental delay/intellectual disability, behavior problems, autistic features, speech delay, epilepsy, and movement disorders. They are diagnosed by abnormal levels of urinary creatine and/or guanidinoacetate (GAA). There may be a marked reduction of the creatine signal peak on proton magnetic resonance spectroscopy (MRS).

Oral supplementation of creatine monohydrate (400 mg/day) is used to restore cerebral creatine levels. High-dose L-ornithine supplementation and substrate deprivation via an arginine-restricted diet help reduce GAA levels.

Lysosomal Storage Disorders

Lysosomal storage disorders presenting with seizures in this age group include conditions such as; neuronal ceroid lipofuscinoses (NCL), gangliosidosis (GM1, GM2), Niemann-Pick disease, Gaucher's disease and sialidosis. The early features are cognitive decline and seizures, while motor regression occurs later. Gangliosidosis, Niemann-Pick disease, Gaucher's disease and sialidosis are characterized by the presence of hepatosplenomegaly in addition to seizures and cognitive decline. Coarse facies are noted in GM1 gangliosidosis. Biochemical assays of lysosomal acid hydrolases in white cell pellets, skin fibroblasts can help the diagnostic process, while confirmation of pathogenic mutations is by molecular genetic testing.

Mitochondrial Disorders

Mitochondrial disorders can present in any age wherein seizures may be preceded by or associated with other symptoms such as failure to thrive, developmental delay, ataxia, vision impairment, deafness and evidence of multiorgan involvement. Epilepsy is a frequent manifestation, with seizures reported to occur in 35% to 60% of individuals with biochemically confirmed mitochondrial disease. The MRI may show signal abnormalities in the basal ganglia and/or cerebellum, cerebral and/or cerebellar atrophy and white matter abnormalities. MRS studies may show an elevated lactate peak in affected regions of the brain.

In suspected mitochondrial epilepsies, diagnosis requires testing of blood and CSF lactate (which may be variably elevated), MRI and MRS of the brain, muscle biopsy (histology may show ragged red fibers and cytochrome oxidase (COX) negative fibers) and analysis of the respiratory chain enzymes on the muscle biopsy. Further genetic testing is guided by the results of the respiratory chain enzyme testing on the muscle biopsy. Treatment is generally supportive and symptomatic. The use of sodium valproate must be avoided in all patients with suspected mitochondrial epilepsies.

Epilepsies Associated with IEM Presenting in Adolescence and Adulthood

Epilepsies associated with IEM presenting in this age group can be divided into 2 major groups: Progressive myoclonic epilepsies and Other epilepsy types.

Clues to an underlying IEM include episodes of encephalopathy (especially during periods of stress and intercurrent infections, vomiting, ataxia, movement disorders, hepatic involvement, organomegaly, and vision and hearing impairment.

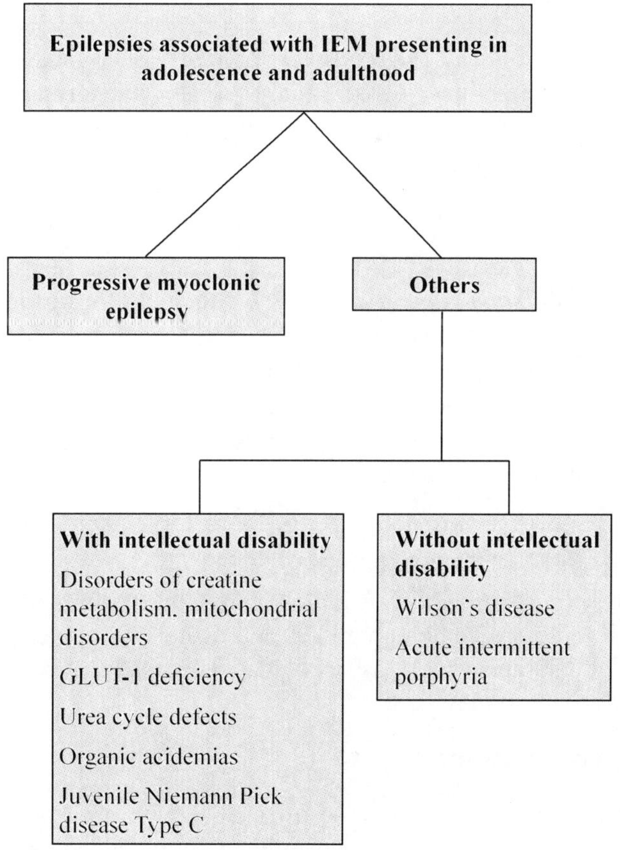

Approach to Diagnosis of IEM Associated Epilepsy

IEM are a rare cause of epilepsy, accounting for about 5-7% in retrospective studies; but must be considered when clinical clues are present.

History

- Details of the pregnancy, delivery and postnatal factors.
- History of excessive fetal movements.
- The age of onset of symptoms.
- The age of onset of seizures, the type of seizures and relationship with the sleep wake cycle and food intake.
- Presence of hiccups along with encephalopathy.
- A detailed family history and a three-generation pedigree with relevant information should be assembled.
- Development along with developmental arrest or regression after the onset of seizures.
- Presence of autistic features.

Examination

- *Craniofacial dysmorphic features* (chromosomal abnormalities, peroxisomal disorders, abnormal fat pads in congenital disorders of glycosylation).
- *Head circumference.*
- *Skin and hair* abnormalities (Menke's disease, biotinidase deficiency).
- *Ophthalmological evaluation* to look for features of pigmentary retinopathy (NCL, mitochondrial disorders), macular cherry red spots (gangliosidosis, Niemann-Pick disease), lens dislocation (sulfite oxidase deficiency), and cataract (serine biosynthesis defects).
- *Systemic examination* to look for organomegaly (storage disorders) must be done.
- *Neurological examination* must be performed to assess tone abnormalities, and associated movement disorders such as dystonia, choreoathetosis and stereotypies.

Investigations

The investigative work up of a child with a suspected IEM with epilepsy is a combination of biochemical, neuroimaging, EEG, tissue biopsies (e.g., muscle biopsies in suspected mitochondrial disorders) and molecular genetic testing.

Biochemical Investigations

- Blood glucose, electrolytes (calcium, magnesium), lactate, arterial blood gas, ammonia and urine ketones are the first line investigations.
- Plasma acylcarnitine, amino acid and urinary organic acid profile.
- Total homocysteine levels (MTHFR deficiency) and biotinidase enzyme assay.
- Lumbar puncture for brain neurochemistry.

EEG

EEG helps to clarify the seizure type and the type of epileptic encephalopathy. A video-EEG is preferable over a routine EEG, especially when there are frequent seizures. A sleep and awake record must be obtained, lasting 45-60 min, in order not to miss abnormalities.. Photic stimulation must be done, as it is frequently elicits abnormal photoparoxysmal. The abnormalities seen in EEG are not specific but some abnormalities such as burst suppression may suggest of an underlying IEM. A comb-like rhythm has been described in MSUD. The presence of rhythmic high-amplitude delta with superimposed (poly) spikes (RHADS) in a child with status epilepticus is a pointer towards the presence of Alpers disease.

Neuroimaging Studies

MRI of the brain must be performed in all children with epilepsy and suspected IEM. The features to be noted while evaluating an MRI for suspected IEM include signal abnormalities in the cortex, basal ganglia, brainstem, dentate nucleus, any diffusion restriction, white matter signal abnormality and its pattern, and presence of any cerebral malformations.

MRI may show symmetrical basal ganglia signal abnormalities in organic acidemias and mitochondriopathies. A proton MR spectroscopy performed simultaneously is of diagnostic value in many IEMs such as glycine encephalopathy, creatine deficiency syndromes, maple syrup urine disease (leucine peak), and mitochondriopathies (elevated lactate). The presence of cortical dysgenesis or malformation of cortical development may be seen in Zellweger syndrome.

Genetic Testing

When a particular disorder is suspected based on the clinical phenotype and results of biochemical testing, molecular genetic testing for pathogenic mutations must be performed to confirm the diagnosis and aid in genetic counseling.

If no diagnosis is reached, targeted next generation sequencing gene panels for epileptic encephalopathy should be performed. complex deficiency. Forty-five percent of patients obtained a genetic diagnosis by targeted next-generation sequencing epileptic encephalopathy panels. All the patients with IEM in this series had either clinical (e.g., Menkes disease with brittle hair) or biochemical features (e.g., GLUT1 deficiency with low CSF glucose level) suggestive of the underlying disorder.

Next generation sequencing technologies, using whole exome sequencing (WES), and whole genome sequencing (WGS) may be considered in patients in whom the diagnosis has not been made by the above-mentioned strategies.

Tissue Biopsies

Invasive procedures such as skin and muscle biopsies are generally reserved until the later stages of investigation when biochemical and genetic testing have proven unhelpful. Ultrastructural abnormalities in the skin and muscle may reveal diagnostic clues to inborn errors of metabolism. Biochemical assays on fresh muscles are necessary to diagnose defects in the respiratory chain, while many specific enzyme assays can be carried out in fibroblast cultures.

Treatment

Specific treatments where available should be instituted.

A sequential therapeutic trial with vitamin B_6, folinic acid and pyridoxal phosphate should be instituted early in all babies with epileptic encephalopathy and poor response to antiepileptic treatment.

Biotin should be added in babies with refractory seizures and alopecia and seborrheic dermatitis.

Patients with thiamine transporter deficiency due to mutations in *SLC19A3*, benefit from treatment with thiamine (200-300 mg/day) if started immediately on the basis of clinical manifestations.Thiamine may also be beneficial for seizures in late-onset pyruvate dehydrogenase complex deficiency.

Ketogenic diet is useful in refractory epilepsy and super refractory status epilepticus, irrespective of etiology however, disorders which may worsen on starting the ketogenic diet must be excluded first. These include β-oxidation defects, disorders of ketolysis and gluconeogenesis.

In IEM where no specific treatments exist, symptomatic treatment is with anti-epileptic drugs. Conventionally used anti-epileptic drugs can be used in most patients. Sodium valproate needs to be used with caution. Sodium valproate is generally contraindicated in mitochondrial disorders and urea cycle defects because of the risk of hyperammonemia.

Steroids are useful in many epileptic encephalopathies but they must be used with caution as they alter metabolic pathways and could therefore be poorly tolerated.

Newer treatments are on the horizon for many IEM that orphan disorders. These may involve repurposing known molecules, developing fusion proteins that navigate across the blood brain barrier, chaperones, gene replacement and enzyme replacement therapies, that will no doubt bring new hope for future outcomes of presently untreatable conditions.

Suggested Reading

- Campistol J, Plecko B. Treatable Newborn and Infant Seizures Due to Inborn Errors of Metabolism. Epileptic Disord 2015: 17:229-42.
- Mercimek-Mahmutoglu S, Patel J, Cordeiro D, Hewson S, Callen D, Donner EJ, Hahn CD, Kannu P, Kobayashi J, Minassian BA, et al., Diagnostic Yield of Genetic Testing in Epileptic Encephalopathy in Childhood. Epilepsia 2015: 56:706-16.
- Pascual JM, Campistol J, Gil-Nagel A. Epilepsy in Inherited Metabolic Disorders. Neurologist 2008:14:S2-S14. doi: 10.1097/01.nrl.0000340787.30542.41.
- Prasad AN Hoffmann GF. Early Onset Epilepsy and Inherited Metabolic Disorders: Diagnosis and Management. Can. J. Neurol. Sci. 2010;37:350-58. doi: 10.1017/S0317167100010246.
- Sharma S, Kumar P, Agarwal R, Kabra M, Deorari AK, Paul VK. Approach to Inborn Errors of Metabolism Presenting in the Neonate. Indian J. Pediatr 2008;75:271-76. doi: 10.1007/s12098-008-0058.
- Sharma S and Prasad AN. Inborn Errors of Metabolism and Epilepsy: Current Understanding, Diagnosis and Treatment Approaches. International Journal of Molecular Sciences 2017:18(7):1384.

23 Chapter

REFRACTORY EPILEPSY IN CHILDREN

Satinder Aneja, Puneet Jain

Approximately one-third of children with epilepsy develop drug-refractory epilepsy. The identification of refractory epilepsy can have broad implications regarding education, social functioning and recreational activities of the child. This review briefly discusses the definition, mechanisms, investigations and treatment modalities available for a child with refractory epilepsy.

DEFINITION

Terms 'refractory', 'intractable', 'drug-resistant', 'pharmaco-resistant' have been used interchangeably in literature. Broadly, refractory epilepsy may be defined as failure of complete or acceptable control of seizures in response to the anti-epileptic drugs. The definition is still evolving.

Recently, International League Against Epilepsy (ILAE) proposed a consensus definition for drug-resistant epilepsy. However, for routine use, failure of seizure-control despite trial of two appropriate AED regimens at maximum tolerated doses should be considered as drug-refractoriness and is highly likely to indicate failure with subsequent AED trials.

'*Pseudo*' or '*apparent*' refractoriness should be excluded before a diagnosis of refractory epilepsy. The factors to be considered includes appropriateness of the drug for the epilepsy syndrome, compliance, 'seizure mimickers', adequate dosing and trial and drug interactions.

EPIDEMIOLOGY

The refractory epilepsy is seen in 9-23% of children with epilepsy. Few studies have also explored the factors which may predict intractability. Younger age at onset, neonatal status epilepticus, high initial seizure frequency, failure of response to first anti-epileptic drug, specific epilepsy syndromes (infantile spasms, Lennox-Gastaut syndrome), mixed seizure types, symptomatic/cryptogenic etiology, history of febrile seizures, history of status epilepticus, abnormal neurological status and abnormal neuroimaging are important factors which may predict drug-refractoriness. EEG features like diffuse slowing and focal spike-wave discharges have also been reported to be independent predictors of intractability.

The natural history of childhood epilepsies is complex. The 'Refractoriness' may not be a permanent state. The focal epilepsies may show late onset of refractoriness as compared to epileptic encephalopathies and other secondarily generalized epilepsies which show early drug refractoriness.

ETIOLOGY

The etiologies of refractory epilepsy in children are diverse. Table 23.1 lists the common etiologies of refractory epilepsy. In developing countries like India, the etiology of refractory epilepsy may differ from the western literature. The adverse peri-natal events (48%) and CNS infection sequelae (24%) were the major causes of refractory epilepsy in one study from India (Chawla *et al.*).

The search for an underlying etiology is pivotal as it may guide the medical or surgical treatment of the child and also aid in parental counseling.

The identification of a particular epilepsy syndrome is critical as it has implications for management and

Table 23.1: Common Etiologies of Refractory Epilepsy in Children

Epilepsy syndromes*
- Ohtahara syndrome
- Early myoclonic encephalopathy
- Epilepsy of infancy with migrating focal seizures
- West syndrome
- Dravet syndrome
- Lennox-Gastaut syndrome
- Epilepsy with Myoclonic-Astatic epilepsy
- Epileptic encephalopathy with continuous spike and wave during sleep (CSWS)

Structural
- *Malformations:* Lissencephaly, Neuronal heterotopias, Polymicrogyria and Schizencephaly, Focal cortical dysplasia, Hemimegalencephaly, Holoprosencephaly
- *Neurocutaneous syndromes:* Tuberous Sclerosis complex, Sturge Weber syndrome, Hypomelanosis of Ito, Incontinentia pigmenti, Epidermal nevus syndrome
- *Infectious/Inflammatory:* Post-meningitis / encephalitis epilepsy, Rasmussen encephalitis, Hypoxic ischemic encephalopathy, Stroke
- *Tumors:* Dysembryoblastic Neuroepithelial tumor (DNET), ganglioglioma, low grade astrocytoma, hypothalamic hamartoma, Mesial temporal sclerosis

Metabolic

Potentially Treatable
- Antiquitin deficiency (Pyridoxine dependent epilepsy)
- Biotinidase deficiency
- GLUT1 deficiency syndrome
- Creatine deficiency
- Serine biosynthesis deficiency

Others
- Organic academia, Urea cycle disorders, Aminoacidopathies
- Peroxisomal disorders, Non-ketotic hyperglycinemia
- Molybdenum cofactor deficiency, sulfite oxidase deficiency
- Mitochondrial disorders including Alpers syndrome
- Menkes disease, GABA neurotransmitter defects
- Congenital disorders of glycosylation
- Progressive myoclonic epilepsies

Genetic
- *Chromosomal:* 1p36 deletion, 4p Syndrome, Ring chromosome 14 and 20, Inv dup 15 syndrome, Down syndrome, Angelman syndrome
- *Syndromic:* Pitt Hopkins syndrome, Mowat Wilson syndrome, PEHO syndrome
- *Specific genes:* MeCP2, CDKL5, FOXG1, SLC25A22, SPTAN1, STXBP1, ARX, KCNJ11, SCN1A, SCN1B, SCN2A

Miscellaneous
- *Fever-related epilepsies:* Febrile infection-related epilepsy syndrome (FIRES), Idiopathic hemiconvulsion-hemiplegia syndrome
- *Autoimmune epilepsies:* NMDA, VGKC complex, GAD

GAD: Glutamic acid decarboxylase; NMDA: N-methyl-d-aspartate; PEHO: Progressive encephalopathy with edema, hypsarrhythmia and optic atrophy syndrome; VGKC: Voltage-gated potassium channel.

*They have diverse etiologies.

counseling. For example, epileptic spasms in a normal or a delayed infant with/without neuroregression and hypsarrhythmia/variants on EEG suggest West syndrome. Refractory polymorphic seizures (predominantly tonic) in 3-5 years age group with cognitive decline and characteristic EEG features (slow spike-wave discharges and paroxysmal fast activity) are characteristic of Lennox-Gastaut syndrome. An infant presenting with frequent febrile seizures (mainly clonic), with subsequent evolution to refractory multiple seizure types (myoclonic/absences/focal) with neurocognitive deterioration, may have Dravet syndrome. The use of appropriate anti-epileptic drugs with realistic seizure-control goals is warranted in these conditions.

CLINICAL EVALUATION

The history and physical examination are the basic tools in the evaluation of a child with refractory epilepsy. Table 23.2 lists the salient points to be included in the clinical evaluation.

Table 23.2: Clinical Evaluation of A Child with Refractory Epilepsy

History
- Age of onset of seizures
- *Accurate description of seizure:* Pre-ictal, ictal, post-ictal; precipitating events
- Seizure types, evolution
- Relation to fever
- Previous history of febrile seizures (simple/complex)
- *Anti-epileptic drugs:* Names, dosages, duration, compliance, response, adverse effects

Developmental trajectory: Normal, stagnation, regression

Pointers towards inborn error of metabolism

Comorbidities

Detailed birth and peri-/antenatal history

Previous history of trauma/CNS infection

Family history

Examination
- *Anthropometry:* Failure to thrive, Head circumference, Facial dysmorphism
- Neurocutaneous features
- Detailed neurological and systemic assessment

INVESTIGATIONS

Electroencephalography (EEG)

A prolonged scalp EEG recording in a child with refractory epilepsy is invaluable and often rewarding. The aims of the EEG recording are epilepsy syndrome classification (e.g., Lennox-Gastaut syndrome, West syndrome), localization in cases of focal epilepsy, diagnosis of non-convulsive status epilepticus (commonly seen in many catastrophic childhood epilepsy syndromes) and evaluate the suspected non-epileptic events which may contribute to 'pseudo' refractoriness. It is especially useful in neonates to evaluate suspected subtle seizures and non-epileptic paroxysmal movements like reactive myoclonus. Figure 23.1 shows the EEG features in common drug-refractory epilepsy syndromes.

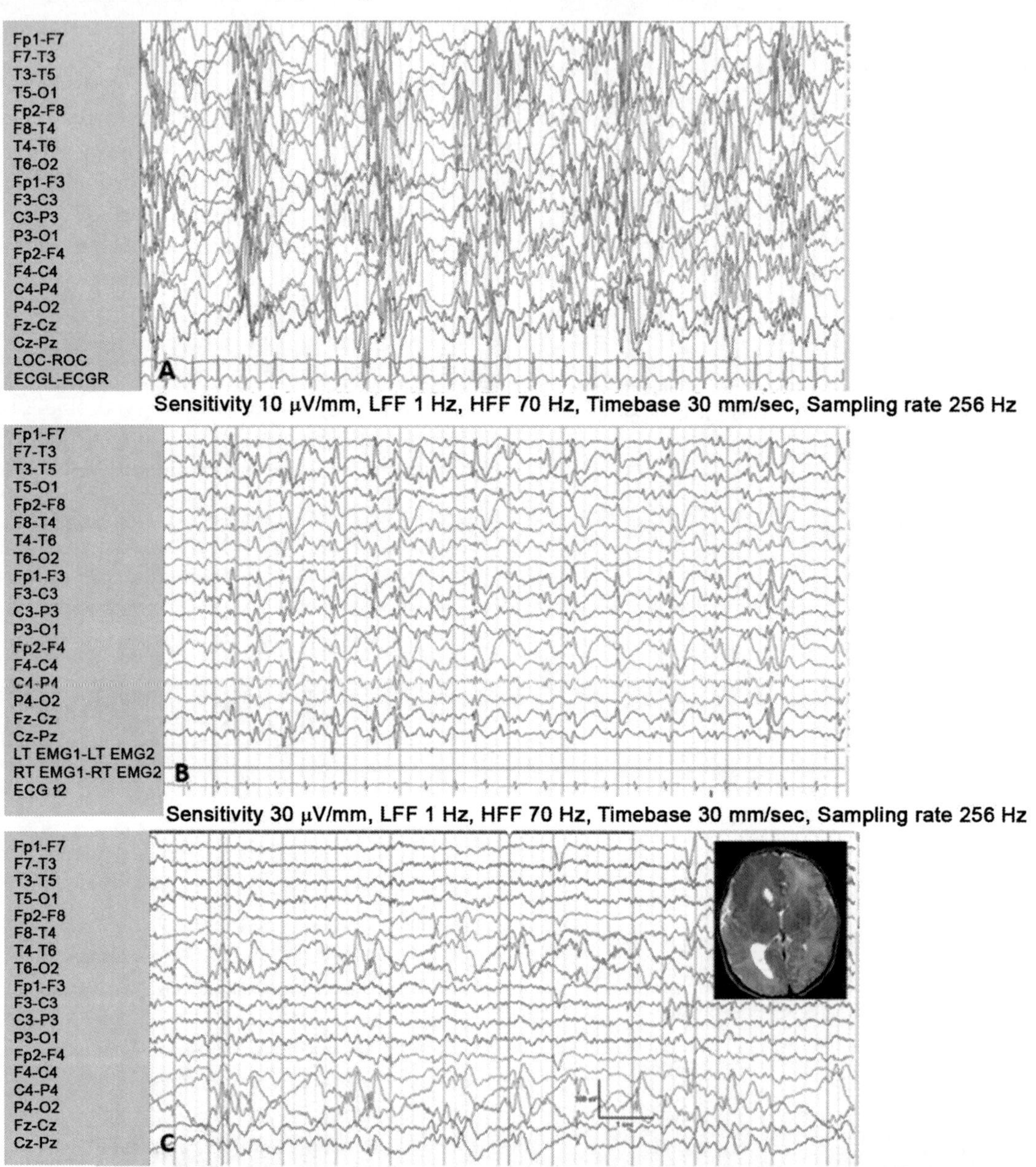

A – Modified hypsarrhythmia in West syndrome: The sleep record shows bursts of generalized synchronous and asynchronous high amplitude slow waves interspersed with spikes followed by electro-decremental response; B – EEG findings in Lennox-Gastaut Syndrome during sleep: There is nearly continuous 1-2 Hz bilateral synchronized spike wave discharges during the sleep (slow spike waves); C – EEG finding in an infant with early onset drug refractory left focal seizures; note very frequent spike/sharp waves over the right hemisphere and occasional spike waves over the left hemisphere. MRI brain showed right hemi-megalencephaly. The child underwent functional hemi-spherectomy at 13 months of age with significant reduction in seizure frequent post-surgery and considerable developmental gains.

Fig. 23.1: EEG in refractory epilepsy

The yield of the EEG recording can be increased by extending the duration of recording, inclusion of the video component or admitting for prolonged inpatient video-EEG monitoring (Long Term Monitoring; LTM). A sleep EEG recording is a must. The natural sleep is preferred but if sedation is required, it is prudent to record arousal at the end of the recording.

The scalp EEG has numerous limitations (e.g., records activity only from the cerebral convexities, artefacts). The invasive EEG recordings are used only when non-invasive methods (scalp EEG/neuroimaging/magneto-encephalography) fail to localize the ictal onset zone sufficiently. It may also be helpful when the epileptogenic lesion is very close to the eloquent cortex.

Neuroimaging

The advances in neuroimaging have revolutionized the management of pediatric epilepsy. The detailed discussion of the newer imaging modalities is beyond the scope of this article and has been reviewed recently.

The role of computed tomography (CT) head is limited. It may aid in diagnosis of disorders like neurocysticercosis, intrauterine infections, neurocutaneous syndromes like Sturge-Weber syndrome and Tuberous Sclerosis Complex and tumors like dysembryoplastic neuroepithelial tumors (DNET).

Magnetic Resonance Imaging (MRI) of the brain is the modality of choice in the initial investigation of a child with refractory epilepsy. As per ILAE recommendations, the following MRI sequences should be performed: thin slice (4-5 mm) volumetric T1-weighted gradient-recalled echo sequence, axial and coronal T2-weighted sequence, fluid attenuated inversion recovery (FLAIR) sequence and high resolution oblique coronal T2-weighted imaging of the hippocampus. Gadolinium contrast may be required where tumors, vascular malformations, inflammation or infectious etiologies are suspected on non-contrast studies. 3T-MRI brain provides improved image signal-to-noise and contrast-to-noise ratios as compared to the conventional 1.5T-MRI brain. It may increase the yield of neuroimaging and is especially useful in cases of suspected malformations of cortical development.

A systematic approach to the visual assessment of the MRI images is essential even in the presence of the obvious lesion as dual pathology (association of two potentially epileptogenic lesions, hippocampal and extra-hippocampal) is not uncommon. Further, mild focal cortical dysplasia may be missed on structural imaging. If the initial MRI brain was normal in a child with refractory epilepsy, a repeat MRI may be rewarding especially if the initial study was inadequate, was done at a younger age (immature myelination) or for disorders with progressive radiological findings like Rasmussen encephalitis.

Functional neuroimaging is usually warranted in all possible epilepsy surgery cases, especially with normal structural imaging or discordant radiological and clinico-EEG features. The functional imaging modalities may include Inter-ictal Positron Emission Tomography (PET), Ictal and Inter-ictal Single-photon emission CT (SPECT) and Subtraction Ictal SPECT co-registered with MRI (SISCOM). Functional MRI is also used to lateralize/localize language especially in children with lesions over the dominant hemisphere. The detailed discussion of the functional imaging and other pre-surgical work-up is beyond the scope of this chapter.

Magnetoencephalography

Magnetoencephalography (MEG) is an important tool in the presurgical evaluation of patients with drug-refractory epilepsy. MEG detects magnetic fields produced by the brain's electrical activity. MEG can only detect electrical sources that are tangential to the skull surface. This is in comparison to EEG which detects only radially oriented electrical sources. Thus, the two modalities complement each other. MEG signals in combination with source modeling techniques can yield vital information regarding the underlying epileptogenic zone. MEG evaluation is particularly useful in children with non-lesional neocortical epilepsy. In these cases, MEG spike sources can guide pre-surgical and perioperative invasive monitoring.

Metabolic Work-Up

Refractory seizures may be seen in diverse neurometabolic disorders (Table 23.1). The epileptogenesis in these disorders may be secondary to lack of energy, intoxication, impaired neuronal function, disturbances of the neurotransmitter system or associated cerebral malformations.

The metabolic work-up may also be warranted in children planned for dietary therapies.

The metabolic screen should include blood gas analysis, arterial lactate, blood sugar, ammonia and urinary ketones. Further investigations should be guided by the clinical suspicion. These may include tandem mass spectroscopy, urine gas chromatography-mass spectrometry, long chain fatty acids (peroxisomal disorders), urine mucopolysaccharides/oligosaccharides, urine sulphite test (sulphite oxidase deficiency), enzyme assays for lysosomal disorders, plasma/urine creatine, transferrin isoelectrophoresis (congenital disorders of glycosylation), serum copper and ceruloplasmin (Menkes disease), CSF sugar, lactate and neurotransmitter profile, skin and muscle biopsies.

Genetic Testing

The presence of suggestive features like dysmorphism, microcephaly, growth retardation, intellectual disability and hypotonia may indicate an underlying genetic syndrome. Currently, the genetic testing is most useful for Dravet and related syndromes, infantile spasms without any obvious etiology, epilepsy with brain malformations, epilepsy with intellectual disability or dysmorphism.

Karyotype remains helpful to identify chromosomal rearrangements like balanced translocations or ring chromosomes and aneuploidy. Patients with associated dysmorphism and/or multiorgan dysfunction may have higher test yields.

Genomic Microarray has higher yields in patients with associated dysmorphism, congenital anomalies or neuropsychiatric features. It detects larger copy number variations (> 100-300 Kb). Rare copy number variations (CNVs) represent variations in genomic DNA sequence of at least 1 Kb in length seen in < 1% of the population. They are reported to account for 10% of childhood epilepsies and up to 5% of epileptic encephalopathies. They are not detected by routine karyotyping.

Fluorescence in situ hybridization (FISH) analyses specific chromosome portions and is required for the diagnosis of various microdeletion syndromes/duplication. MLPA (multiplex ligation-dependent probe amplification) is used to identify intragenic deletions or duplications. Single gene sequencing detects changes in a single gene (point mutations, exonic deletions, small CNV) and may be warranted if one encounters a classical genetic phenotype.

Next generation sequencing is another useful, cost-effective method and analyses large number of DNA segments (usually exons) of a selected group of genes organized in panels. Whole exome/genome sequencing are not available widely at this time-point and are expensive. Further, ever-increasing reports of "variants of unknown significance" further complicates the diagnosis and genetic counselling.

Genetic testing has limited role in focal epilepsies. It may be considered in familial cases (Familial focal epilepsy with variable foci, frontal lobe epilepsy, genetic epilepsy with febrile seizures plus, autosomal partial epilepsy with auditory features). It may be worthwhile in sporadic cases like epilepsy-aphasia syndrome or clustering of febrile seizures in first 3 years of life. In other situations, the role of testing in focal epilepsies is unclear.

TREATMENT

The goals of treatment of children with refractory epilepsy include 'realistic' seizure control with minimal adverse effects of the administered drugs with improvement in overall quality of life. This should be coupled with early identification of potential candidates for non-pharmacological therapies. The treatment revolves around three modalities: pharmacotherapy, epilepsy surgery and alternative measures (like dietary therapy, vagus nerve stimulation).

Pharmacotherapy

The decision to start a particular anti-epileptic drug is largely empirical and rarely evidence-based. The selection should be based on the patients' characteristics (age, sex, comorbidities, co-medications), seizure type or epilepsy syndrome, previous responses and adverse effects to AEDs and the expected response from the remaining untried drugs. A realistic goal with regard to seizure reduction should be set and 'overtreatment' (unnecessary or excessive AED load in the management of epilepsy leading to a suboptimal risk-to-benefit ratio) be avoided.

Polytherapy: Monotherapy with anti-epileptic drugs (AEDs) is often desirable. But as noted earlier, about a third of patients with epilepsy will be drug-refractory, polytherapy with the anti-epileptic drugs is often unavoidable. The main goal of polytherapy is to achieve realistic seizure control (total elimination or seizure reduction based on the etiology) with minimal adverse effects and least impact on the quality of life.

Irrational polytherapy may result from inadequate knowledge of the mechanisms of action of various AEDs, their pharmacokinetic and pharmacodynamic interactions, inappropriate diagnosis of epilepsy syndrome with use of inappropriate AED and unrealistic seizure reduction goals. It is often prudent to combine drugs with different mechanisms of action.

Further, an appropriate diagnosis of the epilepsy syndrome is pivotal for the pharmacotherapy with use of appropriate AEDs. Phenobarbitone, phenytoin, carbamazepine, vigabatrin and gabapentin may exacerbate absence and myoclonic seizures (including epileptic spasms). Benzodiazepines may worsen tonic seizures. Carbamazepine and lamotrigine may worsen Electrical status epilepticus during sleep (ESES) spectrum epilepsies.

Few guiding tips for polytherapy includes: Adequate trial of a single AED (dose and duration), combine drugs with different mechanisms of action, inclusion of at least one broad spectrum AED in the regimen, avoiding combination of drugs with prominent sedative effects, trial of different dual drug therapies before adding a third drug, slow titration of a new drug, reduction of the dose of the older drug once the goal of seizure reduction is achieved with the new drug and exclusion of the causes of 'pseudo' refractoriness. Always consider non-pharmacological options of treatment as children who have failed the first anti-epileptic drug, are less likely to respond to subsequently added drugs.

Treatment of Non-Convulsive Status Epilepticus (NCSE): NCSE may be commonly seen in some epilepsy syndromes [like Lennox-Gastaut syndrome (LGS), Doose syndrome, Dravet syndrome, etc]. Oral or intravenous benzodiazepines are usually the first step. It is to be noted that benzodiazepines may precipitate tonic status in children with LGS and hence should be used with caution. Oral steroids, intravenous pulsed methylprednisolone or adrenocorticotrophin hormone may be tried in children who fail treatment with benzodiazepines. Carbamazepine, phenytoin and phenobarbitone must be avoided in these situations.

Metabolic Treatment: Empiric trials of biotin, pyridoxine, pyridoxal phosphate (not available in India) and folinic acid should be considered in all neonates with refractory seizures. Other epilepsies responsive to metabolic treatment are shown in Table 23.3.

Table 23.3: Metabolic/Genetic Epilepsies with Possible Treatments

Effect on ion channels

- Dravet syndrome (SCN1A) – Avoidance of sodium channel blockers
- SCN8A related epileptic encephalopathy – Carbamazepine, Phenytoin [sodium channel blockers]
- KCNQ2 related epileptic encephalopathy – Retigabine [Potassium channel openers] or Carbamazepine [sodium channel blockers]
- KCNT1 related migrating partial epilepsy of infancy–Quinidine [Gain of function mutations being treated by partial channel antagonist]

Contd.

Contd.

- GRIN2A related epileptic encephalopathy – Memantine [NMDA (N-methyl-d-aspartate) receptor antagonists]

Alternative energy source

- GLUT-1 deficiency syndrome (SLC2A1 gene) – Ketogenic Diet

Modulate epileptogenesis

- Tuberous sclerosis complex (TSC1/2) – mTOR inhibitors (Rapamycin/analogs)

Modulating biochemical pathways

- Pyridoxine dependency (ALDH7A1) – B6 vitamin
- Biotinidase deficiency (BTD) – Biotin
- Cerebral folate deficiency (FOLR1) – Folinic acid
- Creatine deficiency syndromes (SLC6A8, GATM, GAMT) – Creatine, other amino acid supplementation (glycine, arginine, ornithine) or restriction (arginine)
- Serine biosynthesis defects (PHGDH, PSAT1, PSPH) – Serine, glycine

Therapeutic Drug Monitoring (TDM): The routine monitoring of plasma concentrations is costly and does not add any useful information. The drug monitoring may be useful to assess compliance and to explain recent changes in seizure frequency or drug tolerability, particularly in children on polytherapy where the problematic drug is unclear. It may also be prudent to test children when changes in the drug pharmacokinetics are expected like with hepatic or renal failure or gastrointestinal problems affecting drug absorption.

The blood samples should be drawn at a steady state, which occurs at 4-5 half lives after treatment initiation or dose modification. The ideal sampling time for all AEDs is drug fasting in the morning. If drug toxicity is suspected, then one sample is drawn at the time of the trough and the second sample at the time of suspected concentration-related symptoms.

Epilepsy Surgery

Epilepsy surgery can be performed effectively and safely in young children. It often results in reduction in seizure frequency/seizure freedom, improvement in quality of life and probably reversal of developmental stagnation. With over 500,000 potential epilepsy surgery candidates in India, not more than 200 epilepsy surgeries per year in handful of centers are being performed today.

As per ILAE guidelines, the potential candidates for epilepsy surgery evaluation include children with uncontrolled or disabling (including medication side effects) seizures, children with epilepsies that cannot be assigned to an electro-clinical syndrome but with stereotyped, lateralized or focal seizures or in whom the MRI reveals a lesion amenable to surgical removal. The detailed pre-surgical evaluation is beyond the scope of this article. It includes video-EEG, structural and functional neuroimaging, magnetoencephalography and neuropsychological testing. There is a need to identify the potential candidates early with prompt referral to an epilepsy surgery centre.

Role of Dietary Therapies

The ketogenic diet (KD) is a high fat, low carbohydrate, and restricted protein diet and is an effective non-pharmacological treatment for refractory epilepsy. It should be considered earlier as an option for treatment of drug-refractory epilepsy. It is specifically the treatment of choice for GLUT1 deficiency syndrome and pyruvate dehydrogenase deficiency. The contraindications are few and include mitochondrial β-oxidation defects, primary carnitine deficiency, carnitine palmitoyltransferase I or II deficiency, carnitine translocase deficiency, pyruvate carboxylase deficiency and porphyria. It is usually well tolerated and the adverse effects may include gastrointestinal (vomiting, constipation, diarrhea, abdominal pain), hyperuricemia, hypocalcemia, acidosis, renal calculi, growth retardation and prolonged QT interval.

More liberal varieties of the classical KD have been developed and these include Modified Atkins Diet, Low glycemic index diet and Medium Chain Triglyceride (MCT)-KD. They have an efficacy close to the classical KD.

Neurostimulation

Vagus Nerve Stimulation (VNS) therapy stimulates the left vagus nerve. The impulses ascending along the vagus nerve reach the nucleus of tractus solitaries with subsequent spread to limbic, reticular and autonomic regions and brainstem nuclei, which may influence various neurotransmitter systems.

The optimal VNS settings are still unknown. Useful starting settings may include an output current of 0.25 mA (target 1.5-2 mA), 30 Hz signal frequency, 500 microseconds pulse width (may use 250 microseconds in adolescents depending on tolerability), on-time of 30 seconds and off time of 5 minutes. Newer devices which detect changes in heart rate (usually associated with seizures) and give automatic stimulations (above the baseline cycle) are also available.

VNS may be considered as adjunctive treatment for children with refractory partial or generalized epilepsy if they are poor surgical candidates or have had unsuccessful surgery. Its complications are uncommon and minor and may include infections, lead fractures, throat discomfort, hoarseness, coughing, increase in drooling or dysphagia and sleep apnea.

Deep Brain Stimulation (DBS) uses chronic electrical stimulation applied to deep nuclei with widespread connections. Centromedian and Anterior nucleus of thalamus have been used as targets for DBS in refractory epilepsy patients.

Responsive Neurostimulator System (RNS) is a closed-loop system which can detect spontaneous seizures and has the ability to respond automatically with electrical stimulation to interrupt the seizure patterns. The device is implanted in the skull and is connected to one or two intracranial depth or strip electrodes. It senses and records brain activity through depth and/or subdural cortical strip leads that are placed at that patient's seizure focus. Seizure detection is tailored to the patient's individual ictal electrographic patterns. The stimulation is also adjustable in terms of frequency and amplitude. It is usually useful in children with drug refractory epilepsy who are not surgical candidates and have 1-2 epileptic foci.

Comprehensive Care

A multidisciplinary team comprising pediatrician/pediatric neurologist, psychologist, rehabilitation, ophthalmologist, ENT specialist, trained nursing, dietician, social worker and public support, is required for the comprehensive care of children with refractory epilepsy. There is a profound impact on the social functioning, education and recreational activities.

The periodic screening for various comorbidities like tone abnormalities, contractures, vision/hearing deficits, dental hygiene, difficulty in feeding/malnutrition, sleep disorders and behavioral disorders, and adverse effects of the anti-epileptic drugs is warranted. The compliance with the drug therapy is to be emphasized. The triggering factors (e.g., sleep deprivation, fever, trauma) should be avoided if possible. There is no restriction on watching television or videogames provided the child sits at maximum distance possible from the screen and there is additional lighting in the room.

Children with epilepsy are believed to be at higher risk of incurring accidental injury than those without seizures. Supervision while sleeping and bathing is necessary. Swimming should be avoided till 3 months of seizure freedom. Protective helmets may be recommended for poorly controlled generalized epilepsies to avoid head injuries. Children on long-term AEDs especially phenobarbitone, phenytoin, carbamazepine and valproate should receive adequate vitamin D (400 IU/day) and calcium. Periodic screening of serum 25 (OH) Vitamin D should be considered.

Sudden Unexpected Death in Epilepsy (SUDEP)

SUDEP is rare in children with epilepsy. The adult studies have identified many risk factors for SUDEP and include high seizure frequency especially generalized tonic-clonic seizures, polytherapy, early onset of epilepsy (<15 years) and associated intellectual disability. SUDEP is not easy to prevent especially in children with refractory epilepsy. The rational use of AEDs and early referral for non-pharmacological modalities would be prudent.

CONCLUSIONS

The refractory epilepsy is a major source of morbidity in children. An approach to a child with refractory epilepsy is shown in Figure 23.2. A detailed clinical evaluation followed by a meticulous search for an underlying etiology especially potentially treatable causes, is imperative. Rational use of anti-epileptic drugs, early referral of potential candidates for epilepsy surgery and early consideration for non-pharmacological options like dietary therapies is warranted. Newer therapeutic options are exciting but require further development and clinical experience. The pharmacogenetics may improve our understanding of the refractory epilepsy and aid in devising rational therapeutic strategies.

Suggested Reading

- Berg AT, Levy SR, Novotny EJ, Shinnar S. Predictors of Intractable Epilepsy in Childhood: A Case-Control Study. Epilepsia 1996;37:24-30.
- Berg AT, Vickrey BG, Testa FM, et al. How Long Does It Take for Epilepsy to Become Intractable? A Prospective Investigation. Ann Neurol 2006;60:73-79.
- Berg AT. Identification of Pharmacoresistant Epilepsy. Neurol Clin 2009;27:1003-13.
- Bernasconi A, Bernasconi N, Bernhardt BC, Schrader D. Advances in MRI for "Cryptogenic" Epilepsies. Nat Rev Neurol 2011;7:99-108.
- Brodie MJ, Sills GJ. Combining Antiepileptic Drugs–Rational Polytherapy? Seizure 2011;20:369-75.

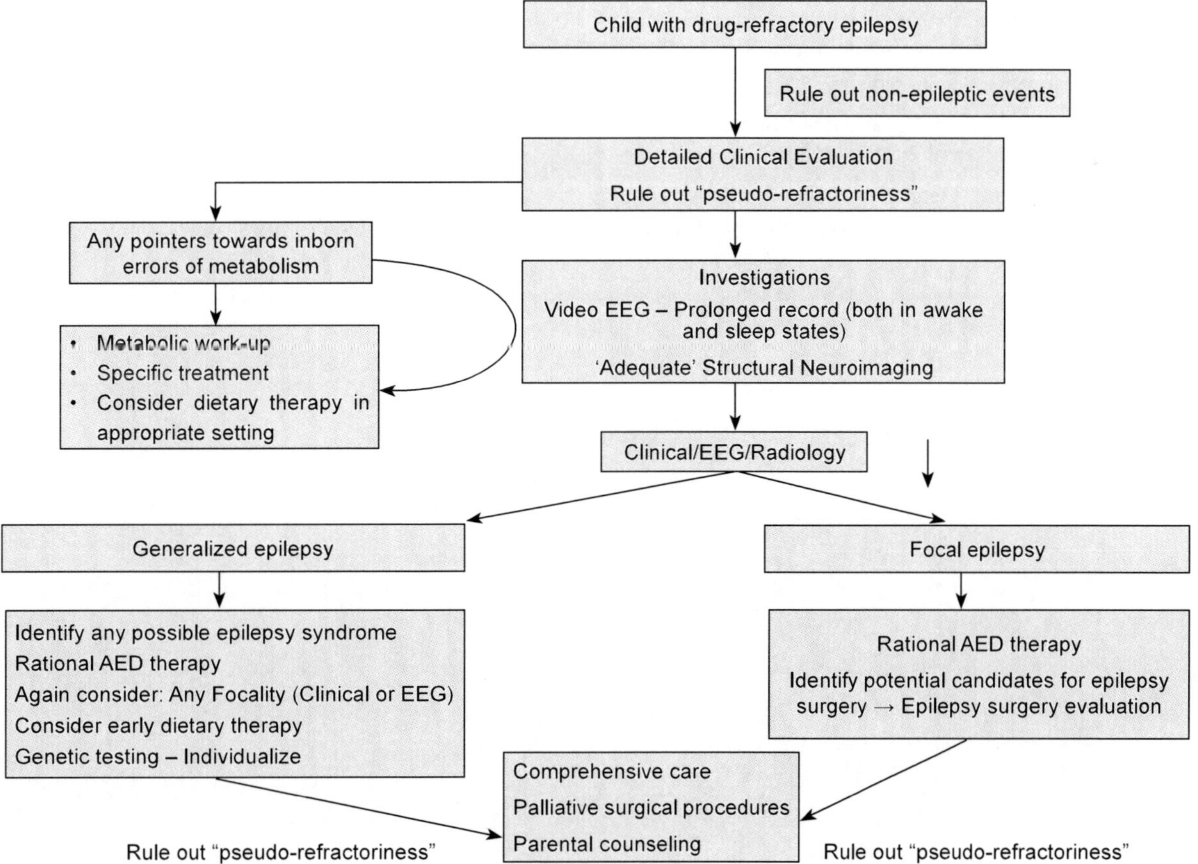

Fig. 23.2: Approach to a child with refractory epilepsy

- Chawla S. Aneja S. Kashyap R. Mallika V. Etiology and Clinical Predictors of Intractable Epilepsy. Pediatr Neurol 2002 September:27(3):186-91.
- Cross JH. Jayakar P. Nordli D. et al. Proposed Criteria for Referral and Evaluation of Children for Epilepsy Surgery: Recommendations of the Subcommission for Pediatric Epilepsy Surgery. Epilepsia 2006:47:952-59.
- Depondt C. The Potential of Pharmacogenetics in the Treatment of Epilepsy. Eur J Paediatr Neurol 2006:10:57-65.
- Devinsky O. Sudden. Unexpected Death in Epilepsy. N Engl J Med 2011:365:1801-11.
- Duncan JS. Imaging in the Surgical Treatment of Epilepsy. Nat Rev Neurol 2010:6:537-50.
- French JA. Faught E. Rational Polytherapy. Epilepsia 2009:50 Suppl 8:63-68.
- Gaillard WD. Chiron C. Cross JH. *et al.* Guidelines for Imaging Infants and Children with Recent-Onset Epilepsy. Epilepsia 2009:50:2147-53.
- Jain P. Sharma S. Tripathi M. Diagnosis and Management of Epileptic Encephalopathies in Children. Epilepsy Res Treat 2013:2013:501981.
- Kossoff EH, Zupec-Kania BA, Amark PE, et al. Optimal Clinical Management of Children Receiving the Ketogenic Diet: Recommendations of the International Ketogenic Diet Study Group. Epilepsia 2009:50:304-17.
- Kossoff EH. Intractable Childhood Epilepsy: Choosing Between the Treatments. Semin Pediatr.
- Kotagal P Neurostimulation: Vagus Nerve Stimulation and Beyond. Semin Pediatr Neurol 2011:18:186-94.
- Kwan P. Arzimanoglou A. Berg AT. *et al.* Definition of Drug Resistant Epilepsy: Consensus Proposal by the Ad Hoc Task Force of the ILAE Commission on Therapeutic Strategies. Epilepsia 2010:51:1069-77.
- Kwan P. Brodie MJ. Early Identification of Refractory Epilepsy. N Engl J Med 2000:342:314-19.
- Levy RG. Cooper PN. Giri P. Ketogenic Diet and Other Dietary Treatments for Epilepsy. Cochrane Database Syst Rev 2012:3:CD001903.
- Morris GL 3rd. Gloss D. Buchhalter J. Mack KJ. Nickels K. Harden C. Evidence-based Guideline Update: Vagus Nerve Stimulation for the Treatment of Epilepsy: Report of the Guideline Development Subcommittee of the American Academy of Neurology. Neurology 2013: August 28.
- Nashef L. So EL. Ryvlin P. Tomson T. Unifying the Definitions of Sudden Unexpected Death in Epilepsy. Epilepsia 2012:53: 227-33.
- Noachtar S. Rémi J. The role of EEG in Epilepsy: A Critical Review. Epilepsy Behav 2009:15:22-33.
- Pal DK. Pong AW. Chung WK. Genetic Evaluation and Counseling for Epilepsy. Nat Rev Neurol 2010:6:445-53.
- Radhakrishnan K. Epilepsy Surgery in India. Neurol India 2009:57:4-6.
- Raspall-Chaure M. Neville BG. Scott RC. The Medical Management of the Epilepsies in Children: Conceptual and Practical Considerations. Lancet Neurol 2008:7:57-69.
- Salmenpera TM. Duncan JS. Imaging in Epilepsy. J Neurol Neurosurg Psychiatr 2005:76 Suppl 3:iii2–iii10.
- Sisodiya S. Etiology and Management of Refractory Epilepsies. Nat Clin Pract Neurol 2007:3:320-30.
- Wolf NI. Bast T. Surtees R. Epilepsy in Inborn Errors of Metabolism. Epileptic Disord 2005:7:67-81.

24 Chapter

CONVULSIVE STATUS EPILEPTICUS

Bibek Talukdar, Rahul Jain

Convulsive status epilepticus (CSE) is the most common type of status epilepticus in children. It continues to be an important cause of morbidity and mortality and often results in long-term neurological sequelae. The problems associated with management has made Convulsive status epilepticus an area of extreme interest and continuing research.

The incidence of convulsive status epilepticus in children is not known, although the incidence of status epilepticus (SE) as a whole, that includes both convulsive and non-convulsive status epilepticus, is reported to be around 18-23 per 100,000 children per year.

Definitions

Status epilepticus is basically a prolonged and protracted seizure that is difficult to control with currently available drugs and other measures. Traditionally, status epilepticus was defined in two different manners. Conceptually, it was defined as a 'a condition characterized by an epileptic seizure that is sufficiently prolonged or repeated at sufficiently brief intervals so as to produce an unvarying and enduring epileptic condition'. Operationally, it was defined as a seizure lasting for more than 30 minutes, based on the premise that irreversible neuronal injury can occur if a seizure persists beyond this time.

Towards the end of 20th century, it was felt that the defining duration should be lowered, as many patients who convulse beyond 5-10 minutes continue to do so after 30 minutes and there is need for early treatment. In 1999, Lowenstein *et al.* came up with a new operational definition of status epilepticus according to which status epilepticus was defined as five or more than five minutes of continuous seizures or one or more discrete seizures between which there is incomplete recovery of consciousness. This definition continues to be commonly used today. The American Epilepsy Society has also defined CSE in the same way (AES guideline, 2016).

The International League Against Epilepsy (ILAE) has recently proposed a new definition that has both conceptual and operational dimensions. It is a condition resulting either from the failure of the mechanisms responsible for seizure termination or from the initiation of mechanisms which lead to abnormally prolonged seizures (after time point t1). It is a condition that can have long-term consequences (after time point t2), including neuronal death, neuronal injury, and alteration of neuronal networks, depending on the type and duration of seizures (Trinka *et al.*, 2015). Time point t1 is the time at which treatment should be started and is currently accepted as 5 minutes for generalized seizures. Time point t2 determines how aggressively this condition should be treated to prevent long-term consequences and is currently accepted as 30 minutes for generalized seizures. For focal seizures with impaired consciousness, t1 and t2 are accepted as 10 and 60 minutes, respectively.

A substantial number of cases do not respond and becomes extremely difficult to treat. The term 'Refractory status epilepticus' is sometimes used for a seizure that continues after using a benzodiazepine and one other anti-epileptic drug (AED). The term 'Super refractory / malignant status epilepticus' is reserved for seizures that continues beyond 24 hours despite the use of anesthetic agents.

Classification

Based on the clinical manifestations and semiology, convulsive status epilepticus has been classified by ILAE as:

(a) Generalized convulsive status epilepticus.

(b) Focal onset evolving into bilateral convulsive status epilepticus; and

(c) Unknown whether focal or generalized (Trinka *et. al.*, 2015). Generalized convulsive status epilepticus is the most common type.

Aetiology of CSE has currently been categorized as *'known or symptomatic'* and *'unknown or cryptogenic'* by ILAE. Known disorders include acute, remote, progressive and defined electroclinical syndromes.

Systematic prospective studies showing the aetiology of CSE in Indian children are scarce. The common and important etiological diagnosis of CSE (diagnosed using the recent operational definition given by Lowenstein *et al.*) in children based on findings of two recent prospective studies (n=132) done in our centre at CNBC were as follows: *Acute disorders* –febrile seizure in 24 (18.18%),viral encephalitis in 8 (6.06%), acute bacterial meningitis in 4 (3.03%), tubercular meningitis in 2 (1.51%), cerebral malaria in 2 (1.51%), septicemia in 1 (0.75%), neurocysticercosis in 7 (5.30%), hypertensive encephalopathy (associated with renal artery stenosis) in 1 (0.75), *Remote disorders* – cerebral palsy in 19 (14.39%), intellectual disability in 3 (2.27%), microcephaly in 2 (1.51%), lissencephaly in 1 (0.75%), post encephalitic sequelae in 1 (0.75%), *Progressive disorders*–neurodegenerative disorders (advanced cases of leukodystrophy) in 3 (2.27%), brain tumour in 1 (0.75%), *SE in defined electroclinical syndrome* – epilepsy (presumed genetic) in 29 (21.96%). Diagnosis of viral encephalitis was based on clinical and extensive investigational findings except virologic confirmation. It was interesting to find that CSE in all the cases of febrile seizure occurred with their first febrile episode. Exact etiological diagnosis of status epilepticus in children however is not always easy because of lot of overlap of pathologies It is important to judge which one could be the primary pathology causing the CSE.

In an earlier retrospective study form India on SE in children admitted into PICU (n=30) (Gulati *et al.*, 2005), the important etiologies observed were–known seizure disorder in 14 cases, acute symptomatic disorders in 12 cases, febrile status epilepticus in 3 cases and idiopathic in 1 case. The acute symptomatic cases were – intracranial bleed in 1, superior sagittal sinus thrombosis in 1, tuberculous meningitis in 1, viral encephalitis in 1, pyogenic meningitis in 1, septic shock in 2, chronic renal failure in 2, aspiration pneumonia in 2 and Stevens-Johnson syndrome in 1.

In some patients with status epilepticus who were previously healthy even extensive diagnostic workup fails to identify the etiology. Some of these cases are preceded by a febrile illness. To categorize these patients, ILAE has come up with two new names with their definitions. New-Onset Refractory Status Epilepticus (NORSE) has been defined as a clinical presentation, not a specific diagnosis, in a patient without active epilepsy or other pre-existing relevant neurological disorder, with new onset of refractory status epilepticus without a clear acute or active structural, toxic, or metabolic cause. This includes patients with viral or autoimmune causes. If no cause is found after extensive evaluation, this is considered 'cryptogenic NORSE' or 'NORSE of unknown etiology'. Febrile Infection-Related Epilepsy Syndrome (FIRES) has been defined as a subcategory of NORSE that requires a prior febrile infection, with fever starting between 2 weeks and 24 hours prior to onset of refractory SE, with or without fever at onset of SE.

Pathophysiology

The exact mechanism of development of status epilepticus remains elusive and mostly hypothetical. Seizure is believed to result from imbalance between excitation and inhibition of cerebral neurones, so that there is excessive and abnormal discharge of cerebral neurones that precipitates a seizure and/or failure of the mechanism that normally terminates an isolated seizure. Important factors responsible for increased excitation are:

(a) Increased activation of NMDA receptors that modulated the production of glutamate, the most important neurotransmitter of the brain; and

(b) Increased synchrony/activation of excitatory collaterals. Gap junctions on cortical neurones also facilitate synchronization. Important factors responsible for termination of seizure primarily is increase in GABA mediated inhibitory synaptic transmission.

The proposed mechanism that leads to continuation of the seizure resulting in status epilepticus are:

(a) Constant activation of hippocampus.

(b) Loss of GABA mediated inhibitory synaptic transmission; and

(c) Glutaminergic excitatory synaptic transmission.

The important pathology that results from SE are multimodal. In the early stage there is massive release of catecholamines tachycardia, arrhythmia, hypertension, systemic and pulmonary and increased left atrial pressure leading occasionally to pulmonary edema. Subsequently there may occur hypotension if SE continues beyond 30 minutes, more so beyond 120 minutes. In our recent studies, we found hypertension in 1.21% and marked hypotension 4.54% and shock in 9.84% cases. Respiratory failure and lactic acidosis can occur resulting in metabolic acidosis. There may be hyperpyrexia and also leucocytosis that may be misdiagnosed as infection. Blood glucose may be elevated, and later hypoglycemia can occur. CSF pleocytosis can occur in about 20% of cases. Severe status can lead to rhabdomyolysis and even renal failure. In the initial phase cerebral blood flow increases that, if severe, may result in cerebral edema, that may precipitate and aggravate seizure.

The physiological changes occurring during episodes of status epilepticus can result in pathological changes. Occasional reports have described acute changes in hippocampus, amygdala, thalamus, basal ganglia, cerebellum and neocortex.

Treatment

The mortality and the mortality are due to the acute CNS insult that results during an attack of status epilepticus. These attacks result in metabolic and systemic disturbances in the form of abnormally high demands for oxygen and glucose, abnormal temperature regulation, acid-base disturbance, electrolyte disturbance, autonomic disturbances and even raised intracranial pressure. Varying degrees of neuronal damage and loss occurs depending upon the duration of the status epilepticus. All these need to be considered in management.

The treatment of status epilepticus thus involves not only the stopping of the seizure, but also taking care of the metabolic and systemic disturbances. The first and most important step should be the maintenance of the airway, circulation and blood pressure and a quick assessment of the general condition and looking for the possible cause. Clearing the airway, lateral positioning and insertion of plastic airway for maintaining the patency of the airway if needed are priority. Starting an IV line, taking a few important blood samples and starting maintenance fluid should be done simultaneously. Shock, if present, should be managed urgently. Oxygen should be administered to all cases. The initial samples should include at least blood counts, blood sugar, serum electrolytes, blood gas, serum calcium, LFT, KFT and blood culture. Anti-epileptic drug level should also be done in known epileptics. Some patients will require additional investigations like lumbar puncture, neuroimaging, coagulation profile, IEM screening, etc. depending on clinical suspicion, which may be done later or as needed.

During management it is extremely important to keep monitoring the child's vital signs, i.e., pulse, respiration, blood pressure and temperature; mechanical monitors are extremely useful here. Appropriate remedial measure for any disturbance found during monitoring should be undertaken. Maintenance of a stable hemodynamic state is extremely important since the cerebral perfusion and oxygenation are extremely important issues. While the seizure activity is going on, respiratory complications even arrest can occur at any time and one has to remain alert to tackle these and be ready for intubation. Hypotension or hypertension can be due to vasomotor imbalance or side effects of drugs especially phenytoin and phenobarbitone and need to be managed as needed. Hyperpyrexia due to vasomotor instability or excessive muscle contractions also needs to be treated urgently since this will increase the metabolic demands tremendously.

Treating urgently any biochemical derangement is extremely important. Some cases respond dramatically to such measurers, i.e., hypoglycemia, hypocalcemia. At times, AED also may be avoided. Waiting for report is cut short. Treating urgently any treatable cause is another important area, a common example is acute bacterial meningitis. These measures should help in quicker control of CSE.

Drugs Used in Convulsive Status Epilepticus

Quite a number of drugs have been used in CSE. However, few drugs continue to hold ground till today. These are benzodiazepines, phenytoin or fosphenytoin, phenobarbitone, and sodium valproate. Of late levetiracetam also has been found to be quite useful.

Benzodiazepines are rapid acting and used as first line drugs. The commonly used benzodiazepines are diazepam (0.3 mg/kg/dose IV slowly) and lorazepam (0.1 mg/kg/dose, IV slowly). Lorazepam is often recommended as the preferred agent. A prospective randomized controlled trial of 178 children with SE showed that lorazepam (0.1 mg/kg) was as safe and effective as diazepam (0.2 mg/kg) and phenytoin (18 mg/kg) combined. Other studies have shown that the two drugs are not different. Immediate side effect that needs to be monitored is respiratory depression and hypotension.

If intravenous access is not available, the use of buccal midazolam (0.2 mg/kg), intranasal midazolam (0.2 mg/kg), or intramuscular midazolam (0.2 mg/kg) are good alternatives. Rectal diazepam is another option. Some studies have indicated that buccal midazolam and intranasal midazolam and may be more or equally effective than rectal diazepam (0.2-0.5 mg/kg). For refractory status epilepticus, midazolam infusion (0.15 mg/kg slow IV followed by infusion at the rate of 1 microgram/kg/min) is used as the preferred agent. In case of persistence of seizures, dose is hiked by 1 microgram/kg/min every 15 minutes to a maximum of 15 microgram/kg/min. Before each increment in dose, additional bolus of 0.15 mg/kg is recommended in order to achieve the desired drug levels.

Phenytoin is used in dose of 15-20 mg/kg/dose at a rate of 1 mg/kg/min. Immediate side effects that can occur and needs monitoring are respiratory depression, hypotension and cardiac arrhythmia. Fosphenytoin (20 mg PE/kg) is an alternative to phenytoin. It can be given at a faster rate (100-150 mg PE/minute) and can be used intramuscularly.

Phenobarbitone is used in a dose of 20 mg/kg/dose, at a rate of 50 mg/min. Immediate side effects that can occur and needs monitoring is respiratory depression and hypotension.

Valproic acid is used in a dose of 20 mg/kg/dose IV, slowly. No significant side effect has been reported. Valproic acid should be avoided in children under the age of 2 years, receiving anti-convulsant polytherapy, hepatic dysfunction and suspected mitochondrial disorder.

Levetiracetam has been found to be useful in several retrospective studies. It has been used in a dose of 20-30 mg/kg. Side effects are few. As this drug does not have hepatic metabolism, it may be useful in patients with liver dysfunction, metabolic disorders, or at risk for major drug interactions.

Treatment of status epilepticus needs special attention and use of defined protocol. The drugs used for controlling an acute attack are also used for CSE, however in specific sequences, considering the emergency nature of the condition, so that the seizure can be aborted as quickly as possible. Quite a number of **guidelines/protocols/algorithms** are available for treatment of SE. We use a protocol based on the American Epilepsy Society (AES, 2016) algorithm, however, modified to suit our condition, keeping in mind availability of drugs, as shown in the inset.

After the use of benzodiazepines as first line agents, there is no consensus on the choice of second line drug in patients with continuing seizures. Studies have shown that phenytoin, valproic acid, levetiracetam and phenobarbitone are all equally efficacious; however, the incidence of side effects in the form of lethargy is more common after phenobarbitone.

If seizure persists after the second drug (refractory status epilepticus), then another drug (not used earlier) may be tried or patient can be directly started on midazolam infusion. In resource constraint settings trial of another second-line drug is justified before starting midazolam. Most of the patients will need assisted ventilation at moderate doses of midazolam. Other anesthetic agents that have been used as continuous infusion in refractory status epilepticus are diazepam, phenobarbitone, propofol and thiopental. Diazepam is less efficacious than midazolam. The efficacy of other three anesthetic agents is almost equal to midazolam; however, the mortality has been shown to be minimal with midazolam. Propofol is also not preferred in children because of the risk of propofol infusion syndrome.

Other drugs and therapeutic modalities that have been tried with limited success in patients with refractory status epilepticus or seizures after withdrawal of anesthetic agents includes ketamine infusion, oral topiramate, oral perampanel, brexanolone infusion, ketogenic diet, therapeutic hypothermia, epilepsy surgery and electroconvulsive therapy. Pyridoxine, given intravenously, also have been found to be useful at times.

In a known epileptic patient who is already on anti-epileptic drugs, the same drugs should not be used if the patient is on more than 50% of the maximal dose of that drug. If patient is on lower doses, then loading with half the dose can be done.

Protocol for Treatment of Status Epilepticus in Children

#On arrival at emergency, a quick clinical assessment is done and vital signs and oxygen saturation (through pulse-oximetry) and blood glucose (through strip test) is recorded. An intravenous line is started, and blood samples taken for hemogram, sugar, electrolytes (Na^+, K^+ and Cl^-), calcium, urea, creatinine and antiepileptic drug levels (in known epileptics). Oxygen is administered to all the cases. Insertion of oral airway, oropharyngeal suctioning and artificial ventilation is resorted to as needed.

#Sequence of anticonvulsant drug use is as follows:

*Intravenous lorazepam 0.1 mg/kg/dose, maximum 4 mg/dose is administered slowly. The dose is repeated once *if seizure is not controlled in 5 minutes.* In case lorazepam is not available intravenous diazepam or intravenous phenytoin is used. Diazepam is administered in a dose of 0.3 mg/kg slowly, which is repeated once as needed.

*If convulsions do not stop, phenytoin is started in the dose of 15-20 mg/kg diluted in normal saline at the rate of 1mg/kg/min. Phenytoin is repeated once after 20 minutes if convulsions persist.

*If convulsions continue to occur, phenobarbitone is started in the dose of 20 mg/kg at the rate of 50 mg/min. Phenobarbitone is repeated once after 20 minutes if there is no response.

*If convulsion persists, midazolam infusion will be started in a dose of 0.15 mg/kg bolus followed by infusion at the rate of 1 μg/kg/min; it is titrated every 15 minutes to the maximum dose of 15 μg/kg/min.

*If convulsions still persist, other pharmacologic agents are tried, not uniformly, however, that include sodium valproate, levetiracetum, pyridoxine, propofol and thiopentone.

#Monitoring of vital signs, oxygen saturation and side effects of antiepileptic drugs are done all throughout. Response is recorded after administration of each drug. All cases are initially kept on intravenous fluid.

Outcome

Mortality continue to occur in convulsive status epilepticus, incidence being variable from centre to centre and type of study. Mortality report of 0-30% (average 11.3%) can be seen in some retrospective studies, 0-25% (average 12.3%) in a few prospective studies and 3% in a population based study. We had a mortality of 8% in our centre. Mortality in status epilepticus thus continues to be worrisome. Certain factors may influence control and outcome of CSE, one important factor being prolonged duration of convulsion before arriving at hospital (Talukdar *et al.*, 2019). This is of importance in resource poor setting as in developing countries specially concerning the rural/peripheral areas. Mortality and morbidity have been shown to be higher in children from rural location (Molinero *et al.*, 2009). Whenever an episode of convulsion starts the patient should be transported to the nearest hospital/treatment facility as quickly as possible. A good transport network for such cases should be useful.

Preventing Development of Status Epilepticus

Quickly aborting an attack of convulsion should prevent it from progressing into CSE. Here use of buccal midazolam (0.2 mg/kg), intranasal midazolam (0.2 mg/kg) rectal diazepam (0.3 mg/kg) has been shown to be efficacious in several studies. Of late intranasal lorazepam (0.1 mg/kg) has also been found to be useful. These can be used by parents at home. Parents of children who frequently get recurrent convulsions can be trained in the technique of administration and also monitoring for side effects like respiratory depression. These can be used even at peripheral centres and other treatment facilities where getting intravenous access is difficult.

Suggested Reading

- Abend NS and Tobias LT. Paediatric Status Epilepticus Management, Curr Opin Pediatr 2014;26:668-74.
- Asadi-Pooya AA, Poordast A. Etiologies and Outcomes of Status Epilepticus in Children, Epilepsy Behav 2005:7(3):502-05.
- Chin RF, Neville BG, Peckham C, Bedford H, Wade A, Scott RC. Incidence, Cause and Short-term Outcome of Convulsive Status Epilepticus in Childhood: Prospective Population Based Study, Lancet 2006:368:222-29.
- Evidence-Based Guideline: Treatment of Convulsive Status Epilepticus in Children and Adults: Report of the Guideline Committee of the American Epilepsy Society, Epilepsy Currents, Vol. 16, No. 1 (January/February) 2016;48-61.
- Eriksson KJ, Koivikko MJ. Status Epilepticus in Children: Aetiology, Treatment and Outcome, Dev Med Child Neurol 1997;39:652-58.
- Gaspard N, Hirsch LJ, Sculier C, *et al.* New-onset Refractory Status Epilepticus (NORSE) and Febrile Infection-related Epilepsy Syndrome (FIRES): State of the Art and Perspectives. Epilepsia 2018:59(4):745-52. doi:10.1111/epi.14022.
- Gulati S, Kalra V, Shridhar MR. Status Epilepticus in Indian Children in a Tertiary Care Center: Clinical Profile and Immediate Outcome, Indian J Pediatr 2005:72:105-08.
- Hussain N, Appleton R, Thorburn K. Aetiology, Course and Outcome of Children Admitted to Paediatric Intensive Care with Convulsive Status Epilepticus: A Retrospective 5-year Review, Seizure 2007:16:305-12.
- Ibrahim SH, Yezdan MA, Nizami SQ. Status Epilepticus in Children: A Five Year Experience at Aga Khan University-Hospital. JPMA 2003:53:597-99.
- Kravijanac R, Jovic N, Djuric M, Jankovic B, Pekmezovic T. Outcome of Status Epilepticus in Children Treated in the Intensive Care Unit: A Study of 302 Cases, Epilepsia 2011:52(2):358-63.
- Lahat E, Goldman M, Barr J, Bristrizter T, Berkovitch RM. Comparison of Intranasal Midazolam with I.V. Diazepam for Treating Febrile Seizures in Children: Prospective Randomized Study, BMJ 2000:321:83-86.
- Lin KL, Lin JJ, Hsia SH, Wu CT, Wang HS. Analysis of Convulsive SE in Children of Taiwan, Pediatr Neurol 2009:41(6):413-18.
- Lowenstein DH, Blek T, Macdonald RL. It's Time to Revise the Definition of Status Epilepticus, Epilepsia 1999;40:120-22.
- Mazarati AM, Baldwin RA, Sankar R, Wasterlain CG. Time-Dependent Decrease in the Effectiveness of Antiepileptic Drugs During the Course of Self-sustaining Status Epilepticus, Brain Res 1998:814(1-2):179-85.
- Mbodj I, Ndiaye M, Sene F, Salif Sow P, Sow HD, Diagana M, Pierre Ndiaye I, Gallo Diop A. Treatment of Status Epilepticus in a Developing Country, Neurophysiol Clin 2000;30(3):165-69.
- Molinero MR, Holden KR, Rodriguez LC, Collins JS, Samra JA, Shinnar S. Pediatric Convulsive Status Epilepticus in Honduras, Central America, Epilepsia 2009;50:2314-19.
- Neville BG, Chin RF, Scott RC. Childhood Convulsive Status Epilepticus: Epidemiology, Management and Outcome, Acta Neurol Scand Suppl 2007;186:21-24.
- Noe KH, Manno EM. Mechanisms Underlying Status Epilepticus, Drugs Today (Barc) 2005;41:257-66.
- Raspall CM, Chin RF, Neville BG, Bedford H, Scott RC. The Epidemiology of Convulsive Status Epilepticus in Children: A Critical Review, Epilepsia 2007:48:1652-63.
- Serino D, Santarone ME, Caputo D, Fusco L. Febrile Infection-Related Epilepsy Syndrome (FIRES): Prevalence, Impact and Management Strategies, Neuropsychiatr Dis Treat 2019 July 9;15:1897-1903, doi: 10.2147/NDT.S177803, eCollection 2019.
- Singh RK, Stephens S, Berl MM, Chang T, Brown K, Vezina LG, Gaillard WD. Prospective Study of New-Onset Seizures Presenting as Status Epilepticus in Childhood, Neurology 2010;74:636-42.

- Scott SC. Besag FM. Boyd SG. Berry D. Neville BG. Buccal Absorption of Midazolam: Pharmacokinetics and EEG Pharmacodynamics. Epilepsia 1998:39:290-94.
- Scott RC. Besag FMC. Neville BGR. Buccal Midazolam and Rectal Diazepam for Treatment of Prolonged Seizures in Childhood and Adolescence: A Randomized Trial. Lancet 1999:353:623-26.
- Trinka E. Cock H. Hesdorffer D. Rosetti AO. Scheffer IE. Shinnar S. Shorvon S. Lowenstein DH. A Definition and Classification of Status Epilepticus–Report of the ILAE Task Force on Classification of Status Epilepticus. Epilepsia 2015: 1-9. doi: 10.1111/epi.13121.
- Talukdar B. Chakravarty B. Efficacy of Buccal Midazolam Compared to Intravenous Diazepam in Controlling Convulsions in Children: A Randomized Controlled Trial. Brain and Development 2009:31:744-49.
- Talukdar B. Bansal S. Jain R. Factors Influencing Control of Convulsive Status Epilepticus in Children. Indian J Child Health 2019:6(5):217-20.
- Ud Din MA. Study of Clinical Course and Outcome of Convulsive Status Epilepticus. A Thesis Submitted to the National Board of Examinations. New Delhi. 2018.
- Wasterlain CG. Fujikawa DG. Penix L. Sankar R. Pathophysiological Mechanisms of Brain Damage From Status Epilepticus. Epilepsia 1993:34:S37-53.

25 Chapter

CLINICAL PHARMACOLOGY OF ANTIEPILEPTIC DRUGS (AEDs)

Sangeeta Sharma

Epilepsy, a chronic disease occurs in approximately 1% of the population with a lifetime prevalence of a single seizure of approximately 9%. Antiepileptic drugs (AEDs) are the mainstay of treatment as considerable progress has been made in the pharmacological treatment of epilepsy, due to improved knowledge of the clinical pharmacology of individual drugs, factors affecting response and need for drug treatment, and development of promising new agents. The primary goals of treatment are to achieve complete seizure freedom, ideally without adverse events, reduce morbidity and mortality, and improve quality of life. Antiepileptic drugs (AEDs) are effective, in about 80% of these patients, but remaining patients are difficult to treat. Therefore, there is a continuing need for newer drugs or the modified versions of old drugs in order to render all patients free of seizures.

Understanding the mechanism of action and pharmacokinetics of antiepileptic drugs (AEDs) is important in clinical practice so that they can be used effectively, especially in multi-drug regimens. Each antiepileptic drug has a characteristic pharmacokinetic profile, and their unique properties must be considered when selecting the optimal agent for a particular patient. The ultimate choice of an AED for any individual patient with newly diagnosed or untreated epilepsy should include consideration of the strength of the evidence for efficacy and effectiveness for each AED along with other variables such as the AED safety and tolerability profile, pharmacokinetic properties, formulations, and cost.[1-2]

MECHANISM OF ACTION

Many structures and processes are involved in the development of a seizure, including neurons, ion channels, receptors, glia, and inhibitory and excitatory synapses. The AEDs are designed to modify these processes to favour inhibition over excitation in order to stop or prevent seizure activity. The narrow spectrum AEDs mostly work for specific types of seizures (such as partial, focal, or absence, myoclonic seizures). Broad spectrum AEDs, additionally have some effectiveness for a wide variety of seizures (partial plus absence myoclonic seizures) (Box 25.1 and 25.2). Some types of seizure are difficult to treat with any AED.

Box 25.1: Spectrum of Antiepileptic Activity of Antiepileptic Drugs

Narrow-spectrum AEDs	Broad-spectrum AEDs
Phenytoin	Valproic acid
Phenobarbital	Lamotrigine
Carbamazepine	Topiramate
Oxcarbazepine	Zonisamide
Gabapentin	Levetiracetam
Pregabalin	Clonazepam
Vigabatrin	Clobazam
Tiagabine	Felbamate

Box 25.2: Generations of Antiepileptic Drugs

First-Generation AEDs	Second-Generation AEDs	Third-Generation AEDs
Phenobarbital	Felbamate	Lacosamide
Phenytoin	Gabapentin	Rufinamide
Ethosuximide	Lamotrigine	Eslicarbamazepine
Carbamazepine	Topiramate	Stiripentol
Valproic acid	Tiagabine	Brivaracetam
	Levetiracetam	Retigabine
	Oxcarbazepine	Selectracetam
	Zonisamide	Perampanel
	Pregabalin	

The AEDs can be grouped according to their main mechanism of action, although many of them have several actions and others have unknown mechanisms of action. The main groups include sodium channel blockers, calcium current inhibitors, gamma-aminobutyric acid (GABA enhancers, glutamate blockers, carbonic anhydrase inhibitors, hormones, and drugs with unknown mechanisms of action. Phenytoin (PHT), carbamazepine (CBZ), valproic acid (VAP), and lamotrigine (LTG) block sodium channels and inhibit the generation of action potentials. Their effect is 'use dependent' that is related to their selective binding and prolongation of the inactivated state of the sodium channel. They decrease neurotransmission by actions on prejunctional neurons. Valproic acid at higher concentrations reduces low-threshold T-type Ca^{2+} current. Ethosuximide like valproic acid reduce the low–threshold Ca^{2+} current provides the pacemaker activity in the thalamus. Barbiturates and benzodiazepines facilitate GABA-mediated inhibition of neuronal activity.

For the past several decades, seizures and epilepsy have been treated with first line AEDs and have been the mainstay in management of both acute and chronic seizures. Since 1993, however, several novel AEDs have been introduced. These drugs were developed in an attempt to overcome the limitations of first line AED therapy. The first line AEDs are associated with a number of systemic and cognitive adverse effects. Some side effects are minor and transient; others are rare, idiosyncratic reactions with serious implications. The complex pharmacokinetic and pharmaceutical properties of first line AEDs make administration difficult at times. Many of these drugs are potent enzyme inducers or inhibitors, and significant drug interactions occur when they are co-administered with hormones or other medications.[3]

The new AEDs compounds are chemically unique, structurally unrelated to the first line AEDs and different from one another (Box 25.2). The new AEDs have less frequent interactions, leading to improved tolerability with co-medication. Potential advantages and disadvantages compared with first line AEDs are discussed in the chapter. Table 25.1 summarize indications, advantages and disadvantages of commonly used first line and newer antiepileptic drugs. Table 25.2 summarizes pharmacokinetic information about AEDs respectively. Table 25.3 shows doses and dosage forms of commonly used AEDs.

First Generation AEDs

Phenobarbital (PHB) has been used to treat primary tonic-clonic generalized seizures, myoclonic seizures, and partial seizures. It has an efficacy similar to phenytoin and carbamazepine. The drug can also be used in neonatal seizures. It has also been used to treat primary tremor.[4]

Phenobarbital is rapidly and completely absorbed following oral doses. Phenobarbital is bound about 55% to plasma proteins and is distributed widely throughout the body. It is about 60% to 80% metabolized in the liver by CYP2C9 and CYP2C19, and then undergoing further metabolism by glucuronidation. The half-life of phenobarbital ranges between 72 and 125 hours. Since it takes three weeks to get to steady state, dose changes must be made very gradually. The metabolism of phenobarbital may be induced or inhibited[4,5] PHB is a powerful inducer of the hepatic microsomal enzymes PHB increases the metabolism of estrogen, steroids, warfarin, CBZ, diazepam, clonazepam and VPA. Its effect on PHT is unpredictable. Metabolism of PHB is inhibited by PHT, VPA, felbamate, and dextropropoxyphene. Enzyme inducers, such as rifampicin, decrease PHB levels.

The use of phenobarbital is restricted due to its significant number of side effects. The most important adverse effects are cognitive and behaviour alterations. Children are more likely to exhibit behavioural changes (i.e., paradoxical hyperkinesis). Sedation is prominent, particularly at the beginning of therapy, and usually subsides with treatment. Other common adverse effects include psychomotor slowing, poor concentration, depression, irritability, ataxia, and decreased libido. Long-term use of PHB may be associated with coarsening of facial features, osteomalacia, and Dupuytren contractures. Folate deficiency, megaloblastic anemia, and idiosyncratic skin reaction are rare.[4,6] Hepatitis has been reported secondary to an immune-mediated process. It has been associated with an increase in falls in the elderly.

Table 25.1: Antiepileptic Drugs: General Information

Drug name	Indications	Most common adverse effects	Major toxic effects[1]	Advantages	Disadvantages
Carbamazepine (CBZ)	Complex partial, generalized tonic-clonic seizures; in combination for multiple seizure types	Nausea, vomiting, drowsiness, dizziness, ataxia, vertigo, diplopia, rash. *GI transit time can affect concentrations when sustained-release preparation is used*	Chronic toxicity leads to seizures. Hematologic dyscrasias, aplastic anemia possible (1/200,000–1/600,000)	Known mechanism Modified release preparation available	Autoinduction resulting in 50% ↓ in levels in 1st few weeks, the $t_{1/2}$ ↓es and $t_{1/2}$ at start will be ~36 h, will \$ to 10–20 hours with autoinduction, and will ↓ further to 8-12 hours if PHB or PHT is added

Contd.

Contd.

			Hepatic failure, Stevens-Johnson, leukopenia		Enzyme inducer affects metabolism of other AEDs; CYP3A4 inhibitors ↓CBZ levels; Neurotoxic; Rarely idiosyncratic reactions (aplastic anemia, hyponatremia, impaired renal function)
Phenobarbital (PB)	Generalized tonic-clonic, partial seizures	Sedation; also nystagmus, ataxia. Habituation to all effects but respiratory depression. Cognitive decline, hyperactivity in children	Life-threatening respiratory depression	Long half life; Known mechanism Cheap	Adverse effects: Physical dependence and withdrawal seizures on long term use; rare idiosyncratic skin reactions; Enzyme inducer
Phenytoin (PHT)	Primary drug for all types of seizures except absence seizures	CNS: Nystagmus, ataxia, impaired concentration; also headache, drowsiness, seizure, rash. Systemic adverse effects Nausea and vomiting. Chronic use leads to osteoporosis, gingival hyperplasia, acne, or hirsutism in ~50% of patients	Stevens-Johnson, seizure lymphadenopathy, hematologic dyscrasias, aplastic anemia	Known mechanism Lacks neuropsychiatric effects	CNS and systemic adverse effects and long-term use: Elimination of PHT is not first order, $t_{½}$ changes as concentration changes and #es in the elderly. PHT rate of elimination correlated with age: Children under 5 have a significantly more rapid elimination than older children and adults; neonates have a highly variable rate of elimination; Many drug interactions as PHT is a potent enzyme inducer and highly protein bound
Valproic acid (VAP)	Simple and complex absence seizures, complex partial seizures, tonic-clonic seizures, and multiple seizures in combination	Nausea, vomiting, abdominal cramps, somnolence, dizziness most common; malaise, weakness, lethargy, facial edema, anorexia, weight gain. Inhibits platelet aggregation, which may increase bleeding time. Side effects profile may change for valproic acid versus divalproex sodium	Hepatic dysfunction, pancreatitis, metabolic disturbances (e.g., hyperammonemia) nystagmus, headache, ataxia, tremor, hallucinations, or changes in vision	Lacks neuropsychiatric side effects; efficacy against some comorbidities (bipolar disorder)	Enzyme inhibitor; significant variation in the half-life. In children and patients taking enzyme-inducing drugs has a short half-life and more frequent dosing is required
Gabapentin (GBP)	Adjunctive treatment for partial seizures	Fatigue, somnolence, dizziness, ataxia		Well tolerated; No idiosyncratic reactions; No drug interactions; Rapid titration; Effective against some comorbidities (neuropathic pain)	Unknown mechanism; Variable absorption; Weight gain; Limited spectrum of activity; no drug interactions; can be used in comorbidities such as neuropathic pain

Contd.

Contd.

Lamotrigine (LTG)	Adjunctive treatment for partial seizures in adults	CNS depression, rash, abnormal thinking, diplopia, dizziness, ataxia, nausea, nervousness, somnolence, vomiting	Stevens-Johnson syndrome (1/3000)	Good CNS profile: Twice daily dosing: Broad spectrum: Predictable kinetics: efficacy against some comorbidities (bipolar disorder)	Unknown mechanism: Slow titration: CNS adverse effects, Stevens-Johnson: drug interactions CBZ and other enzyme inducers/inhibitors: may aggravate severe myoclonic epilepsy
Topiramate (TPM)	Adjunctive treatment for partial and generalized seizures in adults	Psychomotor slowing, concentration/speech difficulty, somnolence, fatigue.	Erythema, Hepatic failure, Hyperthermia, Hypokalemia, Neuropathy, Toxic epidermal necrolysis	Low allergenic potential: High efficacy: No idiosyncratic reactions: Efficacy against comor-bidities (binge eating disorder)	Slow titration, low allergenic potential, no idiosyncratic reaction: CNS adverse effects: Drug interactions with oral contraceptives: thrice daily dosing: effective against comorbidities such as binge eating
Felbamate (FBM)	Severe and/ or refractory epilepsies (Lennox-Gastaut syndrome	Anorexia, vomiting, insomnia, somnolence	Risk of severe adverse effects– aplastic anemia, hepatic failure	Broad spectrum	Unknown mechanism: Multiple dosing: drug interactions
Tiagabine (TGB)	Adjunctive treatment for refractory partial with /without secondary generalization in 12 years and older patients	Most common dizziness, fatigue, generalized muscle weakness, nervousness, tremor, abnormal thinking, depression, aphasia, and encephalopathy; Also abdominal pain, knee buckling, and seizures in patients without epilepsy	Hepatic toxicity	Known mechanism: no idiosyncratic reactions; Low allergenic potential; no interference with hepatic enzymes; no effect on first line AEDs levels	Limited spectrum; Slow titration; Dizziness; Tiagabine metabolism induced significantly by first line AEDs; to be used with caution in patients with history of status epilepticus; Contraindicated in severe hepatic impairment, pregnancy and lactation
Levetiracetam (LEV)	Adjunctive treatment for refractory seizures with/ without secondary generalization	Most common headaches, somnolence, asthenia, dizziness, vertigo, and; vomiting is seen commonly in children and adolescents. Psychiatric and behavioural events such as emotional lability, nervousness, and hostility also reported	Depression, suicidal ideation, seizures that are different, infection, double vision, rashes	Well tolerated; Rapid titration; no drug interactions; twice a day dose	Exact mechanism of action not known; dose to be reduced in impaired renal function
Vigabatrin (VGB)	Adjunctive treatment for partial with / without secondary generalization refractory to all other drugs; infantile spasms (West syndrome)	Common adverse effects are headache, somnolence, fatigue, dizziness, convulsion, and hyperactivity in children; Minor adverse effects, usually at the onset of therapy are fatigue, headache, dizziness, increase in weight, tremors	Retinal toxicity	Ease of titration; No important drug interactions; Good efficacy in infantile spasms; little effect on cognition	Use restricted; Visual field defects; Vision loss onset is unpredictable at any time during treatment, therefore, regular vision testing is recommended for all patients; limited spectrum; weight gain

Contd.

Contd.

Zonisamide (ZNS)	Adjunctive treatment of refractory partial and generalized seizures in 16 years or older reported. Oligohidrosis, sometimes resulting in heat stroke and hospitalization, is seen in pediatric patients	Most common fatigue, dizziness, somnolence, anorexia, psychomotor slowing and ataxia. Renal stones, anorexia, weight loss, also aplastic anemia, and other blood dyscrasias	Stevens-Johnson syndrome, toxic epidermal necrolysis, fulminant hepatic necrosis, agranulocytosis	Twice daily dosing; does not induce its own metabolism; does not alter drug metabolism of other drugs	Slow titration; CNS adverse effects and allergic reactions; Cognitive impairment is dose dependent; The half-life is shorter in patients taking enzyme-inducing drugs such as phenytoin and carbamazepine

GI, gastrointestinal; CBC, complete blood count and CNS, central nervous system.

1. All anticonvulsant drugs are Category C/D: use in pregnancy only when benefit outweighs the risk. Teratogenesis occurs with all AEDs and is estimated to have an incidence of 2–4%. Risk of neural tube defects (highest with valproate (~1%) and carbamazepine (~0.5%)). Teratogenic effects of new anticonvulsant medications are expected to be similar. Patients who become pregnant should be informed of the risks and referred for advice and counselling and antenatal screening. Neural tube defect incidence can be lessened through folic acid supplementation before and during pregnancy. For neonatal bleeding associated with CBZ, PHB and PHT prophylactic Vitamin k for neonate and the mother before delivery. However, AEDs can be continued during breastfeeding. Teratogenic effects of new anticonvulsant medications are expected to be similar.
2. Because of their relatively high metabolic rate, children require high dosages of antiepileptic drugs in relation to their body weight. Therapeutic drug level monitoring of AEDs is particularly important in children, but must keep in mind that the therapeutic range is a relative concept only since levels are affected by several factors. TDM is not widely practiced for the newer AEDs, there are no generally accepted target ranges for any of these drugs, and for most a wide range in serum concentration is associated with clinical efficacy.

Table 25.2: Antiepileptic Drugs: Pharmacokinetic Information

Name of the drug	Oral bioavailability	Serum protein binding (%)	Time to peak concentration (hour)	Serum half-life (hour)	Reference range in serum (mg/l)
First line AEDs					
Carbamazepine	>70	75	4-8	10-20[1]	4-10
Oxcarbazepine	90	40	3-6	8-15[a]	3-35
Phenobarbitone	>95	50	4-12	90-110[2]	10-25
Phenytoin	90	>95	4-12	6-24[3]	10-120
*Primidone	>90	20	2-4	10-20	8-12
Valproic acid	>95	>90	1-4	11-17[4]	30-100
****Second line/Newer AEDs**					
Elsicarbamazepine	≥80	30	1-4	20-24	Not established
Gabapentine	<60	0	2-3	5-9	2-20
Felbamate	>90	25	2-6	16-22[a]	30-60
Lacosamide	≥95	15	0.5-4	12-13	5-15
Lamotrigine	≥95	55	1-3	15-35[a,b]	3-14
Levetiracetam	≥95	0	1	6-8	12-46
Pregabalin	≥90	0	1-2	5-7	2.8-8.3
Rufinamide	85	30	5-6	8-12[a]	3-30
Stiripentol	≥90	99	1-2	Variable	4-22
Tiagabine	≥90	96	1-2	5-9[a]	0.02-0.2
Topiramate	≥80	15	2-4	20-30	5-20

Contd.

Contd.

Vigabatrin	≥60	0	1-2	5-8	0.8-36
Zonisamide	≥65	50	2-5	50-70[a]	10-40

* Primidone is metabolized to phenobarbital. Both drugs should be monitored and concentrations evaluated in light of the patient's response.

** TDM is not widely practiced for the newer AEDs, there are no generally accepted target ranges for any of these drugs, and for most a wide range in serum concentration is associated with clinical efficacy. Furthermore, a considerable overlap in drug concentrations related to toxicity and non-response is reported.

Time to steady state concentration is ~5 $t_{1/2}$.

[1] Carbamazepine half-life variable 24–48 hours, decreases to 10–30 hours due to autoinduction, i.e., CBZ induces its own metabolism ~2-fold in the 1st 1–2 weeks of therapy, the $t_{1/2}$ decreases and $t_{1/2}$ at start will be ~36 hours, will decrease to 10–20 hours with auto-induction, and will decrease further to 8–12 hours if phenobarbitone and phenytoin is added.

[2] Phenobarbitone Serum half-life in infants and children is 40-70 hours; neonates is 67-90 hours.

[3] Phenytoin exhibits Zero-order kinetics, half-life varies with drug conc. 6–60 hours adult; 7–29 hours child; infant 2-7 hours; neonate 15-105 hours. Since elimination of PHT is not first-order, $t_{1/2}$ not a very useful concept: It changes as concentration changes and is increased in the elderly. PHT rate of elimination appears to be correlated with age: Children under 5 have a significantly more rapid elimination than older children and adults; neonates have a highly variable rate of elimination.

Fosphenytoin, a pro-drug for PHT, is converted to PHT with a 15-minute half-life. Drug monitoring of PHT concentrations after use of the pro-drug requires that 2 hours elapse from the end of an IV infusion and 4 hours from an IM injection before samples are obtained the time taken to convert to PHT. Once converted, pharmacokinetic data are the same as for PHT.

[4] There is significant variation in the half-life of this drug. Generally, in children and patients taking enzyme-inducing drugs, valproic acid has a short half-life and more frequent dosing is required. 17–40 hours infants; 7–13 hours children.

[a] Serum half-life significant decreased with concomitant therapy with liver enzyme inducers (rifampin, carbamazepine, phenobarbital, phenytoin, St. John's wort).

[b] Serum half-life significantly increased with concomitant therapy with valproic acid.

Table 25.3: Doses and Dosage Forms of Antiepileptic Drugs

Name of the drug	Dosage form and strength	Initial dose (daily)	Maintenance dose (mg/d)	No. of daily doses	Therapeutic levels and other monitoring
*Phenytoin	Inj 50 mg; Syp/susp 25 mg/ml; Cap 25/100 mg; Parenteral 50 mg/ml for IV injection	5-6 mg/kg	4-8 mg/kg; 300 mg/d max	1-2	10-20 mg/l; infant 6-11 mg/l
Phenobarbital	Tab 30/ 60 mg; Syp 20 mg/5 ml; Parenteral 30/ 60/200 mg/ml fro IV or IM injection	3-6 mg/kg; 30-60 mg once a day. Titrated slowly up to 240 mg per day	30-120 mg	2-3	15-40 mg/l; infant: 20-60 mg/l
Carbamazepine	Tab 100/200/400 mg; SR; Kid tab 100 mg	10-30 mg/kg; starting with 200 mg twice a day and increase by 200 mg daily each week to about 400 mg three times a day	800-1000 mg/day	2-3	6-12 mg/l; Hepatic and renal function and baseline CBC
Oxcarbamazepine	Tab 150/300 mg; Susp 300 mg/5 ml	5-8 mg/kg	10-30 mg/kg/day	2	3-35 mg/l; Not routinely warranted
Primidone	Tab 50/250 mg; 250 mg/5 ml suspension	12-25 mg/kg (>8 y 100 mg; <8 y 50 mg) at bed time	>8 y 250 mg; <8 y 125 mg	3-4	

Contd.

Contd.

Valproate	Tab 200/300/500 mg; CR 200/300/500 mg; SR 200/500 mg; Parenteral 100 mg/ml in 5 ml vial for IV injection	10-60 mg/kg; 20 mg/kg (<20 kg) 400 mg/d (>20 kg)	35 mg/kg max	2	50-100 mg/l; Hepatic function should be checked at frequent intervals first 6 months of therapy
Levetiracetam	Tab 250/500 mg; Syp 500 mg/5 ml; Inj. 500 mg/5 ml for IV administration	***10 mg/kg/day Children 1 month to <6 months:*** Immediate release: 14 mg/kg/day; ***Children 6 months to <4 years:*** Immediate release: 20 mg/kg/day; 50 mg/kg; ***Children 4 to less than 16 years:*** Immediate release: 20 mg/kg/day. ***Children 16 years and older:*** Immediate release: Initial: 1000 mg/day	***20-60 mg/kg/day Children 1 month to <6 months*** 14-42 mg/kg/day; ***Children 6 months to <4 years:*** 20-50 mg/kg/day ***Children 4 to less than 16 years:*** 20-60 mg/kg/day. Reduce daily dose in patients who cannot tolerate this dose ***Children 16 years and older:*** 1000-3000 mg/day; Dose increment every 2 weeks. Do not crush tablet	2	6-45 mg/l; reduce dose in impaired renal function
Gabapentin	Cap/Tab100/300/400/600/800 mg; Oral sol 250 mg/5 ml	15 mg/kg	30-60 mg/kg	3	Not determined
Lamotrigine	Tab 5/25/50/100 mg; dispersible tab	0.5 mg/kg	3-8 mg/kg; max 400 mg/d	2	Not determined
	With enz inducing drugs	2 mg/kg	5-15 mg/kg	2	
	With valproate	0.2 mg/kg	1-5 mg/kg	1-2	
Tiagabine	Tab 4/12/16/20 mg	4 mg/d (>12 y)	32 mg/d max	1	20-200 ng/ml; patients with hepatic dysfunction need slower and more cautious dose titration
Felbamate	Tab 400/600 mg; Susp 600 mg/5 ml	15 mg/kg	30-45 mg/kg	3-4	Requires close monitoring for adverse effects
Topiramate	Tab 25/50/100/200 mg	1-3 mg/kg	5-9 mg/kg	2	Not determined
Vigabatrin	Tab 500/750 mg; Powder 500 mg Sachet	20-50 mg/kg	50-100 mg/kg; 150 mg/d max	2	Not determined; Vision testing is required at baseline and then at least every 3 months; discontinue if no response in 2 weeks
Pregabalin	Cap 75/100/150/300 mg	150-300 mg (adults)	600 mg max	2-3	
Zonisamide	Cap 25/50/100 mg	2–4 mg/kg 100 mg (>16 y)	4–8 mg/kg/day; max 400 mg	1-2	Not determined; Toxic Level: > 80 mcg/ml; titrate dose more slowly in liver dysfunction

*Brand interchange is not permitted because of potential bioavailability differences.

Phenytoin (PHT) is one of the most widely used first line drug in the treatment of primary tonic-clonic seizures, especially status epilepticus, and partial seizures, but has no documented effect against absence or myoclonic seizures or in Lennox-Gastaut syndrome. It has been widely used in a variety of psychiatric disorders including psychoses, mood disorders and aggression.[7]

This drug is highly effective and economical for the patient; however, tolerability of the drug is a problem. Phenytoin alters brain cell sodium channels, which has the effect of limiting rapid firing of the brain cells, limits development of maximal seizure activity, and reduces the spread of seizures. It also demonstrates an inhibiting effect on calcium channels and the sequestration of calcium ions in nerve terminals, thereby inhibiting voltage-dependent neurotransmission at the level of the synapse. Usual adult dose is 300-400 mg per day. Loading dose of PHT can be given by IV route in an emergency. Phenytoin has saturable absorption, e.g., doses of 20 mg/kg given as a single dose result in lower concentrations than four equally spaced doses of 5 mg/kg. Doses higher than 400 mg should be given in at least two equally divided doses. Phenytoin also displays Michael's-Menten pharmacokinetics, which means that the metabolism of the drug saturates.[7] When the metabolism saturates, any additional drug that is administered remains in the circulating blood and is available for transport to the receptor sites. This saturation of metabolism occurs at doses that are used clinically and is unpredictable. The result is that a small change in dose may result in a significantly greater proportional change in serum concentration with possible toxicity. Dosage titration must be done carefully with close patient monitoring. The target serum level is 10-20 mg/l.

The enzymes responsible for the metabolism of phenytoin are CYP2C9 and CYP2C19. Among all AEDs, PHT has one of the most problematic drug interaction profiles. PHT itself is a strong inducer of hepatic enzymes and alters levels of other drugs Phenytoin induces the metabolism of other drugs. It decreases levels of CBZ, VAP, PHB, Clonazepam, LTZ, OXC, felbamate, tiagabine, topiramate and zonisamide. It inhibits dicumarol, warfarin and corticosteroids; clotting factors and immunosuppressants must be monitored and doses adjusted accordingly. Other drugs whose levels are reduced by PHT and require monitoring and adjustment include furosemide, cyclosporine, folate and praziquantel. Levels of chloramphenicol and quinidine are elevated by PHT. Other drugs that significantly increase PHT levels are isoniazid, cimetidine, chloramphenicol, dicumarol and sulfonamides. Levels of PHT are decreased by rifampicin, alcohol (chronic abuse), aminophylline, antacids containing calcium (if taken together), ciprofloxacin, folic acid, methotrexate, sucralfate and vinblastine, warfarin, dicumarol, oestrogen, vigabatrin and amiodarone. PHT is about 90% bound to plasma proteins. Also lowers concentration of oestrogen, itraconazole, rifampicin, digoxin, dicumarol, furosemide, cyclosporine, folate, and praziquantel requiring monitoring and dose adjustment.

Phenytoin has been associated with side effects that are concentration dependent, duration of dosing dependent and idiosyncratic[4,6] Commonly observed adverse effects are unsteadiness and moderate cognitive impairment. CNS effects occur particularly in the cerebellum and the vestibular system, causing ataxia and nystagmus (associated with higher serum concentrations).Though PHT is not a generalized CNS depressant, causes some degree of drowsiness and lethargy. Phenytoin may cause rash and sometimes even the fatal Stevens-Johnson syndrome. The long-term adverse-effect profile (e.g., gingival hyperplasia and coarsening of the facial features in women) makes its use less desirable than CBZ in some patients. Long-term use of PHT has been associated with osteoporosis; therefore, must be used with caution in susceptible populations, and routine screening must be performed to detect the condition early. Most commonly associated adverse effects include nausea and vomiting, rash, blood dyscrasias, headaches, vitamin K and folate deficiencies, loss of libido, hormonal dysfunction, and bone marrow hypoplasia. When given during pregnancy, PHT, like other AEDs, can cause cleft palate, cleft lip, congenital heart disease, slowed growth rate and mental retardation.

Despite the difficult pharmacokinetics and the adverse effects, this drug is used widely. Its main advantages are once-daily dosing, the good efficacy, the extensive clinical experience, the possibility of monitoring the plasma levels, and the availability of a parenteral preparation.

Fosphenytoin sodium is a prodrug intended for parenteral administration. Its active metabolite is PHT. It is safer and better tolerated than PHT and can be infused 3 times faster than intravenous PHT, however, fosphenytoin is much more expensive than PHT. Fosphenytoin is indicated for treatment of status epilepticus. Cardiovascular depression and hypotension may occur with fosphenytoin but to a lesser extent than with PHT. These adverse effects usually are related to the rate of infusion. Slower infusion is recommended in susceptible patients.

Fosphenytoin, a pro-drug for PHT, is converted to PHT with a 15-min half-life. Drug monitoring of PHT concentrations after use of the pro-drug requires that 2 hours elapse from the end of an IV infusion and 4 hours from an IM injection before samples are obtained the time taken to convert to PHT. Once converted, pharmacokinetic data are the same as for PHT.

Carbamazepine (CBZ) CBZ is a major first-line AED for simple, complex, and secondarily generalized seizures and primary tonic-clonic seizures in both adults and children but can worsen atypical absence, myoclonic seizures. In children with Lennox-Gastaut syndrome, it exacerbates certain seizures such as myoclonic and drop attacks. It was initially developed for the treatment of trigeminal neuralgia and later developed as an AED. It is also effective for bipolar depression.[4,6-7] The drug is highly effective and well tolerated. Carbamazepine affects sodium channels, and inhibits rapid firing of brain cells. The major disadvantages of this drug are transient adverse dose-related effects and occasional toxicity. Usual adult dose is 400 mg three times a day starting with 200 mg twice a day and increase by 200 mg daily to about 400 mg three times a day each week.

Since carbamazepine has a slow rate of dissolution, the immediate-release tablets have slow and sometimes erratic absorption. Absorption from the extended-release formulations has less fluctuations and lower peaks and higher troughs, which should result in better efficacy with lower side effects.[8] The chewable tablet is absorbed at the same rate as the immediate-release tablet, whereas the suspension is absorbed faster. CYP3A4 is the primary enzyme for epoxidation. Interestingly, carbamazepine induces its own metabolism and thus the half-life of carbamazepine is significantly shorter after repeated dosing. Auto-induction is usually complete by 2-3 weeks, although it can take longer in some individuals.

Thus, the change in serum concentration is less than the proportional change in dose. The protein binding of carbamazepine ranges between 10% and 50%.[4,6,9,10] Carbamazepine may induce the metabolism of other drugs and its metabolism may be induced and inhibited.[4,5,9,10] Several drugs, such as macrolide antibiotics (erythromycin and clarithromycin), isoniazid, chloramphenicol, calcium channel blockers, cimetidine, and propoxyphene, inhibit the hepatic enzyme cytochrome CYP3A4, which is responsible for the metabolic breakdown of CBZ, thereby raising its levels. Phenobarbital, phenytoin, felbamate, and primidone also lower its levels through CYP3A4. Toxic symptoms or breakthrough seizures may occur if the dose of CBZ is not adjusted. Grapefruit juice and St. John's wort are inducers of CYP3A4 and can decrease CBZ levels. Drug-induced changes in carbamazepine kinetics are particularly pronounced in children.

The most common side effects associated with carbamazepine involve the CNS, e.g., diplopia, dizziness, headache, nausea, vomiting, sedation and lethargy. These side effects have been associated with peak concentrations; extended-release formulations that lower the peak may decrease the incidence of these adverse events. Also slow titration reduces the side effects and have a better tolerance. CBZ causes a rash, sometimes even the fatal Stevens-Johnson syndrome. People of Asian descent with HLA-B*1502 antigen are more at risk. Pharmacogenetic testing for this allele may be useful in patients of South Asian descent who are being considered for therapy with carbamazepine.[10] Other side effects include hyponatremia, and, very rarely, bone marrow suppression.[4,6]

Oxcarbamazepine (OXC): OXC is a structural analogue of carbamazepine. It is functionally a prodrug that undergoes presystemic reduction to 10,11-dihydro-10-hydroxy-carbamazepine, which is known as the monohydroxylated derivative (MHD). MHD is the active form of oxcarbazepine. The mechanism of action and spectrum of activity of oxcarbazepine are similar to that of carbamazepine. It is used in the treatment of partial, primary generalized tonic-clonic seizures as monotherapy or adjunctive therapy but may aggravate myoclonic or absence seizures.[7] Oxcarbazepine also has been used to treat acute mania and for the prophylaxis of bipolar disorders and neuropathic pain.

It was developed in an attempt to maintain the benefits of CBZ while avoiding its auto-induction and drug interaction properties. OXC does not produce the epoxide metabolite, which is largely responsible for the adverse effects reported with CBZ. Like CBZ, OXC blocks the neuronal sodium channel during sustained rapid repetitive firing. It is at least as effective, and a usual adult dose is 600 mg twice a day. OXC may have fewer side effects, except for more risk for hyponatremia. Allergic rash is similar to the one caused by CBZ but idiosyncratic reactions appear to be less common than with CBZ. It is more expensive than generic carbamazepine. Dose-related adverse effects include fatigue, headache, dizziness and ataxia.

Peak concentrations of oxcarbazepine occur in 1-3 hours and peak concentrations of MHD occur in 4-6 hours. There is an increase in the area under the curve (AUC) of MHD when oxcarbazepine is given with a meal that is high in fat or protein. Some MHD is excreted unchanged in the urine and some is further metabolized by glucuronide conjugation or hydroxylation. The clearance of MHD is decreased in patients with impaired renal function. Substitution for CBZ can be made abruptly with an OXC-to-CBZ ratio of 300:200.[4,10,11] The drug interaction profile of oxcarbazepine is complex. Unlike carbamazepine, oxcarbazepine does not induce its own as seen with carbamazepine metabolism as seen with carbamazepine. Although the conversion of oxcarbazepine is neither inhibited nor induced, the further metabolism of MHD may be altered by other drugs. For example, verapamil has been reported to decrease the AUC of MHD by 20%. Also, oxcarbazepine or MHD will interact with other drugs. Oxcarbazepine will significantly reduce the bioavailability of oral contraceptives. The drug has been reported to decrease the concentrations of carbamazepine and lamotrigine while increasing the concentrations of phenytoin and phenobarbital.[4,7,10,11]

The side effect profile of oxcarbazepine is similar to that of carbamazepine although oxcarbazepine has been reported to be better tolerated than carbamazepine The most frequently reported side effects include somnolence, sedation, headache, dizziness, vertigo, ataxia, nausea, vomiting, fatigue, abnormal vision and diplopia. There is a higher incidence of hyponatremia with oxcarbazepine than with carbamazepine, which can be corrected by fluid restriction.[10] Hyponatremia is uncommon in children younger than 17 years but it occurs in 2.5% of adults and 7.4% of the elderly. There is a cross-reactivity of 25% to 31% for rash between carbamazepine and oxcarbazepine. However, idiosyncratic reactions appear to be less common than the CBZ.[4,10,11]

Valproic acid (VPA) VPA is one of the most commonly used a broad-spectrum AED and is the drug of choice for all types of generalized seizures including absence, myoclonic and partial seizures. Also, it is a first line drug in photosensitive epilepsy and Lennox-Gastaut syndrome. It is a second choice in the treatment of infantile spasms. It is also effective in prevention of recurrence of febrile seizures. Valproic acid has been approved for the prophylaxis of migraine headaches and bipolar disorder.[4,6,13,14] VPA has effects on GABA in very high doses, and a neurotransmitter called NPY to block seizures, and may be also on calcium channels. The usual adult dose is 500-1500 mg/day. Intravenous VPA is useful in patients when oral administration is not possible and when rapid IV loading is necessary. An extended release form can be taken once a day. Rapid titration usually is well tolerated. In children, the usual dose is 20 mg/kg/day and the maintenance dose is 40 mg/kg. Serum level has poor correlation with clinical effect and has significant daily fluctuations.

Valproic acid is well absorbed following oral administration and has a bioavailability of greater than 90% compared with an IV dose. The rates of absorption differ depending on the formulation that is used. The syrup and soft gelatin capsule are absorbed rapidly. The enteric-coated tablet was designed to reduce the gastrointestinal (GI) side effects by delaying the release of valproic acid until it reaches the small intestine. IV formulation of valproic acid is used in status epilepticus, acute persistent migraine headache and acute mania.[4,15]

One of the metabolites of valproic acid, the 4-ene-valproic acid, has been associated with liver toxicity. Valproic acid is about 90% bound to albumin at concentrations up to about 75 mcg/ml.[4,12] The meta-bolism of valproic acid is subject to induction and inhibition by other drugs. Valproic acid is an enzyme inhibitor, especially of CYP2C9, epoxide hydroxylase, and UDPglucuronosyltransferase (UDPGT).[4,10] It increases plasma levels of free fractions of PHT, PHB, CBZ epoxide and Lamotrigine. It decreases total PHT levels. The levels of VPA are decreased by enzyme inducing drugs and are increased by felbamate and clobazam.

Dose-related adverse effects include nausea, vomiting (mainly during initiation of therapy and improved by administration of enteric-coated preparations), tremor, sedation, confusion or irritability, hair loss and weight gain. Metabolic adverse effects include hypocarnitinemia hyperglycinemia, and hyperammonemia. Severe sedation or even coma may result from hyperammonemia, typically with normal liver function tests. VPA belongs to category D, therefore, should not be used in women of childbearing age unless the drug is essential to the management of seizures, or for manic episodes associated with bipolar disorder. Treatment with first trimester of pregnancy is associated with 1-2% risk of the neural tube defects in the newborn. Adverse endocrine effects include insulin resistance and change in sex hormone levels causing anovulatory cycles, amenorrhea, and polycystic ovary syndrome, therefore should be given cautiously in adolescent girls. Bone marrow suppression with neutropenia and allergic rashes are rare. The most serious idiosyncratic adverse effect is hepatotoxicity observed mainly in patients younger than 2 years who are on polytherapy and/or have inborn errors of metabolism. Other idiosyncratic side effects include thrombocytopenia, pancreatitis and polycystic ovary disease.[4,7,10,13]

VPA is a potent inhibitor of both oxidation and glucuronidation. It increases plasma levels of free fractions of PHT, PHB, CBZ epoxide and LTG. It reduces the total PHT level. The levels of VPA are decreased by enzyme-inducing drugs and are increased by felbamate and clobazam.

SECOND-GENERATION AEDS

Felbamate (FLB)

Felbamate is effective in the treatment of complex partial seizures in patients with Lennox-Gastaut syndrome.[16] It is not indicated for nonepileptic conditions. Its use is restricted to patients with refractory severe partial epilepsy or Lennox-Gastaut syndrome because of its potentially fatal toxic effects (aplastic anemia and hepatotoxicity) mainly caused by its metabolite.[7]

Felbamate is rapidly and well absorbed following oral administration. About 40% to 50% of a dose is excreted unchanged in the urine with the rest being metabolized by the liver. The isoenzymes involved in felbamate metabolism are CYP3A4, CYP2E1 and UDPGT.[3,4,6,10,17] Inducers of hepatic metabolism increase the metabolism of felbamate, while valproic acid inhibits the metabolism. Children clear felbamate approximately 20-65% faster than adults.[10,18] In children, the recommended dose is 15 mg/kg with weekly increments upto 45-80 mg/kg. Adverse effects involve decreased appetite, nausea, vomiting, insomnia, dizziness, somnolence and headache, rare but life threatening adverse effects are aplastic anemia and hepatic failure limiting its use in refractory epilepsy only. Close monitoring of liver function and blood counts are advised during felbamate therapy, with the goal to discontinue therapy if any signs of bone marrow or liver damage appear.

Gabapentin (GBP)

Gabapentin has been used primarily as adjunctive or monotherapy to treat partial seizures but is ineffective in myoclonus and in most generalized seizure disorders.[7] The drug appears to have only a modest efficacy particularly at lower doses. Nonepilepsy indications for the use of gabapentin are neuropathic pain and other pain syndromes. It has also been used in spasticity, restless legs syndrome, tremors, mood disorders and anxiety.[4]

Following oral administration, GBP is actively absorbed. Although most drugs are passively absorbed, GBP binds to an L-like amino acid transporter resulting in decreased GBP bioavailability as the dose is increased. Many patients with epilepsy may require higher doses. The higher doses have a lower bioavailability, necessitating giving smaller doses more frequently. A high protein meal may increase the bioavailability of GBP. Gabapentin is not metabolized and is completely eliminated by renal elimination. Patients with decreased renal function will have a decreased clearance of GBP. Gabapentin does not bind to plasma proteins. Because GBP is not metabolized by the liver and does not bind to plasma proteins, it is not associated with any significant drug interactions. GBP does not induce or inhibit drug-metabolizing enzymes.[4,10,11]

The most common side effects are dizziness and somnolence and tolerance to these effects may develop with continued dosing. Other less common side effects are ataxia, fatigue, headache, tremors and diplopia. Behavioural disturbances, especially aggressive behaviour, have been reported in children.[4,11] TDM is not usually necessary for gabapentin therapy other than to adjust dosing in patients with impaired kidney function or to assess adherence to therapy,[10,19] rarely hepatotoxictiy has been reported. In children, the starting dose range from 10-15 mg/kg in three divided doses and effective dose is 25-35 mg/kg/day. Infants and children require higher dose by 33% compared to older children.

Lamotrigine (LTG)

Lamotrigine is a broad-spectrum AED and is effective in all seizure types including partial seizures with or without secondary generalized seizures and primary generalized tonic-clonic seizures. It is an effective adjunct to refractory partial and generalized epilepsy. It is particularly useful in typical and atypical absence seizure in Lennox-Gastaut syndrome and in children with myoclonic-astatic epilepsy. It is also useful as a first line agent in children with idiopathic generalized epilepsy.[16] In bipolar disorder it has been used as a mood stabilizer.[4,11,12] Lamotrigine acts by blocking the voltage dependent sodium channels and thus blocks the release of glutamate through stabilization of presynaptic membrane.

Lamotrigine is started at 1-2 mg/kg followed by slow increment in dose biweekly to 3-8 mg/kg/day. The drug dosage is reduced to half when used in combination with valproate as the latter prolongs the half life of lamotrigine.

Absorption following an oral dose is rapid and complete, achieving a bioavailability of about 98%. The administration of LTG with food decreases the rate, but not the extent of absorption. The half-life is widely variable ranging from 30 hours to 2 weeks. However, the half-life is shorter in patients taking enzyme-inducing drugs such as phenytoin and carbamazepine and much longer in patients taking enzyme-inhibiting drugs such as valproic acid, thereby producing a marked elevation in LTG levels, therefore, lower doses of LTG should be prescribed. In children on valproic acid, the starting dose is 0.15 mg/kg; with concomitant enzyme inducers, the starting dose is 0.6 mg/kg and as monotherapy starting dose is 0.4 mg/kg. Similar to carbamazepine, lamotrigine shows the phenomenon of auto-induction during chronic therapy. Autoinduction is usually complete within two weeks, with a ~20% reduction in steady-state serum/plasma concentrations if the dose is not increased.[10] Ethinyl estradiol-containing oral contraceptives also significantly increase the clearance of lamotrigine resulting in a decrease in the concentrations of lamotrigine by 50% with an increase in seizures. However, it does not interfere with the efficacy of oral contraceptives or warfarin.[7] Lamotrigine does not significantly alter the metabolism of other drugs. It is about 55% bound to plasma proteins.[4] Severe renal failure increases the serum half-life to ~50 hours in patients. The clearance of lamotrigine is higher in children and much higher (~300%) in pregnancy.[18]

Different from most AEDs, LTG produces few CNS side effects. The most common dose related side effects associated with lamotrigine somnolence, sleep disturbances, dizziness, diplopia, ataxia, nausea and vomiting. Serious side effects of lamotrigine which often require drug withdrawals include skin rash progressing to Stevens-Johnson syndrome and toxic epidermal necrolysis. The risk factors for neurotoxicity and skin rash are young age, large initial doses, rapid escalation, and concurrent use of valproic acid[3,4,11,16] The rash begins as a maculopapular rash but may progress to Stevens-Johnson syndrome. The incidence of the rash is reported to be higher in children due to increased formation of intermediate of LTG.[20]

Low incidence of congenital malformations is reported on exposure of pregnant patients, thus making it as a one of the preferred treatments during pregnancy.

Topiramate (TPM)

Topiramate is a useful adjunct in refractory partial or generalized epilepsy and other epileptic syndromes, Lennox-Gastaut syndrome, infantile spasms, generalized epilepsy of infancy and myoclonic–astatic epilepsy. Topiramate adjunctive therapy may be efficacious for juvenile myoclonic seizures in adults and children.[16] Topiramate also is used for prophylaxis of migraine, diabetic neuropathy, essential tremors and bipolar disorder.[4] Topiramate is a broad spectrum AED and has several mechanisms, including blocking the enzyme carbonic anhydrase. Usual adult dose is 150-200 mg twice a day, dose titrated slowly. In children is 1-3 mg/kg/day divided into two daily doses and dose increased bi-weekly to 3-8 mg/kg/day.[16]

Topiramate is rapidly absorbed and has a bioavailability of 81% to 95%. Administration with a high-fat meal decreases the rate, but not the extent, of absorption. The half-life of topiramate in patients on monotherapy with normal renal function is lower and ranges between 20 and 30 hours to 12 hours in patients taking enzyme-inducing AEDs. Patients who have impaired renal function have a decreased clearance of topiramate. A 50% dose reduction is recommended for patients with moderate-to-severe renal dysfunction. Topiramate is only about 15% bound to plasma proteins.[4,10,21] Children eliminate topiramate faster than adults and elimination rate decreases progressively with age until puberty, presumably due to age-dependent changes in the rate of drug metabolism. As a result of this, younger patients require higher dosages to achieve serum topiramate concentrations comparable with those found in older children and adults. Enzyme-inducing co-medication decreases serum topiramate concentration by approximately one-half and one-third in children and adults, respectively.

The addition of topiramate to patients taking phenytoin results in upto 25% increase in phenytoin concentration as topiramate inhibits CYP2C19, which is one of the enzymes associated with the metabolism of phenytoin. Topiramate may increase the formation of the 4-ene metabolite of valproic acid and increases the clearance of ethinyl oestradiol in a dose-dependent manner.[4,5]

Topiramate has good safety with no evidence of life threatening adverse effects or organ toxicity. The most frequently reported side effects are ataxia, poor concentration, confusion, dysphagia, dizziness, fatigue, paresthesia, somnolence, word-finding difficulties and cognitive slowing. These effects are enhanced with large initial doses and by rapid dosage titration. Other side effects reported with administration of topiramate are anorexia, weight loss, renal stones, metabolic acidosis, open-angle glaucoma, and decreased sweating.[4,5] Monitor children on combination of topiramate and valproate for signs of encephalopathy resulting from hyperammonemia.[10]

Tiagabine (TGB)

Tiagabine is primarily used to treat refractory partial seizures with or without secondary generalization as add-on therapy. Tiagabine has also been used in the treatment of pain, spasticity, the prophylaxis of migraine headaches, and in bipolar disorder.[4,5,21]

Peak concentrations of tiagabine occur in less than two hours. Tiagabine is rapidly absorbed with high bioavailability. The administration of tiagabine with food reduces the rate, but not the extent, of absorption. This agent is extensively metabolized with less than 2% being excreted unchanged. Although the metabolism of tiagabine has been attributed to CYP3A4, this has been questioned because erythromycin, a potent inhibitor of CYP3A4, does not affect the pharmacokinetics of tiagabine. Tiagabine may undergo enterohepatic recirculation. The half-life of this agent is 5-9 hours, but is shorter (2-4 hours) in enzyme-induced patients.[4,10,21] The serum half-life increases to 12-16 hours in severe liver failure.[10] Children have higher clearance than adults. Renal dysfunction does not significantly impact the pharmacokinetics of tiagabine. Tiagabine does not affect the metabolism of other drugs. Although tiagabine is highly protein bound (>95%). The metabolism of tiagabine can be altered by concomitant therapy with liver enzyme inhibitors or inducers. The inter-individual variation in hepatic metabolism and extensive binding of tiagabine to plasma proteins further makes tiagabine a candidate for TDM and be clinically useful.

The most frequently reported side effects are dizziness, fatigue, generalized muscle weakness, nervousness, tremor, abnormal thinking, depression, aphasia, and encephalopathy. Tiagabine has also been associated with abdominal pain, knee buckling and seizures in patients without epilepsy. Nonconvulsive status epilepticus has been reported in patients with epilepsy. Therefore, TGB should be used with caution in patients with a history of status epilepticus. TGB is contraindicated in severe hepatic impairment, pregnancy and lactation.[4,10,21]

Levetiracetam (LEV)

Levetiracetam is broad spectrum AED effective as adjunctive therapy for refractory partial-onset seizures, primary generalized tonic-clonic seizures, and myoclonic seizures of juvenile myoclonic epilepsy.[16,20] Intravenous preparation has recently shown efficacy in neonatal seizures and status epilepticus. In addition, it has been found equivalent to controlled release carbamazepine as first-line therapy for partial-onset seizures, both in efficacy and tolerability. LEV is a novel AED which selectively inhibits high-voltage-activated calcium channels and reduces calcium release from intraneuronal stores and binds to specific targets (SV2A proteins) and acts through a mechanism that is distinct from any other currently available AED. Its pharmacokinetic profile allows easy titration with little risk for drug interactions. Pediatric dose start from 10 mg/kg/day in two divided doses and increase by 10-20 mg/kg every two weeks to a maximum dose of 40-60 mg/kg/day.[16] In children more than 4 years of age, treatment is initiated with 20 mg/kg in two divided doses and increased every 2 weeks by 20 mg/kg upto 60 mg/kg. It is not approved for children less than 4 years.

Levetiracetam shows low binding to serum proteins and has linear pharmacokinetics. Peak concentrations of levetiracetam are reached in about one hour. The apparent bioavailability is 100%. The administration of levetiracetam with food decreases the rate, but not the extent, of absorption. About 66% of a dose is excreted unchanged in the urine. Therefore, the dose should be altered for patients with impaired renal function. The half-life of this agent ranges between 6-8 hours in healthy subjects. Levetiracetam does not affect the metabolism of other drugs and does not bind to plasma proteins. No drug interactions have been reported with levetiracetam.[4,10,18,19,21,22,23] The serum half-life of levetiracetam is shorter in adult (6-8 hours) compared to neonates (16-18 hours).[19] Clearance of levetiracetam increases significantly in pregnancy, with an approximately 60% decrease in serum concentrations.[24] For therapeutic drug monitoring while collecting samples serum or plasma should be separated from whole blood rapidly, as *in vitro* hydrolysis of levetiracetam can occur in the blood tube and thus lead to artifactually low concentrations.[25] Levetiracetam distribute extensively into saliva, with salivary concentrations usually being slightly higher than serum concentrations in patients receiving chronic therapy.

The most common side effects associated with levetiracetam include somnolence, asthenia, dizziness, vertigo and headaches. Psychiatric and behavioural effects such as emotional lability, nervousness, and hostility have been reported particularly in children. The side effects associated with levetiracetam are not dependent on the rate of dosage titration. Therefore, it may be started at doses that are clinically effective and rapidly titrated to the patient's response.[4,17] As adjunctive therapy, LEV appears to be safe and effective for the treatment of pediatric epilepsy. It has been well tolerated in pediatric studies with an AE profile similar to that demonstrated in adults. Somnolence is the most commonly reported AE across all pediatric studies, and behavioural events were among the most common types of AEs in open-label studies. Improvements in behaviour and cognition were also frequently reported. The relative risk of neuropsychiatric AEs appears similar in children compared with adults.

Vigabatrin

Vigabatrin is a "designer drug", made to block metabolism of GABA, the brain's main inhibitory neurotransmitter. VGB is the drug of choice in infantile spasms, particularly in patients with tuberous sclerosis and it may be considered as a first line treatment in other patients with infantile spasms in whom the use of hormonal treatment (corticosteroids, ACTH) is contraindicated.[16] It has shown efficacy as add-on therapy in the treatment of partial seizures and secondary generalized seizures. It is less effective against primarily generalized tonic-clonic seizures and also may worsen myoclonic seizures or generalized absence seizures. Like TGB, VGB has been reported to cause absence status. Patients with myoclonus or Lennox-Gastaut syndrome do not respond well to VGB.[7] Its use is restricted because of its adverse visual effects – development of bilateral concentric peripheral visual field constriction in 20-40% patients.[16] On long-term use retinal toxicity can result in permanent loss of peripheral vision, therefore, regular vision testing is recommended for all patients. Vision loss onset is unpredictable and can occur within weeks of starting treatment, or sooner, or at any time during treatment (even after months or years), and possibly after vigabatrin is discontinued.[16] Weigh the risks and benefits before starting vigabatrin treatment since infantile spasms comprise a severe epileptic encephalopathy with poor developmental outcome if uncontrolled. Vigabatrin precipitates myoclonic seizures and absence seizures.[16, 26]

In children, starting dose is 40 mg/kg/day and a maintenance dose of 80-100 mg/kg/day. In infantile spasms, the dose of 100-200 mg/kg/day may be necessary. The response in infantile spasms is observed in 1-2 weeks but can be continued only for few months to reduce the chances of visual field defects. It must be discontinued slowly to avoid rebound seizures. If no response is seen in 2 weeks vigabatrin should be discontinued. In infants with good response consider stopping the drug after 6 months. VGB has a wide range of serum/plasma concentrations (0.8-36 mg/l) and is associated with successful treatment with vigabatrin due to the irreversible action of vigabatrin on its molecular target.[10]

VGB is highly water soluble but only slightly soluble in ethanol. It is absorbed rapidly following oral ingestion, with an oral bioavailability of 100%. Time to peak concentration is approximately 2 hours, and the volume of distribution of the drug is 0.8 L/kg. About 10% of the plasma concentration is found in CSF. Only a small fraction crosses the placenta. VGB is excreted in urine (up to 95%) with a half-life of 4-7 hours. In elderly patients, clearance is reduced and the half-life may double. VGB does not induce the activity of hepatic enzymes. Correlation between plasma levels and clinical effect is poor.[7,10]

VGB can reduce plasma concentration of PHT by 25%. This probably is mediated by decreased absorption; however, the exact mechanism is unknown. No other pharmacokinetic or pharmacodynamic interactions are present. Usually adult dose is 500-1500 mg twice a day. Vigabatrin plasma levels show wide inter-patient variability, and co-administration with carbamazepine increases vigabatrin's clearance. While there is no relationship between plasma level and anti-epileptic effect, abnormally high levels of the drug may increase toxicity.

The most common adverse effect is drowsiness. Other important adverse effects include neuropsychiatric symptoms, such as depression, agitation, confusion and, rarely, psychosis. Minor adverse effects, usually at the onset of therapy, include fatigue, headache, dizziness, weight gain, tremor. VGB has little effect on cognitive function. Acute hypersensitivity or idiosyncratic immunological adverse effects are extremely rare.[7]

Zonisamide (ZNS)

Zonisamide is a broad-spectrum AED, is a sulphonamide derivative and has been used as adjunctive therapy of a variety of seizure types including partial, primary generalized tonic-clonic, absence, atonic, and myoclonic seizures for patients who are above 12 years.[4,7,15] It is useful as a second-line agent for infantile spasms, Lennox-Gastaut syndrome, and juvenile myoclonic epilepsy.[16] It has also been used to facilitate weight loss and to treat pain and a variety of psychiatric disorders. Zonisamide is available in a capsule dosage form that can be opened and put in solution or be sprinkled. It acts through multiple actions such as facilitation of dopaminergic and serotoninergic neurotransmission through the blockade of T-type calcium channels, prolongation of sodium channel inactivation and as a weak inhibitor of carbonic anhydrase.[10]

The usual starting dose is 2-4 mg/kg/day, and the maintenance dose is 4-8 mg/kg/day divided once or twice daily. Usual adult dose is 100-300 mg twice a day, dose titrated slowly. Zonisamide is metabolized in the liver, dose should be titrated more slowly in patients with liver dysfunction. About 70% of ZNS is metabolized and about 30% is eliminated unchanged in the urine. The hydroxylation of this agent is facilitated by CYP3A4 with some contributions from CYP2D6, CYP2C19, and CYP3A5. Zonisamide does not induce its own metabolism or inhibit hepatic metabolism. Zonisamide is absorbed quickly and completely when administered orally reaching a peak levels in 2-4 hours. Zonisamide, however, does not affect the metabolism of other drugs. About 40% to 60% of this agent is bound to serum albumin. ZNS exhibits a linear dose/plasma concentration at doses of 100-400 mg.[4,6,10] It has a half life of 50-60 hours but decreases to 25-35 hours in patients concomitantly taking enzyme inducers such as carbamazepine or phenobarbital. On the other hand, liver enzyme inhibitors such as ketoconazole and valproic acid may prolong zonisamide half-life.[10]

The most frequently reported side effects associated with zonisamide include fatigue, dizziness, somnolence, anorexia, psychomotor slowing and ataxia. Although the incidence of severe skin rash is very low, people with a true sulpha allergy should take the drug with caution. Zonisamide has also been associated with renal stones, anorexia, weight loss, and oligohidrosis (decreased sweating).[4,7] Zonisamide is similar in its coverage and adverse effects to topiramate, except glaucoma is not usually listed. Cognitive impairment is dose dependent and less than with topiramate.

Pregabalin (PGB)

Pregabalin (PGB) is a drug with a unique mechanism of action and a favourable side-effect profile and an advantageous pharmacokinetics including high bioavailability, low binding to plasma proteins, minimal metabolism, and no significant drug-drug interactions.

The drug has been shown to be a highly effective adjunctive treatment in patients with partial seizures.[7] Pregabalin is related to gabapentin, it may be better, more effective against seizures than is gabapentin, and can be given twice a day. It shares many clinical similarities to gabapentin, including widespread use to manage conditions other than epilepsy such as neuropathic pain and fibromyalgia. It has a similar adverse effect to gabapentin. Usual adult dose is 150-600 mg twice a day.

The absorption of pregabalin is rapid and extensive. The oral bioavailability is at least 90%. Unlike gabapentin, which has decreased bioavailability with increasing doses, pregabalin does not bind to the L-amino protein carrier system in the gut and the absorption of pregabalin is independent of dose. After single and multiple doses, the AUC and peak concentrations of pregabalin are dose proportional. All doses up to 1200 mg, which is twice the expected total daily dose, have a bioavailability of at least 90%. The absorption of pregabalin is not affected by food. Pregabalin is not extensively metabolized and more than 90% of an administered dose is excreted unchanged in the urine. The dose of pregabalin should be reduced in patients with impaired renal function. Pregabalin does not bind to plasma proteins or induce or inhibit the metabolism of other drugs. It also does not interact with other drugs.[10,27] TDM is routinely not recommended due to its favorable pharmacokinetics other than to adjust dosing during renal failure or to assess compliance. If monitoring is performed, care must be taken in the timing of blood draws for TDM as it has a short half-life of pregabalin (4-6 hours).

The most frequently reported side effects associated with pregabalin are dizziness and somnolence. Other dose related side effects are ataxia, peripheral edema, headache and weight gain. Most were mild to moderate, were dose related, and occurred primarily in the first two weeks of therapy. Rapid withdrawal of pregabalin resulted in anxiety, nervousness, and irritability. Importantly, pregabalin may be dosed rapidly without a significant increase in side effects.[27]

THIRD-GENERATION AEDs

Eslicarbazepine Acetate

It is structurally related to carbamazepine and oxcarbazepine and has been used as adjunctive therapy for adults with partial seizures, however, there is no pediatric experience so far. Unlike carbamazepine, eslicarbazepine does not exhibit auto-induction in metabolism, has low (~30%) binding to serum proteins, and overall has a low potential for drug-drug interactions.[28,29] Eslicarbazepine has an elimination half-life of 20-24 hours during chronic administration.[30] Mild to moderation hepatic failure has minimal impact on the pharmacokinetics of eslicarbazepine.[31] The main route of elimination of eslicarbazepine and other minor metabolites of eslicarbazepine acetate is via the kidneys, with moderate or severe renal failure significantly reducing the clearance of eslicarbazepine. Hemodialysis effectively removes eslicarbazepine and other metabolites of eslicarbazepine acetate.[32] Overall, TDM has a minor role in the therapeutic use of eslicarbazepine given the relatively predictable pharmacokinetics of the drug. TDM for eslicarbazepine may be useful in patients with renal failure.

Lacosamide

It is a novel functionalized amino acid that enhances inactivation of voltage gated sodium channels.[33,34] Lacosamide was approved in Europe in 2008 in patients 16 years and older[35] as an adjunctive treatment of partial-onset seizures. Lacosamide is used in children with refractory epilepsy with 30-50% of children having more than 50% reduction in seizure frequency.[16]

Lacosamide has high bioavailability (~100%) and serum protein binding.[36,37] Approximately 60% of the parent drug is metabolized, mainly by CYP2C19 to an inactive metabolite. The remaining 40% is excreted unchanged by the kidneys. Elimination half-life is approximately 13 hours. Drug-drug interactions involving lacosamide appear to be uncommon.[10,38,39] The predictable pharmacokinetics of lacosamide, along with lack of clinically significant drug-drug interactions, suggests a limited role for TDM in managing lacosamide pharmacotherapy. Consequently, TDM of lacosamide has limited benefit except in patients with severe liver and/or kidney failure, or to assess compliance with therapy.[40,41]

Lacosamide can be administered oral (Tab 50,100, 150, 200 mg; oral solution 10 mg/ml) as well as parenteral (200 mg/20 ml vial) which may have a role in status epilepticus, however, pediatric experience with lacosamide has been limited. Starting dose is 50 mg twice daily. The dosage may be increased by 50 mg twice daily at weekly intervals up to the recommended maintenance dosage of 200 to 400 mg/day, based on response and tolerability and may be taken without regard to meals. In patients with mild or moderate hepatic impairment and **Severe renal function impairment (CrCl less than 30 ml/min) and ESRD** maximum dose is 300 mg/day. It is not recommended in patients with severe hepatic impairment. No dosage adjustment needed in mild to moderate renal impairment.

When switching between the oral and IV route, administer the equivalent daily dose and frequency. Infuse the drug IV over a 30 to 60 min period. Injection may be administered IV without further dilution or may be further diluted with sodium chloride 0.9% injection, dextrose 5% injection, or Ringer's lactate injection. Do not administer if particulate matter, cloudiness, or discoloration is noted. When discontinuing therapy, gradually withdraw over a minimum of 1 week.

Store parenteral lacosamide between 59° and 86°F (Do not freeze). Following dilution, store IV form for up to 24 hours at 59° to 86°F in glass or PVC bags. Discard any unused portion of the injection after 24 hours and oral solution remaining after 7 weeks of first opening the bottle.

Lacosamide may cause dizziness, drowsiness, decreased balance or coordination, and vision changes, nystagmus and are at an increased risk of suicidal thoughts or action. This effect may be worse with alcohol or certain medicines. Dermatological adverse effects include Contusion, pruritus, skin laceration and sometimes may result in a serious and sometimes life-threatening or fatal hypersensitivity reaction. May also cause nausea, vomiting and diarrhea. Lacosamide is generally well tolerated with reports of irritability, oral tics, and prolonged crying as adverse effects in children. Rare but serious side effect seen with lacosamide is prolonged PR interval.[42]

Rufinamide

Rufinamide is a novel anticonvulsant approved for use in Europe in 2007 and in the United States in 2008 for adjunctive use in the treatment of seizures associated with Lennox-Gastaut syndrome in children aged above 4 years.[43] It is likely to be available soon in India. Its mechanism of action is not completely understood, may prolong the inactive state of sodium channels and therefore limiting excessive firing of sodium-dependent action potentials.

Rufinamide is well absorbed (80-90%) following oral administration.[44] The peak exposure to rufinamide may increase significantly when taken with food as compared to an empty stomach. Consequently, patients are often counselled to take rufinamide in the same temporal relation to meals. Rufinamide is extensively metabolized, primarily by carboxyesterases, with only trace amounts of the parent drug excreted in feces or urine. The primary metabolite is inactive and mainly excreted by the kidneys. Hepatic enzyme inducers such as carbamazepine and rifampin increase the excretion of rufinamide.[44] Impaired renal function has minimal effect on clearance of rufinamide; however, increased doses of rufinamide are often needed in patients receiving hemodialysis due to removal of the drug by the dialysis procedure. Although reference ranges for rufinamide have not been well-defined yet, serum/plasma concentrations generally correlate with seizure control, allowing for determination of an individual therapeutic concentration that can be monitored over the course of chronic therapy.[38,44,45] TDM for rufinamide can be especially helpful in patients receiving hemodialysis or who are also taking liver enzyme inducers. The most commonly observed adverse are headache, dizziness, fatigue, somnolence and nausea. Rare but serious side effect seen with rufinamide is arrhythmias (short QT interval).[16]

Stiripentol

Stiripentol is an AED that was originally approved in Europe in 2001 is used as an adjunctive to clobazam and valproate in the treatment of refractory generalized tonic-clonic seizures in patients with severe myoclonic epilepsy in infancy, i.e., Dravet syndrome. It enhances central gamma-aminobutyric acid transmission and inhibits the metabolism of concurrently administered anticonvulsants that are substrates for various cytochrome P450 isoenzymes, such as clobazam.[16]

Stiripentol is rapidly absorbed following oral administration but has overall low bioavailability, in large part due to extensive first-pass metabolism by the liver. The hepatic metabolism of stiripentol is very complex, with at least 5 different metabolic pathways generating over a dozen metabolites. The dosing of stiripentol is further complicated by zero-order (saturation) elimination kinetics, with a marked decrease in clearance with increased dosage. Stiripentol is also highly (>99%) protein bound and prone to drug interactions that can alter the free fraction.[46] A well-defined reference range for stiripentol has not been established, although one study showed that serum concentrations of 4-22 mg/l correlate with control of absence seizures in children.[47] The complex pharmacokinetics of stiripentol (extensive hepatic metabolism, high binding to plasma protein, and saturation kinetics) resemble that of phenytoin.[38] Measurement of the free drug fraction of stiripentol may be clinically useful; however, methods to measure free fractions have not yet been reported. When used in combination AEM therapies, stiripentol may cause drug-drug interactions by inhibiting the metabolism of carbamazepine, clobazam, phenobarbital, phenytoin and valproic acid.[48,49,50]

Retigabine (ezogabine) is a novel investigational AED developed as an adjunctive treatment for partial epilepsy. Retigabine opens voltage-gated KCNQ2/3 and KCNQ3/5 potassium channels leading to cellular membrane hyperpolarization.[16] There is no pediatric experience so far, but retigabine may potentially be a useful agent in the treatment of benign familial neonatal convulsions which is caused by loss of function mutations involving the KCNQ2/3 genes.

Brivaracetam is an analogue of levetiracetam, which has been found useful in adults with photosensitive epilepsy, and as an adjunctive treatment in refractory partial-onset epilepsy. There is no pediatric experience till now.

Ganaxolone is a synthetic analogue of allopregnenolone, a neurosteroid, which is an allosteric modulator of the GABA-A receptor complex. Ganaxolone may also have efficacy for catamenial seizures.

Perampanel is a selective, non-competitive antagonist of a-amino-3-hydroxy 5-methyl-4-isoxazolepropionic acid (AMPA)-type glutamate receptors, currently in clinical development as adjunctive therapy for the treatment of refractory partial-onset seizures.

Learning Disability

More than one in five patients with epilepsy has learning or intellectual disabilities often in tandem with behavioural disorders.[17,51] Important neuropsychiatric comorbidities in children with epilepsy are attention deficit/hyperactivity disorder, autistic spectrum disorders, depression and anxiety, and thought disorders.[52] To avoid further impairing cognition and worsening behaviour, unnecessary polytherapy should be avoided. Paradoxical seizure aggravation has been reported with such drugs as CBZ and benzodiazepines in specific seizures types, and close monitoring is essential during therapy with these AEDs.

SUMMARY

Carbamazepine, phenytoin or valproic acid (sodium valproate) are the first-line drugs, but factors such as adverse effect profiles, age, possibility of pregnancy, and concomitant diseases and medication also should be considered during selection. Most of the newer AED have been tested as add-on therapy in drug resistant epilepsy and are not superior to the first generation AEDs in efficacy. The main advantage of some of the newer agents was their better tolerability and pharmacokinetic profiles compared to the earlier AED, however, higher costs of the newer AEDs limits their wider use, especially in poorer countries.[7,16] Other than oxcarbazepine for partial epilepsy as monotherapy, there is no evidence for the use of the newer AED as monotherapy in new-onset epilepsy in children. Some of the newer AEDs have proven efficacy for some childhood epileptic syndromes and in patients with comorbid conditions such as bipolar disorder, migraine and sleep disturbance. Vigabatrin is the drug of choice for infantile spasms associated with tuberous sclerosis, levetiracetam for juvenile myoclonic epilepsy, rufinamide for Lennox-Gastaut syndrome and stiripentol for Dravet syndrome. Topiramate and zonisamide are good options in patients with infantile spasms who have failed hormonal therapy and vigabatrin. Topiramate is a good add-on drug in patients with epileptic encephalopathies such as Lennox-Gastaut syndrome and myoclonic astatic epilepsy. Lamotrigine, levetiracetam and lacosamide are good add-on drugs for patients with refractory partial seizures. Lamotrigine is also effective in tonic seizures seen in children with Lennox-Gastaut syndrome. Lamotrigine may be considered as monotherapy in adolescent females with idiopathic generalized epilepsy.[16] Among newer AEDs levetiracetam has emerged as effective as adjunctive therapy for refractory partial-onset seizures, primary generalized tonic-clonic seizures, and myoclonic seizures of juvenile myoclonic epilepsy mainly due to pharmacokinetic advantages such as rapid and almost complete absorption, minimal insignificant binding to plasma protein, absence of enzyme induction, absence of interactions with other drugs, and partial metabolism outside the liver and availability of an intravenous preparation for use in status epilepticus.

Certain newer AEDs such as lamotrigine and vigabatrin are known to worsen myoclonic seizures. There is paucity of data on the use of newer AEDs in children from India. As per Indian Guidelines for diagnosis and management of childhood epilepsy, the only newer AED which are recommended for use as monotherapy in new-onset epilepsy are lamotrigine in partial and generalized seizures, and oxcarbazepine in partial seizures.[53] The others are recommended as adjunctive treatment in children who have failed conventional AED.

Intractable epilepsy refractory to appropriate conventional AED is an indication for the newer drugs. Among children presenting with refractory epilepsy, one must always look for causes of pseudo-intractability including possibility of non epileptic event, misdiagnosis of seizure type, and wrong choice of conventional AEDs. These causes must always be thought before using newer AEDs as an adjunct.

The current choice of available AEDs also allows for options for children with concomitant systemic illnesses and comorbidities based on the pharmacokinetic profiles of these drugs.

The Goal of Therapy

The goal of therapy should be complete seizure freedom with a single first line AED taken once or twice a day and without significant adverse effects.

Treatment and selection of an antiepileptic drug (AED) for epilepsy in infancy, childhood, and adolescence should ideally begin after a clear syndromic diagnosis of the patient's seizure disorder. A common cause of failure of the first AED is erroneous diagnosis. The availability of new-generation AEDs has expanded the choice of available agents with comparable efficacy for most syndromes. However, class I or II evidence for efficacy is not available for many syndromes of childhood, and selection must, therefore, be based on efficacy, relative toxicity, and tolerability of AEDs in making the selection especially in view of the age-specific organ toxicities. Further, the use of AEDs in children requires an understanding of their neurobehavioral effects, neuropsychiatric comorbidities such as attention deficit/hyperactivity disorder, autistic spectrum disorders, depression and anxiety, thought disorders etc. Neurobehavioral problems can be exacerbated or ameliorated by specific AEDs. Comorbid migraine in children with epilepsy may benefit from some AEDs. Though newer AEDs may offer significant advantages in terms of impact on body weight, insulin sensitivity, lipid profile, and bone health yet there is a continuing need for the development of newer AEDs that are targeted for the developing brain to improve the efficacy and tolerability of treatment in childhood seizure disorders.

The decision whether to treat a child after an initial unprovoked seizure is an individualized one.

1. **Drug Selection:** Firstly correctly diagnose the type of epilepsy, evaluate need for initiation of AEDs and select most appropriate AED for the type of seizures in convenient once daily dosages to improve compliance. Other considerations include dose formulation, side effect profile, the potential for drug-drug interactions and ease of administration (Box 25.3). Transmucosal AED administration (e.g., rectal diazepam) is an effective and relatively safe emergency home treatment of prolonged or recurrent febrile seizures, prolonged seizures or seizure clusters in settings where intravenous access is not readily available. Thus remains a first line measure in out-of-hospital setting. Buccal midazolam is effective for the emergency treatment of seizures in children.

   Most febrile seizures are brief and would be over by the time a child is brought to the doctor or a health facility. Management includes definitive diagnosis, restraint in investigations, treatment of an acute episode and family counselling. Role of defervescence in preventing febrile seizures is questionable. Prophylaxis for future episodes depends on the assessment of risk factors, e.g., age, nature, and duration of seizures. Most children who have febrile seizures do not develop epilepsy. Prolonged therapy with phenytoin or carbamazepine interferes with cognitive development. Parents may be supplied with rectal preparation of diazepam for acute termination of seizures and management of fever at the first hint of fever and tepid sponging. Consider intermittent prophylaxis during fever with clobazam started on day of fever for 2-3 days.

Box 25.3: Patient and AED Characteristics for Selection of Antiepileptic Drugs

Patient factors	AED characteristics
• Seizure type and syndrome • Age • Gender • Pregnancy potential • Comorbidities	• Spectrum of efficacy • Mechanism of action • Indications (monotherapy vs. polytherapy, children, etc.) • Tolerability/safety profile – short-term and long-term adverse effect profile

Contd.

Contd.

• Co-medications • Individual lifestyle	• Neuropsychological implications and quality of life • Dosing frequency, titration complexity, simplicity of use • Pharmacokinetic considerations, therapeutic range especially in extremes of age group (children, elderly), renal, hepatic impairment • Drug-drug interaction profile • Teratogenic potential (in women of reproductive age group) • Cost of therapy

Status emergency is a medical emergency. Use the least expensive AED (all things being equal, like efficacy). Newer is not always better and second generation AEDs are certainly more expensive (Lamotrigine, Topiramate, Gabapentin).

2. **Monotherapy vs. Polytherapy**

   i. Single-drug therapy is the goal of epilepsy treatment as polypharmacy is not only expensive, but also increases side effects and increases the complexity of adjusting AEDs in the refractory patient. The primary goal is to achieve complete seizure freedom, ideally without adverse effects, reduce morbidity and mortality, and improve quality of life. Most patients are controlled on monotherapy. Remaining patients may require two or more AEDs given together. Combination therapy can result in poor compliance, drug interactions and increased side effects.

   ii. Start with one AED and avoid changing AED so long as seizures are controlled and push the dose to clinical toxicity or seizure control.

   iii. If seizures persist either add another AED or switch to another AED. A second AED is added when initial drug is well tolerated but seizures are not controlled with initial drug. If the initial drug was partially effective, it should be continued until reasonable levels of the new AED are achieved. Attempt tapering the first drug, if seizures are controlled. If the initial AED is ineffective, it can be tapered earlier, as the dose of the second drug is increased. Switch to another AED, if the initial drug is not effective not tolerated well.

   iv. Withdraw AEDs gradually that are not effective.

   v. Arbitrarily never have a patient more than three AEDs.

   vi. Do not use fixed dose combinations medications (e.g., phenytoin with phenobarbital).

   vii. There is no consensus on the number of mono-therapy trials that should be attempted before the combination therapy is introduced. Several combinations should be tested sequentially before adding a third drug. At least two appropriate AEDs at maximally tolerated dose must be used. The dose should be adequately adjusted to maintain blood levels within the so-called "optimal range". Preferably the dose should be kept as low as possible, as long as the clinical control is gained, even if the blood levels remain "subtherapeutic". However, physicians must be aware that, even when the drug is used within the so-called therapeutic range, the control of seizures is the sole criterion of efficacy. Most recurrences occur within 3 months of the first seizure; patients who have had no seizures during that period can probably be maintained on a low dose, regardless of the blood levels. However, if no side effects develop in the absence of control, the dose can be increased cautiously to increase the blood levels above the so-called therapeutic range. Increasing the doses of AEDs to the highest possible level is perhaps safer with the newer antiepileptic agents such as lamotrigine and gabapentin. Ineffective drugs should be withdrawn progressively over 1 to 3 months. Thus, for a brief duration, the two drugs are administered simultaneously. Combination of 3 or more drugs are rarely indicated.

   viii. It is preferable to combine drugs with complimentary or different mechanism of action (such as CBZ and VAP; Phenytoin and phenobarbitone; vigabatrin and lamotrigine). Avoid combinations with similar side effect profile (such as phenobarbital and clonazepam may produce marked sedation; combination of valproate and lamotrigine though is synergistic for efficacy, but is synergistic for side effects, namely tremors). Combination of LTG and CBZs antagonistic. Guidelines for combining AEDs are depicted in Box 25.4 and 25.5. In focal epilepsies, it is now common practice to consider surgery after two or three drugs have failed. To clearly establish the lack of efficacy of drug, serum levels have to be done before it is abandoned.

Box 25.4 Guidelines for Combining Antiepileptic Drugs (AEDs)

- Establish optimal dose of first chosen first-line AED
- Add another alternative first-line AED with different mechanism of action; avoid combining AEDs with similar mechanism of action
- Titrate the dose of alternative AED slowly and carefully
- Reduce dose of first chosen AED
- Replace less effective AED, if response still poor/suboptimal
- Try range of different combination therapies
- Add third adjunctive/add-on AED if still sub-optimal control
- If adjunctive/add-on treatment is not effective or tolerated - consider palliative strategy for refractory epilepsy.

Box 25.5 Different AEDs Targets Suitable for Combination Therapy

1. **Sodium channel blockers**
   a. Fast-inactivated state–phenytoin, carbamazepine, lamotrigine, oxcarbazepine, eslicarbazepine
   b. Slow-inactivated state–lacosamide
2. **Calcium channel blockers**
   a. Low voltage activated channel–ethosuximide
   b. High voltage activated channel–gabapentin, pregabalin
3. **GABA-ergic drugs**
   a. Prolongs chloride channel opening–barbiturates
   b. Increased frequency of chloride channel opening–benzodiazepines
   c. Inhibits GABA-transaminase–vigabatrin
   d. Blocks synaptic GABA reuptake–tiagabine
4. **Synaptic vesicle protein 2A modulation–levetiracetam**
5. **Carbonic anhydrase inhibition–acetazolamide**
6. **Multiple pharmacological targets—sodium valproate, topiramate, zonisamide, felbamate, rufinamide**

Source: Adopted from 63 Brodie Martin J., Sills Graeme J. Combining antiepileptic drugs—Rational polytherapy? Seizure 20 (2011) 369–375. doi:10.1016/j.seizure.2011.01.004

3. **Monitoring**

   i. There are many physiologic differences between neonates, infants, children and adults which can affect the absorption, distribution, metabolism and excretion of antiepileptic drugs. These pharmacokinetic differences may play a part in the age-related differences in the incidence of adverse effects, therefore select dose and monitor these patients accordingly.

   ii. Children on AED should be followed up regularly for compliance, recurrence of seizures and also side effects. Stress on the importance of regular AED usage to avoid loss of seizure control before starting therapy and assess adherence to medication regimens at every visit thereafter. Review diagnosis (confirm diagnosis of true seizure) and adherence to treatment in patients not responding to treatment.

   iii. Monitor growth of the child and suitable adjustment of dose should be done with changing weight.

4. **Therapeutic Drug Monitoring (TDM):** ***Goal of TDM is to ensure that a given drug dosage produces maximal therapeutic benefit with minimal toxic adverse effects.*** Thus, TDM seeks to optimize patient outcome by managing their medication regimen with the assistance of information on the concentration of AEDs in serum or plasma since identification of the optimal dose for an individual on purely clinical grounds can be difficult. These include:

   i. Since AED treatment is prophylactic and seizures occur at irregular intervals, it is often difficult to determine rapidly whether the prescribed dosage will be sufficient to produce long-term seizure control.

   ii. Clinical symptoms and signs of toxicity may be subtle, or difficult to differentiate from the manifestations of underlying disorders.

   iii. There are no direct laboratory markers for clinical efficacy or for the most common manifestations of AED toxicity, such as adverse CNS effects.

   However, monitoring of blood levels of AEDs is not routinely indicated; "Routine" drug levels on controlled, non-toxic patients are not indicated. TDM of AEDs is most likely to be of benefit in situations:

   i. To establish an individual therapeutic concentration in patients with infrequent seizures that has attained seizure control which can be used at subsequent times to assess potential causes for a change in drug response?

   ii. To diagnose clinical toxicity and differentiate between overdose and loss of efficacy.

   iii. To identify therapeutic failure due to under-dosage and in the presence of 'optimal' dosage – fast metabolisers.

   iv. To assess compliance, particularly in patients with uncontrolled seizures or breakthrough seizures.

v. Understanding unexpected seizures or side effects, especially with polypharmacy due to pharmacokinetic interactions which may compromise the adequacy of the therapy.

vi. To guide dosage adjustment in situations associated with increased pharmacokinetic variability (e.g., children, the elderly, patients with associated diseases, drug formulation changes).

vii. When a potentially important pharmacokinetic change is anticipated such as in pregnancy, or drug (when an interacting drug is added or removed) or disease interaction.

viii. To guide dose adjustments for AEDs with dose-dependent pharmacokinetics, particularly phenytoin.

The ideal blood sampling time for all AEDs for TDM is immediately before the next oral dose (trough) after steady state levels are achieved, but if this is not possible, particularly when attending an outpatient clinic, their morning dose should not be delayed for longer than 2 or 3 hours especially for AEDs with short (< 8 hours) half-lives. In such cases sampling time and the time of last dose of medication should be noted. Sometimes, both trough and peak levels or in conjunction with the appearance of symptoms suggestive of transient concentration-related toxicity) could be valuable to optimize the dosing schedule. During overdose/toxicity, sampling should be undertaken as soon as the patient presents at casualty. Further repeat sampling might be necessary, depending on the timing of the overdose, patient's condition and treatment given.

Guide to dosing in children is based predominantly on drug half-life and dosage should be individualized based on response to medication. AED levels can never substitute for clinical judgment. **Treat the patient and not the level, drug level is a guide only.** The quoted "therapeutic" range of blood levels for AEDs is a compromise between toxicity and efficacy (Table 25.2).

5. **Prognosis and comorbidities:** The long-term prognosis for seizure cessation tends to be better in children than adults, particularly those who are neurologically intact.[54] Favourable outcomes seen with early seizure control, younger age of onset, and an absence of underlying brain disorder. On the other hand, status epilepticus, severely abnormal EEG patterns, including West syndrome and Lennox-Gastaut syndrome are more common in children. The detrimental effects of AEDs are probably also greater in the immature and rapidly developing child's brain.

   Significant impact on quality of life seen in patients with epilepsy due to psychological, behavioural, cognitive, neurologic, academic, and social problems caused by their seizures or by their chronic neurologic condition, independent of the seizures.[55-60]

6. **Discontinuing Antiepileptic Drugs:** Treatment of epilepsy usually is prolonged ranging from a minimum duration of 1-2 years to life-long, depending on the cause and type of seizures.

Consider withdrawal of AED therapy in most children after two years without seizures regardless of the etiology of the seizures. The likelihood of recurrence after a two-year period without seizures is approximately 30 to 40%.[61,62] Children with neurologic deficits should also be considered for AED withdrawal if they have been seizure-free for an extended period of time. Abrupt cessation of antiepileptic drugs is always risky and may precipitate not only a return of seizures, but even a bout of prolonged or status seizures. Therefore, withdrawal should be gradual, tapering the AED in fraction, over a period of 3-6 months or even more depending on the dose and number of AEDs. In particular, benzodiazepines and barbiturates are associated with withdrawal seizures and should be discontinued very gradually.

References

1. Glauser T, Ben-Menachem E, Bourgeois B, Cnaan A, Chadwick D, Guerreiro C, Kalviainen R, Mattson R, Perucca E, Tomson T. ILAE Treatment Guidelines: Evidence-Based Analysis of Antiepileptic Drug Efficacy and Effectiveness As Initial Monotherapy for Epileptic Seizures and Syndromes. Epilepsia 2006;47:1094-120.
2. Edward Faught. Pharmacokinetic Considerations in Prescribing Antiepileptic Drugs. Epilepsia 2001;42(S4):19-23.
3. Joseph I Sirven, MD Joyce D Liporace, MD. New Antiepileptic Drugs: Overcoming the Limitations of Traditional Therapy. Postgraduate Medicine 1997;101.
4. Anticonvulsants. Drugs Facts and Comparisons, 2017.
5. Perucca E. Clinically Relevant Drug Interactions with Antiepileptic Drugs. Br J Clin Pharmacol 2006;61:246-55.
6. Drugs Effective in the Therapy of the Epilepsies. In: Goodman and Gilman's The Pharmacological Basis of Therapeutics. 11th Edition. Laurence Brunton, Bruce A. Chabner, Bjorn Knollman (eds) 2011.
7. Johannessen SI, Battino D, Berry DJ, Bialer M, Kramer G, Tomson T, Patsalos PN. Therapeutic Drug Monitoring of the Newer Antiepileptic Drugs. Ther Drug Monit 2003;25:347-63.
8. Ficker DM, Privitera M, Krauss G, Kanner A, Moore JL, Glauser T. Improved Tolerability and Efficacy in Epilepsy

Patients with Extended-release Carbamazepine. Neurology 2005:23:65:593-95.

9. Antiepileptic Drugs–Best Practice Guidelines for Therapeutic Drug Monitoring: A Position Paper by the Subcommission on Therapeutic Drug Monitoring. ILAE Commission on Therapeutic Strategies. Epilepsia 2008:49:1239-76.

10. Matthew D Krasowski (2011). Therapeutic Drug Monitoring of Antiepileptic Medications. Novel Treatment of Epilepsy. Prof. Humberto Foyaca-Sibat (Ed.). ISBN: 978-953-307-667-6. InTech. Available from:http://www.intechopen.com/books/novel-treatment-of-epilepsy/therapeutic-drug-monitoring-of-antiepilepticmedications

11. Garnett WR. Carbamazepine. In: Murphy JE. Edition. Clinical Pharmacokinetics. 3rd Edition. Bethesda MD:ASHP 2005: 103-24.

12. Battino D. Estienne M. Avanzini G. Clinical Pharmacokinetics of Antiepileptic Drugs in Pediatric Patients. Part II. Phenytoin. Carbamazepine. Sulthiame. Lamotrigine. Vigabatrin. Oxcarbazepine and Felbamate. Clin Pharmacokinetics 1995:29: 341-69.

13. Perucca E Pharmacological and Therapeutic Properties of Valproate: A Summary after 35 years of Clinical Experience. CNS Drugs 2002;16:695-714.

14. Gidal BE. Valproic Acid. In: Murphy JE. Edition. Clinical Pharmacokinetics. 3rd Edition. Bethesda. MD: ASHP: 2005: 335-48.

15. Ramsay RE, Cantrell D, Collins SD, *et al.* Safety and Tolerance of Rapidly Infused Depacon: A Randomized Trial in Subjects with Epilepsy. Epilepsy Res 2003:52:189-201.

16. Aneja S and Sharma S Newer Anti-epileptic Drugs. Indian Pediatr 2013:50:1033-40.

17. Perucca E. An Introduction to Antiepileptic Drugs. Epilepsia. 2005;46 (Suppl 4):31-37.

18. Perucca E. Clinical Pharmacokinetics of New-Generation Antiepileptic Drugs at the Extremes of Age. Clinical Pharmacokinetics 2006;Vol. 45:351-64.

19. Patsalos PN. Berry DJ. Bourgeois BFD. Cloyd JC. Glauser TA. Johannessen SI. Tomson T. Perucca E. Antiepileptic Drugs – Best Practice Guidelines for Therapeutic Drug Monitoring: A Position Paper by the Subcommission on Therapeutic Drug Monitoring. ILAE Commission on Therapeutic Strategies. Epilepsia 2008;49:1239-76.

20. Anderson GD. Children Versus Adults: Pharmacokinetic and Adverse-Effect Differences. Epilepsia 2002;43(Suppl 3): 53-59.

21. Perruca E. Pharmacokinetic Variability of New Antiepileptic Drugs at Different Ages. Ther Drug Monit 2005;27:714-17.

22. Bassel Abou-Khalil. Levetiracetam in the Treatment of Epilepsy. Neuropsychiatr Dis Treat 2008:4:507-23.

23. Perucca E. Johannessen SI. The Ideal Pharmacokinetic Properties of An Antiepileptic Drug: How Close Does Levetiracetam Come? Epileptic Disord 2003:5Suppl1:S17-26.

24. Tomson T. Battino D. Pharmacokinetics and Therapeutic Drug Monitoring of Newer Antiepileptic Drugs During Pregnancy and the Puerperium. Clin Pharmacokinet 2007:46:209-19.

25. Patsalos PN. Ghattaura S. Ratnaraj N. Sander JW. *In situ* Metabolism of Levetiracetam in Blood of Patients with Epilepsy. Epilepsia 2006:47:1818-21.

26. Plant GT. Sergott RC. Understanding and Interpreting Vision Safety Issues with Vigabatrin Therapy. Acta Neurol Scand Suppl 2011:57-71.

27. Ben-Menachem E. Pregabalin Pharmacology and Its Relevance to Clinical Practice. Epilepsia 2004:45(Suppl 6):13-18.

28. Almeida L. Nunes T. Sicard E. Rocha JF. Falcao A. Brunet JS. Lefebvre M. Soares-da-Silva P. Pharmacokinetic Interaction Study Between Eslicarbazepine Acetate and Lamotrigine in Healthy Subjects. Acta Neurologica Scandinavica 2010:121:257-64.

29. Bialer M. Johannessen SI. Levy RH. Perucca E. Tomson T. White HS. Progress Report on New Antiepileptic Drugs: A Summary of the Ninth Eilat Conference (EILAT IX). Epilepsy Research 2009:83:1-43.

30. Almeida L. Falcao A. Maia J. Mazur D. Gellert M. Soares-da-Silva P. Single-dose and Steady-State Pharmacokinetics of Eslicarbazepine Acetate (BIA 2-093) in Healthy Elderly and Young Subjects. Journal of Clinical Pharmacology 2005: 45:1062-66.

31. Almeida L. Potgieter JH. Maia J. Potgieter MA. Mota F. Soares-da-Silva P. Pharmacokinetics of Eslicarbazepine Acetate in Patients with Moderate Hepatic Impairment. European Journal of Clinical Pharmacology 2008:64:267-73.

32. Maia J. Almeida L. Falcao A. Soares E. Mota F. Potgieter MA. Potgieter JH. Soares-da-Silva P. Effect of Renal Impairment on the Pharmacokinetics of Eslicarbazepine Acetate. International Journal of Clinical Pharmacology and Therapeutics 2008: 46:119-30.

33. Curia G. Biagini G. Perucca E. Avoli M. Lacosamide: A New Approach to Target Voltage-Gated Sodium Currents in Epileptic Disorders. CNS Drugs 2009;23:555-68.

34. Perucca E. Yasothan U. Clincke G. Kirkpatrick P (2008b). Lacosamide. Nature Reviews Drug Discovery. Vol. 7. No. 12. 2008(December):973-74.

35. Chung S. Sperling MR. Biton V. Krauss G. Hebert D. Rudd GD. Doty P. Lacosamide as Adjunctive Therapy for Partial-Onset Seizures: A Randomized Controlled Trial. Epilepsia 2010:51:958-67.

36. Ben-Menachem. E Biton. V Jatuzis D. Abou-Khalil B. Doty P Rudd. GD. Efficacy and Safety of Oral Lacosamide as Adjunctive Therapy in Adults with Partial-onset Seizures. Epilepsia 2007:48:1308-17.

37. Luszczki JJ. Third-Generation Antiepileptic Drugs: Mechanisms of Action. Pharmacokinetics and Interactions. Pharmacological Reports 2009:61:197-216.

38. Beydoun A, D'Souza J, Hebert D, Doty P. Lacosamide: Pharmacology, Mechanisms of Action and Pooled Efficacy and Safety Data in Partial-Onset Seizures. Expert Review of Neurotherapeutics 2009:9:33-42.

39. Johannessen Landmark C, Patsalos PN. Drug Interactions Involving the New Second- and Third-Generation Antiepileptic Drugs. Expert Review of Neurotherapeutics 2010:10:119-40.

40. Cross SA, Curran MP. Lacosamide: In partial-Onset Seizures. Drugs 2009:69:449-59.

41. Thomas D, Scharfenecker U, Nickel B, Doty P, Cawello W, Horstmann R. Low Potential for Drugdrug Interaction of Lacosamide. Epilepsia 2006:47Suppl:200.

42. Buck ML, Goodkin HP. Use of Lacosamide in Children with Refractory Epilepsy. J Pediatr Pharmacol Ther 2012: 17:211-19.

43. Wier HA, Cerna A, So TY. Rufinamide for Pediatric Patients with Lennox-Gastaut Syndrome: A Comprehensive Overview. Pediatr Drugs 2011:13:97-106.

44. Perucca E, Cloyd J, Critchley D, Fuseau E (2008a). Rufinamide: Clinical Pharmacokinetics and Concentration-Response Relationships in Patients with Epilepsy. Epilepsia 2008:49:1123-41.

45. Wheless JW, Vazquez B. Rufinamide: A Novel Broad-Spectrum Antiepileptic Drug. Epilepsy Currents 2010:10:1-6.

46. Lacerda G, Krummel T, Sabourdy C, Ryvlin P, Hirsch E. Optimizing Therapy of Seizures in Patients with Renal or Hepatic Dysfunction. Neurology 2006:67:12Suppl4:S28-33.

47. Farwell JR, Anderson GD, Kerr BM, Tor JA, Levy RH. Stiripentol in Atypical Absence Seizures in Children: An Open Trial. Epilepsia 1993:34:305-11.

48. Levy RH, Loiseau P, Guyot M, Blehaut HM, Tor J, Moreland TA. Stiripentol Kinetics in Epilepsy: Nonlinearity and Interactions. Clinical Pharmacology and Therapeutics 1984: 36:661-69.

49 Tran A, Rey E, Pons G, Rousseau M, d'Athis P, Olive G, Mather GG, Bishop FE, Wurden CJ, Labroo R, Trager WF, Kunze KL, Thummel KE, Vincent JC, Gillardin JM, Lepage F, Levy RH. Influence of Stiripentol on Cytochrome P450-Mediated Metabolic Pathways in Humans: In Vitro and in Vivo Comparison and Calculation of in Vivo Inhibition Constants. Clinical Pharmacology and Therapeutics 1997:62: 490-504.

50. Tran A, Vauzelle-Kervroedan F, Rey E, Pous G, d'Athis P, Chiron C, Dulac O, Renard F, Olive G. Effect of Stiripentol on Carbamazepine Plasma Concentration and Metabolism in Epileptic Children. European Journal of Clinical Pharmacology 1996:50:497-500.

51. Brodie MJ, French JA. Management of Epilepsy in Adolescents and Adults. Lancet 2000:356:323-29.

52. Sankar R. Initial Treatment of Epilepsy with Antiepileptic Drugs: Pediatric Issues. Neurology 2004 November 23:63(10 Suppl 4):S30-39.

53. Expert Committee on Pediatric Epilepsy, Indian Academy of Pediatrics. Guidelines for Diagnosis and Management of Childhood Epilepsy. Indian Pediatr 2009:46:681-98.

54. Chin RF, Cumberland PM, Pujar SS, *et al.* Outcomes of Childhood Epilepsy at Age 33 Years: A Population-based Birth-Cohort Study. Epilepsia 2011:52:1513.

55. Geerts A, Brouwer O, van Donselaar C, *et al.* Health Perception and Socioeconomic Status following Childhood-Onset Epilepsy: The Dutch Study of Epilepsy in Childhood. Epilepsia 2011:52:2192.

56. Alfstad KÅ, Clench-Aas J, Van Roy B, *et al.* Psychiatric Symptoms in Norwegian Children with Epilepsy Aged 8-13 Years: Effects of Age and Gender? Epilepsia 2011:52:1231.

57. Stevanovic D, Jancic J, Lakic A. The Impact of Depression and Anxiety Disorder Symptoms on the Healthrelated Quality of Life of Children and Adolescents with Epilepsy. Epilepsia 2011:52:e75.

58. Rantanen K, Eriksson K, Nieminen P. Cognitive Impairment in Preschool Children with Epilepsy. Epilepsia 2011:52:1499.

59. Taylor J, Jacoby A, Baker GA, Marson AG. Self-Reported and Parent-Reported Quality of Life of Children and Adolescents with New-Onset Epilepsy. Epilepsia 2011:52:1489.

60. Russ SA, Larson K, Halfon N. A National Profile of Childhood Epilepsy and Seizure Disorder. Pediatrics 2012:129:256.

61. Greenwood RS, Tennison MB. When to Start and Stop Anticonvulsant Therapy in Children. Arch Neurol 1999; 56:1073.

62. Sillanpää M, Schmidt D. Prognosis of Seizure Recurrence After Stopping Antiepileptic Drugs in Seizure-Free Patients: A Long-term Population-based Study of Childhood-Onset Epilepsy. Epilepsy Behav 2006: 8: 713. Brodie MJ, Sills GJ., Combining Antiepileptic drugs–Rational Polytherapy? Seizure. 20(2011): 369-375. doi:10.1016/j.seizure.2011.01.004.

26 Chapter

APPROACH TO DIAGNOSIS AND MANAGEMENT OF CHILDREN WITH SEIZURES AND EPILEPSY

Bibek Talukdar

Seizures and epilepsy are probably the most common neurological problems in Pediatrics. Despite being so common, many issues continue to plague the diagnosis and management of this entity in a developing country like India.

Definitions

Seizure: An epileptic seizure is a transient occurrence of signs and/or symptoms due to abnormal excessive or synchronized neuronal activity in the brain (Fisher *et al.*, 2014).

Epilepsy: Epilepsy is a disorder of the brain characterized by an enduring predisposition to generate epileptic seizures, and by the neurobiologic, cognitive, psychologic, and social consequences of this condition (Fisher *et al.*, 2014).

Acute Symptomatic Seizure: Seizures occurring after an acute disorder associated with abnormal hyperactivity of cerebral neurons. Some common such disorders are hypocalcemia, hypernatremia, stroke, CNS infections like meningitis and encephalitis.

Unprovoked Seizure: Seizure that is not acute symptomatic.

Operational Definition of Epilepsy: Epilepsy is considered to be present in prsesnce of any of the following conditions as per the current propositions by the International League Against Epilepsy (ILAE) (Fisher *et al.*, 2014).

1. At least two unprovoked (or reflex) seizures occurring >24 hours apart.
2. One unprovoked (or reflex) seizure with a probability of further seizures similar to the general recurrence risk (at least 60%) after two unprovoked seizures, occurring over the next 10 years.
3. Diagnosis of an epilepsy syndrome.

Epilepsy is considered to be resolved for individuals who had an age-dependent epilepsy syndrome but are now past the applicable age or those who have remained seizure-free for the last 10 years, with no seizure medicines for the last 5 years (Fisher *et al.*, 2014).

Seizures/epilepsy can be just a one-time event, while many continue to have recurrences again and again. Epilepsy needs prolonged antiepileptic drug (AED) therapy that may even be life-long. Prolonged AED therapy is often associated with problems like development of adverse side effects, compliance related issues that often leads to poor control and these need careful handling for good result.

Etiology

Cause of seizure is not always easy to diagnose. In many cases it remains unknown all through. In many cases the disorder shows familial tendency without any clear genetic entity that can be incriminated. It is often associated with structural lesions in the brain, the incidence of which it seems to be high in developing country like India likely to be due to high incidence of perinatal and postnatal CNS insults like HIE and neurologic infections (Kapoor *et al.*, 1998). The common problems associated with seizures and epilepsy, i.e., etiology, that we encounter are shown in the Table 26.1. Overlapping of etiology, a child having more than one cause, is common in our experience.

Table 26.1: Etiology of Seizures/Epilepsy

• *Developmental disorders* of the CNS–congenital malformations, chromosomal anomalies, genetic disorders • *Prenatal, intranatal and neonatal* (PIN) problems–congenital infections, birth trauma, birth anoxia • *CNS infections*, i.e., meningitis, encephalitis, brain abscess, neurocysticercosis, cerebral malaria • *Head trauma* • *Febrile seizure* • *Asphyxiation*, i.e., drowning • *Metabolic disorders* like hypoglycemia, hypocalcemia, hypo or hypernatremia, inborn errors of metabolism	• *Intracranial hypertension* associated with conditions like tumour, abscess, hydrocephalus, cysts, neurocysticercosis • *Cerebral vascular disorders* like stroke, bleed, arteriovenous malformations • *Sequelae* of PIN insults, past CNS infections and trauma and other past CNS insults, metastatic lesions • *Encephalopathies* ADEM, postinfectious, cerebral palsy, associated with systemic disorders like hepatic, uremic • *Neurocutaneous syndromes* • *Neurometabolic disorders* • *Neurodegenerative disorders* • *CNS toxicity*, i.e., lead poisoning, drugs like aminophylline

ILAE (Scheffer, 2017) currently has put forward a classification of etiology of epilepsy as follows:

1. Genetic.
2. Structural.
3. Metabolic.
4. Infectious.
5. Immunologic; and
6. Unknown.
   - **Genetic** causes are the direct result of a known or presumed genetic defect(s) in which seizures are the core symptom of the disorder. The genetic defect may arise at a chromosomal or molecular level.
   - **Structural** causes are congenital or developmental malformations, stroke, tumour and other acquired brain anomalies.
   - **Metabolic** causes are usually the inborn errors of metabolism.
   - **Infective** causes are various CNS infections like meningoencephalitis.
   - **Immunologic** causes are immunologic disorders like Rasmussen syndrome, anti-NMDA receptor mediated encephalitis etc.
   - **Unknown** causes are those where the etiology is unclear.

Approach to Diagnosis

a. *Establishing that the event is a seizure*

Diagnosis of seizure is primarily clinical. The event is usually witnessed by the parents first and lot depends on their description. Large majority of seizures occur at home and parents/attendant are the only witness. One has to depend quite a lot on observations of the parents.

Clinicians witness many attacks when the cases reach hospital in active seizure. Video recording of the events by the parents have been of great help. After noting down carefully the characteristics/semiology of the event, the clinician can confirm that it is a seizure.

While attempt is being made to diagnose seizure, it is important to keep in mind of certain events/abnormal movements that look like seizure but really it is not. These are often termed as **seizure mimickers;** these are non-epileptic events looking like seizure. However most of these can be ruled out clinically if one takes note of proper seizure characteristics / semiology and the ILAE classification of seizures. Some of the common seizure mimickers that we see in our practice are shown in the Table 26.2. Some important clinical tips how to exclude these are also shown in the same table. Occasional case however may be difficult to diagnose clinically and may need investigations like EEG. Excluding these conditions however is not always easy and may need other investigations and even prolonged follow-up.

The relatively common ones that we find are syncope, breath-holding spell and pseudo-seizure. In *syncope*, the sequence of events is loss of consciousness, fall and then regaining of consciousness and getting up. There is, almost always, a precipitating event like prolonged standing and getting up suddenly from sitting or lying position. The loss of consciousness is gradual, brief, and appears incomplete unlike GTCS

Table 26.2: Common Seizure Mimickers in Children and Important Differentiating Features

Events mimicking seizure	Clnical pointers to diagnosis
Breath-holding spell	Event precipitated by crying, usually vigorous, showing frustration. Holds breath in expiration followed by occasional jerk
Vasovagal attacks	Usually follows prolonged standing, i.e., prayer at school in the morning
Pseudoseizures	Event does not follow the semiology/pattern of any seizure/movement can be modified by suggestion: psychological abnormality in the child, family or environment. No injury
Prolonged QT syndrome	Sudden attack of fall/semiology does not follow clear pattern of any seizure/ pallor, sweating, cardiac arrhythmia
Hypercyanotic spell – cardiac	Severe breathing difficulty followed by cyanosis and then the event, cardiac murmur
Pallid syncopal attacks	Sudden / quick development of pallor
Shuddering attacks	Acute onset shivering of head, neck, trunk, limbs/brief, mostly in infants/not fitting into any clear seizure type
Reflex anoxic spell (temporary asystole of reflex origin)	Often precipitated by bumps to head or fall/pallor, loss of muscle tone, even consciousness/may develop stiffening, clonic movement/quick recovery
Gastroesophageal reflux	Sudden change in posture, colour, arching of back/common in infants and in CP
Sleep myoclonus	Jerks during sleep; no other manifestation of seizure
Benign myoclonus of infancy,	Baby otherwise normal
Sleep walking (somnambulism)	No abnormal movement or other features of seizure
Benign paroxysmal vertigo	Clear history of virtigo
Night terror	No abnormal movement fitting into any seizure type
Temper tantrum / rage attacks	No abnormal movement fitting into any seizure type

where it is usually abrupt. Giddiness and blackening of eyes often precede the loss of consciousness. The fall is gradual unlike the sharp fall seen in GTCS/focal seizure. There is hardly any tonic or clonic movement and if at all it is there, is not sustained. Also there is no post ictal phase. Facial pallor and sweating are common. Associated phenomena of GTCS are not seen.

The typical sequence of events in *breath-holding spell* is that the infant cries and cries, holds breath, occasionally develops cyanosis, sometimes throws a few clonic jerks followed by recovery. The sequence of event is precipitated by crying following same stimulus for it. Such a sequence of event is not seen in GTCS.

Pseudo-seizure, also referred to as pseudoepileptic seizure, nonepileptic seizure, hysterical seizure and psychogenic seizure, is common in older children and adolescents. The most important point which helps in differentiating it from GTCS is that the typical sequence of events of GTCS is not seen in pseudo-seizures. Motor movements and other events are often bizarre, vary from attack to attack in the same child in case of recurrences, and can be influenced by suggestions. Associated phenomena like frothing, injury, incontinence etc are also not seen in pseudo-seizures. History and examination frequently reveal psychological disturbance in the child, in the family or in the child's environment, i.e., bullying in school.

In differentiating seizure mimickers from true seizures, *accurate history of the sequence of the events* occurring during the attack of seizure is most important. Most of the disorders have their own typical clinical features. A normal EEG is helpful in excluding seizure mimickers, although not always. Serum prolactin level that rises to high levels during attack of GTCS is also helpful in diagnosis if can be done within an hour, although false positive results are also seen specially in presence of hypoxia. However, both EEG and serum prolactin levels have their limitations, epileptiform discharges in EEG is sometimes seen in normal population and prolactin levels can be false positive; these tests also may not always be positive.

Picking up abnormalities in EEG is also a matter of chance. Most of the conditions of seizure mimickers can be diagnosed by thoughtful clinical history and examination and little bit of follow-up.

It is, however, extremely important to rule out seizure mimickers. Otherwise many children will be unnecessarily subjected to prolonged AED therapy with its attendant side effects and other disadvantages. Not only that the patient will unnecessarily get the label of epilepsy with its profound psychosocial ramifications. Epilepsy has been shown to be overdiagnosed in about 20-25%. Common conditions misdiagnosed as epilepsy have been reported to be syncope in 44%, psychiatric disturbances in 20%, BHS in 11% and the main reasons for misdiagnosis were inadequate history, presence of family history and history of febrile seizures. About 10-20% of cases referred to as refractory epilepsy actually was found to have non-epileptic events/attacks (Metric *et al.*,1991).

b. *Classifying the seizure*

Once it is established clinically that the event is a seizure, it should be classified according to ILAE classification for proper management. EEG is needed for classifying the seizure and seizure type properly. ILAE currently has classified seizure and epilepsies as follows: (Fisher *et al.*, 2017)

Seizure Types

a. Focal onset (aware/impaired awareness).

b. Generalized onset.

c. Unknown onset.

All these categories can have motor or non-motor onset. Focal non-motor onset can have automatism, behavior, cognitive, emotional and sensory symptoms; Generalized non-motor onset are absence seizures and unknown non-motor seizures are behavior arrest.

Focal onset seizure can evolve into bilateral tonic clonic. Some of the unknown onset cases can remain unclassified.

Epilepsy Types

Focal, Generalized, Combined Generalized and Focal, Unknown.

Epilepsy Syndromes

Otahara syndrome, Dravet syndrome, infantile spasm, Lennox-Gastaut Syndrome, Landau Kleffner syndrome, juvenile myoclonic epilepsy and so on.

c. *Case work-up*

After making a diagnosis of seizure/epilepsy clinical work-up should be done to establish the cause for appropriate treatment. It is important to understand that treatment of seizures and epilepsy is not just antiepileptic drug. No stone should be left unturned to find the cause; finding a treatable cause may lead to specific treatment and permanent cure. Common example is some metabolic seizure. The work-up should include detailed history, thorough physical examination, appropriate investigation guided by clinical suspicion.

History

It should start with: (a) Prenatal–perinatal problems followed by (b) Postnatal development. In our experience we find so many epileptics having prenatal intranatal and neonatal (PIN) problems. The author strongly feels that PIN problems like bad obstetrical history, hypoxic ischemic encephalopathy, neonatal sepsis, neonatal seizures, congenital infections, that are so common in our country, are important cause of seizures and epilepsy in developing countries like ours. Neurodevelopmental delay seen during the postnatal period and through infancy and early childhood are also frequently associated with seizures and epilepsy in our experience. Other essential history that needs evaluation are: (c) Postnatal and past history of CNS insult like (meningitis, encephalitis, trauma, asphyxia, poisoning), (d) Family history of seizures (suggestive of genetic and metabolic epilepsies), (e) Socio-economic status (epilepsy in our experience is common amongst the lower socio-economic strata of our population that is likely to be due to higher incidence of PIN problems and postnatal and past CNS insults). These areas in evaluation of history are extremely important in work-up of a case of seizure and epilepsy. In our experience final diagnosis in good majority of cases is based on history alone all other work-up including examination and investigations being negative.

Examination

A child with seizures should undergo detailed clinical examination special emphasis on certain clinical findings that are commonly seen in epileptics like small head, craniostenosis, hydrocephalus, neurocutaneous stigmata, dysmorphism and other congenital malformations, neurological deficits (like focal deficits–paraplegia, hemiplegia, cranial palsy), cognitive dysfunction, behavior problems, speech, hearing and visual deficits, murmur, hepatosplenomegaly.

Investigation

Investigating a child with seizures and epilepsy is often foxed with the question of how much to investigate and what to investigate. This is more so if it is the first seizure. Investigation in these cases is aimed at establishing further that the event is an epileptic seizure and at finding some clue to etiology that may be treatable completely or partially.

Electroencephalogram (EEG)

Is should be done in all cases suspected to have epileptic seizure. An abnormal EEG showing epileptiform activity, further confirms that the event is an epileptic seizure. It also confirms the type of seizure/epilepsy and helps in categorizing the seizure according to ILAE classification. Abnormalities in EEG may be detected during recording (ictal EEG) or at other times (inter-ictal EEG). EEG however may not always be positive even in cases with typical history. With prolonged recording it may be positive in about 60-80% cases. It is to be remembered however that EEG can be abnormal in about 5-8% of normal population; thus EEG finding has always to be correlated clinically. Video-EEG and ambulatory EEG has important role in difficult epilepsies.

Neuro-Imaging Studies (CT/MRI)

Many structural lesions of the brain that cause seizures can be picked up by imaging techniques like CT and MRI scans and even ultrasound in the infant. Imaging studies looking for an etiology are commonly done investigations in our country and is probably not unjustified as intra-cranial structural lesions are relatively more common in seizures / epilepsy in our country. In infants with open fontallae cranial ultrasonography is also useful at times. In our experience imaging gives useful finding if there are abnormal neurological findings in history like PIN problems, postnatal CNS infections, neurodevelopmental delay and cerebral palsy, focal seizure, focal deficit and congenital malformations.

In an evaluation study by ILAE subcommittee on usefulness of imaging in pediatric epilepsy, based on published report, Gailard *et al.*, (2009) observed that Imaging provides important contributions to establishing etiology, providing prognostic information, and directing treatment in children with recently diagnosed epilepsy. They observed imaging to be abnormal in 50% of focal seizures, to give useful information on etiology or focus in 15-20% instances and also that in 2-4% instances it altered immediate medical management. They concluded that Imaging is recommended when localization-related epilepsy is known or suspected, when the epilepsy classification is in doubt, or when an epilepsy syndrome with remote symptomatic cause is suspected. When available, MRI is preferred to CT because of its superior resolution, versatility and lack of radiation.

Screening for inborn errors of metabolism (IEM) is often resorted to; however, it is well established that yield as a cause of epilepsy is quite low at present. It may be done in presence of strong suspicion of IEM based on features like deterioration of a baby after a period of apparent normalcy, parental consanguinity, history of abortion, family history of neonatal death, persistent/recurrent vomiting that is unexplained, severe/difficult metabolic acidosis, resistant/recurrent hypoglycemia, peculiar odour of body secretions like sweat and urine, dysmorphism and encephalopathy that are well-established (Nichole *et al.*, 2012).

Genetic studies also similarly has a low yield as a cause of epilepsy except in cases having clear clinical findings of genetic abnormality/syndromes. In other cases it may be done when there is strong suspicion of some genetic pathology as indicated by features like history of abortion, strong family history, dysmorphism and neurocutaneous stigmata. Genetic testing is indicated in epilepsy where clear genetic etiology has been established like benign familial neonatal convulsion, benign familial infantile convulsion, X-linked infantile spasm, glucose transporter deficiency syndrome, pyridoxine dependent seizure, pyridoxal phosphate responsive seizure, folate deficiency, Dravet syndrome, GEFS +, EFMR, PME, some focal epilepsies and epileptic encephalopathies (Ream *et al.*, 2015).

Other investigations should be done according to clinical suspicion. While investigating, it is always important to keep in mind the classification and etiology of seizures and epilepsy; this helps in making a proper planning of investigations so that there is no witch-hunt.

Approach to Treatment/Management

Once the diagnosis of seizure and epilepsy is established and even the cause, the next question is treatment. Presentation of seizures and epilepsy is in the form of an acute attack or recurrent attacks. Treatment thus involves two aspects:

(a) Managing an acute attack; and

(b) Preventing recurrent attacks.

In both the situations treatment need is of anti-epileptic drugs besides treating the cause and other comorbidities. The attack may be mild and self aborting or may be severe, i.e., status epilepticus. Recurrent seizures/epilepsy needs prolonged anti-epileptic drug (AED) therapy aimed at preventing recurrences (anti-epileptic drug prophylaxis).

a. Treatment of An Acute Attack

Focal and generalized seizures, specially tonic and tonic-clonic seizure commonly present with acute attacks. These are usually managed with conventional anti-convulsants. Common drugs used to control such acute attacks are benzodiazepines (diazepam, lorazepam, midazolam) carbamazepine, phenytoin, phenobarbitone, valproate and levetiracetum.

Genearalized tonic-clonic seizures and focal seizures at times presents as status epilepticus (SE) that is a medical emergency as it is associated with significant morbidity and also mortality. Seizures of any etiology can progress to SE. Apparently brief seizure also can progress to SE. Treatment of status epilepticus needs special attention and use of defined protocols (referred to the chapter). Non-convulsive status epilepticus (NCSE) also occur in a small proportion of cases in children and needs to be managed appropriately; absence status is the most common.

b. Treatment of Recurrent Attacks/Epilepsy

1. **Decision on Starting Prophylactic AED:** Preventing recurrences in epilepsy is needed for the reasons like:

   (a) Reduce psychosocial problems associated with it.

   (b) Helping in reducing comorbidities like cognitive and behavior problems associated with it.

   (c) Avoiding some dangers, although remote, like serious injury during an acute attack like fall from height, getting burnt in case of an attack occurring near a fire, getting drowned in case of an attack occurring while swimming.

   (d) Risk of neurologic sequel and even mortality in case an attack progresses into status. Prolonged use of anticonvulsant drugs leads to suppression of epileptogenic activity in brain, which if successfully permanent, results in cure.

AEDs *is usually not started after a single attack* seizure as it has been observed that in about 50%-70% of instances the seizures do not recur and chronic AED therapy is associated with many disadvantages like:

(a) Subjecting the child to side effects of AEDs specially cognitive dysfunctions and behaviour disturbances that are totally unwanted for the developing brain.

(b) Need for prolonged medication and hence subjecting the child to the side effects of the AEDs for prolonged period of time, may be several years.

(c) With starting of AED the child gets the label of epilepsy, the disorder associated with a variety of psychosocial afflictions as already highlighted. Therefore starting AED after the first attack means subjecting many children to the disadvantages of chronic AED therapy unnecessarily many of whom would never have a recurrence. However, as per a new guideline by ILAE, AED may be started after the first attack if the chances of recurrence of seizure is high, i.e., probability of further seizures similar to the general recurrence risk (at least 60%) after two unprovoked seizures, occurring over the next 10 years (Fisher 2014). Such risk is exemplified as follows–single seizure occurring after a stroke or say focal cortical dysplasia. Thus instating AED prophylaxis after a single seizure has to be individualized.

Seizures associated with acute systemic illness like meningitis, encephalitis, trauma, stroke etc. (acute symptomatic seizure) where AED was started during the acute event, need not routinely be followed by prolonged AED prophylaxis and may be withdrawn soon if there is no recurrence of seizure. In cases of GTCS with *infrequent recurrences* where the attacks are widely spaced (i.e., several years) it may probably be better to wait and not to start AED prophylaxis if the child is developing normally. This should however be done after explaining the facts to the parents and orienting them to the initial management of an attack in the event of a recurrence. These children must be kept under close follow-up and if recurrences start becoming frequent AED therapy should be initiated. However in a small proportion of cases of generalized tonic clonic seizure there is a chance of sudden death (SUDEP) and many feel that in these cases prophylactic AED may be started.

2. **Selection of AED:** Many AEDs are available for prophylaxis (*see the chapter on drugs and doses.....*). However, trials of these drugs in Pediatrics are not sufficient. Level of evidence for most of the drugs is poor for (Glauser 2013). As commented upon by Glauser al (2013) there is alarming lack of properly conducted RCTs in seizures pediatric age group, the situation being dismal. There is not a single class I and class II study of AEDs in pediatric epilepsy. Thus it is difficult to have a rational approach to AED therapy in this age group. Many newer AEDs have come up in recent times that have been found to be effective in different types of seizures/epilepsies. However, trial of these drugs in children again is insufficient. Based on some trials, clinical experience and also adult experience, several drugs have been in use for AED prophylaxis in different types of epilepsy in pediatrics. AEDs found to be useful in different types of seizures are shown in the Inset 26.1. (The reader also referred to chapter on drugs and doses and related chapter on different types of epilepsy and epilepsy syndromes).

   All the AEDs show efficacy against different types of seizure. Despite being effective against several seizure types most of the AEDs display better effectiveness against one or two types of seizures and this should be kept in mind. It is also important to be well versed with the dose and side effects of the drugs. Selection of AED is primarily based on:

   (a) Seizure type related to efficacy.

   (b) Side effects.

   (c) Availability and also.

   (d) Cost.

Inset 26.1: AED Useful in Different Types of Seizures and Epilepsies and Epilepsy Syndromes seen Commonly in our Setup

- **Tonic, clonic and tonic-clonic seizure:** Carbamazepine, phenobarbitone, phenytoin, topiramet, valproic acid, oxcarbazepine, lamotrigine, levetiracetum, zonisamide, clobazam.
- **Focal seizure:** Carbamazepine, phenobarbitone, phenytoin, topiramet, valproic acid, oxcarbazepine, lamotrigine, levetiracetum, zonisamide, clobazam, felbamet.
- **Absence seizure:** Valproic acid, ethosuccimide, lamotrigine, zonisamide, clobazam.
- **Myoclonic seizures:** Valproic acid, levetiracetum, topiramet, zonisamide, clobazam.
- **Atonic seizures:** Valproic acid, zonisamide, clobazam.
- **Benign epilepsy with centrotemporal spikes:** Carbamazepine.
- **Lennox-Gastaut Syndrome:** Valproic acid, topiramet, lamotrigine.
- **Juvenile myoclonic epilepsy:** Valproic acid, levetiracetum.
- **Infantile spasms/West syndrome:** ACTH, prednisolone, vigabatrine, valproic acid, lamotrigine, zonisamide, felbamet.

Age and sex also sometimes need to be considered. It is extremely important to choose the right drug for the seizure type in concern in right dose. For example, phenytoin is not effective in myoclonic seizures and should not be used here. It is also preferable to initiate treatment with time tested AEDs, like phenytoin, carbamazepine, sodium valproate, as one is dealing with a chronic problem needing prolonged treatment. Other drugs including newer AEDs may be used as necessary.

AEDs with too many *side effects* or significant, or serious side effects, also should be avoided as far as possible and if used at all for unavoidable reasons, there should be close monitoring. Phenobarbitone despite being a good AED for GTCS, is not preferred in the children because of the side effects of cognitive dysfunctions, hyperactivity and other behaviour disturbances that are detrimental to learning. Sodium valproate, may cause hepatotoxicity in infants and young children <2 years and needs to be used with caution.

If the parents cannot afford a *costly drug* it should not be prescribed, this may result in interruption in treatment; epilepsy needs prolonged and uninterrupted AED therapy. Sudden interruption may lead to recurrence of seizure and even status epilepticus. Every recurrence further delays the chances of withdrawal of AED; one expects the patient to remain seizure-free for 2-3 years continuously before withdrawing AED.

Age and sex also sometimes matter in selection of AEDs. Efficay and toxicology of many AEDs has not been established well in infants and young children, i.e., most of the newer AEDs and such drugs should be used with caution in this age group. Because of too many cosmetic side effects like gum hyperplasia, acne and hirsuitism, phenytoin not preferred in adolescent girls.

3. **Initiation, Maintenance and Monitoring:** Treatment is *initiated with one AED* (the one that is selected) in its lowest therapeutic dose. In case of recurrence of seizure the dose should be increased gradually in steps until seizure is controlled or maximum prescribed therapeutic dose is reached. *Stepping up should be systematic; we prefer an increment of 25–50% of the dose the child is receiving* at intervals of 2-4 weeks depending upon frequency of recurrence. For practical reason we prefer to make the dose a round figure. We find that too much of fractionations of the tablet or syrup is difficult for the parents and this often results in under-dosing and consequent recurrence of seizure and apparent poor control. For administration of syrups use of syringe should be insisted upon.

   If one drug fails to control the seizure, despite trial for about two months in its maximum therapeutic dose or maximum tolerated dose for proper drug action, then one may think of starting a second drug, again in its lowest dose with gradual stepwise increase to its maximum. Most cases however can be controlled with one drug (*monotherapy*). When a second drug is added one should be careful of *drug-interaction* which may worsen the seizure control. Drug interactions occur when more than one drug is used sharing the same/similar metabolic pathway and it is obviously seen in cases on multiple drugs (*Polytherapy*). It common in situations with use of hepatic enzyme inducers like phenytoin, phenobarbitone and carbamazepine. Drug interactions can result in increase or decrease in the blood level of the drug already in use. Use of more than one drug is often associated with more problems like deterioration of seizure control due to drug interaction and addition of new side effects of the newly added drug. If seizure control is achieved with the second drug, then effort should be made to gradually taper off and withdraw the first drug that had failed to control the seizure. Sometimes, however, it is difficult to withdraw the earlier drug because of recurrence of seizure while attempting to withdraw it, then it may be continued. Controlling with one drug, i.e., *monotherapy should however be the aim*. Seizure control often takes time and needs patience on the part of both the physician and the parents. A small proportion of cases however do not respond despite trial more than one AED, and gradually slips into what is called difficult to control or intractable epilepsy and they need special management approach.

   A child on AED prophylaxis should be *followed up regularly* preferably at one center to avoid unwarranted manipulation of drug and dose that is so common in our country. We often find cases referred to us for poor control who are on several AEDs mostly in inadequate dose, most get settled with ultimately one drug. At every follow-up visit, records should be made of weight of the child, drugs, dose, compliance, side effects and any recurrence of seizure. Parents should be advised to maintain a seizure diary. We find video recording of the events at home by parents in mobile phones is quite useful and should be encouraged. It is also important to emphasize the importance of strict compliance. Poor compliance is the single-most important cause of continuing recurrence of seizure in epileptic patients and every effort should be made to ensure compliance in terms of proper dosing in terms of accuracy and timing, and not missing doses.

   In cases where seizure is not being controlled/deterioration in control despite apparently adequate therapy, one should suspect unexplained drug toxicity (specially in patients on polytherapy) and non-compliance. *AED blood level estimation* may be done in such situation if facilities exist. Drug level however should be interpreted with caution. Attainment of therapeutic level is not always necessary for seizure control. It is to be remembered that treatment of epilepsy is treatment of symptoms and not the blood level. We find it to be most useful in management of cases on polytherapy who are continuing to throw seizures and in situations where drug toxicity is suspected.

   Parents should also be advised about what to do in case of recurrence of an attack at home like placing the child in a safe place, placing the head in lateral decubitus, loosening the cloths, not putting anything in the mouth, careful cleaning of the mouth in case of excessive salivation and looking for medical help if the seizure is prolonged beyond 5.

AED prophylaxis for epilepsy has to be *prolonged and uninterrupted.* This should be explained to the parents once a decision to put a child on AED prophylaxis has been taken. Interruption of treatment often results in recurrence of seizure, even a status epilepticus, to the great dismay of the parents and further prolonging of the duration of prophylaxis. These facts should be impressed upon the parents. Continuous treatment is important; if the child is out of station, the parents should ensure the drug / drugs is also carried along with. AED prophylaxis is usually needed for 2-3 years.

Emotional support to the parents and the family are integral part of management of epilepsy. During the visits psychosocial problems and the certain general aspects that often perturb the parents need to be taken care of. General activities should be encouraged depending upon the abilities of the child and also seizure control. Some activities like swimming, playing at heights, playing near fire, crossing the road etc may need some supervision depending on seizure control. Schooling also should be encouraged depending upon seizure control and also intelligence. All doubts about epilepsy that parents often harbour, should be resolved at the time of diagnosis and starting therapy. These measures will ensure proper parental co-operation that is vital for successful treatment of epilepsy.

4. **Duration of AED Therapy and Withdrawal of AED:** Currently epilepsy is considered to be resolved if a person has remained seizure-free for the last 10 years and off anti-seizure medication for the last 5 years (Fisher 2014). Withdrawal of AED is considered if the child is *seizure free for 2-3 years* after starting the prophylaxis (Shinner *et al.*). In our center we consider withdrawal of AED after the child is seizure free for 2 years. Withdrawal of AED should be slow and gradual and never abrupt. Abrupt withdrawal often leads to quick fall of AED blood level and recurrence of seizure, even a status epilepticus. The period of tapering should be spread over 3-6 months and even more according to situation, i.e., patients on polytherapy will need longer time. We use a schedule of tapering and withdrawal similar to stepping up, i.e, 25-50% of the doses every 2-4 weeks. We use relatively slower tapering in cases on polytherapy. If a child is on polytherapy, we start tapering with the drug that was started last. Complete withdrawal of AEDs in cases on polytherapy takes time.

   Withdrawal of AED is usually smooth in most of the cases of epilepsy. However, a small proportion of cases have recurrences after withdrawal. One or two recurrences may be acceptable, if however there are more than one recurrence AED prophylaxis has to be restarted.

5. **Treatment of the Cause:** All throughout the course if a treatable cause is discovered, it should be treated. It is important to keep in mind that a cause may surface at any time during the course.

6. **Neurosurgical Consultation:** Epilepsy surgery has a role in certain cases of carefully selected epilepsy. Effectiveness of surgical treatment depends on type of epilepsy, underlying pathology, and accurate localisation of the epileptogenic focus by various clinical, neuroimaging, and neurophysiological investigations. Surgery has been found to be useful in epilepsy with well localized structural lesion. The benefit is in terms of with reasonably good seizure control and minimizing adverse effects of drugs (Kellermann TS, 2016).

Suggested Reading

- Berg AT, Berkovic SF, Brodie MJ, Buchhalter J, Cross JH, van Emde BW, Engel J, French J, Glauser TA, Mathern GW, Moshe SL, Nordli D, Plouin P, Scheffer IE. Revised Terminology and Concepts for Organization of Seizures and Epilepsies: Report of the ILAE Commission on Classification and Terminology, 2005-2009. Epilepsia 2010;51:676-85.
- Degen R, Degen HE. Sleep and Sleep Deprivation in Epileptology. In: Degen R, Neidermyer E (Eds). Epilepsy: Sleep and Sleep Deprivation, Amsterdam, Elsevier 1984;273-86.
- Egg-Olofson Eeg-Olofsson O, Petersen I and Sellden U. The Development of the Electroencephalogram in Normal Children From the Age of 1 Through 15 Years. Paroxysmal Activity, Neuropediatric 1971;2:374-404.
- Evidence-Based Guideline: Treatment of Convulsive Status Epilepticus in Children and Adults: Report of the Guideline Committee of the American Epilepsy Society, Epilepsy Currents, Vol. 16, No. 1 (January/February) 2016;48-61.
- Fisher RS, Chan DW, Bare M et al. Capillary Prolactin Measurement for Diagnosis of Seizures. Ann Neurol 1991;29: 187-90.
- Fisher RS, Helen Cross H, French JA, Higurashi N, Hirsch E, Jansen FE, Lagae L, Moshe SL, Peltola J, Perez ER, Scheffer IE, Zuberi SM. Operational Classification of Seizure Types

by the Internal League Against Epilepsy: Position Paper of the ILAE Commission for Classification and Terminology. Epilepsia 2017:58(4):522-530. doi: 1111/epi.13670.

- Gaillard WD. Chiron C. Helen Cross J. Simon Harvey A. Kuzniecky R. Lucie Hertz-Pannier L and L. Gilbert Vezina L for the ILAE. Committee for Neuroimaging. Subcommittee for Pediatric Neuroimaging. Epilepsia 2009:50(9):2147-53. doi: 10.1111/j.1528-1167.2009.02075.x.
- Glauser T. Ben-Menachem E. Bourgeois B. Cnaan A. Guerreiro C. Ka¨lvia¨inen R. Mattson R. French JA. Perucca E. Toson T for the ILAE subcommission on AED guidelines. Updated ILAE evidence review of antiepileptic drug efficacy and effectiveness as initial monotherapy for epileptic seizures and syndromes. Epilepsia 2013:54(3):551-563. doi: 10.1111/epi.12074.
- Holmes GL. Diagnosis and Management of Seizures in Children. Philadelphia. WB Saunders Company 1987;163-71.
- Kapoor M. Talukdar B. Choudhury V. Puri V. Rath B. Intracranial Structural Lesions In Young Epileptics: A computed tomographic study. Indian Pediatrics 1998:35:537-41.
- Kellermann TS. Wagner JL. Smith G. Karia S. Eskandari R. Surgical Management of Pediatric Epilepsy: Decision-Making and Outcomes. Pediatr Neurol 2016 November;64:21-31. doi: 10.1016/j.pediatrneurol 2016.06.008. Epub 2016 July 5.
- Metrick ME. Ritter FS. Gates JR et al. Non-Epileptic Events in Childhood. Epilepsia 1991:32:322-28.
- Moshe SL. Perucca E. Scheffer IE. Tomson T. Watanabe M and Wiebe S. A Practical Clinical Definition of Epilepsy. Epilepsia 2014:55(4):475-82. doi: 10.1111/epi.12550.
- Nichole L. Rahman S. Footit EJ. Varadkar S. Clayton PT. Inborn Errors of Metabolism Causing Epilepsy. Developmental Medicine and Child Neurology: DOI: 10.1111/j.1469-8749.2012.04406.x.
- Nicole I Wolfl. Thomas Bast. Robert Surtees. Epilepsy in Inborn Errors of Metabolism. Epileptic Disord 2005:7(2):67-81.
- Obeid M1. Mikati MA. Expanding Spectrum of Paroxysmal Events in Children: Potential Mimickers of Epilepsy. Pediatr Neurol 2007 November;37(5):309-16.
- Rahman S. Footit EJ. Varadkar S. Clayton PT. Inborn Errors of Metabolism Causing Epilepsy. Developmental Medicine and Child Neurology: DOI: 10.1111/j.1469-8749.2012.04406.x.
- Ream MA. Patel AD. Obtaining Genetic Testing in Pediatric Epilepsy. Epilepsia 2015:56(10):1505-14. doi: 10.1111/epi.13122.
- Scheffer IE. 1Berkovic S. Capovilla G. Connolly MB. French J. Guilhoto L. Hirsch E. Jain S. Mathern GW. Moshe SL. Nordi DR. Perucca E. Tomson T. Wiebe S. Zhang YH. Zuberi SM. ILAE Classifications of Epilepsies: Position Paper of the ILAE Commission for Classification and Terminology. Epilepsia 2017:58(4):512-21. doi: 10.1111/epi.13709.
- Shinnar S. Berg AT. Moshe SL et al. Risk of Seizure Recurrence Following a First Unprovoked Seizure in Childhood. A Prospective Study. Pediatrics 1990:85:1076-85.28.
- Wyler AR. Hermann BP. Epilepsy Surgery. Stoneham MA. Butterworth-Heinemann. 1994.

27 Chapter

CEREBRAL PALSY

Pratibha Singhi, Arushi Gahlot Saini

Cerebral palsy (CP) is a persistent disorder of posture and/or movement, due to a non-progressive damage to the developing brain. It has recently been defined as "a group of disorders of development of movement and posture, causing activity limitation that is attributed to non-progressive disturbances that occurred in the developing fetal or infant brain". The motor disorders of CP are often accompanied by disturbances of sensation, cognition, communication, perception, behavior or seizure disorders.[1] There is no exact upper age-limit for the above definition. Although the brain injury in CP is non-progressive, the motor disorder and comorbidities evolve over time and the clinical presentation may vary accordingly.

Incidence

CP is the most common physical disability in childhood, occurring in 2-2.5/1000 live births.[2] As there are no national registries, population-based studies contribute to the prevalence rates. Rates of CP in India have been estimated to be around 2-2.8/1000 births overall[2,3] and 1.2/1000 population from rural areas in India.[4] Spastic CP is the most common type and accounts for 60-70% of all cases.[5] Spastic diplegia is commoner in the developed countries due to increasing survival of preterm babies and advances in maternal and neonatal care. Studies from North India indicate an increasing proportion of diplegia (22% to 35%) and reduction in quadriplegia (61% to 51%) over the last decade.[5]

Etiology and Risk Factors

CP is not a single disease and not caused by a single factor; it is an umbrella term that encompasses a large number of heterogeneous conditions resulting in a non-progressive central motor deficit. A 'web of causation' denoting interaction of multiple genetic and environmental risk factors explains the etiopathogenesis of CP. The relative contribution of prenatal, perinatal and genetic factors has been debated and varies across the developed and developing countries.[6] The etiology is congenital in more than a half; nearly one-fifth of the cases are due to acquired causes such as central nervous system (CNS) infections, hyperbilirubinemia, late hemorrhagic disease of newborn or intracranial bleeds, hypoglycemia and head injury; and another one-fifth are due to combined congenital and postnatal causes. Upto 10% of CP cases are due to genetic causes[7,8] and 11-15% of children with CP have at least one co-existing congenital anomaly.[9]

An increased prevalence of CP has been associated with decreasing birth weight or gestational age. The risk in infants born < 28 weeks gestation is about 100/1000 survivors and 1/1000 in term-born infants.[10,11] The corresponding pathological lesions in the preterm babies are either periventricular leucomalacia or periventricular hemorrhagic venous infarcts. Ultrasonographic detection of hypoechoic periventricular areas has been found to be a strong predictor of later development of motor dysfunction in these preterm babies.[12] The prevalence of CP in children born after *in vitro* fertilization is around 4.4/1000 births.[13] Maternal intrapartum fever, chorioamnionitis and elevated serological markers of inflammation in the fetus/newborn have been associated increased risk of CP.[6] The exact contribution of perinatal asphyxia to CP is controversial. Epidemiological studies from the developed world suggest that 6-28% children with CP may be due to birth asphyxia. However, birth asphyxia is implicated strongly in developing countries in 20%-50% of cases.[5,14,15] CP due to CNS infections constitutes 57% and that due to bilirubin-encephalopathy accounts for nearly 30% of the acquired causes.[5,16] Unconjugated bilirubin damages mitochondria and is toxic to neurons and astrocytes. Hyperbilirubinemia has been causally linked with intellectual impairment, choreoathetoid CP, gaze palsies, and sensorineural hearing loss, deficits in attention and learning.[16] Although kernicterus is no longer seen in most developed countries, it continues to be the predominant cause of dyskinetic CP in many developing countries. The various neonatal factors predisposing to CP studied in the Indian scenario are shown in Table 27.1. The clinicopathological correlates of CP are provided below (Table 27.2).

Table 27.1: Neonatal Factors Predisposing to Cerebral Palsy in India[5,15]

	CP cases (n=1212)	%
Birth asphyxia	630	51·98%
Low birth weight	459	37·87%
Neonatal jaundice	426	35·14%
Neonatal sepsis	371	30·6%
Neonatal seizures	326	26·9%
Prematurity	294	24·3%
Twin gestation	41	3·4%

Table 27.2: Some Cliniciopathological Correlates of CP[17]

CP subtype	Pathology	Underlying etiology/risk factors
Spastic diplegia	• Periventricular leucomalacia • Periventricular while matter injury	• Prematurity
Spastic quadriplegia	• Multicystic encephalopathy with cortical atrophy • Selective neuronal necrosis • Parasagittal neuronal injury • Cerebral malformations	• Perinatal/late intrauterine hypoxic ischemic events • Genetic
Dyskinetic	Basal ganglia • Status marmoratus • Bilirubin deposition	• Perinatal asphyxia • Neonatal hyper-bilirubinemia
Spastic hemiplegia	• MCA territory infarction/ injury • Cerebral malformations	• Perinatal arterial ischemic stroke • Genetic
Ataxic, hypotonic	• Cerebellar lesions • Hydrocephalus	• Prenatal (genetic)

Classification

Several classifications have been proposed; none is perfect.[1] A simple classification is based on the type of neuromuscular defect into (i) Spastic (ii) Dyskinetic (including both dystonic and choreoathetotic) (iii) Ataxic (iv) Hypotonic and (v) Mixed. Based on topography, it may be further categorized into (a) Quadriplegia (b) Diplegia and (c) Hemiplegia.

Clinical Characteristics

Spastic CP is the most common and accounts for 60-70% of all cases. It is characterized by upper motor neuron signs, viz., clasp-knife hypertonia, exaggerate muscle stretch reflexes and upgoing plantar reflexes.

- **Spastic quadriplegia:** This is the most severe form of CP. All the four limbs are involved–the arms being either equally or more involved than the legs. One side may be more affected than the other. The term bilateral or double hemiplegia has been applied to the cases where arms are more severely affected than the legs and there is pseudobulbar palsy. However, this distinction is not practically significant. These infants have significantly delayed development and spasticity severe enough to cause arching of the back (Fig. 27.1). Scissoring of the legs may be obvious or may be seen when the infant is suspended from under the arms (Fig. 27.2). Independent walking if achieved develops very late. The feet are held in a position of

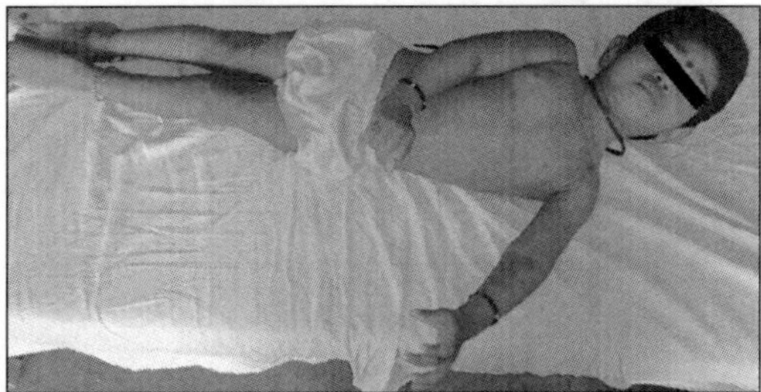

Fig. 27.1: Child with spastic quadriplegia and severe intellectual impairment

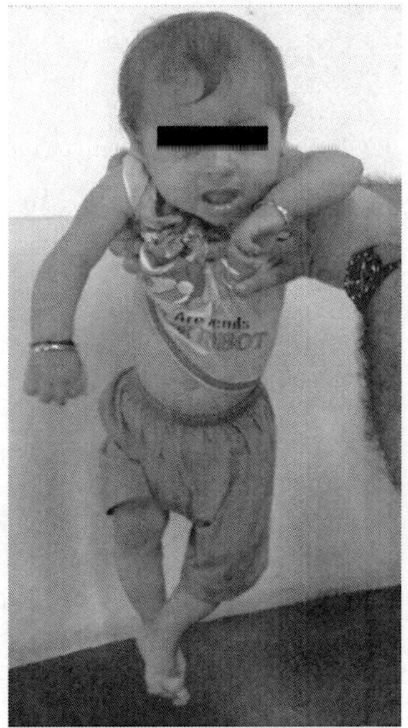

Fig. 27.2: Eleven-month-old infant showing scissoring of legs on being suspended from under the arms

equinovarus and the child walks on tip-toes. In older children, the arms are internally rotated, elbows extended or tightly flexed and hands fisted. Flexion contractures of the knees and elbows often develop. These children generally have multiple associated problems which include mental retardation, seizures, swallowing difficulties, speech problems and visual and hearing deficits.

- **Spastic diplegia:** This term is used when the lower limbs are involved substantially more than the upper limbs. Arm signs vary from minimal to severe. Locomotor development is more impaired than manipulative skills (Fig. 27.3). In severe cases there is disuse atrophy of the lower extremities, development of upper torso remains normal. Intellectual development may also be within normal limits. Spastic diplegia has a strong association with preterm birth and periventricular leucomalacia.

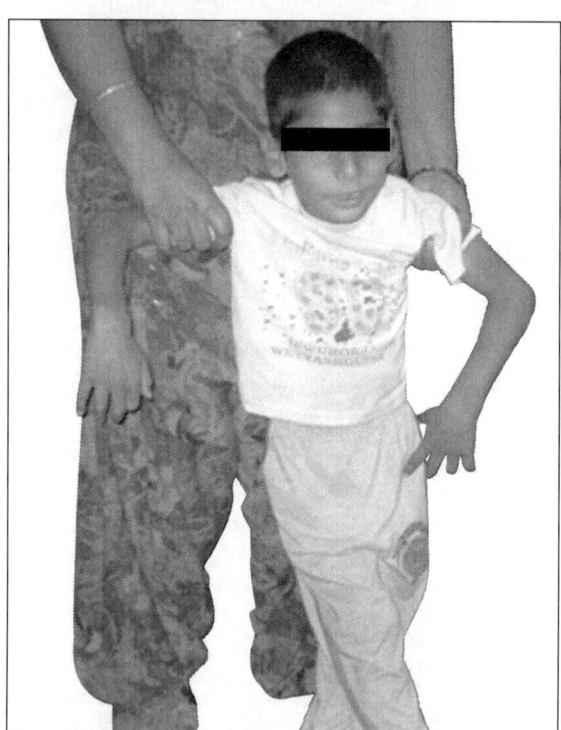

Fig. 27.3: Child with spastic diplegia showing scissoring of legs and locomotor impairment

- **Spastic hemiplegia:** The term refers to upper motor neuron involvement of the face, arm and leg on one side of the body. Usually the arm is more severely affected than the leg. Right sided hemiplegia occurs more frequently than the left–the reasons for this are not yet clear. In early infancy these children may appear to be developmentally normal except for asymmetry wherein the affected hand shows paucity of movements and fisting. A definite hand preference below 12 months of age should alert one to the possibility of hemiplegia. Since the leg is less severely affected, its abnormality may not be noticed until later. An externally rotated position of the lower limb in the supine position is a sensitive early sign of hemiplegia. Sitting and crawling are not much delayed, but walking is generally delayed by 2-3 months. In severe cases, as the child gets older, the arm is held adducted, flexed and internally rotated at the shoulders, with the elbow flexed, forearm pronated, wrist flexed and the thumb adducted. The leg is held adducted, semiflexed at the knee and plantar flexed at the ankle. Vasomotor changes are seen on the affected side and growth arrest eventually occurs. Contractures may develop. Cortical sensory deficits and homonymous hemianopia may be present. Mild cases are missed by parents and sometimes, even by doctors. They may present only around school age with clumsiness or educational problems. Careful examination reveals mild involvement of one side of the body; on simultaneous examination of both hands, the thumb nails are smaller on the affected side (Fig. 27.4).

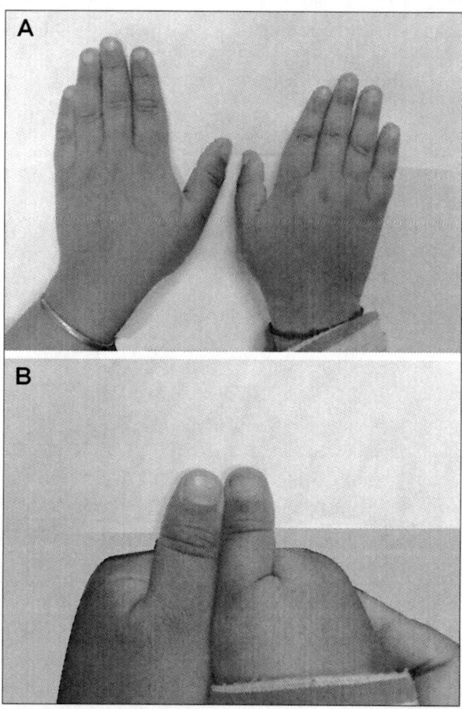

Figs. 27.4 (A and B): Child with right hemiplegic CP showing asymmetry of hands and nail growth with reduced bulk on right side

In Western countries, spastic hemiplegia is reportedly the most common type of CP seen among children born at term. However, in our experience as well as those of others from India and other developing countries, spastic quadriplegia is the most common, followed by diplegia and hemiplegia.[5,15] Although spastic monoplegia and triplegia have been described, they probably represent an evolution of the above forms. Involvement of one limb may be so mild that it is perhaps missed. Pure paraplegia of cerebral origin is extremely rare–a spinal lesion is most likely in such cases.

- **Dyskinetic CP:** This form is characterized by involuntary movements–chorea and/or athetosis, and changes in muscle tone, hence the name dystonia. It is caused by predominant damage to the basal ganglia and extrapyramidal system. Kernicterus and perinatal hypoxia are the most important causes. With aggressive control of neonatal hyperbilirubinemia, this type of CP has become uncommon in Western countries; however it continues to be prevalent in our country.[16]
- These infants are generally hypotonic with marked head lag, drooling and feeding difficulties. The asymmetric tonic neck reflex (ATNR) is prominent (Fig. 27.5) and the postural reflexes appear late. Athetosis becomes apparent generally after one year of age and tends to coincide with the hypermyelination of the basal ganglia, a phenomenon called status marmoratus. The twisting of the hands and flaying of fingers while approaching an object are characteristic (Fig. 27.6). Bizarre writhing movements and facial grimacing occur on attempted movement. Involvement of the oropharyngeal muscles causes speech problems. Standing and walking are markedly delayed and may not be achieved at all. Intelligence is often preserved but because of their severe physical and communication disabilities, these children are mistakenly diagnosed as being mentally retarded.
- **Mixed CP:** The spastic and dyskinetic type of CP often occur together giving rise to a mixed picture with clinical features of both spasticity and dyskinesia.

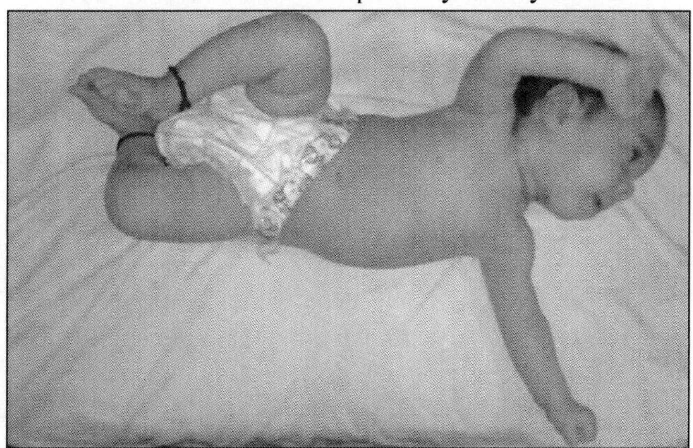

Fig. 27.5: Obligatory ATNR

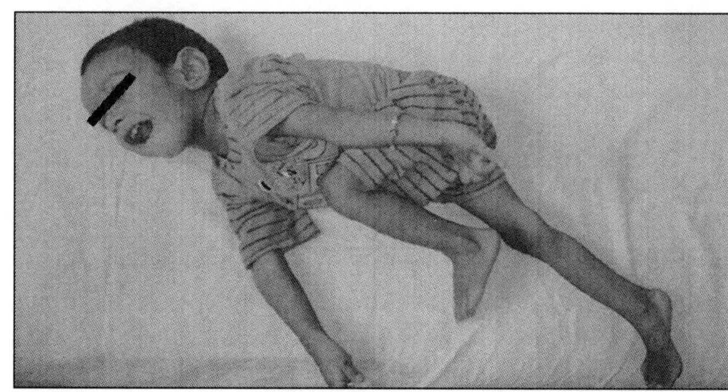

Fig. 27.6: Child with dystonic CP showing bizarre twisting movements and flaying of fingers

- **Ataxic CP:** This occurs due to predominant cerebellar damage. Genetic factors are important in its etiology. These infants are usually hypotonic and inactive and start walking rather late. The gait is ataxic with exaggerated balancing movements of the arms. Cerebellar signs are often present. Nystagmus is however rare. Ataxia may occur in a "pure" or in a "mixed" form with spasticity of the legs (ataxic diplegia). Many of these children have intellectual impairment.
- **Hypotonic CP:** Infants with hypotonia need careful evaluation to exclude neuromuscular disorders. In hypotonic CP, the tone is generally variable, and the muscle stretch reflexes are brisk. Obligatory ATNR and abnormal movement patterns are frequently seen. On follow-up, these children often have dystonia and may subsequently develop dyskinetic, spastic or mixed type of CP.

Associated Problems: Majority of children with CP have one or more associated problems. These need to be actively looked for and managed appropriately (Table 27.3).[18]

Table 27.3: Associated Problems in Children with CP in India[5,15]

Problems (N=1212)	%
Speech problems	84
Microcephaly	64
Visual defect	47
Seizures	44
Malnutrition	43
Mental retardation	39
Feeding problems	19
Hearing problems	14
Behavior problems	14

Diagnosis of CP

Early diagnosis is essential for early intervention. Early identification is ideally done in well-organized follow-up clinics of high-risk babies. Although a number of standardized developmental tests have been available, there is no "diagnostic" test for CP which can be considered as a "gold-standard". Comprehensive neurodevelopmental assessments using standardized methods can be done. However in busy clinics there is often paucity of time for detailed assessment of all babies. The Infant Motor Screen is a screening tool devised for identification of high risk preterm infants in need for detailed neuromotor assessment. We have found it to be highly specific and sensitive for early diagnosis of CP in both preterm and term babies. At places where organized neonatal follow-up services do not exist, the clinician has to use his clinical acumen of developmental testing when the baby is brought to him. Children with severe forms of CP can be easily recognized in infancy. It is the milder forms that need expertise to recognize the problem early. A constellation of certain signs may help in reaching an early diagnosis of CP (Table 27.4).

Table 27.4: Signs Useful in Early Diagnosis of CP[18]

Warning signs

- Lack of alertness
- Decreased spontaneous motility
- Stereotyped abnormal movements
- Reduced or poor quality of sleep

Abnormal signs

- Reduced head circumference/fall off in growth
- Constant fisting with adduction of thumb beyond 2 months
- Delayed social smile
- Primitive reflexes persisting beyond 6 months
- Obligatory ATNR
- Delayed appearance of postural reflexes and developmental milestones
- Persistent tone abnormalities (Fig. 27.7)
- Persistent asymmetry in posture, movement and reflexes

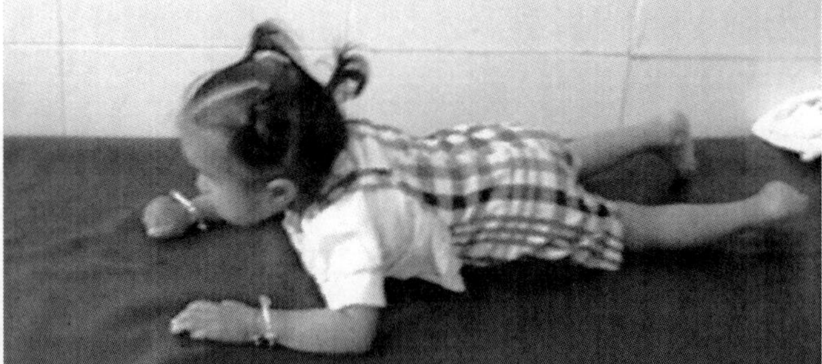

Fig. 27.7: Child with extensor hypertonia of the back muscles–An early warning sign of CP

A reduced head circumference at birth or in infancy, and/or a fall of head growth indicative of secondary microcephaly are strong predictors of CP. Tone abnormalities alone should be interpreted with caution, and reassessed after a few months, as "transient neuro-motor anomalies" may be seen in the first year of life and may lead to overdiagnosis of CP. However, persistent excessive extensor tone and opisthotonus are important early indicators of CP. A reduced popliteal angle (angle of the tibia to the femur when the hip is flexed and knee extended) indicated lower limb hypertonia. If the popliteal angle on one side is less than the other, it is suggestive of hemiplegia.

Early diagnosis of hearing deficits and visual problems is important. Brainstem auditory evoked responses (BSERA) should be done in infancy when audiometry is not possible. Observation of visual fixation, pursuit and use of simple charts for visual acuity can give important information about the integrity of visual pathways. Ideally, all children with CP should have an ophthalmological examination and hearing assessment.[19]

The diagnosis of CP should be made only after ensuring that the motor disorder is non-progressive and is of central origin. Slowly progressive, early onset degenerative disorders like Krabbe's disease, metachromatic leuko-dystrophy, Tay Sach's disease etc. may be mistaken for CP. It is therefore imperative to reassess the child over a period of time.

The dyskinetic, hypotonic and ataxic forms of CP are particularly liable to cause confusion. Neuromuscular disorders and other causes of ataxia should be excluded. Careful history and clinical examination along with appropriate investigations are needed. It must also be remembered that the clinical pattern of CP evolves over a period of time. The clinician need not feel compelled to give a diagnostic label at the first examination. Also, he should not hesitate to change it, if so needed after periodic assessment.

Assessment and Management–General Principles

Comprehensive assessment of a child with CP is essential to plan appropriate treatment. A multidisciplinary team comprising a neuro-developmental pediatrician as the team-leader, physiotherapist, occupational therapist, clinical psychologist, speech pathologist, orthopedic surgeon, otorhinolaryngologist, ophthalmologist, teacher, play therapist and social worker is required, preferably under one roof. The pediatrician's initial role consists of making a correct diagnosis, determining the etiology, and identification of the type, extent and severity of the neuromotor deficit as well as of associated problems.[19] The management of a child with CP starts with:

- **Breaking the news:** This is a very sensitive issue. The disclosure is best done by a senior experienced doctor in a comfortable environment, free of interruptions and distractions and in the presence of both parents.[20] A full account of the condition and possible associated problems should be explained to the parents in a simple and compassionate way preferably in their language.
- **Comprehensive assessment and appropriate treatment plan:** All children with CP must have evaluation of their motor, sensory and cognitive functions, hearing and speech, vision, behavior problems, feeding and nutrition, mobility, functional capacity and specific physical limitations. Pediatrician should then prepare a **"functionally-oriented" plan of management** suited to the child for short-term, implement treatments and follow the progress over long-term.
- **Physiotherapy:** Physiotherapy, especially when started early in life helps in promoting normal motor development and prevents deformities and contractures. In the young child, it aims at reducing abnormal patterns of movement and posture and promoting the normal ones so as to enable the child to gain maximal functional independence. A number of techniques have been used for this purpose (Table 27.5). In our country the neurodevelopmental technique of Bobath is commonly used. It consists of guiding the child through normal sequences of motor development, inhibition of primitive and abnormal reflexes, reinforcement of normal postural reflexes and facilitation of normal movements.

  The method of conductive education devised by Andreas Peto in Hungary is somewhat different from the others as it is based on the philosophy of 'learning' by the child and not on 'providing therapy'. Homogenous groups of children with motor disorders are given education by specially trained 'conductors', generally in residential setting. The method has been evaluated in some countries.

  There has been recent emphasis on activity-based training and muscle-strength training for children with cerebral palsy. There is some evidence of benefit for constraint-induced movement therapy and bimanual intensive training in children with hemiplegic CP.[21]

  There is no scientific evidence to prove the superiority of one method over another and an "eclectic" approach is often adopted to meet an individual child's needs.

Table 27.5: Principles of Various Treatment Methods Used for CP

Method	Principle
Bobath	Neurodevelopmental approach, inhibition of abnormal reflexes and facilitation of normal movements
Vojta	Stimulation of trigger points to produce reflex reactions and movement patterns
Peto	Achievement of "orthofunction" through conductive-education, imparted in group setting by specially trained 'conductors'
Kabat	Proprioceptive neuromuscular facilitation of movements
Temple Fay and Doman-Delacato	Passive and active stimulation of progressive Phylogenetic movement patterns
Phelps	Muscle strengthening and re-education
Rood	Sensory stimulation for movement in an ontogenetic developmental sequence

- **Occupational therapy:** Occupational therapy works in conjunction with physiotherapy. It focuses on activities of daily living such as feeding, bathing, dressing, toilet training etc., teaching co-ordination and sensory perceptual integration and the equipment needed to facilitate these.[22]
- **Play therapy:** It is the use of a natural activity and play with a young child, to help consolidate the levels of development that have been achieved and to encourage the child to move on, to the next level. Playing with a familiar care-giver often reveals a truer picture of the child's abilities.

It must be remembered that giving sessions of therapy is not enough. The important thing is to teach the parents to manage the child properly at home. We use a "Home-based management" program with involvement of the whole family to provide various therapies to the child, with periodic guidance from experts for rehabilitation in resource-constrained settings.[23] All children are evaluated by a dedicated team of experts including pediatric neurologist, therapists, clinical psychologists, ophthalmologists, orthopedicians and otorhinolaryngologist. Parents are taught various therapies and management skills for short period by therapists and advised to practice these at home. They are also taught the correct method of handling and lifting the child; carrying out specific exercises; to break down each activity into its simplest components and make the child practice it in a real life situation. For example, in a child with adductor spasticity, attempts must be made to keep the legs abducted. This can be done by putting a pillow or similar object between his legs while he is lying down or sitting. Similarly, the child should be carried with his legs abducted across, and the back and neck in a flexed posture. Treatment must be incorporated into the pattern of daily life. Parents are taught to break down each activity into its simplest components and make the child practice it in a real life situation. It then is not considered an "exercise" but becomes a way of life. Simple adaptive devices such as angled spoons, two-handled cups etc. can be made to help the child. Similarly, co-ordination and sensory-perceptual integration can be taught and multisensory stimulation provided through peg boards, blocks and other toys of different colours, textures, sizes and shapes, and producing different sounds. This aspect has been discussed and detailed elsewhere.

A number of high-technology devices such as programmed wheel-chairs, electronic feeding devices, various access systems, computerized speech systems and cochlear implants are available for children with CP in Western countries. In our country, very few can have access to such facilities. However, simple low-cost aids and appliances can be made at home as per the requirements of the child. A stiff collar with Velcro adjustment can be used to help neck support. Cloth hammocks can help in keeping the child in a flexed posture. Old stools and boxes can be adapted to provide support during sitting. Parallel bars can be constructed with logs of wood to help gait training. Standing frames and prone boards are a useful intermediate stage in mobilization. A good stable sear with back-support and a detachable table is very helpful for the school-aged children. All these can be made by locally trained carpenters. Manuals are available for guidance on this aspect.

Splints, Casts and Calipers

Light weight splints may at times be required to maintain normal postures. Recently the use of dynamic lycra splints that provide support as well as flexibility is being evaluated. The use of casts is controversial; they may be occasionally needed to prevent deformity. Specially designed shoes, ankle-foot orthoses and calipers may be required to provide stability to the joints in a child who is learning to stand and walk. Splints and casts however, should not be used for prolonged periods of time as they may lead to disuse atrophy of the muscles.

Surgery

Surgery is useful in some children with spasticity, especially where the lower limbs are involved. It should be done with a predefined functional goal, by an experienced surgeon. Tendon lengthening and transfer and availability of intensive physiotherapy is essential. Procedures like injection of dilute alcohol at the motor point of muscles or by the epidural route have been tried but do not provide permanent relief.

Dorsal rhizotomy (Peacock technique) which involves selective resection of posterior nerve roots from L2 to S1; is practiced by some, including a few centers in India. It may be helpful in children with severe lower limb spasticity, with sufficient trunk control and some form of forward locomotion. Its advantages must be weighed carefully against the sensory losses that may occur after the procedure. Postoperatively, intensive physiotherapy is needed.

Thalamotomy for athetoid CP, stereotactic dentatomy and chronic cerebellar stimulation via implanted electrodes have been tried in some cases but are still experimental procedures.

Medications

Drugs are occasionally used in CP for:

(i) **Reducing spasticity:** Proper physiotherapy given regularly considerably reduces spasticity and improves function. A trial of at least 3 months of appropriate physiotherapy should be given in all cases. However, if severe spasticity hampers administration of physiotherapy or if it persists despite an adequate trial of physiotherapy, drugs are occasionally used. Baclofen (GABA-B agonist) is commonly used in a starting dose 2.5 mg/day to maximum of 20-60 mg/d, monitored by clinical response. It is used cautiously in children with seizures as it may provoke them. The common side-effects are weakness, drowsiness, nausea, impaired cognition, orthostatic hypotension, depression and withdrawal syndrome. Intrathecal baclofen has shown good results but requires a special pump. The cost of baclofen implant in India is approximately INR 2.5 lakh and the recurrent drug cost is INR 3000-4000 which lasts for 3-4 months.[24] It can be only used in centers with adequate facilities. Diazepam may be used in cases where anxiety increases spasticity as it facilitates the postsynaptic action of GABA. The dose varies from 0.1-0.8 mg/kg, divided into 3-4 doses. The common side-effects include excessive sedation, increased drooling, cognitive dullness and tolerance. Tizanidine–a centrally acting alpha-2 noradrenergic agonist and dantrolene. Sodium–a direct muscle relaxant may also be used but the experience in children is limited. While using spasticity relieving drugs, one must strike a balance between relaxation and spasticity so that the child does not lose his functional capacity secondary to excessive relaxation. Other options include local chemo-denervation by botulinum–A toxin or phenol injections and neurosurgical interventions such as selective dorsal rhizotomy, selective peripheral neurotomy and orthopedic procedures such as tendon lengthening, transfer and arthodesis.

(ii) **Relief of athetosis and dystonia:** Occasionally levodopa for severe athetosis and carbamazepine or tri-hexyphenidyl for dystonia may be helpful.

(iii) **Control of seizures:** By appropriate anti-epileptic drugs.

(iv) **Control of hyperactivity and aggressive behaviour:** Methylphenidate, and other pharmacological agents may be needed at times.

(v) **Control of excessive salivation:** Atropine and benztropine have been used occasionally for temporary relief.

There is no scientific evidence that the so-called "brain-tonics" are of any benefit for children with CP.

Management of Comorbidities

Almost two thirds of children with CP have associated problems (Table 27.5) which may at times be more disabling than the motor disorder per se. Speech problems (84%), microcephaly (64%), seizures (45%) and intellectual disability (39%) are the common comorbidities (Table 27.3). Interventions such as hearing aids, correction of squint, glasses for refractory errors, speech therapy, behavior modifications and other measures may be needed depending upon the type of problem.

Parent Counseling

This is one of the most important aspects of management of CP because parents are pivotal in the management of their child. Experience, understanding and sensitivity are required for proper counseling. The doctor needs to properly explain the child's condition and help the parents to accept it, guide them regarding proper treatment, address their concerns about the child, try to alleviate the immense psychosocial stress that they face, remove their feelings of guilt and blame and help build positive attitudes. Both the parents, and sometimes the grandparents too need to be counseled together so that they work as a team and avoid blaming each other.

An honest appraisal of child's condition is essential. The clinician should endeavour to provide a balanced account of the child's problem but simultaneously emphasize the child's abilities so as to help channelize the parents' thought process towards positive goals. Parents must learn that treatment is a continuous process; however, it can be broken down into a number of short-constructive goals–attainments of these brings a sense of achievement and a hope of progress. Unfortunately, many misconceptions surround the diagnosis of CP. The parents might get frustrated with slow improvement and try all kinds of alternative therapies which have no evidence of benefit. The pediatrician should have the patience, wisdom and scientific knowledge to explain the futility of various such therapies. Helping the parents accept the limitations of ongoing treatment and the condition and prognosis of their child and at the same time motivating them to continue working with their child is one of the most challenging aspects of management.

Education and Training

These need to be individualized according to the child's abilities, determined after comprehensive assessment. Guidance should be provided to parents regarding availability of appropriate schools and training or rehabilitation centers. Formation of parents groups helps in sharing and providing emotional support for each other. The ultimate aim of management in CP is to help the child achieve his optimal developmental potential and to integrate him as a useful member in the society.

References

1. Bax M, Goldstein M, Rosenbaum P, *et al.* Proposed Definition and Classification of Cerebral Palsy, April 2005. Dev Med Child Neurol 2005;47:571-76.
2. Gladstone M. A Review of the Incidence and Prevalence, Types and Aetiology of Childhood Cerebral Palsy in Resource-Poor Settings. Ann Trop Paediatr 2010;30:181-96.
3. Raina SK, Razdan S, Nanda R. Prevalence of cerebral palsy in children < 10 years of Age in R.S. Pura town of Jammu and Kashmir. J Trop Pediatr 2011;57: 293-95.
4. Razdan S, Kaul RL, Motta A, Kaul S, Bhatt RK. Prevalence and Pattern of Major Neurological Disorders in Rural Kashmir (India) in 1986. Neuroepidemiology 1994;13:113-19.
5. Singhi P, Saini AG. Changes in the Clinical Spectrum of Cerebral Palsy Over Two Decades in North India–An Analysis of 1212 Cases. J Trop Pediatr 2013;59:434-40.
6. Nelson KB. Causative Factors in Cerebral Palsy. Clin Obstet Gynecol 2008;51:749-62.

7. Menkes JH. Flores-Sarnat L. Cerebral Palsy Due to Chromosomal Anomalies and Continuous Gene Syndromes. Clin Perinatol 2006;33:481-501.

8. Gibson CS. Maclennan AH. Dekker GA. *et al.* Candidate Genes and Cerebral Palsy: A Population-Based Study. Pediatrics 2008: 122:1079-85.

9. Rankin J. Cans C. Garne E. *et al.* Congenital Anomalies in Children with Cerebral Palsy: A Population-Based Record Linkage Study. Dev Med Child Neurol 2010: 52:345-51.

10. Glinianaia SV. Rankin J. Colver A. North of England Collaborative Cerebral Palsy S. Cerebral Palsy Rates by Birth Weight. Gestation and Severity in North of England. 1991-2000 Singleton Births. Arch Dis Child 2011;96:180-85.

11. Winter S. Autry A. Boyle C. Yeargin-Allsopp M. Trends in the Prevalence of Cerebral Palsy in a Population-Based Study. Pediatrics 2002;110:1220-25.

12. Kuban KC. Leviton A. Cerebral Palsy. The New England Journal of Medicine 1994:330:188-95.

13. Kallen AJ. Finnstrom OO. Lindam AP. *et al.* Cerebral Palsy in Children Born After *in vitro* Fertilization. Is the risk decreasing? Eur J Paediatr Neurol 2010;14:526-30.

14. Belonwu RO. Gwarzo GD. Adeleke SI. Cerebral Palsy in Kano. Nigeria–A Review. Niger J Med 2009;18:186-89.

15. Singhi PD. Ray M. Suri G. Clinical spectrum of Cerebral Palsy in North India–An Analysis of 1,000 Cases. J Trop Pediatr 2002: 48:162-66.

16. Saini AG. Sankhyan N. Malhi P. *et al.* Hyperbilirubinemia and Asphyxia in Children With Dyskinetic Cerebral Palsy. Pediatr Neurol 2021:120:80-85.

17. Singhi PD. Goraya JS. Cerebral Palsy. Indian Pediatr 1998:35: 37-48.

18. Singhi P. The Child with Cerebral Palsy–Clinical Considerations and Management. Indian J Pediatr 2001;68:531-37.

19. Singhi PD. Cerebral Palsy–Management. Indian J Pediatr 2004:71:635-39.

20. Singhi PD. Counselling the Parents of a Child with Cerebral Palsy. Indian Pediatr 1988:25:368-70.

21. Hoare BJ. Wasiak J. Imms C. Carey L. Constraint-Induced Movement Therapy in the Treatment of the Upper Limb in Children with Hemiplegic Cerebral Palsy. Cochrane Database Syst Rev 2007:CD004149.

22. Ravi DK. Kumar N. Singhi P. Effectiveness of Virtual Reality Rehabilitation for Children and Adolescents with Cerebral Palsy: An Updated Evidence-Based Systematic Review. Physiotherapy 2017;103:245-58.

23. Goswami JN. Sankhyan N. Singhi P. Add-on Home-Centred Activity-Based Therapy vs Conventional Physiotherapy in Improving Walking Ability at 6 Months in Children with Diplegic Cerebral Palsy: A Randomized Controlled Trial. Indian Pediatr 2021.

24. Behari M. Spasticity. Neurol India 2002;50:235-37.

28 Chapter

NON-INFECTIOUS ENCEPHALOPATHIES IN CHILDREN

Arushi Gahlot Saini, Naveen Sankhyan

INTRODUCTION

Consciousness is defined as the arousal and awareness of self and environment. Impaired consciousness thus, implies a significant alteration in the awareness of self and of the environment, with varying degrees of wakefulness (Taylor and Ashwal, 2006). Descriptive terms such as somnolence, stupor, obtundation, and lethargy used to denote different levels of wakefulness are best avoided, given the lack of uniformity in the way these states are defined in the literature. Diseases may alter consciousness by causing various stages of delirium or coma. Delirium (acute confusional state often equated with encephalopathy) is an acute, transient confusional state characterized by global impairment of the sensorium. The patient shows disorientation, amnesia, misperception, hallucinations, delusions, brief attention span, disconnected thoughts, irrational or incoherent mutterings and abnormally decreased or increased psychomotor activity and altered sleep-wake cycles. The encephalopathic patient may return to their previous mental state or may proceed to coma which is sustained pathological unconsciousness resulting from dysfunction of the ascending reticular activating system in the brainstem or bilateral cerebral hemispheres.

Encephalopathy is not a diagnosis but a descriptive term connoting a syndrome of global dysfunction which may be caused by an infectious agent, para-infectious or autoimmune phenomenon, metabolic or mitochondrial dysfunction, brain tumor or increased pressure in the skull, prolonged exposure to toxins, chronic progressive trauma, poor nutrition, or hypoxia-ischemia to the brain (NINDS, 2010). Though signifying diffuse dysfunction, profound encephalopathy may result from small lesions in the upper brainstem. The management of the encephalopathic child is an emergency and presents a challenge in terms of etiological diagnosis, assessment and interventions. Morbidity and mortality in these children is high and prompt recognition and expeditious intervention helps minimize further neurological impairments. We discuss here the common non-infectious causes of encephalopathy in children and an approach to their diagnosis and management. Neuroinfections and neonatal encephalopathies are not covered in this chapter.

Epidemiology

The incidence of non-traumatic coma is 30/100,000 children per year (Wong *et al.*, 2001). Hospital-based studies reveal that central nervous system (CNS) infections constitute nearly two-thirds of the causes of encephalopathy in children followed by toxic-metabolic (Reye's syndrome, hepatic coma, hypoxic encephalopathy, poisoning, snake bite, and diabetic ketoacidosis) in one-fifth (Bansal *et al.*, 2005; Sofiah and Hussain, 1997). Other studies implicate metabolic causes in nearly one-third followed closely by CNS infections (Fouad *et al.*, 2011). Overall, the two major categories of acute encephalopathy in children are CNS infections (Ali *et al.*, 2007; Bansal *et al.*, 2005) and toxic/metabolic causes (Kraus *et al.*, 1984; Tasker *et al.*, 1988). Accidental poisonings are common in young children while intentional poisonings are common in adolescents (Srivastava *et al.*, 2005).

Common Presentations of Encephalopathy

The onset of encephalopathy may be acute or insidious. The defining feature is the presence of an altered mental state, the manifestations of which varies depending on the age of the child, the type and severity of encephalopathy. It may manifest as irritability, developmental regression/stasis, altered sleep-wake cycle, change in personality or behavior, inability to concentrate, progressive loss of memory and cognitive deterioration or reduction in the level of consciousness. Presence of localizing features such as seizures, ataxia, tremors, focal motor signs, or systemic features such as fever, vomiting, lethargy, loss of appetite, headache, presence of abnormal body odors further helps in etiological evaluation. It is important to determine a previously normal neurological status or pre-existing neurological impairment with an "acute on chronic" presentation. Parents' or care-givers' assessment of such children is, thus, crucial.

Non-Infectious Causes of Encephalopathies

Encephalopathy may result from primary/direct insult to the cerebral cortex, diencephalic structures, midbrain or rostral pons; or a secondary manifestation of systemic derangements caused by toxins, metabolic, or endocrine disorders or interplay of multiple interrelated factors in a patient. The differentials are wide and best grouped systematically. Table 28.1 lists the common causes and the important ones are briefly discussed.

Table 28.1: Important Non-Infectious Causes of Encephalopathy in Children

PARAINFECTIOUS/INFLAMMATORY
A. Infection associated encephalopathy
Sepsis-associated encephalopathy*
Toxic encephalopathy (salmonella, shigella, campylobacter, EIEC, cerebral malaria)*
B. Immune mediated
Acute disseminated encephalomyelitis*
Acute necrotizing encephalopathy of childhood*
N-methyl-D-aspartate receptor antibody encephalitis*
Voltage gated potassium antibody encephalitis
Vasculitis/collagen vascular disorders
Hashimoto' encephalopathy
Paraneoplastic
C. Inflammation mediated encephalopathies
Hemiconvulsion-Hemiplegia-Epilepsy (HHE) Syndrome*
Febrile Infection-Related Epilepsy Syndrome (FIRES)*
STRUCTURAL
A. Traumatic (Accidental or Non-accidental*)
Concussion and/or contusion and/or hematoma and/or diffuse axonal injury
B. Hydrocephalus
C. Neoplasms (Primary/Metastatic)
D. Vascular diseases
Cerebral infarction (thrombosis/embolism) (Fig. 28.1)
Intracranial hemorrhage (Fig. 28.2)
Acute complicated migraine
Congenital anomalies of the vascular supply

Contd.

Contd.

TOXIC-METABOLIC
A. Hypoxic/ischemic
Shock
Following resuscitation/cardiorespiratory failure
Near drowning/strangulation
Near miss sudden infant death syndrome
B. Dysmetabolic states
Fluid and electrolyte imbalance (hyponatremia, hypernatremia, hypercalcemia, hypermagnesemia, hypophosphatemia)
Hyper or hypoglycemia
Hyperammonemia (hepatic encephalopathy, urea cycle disorders, Reye's syndrome, drug-induced)
Acidosis (Diabetic ketoacidosis, organic academia, lactic acidemia)
Inborn errors of metabolism*
Endocrine disorders (Diabetic ketoacidosis, Hashimoto's encephalopathy)
C. Organ failures/encephalopathies related to systemic diseases
Hepatic encephalopathy*
Uremia*
Inflammatory bowel disease
Celiac disease/crisis
Hypothyroid coma
D. Toxins and drugs
Drugs (therapeutic including chemotherapy, recreational, industrial)
Heavy metal poisoning
Envenomations
Mushroom and plant intoxication
Carbon monoxide
Alcohol intoxication
E. Nutritional
Thiamine deficiency
Pyridoxine dependency
Folate and B_{12} deficiency
F. Hypertensive encephalopathy*
G. Heat stroke
H. Burn encephalopathy
I. Seizure related
Status epilepticus (convulsive, non-convulsive)
Post-ictal state

* See details in subsequent sections

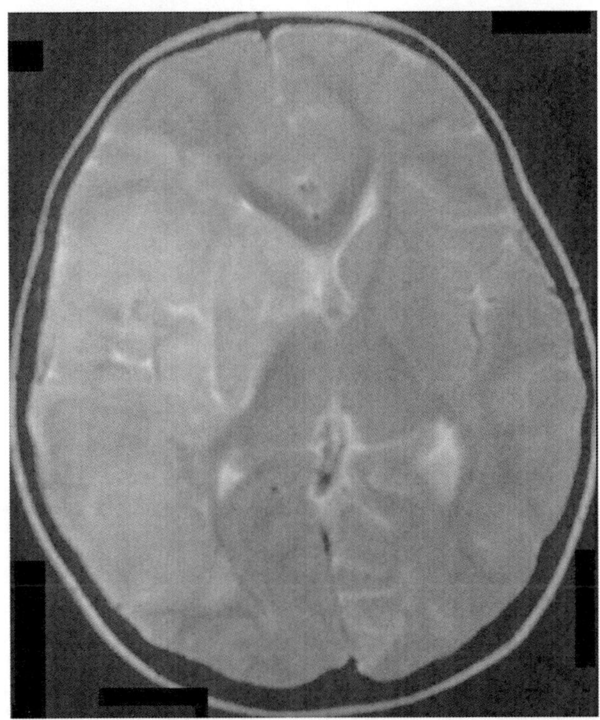

Fig. 28.1: Axial T2W MR image in a 3-year-old boy child with right middle cerebral artery infarction. Note the hyperintense signal and the mild swelling of the affected area

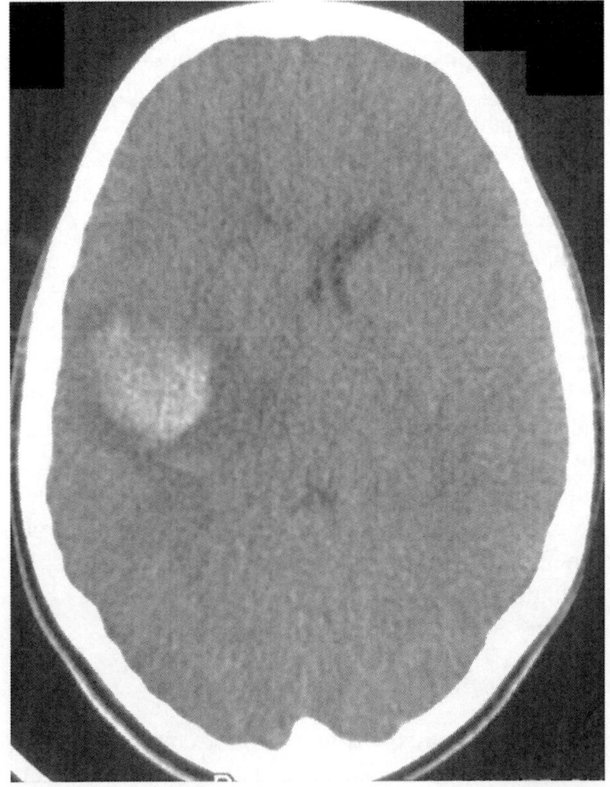

Fig. 28.2: A non-contrast CT of head showing right temporo-parietal intraparenchymal hemorrhage in a 7-year-old girl. Note the surrounding edema and mass effect on the lateral ventricles

APPROACH TO A CHILD WITH ENCEPHALOPATHY

Encephalopathy is a neurological emergency, requiring immediate care and intervention. The basic principles of management are rapid assessment and stabilization, focused clinical evaluation, localization of lesion in the nervous system, and possible clues to etiology and treatment including general and specific measures. The evaluation and treatment have to proceed simultaneously (Table 28.2).

Table 28.2: Steps in Management of Acute Encephalopathy in Children
Step 1: Stabilization
• *Neurological ABCD:* **N**eck stabilization in traumatic brain injuries, **A**irway, **B**reathing, **C**irculation, **D**epth of coma and signs of herniation
• Vascular access and critical sampling
• Correct hypoglycemia, electrolyte imbalances, hyperthermia, acid-base imbalances
• Manage seizures and raised ICP
• Fluid boluses ± inotropes for shock
Step 2: Simultaneous Evaluation
• Assessment of the neurological status, history and examination
• Identification of toxidromes and use of antidotes
• Appropriate empirical antimicrobials/antivirals/antimalarials
Step 3: Investigations and Re-Assessment (Table 28.3)
• *Important etiological investigations:* CSF, CT, Toxic screen
• Reassess the effect of first line measures and investigations
• Manage specific emerging abnormalities from first line investigations
• *Specific treatment:* Insulin, atropine, antivenoms etc.
• MRI brain ± spine
• Electroencephalography
Step 4: Further Investigations and Management
• Metabolic screen for inborn errors of metabolism
• Specific investigations for auto-immune encephalitides/disorders
• Specific CSF markers

At bedside, it may be difficult to differentiate between infectious and non-infectious encephalopathies. The diagnosis may become evident only in retrospect in many cases; however, the critical aspects of early management remain the same. A stepwise approach to relevant investigations in a child with acute encephalopathy is provided in Table 28.3.

Table 28.3: Investigations in a Child with Acute Encephalopathy
First Line Investigations
• Blood glucose
• Complete blood count with PBF
• Coagulogram
• Serum electrolyte levels, calcium and phosphorus
• Renal and liver function tests
• Arterial blood gas analysis
• Blood and urine cultures
• Lumbar puncture and CSF examination
• Neuroimaging
Second Line Investigations (Depend on suspected etiology)
• EEG
• Lactate and ammonia levels
• Urine for reducing sugars and ketones
• Urine and blood samples for amino-acid, organic acid, free fatty acid and carnitine disorders
• Urine toxicology screen
• Glycosylated hemoglobin
• Thyroid function tests and thyroid antibodies
• Urine porphyrins screen
• Vasculitis panel
• Immune mediated encephalopathies panel

History

A careful history should be obtained from the primary caregiver with special emphasis on the events prior to the onset of encephalopathy. Timing and nature of the deterioration and duration of symptoms must be ascertained. History of fever, headache, vomiting, irritability, vision problems, seizures, rash, exposure to drugs or toxins, abnormal body odors, trauma (both accidental and non-accidental, and specifically about any minor, seemingly insignificant head or neck trauma which may lead to carotid artery dissection or stroke in children), animal or snake bite, abuse, child's pre-existing neurological status, birth, developmental and medical history, as well as occupation of the parents must be enquired. A family history of neurological, metabolic, vascular or hematological disease is important, as is a history of parental consanguinity and early childhood or infant deaths. A history of fever or recent illness suggests an acute infectious etiology (sepsis, meningitis, encephalitis), but other disorders where minor febrile illness may precipitate or precede encephalopathy such as ADEM, Reye's syndrome, mitochondrial and other inborn errors of metabolism, due to heat stroke or abnormality of hypothalamic temperature regulatory mechanisms should also be considered.

Examination

Vital signs: Provide important clues to the etiology and severity of encephalopathy. Tachycardia may be the result of fever, hypovolemic or septic shock, heart failure, arrhythmias or toxin exposure. Bradycardia may result from raised ICP or a result of myocardial injury (due to myocarditis, hypoxia, sepsis, or toxins). Tachypnea with increased work of breathing suggests underlying lung pathology; however, quiet tachypnea is indicative of acidosis such as in DKA, uremia, ethylene glycol poisoning or raised ICP. Hypertension may per se cause encephalopathy with or without accompanying intracranial bleeds or may be a compensatory mechanism to maintain cerebral perfusion pressure in raised ICP or stroke. In hypertensive; encephalopathy, there will be diastolic hypertension; left ventricular hypertrophy (on ECG and ECHO), and changes of hypertensive retinopathy. Hypotension due to hypovolemia, sepsis, cardiac dysfunction toxic ingestion, adrenal insufficiency, vasomotor insufficiency may lead to reduced cerebral perfusion and additionally contribute to hypoxic-ischemic encephalopathy.

General physical examination should be thorough and focused for specific possible etiologies. Pallor suggests anemia, shock, hemorrhage or hemolysis; cyanosis suggests poor oxygenation or toxin exposure; lymphadenopathy suggests expansion of reticuloendothelial system especially in infections and malignancies; icterus is indicative of hepatic dysfunction such as in hepatic encephalopathy, complicated malaria, enteric fever; abnormal odor of exhaled breath may suggest underlying DKA, hepatic coma or specific IEMs. The head and scalp should be examined for evidence of head trauma such as cephalhematoma, lacerations or ecchymosis. Any bite marks, rash, petechiae should be carefully looked for especially over hidden sites such as scalp and post-auricular areas. Presence of dysmorphism and neurocutaneous markers may give clues to specific neurological or genetic syndrome especially in children presenting with seizures.

Neurological Examination

Level of consciousness is assessed by body posture, spontaneous motor activity, eye opening and verbalization. Objective scales such as modified GCS for infants and young children must be recorded to document the severity of coma, guide effect of treatment or course of illness.

However, a more detailed description of the child's clinical findings and disability should be recorded for conveying the accurate picture of encephalopathy.

Pupillary abnormalities in size, shape, symmetry and response to light provide clues to brainstem and third nerve dysfunction. Unilateral pupillary dilatation in the comatose patient suggests oculomotor nerve compression from ipsilateral uncal herniation, however, topical administration of mydriatics should be enquired into avoid misinterpretation.

Brainstem function: Intact brainstem function is indicated by the presence of oculocephalic (Doll's eye), oculovestibular, corneal, cough and gagreflexes. Abnormalities of eye position and movement provide additional information. Lateral gaze palsy may signal raised ICP causing herniation with compression of bilateral sixth nerves. Tonic upward gaze may suggest bilateral hemispheric damage. Conjugate lateral deviation of the eyes is a sign either of an ipsilateral hemisphere lesion, a contralateral hemisphere seizure focus, or damage involving the contralateral pontine horizontal gaze center (parapontine reticular formation) (Stevens and Nyquist, 2006).

Motor response: The posture (decerebrate, decorticate, or flaccid) in the bed, positioning of limbs and trunk, spontaneous movements and response to stimulation must be recorded to look for any focal deficits and depth of encephalopathy. Posturing often signals a brainstem herniation syndrome. Presence of tonic-clonic movements or myoclonus signal seizures, dystonias signify extrapyramidal involvement such as in Japanese B encephalitis, tubercular meningitis, and inborn errors of metabolism or metoclopramide toxicity.

Other neurological findings: Fundus examination to look for papilloedema, retinal hemorrhages, and changes of hypertensive retinopathy or underlying neurological illness should always be done. Signs of meningeal irritation may be present in meningitis, encephalitis and subarachnoid hemorrhage. Raised intracranial pressure due to asymmetric, unilateral or generalized pathology may give rise to the various herniation syndromes which need early intervention.

Systemic examination: Chest examination to detect underlying pneumonia, empyema, pneumothorax or space-occupying lesion; the cardiovascular system for congenital or acquired heart diseases or arrhythmias; abdominal examination may reveal hepatosplenomegaly, intra-abdominal mass, fecoliths or fluid. Inspection of genitalia and spine should be followed in quick succession to look for associated malformations or signs of trauma.

Management

Management of children with encephalopathy proceeds simultaneously with evaluation and investigations (Table 28.2). Pediatric intensive care unit care should be sought if there is a suggestion of an unstable airway or organ support is required. In sick children with acute febrile encephalopathy, an empiric course of antibiotics, acyclovir, and anti-malarial agents may be warranted while awaiting results of investigations. Steroids are indicated in conditions such as ADEM, meningococcemia with shock, enteric encephalopathy, tubercular meningitis, and pyogenic meningitis, intracranial bleeds, etc. Specialist consultations must be sought at appropriate levels to direct interventions. After the initial phase, consideration should be given to education and psychological input for the child as well as family support during the ongoing illness period. Few of the treatment options have been discussed in relevant sections below. A synopsis is provided in Table 28.4.

Table 28.4: Specific Management of Non-Infectious Encephalopathy

Seizures	Step-wise treatment of status epilepticus
Trauma	Neck Stabilization Steroids for spinal trauma Neurosurgical intervention: Evacuation of extradural bleed
Ischemic Stroke	Anticoagulation for arterial dissection, venous thrombosis, cardioembolic stroke Aspirin for idiopathic arterial ischemic stroke
Hemorrhage Stroke	Correction of clotting abnormalities Platelet replacement Immunoglobulins (Idiopathic thrombocytopenic purpura) Neurosurgery
Parainfectious/ Demyelination/ Autoimmune Encephalopathies	Immunomodulation (Steroids, Immunoglobulins, Plasmapheresis, other immunosuppressants)
Hydrocephalus	CSF Diversion (Shunt/Ventriculostomy) Treatment of underlying cause such as tumor
Hypertensive Encephalopathy	Antihypertensives (labetalol, sodium nitroprusside)
Toxins	Specific antidotes Anti snake venom Organ support (intubation, anti-arrhythmic, anti-hypertensive, fluid and inotropes, correction of electrolyte, acid-base and clotting derangement, management of hypo/hyperthermia, seizures) Activated charcoal, dialysis

Contd.

Contd.

Metabolic	Dietary restriction Clearance of toxic metabolites (dialysis, sodium benzoate, carnitine) Specific supplementation (thiamine, biotin, arginine) Specific drugs (metabolic specialist)

SELECTED CONDITIONS CAUSING ENCEPHALOPATHY IN CHILDREN

Infection Associated Encephalopathy

Sepsis Associated Encephalopathy (SAE)

Sepsis is often associated with an acute and reversible encephalopathy characterized by alteration in consciousness, awareness, cognition and behavior without focal neurological signs. Additionally, there is diffuse slowing on electroencephalography (EEG), unremarkable findings on cerebrospinal fluid (CSF), and normal brain imaging. The encephalopathy results from diffuse cerebral dysfunction associated with a systemic inflammatory response to infection with no direct CNS infection; hence, the term SAE is preferred over sepsis encephalopathy. SAE is present in more than 70% of patients with severe systemic infection and may even precede the cardinal findings of sepsis (Gofton and Young, 2012). The pathophysiology involves pathogenic activation of neuro-inflammatory pathways leading to alteration of neurotransmission, increase in intracellular calcium, disturbed autoregulation, endothelial activation and blood brain barrier breakdown, mitochondrial dysfunction, oxidative stress and apoptosis of neurons and microglia. Blood brain barrier breakdown can be localized around the Virchow-Robin spaces, predominate in posterior lobes consistent with a posterior reversible encephalopathy syndrome, or may be diffuse in the whole white matter (Iacobone *et al.*, 2009). Clinical features include changes in awareness and consciousness varying from alteration of sleep/wake cycle, disorientation, hallucination, impaired attention, and disorganized thinking to deep coma, and variable motor activity from agitation to hypoactivity. Seizures and myoclonus are infrequent; cranial nerves function is always spared. Pathologically, hippocampal involvement has been correlated to the clinical picture of delirium in SAE (Janz *et al.*, 2010). The diagnosis is one of exclusion and is concluded after CNS infections, metabolic disturbances, respiratory, hepatic or renal insufficiency, drug overdose or thromboembolic phenomenon are excluded. Appropriate laboratory testing including neuroimaging and EEG, may be warranted in the correct clinical context. There is no specific therapy for SAE. Treatment of underlying systemic illness and supportive measures such as control of sepsis, management of organ failure and metabolic disturbances, correction of hypoxia and avoidance of neurotoxic drugs remain the mainstay. There is no current evidence-based role of insulin therapy, activated protein C, or steroids in reducing the incidence or severity of SAE in children. Although SAE is considered reversible phenomenon, features that portend poorer prognosis include GCS<8, burst suppression pattern on EEG and elevated plasma levels of biomarkers (Ely *et al.*, 2001).

Infection Associated Toxic Encephalopathies

Infection associated encephalopathies are considered in those patients in whom the encephalopathy at presentation is associated with evidence of recent or current infection and the other causes have been excluded (Davies *et al.*, 2006). The pathogenic mechanisms linking infection and encephalopathy may be through indirect toxin-mediated mechanisms or other unknown factors. Direct CNS invasion characterized by parenchymal microbial invasion and inflammation is characteristic of neuroinfections and is discussed elsewhere. The pathologic substrate of acute encephalopathy is diffuse or widespread, non-inflammatory brain edema and thus, inflammatory cells are not usually found in the brain or CSF (Takanashi, 2009). The common causes of toxic encephalopathy are enteric toxin producing bacteria and malarial parasites.

Shigella-associated encephalopathy is seen in 12-45% of gastrointestinal infection with Shigella spp. The most common manifestations are confusion, lethargy, hallucinations, seizures and coma (Perles *et al.*, 1995). Encephalopathy is usually reversible, but it may be fulminant. It is possibly mediated by Shigella cytotoxins, which have neurotoxic properties (Goren *et al.*, 1992). A particular form of lethal toxic encephalopathy due to shigellosis characterized by rapid onset of neurological abnormalities with only mild colitis has been named Ekiri syndrome with possible toxin-mediated mechanisms (Pourakbari *et al.*, 2012). Other infections associated with CNS manifestations include Salmonella, Campylobacter, and Enteroinvasive Escherichia coli infections (Ashkenazi *et al.*, 1994; Ephros *et al.*, 1996), but the pathogenesis of encephalopathy is largely unknown.

Typhoid encephalopathy is a manifestation of typhoid fever and may develop in up to 17 percent of patients (Butler *et al.*, 1991). The changes in sensorium typically occur in the 3rd week of illness, though they can occur earlier too. The occurrence of encephalopathy is a grave sign, and a mortality rate as high as 55% has been reported

(Hoffman *et al.*, 1984). Meticulous supportive care, intravenous antibiotics and use of adjunctive intravenous dexamethasone have been shown to reduce mortality (Hoffman *et al.*, 1984).

Cerebral malaria is due to multiple pathophysiological processes, including sequestration, local release of cytokines, blood brain barrier abnormalities, and metabolic derangements. Thus the symptoms of seizures, coma and other signs of neurological impairment are not due to the parenchymal invasion by the organism itself (van der Heyde *et al.*, 2006). The prodrome consists of non-specific signs and symptoms, including fever, anorexia, cough, and vomitings for less than a day followed rapidly by seizures, raised intracranial pressure, signs of brainstem dysfunction, and coma (Birbeck *et al.*, 2010). Early use of intravenous antimalarials, meticulous supportive care and sometimes other measures to reduce parasitemia are needed to save the affected children.

Dengue fever is a viral infection transmitted in urban areas by Aedes aegypti. Hospital-based studies show that 18% of pediatric dengue cases are admitted with neurological involvement (Kankirawatana *et al.*, 2000). The involvement of the CNS has been presumed to be secondary to vasculitis and leaky capillary syndrome with resultant fluid extravasations, cerebral edema, hypoperfusion, hyponatremia, liver failure, and/or renal failure (Kanade and Shah, 2011). As such, it is usually called dengue encephalopathy. However, reports of virus isolation from brain tissue and CSF of patients with neurological symptoms suggest direct virus invasion of the CNS as well (Lum *et al.*, 1996). Treatment is largely supportive. Median coma recovery time for those admitted with encephalopathy is 3.5 days (Solomon *et al.*, 2000).

Immune Mediated Encephalopathies

Acute Disseminated Encephalomyelitis (ADEM)

ADEM is an immune-mediated inflammatory disorder of the CNS, commonly preceded by an infection (70-93%) or vaccination (5%). It is defined as a first clinical demyelinating event with acute or subacute onset encephalopathy, multiple neurological symptoms, and neuroimaging evidence of focal or multifocal hyperintense white-matter lesions, in the absence of previous clinical or radiological evidence of a demyelinating event (Krupp *et al.*, 2007). The duration of the first episode may last as long as three months; hence any relapse within this duration or 4 weeks of tapering steroid treatment is considered "steroid-dependent ADEM" and a part of the initial event itself.

The clinical course is marked by rapid-onset encephalopathy varying from irritability, altered sleep-wake cycle to frank coma, ensuing within two days to 4 weeks of an antigenic challenge. Multifocal neurological deficits appear depending on the location of lesions such as pyramidal signs, acute hemiplegia, quadriplegia, ataxia, ophthalmoparesis, cranial nerve palsies, optic neuritis, seizures, myelitis, speech and sensory impairments. Persistence of fever, headache and meningismus are common in children. MRI is diagnostic and shows large, multiple, patchy, poorly demarcated, asymmetrical areas of T2 and FLAIR hyperintensities (Fig. 28.3) in white-matter with variable contrast-enhancement and deep gray nuclei involvement (Wingerchuk, 2003). Associated spinal cord involvement may be seen in nearly one-fourth of cases. Pulse methyl prednisolone (10 to 30 mg/kg/day up to a maximum dose of 1 g/day) or dexamethasone (1 mg/kg) for 3 to 5 days) followed by oral steroid taper for 4-6 weeks is the first-line treatment (Tenembaum *et al.*, 2007). Improvements with IVIg and plasma exchange have been documented after first line therapy fails.

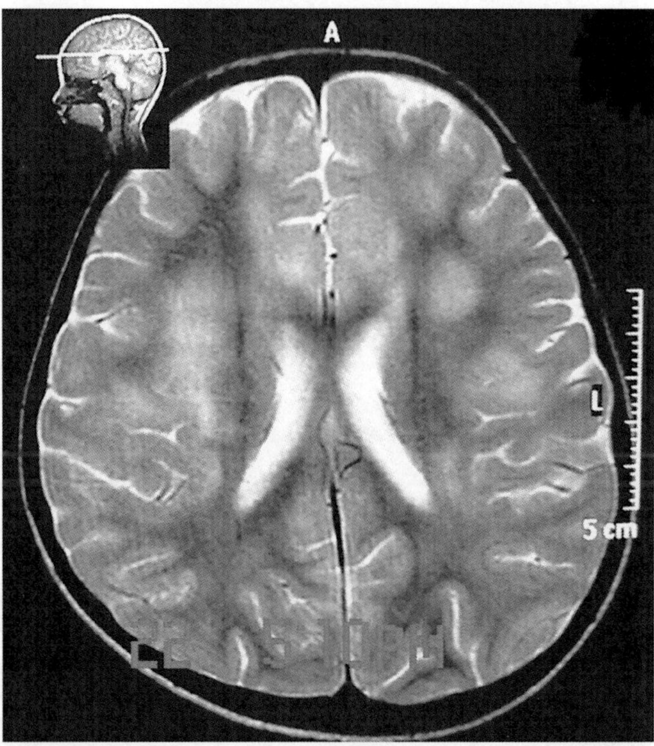

Fig. 28.3: Axial T2W MR image in a child with ADEM showing bilateral, multifocal discrete hyperintense signal changes in areas of demyelination

Acute Necrotizing Encephalopathy of Childhood (ANE)

Acute Necrotizing Encephalopathy of Childhood is a fulminant encephalopathy affecting children under the age of 5 years and characterized by elevated serum transaminases, lack of CSF pleocytosis and bilateral symmetric thalamic lesions often with central hemorrhages and cavitation on neuroimaging (Fig. 28.4). Primarily reported from the Far East, it is an increasingly recognized entity with familial (ANE1) and recurrent cases being linked to mutations in RANBP2 (RAN binding protein 2) (Neilson *et al.*, 2009). The etiology and pathogenesis of this disease are unknown. Although influenza A virus, mycoplasma, herpes simplex virus, and human herpes virus-6 have been reported as common causative agents, it is now believed that this disease is most likely immune-mediated or metabolic (Mizuguchi, 1997). A prodromal viral-like illness followed by rapidly evolving acute encephalopathy within 12-72 hours with vomiting (20%), seizures (40%), decreased level of consciousness (28%), and upper motor neuron signs (66%). Coma may ensue in less than 24 hours. Laboratory and neuroimaging findings help differentiate this condition from other conditions such as ADEM, viral encephalitis, especially Japanese encephalitis, inborn errors of metabolism, hypoxic-ischemic encephalopathy, hemolytic uremic syndrome, toxic encephalopathy, hemorrhagic shock, and Reye's syndrome. Blood biochemistry studies reveal metabolic acidosis, elevated aspartate aminotransferase, alanine aminotransferase,

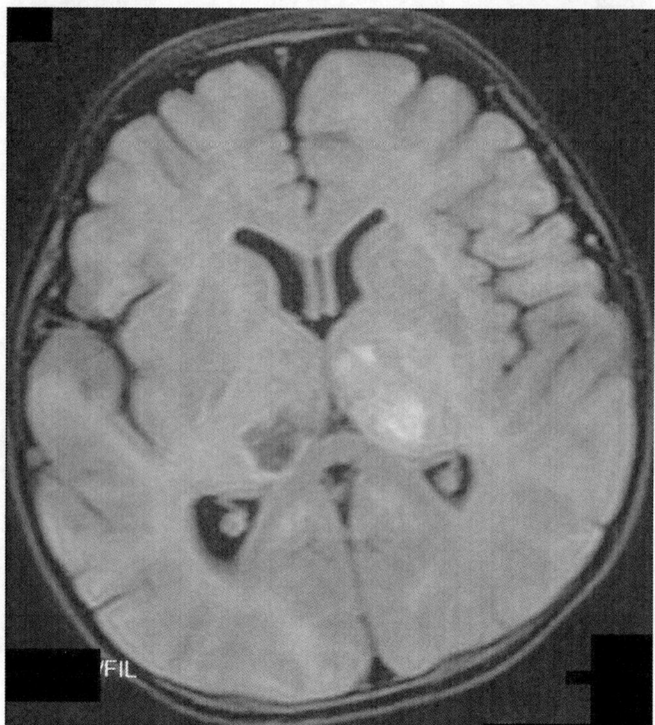

Fig. 28.4: Axial T1W MR image showing left thalamic hyperintensities with hemorrhagic cavitation in the right thalamus in an infant with acute necrotizing encephalopathy (ANE)

and lactate dehydrogenase. Elevations in serum ammonia and bilirubin are uncommon. CSF study shows elevated opening pressure (>15 mm H_2O) and protein (>40 mg/dl) but no cells in the majority. Pathologically, the absence of inflammatory cells in affected brain parenchyma is characteristic, which differentiates this disease from the more common entities of ADEM and acute hemorrhagic encephalitis. Motor deficits such as intention tremor, ataxia, speech impairment, choreoathetosis, spasticity, and focal neurologic signs, including hemiparesis and extraocular motility abnormalities, often develop in the chronic stage. Intravenous pulse steroids within 24 hours of presentation in children have been associated with a more favorable neurological outcome (Okumura *et al.*, 2009). The prognosis of severe ANEC is generally poor; approximately 65% of the affected patients died or were left with severe neurologic sequelae (Wang and Huang, 2001).

Anti-N-Methyl-D-Aspartate Receptor (NMDAR) Encephalitis

Anti-NMDAR encephalitis is a new category of severe yet treatable immune-mediated disorders of young people caused by autoantibodies (IgG1 subclass) against NR1 subunit of the receptor (Dalmau, 2012). With increasing recognition in children, it is postulated to be the most common cause of autoimmune encephalitis after ADEM. NMDA receptors are glutamate-gated Ca^{2+} channels with crucial roles in synaptic transmission and plasticity. Hence overactivity of NMDAR causes excitotoxicity and results in a characteristic neuropsychiatric syndrome. The clinical phenotype in children includes an initial prodromal phase consisting of headache, fever, nausea, vomiting, diarrhea, or upper respiratory-tract symptoms (70%). Within a few days, neuropsychiatric syndrome evolves consisting of behavioral or personality change, decreased sleep, speech regression and seizures; followed by acute encephalopathy alternating between agitation and catatonia, and oro-facial-acral choreoathetoid movement disorder. This is accompanied by dysautonomia, hyperhidrosis, urinary incontinence, persistent pyrexia and central hypoventilation requiring intensive care. Acute viral encephalitis is a close differential diagnosis and needs exclusion. The diagnosis is confirmed by detection of anti-NMDAR antibodies in serum and/or CSF. Additionally, CSF shows moderate lymphocytic pleocytosis, normal or mildly increased protein concentration, and oligoclonal bands (Dalmau, 2012). Post-viral and less commonly, paraneoplastic (commonly ovarian teratoma in older girls) mechanisms for the induction of NMDAR antibodies have been postulated for children. However, no viruses have been isolated and repeated screenings for occult tumors are not recommended in younger children. EEG may be normal, diffusely slow or may show characteristic delta brushes in few patients.

Immunotherapy (IVIg 0.4 g/kg/day for 5 days and methylprednisolone 1g/day for 5 days or plasma exchange) is the mainstay of treatment. If no response is seen after 10 days, second line treatment is begun (Cyclophosphamide 750 mg/m^2 followed by monthly cycles, Rituximab 375 mg/m^2 every week for 4 weeks or both) (Dalmau, 2012; Titulaer *et al.*, 2013). Duration of therapy remains to be determined. Anti-NMDAR encephalitis should be considered in any child with acute behavioral change, seizures, movement disorders with mild fever and CSF lymphocytic pleocytosis, with normal or non-specific MRI changes and unusually prolonged course (Florance *et al.*, 2009).

Inflammation-Mediated Encephalopathies

Hemiconvulsion - Hemiplegia - Epilepsy (HHE) Syndrome

HHE syndrome, along with FIRES and NORSE has been considered a spectrum of inflammation-mediated encephalopathies with difference in clinical expression related to the stage of brain maturation (Nabbout *et al.*, 2011). HHE is an uncommon epilepsy syndrome that follows prolonged, focal, febrile, status epilepticus in infancy and early childhood. The acute stage of the disease begins with a febrile illness with prolonged, predominantly focal, clonic seizures in a child usually younger than four years of age. Motor aphasia may accompany the post-ictal state. This is followed by permanent hemiplegia. Neuroimaging shows acute, unilateral edematous swelling of the epileptic hemisphere (Fig. 28.5) and may cause mass effect on the contralateral hemisphere in severe cases. MR angiography remains normal, and DWI shows evidence of unilateral cytotoxic edema. This initial stage is referred to as HH syndrome (HHS) in the absence of epilepsy. This is followed by a chronic phase characterized by global atrophy of unilaterally affected hemisphere irrespective of the vascular territory (Sankhyan *et al.*, 2008), epilepsy arising within the first 2-3 years of onset and hemiplegia, hence the name HHE. The diagnosis of HHE syndrome is suspected in any child with persistent flaccid hemiplegia after a prolonged febrile status (Auvin *et al.*, 2012). Clinical implications include excluding other causes of acute focal weakness following seizures in a child such as a stroke, neoplasm, focal encephalitis, meningitis and its complications, intracranial abscess, acute disseminated encephalomyelitis, hypoglycemia, mitochondrial disorder

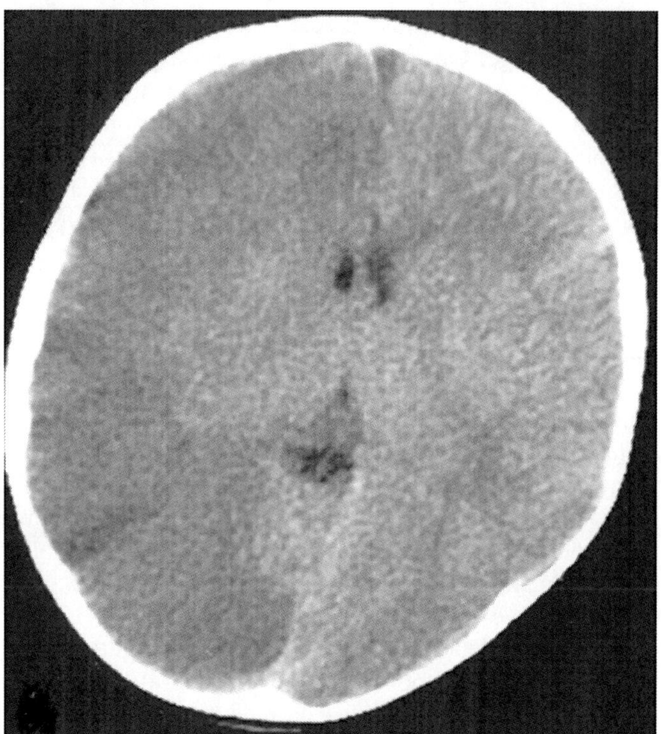

Fig. 28.5: Non-contrast CT head in a 2-year-old child with febrile focal status epilepticus (HHE syndrome). Note the acute hemispheric edema and mass effect on the lateral ventricles. (Compare the area of distribution with Fig. 28.1). The child later had hemispheric atrophy and focal epilepsy

(MELAS), developmental brain malformations and trauma. The pathogenesis is likely interplay between genetic predisposition; viral infection (e.g., influenza, HHV 6) or toxin (theophylline) exposure; excitotoxicity due to prolonged ictal activity; and contributory systemic factors such as fever, cytokine excess, hypoxia and ischemia (Mizuguchi *et al.*, 2007). However, there is currently no explanation of the unilateral involvement of acute edema in HHE syndrome. Possible explanations include altered maturation of corpus callosum, genetic factors (CACNA1A gene) and focal CNS infection by neurotrophic virus (Auvin *et al.*, 2012). Treatment during the early acute phase of the illness is mainly supportive. Most of the patients have severe intellectual disability and variable motor deficits (Mirsattari *et al.*, 2008). Surgical treatment for refractory epilepsy, especially in exclusive temporal lobe involvement may improve quality of life.

Febrile Infection-Related Epilepsy Syndrome (FIRES)

FIRES has also been referred to as new-onset refractory status epilepticus (NORSE), devastating epileptic encephalopathy in school-aged children (DESC), and acute encephalitis with refractory, repetitive partial seizures

(AERRPS). It typically affects children between 4 and 9 years of age. Onset is marked by a nonspecific febrile respiratory or gastrointestinal prodrome followed by encephalitis-like illness with seizures, which rapidly (often <24 hours) exacerbate into either status epilepticus or became frequent requiring high dose barbiturate or midazolam infusion and mechanical ventilation. The seizure types at the onset of the illness are mainly partial or secondarily generalized. The etiology is possibly autoimmune with neuronal hyperexcitability as the leading process rather than cerebral inflammatory damage (van Baalen *et al.*, 2010). Pathologic studies of the brain demonstrated gliosis but no features of encephalitis (van Baalen *et al.*, 2010). CSF may show mild pleocytosis. EEG shows focal, multifocal, or generalized interictal discharges and the ictal onset is usually temporal followed by frontal area (Mikaeloff *et al.*, 2006). Neuroimaging may be normal or show temporal, insular, or basal ganglia hyperintensities in acute stage followed by diffuse brain atrophy in later stages. The epileptic process in FIRES is difficult to control and mostly refractory to AEDs. Ketogenic diet has been shown to be effective in a few case reports (Nabbout *et al.*, 2010). There is not enough evidence to support the use of immune-modulatory therapy. The outcome of FIRES is poor, with death in one-third and refractory epilepsy, mental retardation and learning disabilities in more than two-thirds of the chronic phase patients (Kramer *et al.*, 2005).

Encephalopathy in Organ Failures

Hepatic Encephalopathy

Hepatic encephalopathy is a potentially reversible, neuropsychiatric syndrome resulting from diffuse brain dysfunction due to acute or chronic hepatic failure. The diagnosis requires exclusion of other known metabolic, infectious, intracranial vascular events or space-occupying lesions, which may present in a similar fashion. Acute fulminant liver failure in the absence of early jaundice may mimic drug intoxication and chronic liver failure may mimic a primary psychiatric disturbance due to the associated confusion, delirium and psychosis. The initial stages (stages I–II) are hyperkinetic and agitated and may be followed within hours by stupor with preservation of arousal (stage III), then coma and decorticate or decerebrate posturing (stage IV) (Angel *et al.*, 2008). The pathophysiology of hepatic encephalopathy is not known and has been attributed to elevated arterial and brain ammonia (Butterworth, 2002). Management of the encephalopathy associated with chronic liver failure includes treatment of any intercurrent infection, reversing any inciting triggers such as active gastrointestinal bleed, discontinuation of sedative medication, restriction of dietary protein and lowering blood ammonia (Poh and Chang, 2012).

Uremic Encephalopathy

Uremic encephalopathy is a diffuse, organic brain syndrome that occurs in patients with untreated renal failure due to glomerular, tubular, and parenchymal disturbances, as well as in patients undergoing dialysis. Uremia is linked to accumulation of toxins, anemia, increased inflammatory, and oxidative stress, producing reactive nitrogen species, disturbances in intermediate metabolism with impaired Na1/K1ATPase activity, and accumulation of intracellular Ca^{++}, parathormone and other hormones (Himmelfarb and Hakim, 2003).

Uremic encephalopathy develops in hours to days with fatigue, apathy, restlessness, emotional disturbances, insomnia, impaired memory and cognition, neuroendocrine dysregulation, agitation with aggravation to delirium, delusions, hallucinations, tremor, asterixis and multifocal myoclonus, generalized tonic-clonic seizures, and coma (Brouns and De Deyn, 2004; Lacerda *et al.*, 2010). "Frontal lobe" symptoms are manifest by impaired abstract thinking and behavioral change. Acute uremic encephalopathy reverses with hemodialysis or peritoneal dialysis. Acute encephalopathy can also occur during or immediately after dialysis caused primarily by cerebral edema resulting from overly rapid removal of urea during hemodialysis. This is known as dialysis disequilibrium syndrome and needs meticulous supportive care.

Acute Encephalopathy in Inborn Errors of Metabolism (IEM)

Deterioration of consciousness due to an underlying inherited metabolic disorder often occurs suddenly in a previously healthy child; the early signs may not be so obvious such as excessive drowsiness, unusual behavior or some unsteadiness; the illness may progress rapidly with marked fluctuations; there may be no focal neurological deficits and failure to recognize changes in vital signs may result in deepening of coma. A history of recurrent, unexplained, episodic deteriorations with unprovoked vomitings or impairment of consciousness should be considered as a strong indication for the evaluation of an inherited metabolic disorder. The first step in evaluating such patients is to categorize the presenting symptoms in one of the four common clinical phenotypes: hypoglycemia, intoxication, neurotransmitter defect and cellular energy metabolism defect phenotype. This is followed by routine biochemical tests to further discriminate a possible IEM. Combining the results of these two steps helps in diagnosing an inherited metabolic disorder with further specific testing as required. Importantly, completely normal diagnostic blood tests signify an IEM restricted to the brain compartment and hence, may not completely rule out an IEM.

Hypoglycemia Phenotype: During the intervals between meals, plasma glucose concentration is supported by increased glucose production (glycogenolysis and gluconeogenesis) and decreased peripheral glucose utilization (fatty acid and ketone oxidation). Understandably, hypoglycemia may occur as a result of primary or secondary defects in glucose production (glycogen storage disorders GSD) and defects in fatty acid or ketone oxidation. On the other hand, hyperinsulinism due to inherited or genetic causes leads to increased peripheral uptake and utilization of glucose and suppression of ketogenesis, glycogenolysis, and gluconeogenesis. This deprives the brain of its two primary energy sources: glucose and ketones (Aynsley-Green *et al.*, 2000). The relation of hypoglycemia to the last meal may help in suspecting the defect: onset within 1-2 hours is suggestive of hyperinsulinism; onset after 3-5 hours is suggestive of GSD, particularly type 1; onset after a longer feeding pause, overnight fasting, intercurrent infections is very suggestive of defect in gluconeogenesis or fatty acid oxidation. Hepatomegaly gives a clue towards GSD, gluconeogenetic and fatty acid oxidation disorders. Simultaneously elevated plasma lactate indicates a GSD or gluconeogenesis defect and low urinary ketones indicate a fatty acid oxidation defect.

The common symptoms include irritability, sweating, somnolence, apathy or seizures, especially in infants. Older children may present with hunger, apprehension, jitters, tachypnea, tremor, weakness, drowsiness and progression to coma or risk of permanent neurological damage (Cook and Walker, 2011). Treatment with intravenous glucose should not be delayed while evaluating the cause simultaneously.

Intoxication Phenotype: The common symptoms include nausea, vomiting, anorexia, dehydration, apathy, altered consciousness, hypotonia or spasticity, movement disorders (ataxia and dystonia), convulsions and coma. The common precipitants are an infection or trauma, surgery or substrate load. Signs of other organ dysfunctions may ensue, such as liver dysfunction, abnormal odors form body secretions, skin rash, alopecia, cardiomyopathy, pancreatitis, and bone marrow failure. Hepatomegaly, moderate to severe metabolic acidosis with lactic acidemia and hyperammonemia suggests an underlying organic acid disorder. Marked hyperammonemia with liver dysfunction and respiratory alkalosis suggests a urea cycle defect. Besides the signs of intoxication, and brain edema focal neurological abnormalities may be present, especially with metabolic strokes seen in mitochondrial or urea cycle disorders. Acute encephalopathy without hyperammonemia or significant metabolic acidosis in a child with failure to thrive and mild to moderate psychomotor retardation is typical of MSUD. It presents classically in the newborn period with acute, progressive leucine encephalopathy, maple syrup (burnt sugar) odor from body secretions, and spasticity by the end of the first week of life. Neonates with galactosemia may present with progressive encephalopathy, feed refusal and vomiting, jaundice and severe liver disturbance, and hypoglycemia typically by day 4-5 of life when fed on lactose-containing milks (Segal, 1998). Leigh's disease (subacute necrotizing encephalomyelitis) is a devastating recurrent encephalopathy with progressive psychomotor regression and brainstem dysfunction with necrotic lesions in the basal ganglia (Fig. 28.6), thalami, brainstem and spinal cord (Cook and Walker, 2011). Primary defects of fatty acid oxidation may present with Reye's-like

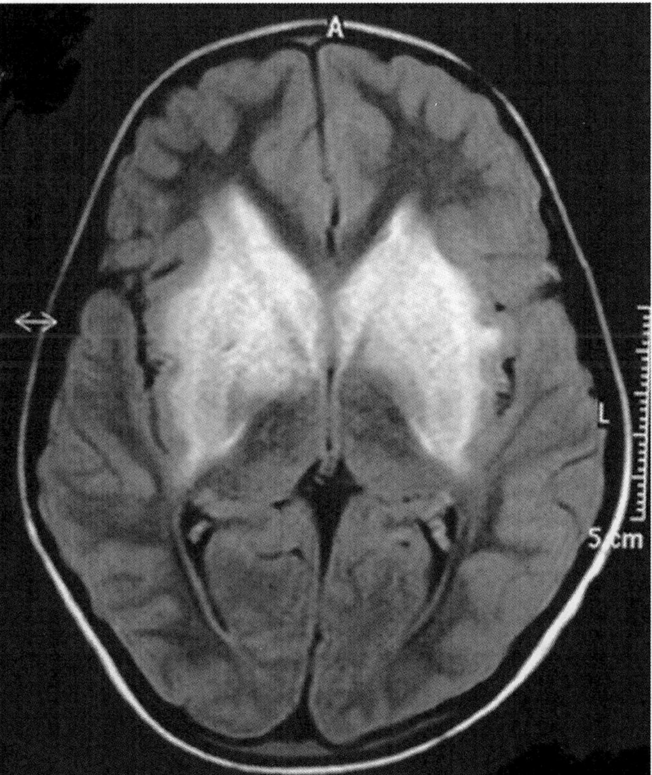

Fig. 28.6: Axial FLAIR MR image showing extensive hyperintense signal changes in bilateral basal ganglia in a child with a suspected inborn error of metabolism

encephalopathy following a mild prodromal illness and poor feeding. Drowsiness and lethargy progress rapidly to stupor and coma, hepatomegaly with hepatocellular dysfunction, hypotonia, hypoketotic hypoglycemia and mild to moderate hyperammonemia. A family history of SIDS or deaths due to cardiac dysrhythmias is highly suggestive.

Neurotransmitter Defect Phenotype: The common clinical symptoms may be limited to the central nervous system, present variably after birth and include convulsions, altered consciousness, movement disorders, abnormal muscle tone and coma. Routine biochemical tests and neuroimaging may be normal. An important differential diagnosis is CNS infections with sequelae and is excluded in the acute state by a normal lumbar puncture. The focus remains on diagnosing the common treatable disorders such as maple syrup urine disease (MSUD), vitamin-dependent epilepsies, glucose transporter defects, and late-onset non-ketotic hyperglycinemia. IEMS presenting as neonatal seizures due to secondary neurotransmitter alterations are many but treatment options are limited and confirmatory investigations are expensive.

Cellular Energy Metabolism Phenotype: Disorders in this category commonly involve several organs with higher metabolic requirements such as the brain, heart, skeletal muscle, liver, kidneys and gastrointestinal tract. Associated lactic acidemia indicates a serious problem in energy-producing processes. The prototypic disorder is mitochondrial encephalopathy (Zeviani and Di Donato, 2004). The common symptoms include hypotonia, skeletal and cardiac myopathies, seizures and multi-organ failure after birth, developmental delay, strokes (especially if recurrent), hypotonia, dementia, oculomotor abnormalities, endocrine, or hearing or feeding problems later; or neuroregression after infection or vaccinations. Defects of pyruvate dehydrogenase, respiratory chain and tricarboxylic acid cycle, may also cause brain damage in utero, and affected newborns may be dysmorphic. Lactate/pyruvate ratio and ketone bodies combined with metabolic tests of blood and urine can support a specific disorder in the group of cellular energy defects. Effective treatments are available for the glycogen storage disorders, gluconeogenic defects and a minority of pyruvate dehydrogenase complex defects.

Hypertensive Encephalopathy

The term "hypertensive encephalopathy" (HTE) signifies alteration of consciousness in hypertensive patients due to diffuse or multifocal CNS dysfunction in the absence of other obvious causes. Significant neurological complications including HTE, may develop in nearly 40% of patients and is related to the rapidity and severity of rise of blood pressure from baseline (Flynn and Falkner, 2009). Due to immature cerebral auto-regulation in younger children, even the mild rise of BP or fluctuations may precede neurological changes. The common clinical manifestations include severe generalized headache, projectile vomiting, meningismus, seizures, vision loss and variable focal neurological deficits. The encephalopathy may vary from confusion, irritability, and lethargy to frank coma. Retinal arteriolar vasospasm on fundus examination is the most reliable sign of HTE. Elevation of blood pressure by four standard deviations above the mean for age signifies HTE rather than due to raised ICP or seizures alone (Proulx *et al.*, 1993). Hypertension associated occipital blindness with other features of encephalopathy and transient motor deficits are termed posterior reversible leukoencephalopathy (PRES) (Fig. 28.7). The syndrome is due to defective cerebral auto-regulation leading to vasogenic edema predominantly in the posterior parieto-occipital cortical and subcortical areas. Other causes of PRES include chemotherapeutic and cytotoxic drugs, infection, shock, nephrotic state and systemic lupus erythematosus.

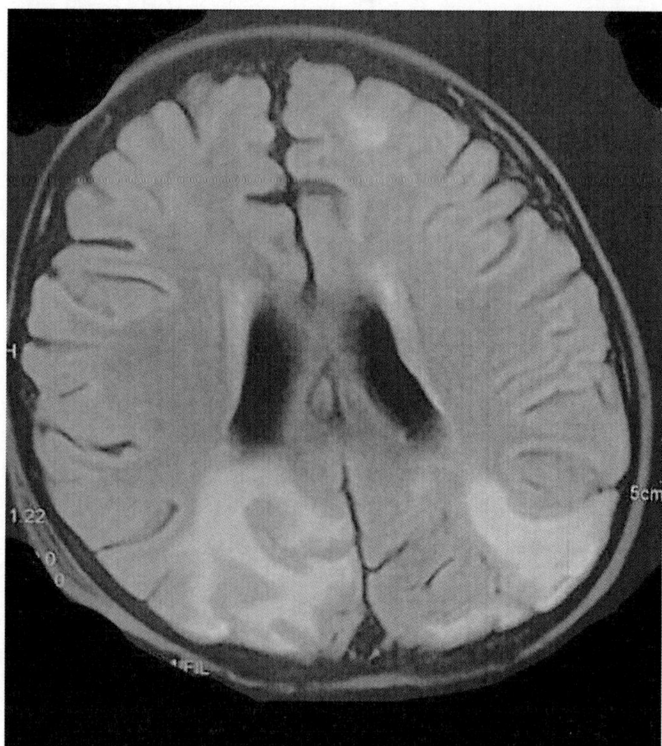

Fig. 28.7: Axial T2W MR image in a child with showing hyperintensities mainly in the parieto-occipital regions suggestive of posterior reversible leukoencephalopathy (PRES) in a child with severe hypertension and acute loss of vision

This form of malignant hypertension is rare in neonates and arises most commonly due to renal failure, congenital adrenal hyperplasia, or renovascular thrombosis. In children up to 1 year of age, coarctation of the aorta, polycystic kidneys, and renal/renovascular diseases predominate. In children older than one year of age, the most common causes of hypertension are inflammatory or infectious parenchymal renal disorders followed by reno-vascular anomalies and tumors such as Wilm's tumor and neuroblastoma. HTE should be suspected in any child with acute or subacute encephalopathy associated with acute hypertension, severe headache and funduscopic evidence of arteriolar spasm. Treatment consists of judicious use of antihypertensive drugs and a controlled lowering of blood pressure. Intravenous antihypertensive medications may be needed in the acute phase followed by oral drugs, partly depending on the underlying etiology of hypertension.

Non-Accidental Head Trauma

Non-Accidental Head Trauma or inflicted head injury is the most common cause of death as a result of physical child abuse. Infants and children may present non-specific neurological features in the absence of history of trauma. It is essential to recognize this condition to prevent misdiagnosis at the initial evaluation and protection and rehabilitation of these children later. The mechanism of cranial injury may be blunt force trauma, shaking or a combination. Infant or child may present with altered consciousness, vomitings, seizures, apnea, breathing difficulty or life-threatening events requiring resuscitation. The absence of a history of trauma has a high specificity (97%) and positive predictive value (0.92) for abusive head injury (Hettler and Greenes, 2003). Other clues in history may be a disproportionate lack of parental concern, history of similar episodes in the past, and changing or evanescent details of the events. The examination may be normal or reveal multiple injury marks in the absence of corroborative history. However, the presence of retinal hemorrhages signals intracranial injury. Associated injuries, especially of the musculoskeletal system, should be looked for (Piteau *et al.*, 2012). The diagnosis requires a high index of suspicion. Intracranial injury with any three of the following, viz., apnea, bruising, long-bone fracture, rib fracture, retinal hemorrhage, or seizures, confers significant probability for Non-Accidental Head Trauma (Maguire *et al.*, 2011). Bleeding diathesis and serious CNS infections must be ruled out by relevant investigations. Neuroimaging is essential in suspected cases to establish the diagnosis, determine the extent and severity of injury and identify impending herniation syndromes. The CT findings significantly associated with inflicted head trauma include multiple subdural hemorrhages of different ages, inter-hemispheric or posterior fossa location, HIE and cerebral edema (Kemp *et al.*, 2011). Skeletal survey to identify pathognomonic skeletal injuries such as posterior rib and metaphyseal fractures aids the diagnosis. Multidisciplinary management including pediatrician, nurse and social worker, child psychologist and counselor, orthopedicians, and neurosurgeons may be needed. Inflicted head injury must be differentiated from accidental injury, birth trauma, bleeding disorders, apparent life-threatening events due to cardiac rhythm disturbances or similar causes, and rare metabolic disorders such as Menkes' disease in males and glutaric aciduria in children with subdural effusions on neuroimaging. Long-term neurological morbidity is significant in the form of motor deficits, blindness, psychomotor delays and intellectual disability (Bonnier *et al.*, 1995).

Prognosis in Children with Acute Encephalopathy

The outcome of children with encephalopathies depends on the etiology, depth and duration of impaired consciousness. Intoxications and infectious encephalopathies have relatively better outcomes, often surviving with no or mild to moderate difficulties only (Grimwood *et al.*, 2000; Lahat *et al.*, 1999). However, prolonged encephalopathy after a hypoxic-ischemic insult carries a poor prognosis (Kriel *et al.*, 1994). Outcomes have been worse in children who were younger, had lower GCS scores on presentation, or absent brainstem reflexes, hypothermia or hypotension (Johnston and Seshia, 1984). In a study of 283 episodes of pediatric coma (defined as GCS <12 for at least 6 hours), mortality at 1 year ranged from 3% (intoxication) to 84% (accident), depending on etiology (Wong *et al.*, 2001). A follow-up of all children for early identification of developmental, learning, behavioral or cognitive problems as well as seizures, motor, visual or hearing sequelae should be done.

CONCLUSION

Non-infectious causes constitute an essential cause of encephalopathy in emergency department. Encephalopathy may result from primary/direct insult to the cerebral cortex, diencephalic structures, midbrain or rostral pons; or a secondary manifestation of systemic derangements or interplay of multiple interrelated factors in a child. Profound encephalopathy may result from even small lesions in the upper brainstem. The management of encephalopathic child in an emergency setting remains a challenge in terms of etiological diagnosis, assessment and interventions. A pragmatic and expeditious approach to diagnostic and therapeutic interventions helps minimize further neurological impairments.

Suggested Reading

- Ali AM, Al-Abdulgader A, Kamal HM and Al-Wehedy A. Traumatic and Non-traumatic Coma in Children in the Referral Hospital, Al-Hasa, Saudi Arabia. East Mediterr Health J 2007: 13(3):608-14.
- Angel MJ, Chen R and Young GB (2008). Handbook of Clinical Neurology (Vol. 90): Elsevier B.V. All rights reserved.
- Ashkenazi S, Yuhas Y, Even-Tov S, Kaminsky E and Danon YL. The Effect of Shiga Toxin and Sonicates of Shigella Isolates from Children with Neurologic Manifestation on Neuroblastoma Cell Lines. Isr J Med Sci 1994;30(8):604-10.
- Auvin S, Bellavoine V, Merdariu D, Delanoe C, Elmaleh-Berges M, Gressens P and Boespflug-Tanguy O. Hemiconvulsion-Hemiplegia-epilepsy Syndrome: Current Understandings. Eur J Paediatr Neurol 2012:16(5):413-21.
- Aynsley-Green A, Hussain K, Hall J, Saudubray JM, Nihoul-Fekete C, De Lonlay-Debeney P, Brunelle F, Otonkoski T, Thornton P and Lindley KJ. Practical Management of Hyperinsulinism in Infancy, Arch Dis Child Fetal Neonatal Ed 2000;82(2):F98-F107.
- Bansal A, Singhi SC, Singhi PD, Khandelwal N and Ramesh S. Non Traumatic Coma, Indian J Pediatr 2005;72(6):467-73.
- Birbeck GL, Molyneux ME, Kaplan PW, Seydel KB, Chimalizeni YF, Kawaza K and Taylor TE. Blantyre Malaria Project Epilepsy Study (BMPES) of Neurological Outcomes in Retinopathy-positive Paediatric Cerebral Malaria Survivors: A Prospective Cohort Study, Lancet Neurol 2010;9(12):1173-81.
- Bonnier C, Nassogne MC and Evrard P. Outcome and Prognosis of Whiplash Shaken Infant Syndrome; Late Consequences After a Symptom-free Interval. Dev Med Child Neurol 1995;37(11):943-56.
- Brouns R and De Deyn PP. Neurological Complications in Renal Failure: A Review, Clin Neurol Neurosurg 2004;107(1): 1-16.
- Butler T, Islam A, Kabir I, and Jones PK. Patterns of Morbidity and Mortality in Typhoid Fever Dependent on Age and Gender: Review of 552 Hospitalized Patients with Diarrhea, Rev Infect Dis 1991:13(1):85-90.
- Butterworth RF. Pathophysiology of Hepatic Ence-phalopathy: A New Look at Ammonia, Metab Brain Dis 2002;17(4):221-27.
- Cook P and Walker V. Investigation of the Child with an Acute Metabolic Disorder. J Clin Pathol 2011;64(3):181-91.
- Dalmau J, Anti-NMDA Receptor Encephalitis: Pathogenic Mechanisms and Treatment Algorithm. Rinsho Shinkeigaku 2012;52(11):978.
- Davies NW, Sharief MK and Howard RS. Infection-Associated Encephalopathies: Their Investigation, Diagnosis and Treatment. J Neurol 2006;253(7):833-45.
- Ely EW, Inouye SK, Bernard GR, Gordon S, Francis J, May L, Truman B, Speroff T, Gautam S, Margolin R, Hart RP, and Dittus R. Delirium in Mechanically Ventilated Patients: Validity and Reliability of the Confusion Assessment Method for the Intensive Care Unit (CAM-ICU). JAMA 2001;286(21): 2703-10.
- Ephros M, Cohen D, Yavzori M, Rotman N, Novic B and Ashkenazi S. Encephalopathy Associated with Enteroinvasive Escherichia coli 0144: NM Infection. J Clin Microbiol 1996; 34(10):2432-34.
- Florance NR, Davis RL, Lam C, Szperka C, Zhou L, Ahmad S, Campen CJ, Moss H, Peter N, Gleichman AJ, Glaser CA, Lynch DR, Rosenfeld MR and Dalmau J. Anti-N-methyl-D-aspartate Receptor (NMDAR) Encephalitis in Children and Adolescents. Ann Neurol 2009;66(1):11-18.
- Flynn JT and Falkner BE. Should the Current Approach to the Evaluation and Treatment of High Blood Pressure in Children be Changed? J Pediatr 2009;155(2):157-58.
- Fouad H, Haron M, Halawa EF and Nada M. Nontraumatic Coma in A Tertiary Pediatric Emergency Department in Egypt: Etiology and Outcome. J Child Neurol 2011;26(2):136-41.
- Gofton TE and Young GB. Sepsis-Associated Ence-phalopathy, Nat Rev Neurol 2012;8(10):557-66.
- Goren A, Freier S and Passwell JH. Lethal Toxic Encephalopathy Due to Childhood Shigellosis in a Developed Country, Pediatrics 1992;89(6 Pt 2):1189-93.
- Grimwood K, Anderson P, Anderson V, Tan L and Nolan T. Twelve Year Outcomes Following Bacterial Meningitis: Further Evidence for Persisting Effects. Arch Dis Child 2000; 83(2):111-16.
- Hettler J and Greenes DS. Can the Initial History Predict Whether a Child with a Head Injury Has Been Abused? Pediatrics 2003;111(3):602-07.
- Himmelfarb J and Hakim RM. Oxidative stress in uremia. Curr Opin Nephrol Hypertens 2003;12(6):593-98.
- Hoffman SL, Punjabi NH, Kumala S, Moechtar MA, Pulungsih SP, Rivai AR, Rockhill RC, Woodward TE and Loedin AA. Reduction of Mortality in Chloramphenicol-Treated Severe Typhoid Fever by High-Dose Dexamethasone. N Engl J Med 1984;310(2):82-88.
- Iacobone E, Bailly-Salin J, Polito A, Friedman D, Stevens RD and Sharshar T. Sepsis-associated Encephalopathy and Its Differential Diagnosis, Crit Care Med 37(10 Suppl) 2009; S331-336.
- Janz DR, Abel TW, Jackson JC, Gunther ML, Heckers S and Ely EW. Brain Autopsy Findings in Intensive Care Unit Patients Previously Suffering from Delirium: A Pilot Study J Crit Care 2010;25(3):538:e537-12.
- Johnston B and Seshia SS. Prediction of Outcome in Non-traumatic Coma in Childhood. Acta Neurol Scand 1984; 69(6):417-27.
- Kanade T and Shah I. Dengue Encephalopathy. J Vector Borne Dis 2011;48(3):180-81.
- Kankirawatana P, Chokephaibulkit K, Puthavathana P, Yoksan S, Apintanapong S and Pongthapisit V. Dengue Infection Presenting with Central Nervous System Manifestation. J Child Neurol 2000;15(8):544-47.

- Kemp AM, Jaspan T, Griffiths J, Stoodley N, Mann MK, Tempest V and Maguire SA. Neuroimaging: What Neuroradiological Features Distinguish Abusive from Non-Abusive Head Trauma? A Systematic Review. Arch Dis Child 2011;96(12):1103-12.
- Kramer NM, Horwitz EM, Cheng J, Ridge JA, Feigenberg SJ, Cohen RB, Nicolaou N, Sherman EJ, Babb JS, Damsker JA and Langer CJ. Toxicity and Outcome Analysis of Patients with Recurrent Head and Neck Cancer Treated with Hyperfractionated Split-Course Reirradiation and Concurrent Cisplatin and paclitaxel Chemotherapy from Two Prospective Phase I and II Studies. Head Neck 2005;27(5):406-14.
- Kraus JF, Black MA, Hessol N, Ley P, Rokaw W, Sullivan C, Bowers S, Knowlton S and Marshall L. The Incidence of Acute Brain Injury and Serious Impairment in a Defined Population. Am J Epidemiol 1984;119(2):186-201.
- Kriel RL, Krach LE, Luxemberg MG, Jones-Saete C and Sanchez J. Outcome of Severe Anoxic/Ischemic Brain Injury in Children. Pediatr Neurol 1994;10(3):207-12.
- Krupp LB, Banwell B and Tenembaum S. Consensus Definitions Proposed for Pediatric Multiple Sclerosis and Related Disorders, Neurology 2007;68(16 Suppl 2), S7-12.
- Lacerda G, Krummel T and Hirsch E. Neurologic Presentations of Renal Diseases. Neurol Clin 2010;28(1):45-59.
- Lahat E, Barr J, Barkai G, Paret G, Brand N and Barzilai A. Long Term Neurological Outcome of Herpes Encephalitis. Arch Dis Child 1999;80(1):69-71.
- Lum LC, Lam SK, Choy YS, George R and Harun F. Dengue Encephalitis: A True Entity? Am J Trop Med Hyg 1996;54(3):256-59.
- Maguire SA, Kemp AM, Lumb RC and Farewell DM. Estimating the Probability of Abusive Head Trauma: A Pooled Analysis. Pediatrics 2011;128(3):e550-64.
- Mikaeloff Y, Jambaque I, Hertz-Pannier L, Zamfirescu A, Adamsbaum C, Plouin P, Dulac O and Chiron C. Devastating Epileptic Encephalopathy in School-aged Children (DESC): A Pseudo Encephalitis. Epilepsy Res 2006;69(1):67-79.
- Mirsattari SM, Wilde NJ and Pigott SE. Long-Term Cognitive Outcome of Hemiconvulsion-Hemiplegia-Epilepsy Syndrome Affecting the Left Cerebral Hemisphere. Epilepsy Behav 2008;13(4):678-80.
- Mizuguchi M. Acute Necrotizing Encephalopathy of Childhood: A Novel form of Acute Encephalopathy Prevalent in Japan and Taiwan. Brain Dev 1997;19(2):81-92.
- Mizuguchi M, Yamanouchi H, Ichiyama T and Shiomi M. Acute Encephalopathy Associated with Influenza and Other Viral Infections. Acta Neurol Scand Suppl 2007;186(45-56).
- Nabbout R, Mazzuca M, Hubert P, Peudennier S, Allaire C, Flurin V, Aberastury M, Silva W and Dulac O. Efficacy of Ketogenic Diet in Severe Refractory Status Epilepticus Initiating Fever Induced Refractory Epileptic Encephalopathy in School age Children (FIRES). Epilepsia 2010;51(10): 2033-37.
- Nabbout R, Vezzani A, Dulac O and Chiron C. Acute Encephalopathy with Inflammation-Mediated Status Epilepticus. Lancet Neurol 2011;10(1):99-108.
- Neilson DE, Adams MD, Orr CM, Schelling DK, Eiben RM, Kerr DS, Anderson J, Bassuk AG, Bye AM, Childs A M, Clarke A, Crow YJ, Di Rocco M, Dohna-Schwake C, Dueckers G, Fasano AE, Gika AD, Gionnis D, Gorman MP, Grattan-Smith PJ, Hackenberg A, Kuster A, Lentschig MG, Lopez-Laso E, Marco EJ, Mastroyianni S, Perrier J, Schmitt-Mechelke T, Servidei S, Skardoutsou A, Uldall P, van der Knaap MS, Goglin KC, Tefft DL, Aubin C, de Jager P, Hafler D and Warman M L. Infection-Triggered Familial or Recurrent Cases of Acute Necrotizing Encephalopathy Caused by Mutations in a Component of the Nuclear Pore, RANBP2. Am J Hum Genet 2009;84(1):44-51.
- NINDS. National Institutes of Health Encephalopathy Information Page 2010; *http://www.ninds.nih.gov/disorders/encephalopathy/encephalopathy.htm.*
- Okumura A, Mizuguchi M, Kidokoro H, Tanaka M, Abe S, Hosoya M, Aiba H, Maegaki Y, Yamamoto H, Tanabe T, Noda E, Imataka G and Kurahashi H. Outcome of Acute Necrotizing Encephalopathy in Relation to Treatment with Corticosteroids and Gammaglobulin. Brain Dev 2009;31(3):221-27.
- Perles Z, Bar-Ziv J and Granot E. Brain Edema: An Underdiagnosed Complication of Shigella Infection. Pediatr Infect Dis J 1995;14(12):1114-15.
- Piteau SJ, Ward MG, Barrowman NJ and Plint AC. Clinical and Radiographic Characteristics Associated with Abusive and Nonabusive Head Trauma: A systematic Review, Pediatrics 2012;130(2):315-23.
- Poh Z and Chang PE. A Current Review of the Diagnostic and Treatment Strategies of Hepatic Encephalopathy. Int J Hepatol 2012;480309.
- Pourakbari B, Mamishi S, Kohan L, Sedighi L, Mahmoudi S, Fattahi F and Teymuri M. Lethal Toxic Encephalopathy Due to Childhood Shigellosis or Ekiri Syndrome, J Microbiol Immunol Infect 2012;45(2):147-50.
- Proulx F, Lacroix J, Farrell CA and Gauthier M. Convulsions and Hypertension in Children: Differentiating Cause from Effect. Crit Care Med 1993;21(10):1541-46.
- Sankhyan N, Sharma S, Kamate M and Subramanian S. Teaching NeuroImage: Hemiconvulsion-hemiplegia-epilepsy syndrome: Sequential MRI Follow-up. Neurology 2008; 71(11):e28.
- Segal S. Komrower Lecture. Galactosaemia today: The Enigma and the Challenge. J Inherit Metab Dis 1998;21(5):455-71.
- Sofiah A and Hussain IH. Childhood Non-traumatic Coma in Kuala Lumpur, Malaysia. Ann Trop Paediatr 1997;17(4): 327-31.
- Solomon T, Dung NM, Vaughn DW, Kneen R, Thao LT, Raengsakulrach B, Loan HT, Day NP, Farrar J, Myint KS, Warrell MJ, James WS, Nisalak A and White NJ. Neurological Manifestations of Dengue Infection Lancet 2000; 355(9209): 1053-59.

- Srivastava A, Peshin SS, Kaleekal T and Gupta SK. An Epidemiological Study of Poisoning Cases Reported to the National Poisons Information Centre, All India Institute of Medical Sciences, New Delhi. Hum Exp Toxicol 2005;24(6): 279-85.
- Stevens RD and Nyquist PA. Coma, Delirium and Cognitive Dysfunction in Critical Illness. Crit Care Clin 2006;22(4):787-804; abstract x.
- Takanashi J. Two Newly Proposed Infectious Encephalitis/ encephalopathy Syndromes. Brain Dev 2009;31(7):521-28.
- Tasker RC, Matthew DJ, Helms P, Dinwiddie R and Boyd S. Monitoring in Non-traumatic Coma, Part I: Invasive Intracranial Measurements. Arch Dis Child 1988;63(8):888-94.
- Taylor D and Ashwal S. Pediatric Neurology: Principles and Practice (4th ed.). Philadelphia Elsevier Publications 2006.
- Tenembaum S, Chitnis T, Ness J and Hahn JS. Acute Disseminated Encephalomyelitis. Neurology 68(16 Suppl 2) 2007:S23-36.
- Titulaer MJ, McCracken L, Gabilondo I, Armangue T, Glaser C, Iizuka T, Honig LS, Benseler SM, Kawachi I, Martinez-Hernandez E, Aguilar E, Gresa-Arribas N, Ryan-Florance N, Torrents A, Saiz A, Rosenfeld MR, Balice-Gordon R, Graus F and Dalmau J. Treatment and Prognostic Factors for Long-term Outcome in Patients with anti-NMDA Receptor Encephalitis: An Observational Cohort Study. Lancet Neurol 2013;12(2):157-65.
- van Baalen A, Hausler M, Boor R, Rohr A, Sperner J, Kurlemann G, Panzer A, Stephani U and Kluger G. Febrile Infection-related Epilepsy Syndrome (FIRES): A Nonencephalitic Encephalopathy in Childhood. Epilepsia 2010;51(7):1323-28.
- van der Heyde HC, Nolan J, Combes V, Gramaglia I and Grau GE. A Unified Hypothesis for the Genesis of Cerebral Malaria: Sequestration, Inflammation and Hemostasis Leading to Microcirculatory Dysfunction. Trends Parasitol 2006;22(11): 503-08.
- Wang HS and Huang SC. Acute Necrotizing Encephalopathy of Childhood. Chang Gung Med J 2001;24(1):1-10.
- Wingerchuk DM. Postinfectious Encephalomyelitis. Curr Neurol Neurosci Rep 2003;3(3):256-64.
- Wong CP, Forsyth RJ, Kelly TP and Eyre JA. Incidence, Aetiology and Outcome of Non-Traumatic Coma: A Population Based Study. Arch Dis Child 2001;84(3):193-99.
- Zeviani M and Di Donato S. Mitochondrial Disorders. Brain 2004;127(Pt 10):2153-72.

29 Chapter

MOVEMENT DISORDERS

N Thilothammal

Pediatric movement disorders (PMD) is a group of disorders that occur in pediatric age. Their main symptoms are pathological movements that cannot be fully initiated, modulated or interrupted voluntarily. Involuntary movements caused by epileptic, cerebellar, pyramidal and neuromuscular disorders are excluded.

NEUROANATOMY AND NEUROCHEMICAL BASIS

Most movement disorders can be attributed to dysfunction of the basal ganglia or to regions of the brain that are intimately interconnected with the basal ganglia. The basal ganglia represent a network that include the striatum (caudate, putamen, nucleus accumbens), the subthalamic nucleus, the globus pallidus (GP), and the substantia nigra.

Most of the movement disorders of basal ganglia origin are circuit disorders that result in impaired ability to facilitate desired movements, inhibit unwanted movements, or both.[1] Lesions or developmental abnormalities in one region can result in dysfunction of the entire circuit. For example, dystonia may result from lesions in striatum (putamen or caudate), globus pallidus, or thalamus.[2] These may subsequently lead to dysfunction in the cerebral cortex and brainstem.

Basal ganglia circuitry is not limited to the motor domain, but also includes circuits involved in cognitive and affective function. Thus, many movement disorders of basal ganglia origin are accompanied by cognitive, affective, or behavioral dysfunction.

Most excitatory synapses of the basal ganglia and its connections use glutamate as neurotransmitter. Dopamine is the major neurotransmitter in the nigrostriatal dopamine system. Other important transmitters in these circuits include GABA, acetylcholine, norepinephrine and serotonin, and most pharmacologic treatments for movement disorders are targeted at these neurotransmitters.[3]

Types of Movement Disorders

By convention, movement disorders are divided into two major categories. The first is hyperkinetic movement disorders, sometimes referred to as dyskinesias. This includes tics, chorea/ballismus, dystonia, myoclonus, stereotypies and tremor. The second category is hypokinetic movement disorders, sometimes referred to as akinetic/rigid disorders.[4] The primary movement disorder in this category is parkinsonism, manifested primarily in adulthood as Parkinson disease or one of many forms of secondary parkinsonism. Hypokinetic disorders are relatively uncommon in children (Table 29.1).

Table 29.1: Phenomenologic Classification of Movement Disorders

Movement Disorder	Brief Description
Tics	Stereotyped intermittent, sudden, discrete, repetitive, nonrhythmic movements, most frequently involving head and upper body.
Chorea/ballismus	Chaotic, random, repetitive, brief, purposeless movements. Rapid, but not as rapid as myoclonus. When of very large amplitude, choreic limb movements often are called ballismus.
Dystonia	Repetitive, sustained, abnormal postures and movements. Abnormal postures typically have a twisting quality.
Myoclonus	Sudden, brief, shocklike movements that may be repetitive or rhythmic.
Stereotypy	Patterned, episodic, repetitive, purposeless, rhythmic movements.
Tremor	Rhythmic oscillation about a central point or position involving one or more body parts.
Parkinsonism	Hypokinetic syndrome characterized by rest tremor, slow movement (bradykinesia), rigidity and postural instability.

DIAGNOSIS OF PEDIATRIC MOVEMENT DISORDERS

History

1. A positive family history suggestive of dominant genetic disorder, or the presence of consanguinity that may suggest a recessive condition, are to be carefully looked for.
2. The presence of perinatal antecedents of neonatal encephalopathy or neonatal icterus is also of interest as it may explain such disorders as athetosis or dystonia.
3. Information about the age or onset of the disorder, its initial manifestations and course (acute onset, slow progression, spontaneous improvement) are essential.
4. Attention should also be given to the possibility of precipitating factors (drugs, infections, muscular exercise) or of aggravating (e.g., effect of fatigue, diurnal fluctuation) or ameliorating factors (e.g., sleep).
5. Photographs and, especially, videotapes of patients are of extreme value and every effort should be made to look at these.
6. Abnormal movements that interfere and those do not interfere with voluntary movements should be noted down. Rigid-hypokinetic syndrome, dystonia, tremor, myoclonus, chorea and ballismus interfere with voluntary movements.Whereas, tics and stereotypies do not interfere with voluntary movements.

Recognition of Abnormal Movement

Attempt is made to recognize the pattern of abnormal movement disorders from the clinical features.

Classify the Movement Disorder

In a primary disorder, the abnormal movements are the sole symptoms where only molecular studies will contribute to the diagnosis. In secondary disorders, abnormal movements are associated with other neurological and/or extra-neurological symptoms and investigations like neuroimaging and biochemical studies are useful diagnostic tools.

Recognize the Unique Features of Abnormal Movements

Each movement disorder may have some peculiar feature and it will be useful in making the diagnosis (Table 29.2).

Table 29.2: Some Peculiarities of the Main Types of Abnormal Movements

Rigid-hypokinetic	**Rarely full syndrome before 12 years of age**
Athetosis	Hand located
Dystonia	Task-specific (writing but not feeding: walking forward but not backward) Sensory tricks 'geste antagoniste' suppress dystonia
Tremor	Other abnormal movements that may be rhythmic: Myoclonus, stereotypies
Myoclonus	Chorea, tics, dystonia may appear as myoclonus
Tics	Are semi voluntary, do not interfere with voluntary movements
Stereotypies	Sometimes can be semi voluntary. Can be non-rhythmic Do not interfere with voluntary movement

CHOREA

Chorea is characterized by frequent, brief, unpredictable, purposeless movements that tend to flow from one body part to another body part. The movements of chorea are more chaotic and less brief and than myoclonus. They are briefer than the sustained contractions of dystonia. When of low amplitude, chorea may cause the appearance of fidgeting, but when they are of large amplitude, chorea can involve dramatic, flinging limb movements. When the amplitude is very large, the term ballismus is used. Choreic movements can be sudden and jerky or continuous and flowing. In the latter case, the term choreoathetosis is used. The term "choreiform" or "minimal chorea" is used to describe the minimal twitching or "piano playing" movements seen in many normal young children when arms are extended during the neurologic examination.[4]

Causes

Chorea can be classified by cause into primary and secondary disorders (Table 29.3). Primary chorea, which is uncommon in childhood, can be caused by benign familial (here-ditary) chorea and Huntington disease. Huntington disease rarely presents in childhood with chorea; juvenile-onset Huntington disease usually is characterized by parkinsonism and dystonia. Most chorea in childhood are secondary.

Table 29.3: Causes of Secondary Chorea

Metabolic	**Toxins**
Hypo/Hypernatremia	Manganese
Hypo/Hyperglycemia	Methanol

Contd.

Contd.

Hypocalcemia	Carbon monoxide
Hyperthyroidism	**Heredodegenerative Disease**
Perinatal Hypoxia-Ischemia	Ataxia telangiectasia
Infectious	Niemann-Pick type C
Rheumatic fever	Gangliosidoses
Human immunodeficiency virus	Lesch-Nyhan disease
Epstein-Barr virus	
Viral encephalitis	
Psychogenic	
Vascular	
Antiphospholipid antibody syndrome	
Stroke	
Global hypoxia	
Moyamoya syndrome	

Sydenham Chorea (Rheumatic Chorea)

Chorea is one of the major Jones criteria for diagnosing acute Rheumatic Fever (ARF). In fact, the presence of chorea without any other criteria is sufficient to make the diagnosis. Although it is widely accepted that chorea can follow group A beta hemolytic streptococci (GABHS) infection, it can be difficult to demonstrate the antecedent infection. Depending on the series, 10% to 40% of children who have ARF have chorea. Sydenham chorea (SC) is most common in children aged 5 to 15 years. There is a 2:1 female predominance after 10 years of age. SC begins several weeks to several months after a GABHS infection.

The onset of symptoms usually is insidious, with gradually progressive clumsiness and behavior change, usually accompanied by emotional lability. After a week or more, choreic movements become more obvious and typically become generalized. There frequently is asymmetry, and in some cases, the chorea can be unilateral. Hypotonia and dysarthria commonly accompany the chorea. Behavioral changes may be striking and include impulsivity, aggression, and obsessive compulsive behaviors. The typical natural history of SC is weeks to months of a waxing and waning course, with ultimate resolution of the chorea. Some individuals have behavioral changes that persist for months. Relapse can occur with or without subsequent GABHS infection.[5]

Diagnosis

It is based on clinical history and can be supported by laboratory data. However, laboratory data should not be viewed as confirmatory. Most affected children have positive serology (antistreptolysin O and antiDNase B antibodies) for GABHS, but more than 25% are serologically negative. Most children who have SC have negative throat cultures for GABHS. Magnetic resonance imaging may show signal abnormalities in the basal ganglia, but diagnostically this technique is neither sensitive nor specific for SC. The presence of carditis or other manifestations of ARF supports the diagnosis of SC. Every child believed to have SC should be evaluated for rheumatic heart disease. Carditis is present in 40% to 75% of children who have SC. Arthritis is less common. SC is usually self limited disorder but recurrences, probably not all related to rheumatic fever, are described in about 40% of the patients.[6]

Treatment

Treatment of SC depends on the impairment or disability associated with the chorea. In many cases, the chorea causes only mild disability, and symptomatic treatment is not required because SC is usually selflimited.

When symptomatic treatment is desired, antiepileptic medications such as carbamazepine or valproate can be effective and usually associated with fewer adverse effects than phenothiazines or butyrophenones. Benzodiazepines and atypical antipsychotics such as risperidone and olanzapine also may be beneficial. Symptomatic treatment for 2 to 4 months generally is sufficient. Some authors have advocated the use of corticosteroids, IVIG, or plasma exchange based on the presumed autoimmune cause. Penicillin prophylaxis to prevent repeated bouts of GABHS is recommended.

Tics

Tics are the most prevalent pediatric movement disorder and is common in boys. It is defined as stereotyped, intermittent, sudden, discrete, repetitive movements which are briefly suppressible and usually associated with a premonitory urge. Movements that involve skeletal muscle are termed "motor" tics; those that involve the diaphragm or laryngeal-pharyngeal muscles, producing a sound, are termed "phonic" or "vocal" tics. Tics occur many times a day, nearly every day. They typically change anatomic location, frequency, type, complexity, and severity over time.

Tics can be classified by mode of manifestation (motor or vocal) and complexity (simple or complex) (Table 29.4). Motor tics can be classified further by speed and quality as clonic (abrupt and fast) or dystonic/tonic (slow and sustained).

Table 29.4: Classification and Diagnosis of Tic Disorders (DSM-IV)

• Transient Tic Disorder (<1 year duration; diagnosis made retrospectively) • Motor • Vocal • Motor and vocal
• Chronic Tic Disorder (>1 year duration) • Motor (common) • Vocal (rare)
• Tourette Syndrome (TS) • Motor and vocal (at some point, but not necessarily, concurrently)

Simple motor tics include blinking, nose twitching, grimacing, neck jerking, shoulder elevation, sustained eye closure, gaze shifts, bruxism, and abdominal tensing. Simple vocal tics include sniffing, throat clearing, grunting, squeaking, humming, coughing, blowing and sucking sounds.

Complex tics appear more "purposeful" than simple tics and may include combinations of movements of multiple body parts. Examples are head shaking, trunk flexion, scratching, touching, finger tapping, hitting, jumping, kicking, and gestures (obscene gestures are termed copropraxia). Complex vocal tics can encompass spoken syllables words or phrases; shouting of obscenities or profanities (coprolalia); repetition of the words of others (echolalia); and repetition of the final syllable, word, or phrase of one's own words (palillalia).[7]

Clinical Features

Median age of onset of tic is about 6 to 7 years. Tic has been reported at 2 years of age. The most common presenting tic is eye blinking. Typically, vocal tics emerge later than motor tics. Tics worsen, with peak severity occurring around 10 to 12 years of age. By age 18 years, approximately 50% of chronic tic disorder patients are tic-free. Tic severity in childhood does not predict adult severity.

Tics frequently are preceded by a premonitory sensation or urge, and performance of the tic usually is followed by a sense of relief. The common occurrence of eye blinking, sniffing, and throat clearing tics preceded by the sensation of an itch leads to the frequent misdiagnosis of tics as allergic symptoms. The premonitory urge is manifested nonspecifically as a sense of anxiety and it may create greater morbidity than the tic itself and, therefore, represents the reason to treat.

Some individuals can suppress tics for limited periods of time. The ability to suppress tics is its unique feature. Voluntary tic suppression often is at a cost of rising anxiety or discomfort and usually requires such active concentration that it may prevent the patient from attending to other tasks. Thus, voluntary suppression is not a useful strategy for managing tics.

A hallmark of tics is variable severity over time. Tics tend to occur in bouts, with interspersed periods of quiescence. Often a pre-existing tic abates as a new tic emerges. Tics tend to wax and wane over weeks to months. Tic severity seems to be modulated by environmental stimuli, stress, intercurrent infection and poor sleep.

Causes of Tics

Most individuals who have tics have a primary tic disorder. Transient tic disorder is the most common; TS is the second most common. Secondary tic disorders do exist, but they are uncommon.

Gilles Dela Tourette Syndrome

Tourette's syndrome (TS) is a familial neuropsychiatric disorder characterized by motor and phonics that begin in childhood. New scientific knowledge in the last decade suggests that TS and related tic disorder are more common and debilitating. TS symptomatology that extends beyond the tic disorder probably include obsessive compulsive disorder, attention-deficit hyperactivity disorder, and anxiety disorders.

Diagnostic Criteria for Tourette's Disorder (DSM-IV-TR™)

a. Both multiple motor one or more vocal tics have been present at some time during the illness although not necessarily concurrently. (A tic is a sudden, rapid, recurrent, non-rhythmic, motor movement or vocalization).

b. The tics occur many times a day (usually in bouts), nearly every day, or intermittently through a period of more than 1 year, and during this period there was never a tic-free period of more than three consecutive months.

c. The onset is before age 18 years.

d. The disturbance is not caused by the direct physiological effects of a substance or disease (e.g., Huntington's disease or post-viral encephalitis).

Tics are very common in children. About 5% of school-aged children have tics, with an estimated prevalence of

4%-19% . The estimated prevalence of TS is 3.0 per 1000, three times more in boys than in girls.[7]

Tics are usually intermittent, but may be repetitive stereotypic. Typically, they are emitted in bouts of several tics, separated by period of normal behavior lasting seconds to hours. Important characteristics of tics include: suggestibility, increases with stress (e.g., test taking) or relaxation, decrease with distraction and concentration, and persist during all stage of sleep. In childhood it is common for tics to increase with intercurrent illness during transitions (e.g., vacation, school year begins/ends, holidays). In about two-thirds of children with TS, the tics will either improve or disappear in early adulthood.

Clinical Management

A multi-modality approach to treatment, education of the family, child and school personnel regarding natural history, prognosis and treatment is essential. The common comorbidities are Attention deficit hyperactive disorder (ADHD), Obsessive-cumpulsive disorder (OCD), learning disabilities, depression, anxiety disorder, and conduct disorders.[7] Medications may be necessary if tics are painful, socially embarrassing, or interfere with concentration during school or employment. The initiative pharmacotherapy is a highly individualized matter of clinical judgment.

Pharmacological Treatment for Tics

Neuroleptic drugs have a tic-reducing effect by blocking dopamine receptors. Neuroleptics been reported to be successful for approximately 70%-80% of treated patients.[8] Haloperidol is initiated at low doses (0.25-0.5 mg) and gradually titrated to 1-5 mg. It is usually dosed to minimize day time sedation. A liquid form haloperidol (2 mg / ml) is available for children.

Pimozide therapy can be started at 0.5-1 mg given at bedtime and is typically dosed at 2-4 mg /day. Fluphenazine is also efficacious and may produce fewer side effects than haloperidol or pimozide.[9] Chronic therapy with a neuroleptic produced better long-term tic suppression than did a short course used to control acute exacerbations. Since tics have been reported to increase after discontinuing neuroleptics, a slow taper is recommended than abrupt cessation.

Newer "atypical" antipsychotics have gained increased usage because they cause fewer motor side effects than the typical ones. Risperidone (Risperdal) is effective for TS begin with 0.5 mg at bedtime and titrate up to 4 mg for clinical effect.[10] Olanzepine significantly reduces aggression and tic severity in TS.[11]

Alpha agonists, clonidine and guanfacine are considered as first line medications in tic management. They are useful for children who are extremely hyperactive, energetic, impulsive, and disinhibited. Clonidine is more useful than methylphenidate.[12,13] The most common side effects of clonidine are sedation, irritability dizziness, headache, dry mouth and insomnia. Begin with a 0.05 mg (1/2 tablet) dose and increase to a total daily dosage of 0.2-0.45 mg for school-age children. It may take up to two months before obtaining maximum clinical effect.[14] Since clonidine may cause hypotension, blood pressure should be monitored during dose titration. Sudden withdrawal can lead to a hypertensive crisis, tachycardia, and profuse sweating.

Pediatric Autoimmune Neuropsychiatric Disorders Associated with Streptococcal Infections (PANDAS)

The existence of PANDAS as a separate entity remains the subject of debate as dyskinesias and psychiatric disorders are known to follow streptococcal infections. PANDAS is defined as an abrupt presentation of OCD or tic disorder following streptococcal infection.[15]

Current diagnostic criteria include OCD and/or a tic disorder, pediatric age at onset, episodic course, association with streptococcal infection, and association with neurological abnormalities. Abrupt changes in attention, impaired executive functions, and deterioration in mathematic skills have been reported. Only one study delineates psychiatric manifestations, which were similar to those seen in Tourette syndrome: OCD (56%), ADHD (40%), ODD (40%), depression (36%), and anxiety (28%); aggressiveness, catatonia, eating disorder, enuresis, and encopresis have also been reported.[16,17]

DYSTONIA

Dystonia is a syndrome of sustained muscle contractions, frequently causing twisting and repetitive movements or abnormal postures.

Focal Dystonia: Involvement of a single body part is affected. Almost any part of the body can be affected. Examples of focal dystonia include torticollis and writer's cramp.

Segmental Dystonia: It refers to involvement of more than one adjacent body parts.

Multifocal Dystonia: Involvement of multiple, nonadjacent body parts.

Hemidystonia: Affects only one side of the body.

Generalized Dystonia: It involves the entire body.

These classification schemes are overlapping. For example, childhood-onset primary dystonia frequently starts in the lower extremities, trunk, or arms and most commonly progresses to generalized involvement, with involuntary twisting of nearly all parts of the body. Adult onset primary dystonias more typically are focal or segmental.[4]

Clinical Features

There are several characteristic clinical features of dystonia. Stress exacerbates most forms of dystonia. Dystonia commonly is triggered or exacerbated by attempted voluntary movement and may fluctuate in presence and severity over time. Dystonic contractions resolve during sleep. The dystonic posturing may occur only with selected movements and paradoxically not with others that may use the same muscles. For example, walking forward may elicit severe lower extremity and truncal twisting, yet walking backward, running, or swimming may be completely normal. Individuals who have dystonia often find that touching one part of the body relieves the dystonic spasms; this phenomenon is called a sensory trick or geste antagoniste. For example, rubbing the back of the hand may diminish writer's cramp.[18]

Causes

Primary Dystonias: Those disorders in which dystonia is the only feature or the primary feature, are accompanied only by other movement disorders, and have a specific causative genetic mutation or unknown cause.

Secondary Dystonias: Disorders in which the dystonia is due to another identifiable cause.

The two most important types of primary dystonia in children are dopa-responsive dystonia and idiopathic torsion dystonia associated with the DYT1 mutation. The most important causes of secondary dystonia in children are listed in Table 29.5.

Table 29.5: Causes of Secondary Dystonia in Children
I. Heredodegenerative Disorders
1. Newborn
a. Branched-chain organic acidurias
b. Non-ketotic hyperglycinemia
2. Infant
a. Glutaric aciduria type I
b. Leigh syndrome (subacute necrotizing encephalomyelopathy)
3. Children and Adolescents
– Niemann-Pick disease type C
– Homocystinuria
– Pantothenate-kinase-associated neurodegeneration (Hallervorden-Spatz disease)
– GM1 GM2 gangliosidosis
– Ataxia telangiectasia
– Huntington disease
– Lesch-Nyhan disease
– Metachromatic leukodystrophy
– Methylmalonic academia
– Mitochondrial disorders
– Wilson disease
II. Drugs/Toxins
III. Psychogenic
IV. Structural Brain Lesions
– Acute disseminated encephalomyelitis
– Infection
– Perinatal hypoxia-ischemia
– Stroke
– Tumor

Dopa-Responsive Dystonia

Dopa-responsive dystonia (DRD) is the most common cause of primary dystonia with onset in childhood. This syndrome is characterized by childhood-onset, progressive dystonia that has a sustained, dramatic response to low doses of levodopa. DRD is also known as hereditary progressive dystonia with diurnal fluctuations or Segawa syndrome. DRD typically presents with a gait disturbance due to foot dystonia starting between 1 and 12 years of age. In untreated older children, diurnal fluctuation may develop, with worsening of symptoms toward the end of the day and marked improvement in the morning. The diurnal fluctuation need not be a presenting feature. In late adolescence or early adulthood, features of parkinsonism can develop.[19]

It is important to recognize the entity of DRD because it responds dramatically to low doses of levodopa. DRD frequently is misdiagnosed as cerebral palsy, particularly spastic diplegia, so it is important to develop high index of suspicion for DRD in children who have motor impairment, prominent dystonia, and a slowly progressive rather than static course. With appropriate diagnosis and treatment, affected children can lead normal lives.[19]

Idiopathic Generalized Torsion Dystonia

Childhood-onset idiopathic torsion dystonia, formerly known as dystonia musculorum deformans, is an autosomal dominant condition that has incomplete (30%) penetrance. Genetic studies have found that a GAG deletion at the DYT1 locus on chromosome 9 causes most autosomal dominant, early-onset primary generalized dystonia affecting Ashkenazi Jewish families (90%) and non-Jews (50% to 60%).[20]

In childhood-onset idiopathic torsion dystonia, symptoms usually begin in a limb at a mean onset age of 12.5 years. Onset usually is before 28 years of age, but seldom before age 6 years. The legs generally are affected before the arms, and symptoms typically become generalized within 5 years. Diagnosis is based on identifying a GAG deletion in the DYT1 gene; genetic testing is available commercially.

Treatment

Most types of dystonia are difficult to treat, and often the response is incomplete. The clear exception is DRD, which responds dramatically to low doses of levodopa. For this reason, a trial of levodopa is recommended for all children who have primary dystonia. Because some secondary dystonias also may respond to levodopa, a trial of the drug is recommended for any child in whom dystonia is a prominent component of the neurologic syndrome.

In late infantile and juvenile forms, administration of small doses (3-5 mg/kg/d) of L-Dopa combined with an inhibitor of peripheral decarboxylation usually produces a rapid response which is independent of the delay in initiating treatment.

The anticholinergic medication trihexyphenidyl has been used with good success in some patients who have dystonia. Some patients who were believed to have idiopathic torsion dystonia and experienced a dramatic response to anticholinergic medication have been shown to have DRD due to a GTPCH mutation. Thus, a dramatic response to trihexyphenidyl suggests the possibility of DRD. If there is inadequate benefit from levodopa or trihexyphenidyl, baclofen alone or in combination with trihexyphenidyl may be beneficial. Benzodiazepines also may be beneficial, but often the benefit is limited by adverse effects or tolerance.

Intrathecal baclofen has been found to be effective in dystonia due to cerebral palsy, but adverse effects are frequent and can be serious. An adequate trial of oral baclofen before considering intrathecal baclofen is recommended.

Botulinum toxin injections may be highly effective, especially if the impairment or disability can be attributed to a few muscle groups. Stereotaxic neurosurgery may be the most effective treatment for dystonia due to the DYT1 mutation.

Tremor

Tremor is a rhythmic oscillation about a central point or position that involves one or more body parts. Tremor in childhood is not rare and is classified by when it occurs: with rest, intention, or action.[21]

Rest tremor is defined as tremor involving a body part that is inactive and supported against gravity. It is associated most commonly with other signs of parkinsonism, but it may occur in isolation. The most common cause of rest tremor in children is antipsychotic (neuroleptic) medications.

Intention tremor occurs as a moving body part approaches a target and usually is associated with other signs of cerebellar dysfunction. Action tremor occurs during maintained posture, voluntary movement, or both. The most important childhood tremors are action tremors and include physiologic tremor and essential (familial) tremor.[22]

Physiologic tremor is a normal phenomenon, consisting of a 6- to 12-Hz oscillation that usually is noticed by the individual or other observers only under certain conditions. Physiologic tremor may increase with anxiety, excitement, fear, or certain medications, including sodium valproate, theophylline, beta-agonists, corticosteroids, and stimulants. The tremor of hyperthyroidism is an enhanced physiologic tremor.

Essential tremor can begin in infancy or childhood. Essential tremor is present with posture and with action, but it usually is greatest with maintained posture. It typically involves the upper extremities, but may involve the head and neck, voice and legs. By definition, essential tremor is unaccompanied by other neurologic abnormalities, although individuals may have slight clumsiness. Essential tremor is "familial" (autosomal dominant) in about 60% of cases.

When tremor is the only abnormality, it is important to identify potential tremor enhancing medications. The primary laboratory tests to be considered are thyroid function tests. The most effective medications are propranolol (or other beta-blockers) and primidone. Propranalol at the dose of 1-4 mg/kg/day is given. Some patients respond to primidone (150 mg/day up to

500 mg/day) alone or in combination with propranolol. Clonazepam may be effective in some cases.[23]

Myoclonus and Related Disorders

Myoclonus is defined as a sudden, brief, shock-like involuntary movement caused by active muscle contractions (positive myoclonus) or pauses in muscle activity (negative myoclonus).[24]

Myoclonus can be classified in three ways:

1. By clinical presentation.
2. By pathophysiology; and
3. By etiology[25] (Table 29.6).

Table 29.6: Classification of Myoclonus

Clinical Presentation	**Pathophysiology (site of origin)**
Spontaneous	Cortical
Action	Subcortical – brainstem, thalamus
Reflex	Spinal
Generalized	Peripheral
Multifocal	
Segmental	
Focal	**Etiology**
Irregulars	
Repetitive	Physiological
Rhythmic	Essential
Epileptic	
Symptomatic	

Physiological myoclonus occurs in otherwise normal individuals and produces no significant disability. Examples include sleep myoclonus, anxiety or exercise – induced muscle jerks, hiccups, and benign infantile myoclonus during feeding.[26]

Essential myoclonus is either an inherited or sporadic idiopathic neurological disorder, where myoclonus is observed in the absence neurological signs or symptoms. In epileptic myoclonus, seizures and myoclonus dominate the clinical picture. In most varieties, encephalopathy is not present, at least initially.[24] Example includes the "fragments of epilepsy" (i.e., myoclonus arising from isolated spike discharges in the motor cortex) such as myoclonic absence seizures or epilepsial partialis continua, childhood myoclonic epilepsies such as Juvenile Mycolonic Epilepsy of Janz, Benign familial myoclonic epilepsy, and progressive myoclonic epilepsy (Unverricht-Londborg).[24-26]

Factor predicting drug responsiveness is the neurophysiologic origin of the myoclonus.[25]

1. Cortical myoclonus–VPA, clonazepam and piracetam have been suggested as the drugs of first choice, while primidone, Phenobarital and 5-HTP are offered as other treatment options.
2. Brainstem reticular reflex myoclonus–VPA or clonazepam are the recommended drugs of first choice, with 5 HTP listed as a second alternative.
3. Spinal myoclonus–clonazepam is suggested as the treatment of first choice with diazepam, carbamazepine and tetrabenazine offered as alternative.
4. Palatal myoclonus/tremor–phenytoin, carbamazepine, clonazepam, diazepam, trihexiphenydyl and baclofen are all suggested as the drugs of first choice, with 5-HTP recommended as a possible alternative.

STEREOTYPIES

Stereotypies are intermittent, involuntary, repetitive, purposeless, patterned movements that are usually rhythmic. Examples of stereotypies occurring in children are arm flapping, rocking, licking, mouth opening and hand waving.

Stereotypies commonly are associated with mental retardation, autism spectrum disorders, Rett syndrome, and blindness, but they also occur in otherwise normal children. Stereotypies occurring in the absence of other neurologic or behavioral features are likely to be benign. Many other terms have been used to describe stereotypies, including "rhythmic habit patterns", "gratification phenomena" and "motor rhythmias".

Stereotypies usually begin in infancy and, unlike tics, tend not to change in type over time. The course is variable, it may resolve over a short period of time in some children or it may persist for years in others. The movements tend to occur in bouts and usually precipitated by excitement, stress, or fatigue. Stereotypies cease when the child is distracted and often children are not aware of the movements. Stereotypies respond inconsistently to medications such as clonazepam, SSRIs and haloperidol. Medical therapy usually is not indicated.[27]

Drug-Induced Movement Disorders

The most common drug-induced movement disorders are those associated with antipsychotic (neuroleptic) treatment (Table 29.7). These medications are dopamine receptor antagonists and cause both acute and tardive (i.e., "late") syndromes. The acute adverse effects of dopamine antagonists include parkinsonism and acute dystonic reactions.

Table 29.7: Common Drug-Induced Movement Disorders

Medications Reaction	
1. Dopamine antagonists (antipsychotics)	
Haloperidol Pimozide Chlorpromazine Metoclopramide Prochlorperzine Risperidone	Acute dystonic reaction Tardive dyskinesia Withdrawal dyskinesia Parkinsonism Neuroleptic malignant syndrome
2. Antiepileptics	
Phenytoin Carbamazepine Sodium valproate	Chorea Dystonia Tremor
3. Beta-adrenergic agonists	
Metaproterenol	Tremor
4. Amphetamines	Chorea, Tremor
5. Cocaine	Chorea
6. Lithium	Chorea, Tremor

Acute dystonic reactions can occur after a single dose of a dopamine antagonist. The typical acute dystonic reaction involves involuntary gaze deviation (oculogyric crisis), torticollis, and appendicular twisting postures involving axial more than appendicular muscles. It can last for hours, but is treated readily with anticholinergic medications such as diphenhydramine (1 mg/kg per dose every 6 hours) and benztropine (0.5 to 2 mg per day bid).[28]

Neuroleptic Malignant Syndrome

The most severe reaction to dopamine antagonists is the neuroleptic malignant syndrome, which is characterized by hyperthermia, hypertonia, dystonia posturing, tremor, and autonomic instability, and can be fatal. Treatment primarily is supportive and includes fever control and correction of metabolic abnormalities. Dantrolene should be given to diminish excessive muscle contraction. Dopamine agonists such as bromocriptine may be effective. Neuroleptic medications should be discontinued.

Tardive Dyskinesia (TD)

It is uncommon in childhood. The dyskinesia can manifest as any of the hyperkinetic movement disorders. TD typically manifests as an orobuccal-lingual stereotypy, but it can involve other body parts. The risk of TD increases with total dose and treatment duration of antipsychotic medication and with the age of the patient. There is some evidence that children who have had brain injuries are more likely to develop TD.[29,30]

Juvenile Parkinsonism

Parkinsonism with onset before 40 years is classified as the juvenile form. Early parkinsonism has more rigidity than tremor, and the course may be slower than in classic cases. Cases in children and adolescents are exceptional.[31]

Paroxysmal Dyskinesias

Paroxysmal dyskinesias represent a heterogeneous group of diseases with paroxysmal occurrence of dyskinesias including dystonia, chorea, ballism and athetosis. These include Paroxysmal Kinesigenic Dyskinesia (PKD), Paroxysmal Nonkinesigenic Dyskinesia (PNKD), Paroxysmal Exertional Dyskinesia (PED) and Paroxysmal Hypnogenic Dyskinesia (PHD). Detailed history taking can be very revealing to differentiate these disorders.

PKD is usually triggered by sudden voluntary movements, startles and hyperventilation whereas PNKD has spontaneous onset which is provoked by alcoholic beverages, coffee, excitement, stress, exhaustion, tea, beverages with caffeine. PED is induced by exercise. PKD has the shortest duration of attack which lasts for seconds to a few minutes with a frequency of up to 100 per day. A typical attack in PNKD usually lasts for minutes to several hours with a frequency of up to 3 per day. PED does not have more than one attack per day which lasts for 15 to 60 minutes.[32-34] There is mounting evidence that PHD are supplementary sensorimotor area seizures.

The kinesigenic dyskinesias respond extremely well to anticonvulsants in particular to carbamazepine. Anticonvulsants are not beneficial in PNKD and PED. PNKD and PED are sometime sensitive to clonazepam, benzodiazepines, acetazolamide, anticholinergics and neuroleptics.[34]

The Expanding Spectrum of GLUT-1 Deficiency Syndrome

GLUT-1 deficiency syndrome, caused by a mutation in the SCL2A1 gene which encodes for the glucose 1 transporter, is classically characterized by infantile epilepsy, developmental delay, decelerated head growth, acquired microcephaly, cognitive impairment, ataxia and spasticity.[35] Laboratory evaluation shows low CSF glucose levels with normoglycemia and can be confirmed by erythrocyte glucose uptake studies and by GLUT-1 gene mutation analysis.

The most common movement disorders described in GLUT-1 deficiency include ataxia, spasticity, and dystonia and infrequently chorea, myoclonus, dyspraxia, kinesigenic and nonkinesigenic dyskinesia may be seen. While the classic presentation of GLUT-1 deficiency syndrome is more common, GLUT-1 deficiency should be considered in the differential diagnosis of childhood-onset movement disorders including paroxysmal dyskinesias. It is especially important because treatment with the ketogenic diet may lead to symptomatic improvement.[36,37]

Pediatric movement disorder is an expanding area of neurological disorder where recognition of treatable disorder in time and providing appropriate management at correct moment will have an important lasting effect on the personal and social domains of a child.

References

1. JW Mink. "The Basal Ganglia and Involuntary Movements: Impaired Inhibition of Competing Motor Patterns," Archives of Neurology, Vol. 60, No. 10, 2003:1365-68.
2. KP Bhatia and CD Marsden. "The Behavioural and Motor Consequences of Focal Lesions of the Basal Ganglia in Man", Brain, Vol. 117, No. 4, 1994;859-76.
3. J Jankovic and KM Shannon. "Movement Disorders", In: WG Bradley, RB Daroff, GM Fenichel and J Jankovic, Eds., Neurology in Clinical Practice, 5th Edition, Butterworth Heinemann Elsevier, Philadelphia 2008;2081.
4. Fernández-Alvarez E, Aicardi J. Movement Disorders in Children. London: MacKeith Press, 2001.
5. F Cardoso, K Seppi, KJ Mair, GK Wenning and W Poewe, "Seminar on Choreas", Lancet Neurology, Vol. 5, No. 7, 2006: 589-602.
6. I Korn-Lubetzki, A Brand and I Steiner. "Recurrence of Sydenham's Chorea: Implications for Pathogenesis", Archives of Neurology, Vol. 61, No. 8, 2004:1261-64.
7. JM Dooley. "Tic Disorders in Childhood", Seminars in Pediatric Neurology, Vol. 13, No. 4, 2006:231-42.
8. Chappell PB, Leckman JF, Riddle MA. The Pharmacologic Treatment of tic Disorders. In Lewis M and Riddle M (eds). Child and Adolescent Psychiatric Clinic of North America: Pediatric Psychopharmacology, Vol. 4, Philadelphia, WB Saunders 1995;197-215.
9. Singers HS, Gammon K. Haloperidol, Fluphenazine and Clonidine in Tourette's syndrome: Controversies in treatment. Pediatr Neurosci 1986:12:71-74.
10. GR Gaffney, PJ Perry, BC Lund, KA Bever-Stille, Arndt and S Kuperman. "Risperidone versus Clonidine in the Treatment of Children and Adolescents with Tourette's Syndrome", Journal of the American Academy of Child and Adolescent Psychiatry, Vol. 41, No. 3, 2002:330-36.
11. RJ Stephens, C Bassel and P Sandor. "Olanzapine in the Treatment of Aggression and Tics in Children with Tourette's Syndrome: A Pilot Study", Journal of Child and Adolescent Psychopharmacology, Vol. 14, No. 2, 2004:255-66.
12. MM Qasaymeh and JW Mink. "New Treatments for Tic Disorders", Current Treatment Options in Neurology, Vol. 8, No. 6, 2006:465-73.
13. Tourette's Syndrome Study Group. "Treatment of ADHD in Children with Tics: A Randomized Controlled Trial", Neurology, Vol. 58, No. 4, 2002:527-36.
14. Leckman JF, Hardin MT, Riddle MA, *et al.* Clonidine Treatment of Gilles de la Tourette's Syndrome. Arch Gen Psychiatry 1991;48:324-28.
15. ST Shulman. "Pediatric Autoimmune Neuropsychiatric Disorders Associated with Streptococci (PANDAS): Update", Current Opinion in Pediatrics, Vol. 21, No. 1, 2009:127-30.
16. R Kurlan, D Johnson, EL Kaplan and the Tourette Syndrome Study Group. "Streptococcal Infection and Exacerbations of Childhood Tics and Obsessive-Compulsive Symptoms: A Prospective Blinded Cohort Study", Pediatrics, Vol. 121, No. 6, 2008:1188-97.
17. V Gabbay, BJ Coffey, JS Babb, L Meyer, C Wachtel, S Anam and B Rabinovitz. "Pediatric Autoimmune Neuropsychiatric Disorders Associated with Streptococcus: Comparison of Diagnosis and Treatment in the Community and at a Specialty Clinic", Pediatrics, Vol. 122, No. 3, 2008: 273-78.
18. Bressman S. Dystonia update. Clin Neuropharmacol 2000;23: 239-51.
19. Nygaard TG, Marsden CD, Fahn S. Dopa-responsive Dystonia: Long-term Treatment, Response and Prognosis. Neurology 1991:41:174-81.
20. Sanger TD. Toward a Definition of Childhood Dystonia. Curr Opin Pediatr 2004:16:623-27.
21. Jankovic J, Fahn S. Physiologic and Pathologic Tremors: Diagnosis, Mechanism and Management, Ann Intern Med 1980:93:460-65.
22. Pranzatelli MR. Update on Pediatric Movement Disorders. Adv Pediatr 1995:42:415-63.
23. Bain PG, Findley LJ, Thompson PD, *et al.* A Study of Hereditary Essential Tremor. Brain 1994;117:805-24.
24. Fahn S Marsden CD, Van Woert MH. Definition and Classification of Myoclonus. Adv Neurol 1986;43:1-5.
25. Obeso JA. Classification, Clinical Features and Treatment of Myoclonus, In: Watts RL and Koller WC, Editors, Movement Disorders: Neurologic Principles and Practice, McGraw-Hill 1986:541-50.
26. Caviness JN. Myoclonus. Mayo Clin Proc 1996 July;71: 679-88.
27. DS Wolf and HS Singer. "Pediatric Movement Disorders: An Update", Current Opinion in Neurology, Vol. 21, No. 4, 2008:491-96.
28. DL Gilbert. "Drug-Induced Movement Disorders in Children", Annals of the New York Academy of Sciences, Vol. 1142, 2008;72-84.
29. CU Correll and EM Schenk. "Tardive Dyskinesia and New Antipsychotics", Current Opinion in Psychiatry, Vol. 21, No. 2, 2008:151-56.

30. CU Correll and JM Kane. "One-Year Incidence Rates of Tardive Dyskinesia in Children and Adolescents Treated with Second-Generation Antipsychotics: A Systematic Review". Journal of Child and Adolescent Psychopharmacology. Vol. 17. No. 5. 2007:647-56.

31. Aicardi J Diseases of the Nervous System in Childhood. 1st Edition. Oxford. Blackwell Scientific Publications Limited 1992:518-88.

32. Strzelczyk A. Burk K. Oertel WH. Treatment of Paroxysmal Dyskinesias. Expert Opin Pharmacother 2011;12:63-72.

33. Szepetowski P. Rochette J. Berquin P. Piussan C. Lathrop GM. Monaco AP Familial Infantile Convulsions and Paroxysmal Choreoathetosis: A New Neurological Syndrome Linked to the Pericentromeric Region of Human Chromosome 16. Am J Hum Genet 1997:61:889-98.

34. Stanley Fahn. Joseph Jankovic. The Paroxysmal Dyskinesias in Principles and Practice of Movement Disorders. Published by Churchill Livingstone 2008:553-75.

35. Wang D. Pascual JM. Yang H. *et al.* GLUT-1 Deficiency Syndrome: Clinical. Genetic and Therapeutic Aspects. Ann Neurol 2005:57:111-18.

36. Pons R. Collins A. Rotstein M. Engelstad K. De Vivo DC. The Spectrum of Movement Disorders in GLUT-1 Deficiency. Mov Disord 2010:25:275-81.

37. Brockmann K. The Expanding Phenotype of GLUT1-Deficiency Syndrome. Brain Dev 2009:31:545-52.

30 Chapter

DEMYELINATING DISORDERS

C. Leema Pauline

ACUTE DISSEMINATED ENCEPHALOMYELITIS (ADEM)

DEFINITION

Acute disseminated encephalomyelitis (ADEM) is an acute rapidly progressive multi focal demyelinating syndrome of central nervous system that occurs in association with a viral infection (parainfectious/postinfectious encephalomyelitis) or an immunization (post vaccination encephalomyelitis). It is usually a monophasic illness. Clinically, it manifests by rapid development of focal or multifocal neurologic dysfunction.

ADEM and Related Disorders

- ADEM
  - Monophasic para/post infectious or post vaccination demyelination
- Acute hemorrhagic leucoencephalitis
  - Hyperacute form of ADEM
- Clinically isolated forms (CIS)
  - Acute transverse myelitis
  - Optic neuritis
  - Acute cerebellitis
  - Brainstem encephalitis
- Multiphasic ADEM
- Combined central and peripheral demyelinating disorders.

Pathogenesis

Acute Disseminated Encephalomyelitis is likely an autoimmune disorder triggered by environmental stimuli in a genetically susceptible individual. The myelin auto antigens such as myelin basic protein, myelin oligodendroglia protein, proteolipid protein share antigen determinants with infecting pathogens (molecular mimicry). Infection triggered circulating immune complexes or humoral factors may increase vascular permeability.

Pathology

Pathologically ADEM is characterized by perivenular inflammation, edema and demyelination characterized by infiltration of lymphocytes, neutrophils, plasma cells and microglia within the central nervous system.

Clinical Features

Acute disseminated encephalomyelitis mainly affects the children. The mean age of presentation ranges from 5-8 years. Males are commonly affected than females in the ratio of 1:0.8. It typically occurs within 2 days to 4 weeks following a viral infection. Symptoms usually lasts for more than 24 hours, peak at 2-7 days.

Common antecedent infections reported include upper respiratory infection and gastrointestinal infection. The infectious agents commonly implicated include measles, EBV, CMV, HSV, Coxsackie, Hepatitis A, HIV, influenza, VZV and West Nile virus. In some, no preceding illness or initiating event could be identified.

In some, there is a prodromal phase of fever, nausea, emesis, malaise, myalgia which is followed by an abrupt or rapid onset of focal or multifocal symptoms such as encephalopathy ranging from lethargy, somnolence, confusion, irritability, behavioural changes to coma, seizures, nuchal pain and multifocal signs such as cranial nerve palsies (22-45%), bilateral optic neuritis (12-16%), pyramidal signs (60-95%), hemiparesis (76%) and ataxia (18-65%). Movement disorders and sensory deficits are less common. Respiratory failure secondary to brainstem involvement or severely impaired consciousness can occur.

Clinically ADEM is indistinguishable from acute encephalitis. Encephalitis is due to direct invasion of the infectious agent into the meninges and brain parenchyma.

It is characterised by gray matter abnormalities in neuroimaging.

Clinical Criteria to Diagnose ADEM

1. A first polyfocal clinical neurological event with presumed inflammatory demyelinating cause.
2. Encephalopathy that cannot be explained by fever.
3. No new symptoms, signs or MRI findings after three months of the incident ADEM.

Course and Prognosis

Recovery begins within days with complete resolution of symptoms in a few days to weeks or months. Complete recovery is seen in 57-94% of the children. The mortality rate is usually less than 5%, in acute hemorrhagic encephalitis or fulminant variant.

Investigations

Magnetic Resonance Imaging (MRI) brain is more sensitive than computed tomography in showing the lesions. MRI brain shows multiple, multifocal, discrete, patchy, asymmetrical hyperintense lesions in T2 weighted and FLAIR sequences. Acute lesions enhance with gadolinium contrast. Usually the lesions involve the subcortical and deep white matter. The gray matter of the thalami and basal ganglia are involved frequently. At times, the lesions may be large with much surrounding edema causing mass effect called tumefactive demyelination (mass like). Involvement of corpus callosum is less common in ADEM. Meningeal enhancement is unusual. The lesions resolve completely or partially after several months (range 6-18 months). Complete resolution of MRI abnormalities have been described in 37-75% of the patients and partial resolution in 25-53% of the children (Fig. 30.1).

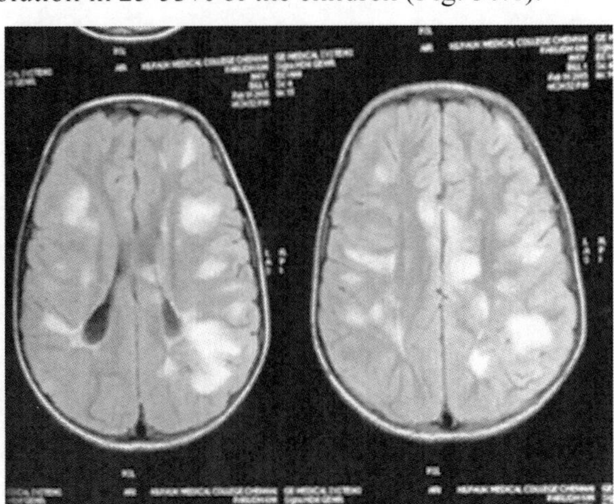

Fig. 30.1

Cerebrospinal fluid shows normal pressure, mild increase in cell count (<100 cells/m^3), moderate increase in protein (<70 mg/dl). CSF oligoclonal bands appear less commonly than multiple sclerosis.

EEG shows background slowing and or bilateral epileptiform discharges.

Risk Factors for Multiple Sclerosis

Increased Risk	Decreased Risk
>10 years of age	<10 years of age
No encephalopathy	Encephalopathy
No precipitating infection	Post infectious presentation
Optic neuritis	Isolated transverse myelitis
Oligoclonal bands in CSF	Fever, seizures, meningismus
Family H/O multiple sclerosis	
Periventricular lesions in MRI	

Differential Diagnosis

ADEM is a diagnosis of exclusion based on clinical and MRI findings.

The differential diagnosis include:

1. Viral encephalitis.
2. Autoimmune encephalitis.
3. CNS vasculitis.
4. Rheumatologic (neuro sarcoid, SLE, Behcet disease).
5. Mitochondrial disorders (POLG, MELAS, Leighs encephalopathy).
6. Leukodystrophies (Alexander, Vanishing White Matter disease).
7. Toxic encephalopathies.
8. Hashimotos encephalopathy.
10. Posterior Reversible Encephalopathy Syndrome (PRES).
11. Neoplasm.
12. Deep cerebral vein thrombosis.

Treatment

The current therapy is high dose corticosteroids– Methyl prednisolone 20-30 mg/kg/day intravenously to a maximum of 1 gm/day for 3-5 days followed by oral steroids taper over a period of 3 weeks if there is incomplete clinical improvement.

Intravenous immunoglobulin 2 gm/kg over a period of 3-5 days, if there is no improvement 2-3 days after completion of steroids can be given.

Longitudinal follow-up MRI should be done once in every 3 months in the first year, then annually until 18 years of age to ensure appearance of no new lesions which would change the diagnosis.

Vaccines are not recommended for 6 months after an attack of ADEM.

ADEM VARIANTS

Acute Hemorrhagic Encephalitis

Also called Weston Hurst disease, it is characterized by acute rapidly progressive fulminant hemorrhagic demyelination of white matter. It is considered as an hyperacute form of ADEM. It is usually associated with death or severe morbidity.

SITE RESTRICTED FORMS

Acute Transverse Myelitis

It is characterized by acute or subacute onset of isolated spinal cord dysfunction. The initial symptoms may be back pain, leg weakness, sensory loss and bladder involvement. Paresis is initially flaccid with hypo or areflexia (spinal shock) followed by spasticity and hyperreflexia. There may be a sensory level.

MRI spinal cord shows intramedullary hyperintense lesions in T2W images with cord edema, which may show enhancement with Gadolinium contrast.

Longitudinally Extensive Transverse Myelitis (LETM) that is involvement of three or more segments, recurrent transverse myelitis, concurrent or sequential optic neuritis should prompt the diagnosis of Neuromyelitis Optica (NMO). Any child presenting with LETM, should undergo serum testing for NMO IgG antibody to rule out Neuromyelitis optica spectrum disorder.

MRI spine sagittal view T2 weighted image showing longitudinally extensive transverse myelitis (Fig. 30.2).

MRI spine T2 weighted image axial view showing hyperintense signals occupying more than two thirds of the cord.

MRI brain screening should be done to look for brain involvement. Visual evoked potentials (VEP) should be done to evaluate subclinical optic nerve involvement.

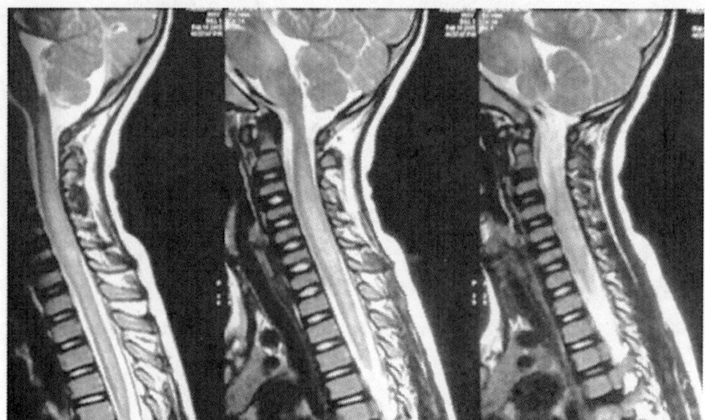

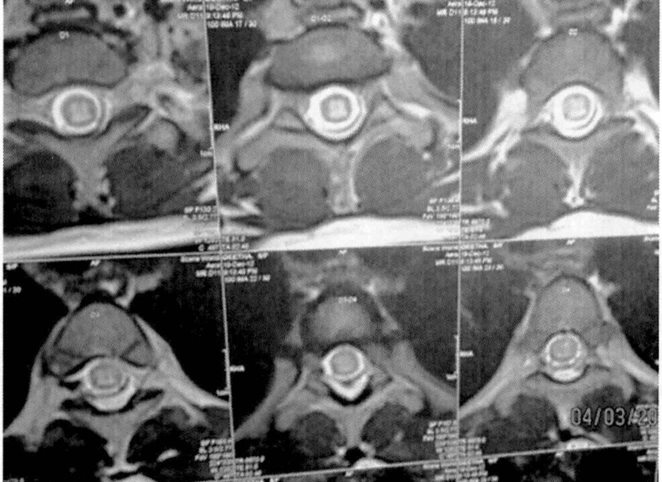

Fig. 30.2

Optic Neuritis

Clinically it presents as acute or sub-acute unilateral or bilateral visual loss. Children usually present with bilateral visual impairment. Typical features include sudden loss of vision, defective colour vision and relative afferent papillary defect (RAPD). Fundus examination may show disc edema.

MRI imaging of optic nerves show abnormalities. Visual evoked potentials show prolonged latencies and reduced amplitudes.

Concurrent or sequential involvement of spinal cord should prompt a diagnosis of neuromyelitis optica. Serum should be tested for NMO IgG antibody.

Optic neuritis is a medical emergency. It should be promptly treated with high dose steroids–Methyl prednisolone intravenously 20-30 mg/kg/day for 3-5 days.

NEUROMYELITIS OPTICA

Neuromyelitis optica is an inflammatory disease primarily affecting the spinal cord and optic nerves, that is clinically and pathologically different from multiple sclerosis. The term Devic disease has been used interchangeably with neuromyelitis optica. Devic and his pupil Gault named the disease as acute optic neuromyelitis.

In 2004, the diagnostic marker of the disease, an autoantibody named NMO IgG, which has high specificity for neuromyelitis optica and neuromyelitis spectrum disorders, was discovered. In 2005, the target antigen of NMO IgG – the predominant water channel of the central nervous system aquaporin 4 was identified. Binding of NMO IgG to aquaporin 4 results in a cascade of biological events resulting in tissue inflammation, edema and demyelination.

Clinical Features

Neuromyelitis optica is marked by acute or subacute onset of optic neuritis and or transverse myelitis. Optic neuritis may be bilateral. Myelitis usually presents with complete transverse myelitis resulting in para/quadriparesis, often a symmetric sensory level and sphincter dysfunction. In contrast, spinal cord lesions are often clinically and radiologically less dramatic with partial transverse myelitis in multiple sclerosis. Encephalopathy, recurrent vomiting can be a part of initial manifestation.

Cerebral lesions may be detected in upto 60% of adult patients in whom they are usually clinically silent, but children with cerebral lesions may present with protean clinical features.

CSF shows a marked elevation of white cell count (often polymorphonuclear) with elevated protein. In contrast to multiple sclerosis, just 6% of pediatric NMO patients have oligoclonal bands in cerebrospinal fluid. Visual evoked potentials show prolonged latency and reduced amplitude.

Neuromyelitis optica may be associated with other autoimmune disorders like Systemic Lupus Erythematosis, Sjögren syndrome, Juvenile Rheumatoid Arthritis and Graves' disease.

Diagnostic Criteria

Diagnosis requires all absolute criterion and one major supportive criteria or two minor supportive criteria.

Absolute Criteria

- Optic neuritis.
- Acute myelitis.
- No evidence of clinical disease outside of the optic nerve or spinal cord.

Major Supportive Criteria

- Negative brain MRI at onset (does not meet criteria for multiple sclerosis).
- Spinal cord MRI with signal abnormality extending over >/=3 vertebral segments.
- CSF pleocytosis of >50 WBC/mm^3 or >5 PMNs/mm^3.

Minor Supportive Criteria

- Bilateral optic neuritis.
- Severe optic neuritis with fixed visual acuity worse than 20/200 in at least one eye.
- Severe, fixed, attack-related weakness (MRC </=2) in one or more limbs.

Treatment

High dose corticosteroids–methylprednisolone intra-venously 30 mg/kg/day to a maximum of 1gm for 5 days is given in the acute stage. If the response is incomplete, plasmapheresis or intravenous immunoglobulin should be considered.

In seropositive cases or in recurrent seronegative NMO, long-term immunosuppression should be initiated to prevent future relapses. Azathioprine, Mycophenolate mofetil, Rituximab and Methotrexate are the options. Interferons are contraindicated as they will worsen the illness.

Families should be educated regarding the long-term side effects of the drugs, immunosuppression, possibility of relapses and the importance of monitoring.

CHILDHOOD MULTIPLE SCLEROSIS

Multiple sclerosis is a chronic inflammatory and degenerative disorder of the central nervous system characterized by dissemination in space and time. It manifests as a relapsing and remitting disease. Symptom onset prior to 18 years of age occurs in about 3-10% of all multiple sclerosis patients. A family history of multiple sclerosis is reported in 5-10% of affected children. Children experience more frequent relapses in the first few years than adults, suggesting that it is highly inflammatory in children. Initial recovery is usually excellent. Most children achieve a complete recovery.

The first attack usually manifests with optic neuritis or monofocal brainstem or polyfocal neurological deficits. Optic neuritis is the first clinical attack in 14-35% of children with multiple sclerosis. It can be unilateral or bilateral. The outcome in children with optic neuritis is usually favourable. Presence of one or more white matter lesions extrinsic to the optic nerve is associated with 60% risk of multiple sclerosis in the following two years.

Isolated acute transverse myelitis with normal brain imaging is usually a monophasic illness. Acute transverse myelitis represents the first clinical attack of multiple sclerosis in only in 10% of children. Spinal lesions are typically small involving less than 3 spinal segments and involve only a portion of the transverse diameter of the cord.

Acute disseminated encephalomyelitis is characterized by polyfocal symptoms with encephalopathy. Nearly 15% of children with an acute ADEM like presentation will ultimately develop multiple sclerosis. However, two or more non ADEM attacks are needed to diagnose definite multiple sclerosis in such children.

The clues that may help to distinguish first attack of multiple sclerosis from ADEM include:

- Absence of a bilateral pattern.
- Presence of black hole.
- Presence of two or more periventricular lesions.
- Involvement of corpus callosum.
- Presence of oligoclonal bands in cerebrospinal fluid.

Neuroimaging and Laboratory Features that Aid in the Diagnosis of Multiple Sclerosis

Atleast two of the following distinguish MS from other non demyelinating controls with 85% sensitivity and 98% specificity (Fig. 30.3).

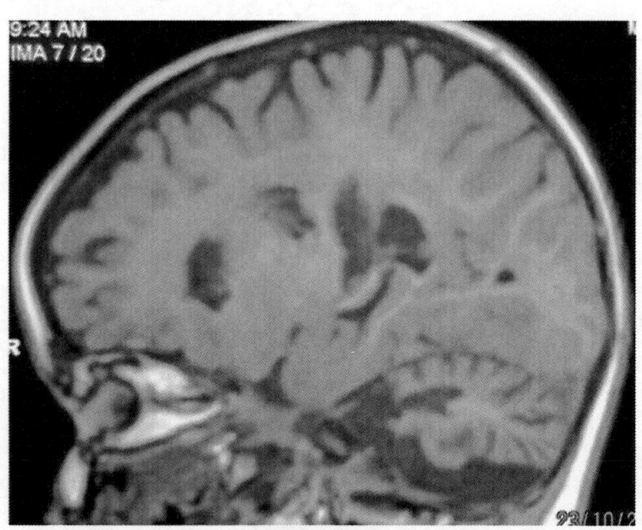

Fig. 30.3

- 1-5 or more lesions.
- More than two periventricular lesions.
- 1 brainstem lesion.

Patients presenting with ADEM phenotypes are to be diagnosed with MS in future, if the brain MRI shows any two of the following:

- Presence of black hole.
- Presence of more than two periventricular lesions.
- Absence of a bilateral diffuse lesion pattern.

Cerebrospinal fluid analysis is the most important laboratory investigation in the diagnosis.

- More than 90% with MS have oligoclonal bands.
- CSF white blood cell count is <50 cells/μl.
- Predominant cells are lymphocytes.

Differential Diagnosis to be Excluded in Pediatric Multiple Sclerosis

1. CNS vasculitis.
2. Collagen vascular disorders.
3. Mitochondrial encephalopathy.
4. Vitamin B_{12} or folate deficiency.
5. Neuro borreliosis.
6. Lymphoma.

Distinguishing Features Between ADEM and MS

Clinical Feature	ADEM	MS
Age group	< 10 years	> 10 years
Sex	Both sexes equally affected	Females more affected
Prior respiratory illness	Present	Absent
Seizures, encephalopathy	Present	Absent
CSF pleocytosis	Common	Never
Oligoclonal bands	Less frequent	More frequent
Course	Monophasic	Relapsing and remitting
MRI brain	Discrete, bilateral lesions at grey white junction	Periventricular, black holes
Deep gray involvement	Common	Not involved
Recovery	Rapid, complete	Variable

Management

Treatment of Acute Relapses

Each relapse should be treated with intravenous methyl prednisolone 20-30 mg/kg/day (up to 1 gm/day) for 3-5 days.

Intravenous immunoglobulin is used as a second line therapy at a dose of 2 gm/kg given over 2-5 days in attacks with inadequate response to corticosteroids or during febrile illness where infection is suspected.

Plasma exchange is reserved for severe relapses that have not responded to steroids or immunoglobulin.

Disease Modifying Therapy

Intramuscular and subcutaneous interferon β1a and subcutaneous interferon β1b appear to be safe and relatively well tolerated in children. International Pediatric Multiple Sclerosis Study Group suggests titration up to 30 μg once weekly for intramuscular interferon β1a and 22 μg 3 times weekly or 44 μg 3 times weekly for subcutaneous interferon β1a and 250 μg for interferon β1b. Side effects include flu like symptoms, leucopenia, thrombocytopenia, anemia, transient elevation of transaminases. Second line therapies include rituximab, natalizumab, mitoxantrone, cyclophosphamide and fingolimod.

Suggested Reading

- Ann Yeh and Bianca Weinstock-Guttman. The Management of Pediatric Multiple Sclerosis: J Child Neurol 2012:27:1384.
- Ascherio A, Munger K. Epidemiology of Multiple Sclerosis. From Risk factors to Prevention. Semin Neurol 2008;28:17-28.
- Dale RC, de Sousa C, Chong WK, Cox TC, Harding B, Neville BG. Acute Disseminated Encephalomyelitis, Multiphasic Disseminated Encephalomyelitis and Multiple Sclerosis in Children. Brain 2000;123:2407-22.
- Dean Wingerchuk, Brenda Banwell, Jeffrey Bennett, Philippe Cabre, William Carroll, Tanuja Chitnis, Jerome De Seze, Kazuo Fujihara, Benjamin Greenberg, Anu Jacob, Sven Jarius, Marco Lana-Peixoto, Michael Levy, Jack Simon, Silvia Tenembaum, Anthony Traboulsee, Patrick Waters, Kay Wellik and Brian Weinshenker. Revised Diagnostic Criteria for Neuromyelitis Optica Spectrum Disorders. Neurology April 8,2014,vol. 82 no. 10 Supplement S63.001.
- Dean Wingerchuk, Brenda Banwell, Jeffrey Bennett, Philippe Cabre, William Carroll, Tanuja Chitnis, Jerome De Seze, Kazuo Fujihara, Benjamin Greenberg, Anu Jacob, Sven Jarius, Marco Lana-Peixoto, Michael Levy, Jack Simon, Silvia Tenembaum, Anthony Traboulsee, Patrick Waters, Kay Wellik and Brian Weinshenker. Revised Diagnostic Criteria for Neuromyelitis Optica Spectrum Disorders. Neurology April 8, 2014 vol. 82 no. 10 Supplement S63.001.
- Gulay Alper. Acute Disseminated Encephalomyelitis: J Child Neurol 2012:27:1408.
- Hynson JL, Kornberg AJ, Coleman LT, Shield L, Harvey AS, Kean MJ. Clinical and Neuroradiologic Features of Acute Disseminated Encephalomyelitis in Children. Neurology 2001: 56:1308-12.
- Krupp LB, Banwell B, Tenembaum S. The International Pediatric MS Study Group. Consensus Definitions Proposed for Pediatric Multiple Sclerosis and Related Childhood Disorders. Neurology 2007;68:S7-12.
- M Alexander, JMK Murthy. Acute Disseminated Encephalomyelitis: Treatment Guidelines Annals of Indian Academy of Neurology Year 2011: Volume 14, Issue 5,60-64.
- M Alexander, JMK Murthy. Acute Disseminated Encephalomyelitis: Treatment Guidelines Annals of Indian Academy of Neurology Year 2011,Volume 14, Issue 5,60-64.
- Menge T, Hemmer B, Nessler S, Wiendl H, Neuhaus O, Hartung HP, *et al.* Acute Disseminated Encephalomyelitis: An Update. Arch Neurol 2005;62:1673-80.
- Menge T, Hemmer B, Nessler S, Wiendl H, Neuhaus O, Hartung HP, *et al.* Acute Disseminated Encephalomyelitis: An Update. Arch Neurol 2005;62:1673-80.
- Saiz A, Zuliani L, Blanco Y, Tavolato B, Giometto B, Graus F. Spanish-Italian NMO Study Group. Revised Diagnostic Criteria for Neuromyelitis Optica (NMO). Application in a Series of Suspected Patients. J Neurol 2007 Sep;254(9):1233-37.
- Saiz A, Zuliani L, Blanco Y, Tavolato B, Giometto B, Graus F. Spanish-Italian NMO Study Group. Revised Diagnostic Criteria for Neuromyelitis Optica (NMO). Application in a Series of Suspected Patients. J Neurol 2007 Sep;254(9):1233-37.
- Sandra Bigi and Brenda Banwell. Pediatric Multiple Sclerosis: J Child Neurol 2012;27:1378.
- Sandra Bigi and Brenda Banwell. Pediatric Multiple Sclerosis: J Child Neurol 2012.
- Tenembaum S, Chamoles N, Fejerman N. Acute Disseminated encephalomyelitis: A Long-term Follow-up Study of 84 Pediatric Patients. Neurology 2002;59:1224-31.
- Tenembaum S, Chamoles N, Fejerman N. Acute Disseminated Encephalomyelitis: A Long-term Follow-up Study of 84 Pediatric Patients. Neurology 2002;59:1224-31.
- Tenembaum S, Chitnis T, Ness J, Hahn JS. Acute Disseminated Encephalomyelitis. Neurology 2007;68:S23-36.
- Til Menge, MD; Bernhard Hemmer, MD; Stefan Nessler, MD; Heinz Wiendl, MD; Oliver Neuhaus, MD; Hans-Peter Hartung, MD; Bernd C. Kieseier, MD; Olaf Stüve, MD, PhD. Acute Disseminated Encephalomyelitis: An Update Arch Neurol 2005;62:1673-80.
- Varina L. Wolf, Pamela J. Lupo and Timothy E Lotze. Pediatric Acute Transverse Myelitis: Overview and Differential Diagnosis: J Child Neurol 2012;27:1426.
- Varina L. Wolf, Pamela J. Lupo and Timothy E. Lotze. Pediatric Acute Transverse Myelitis: Overview and Differential Diagnosis: J Child Neurol 2012;27:11426.

- Wingerchuk DM, Lennon VA, Pittock SJ, Lucchinetti CF, Weinshenker BG. Revised Diagnostic Criteria for Neuromyelitis Optica. Neurology 2006 May 23;66(10):1485-89.

- Wingerchuk DM, Lennon VA, Pittock SJ, Lucchinetti CF, Weinshenker BG. Revised Diagnostic Criteria for Neuromyelitis Optica. Neurology 2006 May 23;66(10):1485-89.

- Wingerchuk DM, Weinshenker BG. Acute Disseminated Encephalomyelitis, Transverse Myelitis and Neuromyelitis Optica. Continuum 2013: Aug;19(4 Multiple Sclerosis):944-67.

- Wingerchuk DM, Weinshenker BG. Acute Disseminated Encephalomyelitis, Transverse Myelitis and Neuromyelitis Optica. Continuum 2013: Aug;19(4 Multiple Sclerosis):944-67.

- Wingerchuk DM, Weinshenker BG. Multiple Sclerosis: Epidemiology, Genetics, Classification, Natural History and Clinical Outcome Measures. Neuroimaging Clin North Am 2000;10:611-24.

- Wingerchuk DM, Weinshenker BG. Multiple Sclerosis: Epidemiology, Genetics, Classification, Natural History and Clinical Outcome Measures. Neuroimaging Clin North Am 2000;10:611-24.

31 Chapter

APPROACH TO PERIPHERAL NEUROPATHIES IN CHILDREN

Vinod Puri, Neera Chaudhry, Ashish Duggal

INTRODUCTION

The causes of neuropathy in children are in general, similar to those in adults but in spite of this the diagnosis of peripheral neuropathy in children is more challenging. Although the symptoms of neuropathy in children are similar to those in adults, evaluation of neuropathy in children becomes more challenging because of difficulties in eliciting a proper history from young children particularly those with developmental delays and inconsistencies in neurological examination. The causes of neuropathy that present in children can broadly be divided into those that are progressive and those that will tend improve over time. Progressive neuropathies include the neuropathies that are hereditary in nature such as the heterogenous group of Hereditary Sensory Motor Neuropathies and some immune mediated neuropathies. Most of the neuropathies that tend to improve with time include acquired neuropathies such as vitamin deficiencies, toxicities, some immune mediated, and focal mononeuropathies. The priority in the diagnosis in neuropathy is to identify treatable, typically acquired conditions. The diagnostic approach of peripheral neuropathies in children often relies on some combination of careful history taking, physical examination findings, a careful determination of family history, electrodiagnostic studies, molecular genetic studies, sural nerve biopsy, and occasionally metabolic laboratory studies.

Epidemiology

The incidence of peripheral neuropathy is not known, but it is a common feature of many systemic diseases. The prevalence of neuropathy was estimated to be 2.4% in a community based study in Mumbai.[1] The prevalence of neuropathy increases with age and is 8% in individuals aged above 55 years.[2] Although the causes of neuropathy are similar in adults and children, the prevalence of individual causes differs in children as compared to adults. In western countries, inherited and metabolic causes represent a much larger proportion of nerve disease in children as compared to immune mediated causes which are more prevalent in adults. In developing countries, however, infectious causes such as tuberculosis, HIV type 1 (HIV-1), leprosy and diphtheria are probably more important than inherited causes.[3,4] In fact worldwide, most common cause of treatable neuropathy is leprosy.[5] Nutritional deficiencies, such as vitamin B_1 and E deficiencies are also an important cause of peripheral neuropathy in children. At the same time, it is possible that because of lack of resources, hereditary disorders–both those of 'pure peripheral neuropathies' and those related to neurodegenerative and systemic diseases are underreported in developing countries. It is believed that in spite of extensive investigations the number of peripheral neuropathies for which an etiology cannot be found ranges from 13 to 22 percent.[6,7]

Anatomy

Neuropathic disorders encompass diseases of the neuron cell body (neuronopathy) and their peripheral processes (peripheral neuropathy). Neuronopathies include anterior horn cell disorders, which are termed motor neuron disease, and dorsal root ganglion disorders, which are termed sensory neuronopathy or ganglionopathy. Peripheral neuropathies can be subdivided into two major categories: primary axonopathies and primary myelopathies. Neuropathies are further subdivided on the basis of the diameter of the impaired axon. Large myelinated axons include motor axons and sensory axons responsible for proprioception, vibration and light touch. Thinly myelinated small diameter axons include sensory fibers responsible for light touch, pain, temperature, and preganglionic autonomic functions. Peripheral nerve damage can comprise a focal lesion of a single nerve (mononeuropathy) or multiple nerves (polyneuropathy).[5]

Peripheral Nerve Maturation

Peripheral nerve myelination is documented as early as by 15 weeks of gestational age. There is a gradual increase in axon diameter and myelin sheath thickness, till adult values are attained at about 4-5 years of age. The results of electrodiagnostic studies have demonstrated that adult nerve conduction velocities are attained by the age of 3-5 years. Normal neonatal nerve conduction velocities are in the range of 20-35 m/s and these values should not be misinterpreted as abnormal.[6,8]

Clinical Evaluation of Peripheral Neuropathy

Symptoms of a peripheral neuropathy are common neurologic complaints. The evaluation process may seem daunting considering the long list of potential underlying causes and formidable number of available diagnostic tests. The evaluation of peripheral neuropathy should begin with the gathering of clinical data including the history of present illness, past medical history, family history, and physical examination. The determination of what of that clinical data is relevant requires knowledge of various diseases and the risk factors for those diseases. This is accomplished in two stages; stage 1 is clinical characterization of the elements of the peripheral nervous system that are involved based on symptoms and signs, and stage 2 is defining the underlying pathology from electrodiagnostic testing.

The first step in diagnosing neuropathy is to establish the clinical diagnosis of neuropathy and rule out cortical, spinal, psychogenic loci. Symptoms of neuropathy may be classified as either negative or positive.[9,10] Positive symptoms reflect inappropriate spontaneous nerve activity, whereas negative symptoms reflect reduced nerve activity.[11] Negative motor symptoms include weakness, fatigue and wasting, while positive symptoms include cramps, twitching and myokymia. The degree of weakness is proportional to the number of axons or motor neurons affected and may not be appreciated until 50% to 80% of nerve fibers are lost while positive symptoms may present earlier in the course of the disease.[12,13] Weakness is often most pronounced in muscles of foot dorsiflexion and eversion and in intrinsic hand muscles such as the first dorsal interosseus, adductor digiti minimi and abductor pollicis brevis. As a result, tripping on the carpet or curb, spraining one's ankle laterally and a high steppage gait are early symptoms of neuropathy in lower limbs. In the hands, symptoms typically involve activities of fine movements, including problems using buttons or zippers and difficulty inserting and turning keys in locks. In lower extremities, weakness usually progresses to muscles of plantar flexion before more proximal muscles become involved.[14] Presence of fallen as well as high arches (due to weakness of extensor muscles) and hammertoes is suggestive of intrinsic foot weakness, a useful clinical sign particularly in patients with hereditary neuropathy. Atrophy is characteristic of chronic disease of the motor neuron or motor axon. Atrophy is more likely to occur in axonal neuropathies and maximum degree of denervation atrophy occurs in 90 to 120 days and reduces muscle volume by 75 to 80 percent after an acute injury. Atrophy frequently occurs in muscles of dorsiflexion, such as the tibialis anterior, in lower extremities, and in intrinsic hand muscles, such as the first dorsal interosseus in upper extremities.[14] Weakness occurs before atrophy in rapidly progressive lesions and atrophy may occur before paralysis in slowly progressing degenerative diseases.

Sensory symptoms should be characterized into those with a positive sensation, such as prickling, tingling, or buzzing, vs those with a negative sensation, such as loss of sensation or imbalance. This differentiation is helpful because presence of positive sensory symptoms often suggest an acquired cause of neuropathy rather than an inherited neuropathy.[15] Common symptoms of small fiber sensory neuropathy include feeling like one's feet are "walking on pebbles or thorns" or difficulties telling with one's feet whether bath water is hot or cold and painful dysesthesias, such as feeling as if one's feet are on fire, on hot coals, or being stuck with pins.[14] Positive sensory symptoms can be present in small fiber neuropathies regardless of whether they are acquired or inherited. Large fiber sensory loss usually causes patients to develop difficulties with balance. When presenting in children with inherited neuropathies, for example, large fiber sensory loss may cause difficulties walking on a balance beam at school or walking across a log over a stream. Because loss of proprioception is also frequently length dependent, children may be able to steady themselves by simply lightly touching a wall with their hand or elbow since nerves from the arm can then provide proprioceptive input to the brain. These problems with balance may be worse in a crowd or at night when vision cannot overcome proprioception loss.[14] Symptoms suggesting autonomic nerve involvement include early satiety, bloating, constipation, diarrhea, impotence, urinary incontinence, abnormalities of sweating (hyperhidrosis, anhidrosis), and lightheadedness associated with orthostasis.

It is also important to be aware of neuropathy mimics or central causes that may present with neuropathy like symptoms. Pseudoneuropathies mimicking the pattern of a polyneuropathy (pseudopolyneuropathies) are most often myelopathies, which can produce distal sensory and sometimes motor dysfunction in a stocking pattern, without telltale features of a sensory level, long tract weakness, sphincter disturbance, or hyperreflexia.[16] The two most common causes of such a presentation are cervical spondylotic myelopathy and spinal multiple sclerosis. Cerebral lesions can also rarely cause a neuropathy like; small cerebral infarcts have rarely simulated ulnar neuropathies and radial neuropathy while bilateral distal leg weakness can rarely be caused by parasagittal lesions.[17]

Further evaluation of neuropathy requires answer to 8 key questions which help in localizing the lesion, allowing the categorization of patients into typical phenotypic patterns and determining the etiology.[18]

Key Question 1: What is the Temporal Evolution?

Key Question 2: What Systems are Involved?

Key Question 3: What is the Distribution of Weakness and Sensory Involvement?

Key Question 4: What is the Nature of the Sensory Involvement?

Key Question 5: Is There Evidence of Upper Motor Neuron Involvement?

Key Question 6: Is There Evidence for a Hereditary Neuropathy?

Key Question 7: Is There a History of Medical Illness or are There Signs Suggesting a Medical Illness Associated with Polyneuropathy?

Key Question 8: Is There Any History of Occupational or Toxic Exposure to Agents Associated with Polyneuropathy?

Key Question 1: What is the Temporal Evolution?

The first and most important question is the temporal profile, i.e., onset, duration, and evolution of symptoms and signs. Neuropathies can be categorized as acute (days to 4 weeks), subacute (4-8 weeks), or chronic (>8 weeks) depending on the onset.[18] A true acute or apoplectic event is rare in neuropathies except in vasculitic mononeuritis multiplex or idiopathic plexopathy.[19] More commonly, acute onset is defined as days to several weeks, and suggests AIDP (Guillain-Barré syndrome), a metabolic event, or a toxic exposure. Polyneuropathies that progress in a stepwise fashion are infrequent and often are associated with a mononeuropathy multiplex pattern. A history of clear remissions and exacerbations suggests CIDP or other form of immune-mediated neuropathy. Hereditary neuropathies have a very slow and insidious onset with a vague recollection of onset of symptoms. It is also important to inquire about preceding or concurrent infections, associated medical conditions, drug use including over-the-counter vitamin preparations (B_6), alcohol and dietary habits.[18,19]

Key Question 2: What Systems are Involved?

It is important to determine if the patient's symptoms and signs are pure motor, pure sensory, autonomic, or some combination of these. Pure motor weakness without any sensory symptoms is most commonly seen in motor neuronopathy or motor neuron disease. Other neuropathic disorders that may present with pure motor symptoms are GBS, CIDP, Lead intoxication, acute porphyria and hereditary motor sensory neuropathy but sensory signs can usually be found on examination in these conditions.[18] Multifocal motor neuropathy is one neuropathy in which there are no sensory signs on examination.[20] In addition patients with pure motor distal weakness with a clinical phenotype of CMT neuropathy but with no sensory involvement are now classified as hereditary motor neuropathy (HMN).[21,22]

On the sensory side, pure sensory neuropathies also are unusual and often suggest a primary process affecting the dorsal root ganglia. These sensory neuronopathies are quite rare and are characteristically seen acutely or subacutely as a paraneoplastic syndrome, postinfectious process, or associated with Sjögren's syndrome or pyridoxine (B_6) intoxication.[23] Most of the neuropathies encountered in clinical practice are sensorimotor in nature. When motor and sensory symptoms are combined, it is helpful to rank them in order of symptom predominance–i.e., motor greater than sensory, or vice versa. This is important because most of the immune mediated neuropathies, such as Guillain-Barré syndrome and chronic inflammatory demyelinating polyradiculoneuropathy (CIDP), produce predominantly motor abnormalities with minimal sensory symptoms. On the other hand sensory complaints predominate in most of the length dependent axonal polyneuropathies, especially those caused by metabolic or toxic disorders.[24] Causes of sensorimotor neuropathy are enlisted in Table 31.1.[25,26] Presence of autonomic features can help in narrowing the differential diagnosis of neuropathy. When complaints do not clearly implicate pathology in the autonomic nervous system, autonomic testing such as bedside orthostatic hypotension or tilt-table testing may be used. Table 31.2 enlists the causes of neuropathies associated with autonomic dysfunction.[25,18]

Table 31.1: Causes of Sensorimotor Neuropathy

1. **Axonal Neuropathies**
   a. Acute/Subacute Onset
   i. Guillain-Barré Syndrome–Acute motor sensory axonal neuropathy (AMSAN) variant (motor predominant).
   ii. Porphyria (motor predominant).
   iii. Critical illness polyneuropathy (motor predominant).
   iv. Tick paralysis (nerve or neuromuscular junction channelopathy).
   v. Toxic, pharmaceutical: Amiodarone, gold salts, nitrofurantoin, vincristine.
   vi. Toxic, heavy metals: Arsenic, mercury, thallium.
   vii. Graft-versus-host disease.
   b. Chronic Onset
   i. **Metabolic/endocrine:** Diabetes, uremia, hypothyroidism, acromegaly, hepatic failure, hypoglycemia/hyperinsulinemia.
   ii. **Nutritional deficiency:** Vitamin B_{12}, folate, thiamine, vitamin E, copper, bariatric surgery (multifactorial), Cuban epidemic optic and peripheral neuropathy (multifactorial).
   iii. **Vascular:** Vasculitis: Systemic (primary or secondary) and nonsystemic, pulmonary failure (chronic hypoxia), polycythemia, large-vessel atherosclerotic vascular disease.
   iv. **Neoplastic (infiltrative):** Leukemia, lymphoma, lymphomatoid granulomatosis, neurofibromatosis 1 and 2.
   v. **Infectious/granulomatous:** Leprosy, Lyme disease, HIV, HTLV-1, HCV, sarcoidosis, Whipple disease.
   vi. **Toxic:** Most peripheral neurotoxic drugs and industrial agents, alcohol, nitrous oxide–associated vitamin B_{12} deficiency.
   vii. **Inflammatory/immune-mediated/connective tissue disorders:** Sjögren syndrome, SLE, RA, scleroderma, mixed connective tissue disease, primary biliary cirrhosis, celiac disease, graft-versus-host disease, hypereosinophilic syndrome.
   viii. **Paraproteinemias:** Amyloidosis (acquired or familial), cryoglobulinemia.
   ix. **Hereditary:** CMT2, abetalipoproteinemia, cerebrotendinous xanthomatosis, choreaacanthocytosis and McLeod neuroacanthocytosis syndromes, adult polyglucosan body disease, adult-onset Tay-Sachs disease.
   x. **Paraneoplastic:** Various tumors.
2. **Demyelinating or Mixed**
   a. Acute/Subacute
   i. GBS (AIDP)
   ii. Diphtheria

Contd.

Contd.

   iii. Toxic/pharmaceutical: Amiodarone, suramin, perhexilene, tacrolimus, L-tryptophan, cytosine arabinoside, bortezomib, tumor necrosis factor-a blockers
   iv. Graft-versus-host disease
   v. Arsenic, acute phase
   vi. n-Hexane (glue sniffer's neuropathy)
   b. Subacute/Chronic
   i. Inflammatory/dysimmune: CIDP
   ii. Dysproteinemias/hematologic disorders/malignancies: cryoglobulinemia, lymphoma
   iii. Hereditary/genetic: CMT1, CMT4, DSD/CHN, CMTX, DI-CMT, lysosomal leukodystrophies (metachromatic leukodystrophy, Krabbe disease), peroxisomal disorders (Refsum disease, adrenomyeloneuropathy), lipoprotein disorders (Tangier disease), transthyretin familial amyloid polyneuropathy, cerebrotendinous xanthomatosis, Cockayne syndrome, xeroderma pigmentosum, mitochondrial disorders (Leigh disease, MNGIE, occasionally MELAS or MERRF), occasionally neurofibromatosis 1 or 2.

Table 31.2: Peripheral Neuropathies with Autonomic Nervous System Involvement

1. Diabetes
2. Amyloidosis–primary (AL) and familial:
   a. *Hereditary disorders:* HSANs, porphyria, Fabry disease, Tangier disease
   b. *Infectious diseases:* HIV, leprosy, diphtheria, Chagas disease, Diphtheria
3. Porphyria
4. Uremia
5. Acute/subacute autonomic neuropathies:
   a. Guillain-Barré syndrome
   b. Paraneoplastic
   c. Autoimmune autonomic ganglionopathy (ganglionic AChR antibodies)
   d. *Connective tissue diseases:* Sjögren's syndrome, Systemic lupus erythematosus, Rheumatoid arthritis, Mixed connective tissue disease
   e. *Viral/postviral:* HSV, EBV, Coxackie B, rubella, mumps
6. Toxins: Vacor, vincristine, heavy metals, alcohol

Key Question 3: What is the Distribution of Weakness and Sensory Involvement?

To make an accurate diagnosis of the cause of neuropathy, it is essential to determine the pattern of weakness and sensory involvement. It should be ascertained whether the weakness is only distal or proximal as well as distal and secondly is the weakness symmetrical or focal and asymmetrical. Based on the distribution of symptoms neuropathies can be characterized into following patterns: symmetric with a length dependent pattern, symmetric with proximal and distal involvement (i.e., length independent pattern) and focal or asymmetric involvement (nerve or plexus pattern). The overall pattern of the polyneuropathy is determined largely by clinical examination and is supplemented and confirmed by electrophysiologic studies. Most axonal polyneuropathies exhibit a distal-to-proximal, dying back pattern, reflecting that the damage to a nerve is length dependent with weakness and sensory symptoms beginning first in the feet symmetrically.[23] The earliest symptoms are usually sensory followed by motor weakness. There is a glove and stocking pattern of sensory involvement so that sensory symptoms appear first in lower limbs distally and then when they have progressed up to the knee level then the upper limbs are involved again in a distal-proximal gradient. This is because; nerve length at knee level is approximately equal to the length innervating the hand. As the polyneuropathy worsens, symptoms may develop over the anterior chest and abdomen, representing distal degeneration of the thoracic intercostal nerves.

Similarly motor weakness is also first observed in the feet first with intrinsic foot muscles being affected first, followed by the peroneal innervated muscles, and then by gastrocnemius-soleus involvement. The anterior tibial compartment is affected before the posterior tibial compartment because the former's nerve supply is longer than the latter by more than 10 cm.[14,25] When all muscle groups below the knee are affected, intrinsic hand muscle involvement starts. Although pure motor distal symmetric weakness is the presentation for hereditary motor neuropathy, rarely it can be caused by distal myopathies and myasthenia gravis. Neuropathies can be differentiated from distal myopathies by examining the extensor digitorum brevis which is preserved in distal myopathies and wasted in polyneuropathies.[27] The second pattern of length independent neuropathy characterized by weakness in both proximal and distal muscle groups in a symmetric fashion is pathologically represented by demyelination at multifocal sites along roots and nerves.[28] The diffuse process may occasionally become manifest in the short cranial nerves, but more commonly, the nerves to the lower extremities are initially involved though a distal predominance may or may not be seen. This occurs because the myelinated axons of the sciatic nerve are longest, contain the most myelin, and are statistically most likely to be involved in a random demyelinating process. However segmental or non-uniform demyelinating neuropathy may affect any nerve segment. Both the segments traversing the subarachnoid space and the most distal segments may be more susceptible to metabolic and immunologic changes because of a weaker blood-nerve barrier and their involvement which may cause a diagnostic confusion with length-dependent neuropathy. This type of involvement is commonly associated with immune mediated or infectious neuropathies and associated with segmental demyelination.[12] The differential diagnosis of length-independent neuropathy includes CIDP and variants (especially multifocal acquired demyelinating sensory and motor neuropathy [MADSAM] variant), Multifocal motor neuropathy, Lyme disease, HIV, diphtheria, sarcoidosis, carcinoma, amyloidosis, lymphoma, porphyria and Tangier disease.[12] The finding of weakness in both proximal and distal muscle groups in a symmetric fashion is the hallmark for acquired immune demyelinating polyneuropathies, both the acute form (GBS) and the chronic form (CIDP).[18,29,30]

In particular, hip flexor weakness is suggestive of CIDP, as it is frequently involved in CIDP and cannot be attributed to L4-S1 compressive polyradiculopathy.[29] The finding of symmetric proximal and distal weakness in a patient who presents with both motor and sensory symptoms is important because it identifies an important subset of patients who may have a treatable acquired demyelinating neuropathic disorder, that is, AIDP or CIDP. On the other hand, if a patient with both symmetric sensory and motor findings has weakness involving only the distal lower and upper extremities, the disorder generally reflects a primarily axonal peripheral neuropathy and is much less likely to represent a treatable entity.[18] There is an important exception to the rule that distal sensorimotor neuropathies are axonal in nature. The acquired demyelinating neuropathies associated with immunoglobulin M–k monoclonal antibodies, which are typically targeted to myelin-associated glycoprotein, have the curious pattern of predominantly distal symmetric sensory loss and weakness, with little or no proximal weakness. This condition known as DADS-M (distal acquired demyelinating symmetric with monoclonal gammopathy) neuropathy is however poorly responsive to immunomodulatory therapy unlike other demyelinating neuropathies.[31]

The presence of any asymmetry is a key finding; it usually excludes a large number of toxic, metabolic, and genetic conditions that usually cause a symmetric pattern. Asymmetry implies the possibility of:

(1) A mononeuropathy multiplex pattern.

(2) A superimposed radiculopathy or entrapment neuropathy; or

(3) A variant of CIDP.[23]

At times it may be difficult to determine whether the neuropathy is symmetric or asymmetric due to clinical progression, so it is best to ask the patient to describe the pattern of onset of symptoms followed by the distribution of subsequent progression. The pattern of a mononeuropathy multiplex is one of the most important patterns to recognize because it has therapeutic implications. Mononeuritis multiplex (MM) type of presentation can occur because of ischemia or infiltration of the nerves. When MM is caused due to ischemia, there is a distinctive clinical presentation with an asymmetric, stepwise involvement of individual cranial and/or peripheral nerves. Over time, a confluent pattern may develop, which may be difficult to distinguish from a generalized polyneuropathy.[23]

Mononeuritis multiplex occurring as a result of ischemia as in various vasculitides is characterized most commonly by a rapid onset of painful weakness in the territory of individual named nerves. Weakness is more striking than sensory loss because of relative resistance of small myelinated and unmyelinated sensory axons to ischemia. Mononeuritis multiplex due to infiltration is characteristically seen in leprosy, besides less common causes such as amyloidosis, sarcoidosis, leukemic and lymphomatous infiltrates, perineural xanthoma, and schwannoma.[25] In leprosy particularly there is early involvement of superficial cooler region cutaneous nerves with predominant sensory symptoms. As the disease progresses, nerve trunk deficits supervene with ulnar nerve proximal to the olecranon groove being most commonly involved. Sensory impairment proceeds in a predictable sequence, with loss of temperature sensation first, followed by pain, and then touch. Sweating is also diminished with sparing of proprioception and vibration.

Another key feature of leprosy is that sensory loss appears in the cooler areas first and the peripheral nerves that are situated in deep tissues under or close to muscles, or warmer areas are not actively involved. Sensory examination of the distal extremities alone in patient with leprosy may result in confusion with a distal sensory polyneuropathy but this can be resolved by an active search for sparing of sensory loss in warmer areas such as axillae, perineum, sternal area, center of the back and webs of the toes or fingers.[32] Hereditary neuropathy with predisposition to pressure palsies (HNPP) or familial brachial plexus neuropathies are also conditions that can present with focal, asymmetric leg or arm weakness much like a mononeuritis multiplex presentation.[33] In contrast to other inherited neuropathies, HNPP often presents with multiple compressive mononeuropathies (e.g., ulnar, median and peroneal nerves). In addition, patients with multifocal motor neuropathy and multifocal acquired demyelinating sensory and motor (MADSAM) neuropathy have distal, asymmetric extremity involvement quite similar to a mononeuritis multiplex pattern but these disorders respond to immunosuppressive therapy.

Focal and multifocal cranial nerve lesions can occur in isolation or in combination with a generalized polyneuropathy and can provide important diagnostic clues to the cause of neuropathy. Cranial nerves tend to be involved later in the evolution of neuropathy (after the limbs), but occasionally the reverse sequence is observed. Isolated or multiple cranial nerve lesions are seen in sarcoidosis, diabetes mellitus, borreliosis, and neoplastic invasion of the meninges or skull base. Table 31.3 enlists the causes of neuropathies in which cranial nerve involvement may be a prominent feature.[12,34]

Table 31.3: Neuropathies with Cranial Nerve Involvement

Neuropathy	Most Commonly Involved Cranial Nerves	Less Commonly Involved Cranial Nerves
Diphtheria	IX	II, III
Sarcoidosis	VII (may be bilateral or recurrent)	I, III, IV, VI
Diabetes	III	II, IV, VI, VII, XII
Guillain-Barre´ syndrome (GBS)	VI, VII	III, IV
Miller-Fisher variant of GBS	III, IV, VI	
Sjögren syndrome	V	
SLE		
Polyarteritis nodosa	VII, III	VIII
Wegener granulomatosis	VIII	VII
Lyme disease	VII, V	All but I
Porphyria	VII, X	III, IV, V, XI, XII
Refsum's disease	I, VIII	
Primary amyloidosis	VII, V, III	VI, XII
Syphilis	III	IV, V, VII, VIII
Arsenic	V	
Leprosy	V, VII	
Vitamin B_{12} deficiency	II	
Copper deficiency	II	
CIDP		III,VII
HIV	VII	

Key Question 4: What is the Nature of the Sensory Involvement?

As mentioned earlier, sensory symptoms in neuropathy can be positive as well as negative (Table 31.4).[9,10,11] Although it is important to ascertain the nature of sensory involvement, complaints of numbness or tingling, and the type of neuropathic pain while implicating sensory involvement, are in general not very helpful in suggesting a specific diagnosis, as these symptoms can accompany many peripheral neuropathies. In addition it may be difficult for many patients to distinguish between uncomfortable tingling sensations (dysesthesias) and pain. Table 31.5 enlists the various terms used to describe pain and abnormal sensations in neuropathic disorders.[35] The sensory examination also can be challenging and confusing because responses are indirect and represent a patient's interpretation of the test and test questions. Sensory examination is obviously less reliable in children because they may not be attentive and may have difficulty in understanding the commands and requirement of tests. Although attempts are made to assess several individual sensory modalities and nerve fiber types, true distinctions may not always be possible.

Table 31.4: Positive and Negative Sensory Symptoms and Signs

Positive Symptoms and Signs		Negative Symptoms and Signs
Large Fiber	Tingling	Ataxia
	Pins and needles	Hyporeflexia or areflexia
		Decreased joint position sensation
		Decreased vibration sensation
Small fiber	Burning	Decreased pain sensation
	Jabbing	Decreased temperature sensation
	Shooting	

Light touch can be tested with a wisp of cotton, tissue paper, a feather, a soft brush, light stroking of the hairs, or even using a very light touch of the fingertip. More detailed and quantitative evaluation can be accomplished using Semmes-Weinstein filaments. These methods employ filaments of different thicknesses to deliver stimuli of varying, graded intensity. Patients who cannot reliably detect application of the 10 g monofilament to designated sites on the plantar surface of their feet are considered to have lost protective sensation. This loss of protective sensation is not equivalent to the total absence of sensation.[11] Vibration threshold can be assessed using a tuning fork. A 128 Hz tuning fork dies out more slowly than a 256 Hz tuning fork and is easier to use. The child must understand the need to indicate complete disappearance. In children and young adults, vibratory stimulus should be appreciated for at least 15 seconds over the great toe. Joint position testing is less sensitive than vibratory testing for large fiber function and may only be impaired in severe cases.[11] Sharp stimulus threshold can be assessed by a patient's ability to distinguish between the lightly applied "pokey" feeling from the sharp end of a safety pin compared with the similarly lightly applied dull end. Reflex testing is also an objective measure of sensory nerve function. The deep tendon reflex is a monosynaptic reflex arc with sensory and motor nerve components, but the arc is much more vulnerable to sensory nerve damage. As has already been mentioned that ankle plantar flexion strength is relatively preserved till late, yet ankle reflexes are lost early on. Ankle reflexes are typically preserved with small fiber neuropathy.

Sensory involvement in neuropathy can occur because of large or small fiber involvement. Although there are examples of large fiber neuropathies and small fiber neuropathies, most sensory modalities (light touch through pain) can be conveyed by both large and small diameter fibers. Further, clinical testing (light touch, stroking, sharp instruments) usually activates a variety of

Table 31.5: Terms Used to Describe Pain and Abnormal Sensations in Neuropathic Disorders

Term	Description
Dysesthesia	An unpleasant abnormal sensation, whether spontaneous or evoked.
Paresthesia	An abnormal sensation which is not unpleasant or painful, whether spontaneous or evoked (for example: feelings of cold, warmth, numbness, tingling, burning, prickling, crawling, heaviness, compression, or itching.
Hyperesthesia	Exaggerated perception of sensation in response to a mild stimulus.
Hyperalgesia	Severe pain in response to a mildly noxious stimulus which is not ordinarily painful.
Allodynia	Condition in which a nonpainful stimulus, once perceived, is experienced as painful, even excruciating.
Hyperpathia	Painful syndrome characterized by an abnormally painful reaction to a stimulus, especially a repetitive stimulus, as well as an increased threshold.
Hypoalgesia	Diminished pain in response to a normally painful stimulus.
Hypoesthesia	Decreased sensitivity to stimulation, excluding the special senses.

receptor types. Thus, distinctions between modalities and fiber types may be more apparent than real. Symptoms of small fiber neuropathies include autonomic dysfunction and a distal sensory deficit, particularly for pinprick, often associated with painful, burning dysesthesias. Neuropathic pain is an important diagnostic feature as presence of pain narrows the diagnostic possibilities and has therapeutic implications as well. Neuropathic pain can be burning, dull, and poorly localized (protopathic pain), presumably transmitted by polymodal C nociceptor fibers, or sharp and lancinating (epicritic pain), relayed by A delta fibers.[18] Pain is often variable, worse at night and following activity, and is also made worse by contact as in causalgia. Besides nerve involvement, pain can also occur because of root or spinal cord involvement as well. In small fiber neuropathy the distribution of pain is usually distal, of the burning type with allodynia. In nerve trunk and root lesions, pain is frequently sharp, stabbing, shooting, and superimposed on a chronic ache, more proximal in location with radiation to distal areas, and may be worsened by maneuvers that stretch or further compress the nerve root. Table 31.6 enlists causes of peripheral neuropathies often associated with pain.[18,25] In children painful neuropathy can be caused by vasculitis, Fabry disease, amyloidosis and HIV-related distal symmetric polyneuropathy. In children another important cause is hereditary sensory and autonomic neuropathy (HSAN). HSAN is a phenotypically and genetically heterogeneous group of disorders characterized by involvement of small-diameter nerve fibers (temperature and pain sensation, autonomic nerves). HSANI which is the most common form is caused by mutations in serine palmitoyltransferase, long chain base subunit 1 gene (SPTLC). Patients typically present within the first two decades of life with distal lower limb sensory loss, and many have neuropathic pain.[36]

Table 31.6: Causes of Small-Fiber, Painful Polyneuropathies: Isolated, Predominant or Associated
1. Cryptogenic sensory or sensorimotor neuropathy
2. Diabetes mellitus
3. Vasculitis
4. GBS
5. Amyloidosis
6. Toxic (arsenic, thallium)
7. HIV-related distal symmetric polyneuropathy
8. Fabry disease
9. Hepatitis C
10. Hereditary sensory and autonomic neuropathies (HSAN)
Contd.
11. Tangier disease
12. Sarcoidosis
13. Celiac disease
14. Erythromelalgia
15. Connective tissue disorders (Sjögren syndrome, SLE)

The other important sensory abnormality that significantly narrows the differential diagnosis is severe proprioceptive loss. Proprioceptive loss can be evident in various neuropathies but when there is a dramatic asymmetric loss of proprioception with significant vibration loss and normal strength, the clinician should immediately consider a sensory neuronopathy (i.e., ganglionopathy). Ataxia and gait difficulty are usually early and prominent complaints but in almost 50% of patients particularly in paraneoplastic cases, upper limbs may be affected first. Light touch and pain sensation are also affected, owing to injury of all sensory cell bodies but pain and temperature loss is much less compared to loss vibration and proprioceptive sensations. The various causes of sensory neuronopathy and other causes of predominantly Large-Fiber, Ataxic Neuropathies are enlisted in Table 31.7.[18] A variant of CIDP termed chronic immune sensory polyradiculopathy (CISP) manifests as a sensory ataxia and clinically resembles a sensory neuronopathy/ganglionopathy with predominant ataxia and asymmetric sensory loss. Normal sensory nerve action potentials (because the lesion is proximal to the ganglion cells) differentiate this disorder from sensory neuronopathy.[37]

Table 31.7: Causes of Predominantly Large-Fiber, Ataxic Neuropathies
1. Sensory neuronopathy (ganglionopathy)
a. Sjögren syndrome
b. Paraneoplastic
c. Idiopathic
d. Toxic: Pyridoxine hypervitaminosis, cisplatin, thalidomide, linezolid, metronidazole, podophyllotoxin, taxanes
e. HIV (rare)
f. Epstein-Barr virus
2. Demyelinating or mixed
a. Acute
i. Ataxic GBS
ii. Fisher syndrome
iii. Diphtheritic neuropathy

Contd.

Contd.

b. Chronic
i. Sensory CIDP
ii. CISP
3. Miscellaneous
a. Tabes dorsalis (dorsal root/posterior columns)
b. Celiac disease
c. HTLV-1 or -2 (tropical ataxic neuropathy)
d. Vitamin deficiencies: B_{12}, B_1, E

Key Question 5: Is There Evidence of Upper Motor Neuron Involvement?

The next key point is to determine any additional involvement of the spinal cord. In patients with symptoms of signs suggestive of lower motor neuron abnormality without sensory loss, the presence of concomitant upper motor neuron signs is the hallmark of ALS. On the other hand, if the patient presents with symmetric distal sensory symptoms and signs suggestive of a distal sensory neuropathy, but there is additional evidence of symmetric upper motor involvement, a clinical diagnosis of Myelo-neuropathy can be made. Conditions known to result in myeloneuropathy include metabolic, inflammatory, infectious, toxic and hereditary disorders (Table 31.8).[18,25] Clinical recognition of a myeloneuropathy may be difficult. A patient may have been previously diagnosed with a peripheral neuropathy or myelopathy in isolation. Symptoms that can be attributed to myelopathy include gait unsteadiness, extremity weakness, bowel and bladder impairment, and sensory symptoms. The diagnostic difficulty arises because many of these findings can occur because of peripheral neuropathy as well.

Secondly when upper motor signs predominate, it may be difficult to appreciate more subtle signs of peripheral neuropathy. The presence of sensory symptoms in both the hands and feet should alert the neurologist to a possible myeloneuropathy. The presence of a Lhermitte sign with precipitation of electrical pain down the spine and into the extremities with neck flexion would also suggest a myelopathy. Other signs of myelopathy include sensory loss with a truncal sensory level, weakness, spasticity, hyperreflexia, and extensor plantar responses. Myelopathies often have more profound proprioceptive loss compared to vibration but this is not absolute. Absent ankle jerk reflexes and distal lower limb atrophy may be the only definite clinical signs of a peripheral neuropathy in a patient with prominent myelopathic findings. Bowel and bladder involvement is less likely to occur in peripheral neuropathic disorders unless peripheral autonomic fibers are involved. Bladder impairment associated with a peripheral autonomic neuropathy is typically characterized as a high-capacity bladder with incomplete bladder emptying or urinary retention. In myelopathy on the other hand, bladder involvement is usually in the form of a low capacity spastic bladder, with symptoms of urgency and sudden uncontrollable evacuation. In spite of all these clinical clues sometimes, EMG testing may be necessary to identify peripheral nerve involvement.[38]

Table 31.8: Causes of Myeloneuropathies
1. **Vitamin/mineral deficiencies:** Vitamin B_{12}, copper, vitamin E, folate, Cuban epidemic (multiple vitamin deficiency)
2. **Toxic:** Nitrous oxide (anesthesia paresthetica), cassava (cyanide), organophosphate insecticides
3. **Inflammatory:** Connective tissue diseases, sarcoidosis
4. **Infectious:** HTLV1, HIV, Lyme disease
5. **Hereditary:** Adrenomyeloneuropathy, "complicated" hereditary spastic paraplegia subtypes, hereditary neuropathies: CMT2A/HMSN-V, CMT2H, CMT2D/dHMN-V, SCA subtypes

Identification of the posterolateral syndrome, which manifests as a sensory ataxia with pyramidal signs, is characteristic of vitamin B_{12} deficiency, copper deficiency, folate deficiency, human T-cell lymphotropic virus (HTLV) and HIV myelopathies. This type of presentation should lead to an intensive search for vitamin B_{12} deficiency (i.e., assessing for elevated serum methylmalonic acid and homocysteine levels), if the B_{12} level is in the lower limit of normal range.[18,38] Demyelinating features on NCS are typical of the hereditary leukodystrophies such as adrenomyeloneuropathy but can also be seen with HIV and HTLV and in rare cases of multiple sclerosis that have signs of central and peripheral nervous system demyelination.[38]

Key Question 6: Is There Evidence for a Hereditary Neuropathy?

Hereditary neuropathies are more common than appreciated and for any polyneuropathy patient, especially when the diagnosis is not clear, particular attention must be paid to family history. A positive family history may be lacking in autosomal recessive or X-linked recessive conditions. In addition patients may not be very forthcoming in giving a positive family history of neuropathy hereditary neuropathies may be subclinical. It has been seen that in large families with known Charcot-Marie-Tooth neuropathy, less than 30% of affected individuals seek medical attention for their symptoms. It is important to inquire in detail about symptoms and signs that may suggest a hereditary neuropathy rather than simply asking about history of a neuropathic or similar disorder (Table 31.9).[19] With the availability of cellular phones with a camera, family members can send photographs of their legs and feet for review. Sometimes it may be beneficial to examine family members, both clinically and with nerve conduction studies and EMG even if they have no symptoms so as to determine whether the underlying etiology of the patient's polyneuropathy is genetic. The possibility of an inherited neuropathy cannot be dismissed even in the face of a truly negative family history because of following reasons: early death of one or both parents, few blood relatives, autosomal recessive disease, and available diagnostic DNA testing have shown that about one third of isolated cases of inherited neuropathies may arise from de novo gene mutations. In the absence of family history factors that may help in deciding that the neuropathy in 'sporadic' patients is hereditary include:[39]

Table 31.9: Family History Questionnaire
1. High arches
2. Curled toes
3. Twist ankles easily
4. Use of cane/crutches
5. Foot surgery
6. Casting of feet as a child
7. Corrective shoes
8. Cramps
9. Skinny legs
10. Numbness feet/hands
11. Difficulty buying shoes
12. Burning of feet
13. Painful feet

- Long, slowly progressive history.
- Presence of foot deformity such as pes cavus in an adult patient.
- Absence of positive sensory symptoms in patients with clear sensory signs.
- Motor conduction velocities are usually uniformly slow in the common hereditary neuropathies as compared to the acquired demyelinating neuropathies.

Patients with hereditary neuropathies have a symmetric, length-dependent pattern of sensory and motor symptoms unlike acquired demyelinating neuropathies which have length independent symptoms. Charcot-Marie-Tooth (CMT) neuropathy refers to a group of inherited disorders characterized by a chronic motor and sensory polyneuropathy. Four major types of CMT are defined based on their inheritance and physiology: the demyelinating autosomal dominant form is CMT1; the axonal autosomal dominant form is CMT2; the autosomal recessive demyelinating form is CMT4; and the X-linked demyelinating form is CMTX. In contrast to CMT, there are a smaller group of inherited polyneuropathies associated with defects of metabolism that have been described. Most are extremely rare and are associated with other systemic abnormalities (Table 31.10).[15,36] In addition neuropathy can be associated with ataxia in autosomal dominant as well as autosomal recessive ataxias. Almost all autosomal recessive cerebellar ataxias have sensory neuropathy or neuronopathy, with associated vibratory and proprioceptive loss and areflexia. In these cases the predominant cerebellar symptoms should usually point to the correct diagnosis.

Table 31.10: Causes of Various Hereditary Neuropathies

Disease	Inheritance	Genetic Defect	Physiology/Pathology/Phenotype
Neuropathies in Which the Neuropathy is the Sole or Primary Part of the Disease			
Charcot-Marie-Tooth Disease (Hereditary Motor and Sensory Neuropathies)			
CMT1 (HMSN I), Subtypes: Median (or ulnar) Nerve Motor Conduction Velocity (MCV) is < 38 m/s			
CMT1A	AD	PMP22 duplication	Demyelinating
CMT1B	AD	MPZ mutation	Demyelinating
CMT1C	AD	SIMPLE/LITAF mutation	Demyelinating
CMT1D	AD	EGR2 mutation	Demyelinating
CMT1E	AD	PMP22 point mutation	Demyelinating
CMT1F/ CMT2E	AD	NEFL Mutation	Demyelinating
CMT2 (HMSN II), Subtypes: Axonal, if the Median MCV is > 38 m/s and Decreased Amplitudes			
CMT2A	AD	MFN2	Axonal
CMT2B	AD	RAB7	Axonal with prominent sensory involvement

Contd.

Contd.

CMT2C	AD	Unknown	Axonal (Vocal cord and diaphragmatic paresis, with sensory Involvement)
CMT2D	AD	GARS	Early hand weakness/wasting
CMT2E	AD	NEFL	Axonal but can have low velocities and early onset severe disease
CMT2F	AD	HSPB1 (HSP27)	Axonal
CMT2L	AD	HSPB8 (HSP22)	Axonal
Dejerine-Sottas disease (HMSNIII)	AR, AD, Sporadic	PMP22, MPZ, EGR2	Demyelinating with extremely low velocities (< 10 m/s), this is no more used in classification of CMTs
CMTX	XLD/XLR	GJB1	Patchy neuropathy, NCV decrease more in males, SNAP and CMAP decreased or absent in lower limbs, Central hearing loss and T2 hyperintense lesions
CMT (CMT4): AR, Demyelinating or Axonal			
CMT4A	AR	GDAP1	Demyelinating or axonal, usually early onset and severe/vocal cord and diaphragm paralysis
CMT4B1	AR	MTMR2	Demyelinating with marked decrease in velocity
CMT4B2	AR	SBF2	Demyelinating with marked decrease in velocity
CMT4C	AR	SH3TC2	Demyelinating with marked decrease in velocity
CMT4E	AR	EGR2	Demyelinating
CMT4F	AR	PRX	Demyelinating
CMT4H	AR	FGD4	Demyelinating
CMT4J	AR	FIG4	Demyelinating
CMT1	AR	PMP22 (point mutation)	Previously labelled DSS/HMSNIII
CMT1	AR	MPZ	Previously labelled DSS/HMSNIII
AR CMT2 (also AR CMT4)			
AR CMT2A	AR	LMNA	Axonal with proximal involvement
AR CMT2B	AR	Unknown	Axonal
AR CMT2	AR	GDAP1	Axonal or demyelinating with early onset and severe/vocal cord and diaphragm paralysis
Intermediate CMT	AD	MPZ, DNM2, YARS (NEFL)	NCVs intermediate between CMT1 and CMT2 (25–45 m/s)
CMT5	AD	MFN2, BSCL2, GJB1	Axonal with decreased SNAPs, Pyramidal involvement: Increased DTR, Babinski sign
CMT6	AD	MFN2	Axonal with preserved NCVs, early onset, optic atrophy with severe visual loss
Hereditary Sensory and Autonomic Neuropathies (HSAN): Predominantly Involve Sensory or Autonomic Axons			
HSANI	AD	SPTLC1	Predominant small-fiber sensory loss, lancinating pain; acromutilation

Contd.

Contd.

HSAN II	AR	HSN2	Infancy, childhood onset; severe sensory loss; acromutilation
HSAN III (Riley-Day syndrome)	AR	IKBKAP	Severe dysautonomia, less profound sensory loss, congenital onset
HSAN IV	AR	NTRK1	Congenital; anhidrosis; recurrent hyper-pyrexia; insensitivity to pain with self-multilation
HSANV	AR	NTRK1	Congenital; HSAN IV with less severe or no anhidrosis and no mental retardation
Distal Hereditary Motor Neuropathy (dHMN): Similar to CMT2 Electrophysiologically but Absence of Clinical Sensory Involvement			
dHMN I	AD	Unknown	Early onset (2–20 years); pronounced weakness and wasting
dHMN II	AD	HSPB8, HSPB1	Later onset (childhood to adulthood)
dHMN III	AR	Unknown	Onset from infancy to young adulthood; slow progression, possible late diaphragmatic involvement
dHMN IV	AR	Unknown	More severe than dHMN III
dHMN V (HMN5A)	AD	GARS	Onset in adolescence; upper-limb predominance
dHMN V (HMN5B)	AD	BSCL2	Upper-limb predominance, spastic paraplegia with distal upper-limb atrophy (Silver syndrome)
dHMN VI (SMARD1)	AR	IGHMBP2	Onset: Congenital to ≤ 2 months, death or respiratory failure at < 3 months
Recurrent Focal Neuropathies			
Hereditary neuropathy with liability to pressure palsies (HNPP)	AD	PMP22 deletion	Nonuniform, distally accentuated demyelination, Focal conduction slowing or conduction block
Hereditary neuralgic amyotrophy (HNA)	AD	SEPT9	Episodes of pain followed by weakness and atrophy, usually involving the brachial plexuses
Familial Amyloid Polyneuropathies			
Transthyretin amyloidosis	AD	Val30Met mutation most common	Progressive, predominant small-fiber and autonomic neuropathy
Apolipoprotein A-1 Amyloidosis	AD	Gly26Arg mutation	Early weakness, predominant nephropathy, limited proteinuria; peptic ulcer
Gelsolin amyloidosis	AD		Corneal dystrophy, progressive cranial poly-neuropathy, mild distal sensory and autonomic polyneuropathy
Disorders of Lipid Metabolism			
Fabry disease	XLR	Alpha-Galactosidase A	Small-fiber sensory and autonomic, decreased plasma or leukocyte α-galactosidase A activity
Metachromatic leukodystrophy (MLD)	AR	Arylsulfatase A	Sensorimotor polyneuropathy, demyelinating–uniform or nonuniform, predominant central features, peri-ventricular and subcortical supratentorial anterior white matter lesions

Contd.

Contd.

Krabbe disease	AR	Galactosylceramidase	Sensorimotor polyneuropathy, demyelinating–uniform, progressive ataxia and spastic paraparesis, optic atrophy
Peroxisomal Disorders			
Refsum disease	AR	Phytanoyl-CoA hydroxylase	Sensorimotor polyneuropathy, demyelinating > axonal–nonuniform, retinitis pigmentosa, ataxia, elevated serum phytanic acid levels
Adrenomyeloneuropathy	XLR	ABCD1 gene	Sensorimotor polyneuropathy, axonal or mixed, myelopathic features restricted to the legs, Adrenal Dysfunction, increased VLCFA
Lipoprotein Deficiencies			
Tangier disease	AR	ABCA1	Mononeuropathy multiplex; syringomyelia-like; sensorimotor polyneuropathy; mixed axonal/demyelinating features, wide range of age of onset, organomegaly, enlarged orange tonsils, very low or absent HDL levels
Abetalipoproteinemia	AR	Microsomal triglyceride transfer protein	Sensory or sensorimotor polyneuropathy, axonal
Miscellaneous Disorders			
Cerebrotendinous xanthomatosis	AR	CYP27A1	Sensorimotor polyneuropathy, axonal or mixed > demyelinating
Porphyrias Associated with Neuropathy			
Acute intermittent porphyria	AD	PBG deaminase	Axonal neuropathy, proximal > distal, Increased ALA, PBG, uroporphyrinogen
Hereditary coproporphyria	AD	Copro-oxidase	Increased ALA, PBG, Uro, Copro
Variegate porphyria	AD	Proto-oxidase	Increased ALA, PBG, Uro, Copro

AD=Autosomal dominant; AR=Autosomal recessive; XLD=X-linked dominant; XLR=X-linked recessive; PMP22=Peripheral myelin protein 22; MPZ=Myelin protein zero; SIMPLE=Small integral membrane protein of lysosome; LITAF=Lipopolysaccharide induced tumor necrosis factor alpha; EGR2=Early growth response 2; NEFL=Neurofilament protein, light polypeptide; MFN 2= Mitofusin 2; RAB7=Member RAS oncogene family; GARS=Glycyl-tRNA synthetase, HSPB1=Heat shock 27 kDa protein 1; HSPB8= Heat shock 22 kDa protein 8; GJB1 =Gap junction protein beta 1; GDAP1=Ganglioside-induced differentiation-associated protein 1; MTMR2=Myotubular in related protein 2; SBF2=SET binding factor 2; SH3TC2=SH3 domain and tetratricopeptide repeats 2; PRX=Periaxin gene; FGD4=FYVE, RhoGEF and PH domain 4; FIG4=FIG4 homolog; LMNA=lamin A/C; DNM2=dynamin 2; YARS=tyrosyl-tRNA synthetase; BSCL2=Berardinelli-Seip congenital lipodystrophy 2(seipin); SPTLC1=Serine palmitoyl transferase; IKBKAP=Inhibitor of kappa light polypeptide enhancer in B cells, kinase complex associated protein; NTRK1=Neurotrophic tyrosine kinase receptor, type 1; IGHMBP2=Immunoglobulin μ binding protein 2; SEPT9=Septin 9; ABCD1=(ATP-binding cassette, subfamily D [ALD], member 1; ABCA1=ATP-binding cassette, subfamily A, member 1; Copro: Coproporphyrinogen; PBG: Porphobilinogen; Uro: Uroporphyrinogen.

Key Question No. 7: Is There a History of Medical Illness or Are There Signs Suggesting a Medical Illness Associated with Polyneuropathy?

Several medical conditions are strongly associated with polyneuropathy and a careful review of systems and examination can go a long way in determining the cause of neuropathy. Most prominent among the systemic conditions are diabetes and other endocrine disorders, cancer, connective tissue disorders, porphyria, vitamin and other deficiency states, and human immunodeficiency virus (HIV) infection. The disease causing neuropathy may be already documented by the time the neuropathy is found or only come to light when the cause of neuropathy is pursued. Given the large number of diseases that can cause neuropathy, the number and kind of tests to be performed should be guided entirely by the clinical picture. Table 31.11 enlists some of the common systemic symptoms and signs that can provide a clue to the cause of neuropathy.[12,23]

Table 31.11: Some Common Systemic Signs and Symptoms Associated with Neuropathy	
Symptom/Sign	**Diseases associated**
Constitutional symptoms (fever, weight loss and malaise)	Underlying malignancy (carcinoma or lymphoma), infection, amyloidosis or diabetes, Collagen vascular diseases
Weight gain	Hypothyroidism
Lymphadenopathy	Lymphoma, metastatic carcinoma and the POEMS syndrome
Abdominal pain	Heavy metal toxicity, Acute intermittent porphyria
Symptoms of gastroparesis such as early satiety, cramps, diarrhea and constipation	Diabetic autonomic neuropathy, sensory ganglionopathies, particularly of the paraneoplastic variety
Jaundice	Hepatitis B or C
Cutaneous Manifestations	
Purpura, livedo reticularis	Necrotizing vasculitis
Raynaud's phenomenon	Sjögren's syndrome or cryoglobulinemia
Hyperpigmentation	POEMS syndrome, Adrenomyeloneuropathy, Arsenic toxicity
Mees' lines	Arsenic or thallium poisoning
Angiokeratoma corporis diffusum	Fabry disease
Skin hypopigmentation, Nodular lesions	Leprosy
Ichthyosis	Refsum disease
Bullous lesions	Variegate porphyria
Alopecia	Thallium poisoning
Curled hair	Giant axonal neuropathy
Pigmentary retinopathy	Refsum's disease, abetalipoproteinemia, hereditary motor and sensory neuropathy type VI, neuropathy, ataxia and retinitis pigmentosa (NARP) syndrome, spinocerebellar ataxia
Renal dysfunction	Fabry's disease, diabetes, or mitochondrial disease
Dry eyes, mouth	Sjögren syndrome
Palpable nerves	HMSN I, Refsum's disease, Dejerine-Sottas disease (HMSN III), leprosy, CIDP

Key Question No. 8: Is There Any History of Occupational or Toxic Exposure to Agents Associated with Polyneuropathy?

Last but not the least, it is always important to ask about occupational and exposure history. Among drugs, most notable are cancer chemotherapeutic agents, which frequently result in polyneuropathy. In addition, a large number of prescription drugs, as well as over-the-counter medicines, can cause polyneuropathy. In developing countries, children could be involved in screen printing or other industries, where chemicals could cause neuropathy.

On the basis of answers to these questions, clinically neuropathies can be divided into following patterns:

- Symmetric proximal and distal weakness with sensory loss (i.e., length independent sensorimotor neuropathy.
- Symmetric distal sensory loss with/without weakness (i.e., length dependent sensorimotor neuropathy).
- Asymmetric distal weakness with sensory loss (i.e., Mononeuritis Multiplex pattern).
- Asymmetric proximal and distal weakness with sensory loss (i.e., Radiculopathy or plexopathy).
- Asymmetric proprioceptive loss without weakness (i.e., Sensory neuronopathy or ganglionopathy).
- Painful small fiber neuropathy with autonomic dysfunction.
- Pure motor neuropathy.
- Myeloneuropathy.

This phenotypic characterization helps in narrowing the differential diagnosis and guides the clinician in further investigations.

Role of Electrophysiology in Diagnosing Neuropathy

The next important step is to determine the nature of neuropathy: demyelinating, axonal or mixed. As an extension of the clinical examination, electrodiagnosis augments the ability to assess the relative motor versus sensory involvement, the severity of the neuropathy, and the distribution of neuropathic dysfunction. In neuropathy, electrodiagnostic evaluation should include a minimum of two limbs. Additional limbs should be evaluated if the initial testing is not sufficiently diagnostic, if there is any clinical or electrophysiologic suggestion of asymmetry or a length-independent process, or if there is a concern regarding multiple diagnoses.

Nerve conduction studies measure conduction along large myelinated motor and sensory nerves. NCS may help determine the relative extent of axonopathy versus myelinopathy (Table 31.12).[40] Slowed conduction velocities (to less than 70% of normal) suggest the neuropathy is primarily demyelinating. Motor nerve conduction velocities measure conduction over the main body of nerves but not their proximal or distal portion. Distal motor latencies and F wave latencies measure velocities over the distal and proximal portions of the nerves. When slowing is roughly the same over the proximal, distal, and main portion of the nerve, the slowing is said to be uniform as seen in inherited myelinopathies. When the slowing is multifocal or asymmetric, either along the same nerve or between different nerves, slowing is said to be non-uniform as seen in acquired neuropathies. In axonal neuropathies, amplitudes of the compound muscle action potential or sensory nerve action potential are reduced without a significant decrease in the conduction velocity (> 70%). Any slowing of conduction in axonal neuropathies is due to loss of the largest and fastest conducting axons. Therefore, the slowing of conduction in axonal neuropathies is less than that seen in demyelinating neuropathies. If all motor nerve fibers were lost except the smallest, even then, it would still conduct at 70% of normal.

Table 31.12: Demyelinating and Axonal Neuropathy

	Demyelinating neuropathy	Axonal neuropathy
Motor Nerve Studies		
CMAP amplitude	Distal amplitudes are preserved but proximal amplitudes may be decreased because of temporal dispersion and conduction blocks	Both distal and proximal CMAP are reduced
CMAP duration	Duration of proximal CMAP is increased	Normal
Conduction velocity	CMAP amplitude is 50–100% of normal then conduction velocity is < 70% of normal If CMAP amplitude is < 50% of normal then conduction velocity is < 50% of normal	When CMAP amplitude is 50-100% of normal conduction velocity is normal or minimally decreased When CMAP amplitude is < 50% of normal then conduction velocity is < 50% of normal, conduction velocity is > 70% of normal
Distal latency	>130% of normal	When CMAP is 50–100% of normal then distal latency is normal When CMPA is < 50% of normal then Distal latency is increased but still < 130% of normal
Conduction block	Present	Absent
Temporal dispersion	Present	Absent
F wave latency	Increased	Mild increase
Sensory Nerve Studies		
SNAP amplitude	↓	↓↓
Conduction velocity	< 50% of normal	> 70% of normal

The needle EMG is also important in analyzing neuropathies. The presence of spontaneous activity, such as fibrillations or positive sharp waves, suggests that there is an acute or active process damaging axons and denervating muscles. If the neuropathy is axonal, the EMG can be of particular help distinguish between symmetric axonal neuropathies or the asymmetric mononeuritis multiplex. The EMG can also help identify whether the neuropathy is chronic. These distinctions are important because they identify potentially treatable neuropathies. However, it is important to realize that interpretation of EMG findings works best when the study is used as an extension of the neurologic exam.

Laboratory and Genetic Testing in Neuropathies

Laboratory testing of blood is often of great value, but only after a particular polyneuropathy has been characterized and placed into one or more potential etiologic subgroups. The tests with the highest yield of abnormality are blood glucose, vitamin B_{12} with methylmalonic acid and homocysteine, and immunofixation electrophoresis (IFE).[18] Vitamin B_{12} deficiency is a common treatable cause of neuropathy. Attention should be paid to the numeric value. When the vitamin B_{12} level is less than 400 pg/ml, the metabolites methylmalonic acid and homocysteine should be tested to increase diagnostic yield. In general the tests should be guided by information gained from clinical and electrophysiological studies.[18] Serum IFE is more sensitive than serum protein electrophoresis in detecting monoclonal gammopathy.[18] Laboratory testing for a distal, symmetric sensory polyneuropathy would be much different than testing for another presentation (e.g., mononeuritis multiplex or length independent demyelinating neuropathy) (Table 31.13).[18,25,41] Laboratory evaluation of suspected vasculitis and connective tissue disorders (e.g., Sjögren syndrome, SLE, rheumatoid arthritis, mixed connective tissue disease, Wegener granulomatosis) may include C-reactive protein, anti-nuclear antibody, double-stranded DNA, rheumatoid factor, proteinase 3, myeloperoxidase, complement, angiotensin-converting enzyme, SS-A and SS-B, hepatitis B and C panels and cryoglobulin.

Table 31.13: Suggested Laboratory Investigations in Various Phenotypic Patterns of Neuropathies

Test ordered	Potential Etiologies in which the investigation may be useful
Mixed Motor Sensory Neuropathies	
Acute Onset	
CSF	Guillain-Barré syndrome, AMSAN
Porphyrins	Porphyria
Heavy metal screen	Arsenic, mercury, thallium
Subacute–Chronic Onset	
Complete blood count, Comprehensive metabolic profile	Uremia, Chronic liver disease, Leukemia, lymphomas or other systemic diseases, Churg-Strauss syndrome
Fasting glucose, 2-h oral glucose tolerance test, HgbA1c	Diabetes
Vitamin B_{12} (methylmalonic acid/homocysteine)	Subacute combined degeneration of cord
ESR	Vasculitis, collagen vascular disease
Serum protein immunofixation electrophoresis (IFE)	Amyloidosis, other paraproteinemias
Thyroid function tests	Hypothyroidism
HCV titer	Hepatitis C
HIV	HIV associated neuropathy
CSF	CIDP, MADSAM, DADS
Serum ACE	Sarcoidosis
SS-A, SS-B, minor salivary gland biopsy	Sjögren syndrome
ANA	SLE
RF, Anti CCP	Rheumatoid arthritis
Abdominal fat pad biopsy	Amyloidosis
Anti-gliadin and tissue transglutaminase antibodies	Celiac disease
ANCA	Wegener's Granulomatosis, Churg-Strauss syndrome, Microscopic polyangiitis
Anti-neural antibodies	MMNCB
Specific genetic testing	Depending on electrophysiology for CMT1, 2, X
Small-Fiber, Painful Polyneuropathies	
Fasting glucose, 2-h oral glucose tolerance test, HgbA1c	Diabetes, Impaired glucose tolerance

Contd.

Contd.

SS-A, SS-B, salivary gland biopsy	Sjögren syndrome
Serum angiotensin-converting enzyme	Sarcoidosis
Serum immunofixation, Quantitative immunoglobulins, tissue biopsy	Amyloidosis
HCV titer, cryoglobulins	Hepatitis C, Cryoglobulinemia
HIV	HIV associated neuropathy
α-galactosidase activity	Fabry's disease
Lipid profile	Tangier disease
Slit skin smears	Leprosy
Transthyretin (TTR) gene sequencing	Familial amyloidosis
Nerve biopsy	In progressive cases with no obvious cause on investigation
Sensory, Large-Fiber, Ataxic Neuropathies	
Vitamin B_{12}, methylmalonic acid, homocysteine	Vitamin B_{12} deficiency
SS-A, SS-B, salivary gland biopsy	Sjögren syndrome
HIV serology	HIV associated neuropathy
VDRL, FTA-Abs or MHA-TP	Tabes dorsalis
Vitamin B_6 levels	Vitamin B_6 toxicity
Gadolinium MRI of nerve roots, CSF	Chronic immune sensory polyradiculopathy
Vitamin E levels	Vitamin E deficiency
Anti-GQ1b	Miller-Fischer syndrome
Anti-gliadin and tissue transglutaminase antibodies	Celiac disease
Anti-sulfatide antibodies	Chronic ataxic neuropathy with ophthalmoplegia, IgM paraprotein, cold agglutinins, and anti-GD1b disialosyl antibodies (CANOMAD)
Predominantly or Isolated Motor Neuropathies	
CSF	GBS, AMAN, Poliomyelitis, Multifocal motor neuropathy
GM1 antibodies	Multifocal motor neuropathy (IgM > IgG), AMAN (IgG > IgM)
Androgen receptor gene	Kennedy disease
Genetic testing for SMA, dHMN	SMA, dHMN
Porphyrins	Porphyria
CMT1/CMT4 genetic testing	CMT1/CMT4
Autonomic Neuropathies	
Fasting glucose, 2-h oral glucose tolerance test, HgbA1c	Diabetes
ANA, RF, anti Ro/La	Connective tissue diseases (SS, RA, SLE, MCTD)
CSF analysis	GBS
HIV	HIV associated neuropathy
Ganglionic AchR antibodies, voltage-gated potassium autoantibodies, GAD-65	Acute autonomic ganglionopathy
Serum immunofixation, quantitative immunoglobulins, serum free light chains, Tissue biopsy: Skin, fat, rectal, or other affected organ	Primary systemic amyloidosis
Porphyrins	Porphyria
α-galactosidase	Fabry's disease
Myeloneuropathy	
Spinal MRI	Concomitant myelopathy and neuropathy
B_{12} level, methylmalonic acid, homocysteine	Vitamin B_{12} deficiency
Serum copper and zinc	Copper deficiency
Genetic testing for HSP	HSP
Very long chain fatty acids	Adrenomyeloneuropathy
ACE/CXR/ chest CT/gallium scan	Sarcoidosis

Contd.

Contd.

ANA, RF, anti Ro/La	Connective tissue diseases (SS, RA, SLE, MCTD)
Serum vitamin E	Vitamin E deficiency
Lipid profile	Cerebrotendinous xanthomatosis, Vitamin E deficiency
Serum angiotensin-converting enzyme, CT chest	Sarcoidosis
HTLV-I serum, CSF	Human T-cell lymphotropic virus type I (HTLV-I) associated myelopathy/ tropical spastic paraparesis
Leukocyte arylsulfatase assay	Metachromatic leukodystrophy
Mononeuropathy Multiplex	
CBC including eosinophil count	Leukemia, lymphomas or other systemic diseases, Churg-Strauss syndrome
CMP for glucose, renal and liver function tests	Diabetes, Uremia, Chronic Viral hepatitis (B and C)
ESR	Collagen Vascular diseases, Vasculitis
RF, ANA, ENA (Ro, La, Sm, RNP, Scl-70)	Connective tissue diseases (SS, Scleroderma, RA, SLE, MCTD)
c-ANCA and p-ANCA	Wegener's granulomatosis, Churg-Strauss syndrome, Microscopic polyangiitis
Hepatitis panel	Hepatitis B and C
Cryoglobulins	Cryoglobulinemia
HIV	HIV associated neuropathy
Urinalysis and CXR	Connective tissue diseases, vasculitis
Angiography or MRA	Polyarteritis nodosa
Chest CT or MRI	Sarcoidosis, Malignancy
Celiac panel	Celiac disease
CSF analysis	CIDP (MADSAM variant), MMN
Anti-GM1 antibody	MMN
Nerve/muscle biopsy	Vasculitis, Sensory perineuritis

CSF analysis is a potentially helpful if not routine test performed in the evaluation of select groups of patients with suspected neuropathies. An abnormality in CSF results implies the existence of pathology in the central nervous system or within the nerve roots. Albuminocytological disassociation in the setting of a peripheral neuropathy implies demyelination of nerve roots, as characteristically seen in both the acute and the chronic inflammatory demyelinating neuropathies. A lymphocytic pleocytosis in the setting of an acute motor neuron syndrome suggests a West Nile, poliomyelitic, or other neurotropic enteroviral infection. A lymphocytic pleocytosis occurring in the setting of an apparent polyradiculopathy with both sensory and motor involvement would suggest neoplastic, inflammatory (such as sarcoidosis), or chronic infection (Lyme's, Tuberculosis) as causes of meningitis.

Genetic testing is most effective when it is tailored to the clinical presentation, inheritance pattern, and electrodiagnostic classification. There are 2 important questions which need to be answered before genetic testing for neuropathies. First is which patients should undergo genetic testing. It is important to counsel the patient and his parents before genetic testing because not all patients with a genetic neuropathy want or need testing to identify the genetic cause of their disease. The ultimate decision to undergo genetic testing rests with the patient or the patient's parents if a symptomatic child is younger than 18 years. Reasons for obtaining genetic testing include: identifying the inheritance pattern of their CMT, making family planning decisions, and obtaining knowledge about the cause and natural history of their form of CMT. On the other hand patients may not want to undergo genetic testing because of high costs of commercial testing and fears of discrimination in the workplace or in obtaining health insurance. It is advisable not to test asymptomatic minors (younger than 18 years) with a family history of

CMT, either by electrophysiology or genetic testing, because of the chance for increased psychological harm to the child.

The second important question is what test to order. Commercially available "CMT panels" are very expensive and include a broad range of genetic tests and are not readily available in resource poor countries like India. Some genes that are tested are very rare or have been described only in single kindreds. Broadly hereditary neuropathies can be divided into one group with slow nerve conduction velocities (NCVs) (less than 38 m/s in upper extremities) and pathologic evidence of a hypertrophic demyelinating neuropathy (CMT type 1), and a second group with relatively normal nerve conduction velocities and axonal degeneration (CMT type 2). The term Dejerine-Sottas syndrome is used to characterize severely affected infants with CMT, independent of their inheritance pattern, and CMT4 is used to describe AR inheritance. In the absence of availability of genetic testing, a tentative diagnosis of the broad categories can be made on clinical and electrophysiological grounds (Table 31.15). In cases with CMT 1–like phenotype, fluorescent in situ hybridization testing for PMP 22 duplication should be done first and if negative then tests for PMP22 point mutation, Cx32, MPZ sequencing can be ordered. In patients with CMT 2–like phenotype, first evaluate for PMP 22 duplication because CMT1A may on occasion have intermediate velocities. If there is no male to male transmission then the next test should be Cx 32, otherwise testing for MPZ and MFN2 should be considered. For most forms of CMT, the acute and chronic care is the same, and predominantly symptomatic so genetic analysis does not add much therapeutically.[36]

Many autoantibodies have been described in association with peripheral neuropathy, but the use of antibody testing in clinical practice remains a matter of some debate. Serum autoantibodies to gangliosides or glycoproteins are implicated in a variety of sensory and motor neuropathy syndromes. Because the cause of acquired neuropathies often is obscure, autoantibody testing can be of great diagnostic value in identifying autoimmune neuropathy. Some tests are important and specific in the appropriate clinical settings, whereas the significance of other antibodies remains unknown.

Nerve Biopsy

A challenge for neurologists is to decide when to perform sural nerve biopsies and how to interpret the results. Nerve biopsies are only indicated in a small number of patients with neuropathy (Table 31.14).[25] Peripheral nerve biopsy is a safe investigation, which, if performed and analyzed in an appropriate setting, can enhance the diagnostic yield of complex patients.[42] However, most guidelines, are adult based and few exist for pediatric population. In general, however, nerve biopsies can be used to determine whether a primary pathologic process, such as vasculitis, is involving endoneurial blood vessels, whether there is an inflammatory process in the nerve, whether there is an infiltrating process or abnormal accumulations of foreign materials, and whether the neuropathy is demyelinating or axonal. In children particularly presence of giant axons could point towards Giant Axonal Neuropathy, CMT2E/CMT1F, CMT4C and 'glue sniffing' neuropathy related to exposure to N-hexane.[43,44,45] Nerve biopsy may also help confirming diagnosis of conditions such as metachomatic leucodystrophy and can often be performed at the time of an orthopedic procedure needed for deformities. In fact in a resource poor setting, nerve biopsy may prove to be more cost effective than genetic analysis for diagnosis of hereditary neuropathies.

Table 31.14: Indications for Nerve Biopsy
Nerve biopsy results show diagnostic abnormalities
1. Vasculitis
2. Amyloidosis
3. Sarcoidosis
4. Hansen's disease
5. Giant axonal neuropathy
6. Polyglucosan body disease
7. Tumor infiltration
Nerve biopsy results show suggestive abnormalities
1. Charcot-Marie-Tooth disease types 1 and 3
2. Chronic inflammatory demyelinating polyradiculoneuropathy
3. Paraproteinemic neuropathy (immunoglobulin M monoclonal gammopathy with anti-myelin-associated glycoprotein antibody)

Conditions that are Associated with Specific Clinical Types of Peripheral Neuropathy in Children

Table 31.15: Causes of Acquired Neuropathies in Children

Disease	Pathology	Comments
Infectious Diseases		
Diphtheria	D	Biphasic illness with progressive cranial neuropathy followed by mixed sensorimotor demyelinating peripheral neuropathy. Toxin detection or throat swabs can be used for diagnosis
Leprosy	A	Sensory > sensorimotor, most often involves cutaneous nerves in coolest parts of body, involvement more in lepromatous spectrum
HIV	A,D	Most common is distal sensory neuropathy (axonal), may have an AIDP (especially with early infection) or CIDP like presentation with CSF showing increased WBC. Other patterns may be mononeuritis multiplex or painful polyradiculopathy
Rabies	M	Peripheral neuropathy, with weakness and loss of deep tendon reflexes similar to GBS seen in 20% of children
Lyme disease	A	Focal or multifocal radiculoneuropathy. Facial neuropathy also common
Inflammatory Disorders		
Guillain-Barré syndrome	D,A	Acute onset (< 4 weeks), Demyelinating or axonal variants (AMAN, AMSAN), Regional variants Albuminocytological disassociation
Chronic inflammatory demyelinating polyneuropathy	D	Symmetric motor > sensory, proximal + Distal involvement, slowly progressive or rarely relapsing remitting, conduction block, Albuminocytological disassociation
Rheumatic Diseases		
Churg-Strauss syndrome	A	Triad of allergic rhinitis, asthma and prominent peripheral blood eosinophilia. 20 percent of cases occur in children. **Neuropathy:** Multiple mononeuropathy, distal symmetric polyneuropathy or asymmetric polyneuropathy. MPO-ANCA or P-ANCA positive
Henoch-Schönlein Purpura	A	Rash, arthralgias, abdominal pain and renal disease, peripheral neuropathy is rare
Juvenile idiopathic arthritis	A	Rare feature
Polyarteritis nodosa		Mononeuropathy multiplex (or asymmetric polyneuropathy) with motor and sensory deficits, distal polyneuropathy with progression, Hepatitis B and arteriography shows strictures and aneurysms, biopsy shows polymorphonuclear arteritis with nerve infarction and demyelination
Sarcoidosis	A	Most commonly involved organ is lung, peripheral neuropathy rare in children
Sjögren syndrome		Cranial (most common V), distal sensory, distal sensory-motor, or pure sensory neuronopathy
Systemic lupus erythematosus	A	Peripheral neuropathy affects 2 to 27 percent of patients with SLE, neuropathy rare in children, distal progressive sensory > motor neuropathy, mononeuritis multiplex, AIDP or CIDP like presentation
Wegener granulomatosis	A	Upper, lower respiratory and renal involvement, distal symmetrical polyneuropathy or mononeuropathy multiplex, PR-3ANCA (C-ANCA)
Other Systemic Diseases		
Renal failure		Distal, symmetrical, mixed sensorimotor neuropathy develops only in advanced renal failure and is an indication to initiate dialysis
Liver transplantation	A	CNS manifestations more common
Chronic liver disease	A and D	Polyneuropathy usually mild, sensory or sensorimotor
Bone marrow transplantation	D	More often associated with graft vs host disease
Critical illness polyneuropathy	A	Usually acute or subacute, associated with multiple organ dysfunction, prolonged mechanical ventilation, and sepsis, flaccid paralysis and areflexia
Diabetes mellitus	A and D	Most common cause of chronic polyneuropathy, may be painful, autonomic involvement, mononeuropathies including cranial nerves

Contd.

Contd.

Hypothyroidism	A	Overall neuropathy in 52%, entrapment neuropathy, axonal neuropathy. Usually acute or subacute, but can be chronic
Celiac disease	A	Case reports suggesting the existence of a reversible neuropathy related to celiac disease. Rarely due to vitamin deficiency; might have an autoimmune basis, sensory or sensorimotor neuropathy
Malignancy	A and D	Usually axonal, but sometimes demyelinating polyneuropathy, in children most commonly associated with lymphoma, GBS like presentation, Distal sensorimotor polyneuropathy, Multiple mononeuropathy, Progressive polyradiculoneuropathy, subacute motor neuronopathy
Hepatitis B	A	Neuropathy associated with PAN
Hepatitis C	A	Associated with cryoglobulinemia
Nutritional Diseases		
Vitamin B_1 (thiamine) deficiency	D	Sensorimotor, distal, axonal peripheral neuropathy often associated with calf cramps, Muscle tenderness and burning feet
Vitamin B_6 (pyridoxine) deficiency	A	Peripheral neuropathy may occur in adolescents, although not in younger children
Vitamin B_{12} (cobalamin) deficiency	A	Neuropathy may be overshadowed by myelopathy (subacute combined degeneration), sensory
Vitamin E (tocopherol) deficiency		Sensorimotor neuropathy late in the course of vitamin E deficiency, loss of vibration and position sense, loss of reflexes and generalized weakness
Medications		
Antibiotic agents	A	Penicillin, sulphonamide, chloramphenicol, metronidazole and isoniazid. Paresthesias, motor weakness, and/or sensory abnormalities
Dapsone	A	Nearly pure motor with predominant arm, hand weakness
Metronidazole	A	Mainly large fibre; dose related
Antiretroviral agents	A	Predominantly by sensory symptoms, Painful; dose-limiting; "coasting" can occur
Vincristine	A	Onset with sensory symptoms in hands more so than in feet; if weakness occurs, medication should be stopped; autonomic neuropathy (gastroparesis, constipation, urinary retention) frequent
Cisplatin	A	Severe large-fibre sensory neuropathy; dose related; coasting can occur; also ototoxicity and nephrotoxicity
Phenytoin	A	Rare and only after decades of use, sensory or sensorimotor
Toxins		
Arsenic	A, may have D	Onset with painful sensory symptoms followed by weakness; prominent systemic effects (gastrointestinal symptoms, anemia) and skin/nail changes (Mees lines); acute intoxication may cause a Guillain-Barré syndrome-like polyneuropathy with proximal nerve demyelination; however, most acute and chronic intoxications cause a distal symmetrical axonal polyneuropathy
Lead	A	Primarily motor neuropathy; arms (wrist drop) affected more than legs; occurs with systemic effects (gastrointestinal symptoms, anemia), neuropathy less common in children
Mercury	A	Predominantly motor neuropathy; can mimic Guillain-Barré syndrome; might occur with CNS effects (lethargy, emotional lability and tremor)
N-hexane (glue sniffing)	A and D	Exposure via inhalation such as inhalational abuse of gasoline or glue; progressive sensory neuropathy followed by distal weakness, severe, may be painful; coasting
Organophosphorus esters	A	Neuropathy is delayed by 10–20 days after exposure; also myelopathy with lower limb spasticity and loss of proprioception
Thallium	A	Painful sensory symptoms prominent; occurs with systemic effects (gastrointestinal symptoms, anemia); alopecia is hallmark but does not occur until 2–3 weeks after exposure
A: Axonal, D: Demyelinating, M: Mixed		

Table 31.15 enlists some of the acquired conditions that can cause peripheral neuropathies in children and their important clinical findings. Most of the conditions are also prevalent in adults. As mentioned earlier infection related neuropathies are an important subgroup in children. A child with diphtheria would be notable for their respiratory signs and the characteristic gray pharyngeal membrane with neuropathy having a biphasic course. Initially palatal and posterior pharyngeal wall paralysis develops within 2 weeks of onset of illness followed 6-7 weeks later by a mixed sensorimotor demyelinating peripheral neuropathy.[46] A child with AIDP typically has an ascending evolution of paralysis compared in contrast to the descending paralysis seen in diphtheria. Episodic neurological crises should draw attention to underlying metabolic derangements such as porphyria or tyrosinemia type 1. The most important disorders to consider in children with a mononeuritis multiplex like presentation would be leprosy in endemic regions, and malignancies. Leprosy is considered the most common treatable peripheral neuropathy in the world; there are an estimated 3 million adults and children with leprosy-related neuropathy.[47] Children with HIV infection are often affected by peripheral neuropathy. Types of neuropathy include distal symmetrical polyneuropathy, mononeuritis multiplex, inflammatory demyelinating polyneuropathy and progressive polyneuropathy.[48]

Peripheral neuropathy in children with HIV has not been extensively studied, but is also described in the form of AIDP at the time of seroconversion as an immune reconstitution phenomenon, and in relation to secondary infection with Cytomegalovirus. In differentiating between AIDP in children who are not infected with HIV and those undergoing seroconversion, CSF findings are important since in the former albumin–cytologic dissociation will be present in contrast to acute HIV seroconversion, which will have pleocytosis (>50 cells/mm^3). Another important condition is sickle cell-related sensory neuropathy. Chronic inflammatory demyelinating polyneuropathy (CIDP) is a rare acquired disorder of peripheral nerves and nerve roots. Although the incidence of CIDP in children is unknown, it is thought to be the most common acquired treatable polyneuropathy in children.

In children, neuropathies can be associated with central nervous system abnormalities as well.[49] Children with central involvement should be further subdivided into those with predominantly white and those with gray matter disease. White matter disorders will be dominated by the leukodystrophies, especially metachromatic leukodystrophy and Krabbe disease. Gray matter diseases include mitochondrial disorders (Leigh disease) and neuroaxonal dystrophy. Friedreich's ataxia (FA) is an important cause of neuropathy combined with CNS disease. FA has a typical phenotypic presentation with a sensory ataxia and loss of deep tendon reflexes, related to loss of large myelinated sensory fibers and cerebellar features in the form of truncal ataxia, dysarthria and oculomotor disturbances in the form of square wave jerks and fixation instability.

CONCLUSION

Although the causes of neuropathy in children are similar to that seen in adults with minor variations, diagnosis is more challenging because of difficulties in eliciting a proper history and conducting a reliable neurological examination. Still the best approach is to conduct relevant investigations in a structures manner depending on the type of neuropathy, rather than using a shotgun approach. Classifying the neuropathy into one of the phenotypic classes goes a long way in arriving at the correct etiological diagnosis. In spite of all efforts, it may not be possible to accurately diagnose a neuropathy in up to one fourth of cases.

References

1. Bharucha NE, Bharucha AE, Bharucha EP. Prevalence of Peripheral Neuropathy in the Parsi Community of Bombay. Neurology 1991;41(8):1315-17.
2. Martyn CN, Hughes RA. Epidemiology of Peripheral Neuropathy. J Neurol Neurosurg Psychiatry 1997;62:310-18.
3. You D, Wardlaw T, Salama P, Jones G. Levels and Trends in Under-5 Mortality, 1990-2008. Lancet 2010;375(9709):100-03.
4. Ndiaye IP, Ndiaye MM, Mauferon JB, Diagne M, Diop AG. Etiological Aspects of Polyneuritis in Senegal. Dakar Med 1989;34(1-4),68-71.
5. Nations SP, Katz JS, Lyde CB, Barohn RJ. Amersterdam, The Netherlands: Excerpta Medica 1990:273-82.
6. Dyck PJ, Oviatt KF, Lambert EH. Intensive Evaluation of Referred Unclassified Neuropathies Yields Improved Diagnosis. Ann Neurol 1981;10:222-26.
7. Lubec D, Mullbacher W, Finsterer J, Mamoli B. Diagnostic Work-up in Peripheral Neuropathy: An Analysis of 171 Cases. Postgrad Med J 1999;75:723-27.
8. García A, Calleja J, Antolín FM, Berciano J. Peripheral Motor and Sensory Nerve Conduction Studies in Normal Infants and Children. Clin Neurophysiol 2000 Mar;111(3):513-20.
9. Sivak M, Ochoa J, Ferna´ndez J. Positive Manifestations of Nerve Fiber Dysfunction: Clinical, Electrophysiologic, and Pathologic Correlations. In: Brown W, Boulton C, Eds. Clinical Electromyography, 2nd Edition, Boston, MA: Butterworth-Heinemann 1993;117-47.

10. Apfel SC, Asbury AK, Bril V, Burns TM, Campbell JN, Chalk CH, *et al*. Ad Hoc Panel on Endpoints for Diabetic Neuropathy Trials. Positive Neuropathic Sensory Symptoms as Endpoints in Diabetic Neuropathy Trials. J Neurol Sci 2001;189(1-2):3-5.

11. Bromberg MB. An Approach to the Evaluation of Peripheral Neuropathies. Semin Neurol 2010;30:350-55.

12. Alport AR, Sander HW. Clinical Approach to Peripheral Neuropathy: Anatomic Localization and Diagnostic Testing. Continuum Lifelong Learning Neurol 2012;18(1):13-38.

13. Carleton S, Brown W. Changes in Motor Unit Populations in Motor Neurone Disease. J Neurol Neurosurg Psychiatry 1979;42:42-51.

14. Shy ME, Lewis RA. An Approach to Patients with Peripheral Neuropathy. Continuum Lifelong Learning Neurol 2003;9(6): 11-35.

15. Pareyson D, Marchesi C. Diagnosis, Natural History and Management of Charcot-Marie-Tooth Disease. Lancet Neurol 2009;8:654-67.

16. Herskovitz S, Verghese J, Schaumburg HH. Pseudoneuropathy: A Review of 22 Cases (Abstract). Neurology 1999;52(2):A286.

17. Phan TG, Evans BA, Huston J. Pseudoulnar Palsy from A Small Infarct of the Precentral Knob., Neurology 2000; 54:2185.

18. Barohn RJ, Amato AA. Pattern-Recognition Approach to Neuropathy and Neuronopathy. Neurol Clin 2013;31:343-61.

19. Bromberg MB. An Approach to the Evaluation of Peripheral Neuropathies. Semin Neurol 2005;25(2):153-59.

20. Katz JS, Wolfe GI, Bryan WW, Jackson CE, Amato AA, Barohn RJ. Electrophysiologic Findings in Multifocal Motor Neuropathy. Neurology 1997;48:700-07.

21. Workshop Report. 2nd Workshop of the European CMT Consortium: 53rd ENMC International Workshop on Classification and Diagnostic Guidelines for Charcot-Marie-Tooth Type 2 (CMT2-HMSN II) and Distal Hereditary Motor Neuropathy (Distal HMN-Spina CMT), 26-28 September 1997, Naarden, The Netherlands. Neuromuscul Disord 1998; 8:426-31.

22. Nanjiani Z, Nations SP, Elliott JL, *et al*. Distal Hereditary Motor Neuropathy: A Distinct Form of Charcot-Marie-Tooth Disease. J Child Neurol 2000;15:200-2001.

23. Polyneuropathy. In: Preston DC, Shapiro BE, Eds. Electromyography and Neuromuscular Disorders, Clinical-Electrophysiological Correlations, 2nd Ed. Philadelphia: Butterworth-Heinemann Elsevier 2005;389-420.

24. Burns JM, Burns TM. An Easy Approach to Evaluating Peripheral Neuropathy. Ask What, Where, When and in What Setting to Narrow Your Search. J Fam Pract 2006;55(10): 853-61.

25. Evaluation and Management of the Patient with Peripheral Neuropathy, In: Herskovitz S, Scelsa SN, Schaumburg HH, Eds. Peripheral Neuropathy in Clinical Practice, 1st Edition, New York: Oxford University Press 2010;24-39.

26. England JD, Asbury AK. Peripheral Neuropathy. Lancet 2004; 363:2151-61.

27. Clarke C, Frackowiak R, Howard R, Rossor M, Shorvon S. The Language of Neurology: Symptoms, Signs and Basic Investigations. In: Clarke C, Howard R, Rossor M, Shorvon S, Eds. Neurology: A Queen Square Textbook, 1st Edition, UK: Blackwell Publishing Ltd 2009;75-107.

28. Mauermann ML, Burns TM. Pearls and Oysters: Evaluation of Peripheral Neuropathies. Neurology 2009;72(6):e28-31.

29. Barohn RJ, Saperstein DS. Guillain-Barré Syndrome and Chronic Inflammatory Demyelinating Polyneuropathy. Semin Neurol 1998;18:49-62.

30. Saperstein DS, Katz JS, Amato AA, Barohn RJ. Clinical Spectrum of Chronic Acquired Demyelinating Polyneuropathies. Muscle Nerve 2001;24(3):311-24.

31. Katz JS, Saperstein DS, Gronseth G, Amato AA, Barohn RJ. Distal Acquired Demyelinating Symmetric (DADS) Neuropathy. Neurology 2000;54:615-20.

32. Britton WJ, Lockwood DN. Leprosy. Lancet 2004;363(9416): 1209-19.

33. Amato AA, Gronseth GS, Callerame KJ, Kagan-Hallet KS, Bryan WW, Barohn RJ. Tomaculous Neuropathy: A Clinical and Electrophysiological Study in Patients With and Without 1.5 Mb Deletions in Chromosome 17 p 11.2. Muscle Nerve 1996;19:16-22.

34. Harati Y, Kwan J, Smyth S. Peripheral Neuropathies and Motor Neuron Diseases, In: Rolak LA, ed. Neurology Secrets, 5th Edition, Philadelphia: Mosby, Elsevier 2010;97-120.

35. Loeser JD and the IASP Taxonomy Working Group. Pain Terms: A Current List with Definitions and Notes on Usage, In: Classification of Chronic Pain: Descriptions of Chronic Pain Syndromes and Definitions of Pain Terms, 2nd Edition, (Revised). Seattle, USA: IASP Press; 2012.

36. Patzko A, Shy ME. Charcot-Marie-Tooth Disease and Related Genetic Neuropathies. Continuum Lifelong Learning Neurol 2012;18(1):39-59.

37. Sinnreich M, Klein CJ, Daube JR, Engelstad J, Spinner RJ, Dyck PJ. Chronic Immune Sensory Polyradiculopathy: A Possibly Treatable Sensory Ataxia. Neurology 2004;63: 1662-69.

38. Goodman BP. Diagnostic Approach to Myeloneuropathy. Continuum Lifelong Learning Neurol 2011;17(4):744-60.

39. Lunn M, Hanna M, Howard R, Parton M, Reilly M. Nerve and Muscle Disease, In: Clarke C, Howard R, Rossor M, Shorvon S, eds. Neurology: A Queen Square Textbook, 1st Edition, UK: Blackwell Publishing Ltd 2009;337-410.

40. Watson JC, Daube JR. Compound Muscle Action Potentials. In: Daube JR, Rubin DI, Eds. Clinical Neurophysiology, Contemporary Neurology Series, 3rd Edition, New York: Oxford University Press 2009;327-68.

41. Levine TD, Saperstein DS. Laboratory Evaluation of Peripheral Neuropathy. Neurol Clin 2013;31:363-76.

42. Hilton DA, Jacob J, Househam L, Tengah C. Complications Following Sural and Peroneal Nerve Biopsies. J Neurol Neurosurg Psychiatry 2007;78(11):1271-72.

43. Yiu EM. Ryan MM. Genetic Axonal Neuropathies and Neuronopathies of Prenatal and Infantile Onset. J Peripher Nerv Syst 2012:17(3):285-300.

44. Fabrizi GM. Cavallaro T. Angiari C. Bertolasi L. Cabrini I. Ferrarini M. *et al*. Giant Axon and Neurofilament Accumulation in Charcot–Marie–Tooth Disease Type 2E. Neurology 2004: 62(8):1429-31.

45. Chang CM. Yu CW. Fong KY. Leung SY. Tsin TW. Yu YL. *et al*. N-hexane Neuropathy in Offset Printers. J Neurol Neurosurg Psychiatry 1993;56(5):538-42.

46. Logina I. Donaghy M. Diphtheritic Polyneuropathy: A Clinical Study and Comparison with Guillain-Barré Syndrome. J Neurol Neurosurg Psychiatry 1999:67(4):433-38.

47. Lancet Neurology. Leprosy As a Neurological Disease. Lancet Neurol 2009:8(3).217.

48. Verma S. Simpson D. Peripheral Neuropathy in HIV Infection. In: Portegies P. Berger J. Eds. HIV/AIDS and the Nervous System. Volume 85. Edinburgh. UK: Elsevier 2007:129-37.

49. Sladky JT. Neuropathy in Childhood. Semin Neurol 1987: 7(1):67.

32 Chapter

GUILLAIN-BARRÉ SYNDROME

C. Leema Pauline

INTRODUCTION

Guillain-Barré Syndrome (GBS) is an acquired disease of the peripheral nerves that is characterized by rapidly progressing paralysis, areflexia and cytoalbumino dissociation. The syndrome was described by Jean Baptiste and Octave Landry in 1859.[1] In 1916, Guillain, Barré and Strohl described cytoalbumino dissociation in the cerebrospinal fluid of two soldiers who presented with paralysis and areflexia. In the post-polio era, it is the most common cause of acute flaccid paralysis.[2]

Etiology

In two thirds of the cases, GBS is preceded by antecedent infections 1-4 weeks before the onset of the illness. It may rarely develop within a day or two or after 4-6 weeks of an acute illness.

Most antecedent illnesses associated with GBS affect respiratory system or gastrointestinal tract. GBS usually follows viral infections such as Epstein Barr virus, Cytomegalovirus, Influenza, Hepatitis A and B, Vaccinia, Variola, Coxsackie, ECHO and HIV. Bacterial infections implicated include Campylobacter jejuni, Mycoplasma pneumonia and Lymes disease. Systemic illnesses associated with GBS are Hodgkin's disease, hyperthyroidism, collagen vascular diseases and sarcoidosis. It has also been described following immunizations (swine flu), bone marrow transplantation, envenomization and drug ingestion (heroin).

The clinical picture produced by these agents are usually identical, although some variation occurs. Patients with preceding Cytomegalovirus infection have a severe course, more frequently develop respiratory insufficiency. GBS can occur with HIV seroconversion. Apart from pleocytosis in cerebrospinal fluid, it is indistinguishable from non HIV GBS clinically and electrophysiologically. Campylobacer jejuni infection is commonly associated with motor axonal form of GBS.

Pathogenesis

The pathogenesis of GBS is multifactorial, with complex interactions involving humoral and cell mediated immunity.

The animal model for GBS is experimental autoimmune neuritis (EAN). The inflammatory response is mediated by T cells against peripheral nerve epitopes. The macrophage are the principal cells that produce demyelination in GBS. It has been suggested that T cells activated by a preceding infection are stimulated by the antigen presenting cells which cause a disruption in the blood nerve barrier by release of inflammatory cytokines such as interleukin-2 and tumour necrosis factor. Cytokines attract macrophages which in turn destroy the myelin sheath.

Humoral factor also are suspected to play an important role in the causation of GBS. Activated complement components attract the macrophages to the nodes of Ranvier which cause detachment of axon from Schwann cells leading onto Wallerian degeneration.

Both demyelination and axonal degeneration can occur with infection due to Campylobacter jejuni. Molecular mimicry between the glycolipids and lipopolysaccharides of C. jejuni underlie the immune mediated injury in these patients. Antibodies to gangliosides GM1 and GD1A are seen in patients with GBS following C. jejuni infection.[3] GQ1B ganglioside antibodies are found in patients with Miller Fisher variant.

The annual incidence is 0.4-1.7 per 100000 population. It can occur at any age including infancy. Though there are documented cases in the newborn period, the syndrome is uncommon in children less than one year of age. There is a slight male preponderance with male to female ratio of 1.5:1. While most of the cases occur sporadically, occurrence of epidemic clusters of GBS has also been described.

Clinical Features

The most common presentation of Guillain-Barré syndrome is the demyelinating form referred to as Acute Inflammatory Demyelinating Polyradiculopathy (AIDP).

Approximately 90% of the patients will follow a fairly typical picture of proximal weakness beginning in the legs and ascending to the arms, although around 10% of patients develop weakness in the arms descending to the lower limbs. Sensory symptoms such as numbness and paresthesia are frequently reported in adults but less frequently in children partly because of difficulty in expressing the subjective symptoms. Eventually both proximal and distal groups of muscles are involved. Relative symmetry of involvement is common. Bilateral facial weakness occurs in about 50% of the patients.[4] Bulbar weakness with reduction in voice volume, difficulty in swallowing, depressed palatal movements, pooling of secretions occur in majority of children with quadriparesis. Extra ocular muscles are affected rarely and if involved Miller Fisher variant has to be thought of. Rarely eighth nerve involvement has been reported. Tendon reflexes are typically absent or depressed with generalized hypotonia. Pain is common and about 10 to 15% exhibit posterior column sensory involvement. Autonomic involvement with blood pressure lability, bladder and bowel involvement, cardiac arrhythmias can occur. Papillodema may occur rarely. Signs of meningeal irritation may dominate the clinical picture.

Nearly 75% of the patients reach a nadir within 7 days of presentation and all would reach the nadir by 4 weeks after the onset. The degree and extent of the progression can be extremely variable, that some may progress rapidly to respiratory failure within days (sometimes hours), while others may have mild progression and may be ambulant throughout.

Recovery usually occurs after a plateau of 1 to 4 weeks after the peak of the illness. Recovery may take several weeks to months.

Acute Motor Sensory Axonal Neuropathy (AMSAN)

Originally described by Feasby and colleagues, acute motor sensory axonal neuropathy presents as a rapidly progressive quadriparesis with areflexia, distal sensory loss and early respiratory insufficiency. Electrophysiological studies show early and rapid decrease or loss of compound muscle action potential and sensory nerve action potential with little or no evidence of demyelination. Pathological specimens have confirmed presence of axonal degeneration with Wallerian degeneration. The occurrence of AMSAN following C. jejuni suggests that molecular mimicry may be the underlying mechanism. AMSAN is characterized by delayed and incomplete recovery.

Acute Motor Axonal Neuropathy (AMAN)

It was originally described in patients from Northern China especially in children. Clinical features include pure motor deficits and no paresthesia or sensory loss. Electrophysiology reveals no sensory nerve involvement or demyelination. In contrast to AMSAN, patients with AMAN tend to have a better prognosis. Some have rapid recovery possibly due to resolution changes at the nodes of Ranvier or regeneration of intramuscular nerve endings.

Miller Fisher Variant

It accounts for nearly 5% of Guillain-Barré syndrome characterized by a triad of ophthalmoplegia, ataxia and areflexia. Around 95% of the patients will have polyclonal antibodies to ganglioside GQ1b which is useful in the diagnosis. Cross reactivity with GQ1b ganglioside has been reported as the reason for the restricted involvement in contrast to molecular mimicry between GM1 antibodies and C. jejuni leading onto classical form of GBS.[5] Cerebrospinal fluid protein is elevated in almost all the patients. Most children make a complete recovery.[6]

Other Variants

- Polyneuritis cranialis.
- Acute sensory variant.
- Acute pandysautonomia variant.
- Pharyngeal-cervical-brachial variant.
- Paraparetic variant.
- GBS with encephalopathy.

Modified Ashburys Criteria for Diagnosis of Guillain-Barré Syndrome[7]

Essential Criteria

- Progressive, symmetric, flaccid motor weakness of more than one limb.
- Areflexia.
- Progression < 4 weeks.

Supportive Criteria

- Sensory symptoms or signs–numbness, tingling, pain.
- Cranial nerve involvement (esp. bilateral VII).
- Autonomic dysfunction–labile BP, cardiac arrhythmias, bladder, bowel involvement.
- Recovery 2-4 weeks after progression.
- Absence of fever at the onset.
- CSF protein elevation with <10 cells/c.mm.
- Demyelination on EMG-NCS.

Points Against the Diagnosis

- Persistent asymmetry.
- Persistent bladder, bowel dysfunction.
- Definite sensory level.
- More than 50 mononuclear cells in CSF.

Exclusion Criteria

- Other causes excluded (diphtheria, porphyria, botulism, toxins etc).

DIAGNOSIS

Diagnosis of GBS is based on the clinical features supported by cerebrospinal fluid examination, electrophysiology and occasionally MRI examination of the spinal roots.

A characteristic finding supporting the diagnosis of GBS is cytoalbumino dissociation or a disproportionate increase in protein in the absence of cells usually after the first week of the illness. Presence of polymorphs in the CSF or a significant pleocytosis should cast doubt about the diagnosis.

Electrophysiology helps to confirm the diagnosis, classify the subtype and to prognosticate. The characteristic findings include asymmetrical, multifocal nerve conduction slowing or conduction block. Findings include prolonged distal latency, reduction in conduction velocity, prolonged F wave velocities, conduction block and temporal dispersion.

MRI examination of the spinal roots may show contrast enhancement.

MANAGEMENT

Supportive Therapy

- Supportive care remains the cornerstone of the treatment.
- All patients with GBS should be hospitalized to observe for further progression of the illness.
- Vital signs should be monitored.
- Watch for respiratory paralysis.
  - Clinically bilateral facial weakness, bulbar palsy, shoulder abductor weakness denotes impending respiratory failure.
  - Forced vital capacity should be measured at least every 8 hours.
  - Intubation and ventilatory assistance if forced vital capacity decreases below 10 ml/kg.
- Monitor the heart rate and BP continuously.
  - Hypertension should be treated by use of short acting anti-hypertensives.
  - Hypotension should be treated by volume boluses rather than pressors.
  - Care should be used while suctioning the airway to prevent the occurrence of asystole or bradycardia induced by vagal stimulation.
- Children with severe disease especially with respiratory insufficiency or autonomic instability need monitoring in Intensive Care Unit.
- Careful nursing for prevention of pressure sores.
- Subcutaneous heparin or leg compressive devices to prevent deep vein thrombosis.
- Pain control with analgesics.
- Physiotherapy to limit contractures and maintain the range of motion.
- Letter boards or electronic devices are mandatory in children who cannot speak to maintain communication.
- Psychological support is crucial for both patients and families.

IMMUNOMODULATING THERAPY

Plasmapheresis

- It involves separation of whole blood into plasma and cellular components. Plasma exchange includes same process with addition of replacement fluids.
- It is carried out using an extra corporeal system with centrifugal force to separate out the blood components. Continuous flow separators are used to separate the blood components which use two venipunctures, one for drawing blood and other for returning it.

- 4-5 sittings of 40-50 ml/kg each upto a total of 250 ml/kg on alternate days.
- Children with mild disease require two sittings of plasmapheresis, whereas with moderate to severe disease may need additional two sittings.[8]
- Plasma has to be replaced with 5% albumin.
- Plasma exchange is recommended in non-ambulant patients within 4 weeks of onset of neuropathic symptoms (Level A class II evidence).[9]
- Tharakan *et al.* and Mehndiratta *et al.* found that small volume plasmapheresis (20-25 ml/kg) is as useful as large volume plasmapheresis.

Disadvantages

- Cannot be carried out in patients with autonomic involvement and cardiovascular instability.
- Complications from central line such as sepsis, thrombosis, bleeding, injury to lung or thoracic duct can occur.
- Not universally available.
- Requires specially trained personnel.

Intravenous Immunoglobulin

Intravenous immunoglobulin is prepared from large pools of plasma. It has shown to shorten the duration of the disease and has become the treatment of choice for GBS.

Dose: 400 mg/kg/day for 5 days.

It is better to give IVIG within 2 weeks of illness onset. Intravenous immunoglobulin is recommended within 2 weeks of onset of neuropathic symptoms (Level A, class II evidence).

Mechanism of Action

The mechanism of action of intravenous immunoglobulin in Guillain-Barré syndrome is speculative. The proposed mechanisms include:

- Binding of anti-idiotypic antibodies.
- Down regulating B cell mediated antibody production.
- Adsorbing the complement.
- Neutralization of pro-inflammatory cytokines.
- Modulation of Fc receptor mediated phagocytosis.

Advantages

- Convenient and safe.

Complications

- Headache, fever, nausea, aseptic meningitis, elevated liver function tests and blood counts and rarely anaphylactic reaction and serum sickness can occur.

RECOMMENDATIONS FOR TREATING GBS

- Treatment with plasmapheresis or IV immunoglobulin hastens recovery from GBS, hence all patients should be treated with either PE or IVIG, even if mild.
- Therapy should be initiated within 2 weeks of onset.
- It is still appropriate to treat patients after 2 weeks, particularly if they are still progressing.
- On the basis of fewer side effects and wider availability, IV immunoglobulin represents the first treatment of choice.
- Plasmapheresis is an alternative, giving 4-5 exchanges over 10-14 days (200-250 ml/kg total).
- Vascular instability, dysautonomia, systemic illness (e.g., Sepsis) or venous access problems are contra-indications to Plasma Exchange. IVIG should be used in this group.
- Patients with GBS variants should be treated in the similar fashion to that for typical GBS.
- There is no justification for using both IVIG and Plasma Exchange in the same patient as sequential treatment with plasmapheresis followed intravenous immunoglobulin does not have a greater effect than either treatment given alone.[10]
- If there is no improvement after 7 days of intravenous immunoglobulin, then a repeat course of immunoglobulin or plasma exchange may be considered.[11]
- Steroids have no role in the management of GBS.

PROGNOSIS

Prognosis of Guillain-Barré syndrome in children is generally good compared to adults. Recovery over a period of several weeks to months is the rule. Nearly 70% of the patients recover. 10-25% will have residual weakness significantly interfering with activities of daily living and 3-5% die usually due to autonomic instability, problems arising out of ventilation.

Poor prognosticating factors include extremes of age, rapid progression, maximal weakness at onset, prolonged ventilatory dependency, autonomic involvement and axonal changes in conduction studies.

Immunizations are not recommended during the acute phase of Guillain-Barré syndrome and probably not for a period of one year following GBS. If GBS has occurred within six weeks of a particular immunization, it is better avoided in future.

References

1. Landry O. Note sur la paralysie ascendante aigue. Gazette Hebdomadaire 1859:6:472.
2. Sejvar JJ, Baughman AL, Wise M, Morgan OW. Population Incidence of Guillain-Barré Syndrome: A Systematic Review and Meta-analysis. Neuroepidemiology 2011:36:123-33 Alter M.
3. Yuki N. Sato S. Fujimoto S *et al.* Serotype of Campylobacter Jejuni, HLA and Guillain-Barré Syndrome. Muscle Nerve 1992: 15:968-69.
4. Chiba A, Kusonoki S, Shimizu T, Kanazawa I, Serum IgG Antibody to Ganglioside GQ1b is a Possible Marker of Miller Fisher Syndrome. Ann Neurol 1992:31:677-79.
5. Koul R. Alfutaisi A. Prospective Study of Children with Guillain-Barré Syndrome. Indian J Pediatr 2008:75:787-90.
6. Asbury AK, Arnason BGW, Karp HR, McFarlin DE. Criteria for Diagnosis of Guillain-Barré syndrome. Ann. Neurol 1978: 3:565-66.
7. Hadden RD. *et al.* Electrophysiological Classification of Guillain-Barré Syndrome: Clinical Associations and Outcome. Ann. Neurol 1998:44:780-88.
8. Guillain-Barré Syndrome Study Group. Plasmapheresis and Acute Guillain-Barré Syndrome. Neurology 1985:35:1096-2104.
9. Van der Meché F. Schmitz P and the Dutch Guillain-Barré Study Group. A Randomized Trial Comparing Intravenous Immune Globulin and Plasma Exchange in Guillain-Barré Syndrome. N Engl J Med 1992:326:1123-29.
10. Chevret S. Plasma Exchange for Guillain-Barré Syndrome. Cochrane Database Syst. Rev 2017;2:CD001798 [PMC free article].
11. Hughes RA, Swan AV, van Doorn PA. Intravenous Immunoglobulin for Guillain-Barré Syndrome. Cochrane Database Syst. Rev 2014;9:CD002063.

33 Chapter

SPINAL MUSCULAR ATROPHY

Sheffali Gulati, Biswaroop Chakrabarty, Rahul Sinha

INTRODUCTION

Spinal muscular atrophy (SMA) is a progressive degenerative disorder affecting predominantly the α motor neurons of the anterior horn cells of the spinal cord and brainstem nuclei.[1] Although the disease entity was first described by Werdnig and Hoffman in the late nineteenth century, the underlying genetic defect was discovered only in 1995.[2-5] The most common form of the disease is caused by mutation in the survival motor neuron (SMN) gene which presents as a proximal predominant muscle weakness and atrophy. However it is divided into various subtypes on the basis of age at presentation and clinical manifestations. Recent years have also seen the emergence of distal predominant SMA which are commonly known as hereditary motor neuropathies. A wide variety of mutations have been described with this latest entity which is entirely different from the classical SMN gene mutation.[6]

EPIDEMIOLOGY

Spinal muscular atrophy is an autosomal recessive disorder with an estimated incidence of 1 in 6000 to 10,000 live births. The carrier frequency described is 1 in 40 to 60.[7,8]

PATHOGENESIS

Classical Proximal SMA

Role of SMN Gene and Protein

Lefevre in 1995 discovered the SMN1 gene in 5q11.2-13.3, which is critical for the survival and functioning of motor neurons.[5] A nearly identical gene called SMN2 is also present in the same region which differs from SMN1gene by 5 nucleotides which includes a translationally silent C → T nucleotide exchange in exon 7 leading to its exclusion in around 90% of SMN2 transcripts.[9] The SMN1 gene encodes a 38 kDa functional protein, whereas only 10-20% of this full protein is expressed by SMN2 gene. The full length SMN protein is present both in the nucleus and cytoplasm.[10] It localises to nucleus (gemini of coiled bodies known as gems), axons, dendrites and to the neuromuscular junction.[11-13]

The most critical function of SMN protein is the formation of small nuclear ribonucleoproteins (snRNP) assembly which is critical to the splicing of gene responsible for motor neuron function.[14] SMN protein also plays active role in motor neuron axonogenesis and formation of neuromuscular junction.[15] Stasimon, a protein involved in motor neuron function and synaptic transmission is also regulated by SMN protein.[16]

The underlying defect in SMA is large deletions involving exon 7 and 8 in SMN gene.[6] About 96% of the patients have homozygous SMN disruption secondary to deletion or conversion to SMN2 and 3% are heterozygotes for one SMN1 allele and subtle intragenic mutations. Loss of SMN1 is central to the pathogenesis of SMA whereas severity is determined by the number of copies of SMN2 available.[17]

Role of Apoptosis

The SMN protein interacts with various proteins involved in regulation of apoptosis which includes caspase-3. Bcl-2, ZPR-1 and p53 with an overall effect of inhibiting apoptosis. Thus a dysfunctional and deficient SMN protein would trigger the proapoptotic cascade.[10] The neuronal apoptosis inhibitory protein (NAIP) gene is located adjacent to the SMN gene. The severe forms of SMA are associated with deletions in this gene as well. NAIP directly inhibits propapoptotic enzymes caspase 3 and 7.[18-20]

Other Rare Proximal Variants of SMA

Other genetic defects involving Ubiquitin activating enzyme 1 (UBE1), Vaccinia related kinase 1 (VRK1), cytochrome oxidase 2, androgen receptor and vesicle associated membrane associated protein have also been implicated in pathogenesis of rare variants of proximal SMA.[21-25]

Distal SMAs (Hereditary Motor Neuropathies)

The mutations implicated in its causation include genes coding for heat shock proteins, glycyl t RNA synthetase, dynactin, cation channelopathy, copper transporting ATPases and immunoglobulin binding proteins.[26-38]

The various genetic defects involved in causation of various forms of SMA have been tabulated (Table 33.1).

Clinical Features

Classical Proximal SMA

This entity is divided into four subtypes on the basis of age at onset and best motor milestone achieved.

Type 1 SMA (Werdnig Hoffman Disease)

This is characterised by onset before the age of 6 months, inability to sit unsupported and death by the end of 2nd year of life. Clinically they have generalised paucity of movements, more involvement of proximal musculature and lower limbs, respiratory muscle weakness (involvement of intercostals with sparing of diaphragm), bulbar dysfunction, tongue fasciculations, spared facial muscles, profound peripheral hypotonia, areflexia and intact sensory system.[17] Aspiration pneumonia is the most common cause of mortality. On the basis of clinical severity, SMA type 1 is further subdivided into 3 types, viz., severe neonatal onset, onset between 1 and 2 months age and onset between 2 and 6 months age.[39] Patients with the last subtype usually can hold their neck and sit with support. A severe variant of this form is SMA 0 which has prenatal onset with congenital contractures and flail ribs.[40]

There is growing evidence in recent years of associated atrial and ventricular septal defects in severe forms of SMA 1. There are reports of autonomic insufficiency as well leading to arrhythmias and sudden cardiac death.[17,41]

Type 2 SMA

This group of patients usually have onset of symptoms between 6 and 18 months of age. The best achieved motor milestone is standing with support. Clinically there is bilateral upper limb polyminimyoclonus, joint contractures and kyphoscoliosis. Bulbar dysfunction is milder compared to type 1. Severely affected patients may require ventilator support consequent to respiratory failure.[17]

Type 3 SMA (Kugelberg Welander Disease)

This group represents a clinically heterogenous spectrum with those retaining the ability to walk who have an onset after 3 years of age and those who have onset before 3 years of age are less likely to walk. Some of them may require wheelchair assistance.[17,42]

Type 4 SMA

These patients are characterised by an adult onset (beyond 18 years) and relatively milder clinical course. They don't have weakness of respiratory muscles.[17]

The clinical features of other proximal SMAs and HMNs have been enumerated in Table 33.2.[21-38]

Table 33.1: Genetic Basis of Spinal Muscular Atrophy Spectrum Disorders

Type of Spinal Muscular Atrophy	Inheritance	Causative gene
Proximal subtype		
Proximal SMA	AR	SMN1
Infantile SMA with arthrogryposis	X-linked	Ubiquitin activating enzyme 1
SMA with pontocerebellar hypoplasia	AR	Vaccinia related kinase 1
SMA type 1 phenotype due to mitochondrial dysfunction	AR	Synthesis of cytochrome oxidase 2
Spinal and bulbar muscular atrophy	X-linked	Androgen receptor
Adult onset proximal SMA	AD	Vesicle and membrane associated protein
Distal SMA (HMN)		
HMN2A	AD	Heat Shock Protein 8
HMN2B	AD/AR	Heat Shock Protein B1
HMN2C	AD	Heat Shock Protein B3
HMN4	AR	Pleckstrin homologous G protein
HMN5A	AD	Glycyl t-RNA synthetase

Contd.

Contd.

HMN5B	AD	Congenital lipodystrophy type 2
HMN7B (Distal spinal and bulbar muscular atrophy with vocal cord paresis)	AD	Dynactin
Scapuloperoneal SMA	AD	Cation channel transient receptor
Distal SMA	X-linked	ATP7A Copper transporting protein
Spinal muscular atrophy with respiratory distress 1	AR	Immunoglobulin binding protein

SMA: Spinal muscular atrophy, AD: Autosomal dominant, AR: Autosomal recessive, SMN: Survival motor neuron, HMN: Hereditary motor neuropathy, ATP: Adenosine triphosphate.

Table 33.2: Clinical Features of Rare Proximal SMAs and Entire Spectrum of Distal SMAs

Rare Proximal SMAs		
1.	Infantile SMA with arthrogryposis	Similar to classical proximal SMA with early contractures
2.	SMA with pontocerebellar hypoplasia	Microcephaly, upper limb ataxia and arthrogryposis, infantile onset
3.	Mitochondrial etiology	Similar to SMA type 1 with additional cardiomyopathy and lactic acidosis
4.	SBMA	Only adult males, flaccid quadriparesis with facial and bulbar weakness, perioral and tongue fasciculations, hyperCKemia, gynaecomastia, androgen resistance, reduced fertility
5.	Adult onset SMA (allelic with ALS)	Proximal gradient adult onset weakness
Distal SMAs (HMNs)		
1.	HMN2A (allelic with CMT2L)	Adult onset, distal predominant weakness, occasional diaphragmatic and vocal fold weakness
2.	HMN2B (allelic with CMT2F)	Distal gradient adult onset weakness
3.	HMN2C	Distal gradient adult onset weakness
4.	HMN4	Childhood onset diffuse weakness without bulbar involvement
5.	HMN5A	Distal arm involved more than leg, thenar and first dorsal interossei affected first, adult onset
6.	HMN5B	Variable age at onset, progression from arms to legs, loss of vibration sense in legs
7.	HMN7B	Adult onset, hand weakness followed by legs, bulbar, facial and vocal fold paresis
8.	Scapuloperoneal SMA (allelic with CMT2C)	Characteristic distribution of weakness, congenital absence of bone, muscle atrophy, laryngeal weakness
9.	Distal SMA	Only men, variable age at onset
10.	SMARD1 (HMN6)	Onset within first 6 months with generalised flaccid weakness with distal weakness and diaphragmatic palsy

SMA: Spinal muscular atrophy, SBMA: Spinal and bulbar muscular atrophy, ALS: Amyotrophic lateral sclerosis, HMN: Hereditary motor neuropathy, CMT: Charcot-Marie Tooth, SMARD: Spinal muscular atrophy with respiratory distress.

Diagnosis

Any patient suspected to have classical proximal SMA on the basis of clinical details should be subjected to genetic testing for SMN1 homozygous deletion. Absence of exon 7 with or without exon 8 deletion is confirmatory for diagnosis of SMA with 95% sensitivity and 100% specificity.[43] In case this is negative, next step should be evaluation of serum creatinine phosphokinase (CPK) followed by detailed electrophysiology (nerve conduction study and electromyogram) and muscle biopsy if required. If electromyogram and or muscle biopsy is suggestive of neurogenic pathology with no evidence of peripheral neuropathy further testing for rare mutations of SMA should be pursued. Multiple ligand probe amplification and real time polymerase chain reaction can identify SMN1 gene copy number and increase diagnostic sensitivity upto 98%.[44] In case of an available SMN1 copy, the undeleted allele's coding region is sequenced which in 2/3rd cases yields a point mutation, insertion or deletion and in remaining 1/3rd, the mutation in deep intronic (usually seen in SMA 3). Sequence analysis of SMN1 gene is also indicated in typical clinical picture with 2 SMN1 copies and consanguineous parents[45] (Fig. 33.1). Details of availability of genetic testing for other rare variants of proximal SMA and distal SMAs are available at the URL http:/ /www.ncbi.nlm.nih.gov/sites/Gene-Tests.[6]

The differential diagnoses include congenital myopathy, early onset variants of CMT (Charcot-Marie Tooth) spectrum, congenital muscular dystrophies and congenital myasthenic syndrome for SMA 1 and 2 whereas the milder and late onset variants have limb girdle muscular dystrophy spectrum as a close clinical mimicker.[17,46]

Management

Consensus guidelines for the management of SMA have been established.[43] The management of SMA involves a multidisciplinary approach. A neuromuscular disorders expert coordinates the entire treatment programme which involves rehabilitation, pulmonary, gastrointestinal, nutritional and orthopedic care.

The muscle weakness in SMA leads to contracture formation and spinal deformity. The consequent restricted mobility leads to osteopenia and fractures.[17] Active muscle training is done for muscle strengthening whereas passive exercises help prevent formation of contractures. Standing position, even with the help of aids should be followed for atleast 2 hours per day. This helps in proper posture maintenance, preservation of respiratory functions and retardation of scoliosis and contracture progression.[47] Continuous physical and occupational therapy is essential for progression of contractures and preservation of range of motion across joints. The joint actions primarily affected by contracture formation are elbow flexion and supination, knee and hip flexion and multiple functions at the ankle joint leading to talipes equinus deformity. Orthotic devices are particularly useful in flexible deformities and retard the progression of contractures. Surgical intervention is in the form of tendon release surgeries are indicated in fixed contractures, mostly in the lower limbs in patients with SMA 2 and 3. However prolonged immobilisation should be avoided post surgery to minimise loss of motor abilities.[48,49]

Around 30-40% and 10-30% SMA 2 and 3 patients respectively are reported to have hip subluxation and dislocation.[50] In view of poor overall prognosis and the morbidities associated with surgery in this disease condition, conservative management is the treatment of choice.[47]

Fractures of the lower limb (supracondylar femur) are common in SMA 2 and upper extremity fractures are more common in SMA 3.[51] Conservative management is the treatment of choice in non ambulatory patients whereas ambulatory patients benefit with surgical intervention and osteosynthesis.[47]

Nearly all SMA 2 and 3 patients have scoliosis, predominantly dorsolumbar.[47] Early and appropriate physiotherapy may retard the development and progression

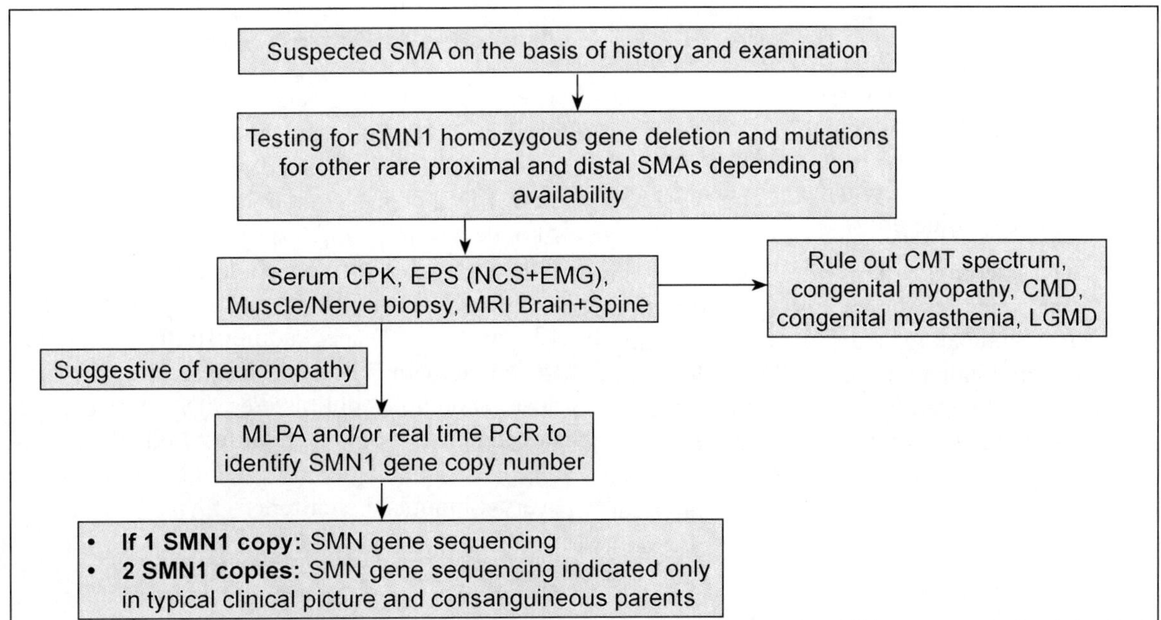

Fig. 33.1: Flowchart depicting diagnostic approach to SMA

of scoliosis.[52] Surgery is indicated at the age of 10-12 years and in non ambulatory patients once Cobb's angle is greater than 20°. Corset therapy is indicated awaiting surgery or if surgery is not done in view of poor general condition or parental refusal.[52,53]

Respiratory involvement is the main cause of morbidity and mortality in SMA, particularly type 1 and 2.[17] The primary underlying mechanism is intercostal muscle weakness and scoliosis leading to hypoventilation, impaired clearance of secretions, recurrent chest infections and atelectasis.[54] Early physiotherapy with respiratory training focussing on muscle strengthening and mechanical cough assisting devices and expectoration techniques is essential for preservation of respiratory function.[55] SMA type 3 patients have less severe involvement manifesting as obstructive sleep apnea, exacerbation during intermittent acute illness and adult onset hypoventilation.[54] Eventually respiratory support is required with declining lung functions. Non-invasive ventilation is the treatment of choice and tracheostomy with invasive ventilation is practised whenever necessary. This causes improvement in overall sleep architecture, day-to-day functioning and life expectancy to some extent.[43]

In view of bulbar and chewing dysfunction, all patients with SMA (particularly type 1) are predisposed to aspiration. Current consensus guideline recommends screening all patients with SMA type 1 for silent aspiration and decision for other types are subject to clinical indicators. Although most of these patients follow lower centiles on the weight chart, abnormal muscle to fat ratio and atrophy of muscles predispose these patients towards obesity. Regular monitoring of body composition and nutritional status is therefore essential. However one must avoid prolonged fasting in these patients due to secondary mitochondrial dysfunction and abnormal fatty acid oxidation. In patients with inadequate intake secondary to bulbar dysfunction, a percutaneous endoscopic gastrostomy should be considered.[43,47]

Post anesthesia complications are common in SMA patients consequent to upper airway obstruction during endotracheal intubation and poor cough leading to hypoventilation and impaired mucociliary clearance causing atelectasis.[56] Preoperative care should include detailed nutritional and gastroesophageal function assessment, cough reflex and respiratory function check in addition to chest X-ray and detailed physical examination.[43, 57]

The essential components of management of SMA is enumerated in Table 33.3.

Table 33.3: Holistic Multidisciplinary Management of SMA

Physical and occupational therapy	• Active and passive muscle training • Prevention of contractures • Orthotics • Surgery
Fractures, subluxation and dislocation	• Conservative management except fractures in ambulatory patients in whom surgery with osteosyntesis may be done
Scoliosis management	• Physiotherapy • Corset • Surgical intervention
Respiratory training	• Early physiotherapy • Expectoration training and cough assistive devices • Noninvasive ventilation • Tracheostomy with invasive ventilation (whenever required)
Nutrition	• Screening for aspiration • Nutrition and body composition assessment • Percutaneous endoscopic gastrostomy
Anesthetic care	• Nutritional and gastroesophageal function assessment • Cough reflex and respiratory function check • Chest X-ray • Detailed physical examination

Advances in Pharmacotherapy

The Spinraza (Nusinersen) is the first FDA approved drug in 2016. Spinraza (Nusinersen) is a survival motor neuron-2 (SMN2)-directed antisense oligonucleotide. It was shown to increase exon 7 inclusion in SMN2 messenger ribonucleic acid (mRNA) transcripts and production of full-length SMN protein. It is supplied as a solution to be administered intrathecally. The recommended dosage is 12 mg (5 ml) per administration. Initiate Spinraza treatment with 4 loading doses. The first three loading doses should be administered at 14-day intervals. The 4th loading dose should be administered 30 days after the 3rd dose. A maintenance dose should be administered once every 4 months thereafter.

The various outcome measures used in research both for understanding the natural history of the disease and for therapeutics have been enumerated in Table 33.4.

Table 33.4: Outcome Measures Applied in Spinal Muscular Atrophy Research

Scale	Measurement of
Myometry	Strength
GMFM	Function
CHOP INTEND	Function
TIMP	Function
HFMS	Function
HFMSE	Function
Six-minute walk test	Function
Pulmonary function tests	Lung function
PedsQL, neuromuscular module	Quality of life

CHOP INTEND: Children's Hospital of Philadelphia infant test of neuromuscular disorders, GMFM: Gross motor function measure, HFMS: Hammersmith functional motor scale, HFMSE, Hammersmith functional motor scale expanded, TIMP: Test of infant motor performance.

Other Agents Increasing SMN2 Gene Expression, SMN Transcription and Translation

Histone deacetylase inhibitors (HDACIs) cause deacetylation of histones, non histones and transcription factors and increase length of SMN2 transcripts.[58] Valproic acid, a HDACI, showed functional improvement in an open label trial, however a phase 2 randomised double blind trial of valproate along with carnitine failed to show any functional improvement.[59,60] Similar results were also seen with sodium 4-phenylbutyrate.[61] Hydroxamic acid has shown increase in SMN2 level in SMA fibroblasts unresponsive to valproic acid, however human trials are yet to be conducted.[62] Nonhistone deacetylase inhibitors like hydroxyurea has shown similar results like valproate whereas albuterol, quinazoline compounds and prolactin have shown encouraging preliminary reports which needs to be investigated further.[63-66]

SMN Protein Stabilising Agents

Geneticin, Indoprofen and Bortezomib have shown encouraging results in mouse models, but these are yet to be replicated in humans.[58,67]

Neuroprotective Agents

Riluzole, a glutamate antagonist, has shown success in mouse models, a phase II multicentre, randomised double blind in humans in SMA 2 and 3 is currently underway.[58] Gabapentin has shown efficacy in limited randomised trials warranting further research.[68] Olesoxime, a novel neuroprotective agent, is currently being evaluated in a multicentric, randomised, double blinded, placebo controlled trial in SMA 2 and 3 patients.[69]

Luteinising Hormone Releasing Hormone Analogue

Leuprorelin, prevents nuclear translocation of abnormal androgen receptor proteins and have shown promise in animal models of spinal and bulbar muscular atrophy. However preliminary human reports are not positive.[6]

Stem Cell Therapy

Pluripotent stem cells have shown promise in initial studies in animal models. However more studies are required to characterise the exact cell type, route of administration and appropriate time of delivery in these patients.[58]

Gene Therapy

The advent of self-complementary adeno associated virus (scAAV) as a vector for gene therapy which is capable of crossing the blood brain barrier has revolutionised the clinical potential of gene therapy in SMA.[70,71] Initial results from animal models are encouraging, although issues like exact route, safety and efficacy need to be addressed by more studies.

Various investigational therapies currently being evaluated in SMA have been tabulated (Table 33.5).

Table 33.5: Investigational therapies in SMA

Histone deacetylase inhibitors	Valproate, Sodium 4-phenyl butyrate, Hydroxamide
Nonhistone deacetylase inhibitors	Albuterol, Hydroxyurea, Quinazoline compounds, Prolactin
Anntisense oligonucleotides	ISIS-SMNRx
Neuroprotective agents	Riluzole, Gabapentin, Olesoxime
Luteinising hormone releasing hormone analogue	Leuprorelin
Stem cell therapy	

Genetic Counselling and Neonatal Screening

Spinal muscular atrophy is one of the most common genetic disorders with a carrier frequency of 1/50. Carrier testing is indicated for parents and siblings of affected child. Prenatal diagnosis is done by chorionic villi sampling between 11-13 weeks of pregnancy as the recurrence risk is 25%. However appropriate counselling should be done stressing upon the sensitivity of molecular testing which is 93-95% and the residual risk of having the mutation. The clinical severity of affected fetus is difficult to predict as the same SMN 2 copy number may be present in more than one subtype. Although no curative therapy exists for SMA, neonatal screening should still be considered. This is because most of the damage in SMA 1 occurs in the first 6 months of life which provides a potential therapeutic window for early intervention.[8]

CONCLUSION

The underlying defective protein in SMA, SMN is a multifunctional protein involved in DNA repair, apoptosis, cell cycle and calcium signalling with motor neuron survival as the major function. Further unravelling of upstream and downstream physiology of SMN protein will lead to better understanding of disease pathology in SMA. Various therapeutic approaches, both SMN dependent and independent, are currently being evaluated which may ultimately help in alleviating the disease.

References

1. Hamilton G, Gilingwater TH. Spinal Muscular Atrophy: Going Beyond the Motor Neuron. Trends Mol Med 2013;13:40-50.
2. Werdnig G. Zwei Frühinfantile Hereditäre Fälle von Progressive Muskelatrophie Unter dem Bilde der Dystrophie, Aber auf Neurotischer Grundlage [Two early infantile hereditary cases of progressive muscular atrophy simulating dystrophy, but on a neural basis; in German]. Arch Psychiatr Nervenkr 1891;22:437-80.
3. Hoffmann J. Über chronische spinale Muskelatrophie im Kindesalter, auf familiärer Basis [On chronic spinal muscular atrophy in childhood, with a familial basis; in German]. Dtsch Z Nervenheilkd 1893;3:427-70.
4. Brzustowicz LM, Lehner T, Castilla LH *et al*. Genetic Mapping of Chronic Childhood-Onset Spinal Muscular Atrophy to Chromosome 5q11.2-13.3. Nature 1990;344:540-41.
5. Lefebvre S, Burglen L, Reboullet S *et al*. Identification and Characterization of a Spinal Muscular Atrophy-Determining Gene. Cell 1995;80:155-65.
6. Wee CD, Kong L, Sumner CJ. The Genetics of Spinal Muscular Atrophies. Curr Opin Neurol 2010;23:450-58.
7. Ogino S, Leonard DG, Rennert H, Ewens WJ, Wilson RB. Genetic Risk Assessment in Carrier Testing for Spinal Muscular Atrophy. Am J Med. Genet 2002;110:301-07.
8. Prior TW, Snyder PJ, Rink BD *et al*. Newborn and Carrier Screening for Spinal Muscular Atrophy. Am J Med Genet 2010;152:1605-07.
9. Lorson CL, Hahnen E, Androphy EJ, Wirth B. A Single Nucleotide in the SMN Gene Regulates Splicing and is Responsible for Spinal Muscular Atrophy. Proc Natl Acad Sci USA 1999;96:6307-11.
10. Anderton RS, Meloni BP, Mastalgia FL, Boulos S. Spinal Muscular Atrophy and the Antiapoptotic Role of Survival of Motor Neuron (SMN) Protein. Mol Neurobiol 2013;47:821-32.
11. Carvalho T, Almeida F, Calapez A, Lafarga M, Berciano MT, Carmo-Fonseca M. The Spinal Muscular Atrophy Disease Gene Product, SMN: A Link Between snRNP Biogenesis and the Cajal (Coiled) Body. J Cell Biol 1999;147:715-28.
12. Pagliardini S, Giavazzi A, Setola V *et al*. Subcellular Localization and Axonal Transport of the Survival Motor Neuron (SMN) Protein in the Developing Rat Spinal Cord. Hum Mol Genet 2000;9:47-56.
13. Broccolini A, Engel WK, Askanas V. Localization of Survival Motor Neuron Protein in Human Apoptotic-like and Regenerating Muscle Fibers and Neuromuscular Junctions. Neuroreport 1999;10:1637-41.
14. Burghes AH, Beattie CE. Spinal Muscular Atrophy: Why Do Low Levels of Survival Motor Neuron Protein Make Motor Neurons Sick? Nat Rev Neurosci 2009;10:597-609.
15. Carrel TL, McWhorter ML, Workman E *et al*. Survival Motor Neuron Function in Motor Axons is Independent of Functions Required for Small Nuclear Ribonucleoprotein Biogenesis. J Neurosci 2006;26:11014-22.
16. Lotti F, Imlach WL, Saieva L *et al*. An SMN-dependent U12 Splicing Event Essential for Motor Circuit Function. Cell 2012;151:440-54.
17. D Amico A, Mercuri E, Tiziano FD, Bertini E. Spinal Muscular Atrophy (Review). Orphanet Journal of Rare Diseases 2011; 6:71.
18. Kesari A, Misra UK, Kalita J *et al*. Study of Survival of Motor Neuron (SMN) and Neuronal Apoptosis Inhibitory Protein (NAIP) Gene Deletions in SMA Patients. J Neurol 2005; 252:667-71.
19. Watihayati MS, Fatemeh H, Marini M *et al*. Combination of SMN2 Copy Number and NAIP Deletion Predicts Disease Severity in Spinal Muscular Atrophy. Brain Dev 2009;31:42-45.
20. Maier JK, Lahoua Z, Gendron NH *et al*. The Neuronal Apoptosis Inhibitory Protein is a Direct Inhibitor of Caspases 3 and 7. J Neurosci 2002;22:2035-43.
21. Ramser J, Ahearn ME, Lenski C *et al*. Rare Missense and Synonymous Variants in UBE1 Are Associated with X-linked Infantile Spinal Muscular Atrophy. Am J Hum Genet 2008; 82:188-93.
22. Renbaum P, Kellerman E, Jaron R *et al*. Spinal Muscular Atrophy with Pontocerebellar Hypoplasia is Caused by a Mutation in the VRK1 Gene. Am J Hum Genet 2009;85: 281-89.
23. Tamopolsky MA, Bourgeois JM, Fu MH *et al*. Novel SCO2 Mutation (G1521A) Presenting as a Spinal Muscular Atrophy Type 1 Phenotype. Am J Med Genet 2004;125:310-14.
24. La Spada AR, Wilson EM, Lubahn DB *et al*. Androgen Receptor Gene Mutations in X-linked Spinal and Bulbar Muscular Atrophy. Nature 1991;352:77-79.
25. Nishimura AL, Mitne-Neto M, Silva HC *et al*. A Mutation in the Vesicle Trafficking Protein VAPB Causes Late Onset Spinal Muscular Atrophy and Amyotrophic Lateral Sclerosis. Am J Hum Genet 2004;75:822-31.

26. Irobi J, Van Impe K, Seeman P, *et al.* Hot-Spot Residue in Small Heat-Shock Protein 22 Causes Distal Motor Neuropathy. Nat Genet 2004;36:597-601.

27. Evgrafov OV, Mersiyanova I, Irobi J, *et al.* Mutant Small Heat-Shock Protein 27 Causes Axonal Charcot-Marie-Tooth Disease and Distal Hereditary Motor Neuropathy. Nat Genet 2004;36:602-06.

28. Kolb SJ, Snyder PJ, Poi EJ, *et al.* Mutant Small Heat Shock Protein B3 Causes Motor Neuropathy: Utility of a Candidate Gene Approach. Neurology 2010;74:502-06.

29. Maystadt I, Rezsohazy R, Barkats M, *et al.* The Nuclear Factor KappaB-Activator Gene PLEKHG5 is Mutated in a Form of Autosomal Recessive Lower Motor Neuron Disease with Childhood Onset. Am J Hum Genet 2007;81:67-76.

30. Antonellis A, Ellsworth RE, Sambuughin N, *et al.* Glycyl tRNA Synthetase Mutations in Charcot-Marie-Tooth Disease Type 2D and Distal Spinal Muscular Atrophy Type V. Am J Hum Genet 2003; 72:1293-99.

31. Windpassinger C, Auer-Grumbach M, Irobi J, *et al.* Heterozygous Missense Mutations in BSCL2 Are Associated with Distal Hereditary Motor Neuropathy and Silver Syndrome. Nat Genet 2004;36:271-76.

32. Puls I, Jonnakuty C, LaMonte BH, *et al.* Mutant Dynactin in Motor Neuron Disease. Nat Genet 2003;33:455-56.

33. Auer-Grumbach M, Olschewski A, Papic L, *et al.* Alterations in the Ankyrin Domain of TRPV4 Cause Congenital Distal SMA, Scapuloperoneal SMA and HMSN2C. Nat Genet 2010; 42:160-64.

34. Deng HX, Klein CJ, Yan J, *et al.* Scapuloperoneal Spinal Muscular Atrophy and CMT2C are Allelic Disorders Caused by Alterations in TRPV4. Nat Genet 2010;42:165-69.

35. Landoure G, Zdebik AA, Martinez TL, *et al.* Mutations in TRPV4 Cause Charcot-Marie-Tooth Disease Type 2C. Nat Genet 2010;42:170-74.

36. Zimon M, Baets J, Auer-Grumbach M, *et al.* Dominant Mutations in the Cation Channel Gene Transient Receptor Potential Vanilloid 4 Cause An Unusual Spectrum of Neuropathies. Brain 2010;133(Pt 6):1798-809.

37. Kennerson ML, Nicholson GA, Kaler SG, *et al.* Missense Mutations in the Copper Transporter Gene ATP7A Cause X-linked Distal Hereditary Motor Neuropathy. Am J Hum Genet 2010;86:343-52.

38. Grohmann K, Varon R, Stolz P, *et al.* Infantile Spinal Muscular Atrophy with Respiratory Distress Type 1 (SMARD1). Ann Neurol 2003; 54:719-24.

39. Bertini E, Burghes A, Bushby K *et al.* 134th ENMC International Workshop: Outcome Measures and Treatment of Spinal Muscular Atrophy, 11-13 February 2005, Naarden, The Netherlands. Neuromuscular Disorders 2005;15:802-16.

40. Felderhoff-Mueser U, Grohmann K, Harder A, Stadelmann C, Zerres K, Bührer C, Obladen M. Severe Spinal Muscular Atrophy Variant Associated with Congenital Bone Fractures. J Child Neurol 2002;17:718-21.

41. Shababi M, Habibi J, Yang HT, Vale SM, Sewell WA, Lorson CL. Cardiac Defects Contribute to the Pathology of Spinal Muscular Atrophy Models. Hum Mol Genet 2010;19:4059-71.

42. Zerres K, Rudnik-Schöneborn S, Forrest E, Lusakowska A, Borkowska J, Hausmanowa-Petrusewicz I. A Collaborative Study on the Natural History of Childhood and Juvenile Onset Proximal Spinal Muscular Atrophy (Type II and III SMA): 569 Patients. J Neurol Sci 1997;146:67-72.

43. Wang CH, Finkel RS, Bertini ES *et al.* Participants of the International Conference on SMA Standard of Care. Consensus Statement for Standard of Care in Spinal Muscular Atrophy. J Child Neurol 2007;22:1027-49.

44. Arkblad EL, Darin N, Berg K *et al.* Multiplex Ligation-Dependent Probe Amplification Improbe Diagnostics in Spinal Muscular Atrophy. Neuromuscul Disord 2006;16:830-38.

45. Cuscó I, López E, Soler-Botija C, Jesús Barceló M, Baiget M, Tizzano EF. A Genetic and Phenotypic Analysis in Spanish Spinal Muscular Atrophy Patients with c.399_402del AGAG, the Most Frequently Found Subtle Mutation in the SMN1 Gene. Hum Mutat 2003;22:136-43.

46. Bodensteiner JB. The Evaluation of the Hypotonic Infant. Semin Pediatr Neurol 2008;15:10-20.

47. Haaker G, Fujak A. Proximal Spinal Muscular Atrophy: Current Orthopedic Perspective. The Application of Clinical Genetics 2013;6:113-20.

48. Fujak A, Kopschina C, Gras F, Forst R, Forst J. Contractures of the Upper Extremities in Spinal Muscular Atrophy Type II. Descriptive Clinical Study with Retrospective Data Collection. Orthop Traumatol Rehabil 2010;12:410-19.

49. Fujak A, Kopschina C, Gras F, Forst R, Forst J. Contractures of the Lower Extremities in Spinal Muscular Atrophy Type II. Descriptive Clinical Study with Retrospective Data Collection. Orthop Traumatol Rehabil 2011;13(1):27-36.

50. Zenios M, Sampath J, Cole C, Khan T, Galasko CS. Operative Treatment for Hip Subluxation in Spinal Muscular Atrophy. J Bone Joint Surg Br 2005;87:1541-44.

51. Fujak A, Kopschina C, Forst R, Gras F, Mueller LA, Forst J. Fractures in Proximal Spinal Muscular Atrophy. Arch Orthop Trauma Surg 2010;130:775-80.

52. Fujak A, Raab W, Schuh A, Kreb A, Forst R, Forst J. Operative Treatment of Scoliosis in Proximal Spinal Muscular Atrophy: Results of 41 Patients. Arch Orthop Trauma Surg 2012;132:1697-706.

53. Fujak A, Ingenhorst A, Heuser K, Forst R, Forst J. Treatment of Scoliosis in Intermediate Spinal Muscular Atrophy (SMA Type II) in Childhood. Ortop Traumatol Rehabil 2005;7:175-79.

54. Schroth MK. Special Considerations in the Respiratory Management of Spinal Muscular Atrophy. Pediatrics 2009; 123(S4):S245-49.

55. Manzur AY, Muntoni F, Simonds A. Muscular Dystrophy Campaign Sponsored Workshop: Recommendation for Respiratory Care of Children with Spinal Muscular Atrophy Type II and III, 13th February 2002, London, UK. Neuromuscul Disord 2003;13:184-89.

56. Graham RJ, Athiraman U, Laubach AE, Sethna NF. Anesthesia and Perioperative Medical Management of Children with Spinal Muscular Atrophy. Paediatr Anaesth 2009;19:1054-63.

57. Iannaccone ST. Modern Management of Spinal Muscular Atrophy. J Child Neurol 2007;22:974-78.

58. Singh P, Liew WKM, Darras BT. Current Advances in Drug Development in Spinal Muscular Atrophy. Curr Opin Pediatr 2013;25:682-88.

59. Kissel JT, Scott CB, Reyna SP, *et al.* SMA Carnival Trial Part II: A Prospective, Single-Armed Trial of L-carnitine and Valproic Acid in Ambulatory Children with Spinal Muscular Atrophy. PLoS One 2011;6:e21296.

60. Swoboda KJ, Scott CB, Crawford TO, *et al.* SMA Carnival Trial Part I: Double-Blind, Randomized, Placebo-Controlled Trial of L-Carnitine and Valproic Acid in Spinal Muscular Atrophy. PLoS One 2010;5:e12140.

61. Mercuri E, Bertini E, Messina S, *et al.* Randomized, Double-Blind, Placebo-Controlled Trial of Phenylbutyrate in Spinal Muscular Atrophy. Neurology 2007; 68:51-55.

62. Garbes L, Riessland M, Holker I, *et al.* LBH589 Induces up to 10-fold SMN Protein Levels by Several Independent Mechanisms and is Effective Even in Cells from SMA Patients Nonresponsive to Valproate. Hum Mol Genet 2009;18: 3645-58.

63. Chen TH, Chang JG, Yang YH, *et al.* Randomized, Double-Blind, Placebo-Controlled Trial of Hydroxyurea in Spinal Muscular Atrophy. Neurology 2010;75:2190-97.

64. Tiziano FD, Lomastro R, Pinto AM, *et al.* Salbutamol Increases Survival Motor Neuron (SMN) Transcript Levels in Leucocytes of Spinal Muscular Atrophy (SMA) Patients: Relevance for Clinical Trial Design. J Med Genet 2010;47:856-58.

65. Van Meerbeke J, Gibbs R, Plasterer H, *et al.* The Therapeutic Effects of RG3039 in Severe Spinal Muscular Atrophy Mice and Normal Human Volunteers. Neurology 2012;78 (Meeting Abstracts 1):SC01.002.

66. Farooq F, Molina FA, Hadwen J, *et al.* Prolactin Increases SMN Expression and Survival in a Mouse Model of Severe Spinal Muscular Atrophy via the STAT 5 Pathway. J Clin Invest 2011;121:3042-50.

67. Porensky PN, Mitrpant C, McGovern VL, *et al.* A Single Administration of Morpholino Antisense Oligomer Rescues Spinal Muscular Atrophy in Mouse. Hum Mol Genet 2012; 21:1625-38.

68. Merlini L, Solari A, Vita G, *et al.* Role of Gabapentin in Spinal Muscular Atrophy: Results of a Multicenter, Randomized Italian Study. J Child Neurol 2003;18:537-41.

69. Trophos Completes Patient Enrolment in Pivotal Efficacy Study of Olesoxime in Spinal Muscular Atrophy, 2012; Available from: http://www.trophos.com/news/pr20110908.htm [Accessed 8 September 2011].

70. Foust KD, Wang X, McGovern VL, *et al.* Rescue of the Spinal Muscular Atrophy Phenotype in a Mouse Model by Early Postnatal Delivery of SMN. Nat Biotechnol 2010;28:271-74.

71. Glascock JJ, Shababi M, Wetz MJ, *et al.* Direct Central Nervous System Delivery Provides Enhanced Protection Following Vector Mediated Gene Replacement in a Severe Model of Spinal Muscular Atrophy. Biochem Biophys Res. Commun 2012;417:376-81.

34 Chapter

NEUROMUSCULAR DISORDERS

V Viswanathan

Muscle disorders in children form a major bulk of cases in any neurology clinic. A unique nature of muscle disorders is that they show wide phenotypic variability even in children with the same disease. The other difficult aspect is that the genotype–phenotype correlation is again very variable. One could come across two children in the same age group with similar genetic abnormality but showing wide variability in the phenotypic expression of the disease and this makes it much more difficult to counsel the families about the future.

The most important aspect in the diagnosis of children with hypotonia and developmental delay is to identify whether the problem is due to a central nervous system disorder or due to a peripheral nervous system disorder. Peripheral nervous system will include the spinal cord, anterior horn cells, peripheral nerves and the muscles along with its appendages. Some disorders can affect both the central and the peripheral nervous system. The next aspect in diagnosis is whether the disease is a progressive or a static condition. Once this is done then it will be easy to decide on the appropriate investigations and the interventional strategies.

Over the last two decades there has been an explosion of knowledge about the various specific proteins responsible for causing different disorders. This has also led the researchers to identify huge number of specific genes responsible for causing the defective proteins. The importance of being specific about the diagnosis is that, now we are able to offer precise counseling and prenatal diagnosis to the families.

EVALUATION OF A CHILD WITH SUSPECTED NEUROMUSCULAR DISEASE

A child suspected to have some neuromuscular disease should undergo good clinical evaluation that is essential for diagnosis. The most important aspects of this evaluation are good history and physical examination. Certain points of diagnostic importance are stated below.

History

1. Age of onset of the problems – since birth or noticed later?
2. What were the presenting symptoms? – Head lag, delay in sitting / standing or abnormal gait patterns, respiratory infection, scoliosis, difficulties in climbing stairs, difficulties in getting up from squatting position, ptosis, slow with writing at school etc.
3. What has happened to the problems – static, improving or worsening?
4. What about his speech, language, understanding, vision and hearing?
5. Any history of frequent breathlessness or fainting.
6. Sleep pattern. Does he sleep well at night or has a disturbed pattern of sleep?
7. Does he complain of any headaches in the mornings?
8. Are there any episodes of vomiting in the mornings?
9. Does he complain of or appear very drowsy during the day time?
10. Is he able to carry on with his usual activities of daily living like brushing, going to toilet, eating etc on his own or does he require help for these?
11. Any family history of premature balding, persons becoming wheel chair bound early in life, early cataracts, persons who have difficulty with day to day activities like opening a bottle, anybody who has died early due to muscle weakness etc. History of consanguinity would also be important to make a note of.

12. History of previous sibling deaths or repeated abortions, decreased fetal movements, polyhydramnios, maternal drug intake particularly thyroxine, steroids etc.
13. The condition of the baby soon after birth including APGAR score, need for resuscitation, oxygen therapy, ventilation would be important.

Examination:

- Alertness – floppy infants are usually alert.
- Facial Dysmorphism – Down syndrome, Prader-Willi syndrome, Zellweger syndrome.
- Myopathic facies, ptosis, eye movements – normal or abnormal.
- Tongue fasciculation – seen in SMA particularly.
- Posture – frog like? Spontaneous activity / movements against gravity?
- Weakness – proximal or distal, any wasting or fasciculation?
- Chest wall movements / breathing pattern – thoraco-abdominal or abdominothoracic – poor chest expansion?
- Shape of chest – bell shaped chest (SMA).
- Tone – pulled to sit – marked head lag, marked hypotonia seen on ventral suspension.
- Deep tendon reflexes – may be present, diminished or even absent.
- Examination of the spine, head circumference and sensation would be important in these children.
- Systems examination – look for any organomegaly – particularly liver (Zellweger syndrome), look for cardiomegaly (Children with Down syndome, Pompe's disease may have congenital heart defects) and respiratory examination – for associated respiratory illnesses in these children due to poor or weak cough, examination of the genitalia for small penile length as in Prader-Willi syndrome.

DISORDERS CAUSING FLOPPY NEONATES AND INFANTS

Down Syndrome

Incidence is about 1:800 live births. Incidence increases with advancing maternal age 1:1528 at age 20 to 1:112 at 40 years of age. Down syndrome is caused by duplication of the genetic material located on the long arm of chromosome 21.[1] The characteristic dysmorphic features are brachycephaly, dysmorphic features, pot belly, acyanotic congenital heart disease, hypotonia, low set ears, short neck, short broad hands, small fingers. Moderate to severe mental retardation is common amongst these children.[2] Hypotonia is profound and many of these children have delayed independent ambulation till about 2 years of age. Epilepsy occurs in about 5 to 6% of these patients.[3] Infantile spasms are frequent. Other important problems that can occur in these children are hypothyroidism, cataracts, intestinal atresias, and recurrent respiratory tract infections.

Hypothyroidism: In its congenital form presents with protruding tongue, pot belly, coarse facial features (Fig. 34.1), wide open anterior frontanelle, hypotonia and early developmental delay. Prolonged physiological jaundice may be there in some. Typically these children have feeding problems and constipation. Mental retardation and global developmental delay eventually follows. Without doubt early detection of the problem and treatment with thyroxine will prevent most of these complications. This is why in many countries neonatal screening for hypothyroidism is done routinely.

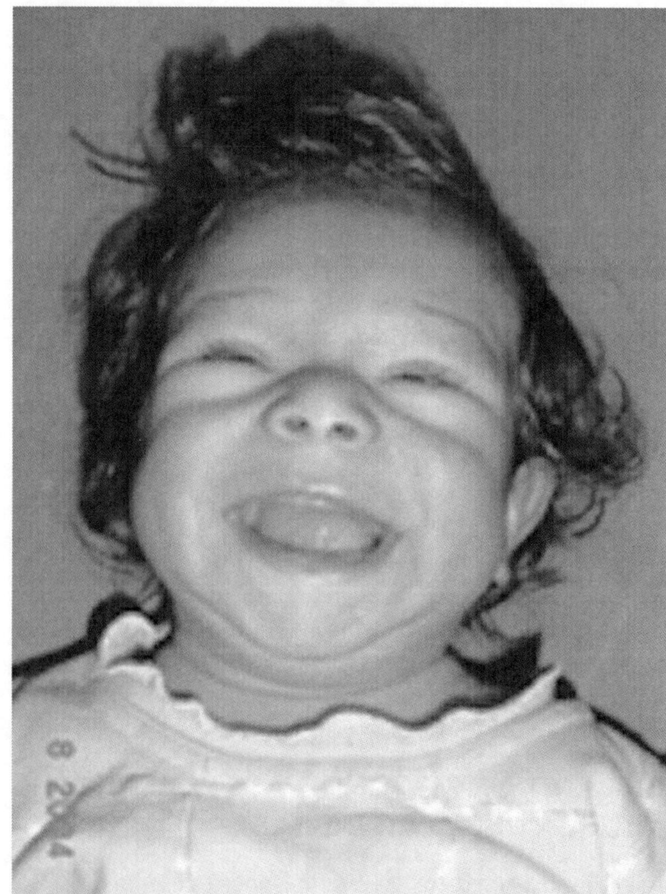

Fig. 34.1: Hypothyroidism (note the coarse facial features, macroglossia)

Spinal Muscular Atrophy – Type 1 (Werdnig Hoffmann Disease)

In 1991 the international SMA consortium subdivided SMA into three types I, II and III.[4] Spinal muscular atrophy type I, type II and type III were mapped to chromosome 5q11.2 – q13.3 locus indicating that they are allelic disorders.[5] The understanding of the genetic locus has helped a lot in prenatal diagnosis.

Spinal muscular atrophy type 1 was found to be the most common cause of floppy infants in a study done on 35 floppy infants from NIMHANS in Bangalore[6] in India. The onset is early either in utero or within the first few weeks of life.[7] Some children appear to be completely normal for a few weeks / months before the onset of weakness. The main clinical characteristics in these children are the profound generalized hypotonia (Figs. 34.2 and 34.3), frog like posture of the limbs, lower limbs are more affected than the upper limbs, proximal more than distal, absent deep tendon reflexes, funnel shaped chest, poor chest expansion, alert baby and fasciculations of the tongue are seen in some. Bulbar weakness with difficulty in sucking and swallowing are seen in others. Contractures are not a feature of severe spinal muscular atrophy. Electromyographic studies in these children show a pattern of denervation with normal sensory and motor conduction velocities.[8] The muscle biopsy provides evidence of skeletal muscle denervation with groups of atrophic and hypertrophic fibres and fibre type grouping.[9] These infants are prone to recurrent respiratory infections and as a result rarely survive beyond the first two years of life.

There is lot of excitement in diagnosis of SMA early in life as there are multiple new therapies that have come up within the last few years including Nusinersen, Onasemnogene abeparvovec and Risdiplam showing some therapeutic benefits in these children, in at least preventing the progression of the disease and improvements in some children.

Congenital Muscular Dystrophy: This disease manifests soon after birth or within the first few months of life. These children also present with severe hypotonia, proximal limb weakness and also have joint contractures affecting the elbows, hips, knees and ankles (Unlike SMA type1 where in contractures are not a feature).

Congenital myopathy: There are various types of congenital myopathies described depending on the structural abnormalities of the muscle fibres visible after staining with histochemical; methods and electron microscopy. The well-known types are central core disease, mini-core disease, nemaline myopathy, myotubular myopathy, congenital muscle fibre type disproportion and other non-specific myopathies. It is difficult to distinguish the various types of congenital myopathy since they may all present as a floppy infant at birth or in early infancy. Some may present later in childhood. The usual clinical features are of hypotonia, weakness, poor spontaneous activity and early motor developmental delay (Fig. 34.4).

It would be important to check the CPK levels in these children who are floppy as some of the congenital muscular dystrophies may also present as floppy infants. All other routine investigations in these children are normal.

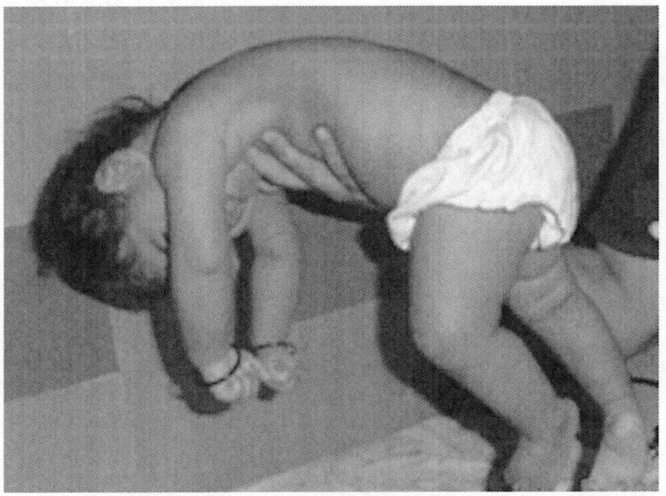

Fig. 34.2

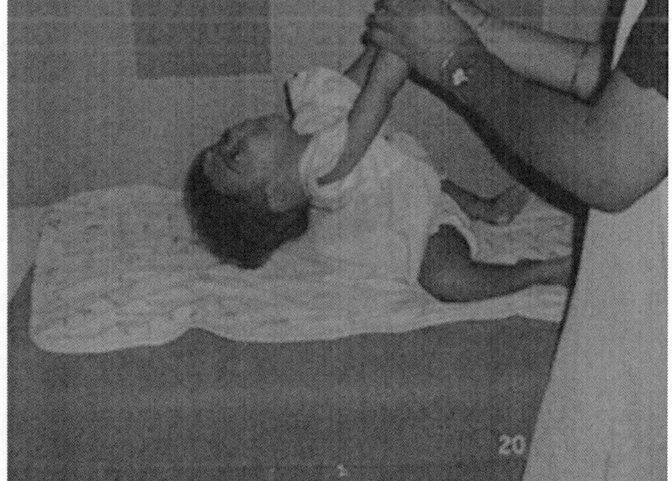

Fig. 34.3

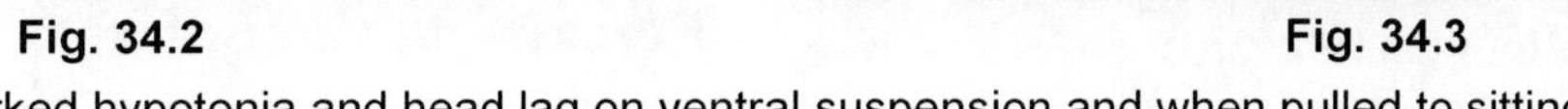

(Marked hypotonia and head lag on ventral suspension and when pulled to sitting)

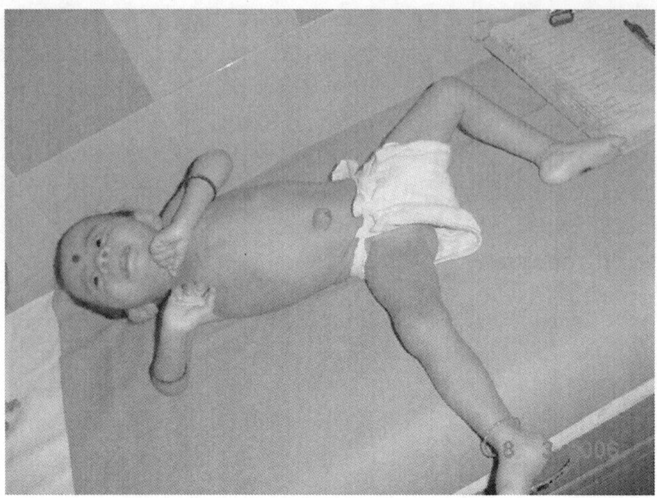

Fig. 34.4: Marked hypotonia, alert child

Central Core Disease: This is the first type of congenital myopathy to be described by Shy and Magee in 1956.[10] The usual clinical feature is that of a mild and relatively non-progressive muscle weakness presenting either in infancy or early childhood. There may be associated hip dislocation, contractures, scoliosis or talipes noticed in these children. The main histological features are the presence of cores within the muscle fibres seen on the NADH-TR preparation. The gene locus has been identified to be on the chromosome 19q13 which codes for the ryanodine receptor 1 protein.[11]

It is estimated that when the muscles from patients with central core disease were analyzed, around 28% of the cases show malignant hyperthermia susceptibility.[12] Maligant hyperthermia is a potentially fatal condition characterized by muscle rigidity and hypermetabolism triggered by certain inhalation anaesthetic agents and depolarizing skeletal muscle relaxants.[13] This needs to be borne in mind and explained to the family about the risks involved in these children in submitting them to general anaesthesia.

Myotubular Myopathies: Myotubular myopathy derives its name from the resemblance of the muscle fibres of the patients to the fetal myotubule present during normal muscle development. There are three well-known forms the X-linked form, the autosomal dominant and the autosomal recessive forms.[14]

Most of these children have early onset weakness, with respiratory difficulty and early motor developmental delay. Ptosis and extraocular muscle weakness may be seen. The disease in general is non-progressive or only slowly progressive. Talipes equino varus, dislocated hips and arthrogryposis may be seen in some children with this condition.

Nemaline Myopathy: The name comes from the rod like inclusions seen on electron microscopy of the muscles in these children. This type of muscle disease is clinically and genetically heterogenous. There are various genetic mutations identified in nemaline myopathy including 1q21-23, 2q21.2-q22 etc. There are six clinical forms of nemaline myopathy recognized[15] which do not appear to have any good correlation with the genetic basis.

1. Floppy infant with facial and respiratory muscle weakness.
2. Severe congenital form.
3. Intermediate congenital form.
4. Milder childhood form.
5. An adult onset type; and
6. A group with features such as cardiomyopathy, ophthalmoplegia or rigid spine. Diagnostic criteria for nemaline myopathy were described in 1996 by Wallgren and Laing[16] depending primarily on the presence of nemaline bodies, pattern of muscle weakness, age of onset, inheritance pattern, laboratory and neurophysiological investigations.

Congenital Muscle Fibre Type Disproportion: This is a description based on the muscle biopsy findings of type 1 fibres being much smaller than the type 2 fibres by more than 12%, in contrast to normal muscle where type1 and type 2 fibres are of approximately equal size.[17] The children with this condition typically present as floppy infants soon after birth and in some, contractures involving the hands and feet are noted. It is not uncommon to find hip dislocation in some of these children. Early motor developmental delay is common. Recurrent respiratory infections are frequent during the first year of life. These features make it difficult to distinguish easily from Werdnig-Hoffmann's disease but that would be important as the children with congenital fibre type disproportion improve after the first two years of life unlike children with Werdnig-Hoffmann's disease who have a poor prognosis.[18] The genetic basis of this disease has not been clearly determined.

Other Types of Congenital Myopathies: Minimal change myopathy, Desminopayhies, hyaline body myopathy, sheroid body myopathy, reducing body myopathy have all been reported.

Peroxisomal Disorders

Zellweger Syndrome cerebro-hepatorenal syndrome):

Facial dysmorphism including high forehead, widely patent frontanelle and sutures, shallow orbital ridges, low nasal bridge, micrognathia and external ear deformity are seen. Neurological manifestations are dominated by severe hypotonia, depressed or absent tendon reflexes and poor sucking and swallowing. Generalized seizures start during the first few days of life. There is global development delay, failure to thrive and retinal degeneration with extinguished ERG, optic atrophy and cataracts may occur. Hepatomegaly and polycystic kidneys are frequent. Stippled calcification is seen in the patella. EEG abnormailities are frequent. CT / MRI may show neuronal migrational abnormalities. Absence of demonstrable peroxisomes in the liver and other tissues with generalized peroxisomal impairment characterizes this disorder.[19]

Prader-Willi Syndrome is characterized by profound hypotonia in the neonatal period, feeding and swallowing problems, dysmorphism. The striking features are the hyperphagia and obesity that develop by the second year of life (Fig. 34.5). Other features are hypogenitalism, cryptorchidism, mental retardation and short stature.[20] The syndrome is associated with an interstitial deletion of chromosome 15q 11-13. The deletion is of paternal origin.[21]

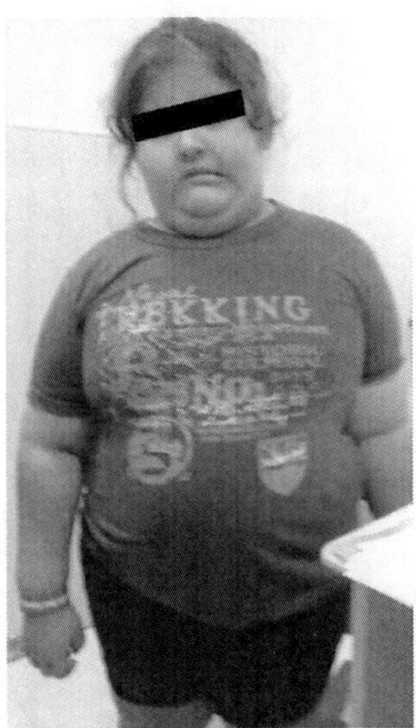

Fig. 34.5: Hyperphagia with truncal obesity

Transient Neonatal Myasthenia is due to transfer of antibodies directed against acetylcholine receptor antibodies from the maternal to fetal circulation.[22] About 10 to 15% of the infants born to myasthenic mothers are affected. Symptoms can occur soon after birth to about 3 days after birth. Hypotonia, facial weakness, poor cry, impaired swallowing and even respiratory distress occur in some requiring ventilation.

Neonatal Myotonic Dystrophy: Hypotonia, facial diplegia, respiratory insufficiency, arthrogryposis are common, usually baby is small for gestational age. The condition is inherited from the mother. Myotonia is rarely observed during infancy and the infant usually dies within the first few weeks after birth.

Pompe's Disease: This is an autosomal recessive disorder caused by a deficiency of the lysosomal enzyme acid alpha glucosidase (GAA).[23] There is a steady accumulation of glycogen in target tissues resulting in organ failure or death. Severity varies by age of onset, organ involvement including degree and severity of muscle involvement (skeletal, respiratory, cardiac) and rate of progression. Recent ACMG guidelines have suggested classifying Pompe's disease into infantile form and a late onset form.[24] The baby with the infantile form shows severe hypotonia and weakness (Fig. 34.6), prominent cardiomegaly, hepatomegaly and die within the first year due to cardiorespiratory failure. The late onset forms tend to be milder and less slowly progressive.

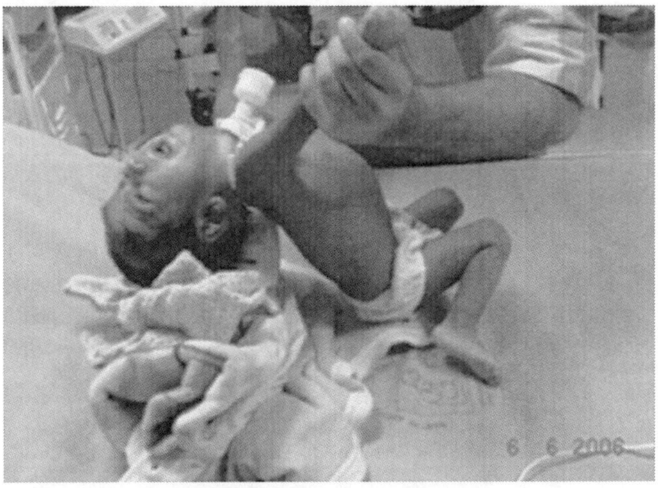

Fig. 34.6: 7-month-old baby with Pompe's disease showing marked hypotonia and has needed a tracheostomy with oxygen for respiratory insufficiency

EXAMINATION OF AN OLDER CHILD WITH SUSPECTED NEUROMUSCULAR DISORDER

- Head circumference (Hydrocephalus may be a feature of Walker Warburg Syndrome – A form of congenital muscular dystrophy).
- Facial dysmorphism (Genetic syndromes – Down, Prader-Willi).
- Facial weakness with loss of naso-labial folds – Congenital myopathy.
- Ptosis +/- ophthalmoplegia (extraocular muscles involvement) – Common in myasthenia, mitochondrial

disorders, may also be seen in congenital myopathy and congenital muscular dystrophies.

- Tongue – Big tongue in Duchenne Muscular dystrophy. Fibrillations in SMA.
- Proximal muscle weakness – Around shoulder and hip girdles seen in most muscular dystrophies and myopathies.
- Scoliosis – Postural / permanent seen in Spinal Muscular Atrophy – Type 2, Duchenne muscular dystrophy, congenital myopathies.
- Depressed or absent tendon jerks – May be feature of all the myopathies and muscular dystrophies or spinal muscular atrophies.
- Gait patterns – Wide based gait – Common in most myopathies, toe walking a feature of Duchenne muscular dystrophy, Walking with feet externally rotated / talipes valgus deformity more common in myopathies.
- Arthrogryposis – Seen in congenital muscular dystrophies.
- Calf muscles – Hypertrophy in Duchenne muscular dystrophy, thinning in Charcot-Marie tooth disease.

SOME OF THE COMMON MUSCLE DISORDERS

Duchenne Muscular Dystrophy: Onset is in early childhood. Toe walking, difficulty in climbing stairs and rising from the floor are early symptoms. Gowers sign is seen due to pelvic weakness. Lordosis (Fig. 34.7) and waddling gait becomes apparent later. Calf hypertrophy and less frequently hypertrophy of vastus lateralis and deltoids may be seen. Many of these children become wheel chair bound by 12 years. Scoliosis and respiratory difficulties occurs usually at this stage. Cardiac involvement is seen towards the later stages. Approximately 20 to 30 % have subnormal range of intelligence quotient. The diagnosis is made based on very high creatine kinase, myogenic pattern on EMG, lack of dystrophin (Figs. 34.8 and 34.9) seen on immunocytochemistry of the muscle biopsy[25] and by genetic testing looking for deletions / translocations in the DMD gene located in the short arm of X chromosome in the band Xp21. At present the need for muscle biopsy has considerably reduced thanks to the advances in the genetic testing methods including MLPA and Next generation sequencing. Prenatal diagnosis and carrier testing are important to prevent recurrence of same disease in the family. There is a lot of phenotypic variability among the

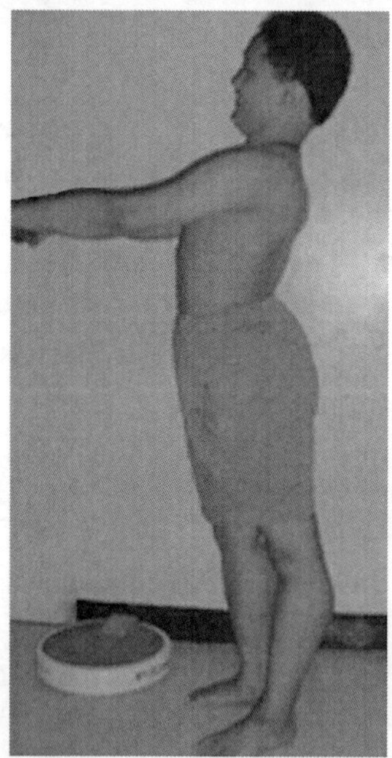

Fig. 34.7: DMD – lumbar lordosis

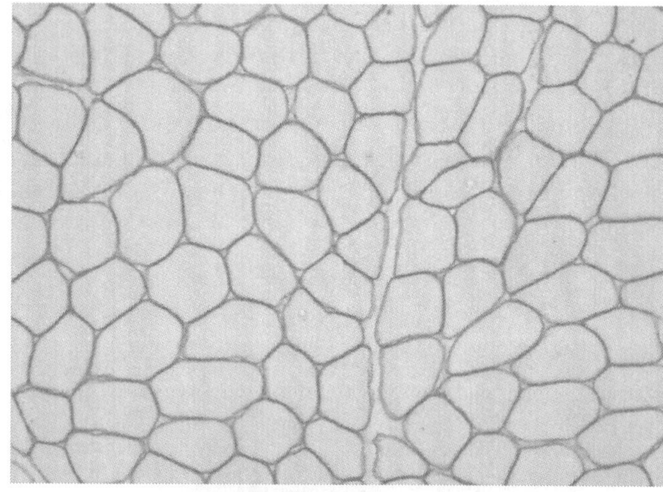

Fig. 34.8: Dystrophin – present
(Courtesy of Dr. Gayathri, NIMHANS)

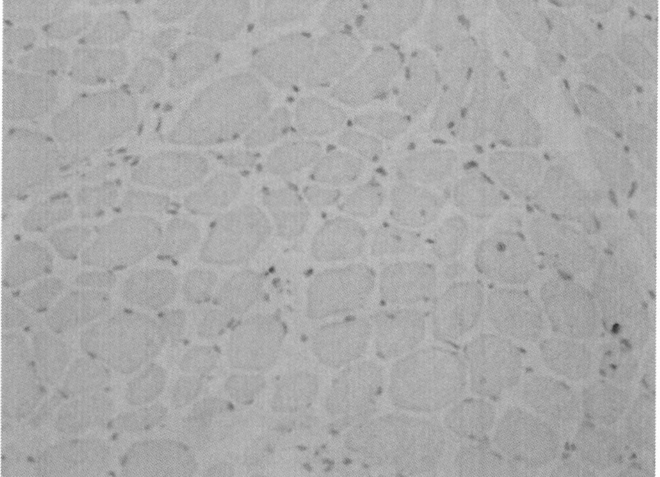

Fig. 34.9: Dystrophin – absent
(Courtesy of Dr. Gayathri, NIMHANS)

children suffering from Duchenne Muscular Dystrophy with some children having early difficulty with walking as compared to the others.[26,27]

In a study performed on Duchenne Muscular Dystrophy in 62 children at Chennai – the age of onset of symptoms was between 61 and 120 months in 58.06% of the cases and in the remaining 41.94% the symptoms started before 60 months. Age at diagnosis in 77.41% of the patients was between 61 and 120 months, 14.51% patients were diagnosed before 60 months and 8.06% after 180 months.[28] The mean age at loss of ambulation was 119 months (range 96 – 168 months). Assessment of the IQ in our patients showed normal IQ (>70) in 80% of the children and the rest 20% had (<70) IQ scores. There was no significant correlation between the location of the genetic deletion and IQ scores [28]. The primary concern is the delay in the diagnosis of the index case as this results in more children being born in the same family with Duchenne Mucsular Dystrophy before genetic counseling could be done. It is also important to counsel the families about the availability of prenatal testing particularly when we have a clear genetic defect identified in the index case.

Becker Muscular Dystrophy: Allelic to Duchenne Muscular Dystrophy. Onset after 5 years up to adolescence. Patients continue to walk well into adulthood. Pseudohypertrophy of calf muscles, pes cavus, Achilles tendon contractures with absent ankle jerks may occur. Dystrophin staining shows about 10 – 40% positive fibres.[29] Creatine kinase is elevated. Many of these patients experience calf pain and muscle cramps after exercise. Cardiac involvement is less common than in Duchenne and is usually a late manifestation.[30]

Limb Girdle Muscular Dystrophies: This is a group of clinically and genetically heterogenous type of muscular dystrophy characterized by weakness and wasting at the shoulder and pelvic girdle. The age of presentation and the severity are also widely variable. There are autosomal dominant and autosomal recessive modes of inheritance seen in Limb Girdle Muscular Dystrophies.

Autosomal Dominant Types of LGMD: The main types of LGMD under this category are classified as LGMD type 1A to 1F.

LGMD Type 1A is primarily an adult onset disease with limb girdle weakness associated with pharyngeal involvement and nasal speech in some. The protein defect has been identified as myotilin[31] in the sarcomere and the gene localized to 5q31. Creatinine phosphokinase levels are usually normal. Contractures and cardiac involvement are not usually seen.

LGMD Type 1B usually begins in childhood starting from the lower limbs and affecting the upper limbs later. Many of these patients present with cardiac involvement in the form of atrioventricular conduction defects[32], dysarrhythmias can lead to sudden death at times. Dilated cardiomyopathy is rarely observed.

The gene locus has been identified to chromosome 1q11-q21 which codes for Lamin A/C component of the nuclear membrane.[33]

LGMD Type 1C has an onset around 5 years of age with calf muscle hypertrophy, proximal muscle weakness and cramping muscle pains after exercise. Clinical examination usually reveals a positive Gowers' sign. There is slow progression of the weakness into adulthood. The CPK is hugely elevated. The genetic locus for this has been mapped to chromosome 3p25 and the protein to caveolin 3 in the sarcolemma.[34] LGMD type 1D,1E and 1F are very rare and occur only in adults.

Autosomal Recessive Type of LGMD: These are generally childhood forms of LGMD that affect both males and females. The course of disease is one of gradual progression over years. Distribution of muscle weakness is typically in the pelvis (80-90% of cases), and later in life, involvement of the shoulder girdle is noted in approximately 30% of cases. Hypertrophy of the calves is absent, in contrast to other forms of muscular dystrophy. The types range from LGMD type 2A to 2I.

LGMD Type 2A: The first symptoms are noticed around 10 years of age with difficulties in running / walking. There is symmetric weakness of the pectoral and pelvic groups of muscles. Toe walking with contractures of the Achilles tendon are seen at an early stage. CPK levels are markedly elevated. The disease progresses slowly and most become wheel chair bound by the time they attain the age of 25 years. The genetic locus is in chromosome 15[35] and the protein product is calpain 3.[36]

LGMD Type 2B: Onset is during early adulthood with weakness involving mainly the proximal muscles in the legs and later progressing to involve the arms over many years. CPK levels are markedly elevated usually. The genetic locus is mapped to chromosome 2p13[37] and the protein product that is deficient is dysferlin.[38]

LGMD Type 2C, 2D, 2E, 2F (Sarcoglycanopathies): These are a heterogenous group of disorders with varying clinical severity. Clinical features are similar to dystrophinopathy with manifestations ranging from very mild to severe. The sarcoglycans that are absent on immunocytochemistry are gamma sarcoglycan in LGMD type 2C.[39] alpha sarcoglycan in LGMD type 2D, Beta sarcoglycan in LGMD type 2E and delta sarcoglycan in LGMD type 2F.[40] In general all these types show similar clinical features with proximal muscle weakness involving the legs as well the arms and showing slow progression over the years. The sarcoglycan proteins on immune-staining can show secondary deficiency in primary dystrophinopathy and so interpretation of the sarcoglycans must be done in the context of the dystrophin protein.[41] Other types of LGMD are extremely rare.

Congenital Muscular Dystrophies

These are a heterogenous group of disorders wherein the presentation is from birth or within the first few months of life with hypotonia, arthrogryposis and associated contractures at various joints. The progression is variable with some remaining static, some showing worsening and some others showing some improvement. CPK is usually elevated 3 to 10 fold.

Merosin Negative Congenital Muscular Dystrophy: This is the most common form of congenital muscular dystrophy showing complete lack of merosin (Fig. 34.10) in the basal lamina on immunocytochemistry.[42] These children usually present with hypotonia (Fig. 34.11) and motor developmental delay. They have normal cognition, vision and hearing. Proximal muscle weakness in the legs and arms are seen with toe walking early. Tightness of the tendo Achilles with contractures may be seen. White matter changes (Fig. 34.12) are seen on the MRI brain[43] in a number of these children but do not appear to be related with any central nervous system dysfunction and over the years the MRI changes appear to remain static.

Most of these children show slow but steady improvement in their motor ability over the years but some may require orthopedic intervention like tendo

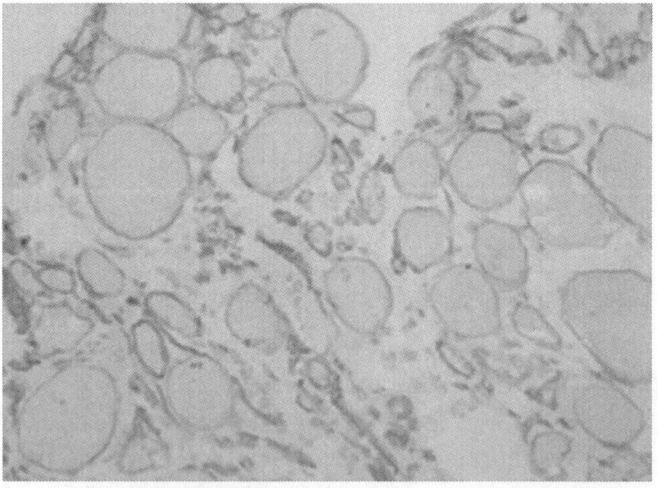

Fig. 34.10: Merosin staining – absent

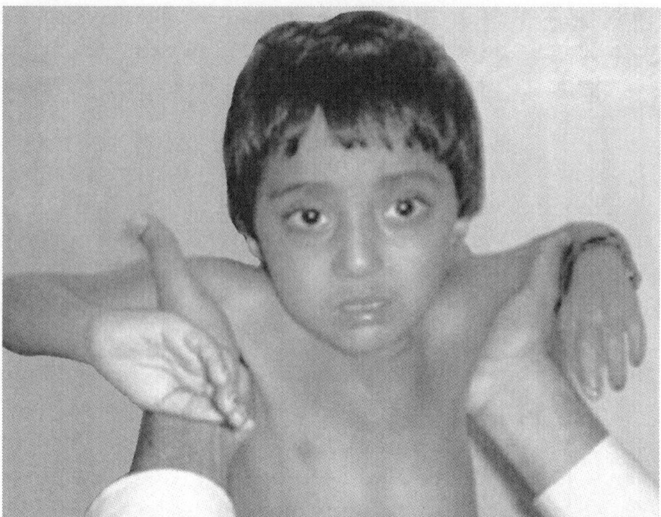

Fig. 34.11: Proximal muscle weakness

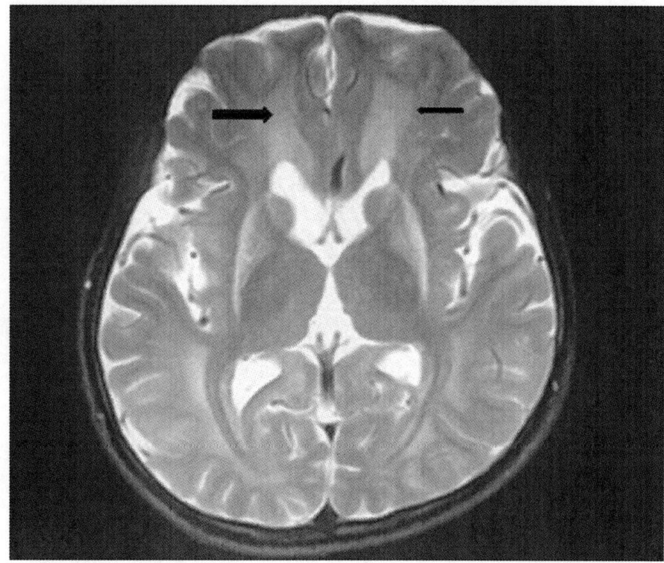

Fig. 34.12: White matter changes on MRI brain scan

Achilles release if there are contractures. Genetic testing shows LAMA 2 gene variant.

Merosin Positive Congenital Muscular Dystrophy: The clinical features are very similar to the merosin negative CMD but tend to be much milder and show no evidence of white matter changes in the brain.

Fukuyama Congenital Muscular Dystrophy: Children with this problem present with marked hypotonia and weakness of early onset, global developmental delay, multiple joint contractures (Fig. 34.13), mental retardation, brain malformations – neuronal migration abnormalities are detectable on CT / MRI brain scans and elevated CPK in the blood.[44] Many of these children progressively worsen in their abilities and die by the time they are 10 years old. The genes underlying this disorder have been implicated in O-linked protein glycosylation: *Fukutin.*[45]

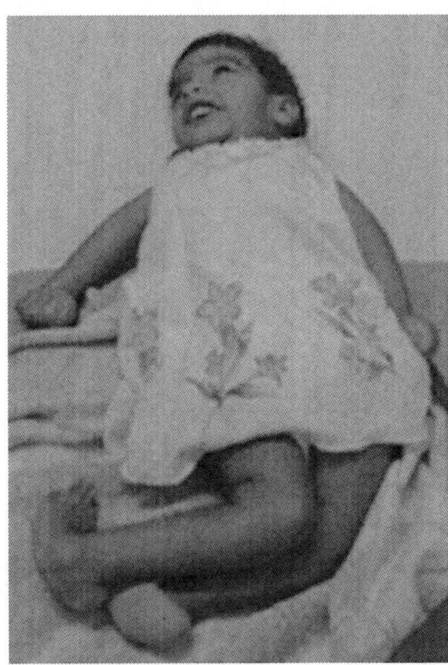

Fig. 34.13: Multiple contractures

Walker Warburg Syndrome: In this condition children at birth are blind, suck poorly, have a weak cry and are markedly hypotonic.[46] The eye abnormalities include anterior chamber abnormalities, corneal opacities and micro or macrophthalmia. Multiple joint contractures are common. Dysmorphism and marked developmental retardation are common. Neuroimaging shows dilated ventricles.[47]

Muscle Eye Brain Disease: These children present with marked hypotonia, muscle weakness, mental retardation and ocular abnormalities.[48] Severe myopia with progressive loss of vision is seen in many of these children. They develop joint contractures and spasticity over the years. Creatinine kinase is markedly elevated.

Neuro-imaging shows cerebral atrophy with dilated ventricles and low density of white matter.[49]

Congenital Myopathies: Hypotonia, proximal muscle weakness, facial weakness, depressed or absent tendon reflexes. No muscle hypertrophy and creatine kinase are normal. Large number of congenital myopathies are known (Discussed previously in this chapter).

Myotonia Congenita: Was described by Thomsen who himself had myotonia congenita. The muscles are unable to relax quickly after a voluntary contraction. The usual age of presentation is around 2 to 3 years of age with history of difficulty in initiating movement soon after a period of rest. The muscle stiffness is usually seen in the legs and in many of these children the calf muscles appear very bulky. The muscle strength is usually increased. The stiffness tends to reduce following activity through the day but is prominent in the mornings soon after waking up after rest. The myotonia tends to get aggravated by cold, fatigue and moods. Clinically myotonia can be demonstrated by opening a clenched hand quickly, tongue or in the eyes by asking them open tightly closed eyes.

There are dominant (Thomsens disease) and recessive (Becker type) described and the recessive type is much more common.[50] Both forms are caused by mutations in the same gene which codes for the major chloride channel of adult human skeletal muscle.[51] Creatinine kinase is usually normal and EMG shows typical myotonic discharges in the skeletal muscles. Many of the children with myotonia congenita can manage without medications but phenytoin or mexiletine can be used if need be.

Paramyotonia Congenita is a much milder form of myotonia and separation of this is only of minor importance as these diseases are benign and respond to the same treatment.[52]

Myotonic Dystrophy is the most common form of muscular dystrophy in adults. Other associated features in adults are baldness, testicular atrophy, posterior cataracts and low intelligence. Cataracts are common in later stages of the disease but may be detected by slit lamp in earlier stages.

Myotonic dystrophy may take various forms in childhood. The classical adult type may be recognized in childhood in affected families. The most severe form of the disease is the **congenital myotonic dystrophy** wherein the baby at birth is noticed to be severely hypotonic, has diminished respiration and swallowing difficulties. There is usually a history of polyhydramnios in the mother during pregnancy. These babies usually die shortly after birth due to respiratory difficulties. Talipes equinovarus deformity of the feet may be seen. Myotonia is not a feature of this condition at this stage and is also not detectable on EMG.[53] The clue to diagnosis comes from examination of the mother who will show sub-clinical or overt features of myotonic dystrophy. The mother may have difficulty in screwing her eyes and burying her eye lashes and she may also show clinical myotonia after clenching her fist.

Myotonic dystrophy is an autosomal dominant disease caused due to a mutation in the length of a polymorphic CTG[5-37] trinucleotide repeat, located in chromosome 19.[54] In classical or adult-onset myotonic dystrophy CTG triplet repeats up to several hundreds may be seen but in congenital myotonic dystrophy expansions greater than 1000 CTG's in blood DNA may be seen.

Myasthenia

Myasthenia is characterized by abnormal fatigue after sustained muscle activity and by improvement after rest. There are three main clinical varieties that occur during childhood.[55]

1. Transient neonatal myasthenia in the infant born to a mother suffering from myasthenia.
2. Congenital or infantile myasthenia.
3. Juvenile myasthenia which is similar to the adult variety.

Transient Neonatal Myasthenia occurs in about 10 to 15% of infants born to myasthenic mothers.[56] This is due to the transplacental transfer of circulating anti-acetylcholine receptor antibodies from the myasthenic mother to the fetus. The symptoms appear within a few hours of birth with feeding difficulties, generalized hypotonia and weakness, breathing difficulties and a weak cry. Very rarely facial weakness and ptosis may be seen. The diagnosis can be confirmed with edrophonium test. The treatment is largely supportive. If the child has respiratory compromise then ventilatory support may be necessary. Tube feeds may be needed during the first few days. Usually the baby recovers over the next few days.

Congenital Myasthenia: These are a group of genetically determined disorders that present over the first few years. They have been classified according to their mode of inheritance, clinical symptomatology and results of investigations.[57,58] The main groups are pre-synaptic defects, pre and post-synaptic defects, post-synaptic defects and partially characterized syndromes. Onset of symptoms is usually after 1 year of age. Ptosis and ophthalmoplegia due to involvement of extra ocular muscles are common. They can progress to cause weakness in the proximal limb muscles and bulbar muscles. Respiratory muscles may be affected in some. The characteristic feature of myasthenia is the variability of the weakness – appear normal on awakening but fatigue and weakness appear following exercise and are more marked towards the end of the day. Diagnosis is confirmed by:

1. Tensilon test (edrophonium chloride test).
2. Repetitive nerve stimulation test showing decrement in amplitude of the muscle action potentials of more than 20% from the third response (between 3 to 20 Hz).
3. Acetylcholine receptor antibodies – present in 80% of juvenile cases but are usually absent in congenital myasthenic syndromes. In a recent study of congenital myasthenic syndrome subjects from many parts of Indian subcontinent were found to have 1267 del G mutation.[59]

Treatment is mainly for symptomatic relief with partial amelioration in some with anti-acetylcholinesterase medication. Thymectomy and immunomodulatory agents have shown no benefit. 3,4-Diaminopyridine was shown to produce additional improvement in some, who were already receiving acetylcholinesterase treatment.[60]

Juvenile Myasthenia: Onset of symptoms is often insidious. The condition usually affects the eye with ptosis with or without ophthalmoplegia. Proximal muscle weakness more in the upper than lower limbs is often seen. In some cases the weakness may involve the face, the jaw, swallowing, speech, neck and trunk (Fig. 34.14).

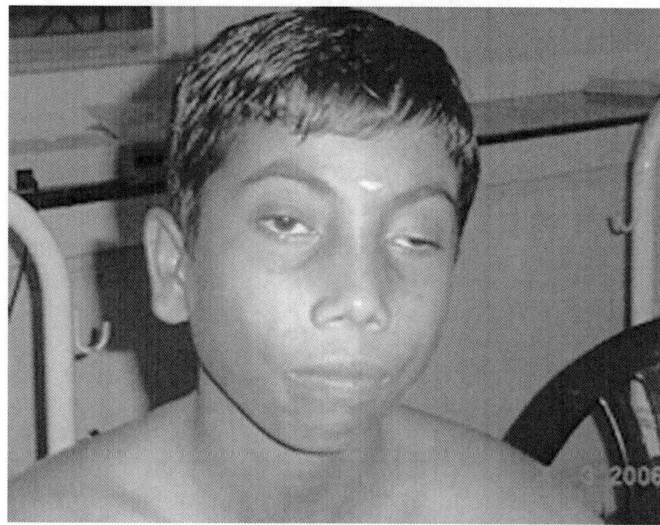

Fig. 34.14: Ptosis with facial weakness

The course tends to be slowly progressive with marked fluctuations. The child tends to be better early in the mornings and after rest but gets worse towards the end of the day. Occasionally other autoimmune disorders like thyroid disease and diabetes may be associated. The best method of confirmation of the diagnosis is by the edrophonium test which produces an immediate response. Anti-acetylcholine receptor antibodies are seen in 80-85% of those with generalized myasthenia but only in about 50% of case of ocular myasthenia.[61] More than 10% decrement in muscle action potential after repetitive stimulation of a nerve suggests easy fatiguability of the muscle. The main drugs that help are neostigmine and pyridostigmine (Fig. 34.15). The size of the individual dose and the frequency of the dosage has to be tailored to the individual patient. The usual starting dose of neostigmine is 0.3 mg/kg every 3 hours and of pyridostigmine is 1.0 mg/kg every 4 hours.[62] Alternate day prednisolone is helpful in some cases.[63] The

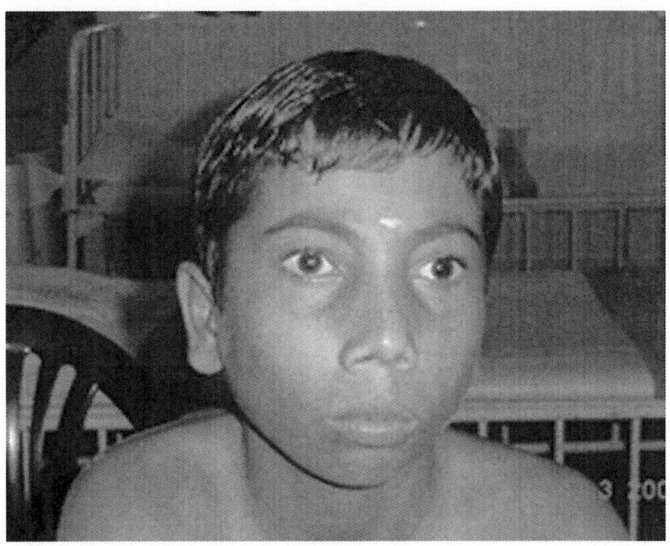

Fig. 34.15: Good eye opening and eye movement after pyridostigmine

other treatments that have been tried are azathioprine, cyclosporin, and intravenous immunoglobulin infusions. Thymectomy is of potential value particularly in adults.

Drugs to be Avoided in Children with Myasthenia

Muscle relaxants like curare, gallamine triethiodide and succinylcholine. Quinine, quinidine and neomycin as they increase the neuromuscular blockade. Morphine is best avoided.

Spinal Muscular Atrophies: Characterized by progressive degeneration of the anterior horn cells of the spinal cord. Most common form is the **SMA type 1 (Werdnig Hoffman disease)** (discussed earlier in this chapter).

SMA Type 2 (Intermediate SMA): Onset is after 3 months of age. Generally insidious, attaining early motor milestones upto sitting but standing does not develop. Excessive curvature of the back is noticed during sitting. Tongue fasciculation may be present. These children show weakness and wasting in both legs and have absent deep tendon reflexes. Contractures and kyphoscoliosis may occur. These children never walk. Genetic diagnosis is confirmatory and the key is to check the SMN 2 copy numbers which are usually 2 to 4 in most of these children.

SMA Type III (Kugelburg Welander syndrome): Onset may be at any age between infancy to early childhood. Weakness predominates in the proximal muscles. Waddling gait is common. Absent knee jerks and preserved ankle jerks are seen in these children. Clinically resemble muscular dystrophies. EMG is very helpful in diagnosis. In these children SMN 2 copy numbers on genetic testing are usually between 3 and above.

Mitochondrial myopathies is a group of disorders characterized by muscle weakness and wasting of muscles appearing usually before the age of 20 years. The inheritance of these disorders is usually from the mother[64] and can be dominant or recessive. Although the disease primarily affects the muscles it can involve the brain, heart, lungs, liver, kidneys and other endocrine organs and so needs close follow-up. Neurological manifestations of mitochondrial cytopathies encompass a diverse group of clinical manifestations including certain defined clinical syndromes and multisystem manifestations.[65]

MERRF–Myoclonic Epilepsy with Ragged Red Fibres is characterized by mitochondrial myopathy with various seizure types (myoclonic epilepsy, generalized tonic-clonic seizure, focal seizures) and variable central nervous system (CNS) dysfunctions ranging from severe CNS dysfunction (deafness, ataxia, spasticity, myoclonus, dementia, pigmentary retinopathy), cardiomyopathy, renal tubular dysfunction and peripheral neuropathy to asymptomatic myopathy with red ragged fibres.[66,67,68] The most constant finding in this condition is the ragged red fibres and the ultrastructurally abnormal mitochondria in the muscle biopsy.

MELAS – Mitochondrial Encephalomyopathy Lactic Acidosis and Stroke Like Episodes: The children may be normal over the first few years with early normal development and then present with recurrent stroke like episodes, seizures and dementia.[69] The symptoms can begin any time between the ages of 3 and 35. The stroke like episodes are characterized by hemiparesis with associated visual problems. Seizures are focal and many times lead to epilepsia partialis continua.[70] Muscle weakness may be mild and short stature, diabetes mellitus, sensorineural hearing loss, mild retinal degeneration and cardiac involvement may be seen.[71,72] Lactate levels in both blood and CSF are high and creatinine phosphokinase levels are inconsistently elevated. Diagnosis can be confirmed genetic testing.

Kearns-Sayre syndrome: Children with this condition have external ophthalmoplegia, retinal degeneration, cardiac conduction defects and sometimes diabetes, deafness and ataxia.[73] These children appear normal at birth and develop ptosis with progressive external ophthalmoplegia during early childhood. Later mild visual loss with pigmentary retinopathy and optic atrophy may occur. Ataxia and mental retardation are often present. Heart block is a late sign and may result in episodes of syncope or even sudden death. Elevated lactate is usually seen in the CSF and serum. CSF protein may be elevated. Muscle biopsy shows ragged red fibres and abnormal mitochondria.

Chronic Progresive External Ophthalmoplegia is a disorder characterized by slowly progressive paralysis of the extra-ocular muscles. Patients usually experience bilateral, symmetrical, progressive ptosis, followed by ophthalmoparesis months to years later.[73] Ciliary and iris muscles are not involved.

McArdles Disease: This is a rare glycogen storage disorder caused by the deficiency of the enzyme myophosphorylase.[74] The main clinical features are cramps on exertion. During childhood the main symptom may be easy fatiguability. Transient myoglobinuria may occur on exertion.

INVESTIGATIONS IN MUSCLE DISEASE

CPK: High in muscular dystrophies but normal in myopathy

EMG: Fasciculations, denervation potentials and high amplitude polyphasic motor potentials are seen in anterior horn cell disorders (SMA), small amplitude polyphasic motor units in myopathy / muscular dystrophy and normal in myasthenia.

Nerve Conduction Velocity: Normal in anterior horn cell disorders and myopathy but decremental response to repetitive nerve stimulation seen in Myasthenia.

Muscle Biposy: This is a very important test of great value in differentiating the various types of myopathies and muscular dystrophies. Immunocytochemistry, enzyme histochemistry and electron microscopy of the muscle specimen may be necessary to make a precise diagnosis. It is therefore very important that we provide all the available history and clinical data to help the pathologist decide on the best diagnostic tool.

Ultrasound of the Muscle: May be of value in selected cases to identify the affected muscle clearly before proceeding with a biopsy.

Magnetic Resonance Imaging: This is being used more and more now to identify the specific group of muscles affected and also to follow-up regarding the degree of involvement of specific muscle groups over a period of time.

THERAPY IN MUSCLE DISORDERS

On the whole the mainstay of therapy is supportive and prevention of secondary problems like contractures, scoliosis, respiratory infections etc. Physiotherapy is the backbone of these disorders. There is of course renewed hope over the last 10 years about the scope for stem cell therapy, gene therapy and certain pharmacological interventions for specific disorders. Enzyme replacement therapy is now available for diseases like Pompe's disease and so needs to be considered.

References

1. Huret JL, Delabar JM, Marlhens F, Aurians A, Berthire M Tanzer, J Sinet PM. 'Downs Syndrome with Duplication of a Region of Chromosome 21 Containing the CuZn Superoxide Desmutase Gene Without Detectable Karyotypnic Abnormality. Human Genetics 1987;75:251-57.
2. Smith GF, Berg JM. Down's Anomaly. 2nd Edition. Edinburgh: Churchill Livingstone 1976.
3. Stafstrom CE, Patxot OF, Gilmore HE, Wisniewskie KE.'Seizures in Children with Down Syndrome: Etiology, Characteristics and Outcome', Dev Med Child Neurology 1991 1991;33:191-200.
4. Munsat TL. Workshop Report, International SMA Collaboration. Neuromuscular Disorders 1991;1:81.
5. Brzustowicz LM, Lehnar T, Castilla LH *et al.* Genetic Mapping of Chronic Childhood Onset Spinal Muscular Atrophy to Chromosome 5q11.2-q13.3, Nature 1990;344:540-41.
6. A Vasant, M Giurie Devi, S Das, Gayathri, Ram Mohan Y. Neuromuscular Disorders in Infancy and Childhood, Neurology India 1997;45:63-68.
7. V Dubowitz, Muscle Disorders in Childhood, 2nd Edition, Chapter 8:328-29.
8. Moosa A, Dubowitz V. Motor Nerve Conduction Velocities in Spinal Muscular Atrophy of Childhood, Arch Dis Childhood 1976;51:974-77.
9. Engel WK. Selective and Non-Selective Susceptibility of Muscle Fibre Types Archives of Neurology 1970;22:97-117.
10. Shy Gm, Magee KR. A New Congenital Non-Progressive Myopathy. Brain 1956;79:610-21.
11. Scacheri PC, Hoffman EP, Fraktin JD *et al.* A Novel Ryanodine Receptor Gene Mutation Causing Both Cores and Rods in Congenital Myopathy, Neurology 2000;55:1689-96.
12. Krivosic-Horber R and Krivosic I. Susceptibility to Malignant Hyperthermia Associated with Central Core Disease. Presse Med 1989;18:828-31.
13. Mark B, Marian S. Central Core Disease, Chapter 13, Neuromuscular Disorders: Clinical and Molecular Genetics, 2nd Edition 277-88.
14. Carina WP, Angus C. Myotubular Myopathy, Chapter B_{12}, Neuromuscular Disorders: Clinical and Molecular Genetics, 2nd Edition 263-76.

15. Ryan MM. Schnell C. Strickland CD. Shield LK. Morgan G. Innacombe ST. Laing NG. Beggs AH. North KN. Nemaline Myopathy: A Clinical Study of 143 Cases. Ann Neurol 2001:50:312-20.

16. Wallgren-Petterson C. Laing NG. Nemaline Myopathy. Neuromuscular Disorders 1996:6:20-28.

17. Brooke MH. A Neuromuscular Disease Characterized by Fibre Type Disproportion. In: Kakulas BA Clinical Studies in Myology. Proceedings of the Second International Congress on Muscle Disease. Perth. Australia 1971 Part 2. Amsterdam. Excerpta Medica ICS 1973: No. 295.

18. V. Dubowitz. Muscle Disorders in Childhood. 2nd Edition. Chapter 3:166.

19. Jean Aicardi. Diseases of the Nervous System in Childhood. Chapter 9:470-71.

20. Butler MG. Meaney FJ. Palmer CG. "Clinical and Cytogenetic Survey of 39 Individuals with Prader-Labhart-Willi Syndrome". American Journal of Medical Genetics 1986:23:793-809.

21. Knoll HM. Nichols RD. Magenis RE. Graham DM. Lalande M. Latt SA. "Angelman and Prader-Willi Syndromes Share a Common Chromosome 15q Deletion but Differ in Parental Origin of the Deletion". American Journal of Medical Genetics 1989:32:285-90.

22. Lefvert AK. Osterman PO. "Newborn Infants Born to Myasthenic Mothers: A Clinical Study and An Investigation of Acetylcholine Receptor Antibodies in 17 Children". Neurology 1983:33:133-38.

23. Hers HG. Alpha Glucosidase Deficiency in Generalized Glycogen Storage Disease (Pompe's disease) Bochem J 1963:86:11-16.

24. Priya S Kishnani. Robert D Steiner. Deeksah Bali *et al.* Pompe Disease Diagnosis and Management Guideline Genetics in Medicine May 2006;Vol 8:No.5:267-88.

25. Hoffman EP. Fischbeck KH. Brown RH. Characterization of Dystrophin in Muscle Biopsy Specimens from Patients with Duchenne or Becker Muscular Dystrophy N Eng J Med 1988; 318:1363-68.

26. Baumbach LL. Chamberlain JS. Ward Ps. *et al.* Molecular and Clinical Correlations of Deletions Leading to Duchenne and Becker Muscular Dystrophies. Neurology 1989:39:465.

27. Koenig M. Beggs A. Moyer M. *et al.* The Molecular Basis for Duchenne vs Becker Muscular Dystrophy: Correlation of Severity with Type of Deletion. American J Hum Genetics 1989:45:498.

28. Saravanan K. A Study of Neuropsychological Profile of Children with Duchenne Muscular Dystrophy – Phenotype and Genotype Correlations – Dissertation Submitted for Diplomate of National Board 2006:43-53.

29. Hoffman EP. Kunkel LM. Angelini C. *et al.* Improved Diagnosis of Becker Muscular Dystrophy by Dystrophin Testing Neurology 1989:39:1011-17.

30. Lazzeroni E. Favaro L. Botti G. Dilated Cardiomyopathy with Regional Myocardial Hypoperfusion in Becker Muscular Dystrophy. International Journal of Cardiology 1989:22:126-29.

31. Hauser MA. Horrigan SK. Salmikangas P. *et al.* Myotilin is Mutated in Limb Girdle Muscular Dystrophy 1A. Hum Mol Genet 2000: September 1:9(14):2141-47.

32. Muchir A. Bonne G. van der Kooi AJ. *et al.* Identification of Mutations in the Gene Encoding Lamins A/C in Autosomal Dominant Limb Girdle Muscular Dystrophy with Atrioventricular Conduction Disturbances (LGMD1B). Hum Mol Genet 2000: May 22:9(9):1453-59.

33. Bonne GB. Di Banletta MR. Varnous S. Mutations in the Gene Encoding Lamin A/C Cause Autosomal Dominant Emery Dreifuss Muscular Dystrophy. Nat Genet 1999:2:285-88.

34. Merlini L. Carbone I. Capanni C. *et al.* Familial Isolated Hyper-CK-aemia Associated with a New Mutation in the Caveolin-3 (CAV-3) Gene. J Neurol Neurosurg Psychiatry 2002 July:73(1):65-67.

35. Fardeau M. Emard B. Mignard C. Tome E. Richard T. Beckemann J. Chromosome 15 Linked to Limb Girdle Muscular Dystrophy–Clinical Phenotype in Reunion Island and French Metropolitan Communities. Neuromucular Disorders 1996:6:447-53.

36. Richard I. Broux O. Allamand V. *et al.* Mutations in the Proteolytic Enzyme Calpain 3 Cause Limb-Girdle Muscular Dystrophy Type 2A. Cell 1995: April 7:81(1):27-40.

37. Bashir R. Strachan T. Keers S. Stepehenson A. Mahjneh I. Marconi G. Nashef L. Bushby KM. A Gene for Autosomal Recessive Limb Girdle Muscular Dystrophy Maps to Chromosome 2p Hum Mol Genet 1994:3:455-57.

38. Bansal D. Miyake K. Vogel SS. *et al.* Defective Membrane Repair in Dysferlin-Deficient Muscular Dystrophy. Nature 2003May8:423(6936):168-72.

39. Noguchi S. McNally EM. Ben Othmane K. *et al.* Mutations in the Dystrophin-Associated Protein Gamma-Sarcoglycan in Chromosome 13 Muscular Dystrophy. Science 1995 November 3:270(5237):819-22.

40. Nigro V. de Sá Moreira E. Piluso G. *et al.* Autosomal Recessive Limb-Girdle Muscular Dystrophy. LGMD2F. is Caused by a Mutation in the Delta-Sarcoglycan Gene. Nat Genet 1996 October:14(2):195-98.

41. Gayathri N. Yasha TC. Santhosh V. Muscle Biopsies for the Diagnosis of Myopathies Reviews in Indian Neurology 2005; 15:283-330.

42. Zhang X. Vuolteenaho R. Tryggvason K. Structure of Human Laminin Alpha 2 Chain Gene (Lama 2). When it is Affected in Congential Muscular Dystrophy J Biochem 1996:271: 27664-69.

43. Van der Knaap MS. Smit LME. Barth PG *et al.* Magnetic Resonance Imaging in Classification of Congenital Muscular Dystrophies with Brain Abnormalities. Ann Neurol 1997:42:50-59.

44. Fernando MST. Pascale G. Michel F. Congenital Muscular Dystrophies. Neuromuscular Disorders: Clinical and Molecular Genetics Ed Alan EH Emerey 1999:Chapter 2:21-57.

45. Kobayashi K. Nakahori Y. Miyake M. *et al.* An Ancient Retrotransposal Insertion Causes Fukuyama-Type Congenital Muscular Dystrophy. Nature 1998:394:388-92.

46. Banker BQ. The Congenital Muscular Dystrophies. In Myology. 2nd Edition (eds A.G. Engel C.Franzini Armstrong). Mcgraw Hill Inc. New York 1994:1275-89.

47. Dobyns WB. Pagon RA. Armstrong D *et al.* Diagnostic Criteria for Walker Warburg Syndrome. American Journal of Medical Genetics 1989:32:195-210.

48. Pihko H. Lappi M. Raitta C. *et al.* Ocular Findings in Muscle Eye Brain Disease: A Follow-up Study. Brain Dev 1995:17: 57-61.

49. Santavuori P. Somer H. Sainio K *et al.* Muscle Eye Brain Disease (MEB). Brain Dev 1989:11:147-53.

50. Thomasen E. Myotonia: Thomsens Disease (Myotonia Congenita). Paramytonia and Dystrophica Myotonica. Universitetsforlaget I Arachus. Denmark 1948.

51. Koch MC. Steinmeyer K. Lorenz. C. *et al.* The Skeletal Muscle Chloride Channel in Dominant and Recessive Human Myotonia. Science 1992:257:797-800.

52. Subramony SH. Malhotra CP and Mishra SK. Distingusihing Paramyotonia Congenital and Myotonia Congenital by Electromyography. Muscle Nerve 1983:6:374-79.

53. Harper PS. Congenital Myotonic Dystrophy in Britain I Clinical Aspects. Archives of Diseases in Childhood 1975:50:505.

54. Brook JD. Mc Currah ME. Harley HG. *et al.* Molecular Basis of Myotonic Dystrophy: Expansion of Trinucleotide (CTG) Repeat at the 3' End of a Transcript Encoading a Protein Kinase Family Member Cell 1992:68:799-808.

55. V Dubowitz. Muscle Disorders in Childhood. 2nd Edition. Chapter 10:398

56. Keesey J. Lindstrom J. Cockeley H *et al.* Anti Acetylcholine Receptor Antibodies in Neonatal Myasthenia Gravis. New England Journal of Medicine 1977:296:55.

57. Engel AG. Congenital Myasthenic Syndromes Myology McGraw Hill. New York 1994:Vol 1:1806-1835.

58. Middleton L.T. Report of the 34th ENMC International Workshop–Congenital Myasthenic Syndromes, Neuromuscular Disorders 1996:6:133-36.

59. Bharti M, David G, Hanns L, Viswanathan V *et al.* Mutation History of Roma/Gypsies American Journal of Human Genetics. October 2004:75(4):596-609.

60. Palace J. Wiles CM and Newsome–Davis J. 3. 4-Diamino-pyridine in the Treatment of Congenital Myasthenia J. Neurol. Neurosurg. Psychiatry 54:1069.

61. V Dubowitz. Muscle Disorders in Childhood. 2nd Edition. Chapter 10:407.

62. V Dubowitz. Muscle Disorders in Childhood 2nd Edition. Chapter 10:409.

63. Newsome-Davis J. Myasthenia Gravis and Related Syndromes In: Walton J. Karpati G. Hitlon Jones D. eds: Disorders of Voluntary Muscle: Edinburgh: Churchill Livingstone 1994: 761-80.

64. Attardi G. Schartz G. Biogenesis of Mitochondria. Ann Rev Cell Biol 1988:4:289-333.

65. Walker U. Collin S. Byrne E. Respiratory Chain Encephalo-myopathies: A Diagnostic Classification. Eur Neurol 1996:36: 260-67.

66. Datta V. Jain P. Mehndirrata MM *et al.* Myoclonic Epilepsy with Red Ragged Fibres. Indian Pediatr 1999:36:817-19.

67. Rowland LP. Blake DM. Hirano M *et al.* Clinical Syndromes Associated with Ragged Red Fibres. Rev Neurol (Paris) 1991: 147:467-73.

68. Sivestri G. Ciafoloni E. Santorelli FM *et al.* Clinical Features Associated with the A-G Transition at Nucleotide 8344 of mt DNA (MERRF mutation). Neurology 1993:43:1200-06.

69. Hirano M. Ricci E. Koingsberger MR *et al.* MELAS: An Original Case and Clinical Criteria for Diagnosis. Neuromuscul Disord 1992:2:125-35.

70. Chevrie JJ. Aicardi J. Goutieres F. Epilepsy in Childhood Mitochondrial Encephalomyopathies: In Wolf P. Dam M. Janz D. Dreifuss F (eds) Advances in Epileptology. 16th Epilepsy International Symposium. New York: Raven Press 1987:181-84.

71. Pavlakis SG. Di Mauro S. De Vivo DC. Rowland LP. Mitochondrial Myopathy. Encephalopathy. Lactic Acidosis and Stroke Like Episodes: A Distinctive Clinical Syndrome: Annals of Neurology 16:481-88.

72. Schapira AHV. Cooper JM. Morgan Hughes JA. Patel SD. Cleeter MJW. Regan CI. ClarK JB. Molecular Basis of Mitochondrial Myopathies: Polypeptides Analysis in Complex 1 Deficiency. Lancet 1:500-03.

73. Moraes CT. Di Mauro S. Zeviani M. *et al.* Mitochondrial DNA Deletions in Progressive External Opthalmoplegia and Kearns-Sayre Syndrome New Engl. J. Med 1989:320(20): 1293-99.

74. Bartran C. Edwards RH. Beynon RJ. McArdles Disease – Muscle Glycogen Deficiency. Biochem. Biophysics. Acta Phosphorylase 1995:1272:1-13.

35 Chapter

TRANSPLACENTAL INFECTIONS

Rashmi Kumar, Chandrakanta

TRANSPLACENTAL INFECTIONS

A number of agents may infect the fetus in utero and produce manifestations in the newborn period or later. These include cytomegalovirus, toxoplasma gondii, Treponema pallidum, rubella virus, parvovirus B_{19}, hepatitis B and C viruses, varicella, herpes simplex type 2, HIV, Zika virus and M tuberculosis. Although HSV, HIV, HBV, HCV, and tuberculosis can result in transplacental infection, the more common mode of infection to the baby is intrapartum (during labour and delivery and passage through infected birth canal) and post natal from contact with infected mother or caretaker.[1] Only those transplacental or intrauterine infections which result in neurological manifestations in the infant (Toxoplasma, rubella, syphilis, cytomegalovirus, herpes, HIV, varicella and Zika virus) will be discussed here. Of these the former 5 are grouped under the TORCH complex.

Common Features About These Transplacental Infections Are:

1. Infections occurring in the mother during pregnancy may affect the fetus. However, if the mother is already immune to the infection, the fetus will not be affected.
2. The time to provide information about these infections is before pregnancy begins, because this is the best time for preventive measures.
3. The first trimester of pregnancy is usually the most dangerous time for the mother to catch these infections because there is a greater risk for the fetus to be affected with developmental defects.
4. Infection in the mother does not always mean that the baby will be affected.
5. Infection in the mother can often be accompanied by very trivial symptoms or be asymptomatic so the condition in the mother can be easily missed.
6. Manifestations of the congenital infection in the baby may be quite different than if the same infection is acquired in the usual way.
7. Some infections can be avoided by the mother through simple measures such an immunization for rubella before pregnancy. Some infections such as syphilis and congenital toxoplasmosis are treatable.
8. Considerable clinical overlap is seen in the manifestations of these various infections. The infection may be asymptomatic at birth or may cause a spectrum of disease ranging from mild disease to severe life threatening illness with multisystem involvement in the newborn. Common signs and symptoms include intrauterine growth retardation, microcephaly, hydrocephalus, intracranial calcifications, chorio-retinitis, cataracts, myocarditis, pneumonia, hepato-splenomegaly, direct hyperbilirubinemia, anemia, thrombocytopenia, hydrops fetalis, petichiae, purpura and vesicles.
9. Many of these agents cause late sequelae, even if the infant is asymptomatic at birth. Adverse outcomes include sensorineural hearing loss, visual disturbances, seizures and neurodevelopmental abnormalities.
10. Common features about their diagnosis is that IgG antibodies against the specific pathogen may be transferred passively from the mother and may be high in the newborn period. Diagnosis has to be established either by demonstration of a rising titre of IgG antibodies or by detection of specific IgM type antibodies. A high cord total IgM level is a non-specific test suggestive of some intrauterine infection in the baby and can be used for screening purposes. However, detection of specific IgM is technically difficult and often false negative. It should not be used to preclude an infection.

Prevalence: Various workers have screened for transplacental infections in different parts of the world. In India, Shanmugam, Raveendranath and Nair (1982) studied prevalence of rubella by hemagglutination inhibition test in 536 and CMV by complement fixation test in 260 pregnant women attending an antenatal clinic.[2] The antibody detection rate was 74.1% for rubella and 85.4% for CMV. CMV was more prevalent in 3rd trimester and in age group 21-25 years while rubella was more during 2nd trimester and in age group 26-30 years. The authors concluded that 26% and 15% of pregnant women were susceptible to rubella and CMV infection respectively. Broor *et al.* (1991) studied 249 infants suspected of having congenital infections by IgM antibodies in serum.[3] Thirty (12%) were positive for rubella and 50 (20%) for CMV. CMV infection was significantly higher in the group presenting with hepatosplenomegaly and rubella in those with congenital malformations. Kaur *et al.* (1999) screened 120 pregnant women for IgM antibodies to toxoplasmosis, rubella, CMV and IgG antibodies to HSV 1 and 2.[4] They found that 112 (93.4%) had evidence of one or more infections. Prevalence of IgG antibodies to HSV was 70% while seropositivity for toxoplasmosis, rubella and CMV was 11.6, 8.3 and 20.8% respectively. Cao, Qui and Zhang (1999) studied TORCH group of infections in relation to abnormal pregnancy outcomes. Rates of active infection (CMV 57.4%, rubella 59.3%, Toxoplasma 11.1% and HSV–2 22.2%) were significantly higher in women with history of abnormal pregnancy outcomes as well as previous TORCH infections and recurrent infections.[5] Camargo Neto *et al.* (2004) screened neonatal dried blood samples for Toxoplasma gondii IgM in 364,130 neonates in Brazil and for cytomegalovirus and rubella IgM and Trypanosoma cruzi IgG in 15,873 neonates. A total of 195 were diagnosed as congenital toxoplasmosis, 16 with CMV and 11 with rubella while 1 neonate and 21 mothers were positive for Chaga's disease.[6] Prabhakar *et al.* (1991) studied seroprevalence of TORCH group of infections in pregnant Jamaican women in 1986 to assess immune/susceptible status. Positivity rates were 57% for T gondii, 69% for rubella, 97% for CMV, 91% for herpes and 4.9% for syphilis.[7] Khan and Kazzi (2000) conducted workup for TORCH infections in 75 infants with intrauterine growth retardation. None of the infants had positive IgM titres for toxoplasma, rubella, CMV or herpes. No infant had elevated total IgM. One infant had positive urine culture for CMV and 2 had abnormal cranial ultrasound – calcifications in one and hydrocephalus in the other. These authors concluded that work up for TORCH infections in all infants with IUGR does not justify the cost.[8] Wang *et al.* (2003) screened 1554 newborns treated in a neonatal intensive care unit in China for TORCH infections by IgM antibodies. Forty-eight had TORCH infection of which CMV, rubella and herpes accounted for 52.1%, 33.3% and 14.6% respectively. No case had toxoplasma infection.[9] Kishore *et al.*, (2011) from Lucknow found ELISA IgM positivity to T. gondii, rubella, cytomegalovirus, herpes simplex virus and B_{19} virus 8.3%, 15%, 30%, 3.3% and 13.6% respectively in 60 women with bad obstetric history (BOH) and pregnancy complications. B_{19} infection caused non immune hydrops fetalis in three cases and cardiac anomaly in one. Cord blood and 33 placental tissues from six malformed newborns tested for B_{19} DNA by PCR were negative.[10] Sen *et al.* (2012) from Varanasi tested sera from women with BOH for TORCH infections. The specific IgM antibodies were found to be positive by ELISA in 74 (19.4%) cases for toxoplasmosis, in 126 (30.4%) cases for the Rubella virus, in 130 (34.7%) cases for CMV and in 151 samples (33.5%) for the HSV-2 infections.[11] The seropositivity in high risk pregnant women for toxoplasma, rubella, CMV and HSV was 28, 84, 92 and 61%, respectively for IgG while it was 6, 3, 4 and 3% for IgG + IgM in a study done by Prasuna *et al.* (2015) in South India.[12]

TOXOPLASMOSIS

Toxoplasma infections are ubiquitous in animals and are one of the most common latent infections of humans worldwide. Throughout the world there are wide regional variations in the prevalence of toxoplasma infections and its seropositivity range from less than 10% to over 90%. High burdens are seen in South America and in some Middle Eastern and low-income countries.[13] Overall prevalence of about 22.4% (8.8-37.3%) has been found in India with IgM positivity rate of 1.43%. Approximately 56,737 to 176,882 newborns in India have a risk of possible congenital infection by toxoplasma.[14]

In a study it was found that maternal infection with T gondii is responsible for 12.5% of fetal wastage in women with bad obstetric history in Pondicherry. High antibody titer by indirect hemagglutination test was found in 13% of habitual abortion cases, 6.7% of sporadic abortion, 8.3% of the congenital anomalies, 13% of stillbirths and 17.2% of premature births.[16] Mohan *et al.* (2002) investigated 500 subjects from each group–rural, urban and urban slum populations of Chandigarh. Overall, 5.4% were positive for IgM and 4.6% to IgG by using microwell ELISA. IgM prevalence was highest in urban slums. Positivity was highest 6-12 years age group.[17] Hingorani *et al.* found Hemagglutination test positivity in 14% of pregnant women with bad and 4.9% of good obstetric history.[18] Chintapalli *et al.* (2013) tested 80 pregnant women with bad obstetric history by ELISA and found 36 (45%) seropositive for Toxoplasma specific IgG antibodies, 16 (20%) seropositive for IgM antibodies and 8 (10%) seropositive for both IgG and IgM.[15]

Toxoplasma gondii is an obligate intracellular protozoan that multiplies only in living cells. Newly infected cats and other Felidae excrete infectious Toxoplasma oocysts in their feces. Humans are infected through ingestion of infected meat containing encysted bradyzoites or by ingestion of oocysts in cat feces. Freezing meat to –20 °C or heating it to 66 °C renders it non-infectious. Infection is not spread from person to person except from mother to infant or rarely through organ transplantation. Tissue cysts which are 10-100 μm in diameter may contain thousands of parasites and remain in tissues especially CNS, skeletal and heart muscle for the life of the host.[19]

In immunologically normal children acute acquired infection may be asymptomatic, cause lymphadenopathy or damage any organ. In immunocompromised children symptoms are related to central nervous system.

Transmission to the fetus usually occurs when infection is acquired in immunologically normal mother during that pregnancy. The average global incidence of congenital toxoplasmosis is about 1.5/1000 live births.[13] The infection may be asymptomatic or produce only mild symptoms in the mother. Of untreated maternal infection acquired in the 1st trimester, approximately 17% of fetuses are infected, usually with severe disease. Of untreated maternal infection acquired in the 3rd trimester, approximately 65% of fetuses are infected, usually with mild or in apparent disease. Overall, the rate of transmission is about 50%.[20]

Congenital infection may present in the newborn period or with late sequelae. In the neonate, infection may result in small for gestational age, prematurity, hydrops fetalis or perinatal death. Other neonatal manifestations include peripheral retinal scars, persistent jaundice, hepatosplenomegaly, anemia, thrombocytopenia and rash. Besides toxoplasma encephalitis may be evident with CSF pleocytosis, convulsions, microcephaly or hydrocephalus and psychomotor retardation. The classic triad of hydrocephalus, chorioretinitis and intracranial calcifications may occur.

Later in infancy, the baby with congenital toxoplasmosis may have skin rashes, which may be fine, punctate, diffuse maculopapular, sharply defined, or diffuse macular. Lymphadenopathy, hepatosplenomegaly, cholestasis, myocarditis, pneumonitis and nephrotic syndrome and endocrine abnormalities may be seen.

Neurologic manifestations vary from massive acute encephalopathy to subtle neurologic syndromes. Toxoplasmosis should be considered in any undiagnosed neurologic disease in infancy especially if retinal lesions are also found. Hydrocephalus may be the sole manifestation of congenital toxoplasmosis. Various seizure types may occur, including massive infantile spasms with hypsarrhythmia. Paralysis of extremities, swallowing difficulty and microcephaly may occur. CSF abnormalities occur in at least one third of infants. CT scan of brain may reveal hydrocephalus, active inflammatory lesions and porencephalic cystic changes. Calcifications may be found throughout the brain but has propensity for caudate nucleus, choroids plexus and subependyma.[20]

Almost all untreated congenitally infected persons will develop chorioretinal lesions by adulthood and half will have severe visual impairment. T gondii causes a focal necrotising retinitis in congenitally infected persons. Any part of the retina may be involved and detachment may occur. Other findings include anterior chamber inflammation, keratic precipitates, iris nodules, posterior synechiae, glaucoma and microphthalmia. Sensorineural hearing loss may occur. Concomitant infection with HIV results in a fulminant encephalitis.[20]

Diagnosis: Acute toxoplasma infection can be diagnosed by isolation of T gondii from blood or body fluids and by demonstration of tachyzoites in tissue sections or cysts in placenta or tissues, by characteristic histologic features in lymph nodes and serology.

Isolation of the organism is done by inoculation of the body fluid, leukocytes or tissue specimen into mice or tissue cultures. Body fluids should be processed and inoculated immediately. Freezing or treatment with formalin kills the organism.

Serology: Many serologic tests are used. The Sabin – Feldman dye test is sensitive and specific and measures IgG antibodies. The IgG – Indirect fluorescent antibody test (IgG-IFA) measures the same antibodies as the dye test and titres of the two tend to parallel. An agglutination test available in Europe uses formalin preserved whole parasites to detect IgM antibodies. This test is accurate, simple and inexpensive. The IgM–IFA test is useful for diagnosing acute infection in older children but is positive in only 25% of congenitally infected babies. The test may yield a false positive result in presence of rheumatoid factor. The IgM ELISA test picks up 75% of congenital infections but false positive results are not uncommon with commercial kits. The IgA ELISA is more sensitive for detection of congenital infection. The immunosorbent agglutination assay (ISAGA) involves trapping of a patient's IgM to a solid surface and use of formalin fixed organisms or antigen coated latex particles. There are no false positives due to rheumatoid factor or antinuclear antibodies. This is a more sensitive test than IgM ELISA and at present the best test for diagnosis of congenital infection. The indirect hemagglutination test (IHA) should not be used for suspected congenital infection because it may be negative for too long a period early in infection. The enzyme linked immunofiltration assay (ELIFA) permits simultaneous study of antibody specificity by immunoprecipitation and characterization of antibody isotypes. This test may be capable of detecting upto 85% of congenital infections in the 1st few days of life. It is still being evaluated. Apart from this, relatively higher level of Toxoplasma antibody in CSF or aqueous humour suggests active CNS or ocular infection. The comparison is calculated as:

C= Antibody titre in body fluid X concentration of IgG in serum

Antibody titre in serum X concentration of IgG in body fluid

Significant levels of C are 8 or more for aqueous humour and 4 or more for CSF.

Toxoplasma antigen can be detected in acute infection but not in chronically infected. Western blot assay in mother and baby's sera can detect congenital infection. Lastly, Polymerase chain reaction (PCR) can be used to amplify Toxoplasma DNA. Detection of a repetitive T gondii gene – the B1 gene in amniotic fluid is the procedure of choice for diagnosing infection of the fetus. Sensitivity and specificity of this test at and beyond 18 weeks gestation are approximately 95%.

At birth when a diagnosis of congenital toxoplasmosis is suspected, the diagnostic studies to be performed are: general ophthalmologic and neurological examinations, CT scan head, isolation of T gondii from placenta, cord blood leucocytes or infant's buffy coat, Toxoplasma specific IgG, IgM, IgA and IgE and total amount of IgG and IgM, CSF analysis for cells, protein and glucose, Toxoplasma specific IgM in CSF, PCR in CSF and CSF inoculation into mice. Presence of Toxoplasma specific IgM in CSF or local production of Toxoplasma specific IgG in CSF establishes the diagnosis of congenital toxoplasma infection.

Treatment: All infected newborns should be treated whether or not clinical manifestations are present. Pyrimethamine plus sulfadiazine or trisulfapyrimidines act synergistically against toxoplasma. Infants should be treated for 1 year with oral pyrimethamine 2 mg/kg/day for 2 days, then 1 mg/kg/day for 2-6 months and then 1 mg/kg given on Monday, Wednesday and Friday. Sulfadiazine or triple sulfonamides (100 mg/kg/day in 2 divided doses) and calcium leukovorin (5-10 mg/kg/day on Monday, Wednesday and Friday). Efficacy of oral prednisolone (1 mg/kg/day in 2 doses) for active chorioretinitis threatening vision is being evaluated.

Treatment of a pregnant woman who acquires infection at any time during pregnancy reduces the chances of congenital infection in the baby.[20] Spiramycin is used for prevention and pyrimethamine plus sulfadiazine when the fetus is found to be or is highly likely to be infected. Pyrimethamine is avoided in the 1st trimester because of its potential teratogenicity.

Prognosis: Early therapy for congenitally infected babies usually cures the manifestations of congenital toxoplasmosis and also reduces sequelae such as cognitive impairment. Hydrocephalus due to aqueductal obstruction may worsen.

Prevention: Pregnant women who do not possess antibodies to T gondii should be counseled to eat well cooked meat and avoid contact with cat excreta. Serologic screening and treatment of pregnant women who acquire infection in pregnancy also reduce the incidence and manifestations of the infection in the baby.

CYTOMEGALOVIRUS INFECTION

Congenital cytomegaloviral (CMV) infection is the most common cause of congenital infections. CMV is the largest of the herpesviruses, with a diameter of 200 nm. Routine serologic tests do not define specific serotypes but restriction endonuclease analysis of CMV DNA shows that although all human strains are genetically homologous, none are identical unless obtained from epidemiologically related cases.[21]

The incidence of congenital CMV infection ranges from 0.2 to 2.4% of all live births, the higher rates occurring among populations with lower socioeconomic standards. The risk of fetal infection is greatest with maternal primary CMV infection (30%) and much less likely with recurrent infection (<1%). Most symptomatic infections are caused by primary rather than reactivated maternal infection. Besides, perinatal infection also occurs through genital tract secretions and breast milk. Virus is detectable in breast milk in 96% of infected mothers, resulting in infection in 38% of babies and symptomatic infection in half of preterm babies.

A study in Brazil on 189 mothers and their newborns yielded a prevalence of congenital CMV infection as 2.6% and prevalence of CMV antibodies in mothers as 95%. None of the 5 infected babies had clinical manifestations at birth, although one had intracranial calcification. A 2nd group of 130 newborns and 74 infants with clinical evidence of congenital disease were also investigated. Congenital CMV was diagnosed in 12 (5.9%) and of these 10 were beyond the neonatal period.[22] Morita *et al.* (1998) conducted a national survey to investigate the prevalence of CMV infection in Japan. A total of 46 cases of CMV were reported for 1992 and 1993. The annual incidence of symptomatic disease was 1.6 cases/100,000 live births.[23] India has a high seroendemicity with almost 99% adults showing IgG antibodies.[27]

Pathology: Cytomegalic cells contain large intranuclear inclusions and smaller cytoplasmic inclusions. These inclusions are pathognomonic for CMV infection. The virus induces focal necrosis in the brain and liver, which may be extensive. Granulomatous change and calcification may be seen.[21]

Manifestations: Symptomatic congenital CMV infection was originally termed cytomegalic inclusion disease. About 5% of congenitally infected infants have severe disease, 5% have mild symptoms and 90% are born with asymptomatic but chronic CMV infection. The manifestations include intrauterine growth retardation, prematurity, hepatosplenomegaly, jaundice, thrombocytopenia, purpura, microcephaly, intracranial calcifications, chorioretinitis, sensorineural hearing loss and increase in CSF protein. CMV infection should be suspected in any newborn with involvement of hepatobiliary, hematopoetic and central nervous systems. CMV infection is probably the leading cause of congenital sensorineural hearing loss which occurs in 7% of infected infants.[21] Pemde *et al.* studied hematologic manifestations of congenital CMV infection in 9 cases. Hepatomegaly was present in all, splenomegaly in 6, peticheal rash in 5, hepatitis in 4 and optic atrophy and corneal opacities in one patient each. Significant pallor, thromocytopenia and evidence of hemolysis were seen in 8, 4 and 4 patients each. Paucity of erythroid and megakaryocytic cells were in 2 of 3 bone marrows examined.[24] Sharma *et al.* described the profile of congenital CMV cases seen in Shimla hills. A study conducted in Brazil found that of 12 newborns with symptomatic CMV infection, 75% had hepatosplenomegaly, and 42% each had jaundice with direct reacting hyperbilirubinemia, and neurologic disease consisting of microcephaly and intracranial calcification.[25]

Diagnosis: The definitive method for diagnosis of congenital CMV infection is virus isolation or PCR performed at or shortly after birth. Urine and saliva are the best specimen for culture. Performing PCR on the dried blood spots (DBS), retrieved in the first week of life is the other option. Infants with congenital CMV infection may excrete virus for several years in the urine. Demonstration of PP65 Antigenaemia assay is also good for diagnosing CMV disease.[27] IgG tests is of little diagnostic value because a positive test may indicate transplacentally transmitted antibodies from the mother. A negative IgG test rules out CMV infection. A rising titre of IgG antibodies is again not helpful because postnatally acquired infection in infancy is common.[21] IgM tests lack sensitivity and are unreliable for diagnosis. However, a study from AIIMS, New Delhi compared IgM ELISA (Mac–ELISA) with nested PCR and found that PCR was highly specific (100%) but less sensitive (95%) than Mac ELISA.[26]

IgM antibody tests and measurement of CMV-IgG avidity can identify women at risk for transmitting CMV transplacentally. Fetal infection can be confirmed by viral isolation from amniotic fluid or PCR in amniotic fluid.[21]

Treatment: Relatively little information exists concerning the use of GCV in the setting of congenital CMV infection. Because some of the neurological sequelae of congenital CMV, particularly sensorineural hearing loss, progress postnatally, the presentation of results from a recently terminated nationwide US collaborative trial are of interest. Intravenous Gancyclovir (GCV) led to improvement or stabilization of hearing in a significant number of 6-month-old infants. Drug related neutropenia was common (63% compared to 21% in control group).[21] Case reports have suggested the efficacy of GCV for acutely ill neonates with life-threatening CMV disease (e.g., pneumonia). More recently there are reports of use of intravenous GCV followed by oral valgancyclovir which have shown encouraging results.[28]

Prognosis: Nearly 90% of symptomatic CMV infants demonstrate central nervous system and hearing deficits in later years. Infants with subclinical infection have a more favorable outlook, but may develop hearing loss in 5-10%, chorioretinitis in 3-5% and developmental delay, microcephaly and neurologic deficits in a smaller proportion.

Prevention: Observational studies have shown beneficial effects after administration of high titer CMV hyperimmunoglobulin to pregnant women with fetal infection or disease subsequent to primary CMV infection.[29] Pregnant women who are seronegative should be counseled regarding good handwashing and avoiding contact with oral secretions of others. Those with suspected recent infection may undergo additional diagnostic evaluation for in utero transmission and fetal infection.

RUBELLA

Rubella or German measles is an acute viral infection characterized by constitutional symptoms, a rash and enlargement of postoccipital, retroauricular and posterior cervical lymph nodes. Rubella virus belongs to togaviridae, is a member of the genus Rubivirus.

Rubella in early pregnancy can cause the congenital rubella syndrome (CRS) – a severe multisystem disease with a wide clinical spectrum. The risk for congenital defects and disease is 70% in the first trimester (90% before 16 weeks of gestation). The risk for congenital defects is low after the 1st trimester but fetal infection may occur. Worldwide, it is estimated that more than 100000 infants are born with congenital CRS each year.[30]

All Indian studies to evaluate the CRS burden are done in symptomatic cohorts of children not in general population. Laboratory evidence of CRS was found in 1-15% of infants suspected to have intrauterine infection. Only 3-10% of suspected CRS cases are ultimately proven to have confirmed CRS with laboratory tests. It accounts for 10-15% of pediatric cataract cases. Laboratory evidence of CRS was present in 10-50% of children with congenital anomalies. In India, 12-30% of women in the reproductive age-group are susceptible to rubella infection.[31]

Manifestations: Congenital rubella virtually affects all organ systems causing intrauterine growth retardation, cataracts, microphthalmos, myocarditis, structural heart defects (patent ductus arteriosus, pulmonary artery stenosis), blueberry muffin skin lesions, sensorineural deafness and meningoencephalitis. Persistent infection causes pneumonia, hepatitis, bone lucencies, thrombocytopenic purpura and anemia. Classical triad of CRS includes cataract (1/3 of cases), sensorineural hearing loss (upto 80%) and congenital malformations (patent ductus arteriosus and pulmonary stenosis in upto 50%). Other late sequelae include motor and mental retardation.[30]

Diagnosis: Diagnosis is made by finding rubella specific IgM in neonatal serum or persistence of rubella IgG antibodies at a higher level and for longer duration than expected from passive maternal antibody. Virus can be detected by PCR or by culture from the infant (nasopharynx, urine or tissues). Virus may be shed from the throat and urine for a year or longer. Fetal diagnosis is possible by isolating virus from amniotic fluid.[30]

Prognosis: Infants with the complete spectrum of congenital rubella syndrome have a bad prognosis. Those born with a few stigma, presumably infected later in pregnancy have a better prognosis. Two thirds of infants with encephalitis have neuromotor deficits including autism.

Prevention: It is important for girls of child bearing age to be immune to the virus. A live attenuated virus vaccine prepared from RA 27/3 strain is available mostly as a combination of Mumps-measles-rubella (MMR). The vaccine induces antibody response in 98% and has protective efficacy of more than 90%. It is contraindicated in pregnancy and if given to adult women, they must be advised against getting pregnant for at least 3 months. In India, coverage of MMR vaccine has been reported as 42%, 30% and 5% from Delhi, Chandigarh and Goa, respectively which is expected to improve with introduction of rubella vaccine in National Immunization Schedule recently.[31] If a seronegative pregnant woman is exposed to rubella, she should be tested after 3-4 weeks and again after 6 weeks for seroconversion. She should be counseled about the risk to the fetus and offered termination of the pregnancy if found positive.[32]

HERPES SIMPLEX VIRUS

Herpes simplex virus (HSV) causes primary infection, non primary infection among humans. HSV is a double stranded DNA containing enveloped virus and has two types–HSV-1 and HSV-2. Neonatal infection is predominantly (75-80%) caused by the HSV-2 as majority of maternal genital tract infection is due to this type.[40]

Worldwide, 50%-90% of adults have antibodies against HSV-1 and 20%-30% against HSV-2. Prevalence is greater in persons having lower socioeconomic status and multiple sex partners. Incidence of neonatal herpes ranges from 1 in 1400 to 1 in 30,000 deliveries.[33] The acquisition of genital herpes during pregnancy has been associated with abortions, prematurity, and congenital and neonatal herpes.[35] Transmission to the neonate can occur in antenatal, natal and postnatal period either by transplacental infection or by ascending infection. Commonly it is due to contact with infected genital tract mucosa or skin during delivery or just after birth. Risk of transmission is higher in case of primary infection (50%) in comparison to recurrent infection (3%) in mother.[40]

Incubation period is 2-12 days, but in newborn clinical manifestations may present at birth and as late as 4-6 weeks postpartum. Communication period in the mother is 7-12 days with primary genital lesions and 4-7 days in recurrent disease. Infected neonates are infectious throughout their illness.[38] Clinical manifestations are different depending on whether infection is acquired in intrauterine period or perinatal period.

Intrauterine HSV Infection: In utero transmission of HSV is uncommon accounts for about 5% of all neonatal disease.[41] Spontaneous abortions have been reported after primary maternal infection before 20th week of gestation. Disease severity may range from localized skin or eye involvement to multi organ disease and congenital malformations. Few patients have chorioretinitis, microphthalmia, microcephaly and hydrancephaly.[39,41]

Perinatal HSV infection: HSV infection in neonatal period is a severe disease if not treated properly. There are three categories of neonatal HSV infection:

1. **Localized Infection:** Localized infection of skin, eyes, and mucus membrane is found in half of the neonates. Vesicles, usually on presenting part of body appear on sixth to ninth day of life. If untreated 5-10% of these neonate develop CNS involvement, ocular complications or disseminated disease.[40]
2. **CNS Infection:** HSV encephalitis develops in 30% of neonate in absence of disseminated disease. This probably result from retrograde axonal spread because transplacentally derived viral neutralizing antibodies may protect neonate from disseminated disease, but have no influence on intraneuronal viral replication.

   Symptoms begin at 10-14 days of life with lethargy, seizures, hypotonia and temperature instability. Skin lesions are present in 40-60% cases. Without treatment 15% die and two third of survivors have long-term sequelae like microcepahly, hydranencephaly, porencephalic cysts, spasticity, chorioretinitis, blindness and learning disabilities.[39, 41]
3. **Disseminated Infection:** It occurs in 20-25% of neonatal HSV infection mostly within one week after birth. Clinically presents as hepatitis, shock, seizures, respiratory distress, pneumonitis and disseminated intravascular coagulation.[40]

Case Definition of Congenital HSV Infection: Isolation of HSV from any site in neonate less than one month of age who has any one of the following:

1. Generalized systemic infection compatible with congenital herpes infection.
2. Focal nervous system disease.
3. Localized infection involving the skin, eyes or mouth.[42]

Diagnosis: Diagnosis is generally confirmed by culture of organism, usually from genital or oral tract lesions and occasionally from brain biopsy in encephalitis. Typing can be done from the culture by direct fluorescent antibody testing. Detection of HSV antigen in lesion scraping by immunologic assays using monoclonal anti-HSV antibodies in either an ELISA or fluorescent microscopy assay is very specific and sensitive test (80-90%).

Tzanck Smear: Cytological examination of the base of skin vesicles, looking for characteristic but non-specific giant cells is only about 50% sensitive. Serology is of little value because specific IgM antibodies may not be detected for upto 3 weeks.

Elevated CSF protein level and pleocytosis are often seen with encephalitis, but it may be normal initially. PCR testing of CSF is a useful diagnostic test. Electroencephalography and CT/MRI are also useful in the diagnosis of HSV encephalitis.

Other laboratory abnormalities seen in disseminated disease include elevated hepatic transaminase levels, direct hyperbilirubinaemia, neutropenia, thrombocytopenia and coagulopathies.[38,40]

Treatment: Intravenous acyclovir (20 mg/kg/dose, 8 hourly) should be started immediately in all suspected HSV cases.[37] Treatment should be continued for 21 days in case of disseminated or CNS infection. For local infection 10-14 days treatment is sufficient. Recurrences of cutaneous lesions are frequent and these can be suppressed by the oral acyclovir therapy (300 mg/m^2 tid PO) for 6 months.

Newer drugs valacyclovir and famcyclovir have no additional advantage. Vidarabine is an alternative drug, but is much less effective and should be used only if the virus is resistant to acyclovir.[38]

Prognosis: Disseminated HSV infection is fatal in up to 80% of newborns; however treatment can decrease its mortality upto 10%. Mortality is around 15% in untreated CNS infections. Acute infection in mother at delivery, prematurity, seizures and disseminated intravascular coagulation are the poor prognostic factors. Recurrent HSV infection in mother and localized skin involvement in a neonate carries lower risk for severe complications. Only 5-10% of neonates with local infection develop complications.[34,36]

Prevention: In presence of active genital lesions in the mother at the time of delivery or culture from the lesions show viral shedding, cesarean section is the preferred mode of delivery. This approach reduces neonatal infection rate from 7.7% to 1.1%. Antiviral suppression therapy during pregnancy is not routinely recommended but few studies have demonstrated that acyclovir decreases viral shedding and need for cesarean section. Use of scalp electrode is contraindicated.[35,40]

SYPHILIS

Syphilis is a sexually transmitted disease caused by a spirochete, Treponema pallidum. Syphilis is common in many developing countries. Maternal infection during pregnancy can cause still birth, hydrops fetalis, premature delivery and congenital syphilis. T. pallidum cannot be cultured in vitro, and requires dark field microscopy or direct immunofluorescent staining techniques.

As per the World Health Organization (WHO), in India, 65.4% women attending antenatal care were tested for syphilis at the first visit and 0.3% were found seropositive for syphilis.[43] Transmission to the fetus is more likely with recent maternal infection, approaching 100% during the primary and secondary stages of syphilis. In late latency stage transmission declines upto 10-30%.[49] The fetus can be affected at any trimester of pregnancy.

Clinical Manifestations: Fetal and perinatal deaths occur in 40% of the affected fetuses. Early manifestations of congenital syphilis (analogous to secondary stage of acquired syphilis) include hepatosplenomegaly, jaundice, hemolytic anemia and lymphadenopathy. Characteristic features are: osteochondritis (pseudoparalysis of Parrot), periostitis, macuopapular rash, rhinitis (snuffles), and condylomata lesions.[48] CNS involvement in the form of meningitis or cerebrovascular disease due to arteritis and thrombosis of vessels, occur during the first few months or years of life. Meningitis usually appears at 3-12 months, whereas vascular syndromes are prevalent during the first 2 years of life. Syphilitic meningitis presents with irritability, apathy, convulsions, vomiting, neck stiffness, bulging fontanel, nerve palsies and optic atrophy. Chronic meningitis can lead to hydrocephalus. Intellectual disabilities are common.[45] Other manifestations are nephritis, nephrotic syndrome, gastroenteritis, pancreatitis, pneumonia, chorioretinitis and testicular masses.

Late manifestations (analogous to tertiary stage of acquired syphilis) appear after 5-25 years of infection and include bone, teeth, and CNS abnormalities. Bones are involved because of recurrent or persistent periostitis leading to frontal bossing, thickened sternoclavicular portion of clavicle, and bowing of tibia (Saber shin). Dental problems are found in the form of Hutchison teeth, mulberry molars and enamel abnormalities. Syphilitic rhinitis leads to saddle nose.[48] Juvenile paresis and mental deterioration are late CNS problems. Spastic limb paresis, seizures, cerebellar signs, taboparesis, cranial nerve palsies, optic atrophy and chorioretinitis are present. Tabes dorsalis is uncommon in children. It presents as failing vision, urinary incontinence, cranial nerve palsies, Argyll Robertson pupil and other papillary abnormalities. Untreated disease progresses to death in 2-5 years.[45]

Diagnosis: Syphilitic infection can be detected by treponemal and nontreponemal tests. These serological tests may be false positive in neonate because of maternal antibodies.

Non-treponemal tests are rapid plasma reagin test (RPR), venereal disease laboratory test (VDRL) and automated reagin test (ART). These tests are useful for initial screening and follow-up after treatment. A positive non-treponemal test should be confirmed by the treponemal tests.

Treponemal tests are: fluorescent treponemal antibody absorption test (FTA-ABS) and treponemal pallidum particle agglutination test (TP-PA). They remain positive even after successful treatment.

CSF abnormal cytology, protein and positive CSF VDRL suggest neurosyphilis. But, CSF VDRL may be false negative also. CSF FTA-ABS is more sensitive test. CSF-RPR should not be used.[44,50]

Other tests are FTA-ABS 19S immunoglobulin M test, IgM immunoblotting of serum, PCR for syphilis, dark field microscopy and gross and microscopic examination of placenta. Detection of specific IgM is the most sensitive serological method, and a positive test should be considered as evidence of a congenital T. pallidum infection.[50]

Treatment: CDC recommends that any infant who shows physical, radiological, or serological evidences of congenital syphilis need treatment. Treatment should also be given to a baby whose mother is having disease relapse, re-infection or untreated syphilis at delivery.[46]

Penicillin is the drug of choice for all stages of syphilis. Other drugs like tetracycline, doxycycline and erythromycin should not be used for congenital syphilis, neuyosyphilis and syphilis during pregnancy. Congenital syphilis is treated by aqueous penicillin G (1-1.5 lac U/kg/day intravenously) or procaine penicillin G (50,000 U/kg intramuscular once a day) for 10-14 days.[46]

Non-treponemal test should be repeated 3 monthly and CSF analysis with CSF VDRL 6 monthly till the findings are normal. Re-treatment is required if: (1) VDRL is positive at 6-12 months of treatment, CSF VDRL is positive at any 6 months interval, and abnormal CSF cell count or protein at 2 years.[49]

Prevention: Routine prenatal screening and adequate treatment of syphilis during pregnancy can prevent congenital syphilis. Screening is done at first antenatal visit. In high risk population repeat screening should be done at 28 weeks of gestation and at delivery. Safer sexual practices may help prevent syphilis during pregnancy.[47]

HUMAN IMMUNODEFICIENCY VIRUS (HIV)

HIV infection is a worldwide problem. First paediatric case was reported in 1983, and this problem is increasing since then.

Agent: HIV belongs to lentivirus, one of a subfamily of retroviruses. This is a cytopathic RNA virus, which binds to the host CD4+ cells. They have a unique enzyme, reverse transcriptase, which copies the viral RNA into DNA. HIV contains a genomic RNA core in centre, outer lipid envelope, and a protein shell in between the two.

Viral genome include: GAG region, POL region and ENV region. They encode for core protein, viral enzymes, and envelope proteins respectively. There are two types of HIV: HIV-1 and HIV-2. Majority of infection (95%) in India is of HIV-1, subtype C.[51]

Epidemiology: According to the report of UNAIDS (United Nations Program on HIV/AIDS) about 1.8 million of children below 15 years of age were affected by HIV worldwide in year 2015.[52] In India 2.1 million people were living with HIV in year 2015 out of which 6.54% were below 15 years of age. About 10,400 children were newly infected during the year.[53] High prevalence states of India are Manipur, Maharashtra, Tamil Nadu, Karnataka, Andhra Pradesh and Nagaland.[52] Congenital and perinatal transmission is responsible for majority (90%) of childhood cases.[51] Others acquired it by parenteral or sexual route. An HIV infected woman can transmit HIV to her fetus or infant before, during, or after birth. Risk of transmission is 30-45% if baby is breast fed, and around 20% when baby is not breast fed by its HIV positive mother.[56] Antiretroviral treatment of mother during pregnancy, caesarean delivery, avoidance of breastfeeding and newborn prophylaxis can reduce this risk to 1%.[52] Risk of transmission is more in presence of any of these risk factors–Low maternal CD4+ count, high level of maternal viraemia, no anteretroviral treatment during pregnancy, prolonged rupture of membranes, instrumentation during delivery, invasive fetal monitoring, intrapartum hemorrhage, preterm and twin delivery, breastfeeding.[57]

Pathogenesis: In initial HIV infection, virus first infects dendritic cells, viraemia is present, and the lymphatic tissue is seeded. CD4+ cells are selectively affected. This intense viraemia cause flu like symptoms within 3-6 weeks from time of infection, but these symptoms are usually absent in children. This viral load declines within 2-4 months because of host immune responses and most of the patients become asymptomatic.

During this latency period (8-12 years in adults), gradual decline in CD4+ cells occurs. Slow disruption of lymph node architecture and degeneration of the follicular dendritic cell network with loss of ability to trap virus, produces high levels of viraemia seen in later stages of disease. This latency period is shorter in perinatally infected children.[58]

Clinical Manifestations: According to progression of disease children may be divided into 3 groups–rapid progressors (manifestations present within few months of life), intermediate progressors (manifestations present after one year), and adult equivalents (present later in life).

Manifestations of pediatric HIV infection and AIDS are different from those of AIDS in adults, and these differences are:

- Overall progression of disease is more rapid in children.
- Immune system is more immature with higher CD4+ counts.
- Parotid swelling and recurrent invasive bacterial infections, and CNS infections are more common in children.
- Disseminated CMV, pneumocystitis carinii pneumonia, herpes and lymphoid interstitial pneumonia occur almost exclusively in children. Cryptococcus, histoplasmosis, toxoplasmosis and disseminated mycobacterium avium complex infections are less common than in adults.
- Peripheral neuropathy, myopathy, Kaposi sarcoma is rare in children.

Common presenting features of pediatric HIV infection are failure to thrive, diarrhea, opportunistic infections and lymphadenopathy. Hepatomegaly, splenomegaly, parotid swelling, lymphoid interstitial pneumonitis and skin manifestations are also common. Nephropathy and cardiomyopathy have been described.

Being a neurotropic virus, primary CNS infection is quite common in HIV infection (50-90%). Neuronal damage is mediated via astrocytes and neurotoxic cytokines. HIV encephalopathy is common in children and usually manifests in the presence of significant immunosuppression and other features of HIV disease such as hepatosplenomegaly and lymphadenopathy. It can be static or progressive and carries a poor prognosis.

HIV encephalopathy presents with developmental delay or regression of milestones. Other manifestations are cognitive impairment, neuropsychiatric problems, weakness, spasticity, hyperreflexia, extrapyramidal signs, cerebellar dysfunction, and acquired microcephaly. Rarely, distal peripheral neuropathy is present. Late signs include emotional liability, hyperactivity and lethargy. Abnormalities detected on neuroimaging are cerebral atrophy, increased ventricular size, basal ganglia calcifications, and leukomalacia. Unusually CNS tumor, opportunistic infection or stroke may present with focal neurological signs and seizures. Opportunistic infections like tubercular meningitis, cryptococcal meningitis, pyogenic meningitis and CNS toxoplasmosis can also give rise to neurological manifestations in HIV infected children.[58-61]

Diagnosis: Age < 18 months: The diagnosis of HIV infection in exposed infants is difficult before 18 months because routine screening tests like rapid test, ELISA will only detect presence of maternal antibodies. Virologic testing with either an HIV DNA or HIV RNA test is recommended at 14 to 21 days of life. It should be repeated at 1-2 months, and 4-6 months of age. First testing can be done at birth in case of high risk of transmission. HIV infection can be definitely excluded in non breast fed babies if two or more HIV NAATs are negative, with one test performed at age 1 month or older and the other test at age 4 months or older, or antibodies against HIV are negative in 2 samples at 6 months of age or older.[52] Child is considered HIV positive if two tests are positive. In case virological diagnosis is not feasible then a presumptive diagnosis of severe HIV disease should be made if infant is serologically positive with:

- Any AIDS-indicator condition; or
- Two or more of following–Oral thrush, Severe pneumonia, Severe sepsis.
- Other supporting factors–Recent HIV-related maternal death; or advanced HIV disease in the mother; CD4 < 20%.

Children ≥ 18 months: They are diagnosed according to adult national testing strategies using antibody tests. Three positive tests or two positive with suggestive symptoms indicate HIV infection in a child. Two positive HIV antibody test results and one negative result (done sequentially) in an asymptomatic child is indeterminate HIV status result and need follow-up.

Infants and children with confirmed HIV infection need a baseline CD4 testing (absolute count and CD4%) and repeat every 6 months or earlier if clinically indicated. All children on ART should have regular clinical, immunological and virological monitoring for early recognition of treatment failure.[62]

Treatment: WHO recommends that antiretroviral therapy (ART) should be initiated in all HIV infected children below 10 years of age irrespective of CD4 counts and clinical stage.[54,55] Priority should be given to children below 2 years of age and to children with advanced disease.[52] For infant not exposed to ART nevirapine (NVP) + 2 nucleoside reverse transcriptase inhibitors (NRTIs) should be given. Infants exposed to maternal or infant NVP or other NNRTI should receive lopinavir/ritonavir (LPV/r) + 2 NRTIs.[63]

Supportive Therapy: At 4-6 weeks of age, all exposed infants should receive cotrimoxazole in the dose of 150-750 mg/m^2/day, in two divided doses until HIV infection can be ruled out.[63] These children required frequent treatment for infections including opportunistic infections. Nutritional support and immunization are important aspects of supportive care. Recommended vaccines are DPT, OPV, IPV, measles, MMR, hibconjugate and hepatitis B, however; live vaccines in symptomatic children need to be withheld.[58]

Prognosis: A high viral load (>100,000 copies/ml) and low CD4+ count (<15%) are poor prognostic indicators. Children with opportunistic infection, encephalopathy, or wasting syndrome have high mortality with 75% dying before 3 years of age. In contrast recurrent bacterial infection and lymphoid interstitial pneumonia carries a much better prognosis with a median survival of 50 and 72 months respectively. Other poor prognostic factors are persistent fever, hepatitis, serious bacterial infections, persistent anemia and/or thrombocytopenia.[58]

Prevention: Voluntary confidential counseling and testing (VCCT) of all pregnant women and proper antenatal treatment of HIV infected women is mandatory to reduce the HIV transmission to newborns. WHO recommends (2016 guidelines) that all HIV infected mothers should receive triple-drug antiretroviral regimen throughout pregnancy, delivery and breastfeeding – continuing for life, regardless of CD4 count and clinical stage.[52] All newborns with perinatal HIV exposure should receive antiretroviral medications in the neonatal period, with the first doses initiated as soon as possible after birth, ideally within 6 to 12 hours following delivery. Nevirapine is given for 6 weeks to non breast fed babies and nevirapine alone or in combination with zidovudine should be given for 12 weeks to breast fed babies. In high risk cases a combination of 2 or three drugs is recommended for prophylaxis. WHO advocates breastfeeding by infected mothers should be continued in developing countries for overall benefit.[63]

VARICELLA

Chickenpox is a common, mild childhood illness caused by varicella zoster virus (VZV), but if develops during pregnancy can lead to serious adverse sequelae such as congenital varicella syndrome (CVS) and neonatal varicella infection in fetus/neonate. VZV belongs to herpes virus family with similarities to herpes simplex virus. It has an envelope and a double stranded DNA genome in center.

Incidence of varicella in pregnancy has been reported to be between 0.1 to 0.7/1000 pregnancies as around 88 to 98% of the population is already seropositive by 20-40 years of age.[64-65] Primary VZV infection in the first two trimesters of pregnancy is associated with intrauterine infection in up to 25% of cases, and CVS in 1-2% of cases. Embryopathy mostly occurs when infection is between 13 and 20 weeks of gestation. First trimester spontaneous abortion is not associated with chickenpox. Maternal Varicella infection in 3rd trimester do not cause CVS but peripartum infection carries 24%-50% chances of neonatal chickenpox.[66-68]

Pathogenesis: The mechanism of congenital malformations caused by varicella zoster virus seems to be due not to fetal varicella but to the development of herpes zoster in utero and to encephalitis associated with herpes zoster. Immature fetal cell mediated immunity is probably responsible for short latency period between primary infection and reactivation. Dermatological pattern of skin lesions, similar to HZ, segmental maldevelopment of the musculoskeletal system and segmental dysfunction of the somatic and autonomic nervous system also support this hypothesis.[69,70] Maternal chickenpox in late pregnancy may result in neonatal chickenpox before passive immunity from mother to baby can be conferred and the cell-mediated immune response of the neonate is unlikely to be sufficient to prevent hematogenous spread of VZV. Infection is acquired by transplacental route, ascending infection or via the neonatal respiratory tract during passage through the birth canal.[71]

Clinical Manifestations: Low birth weight is a constant feature of fetal varicella syndrome with multisystem involvement but some tissues and organs are selectively damaged which include skin, nervous system, eyes, musculoskeletal, gastrointestinal and genitourinary involvement. Skin lesions occur in approximately 70% of cases and limb hypoplasia in 46-72%. Characteristic skin lesions are cicatrical, depressed, pigmented with a dermatomal distribution and zigzag configuration. Limb hypoplasia and skeletal deformities are either due to cicatricial lesions causing reduction abnormalities or secondary to denervation of limb. Neurological abnormalities such as microcephaly, cortical atrophy, seizures, damage to autonomic nervous system and mental retardation occur in 48-62% of cases. Spinal cord atrophy, limb paresis, cerebellar aplasia have also been reported. Survivors may have long-term learning difficulties, deafness and developmental problems. Neurodevelopmental disorders have not been documented in asymptomatic children. Eye disorders such as microphthalmia, chorioretinitis, optic atrophy and cataracts occur in 44-52% of cases. Gastrointestinal, genitourinary tract and the cardiovascular system involvement occur in 7-24% of cases. About 20% of infants with intrauterine acquisition of VZV infection develop neonatal or infantile herpes zoster which is mostly uncomplicated.[72,73]

NEONATAL CHICKENPOX

Chickenpox within 10 days of life suggests intrauterine infection and is associated with 30% mortality, if left untreated. These neonates develop widespread cutaneous and visceral lesions and respiratory distress due to varicella pneumonia. Neonatal varicella due to postnatal exposure is generally a mild disease and rash appear after 13-15 days of appearance of maternal rash.[71]

Diagnosis: Intrauterine varicella infections irrespective of whether or not CVS develops can be confirmed by the detection of VZV DNA by PCR in the fetal or neonatal tissue sample/ amniotic fluid, presence of specific IgM in fetal or cord blood, persistence of specific IgG antibodies beyond six months of age, and development of HZ during infancy. These antibodies are not constantly present and cross reactivity with herpes simplex virus is possible. Viral isolation by culture is often unsuccessful. Antenatal diagnosis by USG is difficult, as often the defects are not present until late in pregnancy.[74]

Varicella infection in neonate can be diagnosed by Tzanck smear, direct fluorescence assay, PCR amplification test, capture IgM assay and a rising titer of IgG antibodies against VZV.[71]

Treatment: No antiviral drug is required for CVS as active viral multiplication is not present. Neonate with chickenpox should be given intravenous acyclovir (500 mg/m^2 every 8 hrly) for 5-7 days or until there is good evidence of crusting and no further lesion formation. Valacyclovir is the other alternative drug. Foscarnet may be given for acyclovir resistant VZV infection. Anti-varicella-zoster immunoglobulin (VZIG) is also advocated by some researchers as the passively administered antibodies can limit the severity of disease.[71,75]

Prevention: Varicella zoster immunoglobulin (VZIG) in a dose 125 U IM must be administered to the newborn if maternal varicella disease began less than 5 days before delivery or within 2 days postpartum to prevent neonatal chickenpox. Post exposure prophylaxis by VZIG is also recommended for pregnant mothers. Vaccination by available live attenuated vaccine is not recommended in pregnancy. Acyclovir should be used to treat varicella during pregnancy.[73,75]

ZIKA VIRUS

Zika virus belongs to genus flavivirus of Flaviviridae family. It is spread by the infected *Aedes* species mosquito bite (*Ae. aegypti* and *Ae. albopictus*). Zika virus was first isolated in Uganda, East Africa in 1947 from a sentinel monkey. Though epidemics of Zika virus are occurring since year 2007 but its association with congenital birth defects and microcephaly was reported only few years back. In year 2016 WHO reported a cluster of microcephaly cases in Brazil and this was found to be associated with the epidemic of Zika virus infection. More than 100 countries are at risk of Zika virus infection. Its seroprevelance among various countries ranges from 1-50%.[76] There are only few reports of Zika virus infection in India. Its outbreak has been reported from Ahmedabad and Krishnagiri district of Tamilnadu in 2017. A 3rd outbreak has recently occurred in Jaipur in 2018.[79]

Pathogenesis: Neuronal progenitor cells in developing brain are the main target of the virus. Proliferation arrest and an increase in the neuronal progenitor cells have been found associated with early infection. Chances of birth defects are more if infection is acquired in first trimester. There is 7-10% risk of birth defects with maternal Zika virus infection highest during the first trimester. About 13-15%, 3.6% and 5.3% newborns are affected with infection during the first, second, and third trimester, respectively.[76,77]

Clinical Features: A wide range of neurological problems can be caused by the congenital Zika virus infection. Microcephaly both proportionate and disproportionate is a prominent feature, which is found in 5.8% of maternal infections. Severe microcephaly occurs in 1.6% newborn when infections occur during first or second trimester. Microcephaly can develop after birth also. Brain calcifications, ventriculomegaly, Lissencephaly, Neural tube defects have been reported in 3.6% of newborns. Other problems are skeletal abnormalities, eye abnormalities, miscarriage and still births.[77]

Typical congenital Zika syndrome is found in 3.1% of newborns which is a distinct pattern of birth defects having these five features (CDC):

1. Severe microcephaly with partially collapsed skull.
2. Decreased brain tissue with a specific pattern of brain damage including subcortical calcifications.
3. Damage to the back of the eye including macular scarring and focal pigmentary retinal mottling.
4. Congenital contractures, such as clubfoot or arthrogryposis.
5. Hypertonia soon after birth leading to restriction of body movement.[78]

Diagnosis: Diagnosis of Zika virus infection is confirmed by either RTPCR or IgM ELISA in blood and urine. IgM ELISA can be false positive due to cross reaction with other viruses. Plaque reduction neutralization test (PRNT) is helpful in detection of cross reactivity. In suspected congenital infection newborn should be investigated within 2 days after birth. RTPCR should be done on both serum and urine, and ELISA on serum. Antenatal detection of virus is done by RTPCR in maternal blood, urine and amniotic fluid but this can be negative or transient also.[76]

Treatment and Prevention: There is no antiviral drug against Zika virus. A good vector control is the only option to decrease risk of maternal Zika virus infection at present. More than 40 vaccines against Zika virus are in pipeline and one DNA vaccine has entered phase 1 clinical trial.[76]

References

1. Stoll BJ. Infections of the Neonatal Infant in Nelson Textbook of Pediatrics Eds Behrmann RE. Kliegman RM. Jenson HB 19th Edition. Saunders 2004:626.
2. Shanmugam J. Rtaveendranath M. Nair VR. Seroprevalence of Rubella and Cytomegalovirus (CMV) Infection in Pregnant Women from Kerela State. J Indian Assoc Commun Dis 1982: 5(3-4):58-63.
3. Broor S. Kapil A. Kishore J. Seth P. Prevalence of Rubella Virus and Cytomegalovirus Infections in Suspected Cases of Congenital Infections. Indian J Pediatr 1991:58:75-78.
4. Kaur R. Gupta N. Nair D. Kakkar M. Mathur MD. Screening for TORCH Infections in Pregnant Women: A Report from Delhi. Southeast Asian J Trop Med Public Health 1999:30: 284-86.
5. Cao Y. Qui L. Zhang Q. Study of the Relationship Between the History of Abnormal Pregnancy and TORCH Infection in Pregnant Women. Zhonghua Fu Chan Ke Za Zhi 1999:34: 517-20.
6. Camargo Neto E. Rubin R. Schulte J. Giugliani R. Newborn Screening for Congenital Infectious Diseases. Emerging Infectious Disease 2004:10:6-11.
7. Prabakar P. Bailey A. Smikle MF. McCaw Binns A. Ashley D. Seroprevalence of Toxoplasma Gondii. Rubella Virus. Cytomegalovirus. Herpes Simplex Virus (TORCH) and Syphilis in Jamaican Pregnant Women. West Indian Med J. 1991:40:166-69.
8. Khan NA. Kazzi SN. Yield and Costs of Screening Growth Retarded Infants for TORCH Infections. Am J Perinatol 2000: 17:131-35.
9. Wang L. Li KH. Liu H. Liu JY. Li YJ. Analysis of Serological Findings and Clinical Manifestations of TORCH Infections in Newborns. Zhonghua Shi Yan Hi Liu Chuong bing Du Xue Zo Zhi 2003:17:283-84.
10. Kishore J. Misra R. Paisal A. Pradeep Y. Adverse Reproductive Outcome Induced by Parvovirus B19 and TORCH Infections in Women with High-Risk Pregnancy. J Infect Dev Ctries 2011 December13:5(12):868-73.
11. Sen MR. Shukla BN. Tuhina B. Prevalence of Serum Antibodies to TORCH Infection in and Around Varanasi. Northern India. J Clin Diagn Res 2012 November:6(9):1483-85.
12. Prasoona KR. Srinadh B. Sunitha T. Sujatha M *et al.* Seroprevalence and Influence of Torch Infections in High Risk Pregnant Women: A Large Study from South India. J Obstet Gynaecol India 2015 October:65(5):301-09.
13. Torgerson R and Mastroiacovo P. The Global Burden of Congenital Toxoplasmosis: A Systematic Review. Bull World Health Organ 2013:91:501-08.
14. Sarman Singh. Congenital Toxoplasmosis: Clinical Features. Outcomes. Treatment and Prevention. Trop Parasitol 2016 July-December:6(2):113-22.
15. Chintapalli S. Padmaja IJ. Seroprevalence of Toxoplasmosis in Antenatal Women with Bad Obstetric History. Trop Parasitol 2013 January:3(1):62-66.
16. Oumachigui A. Bhatia VN. Nayak PN. Toxoplasma Antibodies and Fetal Wastage. Indian J Med Res 1980:71:522-25.
17. Mohan B. Dubey ML. Malla N. Kumar R. Seroepidemiological Study of Toxoplasmosis in Different Sections of Population of Union Territory of Chandigarh J Commun Dis 2002: 34:15-22.
18. Hingorani V. Prakash O. Chowdhry P. Toxoplasmosis: Abortions and Stillbirths. Indian J Med Res 1070:58:967-74.
19. Jones J. Lopez A. Wilson M. Congenital Toxoplasmosis American Family Physician 15th May 2003.
20. Mc Leod R. Remington JS. Toxoplasmosis in Nelson Textbook of Pediatrics Eds Behrmann RE. Kliegman RM. Jenson HB 17th Edition. Saunders 2004:1144.
21. Stagno S. Cytomegalovirus in Nelson Textbook of Pediatrics Eds Behrmann RE. Kliegman RM. Jenson HB 17th Edition. Saunders 2004:1066.
22. Yamamoto AY. Figueiredo LT. Mussi-Pinhata MM. Prevalence and Clinical Aspects of Congenital Cytomegalovirus Infection. J Pediatr (Rio J) 1999:75:23-28.
23. Morita M. Morishimi T. Yamozaki T. Chilon S. Kawana K. Clinical Survey of Cytomegalovirus Infection in Japan. Acta Pediatrica Japan 1998:40:432-36.
24. Pemde HK. Kabra SK. Agarwal R. Jain Y. Seth V. Hematological Manifestations of Congenital CMV Infection. Indian J Pediatr 1995:62:473-77.
25. Sharma R. Bahl L. Goyal A. Sharma A. Sharma M. Thakur JS. Congenital Cytomegalovirus Infection in Shimla Hills. Himachal Pradesh. India. J Commun Dis 1995:27:23-26.
26. Sivakumar R. Singh N. Singh S. Nested Polymerase Chain Reaction in the Diagnosis of Congenital Cytomegalovirus Infection. Indian J Pediatr 2001:68:1043-46.
27. Bhatia P. Narang A. Minz RW. Neonatal Cytomegalovirus Infection: Diagnostic Modalities Available for Early Disease Detection. Indian J Pediatr 2010 January:77(1):77-79.
28. Meine Janson C. Toet MC. Rademaker CMA. Ververs TFF. Gerards LJ. Van Loon AM. Treatment of Symptomatic Congenital Cytomegalovirus Infection with Valganciclovir. J Perinatal Med 2005:33:364-66.
29. Nigro G. Adler SP. Hyperimmunoglobulin for Prevention of Congenital Cytomegalovirus Disease. Clin Infect Dis 2013 December:57Suppl4:S193-95.
30. Maldonado Y. Rubella Nelson Textbook of Pediatrics Eds Behrmann RE. Kliegman RM. Jenson HB. 19th Edition. Saunders 2004:1032.
31. Dewan P. Gupta P. Burden of Congenital Rubella Syndrome (CRS) in India: A Systematic Review. Indian Pediatr 2012: 49(16):377-99.
32. World Health Organization. Rubella Vaccines. WHO Position Paper. Geneva. Switzerland: World Health Organization: 2011: Available at http://www.who.int/wer/2011/wer8629.pdf
33. Avgil M. Ornoy A. Herpes Simplex Virus and Epstein-Barr Virus Infections in Pregnancy: Consequences of Neonatal or Intrauterine Infection. Reprod Toxicol 2006:21:436-45.

34. Whitley RJ. *et al.* Predictors of Morbidity and Mortality in Neonates with Herpes Simplex Virus Infections. N Engl J Med 1991:324:450-54.

35. Kohl S. Herpes Simplex Infections in Newborn. Semin Pediatr Infect Dis 1999:10:154-60.

36. Klimberlin DW. Lin CY. Jacobs RF. *et al.* Natural History of Neonatal Herpes Simplex Virus Infections in the Acyclovir Era. Pediatrics 2001:108:223-39.

37. Klimberlin DW. Lin CY. Jacobs RF. *et al.* Safety and Efficacy of High Dose Intravenous Acyclovir in the Management of Neonatal Herpes Simplex Virus Infections. Pediatrics 2001: 108:230-38.

38. Steve Kohl. Herpes simplex virus. In: Nelsons Textbook of Pediatric. 19th Edition. Eds. Behrman. Kliegman. Jenson. Elsevier 2004:978-82.

39. South MA. *et al.* Congenital Malformation of the Central Nervous System Associated with Genital Type (Type 2) Herpes Virus. J Pediatr 1969:75:13-18.

40. Sharda K Burchett. Viral Infections. In: Manual of Neonatal Care. 7th Edition. Eds. John P Cloherty. Lippincott William and Wilkins. 2011.

41. Hutto C. Arvin A. Jacobs R. *et al.* Intrauterine Herpes Simplex Virus Infections. J Pediatr 1987:110:97-101.

42. Communicable Disease Management Protocol. Congenital/ Neonatal H. Simplex Infection. November 2001. Available at: http://www.gov.mb.ca/health/publichealth/cdc/protocol/congenital.pdf (last accessed on 10/12/2013).

43. Global HIV/AIDS Response–Epidemic Update and Health Sector Progress Towards Universal Access: Progress Report 2011. Geneva: WHO; 2012. Available from: http://www.who.int/reproductivehealth/topics/rtis/GlobalData_cs_pregnany2011.pdf [Last accessed on 2013 Dec 10].

44. Sanchex P J. Laboratory Tests for Congenital Syphilis. Pediatr Infect Dis J 1998:17:70-71.

45. Michelow I C. *et al.* Central Nervous System Infection in Congenital Syphilis. N Engl J Med 2002:346:1792-98.

46. Centers for Disease Control and Prevention. Sexually Transmitted Diseases Treatment Guidelines. 2010. MMWR 2010:59(No. RR-12).

47. Centers for Disease Control and Prevention. Congenital Syphilis. United States. 2000. MMWR 2001:50:573-77.

48. Parvin Azimi. Syphilis. In: Behrman R. Kleigman R. Jenson H. Nelson Textbook of Pediatrics. 19th Edition. Philadelphia: W.B. Saunders Company 2011:978-82.

49. Louis Vernacchio. Syphilis. In: Manual of Neonatal Care. 7th Edition. Eds. John P Cloherty *et al.* Lippincott William and Wilkins 2011:321-27.

50. Herremans T. Kortbeek L. Notermans DW. A Review of Diagnostic Tests for Congenital Syphilis in Newborns. Eur J Clin Microbiol Infect Dis 2010 May:29(5):495-501.

51. Ramalingam S *et al.* Subtype and Cytokine Profiles of HIV Infected Individuals from South India. Indian J Med Res 2005: 121:226-34.

52. http//aidsinfo.nih.gov/contentfiles/lvguidelines/oi_guidelines_paediatrics.pdf. Accessed on 20/11/18.

53. http//www.naco.gov.in/sites/default/files/Annual%20 Report%202015-16_NACO.pdf. Accessed on 20/11/18.

54. http://pib.nic.in/newsite/printrelease.aspx?relid=89785 accessed on 16/12/13.

55. WHO Recommendations on the Diagnosis of HIV Infection in Infants and Children 2010:3.

56. Coust Soudis A. *et al.* Method of Feeding and Transmission of HIV-1 from to Children by 15 Months of Age: Prospective Cohort Study from Durban. South Africa. AIDS: 2001:15: 379-87.

57. Godbole S and Mehendale S. HIV/AIDS Epidemic in India: Risk Factors. Risk Behaviour and Strategies for Prevention and Control. Indian J Med Res 2005:121:356-68.

58. Yogev R. Chadwick E G. Acquired Immunodeficiency Syndrome (Human Immunodeficiency Virus). In: Behrman R. Kleigman R. Jenson H. Nelson Textbook of Pediatrics. 19th Edition. 2011: Philadelphia: W.B. Saunders Company.

59. Dhurat R. Manglam M. Sharma R. Shah NK. Clinical Spectrum of HIV Infection. Indian Pediatric 2000:37:831-36.

60. Merchant RH. Oswal JS. Bhagwat RV. Karkare J. Clinical Profile of HIV Infection. Indian Pediatr 2001:38:239-46.

61. Shankar SK. *et al.* Neuropathology of HIV/AIDS with An Overview of the Indian Scene. Indian J Med Res 2005:121: 468-88.

62. WHO. Manual of WHO Recommendations on the Diagnosis of HIV Infection in Infants and Children. 2010.

63. WHO. Manual of Guideline on Treatment of HIV in Children. 2010 available at http://www.who.int/hiv/topics/mtct/en/ accessed on 16/12/13.

64. Lokeshwar MR. Agrawal A. Subbarao SD. Chakraborty MS. Ram Prasad AV. Weil J. Bock HL. Kanwal S. Shah RC. Shah N. Age Related Seroprevalence of Antibodies to Varicella in India. Indian Pediatr 2000:37(7):714-19.

65. Reynolds MA. Kruszon-Moran D. Jumaan A. SchmidDS. McQuillan GM. Varicella Seroprevalence in the U.S.: Data From the National Health and Nutrition Examination Survey. 1999-2004: Public Health Rep 2010:125(6):860-69.

66. Jones KL. Johnson KA. Chambers CD. Offspring of Women Infected with Varicella During Pregnancy: A Prospective Study. Teratology 1994: 49(1):29-32.

67. Pastuszak AL. Levy M. Schick B. Zuber C. Feldkamp M. Gladstone J. *et al.* Outcome After Maternal Varicella Infection in the First 20 Weeks of Pregnancy. N Engl J Med 1994: 330(13):901-05.

68. Sauerbrei A. Wutzler P. Varicella-Zoster Virus Infections During Pregnancy: Epidemiology. Clinical Symptoms. Diagnosis. Prevention and Therapy. Current Pediatric Reviews 2005:1:205-15.

69. Higa K. Dan K. Manabe H. Varicella-Zoster Virus Infections During Pregnancy: Hypothesis Concerning the Mechanisms

of Congenital Malformations. Obstet Gynecol 1987:69(2) 214-22.

70. Grose C. Congenital Varicella-Zoster Virus Infection and the Failure to Establish Virus-Specific Cell-mediated Immunity. Mol Biol Med 1989:6(5):453-62.

71. Sauerbrei A. Wutzler P. Neonatal Varicella. J Perinatol 2001: 21(8):545-49.

72. Schulze A. Dietzsch HJ. The Natural History of Varicella Embryopathy: A 25-year Follow-up. J Pediatr 2000:137 (6): 871-74.

73. Ronald F *et al.* Varicella Zoster Virus Infection (Chickenpox) in Pregnancy. BJOG 2011September:118(10):1155-62.

74. Kustermann A . Zoppini C. Tassis B. *et al.* Prenatal Diagnosis of Congenital Varicella Infection. Prenat Diagn 1996;16:71-74.

75. Shrim A. Koren G. Yudin MH. Farine D. Maternal Fetal Medicine Committee. Management of Varicella Infection (Chickenpox) in Pregnancy 2012 March:34(3):287-92.

76. David Baud. Duane J Gubler. Bruno Schaub. Marion C Lanteri. Didier Musso. An Update on Zika Virus Infection. Lancet 2017:390: 2099-109.

77. Bruno Hoen. M.D.. Ph.D.. Bruno Schaub. M.D.. Anna L. Funk. M.Sc.. Vanessa Ardillon. *et al.* Pregnancy Outcomes After ZIKV Infection in French Territories in the Americas. N Engl J Med 2018:378:985-94.

78. Congenital Zika Syndrome and Other Birth Defects/Zika and Pregnancy/CDC.https://www.cdc.gov>testing-follow-up. Accessed on 20/11/18.

79. Zika Virus in India: Facts You need to Know–What is Zika? https://economictimes.indiatimes.com accessed on 20/11/18.

36 Chapter

ACUTE BACTERIAL MENINGITIS

Satinder Aneja, Ashok K Patwari

Acute bacterial meningitis (ABM) remains a common life threatening condition in children. Even though the mortality on account of this formidable disease has decreased over the years with the availability of potent antibiotics, a significant number of patients are left with neurological sequelae.[1]

Epidemiology

ABM is essentially a disease of young children mainly due to attenuated immunologic response in this age group. Poor socioeconomic condition, overcrowding, recent colonization with pathogenic bacteria, cerebrospinal fluid (CSF) communications (congenital or acquired) across the mucocutaneous barrier are some of the host factors which increase the risk of meningitis.[2] An increase in bacterial meningitis among recipients of cochlear implants has been reported.[3] Amongst environmental factors exposure to cigarette smoke has been demonstrated to increase the risk of ABM.[4] The widespread use of conjugate vaccine against *Haemophilus influenzae* type B in many developed countries has lead to marked decline in number of cases of meningitis. In countries with routine vaccination against Hib and Strep pneumoniae the median age of ABM has shown an increase with proportionately more cases occurring in adults.[5]

With introduction of Hib vaccination in several parts of India and neighbouring countries the epidemiology of ABM in India is likely to change.

Most cases of ABM are sporadic except meningococcal meningitis which often occurs in epidemic form specially in sub-Saharan Africa and Indian subcontinent. Meningococcal meningitis occurs most frequently in young children with peak attack rates in 6-12 months infants. A second peak occurs in adolescence. Clusters of meningococcal disease among adolescents and young adults have been reported with increasing frequency in the last decade. Disease rates in adolescents are high because this age group has highest rate of carriage of meningococcus. Serogroups A, B and C account for most cases of meningococcal disease throughout the world, with serogroups B and C responsible for the majority of cases in Europe and the Americas and serogroups A and C predominating throughout Asia and Africa.[6] Serogroup A has been associated with all the repeated outbreaks of meningococcal meningitis outbreaks from India, although serogroup B and C have been detected in a few sporadic cases.[7]

Etiology

Any organism can potentially cause meningitis but the usual causative agents of ABM varies with age, immune system and immunization status of the patient. During the first 2 months of life, *Escherichia coli* K1 and other Gram negative enteric bacilli, *Streptococcus agalactiae* and *Listeria monocytogenes* are the usual offending organisms. In children between 2 months and 12 years, bacterial meningitis is primarily due to *H. influenzae* type B (Hib), *Streptococcus pneumoniae (Sp)* and *Neisseria meningitides (Nm).* Hib is the most common etiological organism identified in children less than 2 years in India.[8] Meningitis in infants between the age of 1 and 3 months may be due to pathogens found both in neonates and older children.

In children with severe malnutrition, compromised immunity or anatomical defects, infection can occur with other microbes like *Staphylococcus, Salmonella, Pseudomonas, etc.* Reports from developing countries indicate Hib and Sp account for most of the cases though a sizeable proportion of cases presumed to be bacterial in nature fail to demonstrate any pathogen.[9] Gram negative aerobic organism and Staphylococcal aureus are common pathogens which cause ABM in patients who have undergone neurosurgical procedures while pneumococcus is predominant pathogen in cases with active CSF leak. Ventriculo-peritoneal shunt meningitis is usually due to coagulase-negative staphylococci, Staphylococcus aureus and Pseudomonas aeruginosa.[10]

Pathogenesis and Pathology

The mucosal surfaces in the nasopharynx are the initial site of colonization for the common meningeal pathogens. The exact mechanism by which bacteria invade CNS is not clear. For some organisms, specific surface components as K1 polysaccharide antigen of E. coli are essential for attachment to mucosal surface and specific virulence. Concurrent viral infection of the upper respiratory tract, increases the risk of disease by enhancing the formation and spread of respiratory droplets or diminishing the functional and mechanical integrity of the respiratory mucosa as a barrier to invasion. Bacteria penetrate through (e.g., Nm) or between mucosal epithelial cells (e.g., Hib) and enter sub-epithelial blood vessels to enter blood stream. The bacteria survive in blood stream if it is able to counter the host defence mechanism. From the blood stream the pathogen may cross blood brain barrier to induce ABM. To get across BBB pathogen has to attach to brain microvascular endothelial cells, which is facilitated by receptors for meningeal pathogens found on endothelium in choroid plexus. After attaching itself to endothelial cell the pathogen gains entry to CSF space either by transcellular or paracellular route. Bacterial invasion of meninges may also occur following tympanogenic labyrinthitis even in the absence of significant tympanic membrane pathology or from a contiguous focus of infection, e.g., mastoid or paranasal sinuses or osteomyelitis of skull following neurosurgical procedures.

Once inside the CSF space the bacteria multiply freely because of relative lack of host defense mechanism in this space. The release of bacterial cell components, e.g., lipopolysaccharide of gram negative organism and lipotechoic acid of gram positive bacteria are liberated in CSF during this process of replication stimulates the release of pro-inflammatory cytokines including tumor necrosis factor, interleukin-1, and platelet activating factor. In addition, the complement cascade is activated bringing out inflammation, and activation of granulocytes and platelets. With induction of inflammation, neutrophils migrate into CSF, there is release of reactive oxygen species and nitric oxide and all this adds to the deleterious effect of inflammation on the brain. Inflammatory cells also secrete vascular endothelial growth factor during bacterial meningitis and this may also contribute to blood-brain barrier disruption.[11] The proinflammatory cytokines also play a synergistis role in production of shock.

The fundamental pathological change in ABM is inflammation of leptomeninges with a meningeal exudates of varying thickness encasing the brain. The exudates extends into Virchow Robin spaces along with penetrating vessels. Involvement of vessels leads to phlebitis or arthritis and softening or necrosis of corresponding vascular territory. Cerebral edema develops early in the course of ABM and together with acute hydrocephalus it may be responsible for intracranial hypertension. Intracranial pressure (ICP) is maximally increased within first 48 hours. This in turn impedes cerebral perfusion resulting in neuronal injury. Nearly 30% of infants and children with ABM have decreased cerebral blood flow (CBF) ranging from 30-70%.[12] Transcranial Doppler studies on patients with meningitis show disease related arterial narrowing in approx 50% of cases and this correlates with neurologic impairment.[13]

Clinical Features

Early symptoms of meningitis in young children are often vague and ill defined. In general, younger the infant the more non-specific are the symptoms. History suggestive of upper respiratory infection may be noted in nearly 75% of patients. The main symptoms which are highly suggestive of a diagnosis of ABM in infants are fever (with or without vomiting), alteration of behavior (infant becomes lethargic or drowsy, irritable, feeds poorly), a high-pitched cry, seizures and a full or tense anterior fontanelle. Specific signs of meningeal irritation are hardly ever present in infants.

In older children, classical signs and symptoms of meningitis like fever, headache, vomiting, photophobia, neck stiffness and the meningeal signs are likely to be present. Neck stiffness is the most important of all meningeal signs and earliest to appear. It becomes more marked if tested while the patient sits up with knees extended. Kernig sign and Brudzinski sign are other meningeal signs. The meningeal signs are due to reflex muscle spasm in reaction to pain on stretching of contents of spinal cord. These signs may be absent in comatose patients. A combination model of a history of convulsions, or being lethargic or unconscious, or having a stiff neck, as used in the WHO-Integrated Management of Childhood Illness (IMCI) guidelines, had a sensitivity of 98% and a specificity of 72% to predict meningitis in infants > 2 months.[14]

The second mode of presentation is acute and fulminant in which manifestations of sepsis and meningitis develop rapidly associated with severe brain edema and raised ICP. This type of presentation is seen most often with *N. meningitides*. Petechial hemorrhages appearing on the skin, which rapidly coalesce producing areas of purpura, are considered hallmark of this disease, although they may be seen in meningitis due to other organisms also. Profound hypotension and fatal shock is reported.[15]

Seizures occur in about 30-40% cases of ABM. A high concentration of tumour necrosis factor (TNF) has been associated with occurrence of seizures.[16] Generalized seizures occurring early in disease are of no prognostic significance. Alterations of mental status and reduced level of consciousness is common and may be due to increased intracranial pressure (ICP), cerebritis or hypotension. Papilledema is uncommon in uncomplicated acute meningitis and when present suggests a more chronic process such as presence of intracranial abscess, or subdural empyema. Focal neurologic signs may be due to vascular occlusion, subdural collection or cortical infarction. Overall 14% of children of bacterial meningitis have focal neurological signs.[1]

Reactive thrombocytosis is common during recovery from meningitis and implies favorable prognosis for survival.[17]

Complications

Complications of ABM can develop early in the course of illness or later after several days of therapy or may be noticed on follow-up (Table 36.1).

Table 36.1: Complications and Sequelae of ABM
Complications
Neurological
• Increased ICP
• Seizures
• Subdural effusion/empyema
• Ventriculitis
• Cranial nerve palsies
• Hemi/quadriparesis
• Hearing loss
• Hydrocephalus
Systemic
• Peripheral circulatory failure
• Disseminated intravascular coagulation
• SIADH
• Arthritis
Sequelae
• Epilepsy
• Sensorineural hearing loss
• Visual impairment
• Behavioral problems
• Motor deficits
• Hydrocephalus
• Learning disabilities

Neurological Complications

Neurological complications may be seen in acute stage of disease and later may account for permanent residual deficits. It must be remembered that while most of the neurologic signs seen during acute phase of illness generally disappear, some complications may appear years after recovery. In general the neurologic complications can be attributed to:

(i) Raised intracranial pressure (ICP).

(ii) Parenchymal brain injury and disturbed function of nerves.[18]

Increased intracranial pressure (ICP) is present in almost all cases of ABM initially though only 1-3% of cases have persistent hydrocephalus.[18] Raised ICP as a complication of ABM should be anticipated and treated promptly. Raised ICP is due to multiple factors. There may be cerebral edema due to vasodilatation and breakdown of BBB. Serial CT measurements have demonstrated that ventricles tend to be small initially but with accumulation of purulent exudates in CSF it increases in size and then gradually become normal again weeks after recovery.[19]

When ICP is very high, herniation of brain tissue may occur at the incisura or at foramen magnum. Transtentorial herniation is generally accompanied by oculomotor palsy. Infarction of upper brainstem with severe impairment of motor and sensory function has been as consequence of incisural herniation. Herniation at foramen magnum may lead to sudden respiratory arrest, sudden death or persistent vegetative state. Cerebral herniation following LP is an important contributor to overall mortality.[20] LP should therefore not be done in children with clinical evidence of raised ICP.

Subdural effusion develops in 10-30% of patients with meningitis and are more common in children < 2 years and with *H. influenzae* or pneumococcal meningitis. These effusions are mostly asymptomatic. Reactive effusions usually resolve spontaneously and aspiration is required only in case of increased ICP or a depressed consciousness. Reactive subdural effusions need to differentiated from subdural empyema which more aggressive treatment in repeated aspirations. Neuroimaging is helpful in differentiating the two. On ultrasonography reactive subdural effusion is anechoic while empyema is often hyperechoic convex collection.[21] MRI scans with contrast may offer a more sensitive means of making an early diagnosis of subdural empyema.

Parenchymal central nervous system injury: Though the bacteria do not invade the brain parenchyma some injury to brain or spinal cord may occur. This is usually due to ischemia due to cerebral hypoperfusion secondary to occlusion of vessels due to endarteritis. Raised ICP as well as inflammation is responsible for these changes. Patients with shock or PCF are especially likely to suffer from hypoxia and ischemia and have diffuse neuronal damage. The common manifestation of parenchymal injury are seizures, neurological deficits, alteration of sensorium and sensory deficits like visual impairment.

Seizures occur in about 30-40% of children with meningitis. These may be due to concomitant electrolyte disturbance, raised ICP or parenchymal injury. Rarely ABM may present as status epilepticus.[22] Factors associated with seizures during acute bacterial meningitis include disturbed consciousness on admission, abnormal neuroimaging findings, and low glucose and high concentration of total proteins in cerebrospinal fluid.[23] Children with focal convulsions are more likely to have neurologic sequelae of meningitis. Late onset seizures during the course of illness can occur due to cerebritis, subdural effusion, and vascular thrombosis. Alteration in sensorium is commonly seen in children. A Glasgow coma scale of < 8 is a sign of poor prognosis. Motor deficits may be seen during acute phase of illness.

Brain abscesses are uncommon complication of ABM and are more likely to occur in neonates infectioned with *Citrobacter* or *Proteus* species. Myelopathy may complicate acute meningitis, possibly due to a vasculitis, stroke, autoimmune myelopathy, or direct infection of the spinal cord. Severe necrotizing myelitis and syringomyelia has been observed in cases who have residual flaccid paralysis.[24]

Cranial nerve dysfunction: Meningeal inflammation can affect any cranial as well as spinal nerve in acute phase. This dysfunction is transient and generally does not give rise to sequelae except when 8th nerve is involved. Deafness and loss of vestibular function occurs frequently as a sequelae of bacterial meningitis and concomitant purulent labyrinthitis which may subsequently go on to ossification and irreversible damage. The vestibular dysfunction and ataxia is generally a temporary complication and most patients compensate for any neural injury over a period of time. *Hearing loss* is the most common sequel of ABM. Nearly 10% - 25% of case of survivors are left with permanent sensorineural loss.[2,25] All patients of ABM should have audiologic evaluation after recovery. Visual impairment after ABM is an uncommon complication but may result from endophthalmitis or cortical involvement.

Systemic Complications

Peripheral circulatory failure is a sudden life threatening complication of meningitis. It occurs most commonly with meningococcal infection but can accompany other types of infection. About 15% children with Sp meningitis have been reported to present with shock.[26] Antibiotic therapy may initially aggravate hypotension, hence intensive monitoring is required in the initial period. Other manifestation of acute bacterial sepsis may be seen as coagulopathy, acidosis and hypoglycemia.

Pneumonia, pericarditis and arthritis occur occasionally. *Prolonged fever* (>10 days) is seen in some cases due to intercurrent viral infection, secondary bacterial infection, thrombophlebitis or a drug reaction. Secondary fever that is seen after an initial afebrile period is usually due to nosocomial infection.

Fluid and electrolyte imbalance: Hyponatremia is a frequent finding in patients with meningitis and can be due to volume contraction or SIADH.[27] Syndrome of inappropriate antidiuretic hormone secretion (SIADH) has been reported to occur in 28% of cases of ABM.[28] It leads to cerebral edema and hyponatremic seizures. Cerebral salt wasting is another cause of hyponatremia. It is characterised by extracellular fluid depletion and hyponatraemia caused by progressive natriuresis with concomitant diuresis. Therefore, the cause of hyponatremia should be assessed along with clinical signs of volume depletion or water retention and biochemical parameters, i.e., serum and urine osmolality.

Diagnosis

Outcome of ABM depends heavily on institution of early and appropriate antimicrobial therapy, which would depend on making a diagnosis of ABM and identification of specific pathogen. Confirmation of diagnosis by isolation of causative organism from CSF culture requires 24-48 hours and may be negative in patients who are pretreated with antibiotics. Hence, immediate diagnosis of ABM is generally made by CSF examination.

CSF Examination

The routine evaluation of CSF should include naked eye examination, CSF pressure, microscopy for total and differential cell count, gram's stain, estimation of protein and glucose and CSF culture. Diagnosis of ABM is based on documenting inflammatory response and on tests that demonstrate the specific causative bacterial agent in CSF (Gram's stain, culture, tests for bacterial antigen/DNA). Since the clinical features of ABM are non-specific specially in infants LP should be performed whenever there is suspicion of meningitis. Occasionally, LP may have to be postponed due to cardiorespiratory compromise, signs of increased ICP and infection at the LP site. Clinical signs of raised ICP is a more reliable indicator to withhold a lumbar puncture since even a normal CT scan does not exclude the imminent risk of coning. In case LP is deferred, empirical anti-meningitic treatment should be started after taking blood culture.

The CSF should be examined immediately after doing the LP since the cell count tends to fall over a period of time and may be falsely low after 30–60 min. The normal CSF of children contains less than 6 WBCs/mm^3 and in 95% of cases there are no polymorphonuclear (PMN) leukocytes. Hence, presence of more than a single polymorphonuclear leukocyte in a child over 6 weeks of age is suggestive of ABM. However, CSF lymphocytosis may be a predominant feature in 10-13% of cases.[29] CSF lymphocytosis is believed in represent an early phase of infection and repeat CSF examination in these cases will show a PMN predominance. Prior antibiotic therapy also results in lymphocytosis.

Protein in CSF is raised (normal value 40 mg/dl after 2nd month of life) in all cases of ABM. In patients of ABM, CSF glucose and ratio of CSF to blood glucose (normally about 66%) are low.

Gram stain of the smear is one of the most simple, cheap and rapid diagnostic bedside tool useful for detection of etiological organism. Centrifugation of CSF increases the positivity. Fluorescent staining of bacterial DNA with acridine orange may show the bacterial morphology in cases where Gram stain is negative. Acridine orange staining is superior to Gram stain in pretreated patients. CSF culture provides a confirmatory evidence of ABM and is essential for selecting appropriate antibiotic for the etiological organisms. The rate of bacterial isolation is affected by antibiotic use prior to lumbar puncture, further rate of isolation is increased if direct plating of CSF is done at bedside.

In case LP is traumatic it is recommended to do the cell count and then lyse RBCs with acetic acid and repeat cell count. The ratio of WBCs to RBCs (normal 1:500 to 1:750) can give some indication of the total cell count. A WBC: RBC ratio of < or=1:100 (0.01) has a positive predictive value of 100% for absence of meningitis identified a large group of patients without meningitis.[30] Besides, the biochemical parameters and the Gram stain and culture are not affected by blood in CSF. CSF from a traumatic LP should therefore be interpreted on a combination of factors and the clinician should examine all clinical and laboratory information before opting not to treat a child after a traumatic LP.

Rapid Diagnostic Tests

Several rapid diagnostic tests have been employed for rapid diagnosis of meningitis to guide the treatment of patient. The specific tests are based detection of bacterial antigen or antibody in CSF or other body fluids. Various tests including counter immunoelectrophoresis (CIE), latex particle agglutination (LPA), and enzyme linked immunosorbent assay (ELISA) are used to detect bacterial antigen. LPA is more sensitive than CIE. The sensitivity of CIE can be improved by screening multiple body fluids. LPA kits are commercially available for detecting antigen of Hib, Sp and Nm.

A negative test for bacterial antigen cannot exclude bacterial meningitis since these tests are limited to a few specific pathogens. Due to high cost, these tests should be reserved for patients who have received antibiotics and those in whom Gram's stain is negative.

Amplification of 16 S rRNA gene by PCR of CSF has been developed to diagnose ABM in patients pretreated with antibiotics. A broad range PCR which can detect common pathogens of ABM simultaneously has been reported to have high sensitivity and specificity.[31,32] PCR based detection of Nm antigen in CSF has been found to be useful in patients with meningococcal disease who have been pretreated with antibiotics as bacterial DNA remains in CSF 2-3 days after treatment.[33] However PCR cannot be used routinely because of high cost and need for special laboratories.

Various non-specific markers of inflammation such as C-reactive proteins, CSF lactate, CSF, CPK, TNF α, interleukins and procalcitonin have been investigated to differentiate bacterial meningitis from aseptic meningitis and as markers of severity of ABM with relation to outcome.[34] Leukocyte aggregation score–which is based on percentage of cells aggregated is a rapid and cheap test to distinguish bacterial from viral meningitis. Further studies are required for confirmation of this simple test.[35] However, these tests do not help in confirming the diagnosis and are of no value in choice of therapy.

Despite advancements in lab techniques routine culture of CSF, blood and Gram stain of CSF remain the standard methods of establishing the etiological agent of ABM. Gram stain, LPA and PCR based tests are useful in patients pretreated with antibiotics. These tests can also be helpful in identifying the serotype of Nm in outbreak situation.

Blood Culture: Blood culture is positive in a 2/3rd cases of ABM and should be done in all cases. It is specially useful in cases in whom LP cannot be done or is traumatic.

Smear of Petechial: Smear of petechial lesion (if present) after puncture with a lancet should be made and subjected to Gram stain to see for Nm.

Indications for Repeat Lumbar Puncture

If LP was deferred on admission it should be reconsidered after the patient is stable and attempt made to demonstrate organism on Gram stain or by LPA. Repeat LP are useful to demonstrate improvement, which can be assessed clinically. A repeat spinal tap is therefore not indicated in most of the cases of ABM. It should be done in case of poor clinical response to therapy of 48-72 hours, persistent fever, neonatal meningitis, unusual etiological organism or suspicion of resistance, e.g., Sp. Similarly end of therapy LP is not routinely required if the patient is well and afebrile for preceding 5 days.

Neuroimaging

Sonography in infants with open fontanelle is a non-invasive imaging modality to detect early structural changes and follow-up in ABM. Sonography should be done in all neonates and infants less than 2 months since the risk of complications are higher. Sonography is better than CT in demonstrating intraventricular septae, which has therapeutic implication. Contrast enhanced CT is the preferred modality if sudural empyema or parenchymal damage is suspected. In the early phase of meningitis, the CT findings are mostly normal. Contrast enhanced CT may show beginning meningeal enhancement, which becomes more accentuated in later stages of disease. However, in uncomplicated meningitis radiological evaluation by CT or MRI is not necessary. In complicated cases with seizures and evolving focal signs, neuroimaging is required. MRI is superior to CT in demonstrating parenchymal lesions due to meningoencephalitis or vasculitic complications.[36] These investigations should be considered in patients with:

(i) Signs of raised ICP.

(ii) Focal neurologic deficits.

(iii) Persistent fever.

(iv) Recurrent /focal seizures.

(v) Prolonged coma.

(vi) Increasing head circumference.

Differential Diagnosis

Several diseases particularly aseptic meningitis, tuberculous meningitis, cerebral malaria, brain abscess and lead encephalopathy present with signs and symptoms similar to ABM. A careful examination of CSF, which shows pleocytosis with polymorphonuclear predominance with reduced CSF sugar is highly suggestive of ABM. Gram stain and culture, confirm the diagnosis. It may be difficult to distinguish viral meningitis from ABM since polymorphonuclear predominance may be seen in significant proportion of viral meningitis and there are no specific clinical features. The absence of bacteria/antigen and presence of viral nucleic acid on PCR may help to reliably diagnose enteroviral meningitis. Partial treatment of meningitis with oral and systemic antibiotics often poses a diagnostic problem since CSF is rapidly sterilized though cell count, and CSF biochemical abnormalities persist. In any case, of clinically suspected ABM empiric therapy for ABM should be immediately started and not withheld because of inability to undertake CSF examination or while awaiting the result of investigations.

Both ABM and cerebral malaria are common cause of encephalopathy in tropical countries endemic for falciparum malaria. The finding of malaria parasites in the blood of an unconscious child in areas with high malaria risk is not sufficient to establish a diagnosis of cerebral malaria, and acute bacterial meningitis must be actively excluded in all cases. It is not uncommon to see parasitemia along with ABM.[37]

Management

ABM is a medical emergency and prompt treatment can make the difference on mortality and long-term sequelae. The physician in Emergency room should evaluate the patient for raised ICP, hypotension or impending circulatory failure. In patients with rapidly progressive disease antibiotics should be administered within 30 minutes of presentation along with supportive care. In case LP is contraindicated, blood culture should be taken and empiric antibiotic therapy started. Treatment can be broadly categorized into:

(1) Antibiotic therapy.

(2) Supportive care; and

(3) Adjuvant therapy.

Antibiotic Therapy

The initial antibiotic regimen should be such that covers all the likely pathogens anticipated according to the age of the child, combination should not be antagonistic and it should achieve bactericidal concentrations in the CSF. The three major factors affecting the bactericidal activity of an antibiotic in cerebrospinal fluid are its relative degree of penetration into the CSF, its concentration, and its activity in infected fluid. When the blood-brain barrier is intact, penetration is limited, because transport across cells is minimal. In meningitis, the integrity of the barrier is altered, resulting in increased permeability and enhanced CSF penetration of most antibiotics.

The initial empiric therapy is based on age of the patient and host factors. In countries where Hib has virtually disappeared due to universal immunization and proportion of penicillin resistant pneumococci (PRSP) is high the initial recommended therapy is 3rd generation cephalosporins plus vancomycin.[38] When considering recommendations for empiric vancomycin therapy of presumptive bacterial meningitis, there are two major issues–the probability that an episode of meningitis is pneumococcal, and the local prevalence of cephalosporin resistance or high level resistance to penicillin. In countries like India since the reported rate penicillin resistance of strep pneumonia is low the initial empiric therapy with ceftriaxone/cefotaxime alone is adequate. Third generation cephalosporins cefotaxime and ceftrioxone are the preferred initial antibiotics for meningitis as they are effective against most bacteria causing meningitis including resistant. Slow initial infusions of cefotaxime have been shown to have better outcome as compared to bolus doses.[39] H. influenzae type B and penicillin resistant strains of S. pneumoniae. In neonates during first 2-3 weeks of life a combination of ampicillin and cefotaxime is used as initial empiric therapy. For late onset meningitis it is advisable to add antibiotic which cover staphylococcus and gram negative bacteria–nafcillin plus cefotoxime plus aminoglycoside. In patients with cerebrospinal fluid shunts, broad spectrum antibiotics against Gram positive and Gram negative organisms should be given, such as a combination of vancomycin and ceftazidime. Removal of all components of the infected shunt along with appropriate antimicrobial therapy, appears to be the most effective treatment for CSF shunt infections.

Various antibiotics used in initial therapy and subsequent treatment are shown in Table 36.2.

Table 36.2: Indication for Neuroimaging in Children with ABM

1.	All infants < 2 months
2.	Focal neurologic findings
3.	Seizures 72 hours after start of treatment
4.	Prolonged alteration of sensorium
5.	Persistently abnormal CSF indices
6.	Relapse/recurrence
7.	Persistent fever
8.	Increase in head circumference

Cefepime–an extended spectrum cephalosporin has been used as montherapy in empric treatment of ABM with favorable results.[40] Cefuroxime, cefaperazone, and cefoxitin are not effective in ABM and should not be used. However, due to high cost, combination of penicillin and choramphenicol is often used as initial therapy. Ceftriaxone and cefotaxime have shown to be superior to chloramphenicol in clinical studies and is therefore cannot be recommended as initial empiric therapy.[41] Reports of increase in frequency of resistant Sp are emerging throughout the world. In India, the exact incidence of resistant pneumococci is not known. The data from Vellore suggests that PRSP is not a significant problem in India, but the trends from other Asian countries show an alarming increase in penicillin resistance.[42] Penicillin can no longer be recommended as empiric therapy when Sp is a likely pathogen since this therapy may not be effective for meningitis caused by penicillin resistant strains of Sp. Meropenem has been reported to be as efficacious and safe as cefotaxime as initial therapy for meningitis in a prospective study and can be considered as an alternative treatment.[43]

Subsequent therapy depends on the organism isolated and its antibiotic sensitivity. In patients in whom Gram's stain is positive or antigen is positive but culture is sterile therapy is based on the drug of choice for that pathogen.

For penicillin resistant pneumococci, combination of Ceftriaxone and vancomycin should be used. Addition of rifampicin should be considered in highly resistant strains. Vancomycin is not recommended in the treatment of bacterial meningitis caused by isolates that are susceptible to other agents. Even in patients with meningitis caused by highly penicillin- and cephalosporin-resistant strains, vancomycin should be combined with a 3rd generation cephalosporin and should not be used as a single agent.

There are anecdotal reports of cefotaxime or ceftrioxone failure in the management of Sp meningitis.[44] Meropenem has been used for treatment of penicillin resistant Sp and multi-resistant pseudomonas meningitis. Meningitis caused by gram-negative bacilli that produce extended-spectrum-lactamases or those that may hyper produce–lactamases (i.e., *Enterobacter* species, *Citrobacter* species, or *Serratia marcescens*) are also best treated with a regimen that contains meropenem. Levofloxacin has been found useful for meningitis due to staphylococcal aureus.[45]

Fortunately, resistance to 3rd generation cephosporins by Hib has not emerged. There are reports of Nm resistance to penicillin.[46] For multiple drug resistant staphylococci, vancomycin remains the drug of choice. Other alternative drugs are teicoplanin and lineozolid.

It is recommended that antibiotics be given by intravenous bolus infusion so as to achieve required CSF concentration. The duration of antimicrobial therapy is based on the causative agent, and clinical response (Table 36.3). In patients in whom pathogen is not identified, antibiotics are generally administered for 10 days. A large randomized controlled trial found no significant difference in outcome with shorter duration (5 days) as compared to conventional 10 days of treatment.[47] Longer duration of treatment is required for meningitis in neonates or those caused by staphylococcus, or gram negative bacilli and in cases of complications such as subdural empyema, prolonged fever, persistence of meningeal signs or development of nosocomial infections. In such cases discontinuation of antimicrobial therapy is individualized. End of therapy spinal tap is not required in all cases. It should be done in all cases of neonatal meningitis, patients with unusual organism and in patients with PRSP. The neonate with meningitis due to gram-negative bacilli should undergo repeat LP to document CSF sterilization, because the duration of antimicrobial therapy is determined, in part, by the result of CSF rather by clinical criteria.

Table 36.3: Initial and Subsequent Therapy in Cases of Bacterial Meningitis

(A) Initial Empiric Therapy

Age	*Suspected pathogen*	*Drug of choice**	*Alternative choice*
0-2 months	• Gram negative enteric bacilli	Ampicillin +	Cefotaxime +
	• L. monocytogenes	Cefotaxime	Aminoglycoside
	• Streptococcus agalactae		
2 months to 12 years	• H. influenzae	Ceftriaxone$#	Cefotaxime
	• S. pneumoniae		
	• N. meningitidis		

(B) Subsequent Antibiotic Therapy

Pathogen	*Drug of choice*	*Duration of therapy(days)*
Pathogen Unknown	Ceftriaxone	14
H.influenzae Type B	Ceftriaxone	10
S. pneumoniae		
Penicillin sensitive	Crystalline penicillin	14
Penicillin resistant	Ceftriaxone + Vancomycin	14
N. meningititds	Penicillin G/ceftriaxone	7-10
Staphylococci		
Methicillin susceptible	Oxacillin	3 weeks
Methicillin resistant	Vancomycin + rifampicin	
Pseudomonas	Ceftazidime+ Amikacin	
S. agalactae	Penicillin G/ampicillin ± gentamicin	14
Eschericia coli	Ceftriaxone + aminoglycoside	3 weeks

$ Empiric therapy should consist of ceftriaxone + vancomycin in areas with high rates of Penicillin resistant strep pneumoniae.

In patients with shunts empiric therapy should be vancomycin + ceftazidime.

Supportive Therapy

The first 3-4 days of treatment are critical because life-threatening complications of meningitis occur most frequently during this period. It is advisable to manage infants and children with meningitis with evidence of raised ICP, altered sensorium and signs of reduced perfusion in PICU. Vital signs of patients should be monitored regularly during the first 24-28 hours of treatment. The patient should be kept nil orally to prevent aspiration. Blood urea, blood sugar, blood gases, serum electrolytes, blood and urine osmolality, urine output, body weight should be monitored closely.

Hypovolemia and hypotension should be aggressively treated with normal saline and inotropic support. Maintenance of systemic blood pressure is critical to maintain cerebral blood flow. Concurrence of shock and cerebral edema is a therapeutic challenge. The treatment of shock with fluids and inotropes takes priority in such cases. While optimizing the fluid therapy it is important to recognize that hyponatremia may be due to dehydration or water retention as in SIADH.[48] The circulatory compromise caused by hypovolemia is as dangerous as cerebral edema caused by water retention. Some evidence supports maintaining intravenous fluids rather than restricting them in the first 48 hours in settings with high mortality rates and where children present late. However, where children resent early and mortality rates are lower, there is insufficient evidence to guide practice.[49] Therefore the cause of hyponatremia should be assessed along with clinical signs of volume depletion and biochemical parameters, i.e., serum and urine osmolality.

Intracranial pressure can be reduced by elevating the head end of the bed by 30° to maximize venous drainage. Osmotic diuretics such as Mannitol (0.5-1 g/kg) and oral glycerol are often used to reduce ICP. The only osmotic diuretic to have undergone randomised evaluation is glycerol. Data from trials to date have not demonstrated benefit on death, but it may reduce deafness.

Hyperventilation to maintain the arterial PCO_2 between 27-30 mm of Hg may also be used to reduce ICP. Aggressive hyperventilation may be counter productive as it causes reduction of already compromised CBF with resultant ischemic damage. Early neuro-intensive care using ICP-targeted therapy, mainly cerebrospinal fluid drainage, reduces mortality and improves the overall outcome in adult patients with ABM and severely impaired mental status on admission.[50] A study in adults–we suggest that early ICP-specific treatment in Neuro ICU with CSF-drainage should be considered on admission in patients with ABM and severely impaired mental status.[51]

Seizures are common during the course of bacterial meningitis. Metabolic complications like hyponatremia, hypocalcemia and hypoglycemia must be excluded and specific therapy instituted if present. Immediate management of seizures include intravenous diazepam (0.1-0.2 mg/kg/dose) or lorazepam (0.05 mg/kg/dose). This is followed by a loading dose of phenytoin (15 mg/kg) and the maintenance dose of 5 mg/kg/24 hours for further control of seizures. Phenytoin is preferred over phenobarbitone because it causes less CNS depression and allows assessment of sensorium. Anti-convulsants can be discontinued after a few days unless there is evidence of persistent seizure activity.

Adjunct Therapy

Improvement in our understanding of the pathophysiology of ABM has lead to the development of therapeutic approaches to modulate the inflammatory cascade to reduce the incidence of sequelae and death. Adjunctive anti-inflammatory agents which may be of benefit in treatment of bacterial meningitis include corticosteroids and newer anti-inflammatory drugs which are still in experimental stage.

Corticosteroids have been used with objective of blocking secondary release of cytokines and toxic intermediaries from the brain cells and are also presumed to stabilize altered vascular permeability. A number of trials were conducted in the last 2 decades to evaluate the role of dexamethasone (0.15 mg/kg every 6 hours for 2-4 days). The benefit of dexamethasone use in these studies was only moderate and limited to decrease in frequency of audiologic sequelae in meningitis due to Hib.[52] Corticosteroids significantly reduced hearing loss and neurological sequelae, but did not reduce overall mortality. A meta-analysis supports the use of corticosteroids in patients with bacterial meningitis in high-income countries but found no beneficial effect in low-income countries.[53] With routine vaccination with hib and pneumococcal conjugate vaccine in many countries, the pathogens of ABM may change and the role of Dexamethasone may require further evaluation. The effect of dexamethasone in treatment of neonatal meningitis has not been evaluated. Dexamethasone should not be used if aseptic or non-bacterial meningitis is suspected and if it is started before the diagnosis is established it should be discontinued immediately. Dexamethasone should not be used in partially treated meningitis. The maximum benefit of dexamethasone is obtained when it is given along with the first dose of antibiotics.

Anti-endotoxin antibodies have been produced by monoclonal antibody technology and appear to have beneficial role in ABM caused by gram negative organisms. Monoclonal antibodies against TNF, IL-IB and against CD 18 cells may help in reducing inflammation as shown in experimental studies. Non steroidal anti-inflammatory agent, e.g., indomethacin inhibit synthesis of prostaglandins from arachidonic acid via cycloxygenase pathway and can thereby reduce brain edema. Preliminary results of pentoxifylline-a-methylxanthine phosphodiesterase inhibitor indicate that it reduces some of the inflammatory indices of ABM in animal model. Role of all these is still at experimental stage and further trials are required to define their use in meningitis in humans. Induced hypothermia has been used as a neuroprotective strategy in traumatic brain injury and has been investigated in ABM. In a randomized trial which investigated the effect of hypothermia in severe bacterial meningitis in adults. Moderate hypothermia did not improve outcome in patients with severe bacterial meningitis and was observed to be associated with higher mortality.[54] Acetaminophen as adjuvant therapy did not affect outcome in children with bacterial meningitis.

Prognosis

Acute bacterial meningitis (ABM) in children is associated with a high rate of acute complications and mortality, particularly in the developing countries. Most of the deaths occur during first 48 hours of hospitalization. Case fatality is reported to be 3-6% in developed countries but higher mortality (31%) is reported from developing countries.[56,57] Coma, raised intracranial pressure (ICP), seizures, shock have been identified as significant predictors of death and morbidity.[57]

The prognosis of a patient with pyogenic meningitis depends on many factors including age, causative micro-organism, bacterial density, intensity of host's inflammatory response and time taken to sterilize the CSF. Neurodevelopmental sequelae are seen in 10-20% of patients.[1,18] Baraff *et al.* in a meta-analysis of 19 reports estimated that 83.6% patients had no sequelae.[1] The common sequelae reported were deafness (10.5%), mental retardation (4.2%), epilepsy (4.2%) and motor deficits (3.5%). The sequelae of bacterial meningitis may improve with time and even resolve completely. The potential for recovery is attributed to the plasticity of brain.[55] Focal neurological signs at admission have been found to be reliable predictors of permanent sequelae especially later epilepsy.[59] Persistence of fever, neck rigidity and reluctance to leave the supine position beyond the first week was associated with risk of neurologic complication or sequelae.[60] Prognosis is poorest among infants less than 6 months, in those with delayed sterilization of the CSF, seizures beyond 4th day of hospital stay, coma, focal neurological signs on presentation, infection with Sp, and other organisms like *Salmonella or Pseudomonas infection.*[58]

Prevention

Prevention of ABM is possible with:

(i) Prevention of secondary cases with antibiotic chemoprophylaxis of index case and close contacts; and

(ii) Vaccination of susceptible population with specific vaccines. Vaccination is not a substitute for chemoprophylaxis because secondary cases develop within 2-7 days of presentation of index case and vaccination is not effective in that stage.

Chemoprophylaxis

Rifampicin prophylaxis for Hib is recommended (20 mg/kg daily for 4 days; 10 mg/kg for infants <1 month) for all household contacts, if there is an infant (<12 months) in the household or when a child 1-3 years who is inadequately immunized resides in the house. Prophylaxis for index case is not required for those treated with cefotaxime or ceftrioxone. Ampicillin and chloramphenicol do not eradicate Hib, therefore patients treated with these antibiotic should be given rifampicin before discharge from hospital.

For N. meningitides, chemoprophylaxis is recommended for all close contacts (household contacts, day care contacts and any one exposed to oral secretions) regardless of age and immunization status. Rifampicin (10 mg/kg every 12 hours for 2 days) can be given (Table 36.4). There is concern about emergence of resistance to rifampicin among strains of Nm. This has to be monitored closely with obvious implication for prophylaxis. Ceftriaxone (250 mg intramuscularly as a single dose) and ciprofloxacin (single dose 500 mg) are other effective chemoprophylactic agents.

Table 36.4: Recommended Doses of Antimicrobial Agents in Children with ABM

Total daily dose mg/kg (dosing interval in hours)

Drug	Neonate 0-7 days	Neonate 7-28 days	Infant and children
Ampicillin	150 (8)	200 (6)	300 (6)
Ceftriaxone	–	–	100* (12)
Cefotaxime	100-150 (8-12)	150-200 (6-8)	225-300 (6-8)
Ceftazidime	100-150 (8-12)	150-200 (8)	150-300 (8)
Cefipime	–	–	150 (8)
Meropenem	–	–	120 (8)
Penicillin	0.15 mU (8-12)	0.2 mU (6-8)	0.3 mU (4-6)
Chloram-phenicol	25 (24)	50 (12)	100 (6)
Oxacillin	75 (8-12)	150-200 (6-8)	200 (6)

Contd.

Contd.

Vancomycin	20-30 (8-12)	30-45 (6-8)	60 (6)
Gentamicin	5 (12)	7.5 (8)	7.5 (8)
Amikacin	15-20 (12)	30 (8)	30 (8)
Tobramycin	5 (8-12)	7.5 (8)	7.5 (8)
Rifampicin	–	10-20 (12)	10-20 (12)

* A loading dose of 75 mg/kg may be given at start of therapy

Intrapartum prophylaxis of GBS carriers with penicillin and selective administration of antibiotics to newborns can prevent early onset neonatal GBS meningitis.

Vaccination

Polysaccharide-protein conjugate vaccines are now available to protect against Haemophilus influenzae type B, Neisseria meningitidis serogroups A, C, Y and W and 13 serotypes of Streptococcus pneumonia. These have been incorporated in childhood immunization programs of most developed countries. Hib conjugate vaccine has 70-100% protective efficacy against meningitis due to Hib. Routine immunization with Hib was started in Gambia and despite irregular vaccine supplies there was dramatic reduction in Hib meningitis.[61] Hib vaccination has been incorporated in immunization program in several states of India which will reduce the burden of meningitis in infants. A tenvalent and 13 valent conjugate vaccine against Sp are part of immunization schedule of several countries. For Nm several types of vaccines are available. A tetravalent vaccine against Nm A,C,W135 and Y strains is recommended to vaccinate adolescents and patients with high risk for meningitis (e.g., Sickle cell disease, asplenia etc.). A multicomponent meningococcal group B vaccine (ribosomal deoxyribonucleic acid, component, adsorbed), covering different strains of Men B is also now available.[62]

Universal immunization with Hib, PCV7 and meningococcal vaccine is likely to bring down the incidence of meningitis. Maternal immunization with GBS conjugate vaccine may represent a future strategy to reduce neonatal GBS streptococcal disease.[63] The overall incidence of ABM will fall only if the cost of vaccination is brought down so that it can be given to children all over the world. In the mean time development of new and effective antimicrobial drugs against the ever increasing resistant pathogens is urgently needed.

References

1. Baraff LJ, Lee SI, Schriger DL. Outcomes of Bacterial Meningitis in Children: A Meta-analysis. Pediatr Infect Dis J. 1993;12:389-94.
2. Behrman RE. Acute Bacterial Meningitis Beyond the Neonatal Period. In: Nelson Textbook of Pediatrics. 15th Edition. Eds. Behrman RE, Kleigman RM, Nelson WE, Vaughan VC. Philadelphia. W.B. Saunders Company 1996;707-16.
3. Reefhuis J, Honein MA, Whitney CG, Chamany S, Mann EA *et al.* Risk of Bacterial Meningitis in Children with Cochlear Implants. N Engl J Med 2003;31:349:435-45.
4. Stanwell-Smith RE, Stuart J, Hughes AO, Robinson P, Griffin HB, Cartwright K. Smoking, The Environment and Meningococcal Disease: A Case Control Study. Epidemiol Infect 1994;112:315-28.
5. Thigpen MC, Whitney CG, Messonnier NE, *et al.* Emerging Infections Programs Network. Bacterial Meningitis in The United States, 1998-2007. N Engl J Med. 2011;26;364(21):2016-25. doi: 10.1056/NEJMoa1005384. Pub. Med PMID:21612470.
6. Rosenstein NE, Perkins BA, Stephens DS, Popovic T, Hughes JM. Meningococcal Disease. New Eng J Med 2001;344: 1378-88.
7. Manchanda V, Gupta S, Bhalla P. Meningococcal Disease: History, Epidemiology, Pathogenesis, Clinical Manifestations, Diagnosis, Antimicrobial Susceptibility and Prevention Indian J Med Microbiol 2006;24:7-19.
8. Ramachandran P, Fitzwater SP, Aneja S, *et al.* Prospective Multi-centre Sentinel Surveillance for Haemophilus Influenzae Type B and Other Bacterial Meningitis in Indian Children. Indian J Med Res 2013April;137(4):712-20.
9. Sahai S, Mahadevan S, Srinivas S, Kanungo R. Childhood Bacterial meningitis in Pondicherry, South India. Indian J Pediatr 2001;68:839-41.
10. Filka J, Huttova M, Tuharsky J, Sagat T, Kralinsky K, Kremery V Jr. Nosocomial Meningitis in Children After Ventriculoperitoneal Shunt Insertion. Acta Paediatr 1999; 88(5):576-78.
11. van der Flier M, Stockhammer G, Vonk GJ, Nikkels PG, van Diemen-Steenvoorde RA, van der Vlist GJ. Vascular Endothelial Growth Factor in Bacterial Meningitis: Detection in Cerebrospinal Fluid and Localization in Postmortem Brain. J Infect Dis 2001;183:149-53.
12. Quagliarello VJ, Scheld WM. New Perspectives in Bacterial Meningitis. Clin Infect Dis 1993;17:603-08.
13. Ashwal S, Perkin RM, Thompson JR, Schneider S, Tomesi LG. Bacterial Meningitis in Children: Current Concepts of Neurological Management. In: Advances in Pediatrics. Ed. Barness LA. St. Louis. Mosby Year Book Inc 1993;185-215.
14. Trop Med Int Health. 2002 Sep;7(9):722-31Clinical Predictors of Bacterial Meningitis in Infants and Young Children in the Gambia. Trop Med Int Health 2002 September;7(9):722-31.
15. Talukdar B, Khalil A, Sarkar R, Saini L. Meningococcal Meningitis: Clinical Observations During An Epidemic. Indian Pediatr 1988;25:329-34.
16. Arditi M, Manogue KR, Caplan M, Yoger R. Cerebrospinal Fluid Cachectin/Tumor Necrosis Factor and Platelet Activating Factor Concentrations and Severity of Bacterial Meningitis in Children. J Infect Dis 1990;162:139-47.

17. Kilpi T. Anttila M. Markker JT. Peltola H. Thrombocytosis and Thrombocytopenia in Childhood Bacterial Meningitis. Pediatr Infect Dis J 1992;11:456-60.

18. Dodge PR. Neurological Sequelae of Acute Bacterial Meningitis. Ped Annals 1994;23:101-06.

19. Cabral DA. Flodmark O. Farrel K. Speert DP. Prospective Study of Computed Tomography in Acute Bacterial Meningitis. J Pediatr 1987;111:201-05.

20. Rennick G. Shann F. de Campo J. Cerebral Herniation During Bacterial Meningitis in children. BMJ 1993;306:953-55.

21. Chen CY. Huang CC. Chang YC. Chow NH. Chio CC. Zimmerman RA. Subdural Empyema in 10 Infants: US Characteristics and Clinical Correlates. Radiology 1998 June;207(3):609-17.

22. Chin RFM. Neville BGR. Scott RC. Meningitis is a Common Cause of Convulsive Status Epilepticus with Fever. Arch Dis Child 2005;90:66-69.

23. Chang CJ. Chang HW. Chang WN. Huang LT. Seizures Complicating Infantile and Childhood Bacterial Meningitis. Pediatr Neurol 2004Sep;31(3):165-71.

24. Tu YF. Chang YC. Chen CY. Huang CC. Acute Flaccid Paralysis Due to Myelopathy in Childhood Bacterial Meningitis. Acta Paediatr Taiwan 2004;45(3):158-62.

25. Damodaran A. Aneja S. Malhotra VL. Bais AS. Ahuja B. Taluja V. Sensorineural Hearing Loss Following Acute Bacterial Meningitis. A Prospective Evaluation. Indian Pediatr 1996; 33:763-66.

26. Arditi M. Mason EO. Bradley JS. Tan TQ. Barson WJ. Schutze GE. Wald ER. *et al.* Three Year Multicenter Surveillance of Pneumococcal Meningitis in Children: Clinical Characteristics. and Outcome Related to Penicillin Susceptibility and Dexamethasone Use. Pediatrics 1998;102:1087-97.

27. Laine J. Holmeberg C. Antilla M. Peltola H. Types of Fluid Disorders in Children with Bacterial Meningitis. Acta Pediatr Scand 1991;80:1031-36.

28. Patwari AK. Singh BS. Deb M. Inappropriate Secretion of Antidiuretic Hormone in Acute Bacterial Meningitis. Ann Trop Pediatr 1995;15:179-83.

29. Powers WJ. Cerebrospinal Fluid Lymphocytosis in Acute Bacterial Meningitis. Am J Med1985:79:216-20.

30. Mazor SS. McNulty JE. Roosevelt GE. Interpretation of Traumatic Lumbar Punctures.

31. Wu HM. Cordeiro SM. Harcourt BH. *et al.* Accuracy of Real-time PCR. Gram Stain and Culture for Streptococcus Pneumoniae. Neisseria Meningitidis and Haemophilus Influenzae Meningitis Diagnosis. BMC Infect Dis 2013 January 22:13:26. doi: 10.1186/1471-2334-13-26.

32. Schuurman T de Boer RF. Koostra-SmidAM. van Zwet AA. Prospective Study of Use of PCR Amplification and Sequencing of 16 S Ribosomal DNA from Cerebrospinal Fluid for Diagnosis of Bacterial Meningitis in Clinical Setting. J Clin Microbio 2004:4229:19-25

33. Borrow R. Clause H. Guiver M. Smart L. Jones DM. Kaczmarski EB *et al.* Non-Culture Diagnosis and Serogroup Determination of Meningococcal B and C Infection by A Sialyltransferase (siaD) PCR ELISA. Epidemiol Infect 1997;118:111-17.

34. Jain M. Aneja S. Mehta G. Ray GN. Batra S. Randhava VS. CSF Interleukin-1s. Tumor Necrosis Factor–A and Free Radicals Production in Relation to Clinical Outcome in Acute Bacterial Meningitis. Indian Pediatr 2000;37:608-14.

35. Garty BZ. Berliner S. Liberman E. Danon YL. Cerebrospinal Fluid Leukocyte Aggregation in Meningitis. Pediatr Infec Dis J 1997;16:647-51.

36. Kastrup O. Wanke I. Maschke M. Neuroimaging of Infections. NeuroRx 2005April;2(2):324-32.

37. Berkley JA. Mwangi I. Mellington F. Mwarumba S. Marsh K. Cerebral Malaria Versus Bacterial Meningitis in Children with Impaired Consciousness. QJM 1999March;92(3):151-57.

38. Tunkel AR. Hartman BJ. Kaplan SL *et al.* Practice Guidelines for the Management of Bacterial Meningitis. Clin Infect Dis 2004;39:1267-84.

39. Pelkonen T. Roine I. Cruzeiro ML. Pitkäranta A. Kataja M. Peltola H. Slow Initial β-lactam Infusion and Oral Paracetamol to Treat Childhood Bacterial Meningitis: A Randomised. Controlled Trial. Lancet Infect Dis 2011;11(8):613-21.

40. Saez–Llorens X. O'Ryan M. Cefepime in the Empiric Treatment of Meningitis in Children. Pediatr Infect Dis J 2001;20:356-61.

41. Peltola J. Anttila M. Renkonen OV. *et al.* Randomised Comparison of Chloramphenicol. Ampicillin. Cefotaxime. and Ceftriaxone for Childhood Bacterial Meningitis. Lancet 1989; 1:1281-87.

42. Lee NY. Song JH. Kim S. Peck KR. Ahn KM. Lee SL *et al.* Carriage of Antibiotic Resistant Song JH. Jung SI. KoKS. Kim NY. Son JS. *et al.* A High Prevalence of Antimicrobial Resistance Among Clinical Streptococcus Pneumoniae Isolates in Asia (an ANSORP study). Antimicrob Agents Chemother 2004;48:2101-07.

43. Odio CM. Puig JR. Ferris JM. Khan WN. Rodrigues WJ. McCracken GH Jr. Bradley JS. Prospective. Randomized Investigator–Blinded Study of the Efficacy and Safety of Meropenem vs Cefotaxime Therapy in Bacterial Meningitis in Children. Merpenem Meningitis Study Group. Pediatr Infect Dis J 1999;18:581-90.

44. Bradley JS. Connor JD. Ceftrioxone Failure in Meningitis Caused by Streptococcus Pneumoniae with Reduced Susceptibility to Beta-lactamase Antibiotics. Pediatr Infect Dis J 1991.10:871-73.

45. Saez-Llorens X. McCoig C. Feris JM. Vargas SL. Klugman KP. Hussey GD *et al.* Quinolone Treatment for Pediatric Bacterial Meningitis: A Comparative Study of Trovafloxacin and Ceftrioxone with or without Vancomycin. Pediatr Infect Dis J 2002;21:14-22.

46. Blondeau JM. Ashton FE. Isaacson M. Neisseria Meningitides with Decreased Susceptibility to Penicillin in Saskatchewan. Canada. J Clin Microb 1995.33:1784-86.

47. Molyneux E. Nizami SQ. Saha S. Huu KT. Azam M. Bhutta ZA. Zaki R. Weber MW.Qazi SA. CSF 5 Study Group. 5 versus 10 days of treatment with ceftriaxone for bacterial meningitis

in children: A Double-Blind Randomised Equivalence Study. Lancet 2011 May 28;377(9780):1837-45.

48. von Vigier RO, Colombo SM, Stoffel PB, Meregalli P, Truttmen AC, Bianchetti MG. Circulating Sodium in Acute Meningitis Am J Nephrol 2001:21:87-90.
49. Maconochie IK, Bhaumik S. Fluid Therapy for Acute Bacterial Meningitis. Cochrane Database of Systematic Reviews 2014, Issue 5. Art. No.: CD004786. doi: 10.1002/14651858.CD004786.pub4.
50. Wall ECB, Ajdukiewicz KMB, Heyderman RS, Garner P. Osmotic Therapies Added to Antibiotics for Acute Bacterial Meningitis. Cochrane Database of Systematic Reviews 2013: Issue 3, Art. No.: CD008806. doi: 10.1002/14651858.CD008806.pub2.
51. Glimaˇker M, Johansson B, Halldorsdottir H, Wanecek M, Elmi-Terander A, *et al.* Neuro-Intensive Treatment Targeting Intracranial Hypertension Improves Outcome in Severe Bacterial Meningitis: An Intervention-Control Study. PLoS ONE 2014:9(3):e91976.
52. Lebel MH, Freij BJ, Syrogiannopoulos GA, Chrane DF, Jean HM, Stewart SM, *et al.* Dexamethasone Therapy for Bacterial Meningitis, Results of 2 Double Blind, Placebo Controlled Trials. N Eng J Med 1988:319:964-71.
53. Brouwer MC, McIntyre P, de Gans J, Prasad K, van de Beek D. Corticosteroids for Acute Bacterial Meningitis. Cochrane Database of Systematic Reviews 2010, Issue 9. Art. No.: CD004405, doi: 10.1002/14651858.CD004405.pub3.
54. Mourvillier B, Tubach F, van de Beek D, *et al.* Induced Hypothermia in Severe Bacterial Meningitis: A Randomized Clinical Trial, JAMA 2013 November27:310(20):2174-83.
55. Molyneux EM, Kawaza K, Phiri A, Chimalizeni Y, Mankhambo L, Schwalbe E, Kataja M, Pensulo P, Chilton L, Peltola H. Glycerol and Acetaminophen as Adjuvant Therapy did not Affect the Outcome of Bacterial Meningitis in Malawian Children. Pediatr Infect Dis J 2014 February:33(2):214-16.
56. Mwangi I, Berkley J, Lowe B, Peshu N, Marsh K, Newton CR. Acute Bacterial Meningitis in Children Admitted to A Rural Kenyan Hospital: Increasing Antibiotic Resistance and Outcome, Pediatr Infect Dis J 2002 November:21(11):1042-48.
57. Chinchankar N, Mane M, Bhave S, Bapat S, Bavdekar A, Pandit A, Niphadkar KB, Dutta A, Leboulleux D. Diagnosis and Outcome of Acute Bacterial Meningitis in Early Childhood. Indian Pediatr 2002:39:914-21.
58. Odetola FO, Bratton SL. Characteristics and Immediate Outcome of Childhood Meningitis Treated in the Pediatric Intensive Care Unit, Intensive Care Med 2005;31:92-97.
59. Pomeroy SL, Holmes SJ, Dodge PR, Feigin RD. A Prospective Evaluation of the Neurologic Sequelae of Bacterial Meningitis in Children with Special Emphasis on Late Seizures, N Eng J Med 1990:323:1651-57.
60. Antilla M. Clinical Criteria for Estimating Recovery from Childhood Bacterial Meningitis, Acta Paediatr 1994:83: 63-67.
61. Adegbola RA, Secka O, Lahai G, Lloyd-Evans N *et al.* Elimination of Haemophilus Influenzae Type B (Hib) Disease from The Gambia after the Introduction of Routine Immunisation with a Hib Conjugate Vaccine: A Prospective Study, Lancet 2005;366:101-03.
62. Roderick M, Finn A. Advances Towards the Prevention of Meningococcal Disease: A Multidimensional Story, J Infect 2014 January;68 Suppl;1:S76-82.
63. Paoletti LC, Madoff LC. Vaccines to Prevent Neonatal GBS Infection, Semin Neonatol 2002;7:315-23.

37 Chapter

TUBERCULOUS MENINGITIS

S Mahadevan, R Ramesh Kumar

INTRODUCTION

Tuberculous meningitis (TBM) is the most severe, deadliest and most debilitating form of tuberculosis, disproportionately affects young children particularly in India. TBM kills or disables roughly half of everyone affected. After scrofula (Primary tuberculosis of the lymphatic glands, esp. of the neck), TBM is the most common form of pediatric extra-pulmonary tuberculosis.[1] Pediatrician and Intensivists face substantial challenges in the diagnosis and management of TBM because of disease pathogenesis is poorly understood; rapid, sensitive, and affordable diagnostic tests are not available and even if available not there in primary health care level; and the best management approach in particularly duration, daily versus intermittent therapy has not been established by randomized controlled trials involving children.

Burden of Disease

According to World Health Organization (WHO) global tuberculosis 2014 report, TB is present in all regions of the world and 2013, an estimated 9.0 million people developed TB and 1.5 million died from the disease. More than half (56%) cases were in the South-East Asia and Western Pacific Regions. India alone accounted for 24% of total cases. There were 80000 deaths from TB among HIV-negative children in the same year. In India, there are about ~400 million children who constitute about 34% of the total population.[2] The extent of childhood TB in India is unknown due to diagnostic difficulties; it is estimated to be 10.2% of the total adult incidence.[2]

TBM accounts for 20-45% of all types of TB among children compared with only 3-8% of adult TB. The reported mortality due to TBM ranges from 17-71%[3] and 6.5-60% in recent serious due to improvement in management.[4] Even with antitubercular therapy (ATT), TBM short-term mortality is high, ranging from 20 to 69% with permanent neurological sequelae occurring in 50% of cases.[5] However, the exact prevalence of TBM is unknown in India due to clinical manifestations being non-specific particularly in the early stages of the disease, are also observed in a number of other neuro infections and bacteriological procedures often employed are ineffective and insensitive in the early stages as causative organism are few in the cerebrospinal fluid (CSF).

Risk of TBM Following Mycobacterium Tuberculosis Infection

TBM occurs as a consequence of the lymphohematogenous spread of tubercle bacilli during the primary infection and the formation of small subpial and subependymal foci (Rich foci) in the brain and spinal cord. In some foci rupture and release bacteria into the subarachnoid space causing meningitis. In others, foci enlarge to form tuberculomas without meningitis. The timing and frequency of these events about primary pulmonary infection are dependent upon age and immune status. TBM occurs in children more frequently within two years of primary infection, predominantly under the age of 5 years. In children, dissemination usually occurs early, and the risk of CNS tuberculosis is highest in the first year following infection; in high tuberculosis prevalence countries CNS tuberculosis predominantly affects very young children (<3 years) (Table 37.1).[6] In low tuberculosis prevalence countries, most cases are in adults, often immigrants from areas of high tuberculosis prevalence. Immunosuppressed especially those with HIV infection, are more likely to suffer disseminated disease with CNS involvement. Other risk factors include diabetes mellitus, malignancy, corticosteroid treatment, and agents that block the action of tumor necrosis factor.

Table 37.1: The Risk of Pulmonary and Extrapulmonary Disease (Disseminated TB/TBM) in Children Following Infection with *Mycobacterium Tuberculosis*

Age Group	Pulmonary TB	Disseminated TB/ TBM	Comment
< 1 year	30-40%	10-20%	High rates of mortality and morbidity
1-2 years	10-20%	2-5%	High rates of mortality and morbidity
2-5 years	5%	0.5%	–
5-10 years	2%	< 0.5%	"Safe school years"
> 10 years	10-20%	< 0.5%	Adult-type pulmonary disease

Pathology and Pathogenesis

The necropsy studies done in 1933 are the basis for the recent concepts regarding the pathogenesis of TBM. The development of TBM during initial hematogenous dissemination is the result of the break into the CSF of tuberculomas surrounding the *M. tuberculosis* accumulation in the brain parenchyma and meninges.[7] In children, it is a proven and accepted that hypersensitivity holds a vital part in neuro tuberculosis pathogenesis. The brain's immune system fails to detect the various pathogens and foreign antigens collected in the brain parenchyma. Data collected over a period from patients taking antituberculous therapy, through clinical scrutiny can clarify the development of intracranial tuberculomas or the concept of delayed paradoxical enlargement. Bacterial foray and survival in the host's brain is not only due to the host but also due to the genes and protein-coding of M. tuberculosis. The evolution of effective preventive measures rests mainly on figuring out how the various microbial aspects would affect TBM.

The CSF and BBB (blood-brain barrier) protect the CNS from the general circulatory system (Fig. 37.1 and Fig. 37.2). Despite the efficiency of the barricade, various pathogens – both viral and bacterial, can overpass and instigate encephalitis and/or meningitis.[7] The detailed research by Howard McCordock and Arnold Rich paved way for our present knowledge regarding the TBM's pathogenesis through their autopsy demonstration that the meninges or brain parenchyma of most of the patients suffering from TBM exhibited a caseating focus.

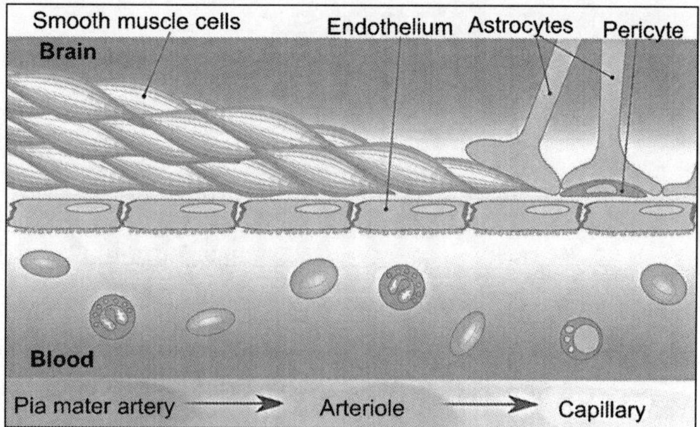

Fig. 37.1: Blood-brain barrier (BBB). This barrier is principally composed of tightly apposed human brain microvascular endothelial cells. Astrocyte processes interspersed with the extracellular matrix support the basal portion of these endothelial cells. Paracellular transport is limited by the presence of endothelial cell tight junctions while transcellular movement is restricted by the relative paucity of endocytic vesicles. Such properties render the barrier impermeable to many large, hydrophilic molecules and circulating pathogens

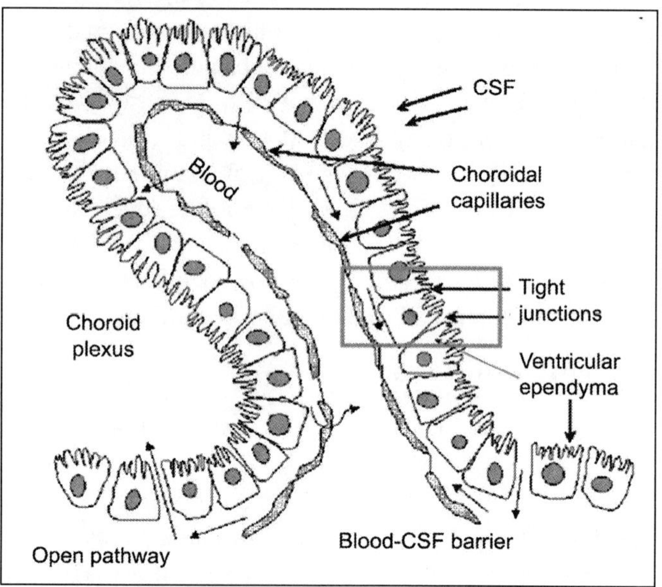

Fig. 37.2: Blood cerebrospinal fluid (CSF) barrier. Provide spatial separation of the circulatory system from the CSF at the choroid plexus. Cells lining the blood-CSF barrier share similar properties to those lining the BBB, with enhanced tight junctions and more stringent regulation of transcytosis

Bacterial colonization in the macrophages within the alveoli due to access of bacilli into lungs as a result of inhalation of contagious drops is the beginning stage of tuberculosis infection. As the active pulmonary disease advances, we can see the bacteria spread into the bloodstream and local lymph nodes, ultimately even spreading over the systemic circulatory system. Widespread bacteremia subsequent to lung diffusion intensifies the chances of developing a subcortical focus in the CNS.[7] A large number of bacilli invasion in the circulatory system aggravates the chances of CNS invasion and ensuing TBM (Fig. 37.3).

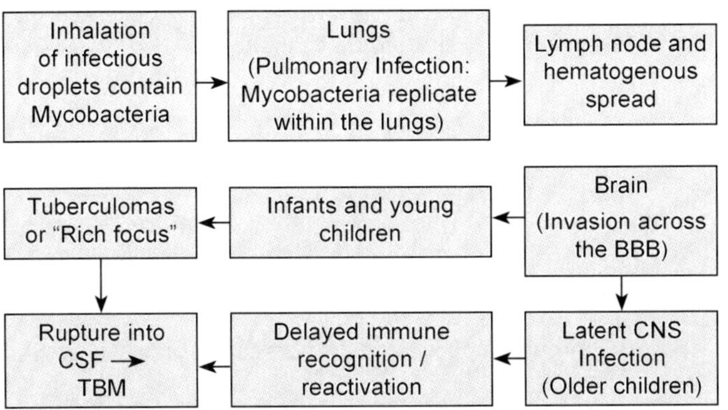

Fig. 37.3: Spread to the central nervous system. The establishment of central nervous system (CNS) tuberculosis occurs after hematogenous dissemination of mycobacteria from the lungs. The mycobacteria invade/traverse the blood-brain barrier and get deposited in the CNS. When deposited in large numbers as part of primary tuberculosis in infants/young children, they may cause TBM and formation of tuberculomas. However, in adults/older children, deposited mycobacteria may not elicit any immune response and cause latent disease until immune recognition/reactivation causes the formation of tuberculomas in the CNS. These tuberculomas may later rupture into the cerebrospinal fluid, leading to severe inflammation and TBM

Causative pathological sequence takes at least three months to develop. Bacterial seeding of meninges and subpial region of the brain leads to the formation of tubercles. Pre-existing caseous lesions (Rich's focus in the cortex or meninges) older than any concurrent miliary TB remain a commonly accepted hypothesis. After the release of bacilli and granulomatous material into the subarachnoid space, a dense gelatinous exudate forms; it is maximally seen in interpeduncular fossa and suprasellar region anteriorly and may extend throughout the prepontine cistern and surround the spinal cord. Within the ventricles, there is ependymitis with a similar exudate. Large caseous plaques deeper in the sulci and direct contact with the exudate with the brain surface cause a border zone hypersensitivity reaction damaging the underlying brain tissue.[8]

The precise pathogenesis of hydrocephalus in TBM is ambiguous. The hydrocephalus development seen in maximum areas are usually interactive in nature and occur due to the elimination of basal cisterns. The cranial nerves and arteries are enclosed by exudate that prevents CSF's flow at the tentorial opening that leads to the hydrocephalus. The various theories suggested being the cause of hydrocephalus TBM would also include the prevention of CSF flow from the fourth ventricle (exit point) to the arachnoid villi (absorption point) – the basic adhesive meningeal reaction, or even eradicating the arachnoid villi.[9] Similar to the TB infection of the body, in the case TB infection in the brain, the incidence of the destructive disease is advocated by the arteries and basal arachnoiditis. Incidences of tuberculomas encourage a forceful body response likely to have a positive clinical outcome.[9]

The pathology of the vessel develops as an outcome of the local immersion exudate. Infiltrative (inflammatory; vasculitic), proliferative and necrotizing processes are the various usual pathologies of vessels. Their contribution either on their own or in-group towards brain damage is doubtful. The duration of the disease is an echo of the comparative incidences of changes in the vessels. Stenosis may develop as a result of initial inflammatory lesions. Two to three weeks later as the exudate thickens and organizes proliferative reactions can be observed.[10]

Proliferative endarteritis (smooth muscle cells, earlier assumed to be fibroblasts) usually visible in the intima from 11th day onwards, collagen (about 45 to 60 days) and elastic fibres (about 16 weeks) are due to chemotherapy-related disease prolongation. This is not due to the treatment as such but can be linked to disease prolongation. Supportive evidence proposes that in the strokes in the earlier stages of the disease may be due to vasospasm and in the later stages of the disease may be due to the proliferation of the intima of the vessels. Vessel appearances are not exclusive to TBM and are often observed in various inflammatory and infectious diseases.[10] Frequent infarction in this period may indicate an underlying role for stenosis of intimal proliferation.

The choroid plexus vessels happen to be secure, but the spinal cord faces the same changes. In case of vessel lesions, we may find Tubercle bacilli specifically in the adventitia, less frequently in media and seldom in the intima. The infarction of deep white matter happens as a result of prominent vasculitis of the penetrating vessels of the carotid territory. The most affected being the proximal portion of the middle cerebral artery in a Sylvian fissure. The various clinical indications are the formation of scars, blood vessel damage due to inflammation, edema exudates that encase the base of the brain. Ruptured mycotic aneurysms, aneurysmal dilatations, and a unique case of granulomatous septic embolism to the basilar artery from endocardial vegetation are few of the rare vascular lesions reported in TBM. All evidence support the fact that majority of the infarcts happen as a result of hemodynamic hypoperfusion due to a various grouping of thrombosis, vasospasm, and intimal proliferation. Even the latest developments in the area of the molecular biology of tuberculosis fail to throw light on TBM vasculopathy. Based on the primary data we can propose that more that brain vessel damage in TBM facilitated by many compounds.[10]

Epigenetics of TB Infection

The concept of epigenetics was first introduced by Waddington in 1942 to describe the interaction between gene and their phenotypic variations. It describes how these mitotic changes in cellular phenotype act at genetic expression potential without altering the DNA sequence in the genome. Epigenetics plays a critical role in the regulation of many cellular processes, including inactivation of X chromosome, conformational stability of chromosomes, chromatin conformation changes, stages of embryonic development and transcriptional activation/ repression. Hence, epigenome the overall epigenetic mark of an organism instructs transcriptional machinery to switch genes on or off to control phenotypic variation that can be directly influenced by host and pathogen.[11]

The interaction of host epigenetic system and *M. tuberculosis* infection is a novel field, and direct evidence is scarce and only a few studies are documented till now. Host cellular transcriptional machinery is modified/activated by tubercle bacilli, or mycobacterial products have been identified recently (Mycobacterial 19-kDa Lipoprotein);[12] early secreted antigenic factor 6 (ESAT-6)[13] (Fig. 37.4). These mycobacterial products are driven by pathogens for the successful establishment of disease pathogenesis in the host. Hence, epigenome the overall epigenetic mark of an organism instructs transcriptional machinery to switch genes on or off to control phenotypic variation that can be directly influenced by host and pathogens. As a result, the epigenetic mark of the host is a readily available target that can be directly altered with the pathogen to introduce phenotypic variations in immune cells.

Clinical Features

Clinical presentation based on the type of involvement of intracranial TB namely TBM, space-occupying lesions (tuberculomas, tubercular abscess), tubercular encephalopathy, and tubercular vasculopathy. Among the intracranial TB, TBM is the most common type encountered in children of our country. Early diagnosis is the key to the satisfactory

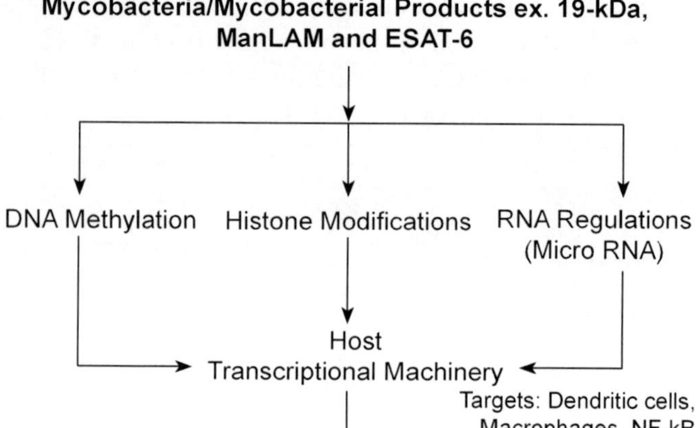

Fig. 37.4: Schematic representation of the interaction between mycobacteria and host epigenome. Host transcriptional machinery is controlled by TB bacilli and induced epigenetic regulation as up and down-regulation of the host key targets via, Histone acetylation, DNA methylation, and miRNAs processes

outcome. It is unfortunate that more than 70% of children are presented to hospitals in later stages of the disease. Infants under five years old are the prime targets of TBM, and often occur within two years of primary infection. Non-specific symptoms including vomiting, headache, anorexia and fever delay TBM diagnosis.

The clinical presentation may be insidious with fever and headache or more subacute with a well-developed meningeal reaction. Prolonged fever, malaise anorexia, weight loss and apathy dominate the picture. Fluctuating mood changes – loss of interest in surrounding and alternating with normal playfulness at times mislead the pediatrician. Apathy recurs, and the vague illness is dismissed as non-specific. The vague illness includes– child prefers to sit in a chair than play; appears cross and irritable, frequently sleeps, restless at night, difficult to wake up in the morning and resents the interference.

TBM is always associated with TB infection elsewhere (miliary, or pulmonary). A timely chest X-ray may prevent the delay in diagnosis. In 50 to 90% of children, we can usually find recent tuberculosis contact along with unusual neurological presentations. Infected children are afflicted with febrile and non-febrile seizures in addition to the focal neurological deficit, most usual being hemiplegia and cranial nerve palsies.

According to Medical Research Council, TBM consists of three stages.[14] Insidious prodromal period, gradual, the fluctuating onset of fever, lassitude, weight loss, behavior changes, headache, and vomiting characterize the **First stage** of the disease (Non-specific febrile illness without neurological signs). Delay in considering the diagnosis during this 1-2 weeks period will be followed by neurologic deficits, loss of consciousness or convulsions. Meningeal signs and fever may be absent in children under two years of age. A few cases (20%) have sudden onset of fever, vomiting, and convulsions with CSF pleocytosis mimicking pyogenic meningitis.

The second stage (Neurological signs without marked changes in sensorium) is ushered into with the finding of a squint or ptosis in the child whose neurologic status was 'apparently normal' during the previous two weeks. Some resistance to neck flexion, sluggish pupillary reaction, positive Kernig's or Brudzinski's sign bulging fontanel are the dominant findings. Since TBM involves the base of the brain, cranial nerve palsies are seen. Involvement of cranial nerves occurs in 20-40% of cases. The sixth cranial nerve is most commonly affected followed by third and fourth cranial nerve. Two-thirds of children reach the hospitals only at this stage when irreversible neurologic damage is evident. The visual deficit is, in general, a result of affection of the optic nerve and its membranes. Optic atrophy and visual deficits occur relatively early in the clinical course and suggest the severity of the disease. Thick exudates or edema around the optic nerve, involvement of visual area of the cortex producing blindness without changes in the optic fundi or involvement of the cranial nerves controlling the muscles of the eye account for the visual loss which is reversible in many. Hemiparesis is secondary to vascular changes, and the deficits may be permanent depending on the area of infarction. Aphasia, facial paralysis, and deafness may also occur. Hydrocephalus is an invariable accompaniment–communicating type is often encountered. Marked peripheral tremors, slurred speech, orofacial movements, athetoid movements of the extremities are seen in children with basal ganglia infarcts (15%).

Unresponsiveness to any stimuli marks the **Third stage** (Major neurological changes with sensorial changes and or coma) of the illness with neurologic signs of opisthotonus, decerebrate rigidity and irregular respirations.

Altered sensorium (25-45%), vomiting (40-45%), convulsion (50-60%) and fever (80-90%) are the various clinical symptoms in children. The various seizures are listed on the basis of their frequency of occurrence–general tonic and clonic seizures, tonic spasms, and focal seizures. A recurrence of neonatal reflexes may be observed even one year later in the progressive stages. In 20% of the TBM cases, there are incidences of quadriplegia and hemiplegia. Cerebral paraplegia and monoplegia are relatively rare. At the beginning or during the disease various movement disorders namely–ataxia, myoclonic jerks, generalized tremors, hemiballismus, athetosis and chorea are reported, frequently in children than adults.

In nearly 25% of TBM cases, we can observe cranial nerve palsies. Due to nerve entrapment in adhesive basal exudates or raised intracranial pressure the following cranial nerves are affected in the following order–sixth, third and fourth cranial nerve. Vision loss is the most certain in case the optic nerve is involved. The various possible mechanisms are – optic nerve granuloma, optochiasmatic arachnoiditis, and third ventricular compression of optic chiasma in patients with large hydrocephalus.

Diagnosis

CSF Study

The definitive diagnosis of TBM can be made by demonstration of mycobacteria in cerebrospinal fluid (CSF), by direct staining or culture. The classical findings in children with TBM include a clear CSF, a relatively low cell count ($< 400 \times 10^6$/l) with an excess of lymphocytes, an accompanying rise in protein concentration (50-200 mg/dl) and a fall in glucose concentration (20-50 mg/dl). Less well known, but nonetheless well documented is the occurrence of polymorphonuclear predominance in a small percentage of cases (8%). Typical, atypical, and normal CSF pictures were obtained in 91%, 6% and 3% of cases respectively of TBM children. CSF may be turbid simulating pyomeningitis, and a "spider web clot" may be seen when CSF is allowed to stand for 5-6 hours. The pellicle indicated the presence of fibrinogen and related to a number of gamma globulins. It is one of the important materials for detection of Acid-Fast Bacilli (AFB). Hemorrhagic CSF due to vasculitis is also encountered. Udani *et al.*[15] had reported normal CSF till the end though the diagnosis was proved at autopsy.

The type of cellular response in the CSF and the trend of changes in cell counts are noteworthy in TBM. Maximum variability of cells in the initial stages of the illness, persistence of polymorphs in the later stages, monocyte-macrophage cells (large cells with indistinct cell margins, abundant cytoplasm and elongated irregular nucleus) have been noted in majority. Neutrophils (60-80%) in the first ten days of the illness, mononuclear cells and macrophages, lymphocytes, later; lymphoid cells, monocytic cells, and macrophages replace them subsequently. Uninterrupted decline (37%), fluctuating downward trend (43%) and fluctuating upward trend (21%) are encountered in the CSF cellular profile in childhood TBM.

Detailed cytological analysis of CSF sediment, follow-up of the dynamics of cellular modifications can suggest a diagnosis of TBM even when the clinical and biochemical findings in the CSF are atypical. The rise in protein concentration (50-200 mg/dl)) accompanies the cellular changes. Xanthochromic fluid with increased protein, normal sugar was found in few percent of cases. Normal CSF glucose cannot be taken to exclude TBM, and 30% of children showed an initial normal CSF glucose. A persistent low glucose level strengthens the diagnosis TBM. Low CSF glucose may occur in mumps meningitis, subarachnoid bleed, and herpes simplex meningoencephalitis. Pia-arachnoiditis elicited by the secretory/excretory mycobacterial proteins (similar to an intrathecal tuberculin reaction), and stage of the disease account for the varied biochemical values and cellular recruitment in the immunologically privileged compartment of CSF.

Rapid return to normal in CSF composition within a few days virtually excludes the diagnosis of TBM. The glucose and cells and proteins return to normal after a few weeks to months. The diagnostic yield of CSF smear and culture has been lower (10-40%). Success in detecting tubercle bacilli in CSF by acid-fast, auramine or fluorescent staining can, in some hands, is increased from the normal average of 10-30% by centrifuging a large volume of CSF (10-20 ml) and carefully examining the sediment under a microscope. Repeated lumbar puncture is a safe treatment for the increased intracranial pressure and increases the chance of detecting the tubercle bacilli. The stage of the disease, extent of pia-arachnoiditis, intrathecal tuberculin reaction elicited by the secretory and excretory proteins of MTB account for the variable profile of the CSF among the children with TBM.

CSF adenosine deaminase activity (ADA): Level of ADA is raised in the CSF of patients with TBM. Lack of specificity has been the major problem: High CSF ADA activity has been reported from patients with lymphomas, malaria, brucellosis and pyogenic meningitides.

Tuberculin Test

An adult source of contact is an important indicator but available in only 25% of cases. Tuberculin test detects hypersensitivity to tuberculin, though not a specific test it is a strong pointer to latent tuberculous infection. Tuberculin test is positive in 50% of children with TBM. In tuberculin negative children, intradermal injection of 0.1 ml of freeze-dried BCG would produce a papule of 5 mm size within 24 hours. Tuberculin negative tests are not uncommon in TBM.

Interferon-Gamma Release Assays (IGRA)

To improve the sensitivity and specificity of tuberculin test, assays that rely on cellular response to specific antigens of MTB have been developed. QuantiFERON (QuantiFERON-TB gold and T-SPOT.TB) is a diagnostic test that quantifies interferon gamma (IFNr) released by sensitized lymphocytes. It is more accurate than skin testing at diagnosing latent tuberculosis and the agreement between Tuberculin test, and QFT is 85%. Whether these assays can be adapted to diagnose active tuberculosis is uncertain.

Serological tests for HIV infection and CD4 cell count are required to the present day increase of AIDS cases globally. Detection of structural cell wall components of MTB in CSF (Tuberculostearic acid) is a fairly sensitive and highly specific test. It requires the use of gas chromatography and mass spectrometry with ion monitoring. Normal sialic acid a level in CSF is useful to differentiate partially treated pyomeningitis due to the inability of MTB to elaborate sialidase.

Enzyme-Linked Immunosorbent Assay (ELISA)

The manifestation of TBM being immunologically directed inflammatory reaction to M. tuberculosis infection, it is logical to look for specific antigen, antibody and immune complexes in the CSF-ELISA tests do provide an adjunct to standard diagnostic procedures in childhood TBM. The use of ELISA as a diagnostic tool offers a lot of scope but caution must be exercised in interpreting the results of the stage of the disease. LAM antigen, 17 KDa antigen and antigen 85 complexes of M. tuberculosis is strong candidate antigens useful in TBM. It must be recognized that immune complexes, optimal selection of antigen/epitopes affect the sensitivity of ELISA tests.

During an infection of CNS with M. tuberculosis many secretory or degradative products of the bacilli occur in the CSF. While the presence of antibodies indicates infection with *M.tuberculosis*, the presence of antigens of *M.tuberculosis* invariably indicates active infection. In the pathogenesis of TBM, the pathogen M. tuberculosis sheds initially antigens or is exposed to immune cells within CNS, in which an immune response occurs; thus it is the antigen that is seen earlier. The rising levels of antibody then start complexing with an antigen that result in a phase where the levels of both will be affected, and detection becomes difficult: later on, it is the antibody that dominates. Thus when the antigen is abundant, there are low levels of antibody because they are being newly synthesized and vice-versa during the later stages. It is imperative that immune complexes (IC) be dissociated besides detection of the antigen and antibody in CSF.

With the development of competition assays, purified and recombinant antigens there are optimism on the role of ELISA tests in TBM. However, as of today there is no single kit for TBM that can universally be recommended that can replace either smear or culture method.

A **dot-immunobinding assay (Dot-Iba)** has been standardized to measure circulating antimycobacterial antibodies to 14 KDa antigen in CSF specimens for the rapid laboratory diagnosis of TBM (with partially treated pyogenic meningitis. The Dot-Iba developed in their laboratory is a simple, rapid, and specific method and, more importantly, is suited for the routine application in laboratories with limited resources. Studies are promising that Dot-Iba can be used as an adjunct to the laboratory diagnosis of TBM, particularly in culture negative TBM patients and also in those clinical situations where no laboratory tests are available to distinguish between TBM and partially treated pyogenic meningitis.

Enzyme Linked Immunospot ELISPOT is immunoassay that detects IFN-r molecule secreted by ESAT-6 specific T cells. ESAT-6 is a secreted antigen specifically expressed by M. tuberculosis complex but absent in strains of M.bovis BCG and most NTM. The available evidence suggests that ELISPOT assay is sufficiently accurate to diagnose tuberculous as a stand-alone technique. In fact, it appears to be superior to assays based on adenosine deaminase and gamma interferon for screening patients and confirming the diagnosis of tuberculosis. Newer diagnostic assays can differentiate T cell response to MTB, NTM or BCG.

Nucleic Acid Amplification (NAA) Assays

Calculation of NAA – commercial nucleic acid amplification using meta-analysis evaluates that the TBM diagnosis were 56% sensitive (95% CI 46 to 66%) and 98% specific (95% CI 97–99%).[16] Commercial NAA tests can only confirm cerebral TB; it cannot rule it out as has been proven by multiple studies.[16] By using large volume (high diagnostic yield) of CSF to facilitate comparison of culture, microscopy and NAA have shown the similarity of NAA and microscopy in TBM diagnosis.[17] After the onset of treatment, there is a rapid decrease in CSF microscopy and culture sensitivity, even after one month of treatment initiation mycobacterial DNA may remain evident.[17] Bacterial detection in the CSF can be improved by quantitative real-time PCR–polymerase chain reaction.[17]

Polymerase Chain Reaction (PCR)

Given the situation of the growth of culture is slow, and microscopy has insufficient sensitivity. PCR is currently the most sensitive and rapid method to detect extrapulmonary M. tuberculosis. Studies comparing conventional IS6110 primers with a new set of primers (TRC 4) which is a consult repetitive element with specificity for MTB complex have shown 80 and 86% levels of concordance with CSF specimen from children with TBM.[18] Recent studies are found that real-time IS6110-PCR is a quick, sensitive and specific test for diagnosing of TBM as compared to microscopy and culture (solid; liquid) methods.[19] Research is needed to simplify PCR converting into a cost effective for diagnosis of TB meningitis. One of the weaknesses in any childhood TBM series reported is the difficulty in confirming the diagnosis. However, these PCR tests can be difficult to implement with appropriately rigorous quality controls in resource-limited, high-burden health care centers, where the need is greatest.

GeneXpert MTB/RIF Test

Staff with minimal training can operate this closed-cartridge based system, capable of producing results in around 2 hours. The Foundation for Innovative New Diagnostics (FIND) conducted extensive evaluation projects in 6 countries, which resulted in WHO's approval in 2010 to use Xpert MTB/RIF test to diagnose pulmonary TB.[20] The presence of M. tuberculosis complex bacilli is detected using a real-time heminested PCR test. The test concurrently determines the vulnerability to rifampin (used as a surrogate marker for MDR–multidrug resistance), by using the five molecular beacons that span the rpoB gene 81-bp rifampin resistance-determining region (RRDR). The test can be used out of the laboratory due to its closed-cartridge system. The use of Xpert MTB/RIF relatively carries a low biohazard risk than smear microscopy as proven by various biosafety studies. The test has revealed sensitivity greater than 90% for culture-positive TB, with a high specificity in sputum samples.

In patients with HIV co-infection, the sensitivity of this test is more than 80%. Use of Xpert MTB / RIF tests on extrapulmonary samples have been extremely successful, with over 80% sensitivity and 100% specificity.[20,21] With a pooled sensitivity of 88% (95% CI, 83 to 92%) and specificity of 98% (95% CI, 97 to 99%), a Cochrane review established and supported the replacement of sputum smear with the Xpert MTB / RIF.[22] Even in low-resource setting this test can be easily and efficiently utilized, this promotes early patient access for precise diagnosis. The overall morbidity due to diagnostic delay, mistreatment or dropout can be successfully reduced.[21]

Radiological Investigations

Most but not all affected children with TBM have abnormal chest X-ray for evidence of thoracic tuberculosis. They include segmental atelectasis, mediastinal, hilar adenopathy, miliary mottling. The most common cerebral CT features of TBM are hydrocephalus (Fig. 37.5) and basal contrast enhancing exudates (Figs. 37.6 and 37.7). Both features are more common in children (80%) than adults (40%). More than 70% develop tuberculomas (Fig. 37.6) during treatment, although the majorities are asymptomatic. CT is useful for infarcts, cerebral edema, hydrocephalus and enhancement of basal meninges. Infarctions most commonly involve the basal ganglia and the territories of the medial striate and thalami perforating arteries. Common sites of exudates are basal cisterns ambient, suprasellar cisterns, and Sylvian fissures. Meningeal enhancement over chiasmatic peri-mesencephalic cisterns and one or both Sylvian fissures are not an accurate diagnostic criterion as they are absent in 20% of cases. Appearance or disappearance of meningeal enhancement did not correlate with the ultimate prognosis.

Areas of low attenuation suggestive infarcts are due to arteritis, areas of increased attenuation with classical target lesion and central low attenuated areas along with localized cerebral edema small disc and ring lesions are encountered in these conditions. Tuberculomas are seen more near the surface of the brain periphery or develop near basal exudates. Tuberculomas lesions can develop while on treatment. An immunological basis is suggested though the reason for this paradoxical phenomenon is not clear. Ring lesions of neurocysticercosis and tuberculomas cannot be distinguished with certainty on CT scan. The combination of hydrocephalus, basal enhancement and infarction was 100% specific and 41% sensitive for the diagnosis of childhood TBM, although pre-contrast hyperdensity in the basal cisterns was the best predictor of TBM. Gadolinium-enhanced magnetic resonance imaging (MRI) was useful in the detection of basilar meningeal enhancement and small tuberculomas. MRI provides a high definition of infratentorial lesions and the early cerebral. However, data regarding the diagnostic sensitivity and specificity of these features are limited. Cryptococcal meningitis, cytomegalovirus encephalitis, toxoplasmosis, sarcoidosis, meningeal metastases, and lymphoma may all produce similar radiographic findings.[17]

Complications

Immediate

Increased intracranial pressure (ICP): In early stages, it is due to the inflammatory process leading to cerebral edema. Decerebration develop due to untreated raised ICP and rostrocaudal transtentorial herniation.

Bilateral visual failure with optic atrophy: Occurs due to arachnoiditis in the cistern of optic chiasma. Blindness can also occur due to compression or ischemia of optic nerves and chiasma. Hydrocephalus and ethambutol are induced disturbance in vision also occur. **Convulsive disorders** are common in children. **Syndrome of Inappropriate Antidiuretic Hormone Secretion (SIADH):** Impairment in consciousness and decerebrate rigidity; other signs of brainstem damage are not found.

Long Term

Other uncommon abnormalities are hemichorea and hypothalamic disorders. Learning disorders and attention deficit disorders. Deafness, Preventable peripheral neuropathy, Relapse of TBM after months or years are noted in some children.

Treatment

Despite the availability of drugs, mortality is still high due to failure to start treatment in early stages of the disease. Therapy should be initiated early (within 48 hours of presentation) whenever an increased index of suspicion is present even if tuberculin reaction is negative, and chest X-ray is normal. In any young infant with the clinical impression of meningitis, in the context of CSF white cell count of $< 500/mm^3$, lymphocyte predominance, hyponatremia and hydrocephalus, empirical antitubercular therapy (ATT) with steroid is justified. Therapy is often decided on any of the following criteria even in tertiary care centers; pending definite microbiological diagnosis:

(a) Epidemiological and other risk factors for TB very high.

(b) CSF picture is compatible.

(c) Neuroimaging studies show hydrocephalus/basal enhancement/tuberculomas. However, there are no published studies that help determine when empirical therapy should be stopped.

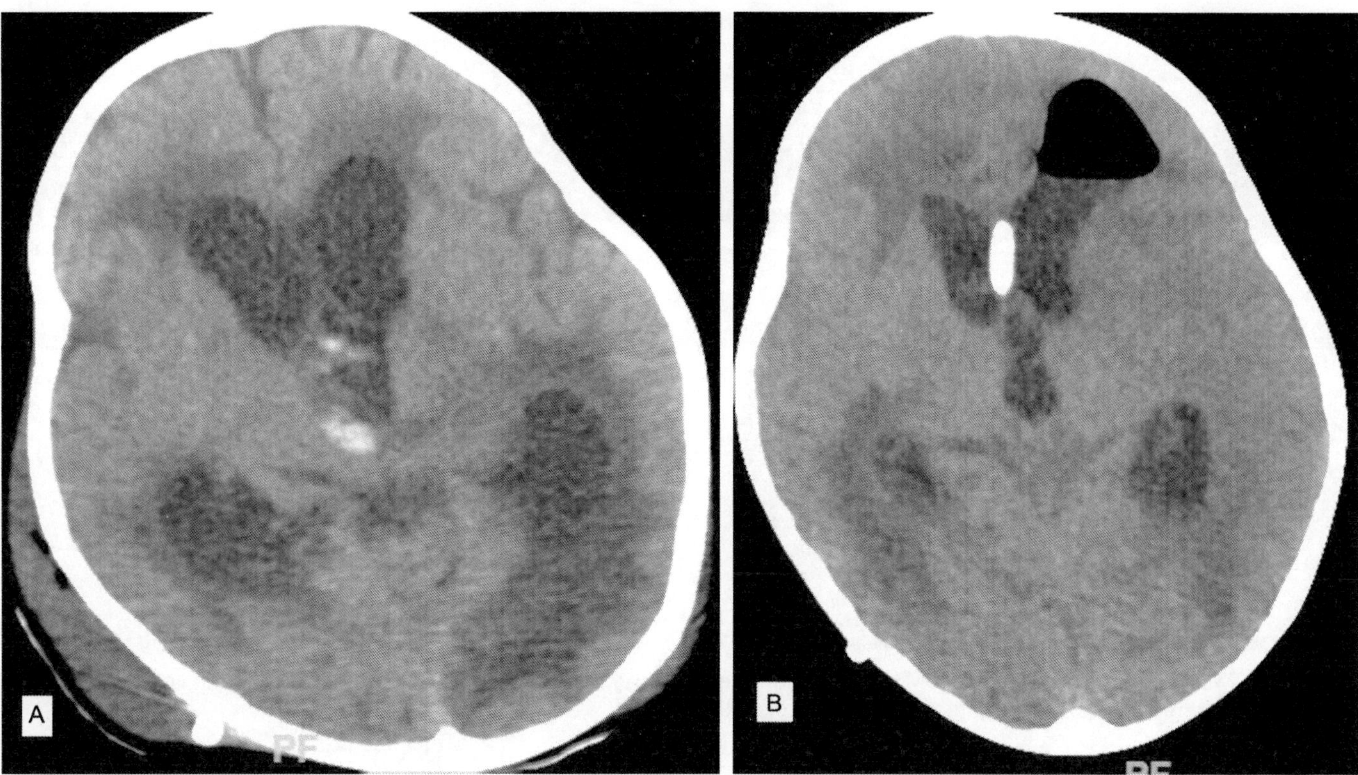

Fig. 37.5: Contrast enhancing computer tomography (CECT) of head, A. Showing communicating hydrocephalus with periventricular ooze and left parietal region infarct. B. Non-contrast CT head showing hydrocephalus with VP shunt in situ/ Periventricular ooze, pneumocephalus (air in the cranial cavity)

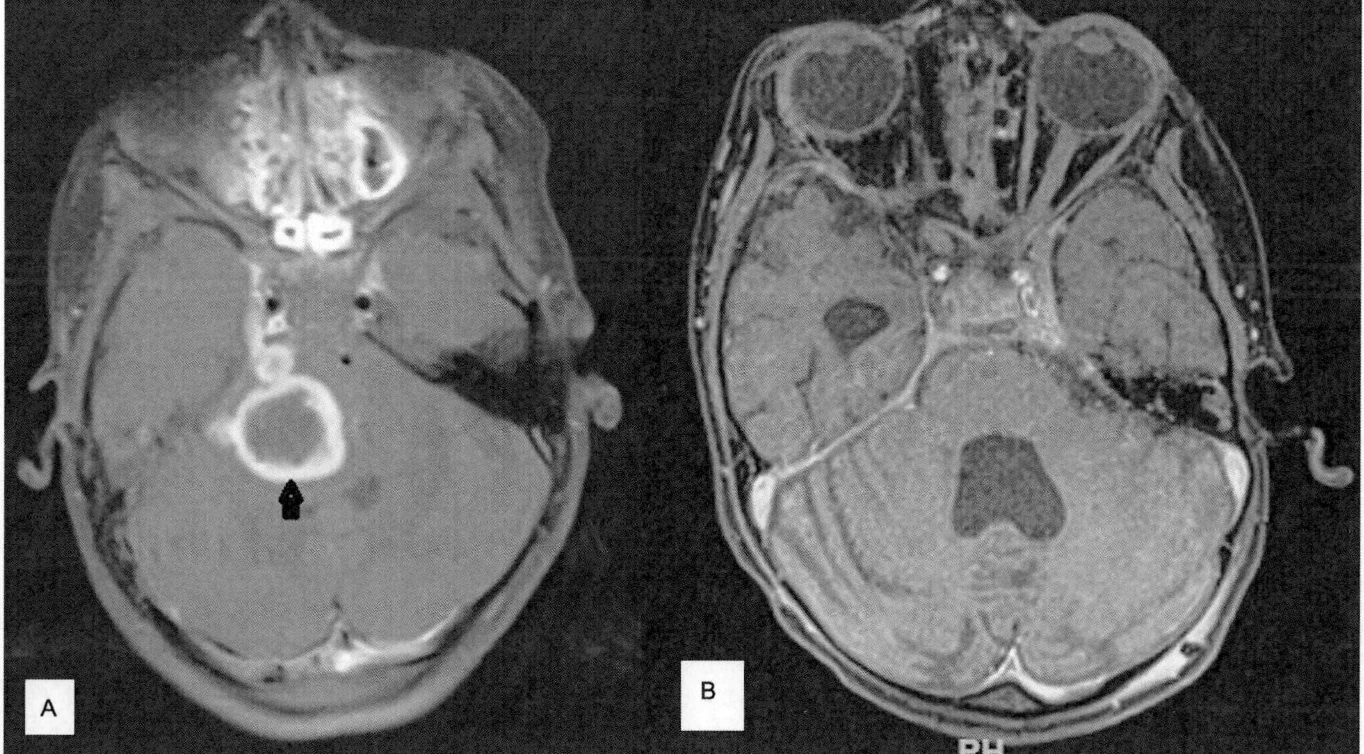

Fig. 37.6: Magnetic resonance imaging (MRI) with Gadolinium contrast imaging, A. Showing ring enhancing lesion (tuberculoma) with perilesional edema (black arrow-head). B. Showing basal exudates

CNS TB

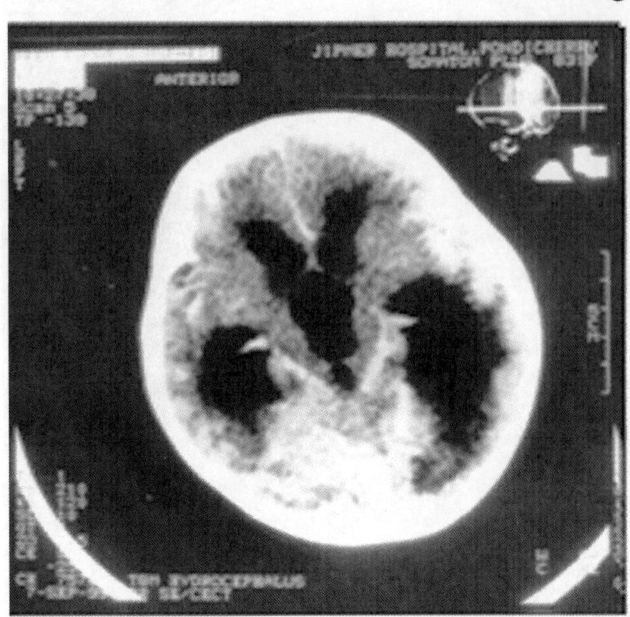

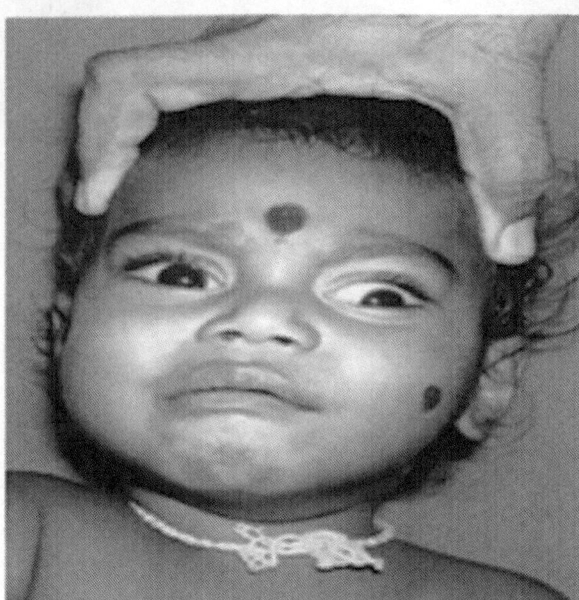

Fig. 37.7: Two-year-old child Stage II TBM with left lateral rectus palsy and Facial palsy. Contrast CT with pan ventriculomegaly/ basal enhancement reflecting exudates and pia arachnoiditis

Drug(s) of Choice and Duration

Chemotherapy for CNS tuberculosis follows the model of short course chemotherapy for pulmonary tuberculosis an intensive phase of treatment, followed by a continuation phase. However, unlike pulmonary tuberculosis, the optimal drug regimen and duration of each phase are not clearly established. Choice of anti-TB drugs has been based on pharmacokinetics and antibacterial properties of the drugs. Isoniazid (H) and Rifampicin (R) are the key components of the regimen. Isoniazid penetrates the CSF freely and has potent early bactericidal activity. Rifampicin penetrates the CSF less well (maximum concentrations around 30% of plasma), but the high mortality from rifampicin resistant TBM has confirmed its central role in the treatment of CNS disease. There is no conclusive evidence to demonstrate that Pyrazinamide (Z) improves the outcome of CNS tuberculosis, although it is well absorbed orally and achieves high concentrations in the CSF. Isoniazid, Rifampicin, and Pyrazinamide are considered mandatory at the beginning of TBM treatment, and some centers use all three drugs for the whole duration of therapy.

To support the fourth drug choice, there are no available data from controlled trials. Streptomycin (S) or Ethambutol (E) is the most common recommendation by the authorities. Both the drugs cannot penetrate the CSF well in the nonexistence of inflammation and are capable of adverse reactions. While treating comatose patients, a major concern is Ethambutol-induced optic neuropathy even when there is a 3% or less incidence rate at the standard dose of 15-20 mg/kg. Ethionamide is a favorable drug advocated in some centers in South Africa as it can penetrate both healthy and inflamed meninges even if it causes severe nausea. There may be a better tolerance towards Prothionamide. The most effectual fourth agent can be fluoroquinolones, even if data about their prolonged use and CSF pharmacokinetics is inadequate. Nevertheless, Ethambutol (the fourth anti-TB drug) must be given in the first two months of intensive chemotherapy. This is because BBB (blood-brain barrier) lets in sufficient quantities of anti-TB drugs to kill the organisms.

British and American Thoracic Societies advise 12 months of treatment for TBM with at least HRZ. Short course chemotherapy is advocated by several groups, but relatively few have been so treated and followed up. Six months treatment is sufficient for TBM with susceptible bacteria. ICMR have compared SHE/RZ thrice a week in the first 2 months of intensive phase–RH for 7 months along with steroids for 6-8 weeks versus SHE/RZ twice a week in first 2 months of intensive phase–RH for 7 months along with steroids for 6-8 weeks. The response to therapy is same in children and adults, but mortality was high despite intensive regimens.

Pyrazinamide 35 mg/kg, INH 10-15 mg/kg and Rifampicin 10 mg/kg are recommended dosages by RNTCP. Our experience suggests that TBM can be safely treated for six months with a high dose of anti-tuberculous drugs 2(SHERZ) 3/4 RZ without overt hepatotoxicity and with low risk of relapse. In those who responded, the improvement of a headache, general well-being, and raised intracranial pressure responded early though slowly. CSF cells returned to normal after few months. However, no studies have compared six months treatment with longer treatment. In HIV-infected children should be similarly treated as meningitis in those not infected. Responses to treatment and outcome are similar in the two groups.

In case of low drug resistance six months of treatment was sufficient for TBM, this was the conclusion of a meta-analysis and systemic review. Due to factors such as undetected drug resistance, CNS drug penetration, patient compliance on response to therapy and uncertain influences of disease severity, many authorities endorse 12 months treatment.[17]

Role of Steroids

Since the 1950s, ATT have been used along with corticosteroids even if their role remains debatable. They decline absorption of anti-tuberculosis drugs into the CNS and cause gastrointestinal bleeding. Use of corticosteroid may save lives, with an increased occurrence of disability among survivors. These fears are yet to be proven.[17] The use of corticosteroids has a biased support, some consider it to improve outcome, and others point to the insufficient evidence. In immunocompromised patients due to HIV infection, the benefits and risks of steroids are not known.

Steroids are beneficial in early phases of the disease goes with evidence of subarachnoid block and impending cerebral herniation, patients with single or multiple tuberculomas with cerebral edema are helped by steroids. Randomized trials from South Africa provided evidence that corticosteroids improved survival in children with severe disease and probably reduced neurologic sequelae. Steroids did not prevent severe disability in survivors. Cochrane systematic review and meta-analysis concluded that corticosteroids are improved outcome in HIV-negative children and adults with TBM, but the benefit of HIV-infected individuals remains uncertain.[23] Lack of comparative data from controlled trials for various corticosteroid treatment schedules forces us to choose the most effective treatment plan for the published trials. A useful treatment is a use of prednisolone 4 mg/kg/24 hours (or equivalent dose dexamethasone: 0.6 mg/kg/24 hours) for four weeks, trailed by a reducing course over four weeks. Corticosteroid breakdown is expedited with the use of rifampicin. Routine adjunctive corticosteroids for all patients with tuberculomas without meningitis, or with spinal cord tuberculosis cannot be recommended due to lack of sufficient evidence. They might be useful in patients with uncontrolled symptoms, on anti-tuberculosis therapy, or who are worsening, or patients with acute spinal cord compression secondary to vertebral tuberculosis. Thalidomide might help patients with non-responsive tuberculomas to anti-tuberculosis drugs and high-dose corticosteroids, but they should not be used for the routine treatment of TBM.[17]

The coma clearance time and ever clearance time were 7-10 days. There is high mortality especially when treatment is only started after reduced consciousness and focal neurological deficits have appeared. Intrathecal injection of steroids is unnecessary.

Management of Complications

Increased intracranial pressure (ICP): ICP is often associated with communicating hydrocephalus caused by basal arachnoiditis. Less commonly it is due to diffuse cerebral edema. Markedly bulging fontanelle or enlarging head size is seldom observed in TBM. ICP is low or only marginally raised. Beneficial results were reported with intrathecal hyaluronidase from a few centers. In children with predominant drowsiness, after adequate conservative measures that include repeated lumbar puncture, isosorbide with or without furosemide, acetazolamide, shunt surgery is indicated. Hydrocephalus is the most common reason for neurosurgical referral in patients with TBM.

Most authorities suggest early ventriculo-peritoneal shunting should be considered in all patients with non-communicating hydrocephalus, although outcomes are variable. Endoscopic third ventriculostomy is as an alternative to shunt surgery. Early temporary external ventricular shunting helps a group of children who develop hydrocephalus after a period of apparent clinical improvement. However, response to external ventricular drainage has failed to predict those who benefit from early shunting. Rarely, tuberculomas coalesce and liquefy to cause tuberculous cerebral abscess that may necessitate surgery. There are various treatment options, including aspiration, repeated aspiration through a burr hole, stereotactic aspiration, and total excision, but there is no consensus as to which is best.

Fluid disturbance: Vomiting, inadequate intake, and SIADH result in fluid and electrolyte disturbance. Judicious use of mannitol and glycerol for decreasing ICP is a must.

Therapeutic Paradox

Cerebral tuberculomas occasionally develop during treatment. These are thick walled nodules in clusters developing on the surface of the brain near basal cisterns. It takes 24 months for these lesions to disappear. Anticonvulsants other than Phenobarbitone are beneficial in the management of convulsions.

Prognostic Factors

The stage of the disease at presentation, younger age, tonic posturing, confusion or lethargy, papilledema, the presence of cranial nerve abnormalities at admission, elevated CSF protein affect the prognosis adversely independently in children with TBM.[24] Reasonable therapy for six to nine months can be ensured by relatives/parental responses, urine color in the morning, pill counts and home visits. Monitoring of liver functions an adverse effect for rifampicin. Monitoring of adverse effects of peripheral neuropathy (INH), hepatitis (Rifampicin), color blindness (Ethambutol) cannot be overemphasized.

Prevention

BCG vaccination among newborns and infants reduces the risk of tuberculosis by over 50% on average. The possible protective effect of BCG may be over helmed by excessive and indiscriminate exposure to disease as in many Indian children. In children with unexplained fever, bursts of irritability and nocturnal wakefulness, timely chest X-ray may prevent the late diagnosis of TBM.

Key Points

- Early diagnosis is highly relevant to treatment and prognosis in TBM.
- Empirical therapy is justified in young infants with the clinical impression of meningitis and reasonably certain evidence in one or more of the following parameters: risk of exposure and infection, CSF picture, neuroimaging abnormalities.
- The search and isolation of AFB in CSF and tissue remain the best rapid diagnostic test for CNS tuberculosis.
- Sensitivity and specificity of Xpert MTB/RIF test on extrapulmonary samples are 80% and 100% respectively.
- Contrast-enhanced CT as part of the dignostic work-up or within two days of treatment, should be done in every patient with neurotuberculosis.
- Drugs should be taken each day either individually or in combination form and patients should be treated for a minimum of 12 months.
- All patients with TBM should receive adjunctive corticosteroids regardless of disease severity at presentation.

References

1. Chiang SS, Khan FA, Milstein MB, Tolman AW, Benedetti A, Starke JR, *et al*. Treatment Outcomes of Childhood Tuberculous Meningitis: A Systematic Review and Meta-analysis. Lancet Infect Dis 2014;14:947-57.
2. Kumar A, Gupta D, Nagaraja SB, Singh V, Sethi GR, Prasad J, *et al*. Updated National Guidelines for Pediatric Tuberculosis in India, 2012. Indian Pediatr 2013;50:301-06.
3. Sharma SK, Mohan A. Extrapulmonary Tuberculosis. Indian J Med Res 2004;120:316-53.
4. Savardekar A, Chatterji D, Singhi S, Mohindra S, Gupta S, Chhabra R. The Role of Ventriculoperitoneal Shunt Placement in Patients of Tubercular Meningitis with Hydrocephalus in Poor Neurological Grade: A Prospective Study in the Pediatric Population and Review of Literature. Childs Nerv Syst 2013; 29:719-25.
5. Piccini P, Chiappini E, Tortoli E, de Martino M, Galli L. Clinical Peculiarities of Tuberculosis. BMC Infect Dis 2014;14:S4.
6. Newton SM, Brent AJ, Anderson S, Whittaker E, Kampmann B. Paediatric Tuberculosis. Lancet Infect Dis 2008;8:498-510.
7. Be NA, Kim KS, Bishai WR, Jain SK. Pathogenesis of Central Nervous System Tuberculosis. Curr Mol Med 2009;9:94-99.
8. Donald PR, Schoeman JF. Tuberculous Meningitis. N Engl J Med 2004;351:1719-20.
9. Goel A. Tuberculous Meningitis and Hydrocephalus. Neurol India 2004;52:155.
10. Lammie GA, Hewlett RH, Schoeman JF, Donald PR. Tuberculous Cerebrovascular Disease: A Review. J Infect 2009;59:156-66.
11. Bayarsaihan D. Epigenetic Mechanisms in Inflammation. J Dent Res 2011;90:9-17.
12. Pennini ME, Pai RK, Schultz DC, Boom WH, Harding CV. Mycobacterium Tuberculosis 19-kDa Lipoprotein Inhibits IFN-gamma-induced Chromatin Remodeling of MHC2TA by TLR2 and MAPK Signaling. J Immunol 2006;176:4323-30.
13. Kumar R, Halder P, Sahu SK, Kumar M, Kumari M, Jana K, *et al*. Identification of A Novel Role of ESAT-6-Dependent miR-155 Induction During Infection of Macrophages with Mycobacterium Tuberculosis. Cell Microbiol 2012;14: 1620-31.
14. STREPTOMYCIN Treatment of Tuberculous Meningitis. Lancet 1948;1:582-96.
15. Udani PM, Dastur DK. Tuberculous Encephalopathy with and without Meningitis. Clinical Features and Pathological Correlations. J Neurol Sci 1970;10:541-61.
16. Dinnes J, Deeks J, Kunst H, Gibson A, Cummins E, Waugh N, *et al*. A systematic Review of Rapid Diagnostic Tests for the Detection of Tuberculosis Infection. Health Technol Assess. 2007;11:1-196.
17. Thwaites G, Fisher M, Hemingway C, Scott G, Solomon T, Innes J, *et al*. British Infection Society Guidelines for the Diagnosis and Treatment of Tuberculosis of the Central Nervous System in Adults and Children. J Infect 2009;59: 167-87.
18. Narayanan S, Parandaman V, Narayanan PR, Venkatesan P, Girish C, Mahadevan S, *et al*. Evaluation of PCR Using TRC(4)

and IS6110 Primers in Detection of Tuberculous Meningitis. J Clin Microbiol 2001;39:2006-08.

19. Chaidir L, Ganiem AR, Vander Zanden A, Muhsinin S, Kusumaningrum T, Kusumadewi I, *et al.* Comparison of Real Time IS6110-PCR, Microscopy and Culture for Diagnosis of Tuberculous Meningitis in a Cohort of Adult Patients in Indonesia. PloS one 2012;7:e52001.
20. Nhu NT, Heemskerk D, Thu do DA, Chau TT, Mai NT, Nghia HD, *et al.* Evaluation of GeneXpert MTB/RIF for Diagnosis of Tuberculous Meningitis. J Clin Microbiol 2014;52:226-33.
21. Boehme CC, Nicol MP, Nabeta P, Michael JS, Gotuzzo E, Tahirli R, *et al.*, Feasibility, Diagnostic Accuracy and Effectiveness of Decentralised Use of the Xpert MTB/RIF Test for Diagnosis of Tuberculosis and Multidrug Resistance: A Multicentre Implementation Study. Lancet 2011;377:1495-05.
22. Steingart KR, Sohn H, Schiller I, Kloda LA, Boehme CC, Pai M, *et al.* Xpert(R) MTB/RIF Assay for Pulmonary Tuberculosis and Rifampicin Resistance in Adults. Cochrane Database Syst. Rev 2013;1:CD009593.
23. Prasad K, Singh MB. Corticosteroids for Managing Tuberculous Meningitis. Cochrane Database Syst Rev 2008;1:CD002244.
24. Mahadevan B, Mahadevan S, Serane VT. Prognostic Factors in Childhood Tuberculous Meningitis. J Trop Pediatr 2002; 48:362-65.

38 Chapter

UNUSUAL MENINGITIS AND OTHER CNS INFECTIONS

Sujata Kanhere

Infection of the central nervous system (CNS), most commonly, manifests as meningitis. In India, acute bacterial (pyogenic) meningitis and tuberculous meningitis account for the majority of CNS infections in children. In recent times, viral meningoencephalitis has seen a seasonal increase during epidemics, in many parts of the country. A number of other organisms can also cause acute or subacute meningitis and this chapter deals with those unusual CNS infections.

Fungi, mycoplasma, protozoa, helminths, other parasites and some noninfectious conditions can cause meningitis in children. Inflammatory involvement of the subarachnoid space with meningeal irritation leads to the classic features of headache, fever and meningismus and pleocytosis in the cerebrospinal fluid (CSF). The most characteristic finding in meningitis due to these agents, as well as viruses, is that the CSF is bacteriologically sterile, hence these forms of meningitis were previously referred to as 'aseptic meningitis'.

FUNGAL MENINGITIS

General Considerations

Many fungi are known to cause CNS infections in children. Fungal CNS infections may present as meningitis, meningoencephalitis, focal lesions, infarcts and abscesses. Meningitis is the most frequent manifestation and can be caused by Candida, Cryptococcus, Coccidioides, Histoplasma and Blastomyces (Table 38.1).

Fungal CNS infections, though uncommon, are usually seen in immunocompromised children. In recent times, this trend is on the increase. However, some fungi (Cryptococcus and Candida spp) can cause infections in healthy children as well as immunocompromised hosts while others cause disease in healthy hosts. When the fungus becomes invasive, it leads to the disseminated form. Dissemination usually occurs from some primary focus of infection, most often, the lungs or skin and sometimes ear, sinus and eye.

Table 38.1: Fungal CNS Infections: Presentation and Treatment

Fungal agent	Common CNS presentation	Treatment
Candida spp	Meningitis	Amphotericin B in neonates
Cryptococcus spp	Meningoencephalitis, mass lesions, abscess	Amphotericin B, 5-Flucytosine, Fluconazole
Coccidioides immitis	Meningitis	Fluconazole or Itraconazole
Blastomycosis dermatitidis	Meningitis, mass lesion in brain or spine	Liposomal Amphotericin B followed by prolonged fluconazole, itraconazole or voriconazole
Histoplasma capsulatum	Meningitis or mass lesion	Amphotericin B followed by itraconazole
Aspergillus spp.	Multiple mass lesions	Voriconazole
Zygomycosis	Mass lesion, invasion from sinuses	Liposomal Amphotericin B
Scedosporium spp	Brain Abscess	Voriconazole

The clinical features of meningitis are variable but most often the course is protracted and prolonged. CSF shows mononuclear (lymphocytic or monocytic) pleocytosis, with low sugar and raised protein. The outcome depends on the causative fungus, the underlying condition and the child's immune status, but fatality in general is high.[1]

Candidiasis

The most common invasive fungal infection in infants and children is Candida spp. However, cerebral candidiasis is rare and seen in only 12% of disseminated candidiasis.

Candidal meningitis results from disseminated infection by Candida albicans occurring in mycelial form and is at times seen in newborn infants in presence of predisposing factors like prematurity, low birth weight, prolonged intravenous catheterization, prolonged ventilatory support, neutropenia, prolonged use of broad spectrum antibiotics and ventriculoperitoneal shunt.[2,3,4,5] The common species are Candida albicans, Candida tropicalis, Candida glabrata and Candida parapsilosis. Candida spreads to the CNS through the hematogenous route, usually from a focus of infection somewhere in the body.

The clinical presentation of candidal CNS disease is mostly as meningitis, which may be masked because of the presence of serious underlying illness or infection. Granulomas and abscesses, usually multiple, may occur in isolation or with meningitis and act as space occupying lesions to cause hydrocephalus, hemiparesis and cranial nerve palsies. Serious complications like intracranial mycotic aneurysms secondary to arterial or venous involvement may occur. Disseminated candidiasis seen with Candida albicans and Candida tropica can cause focal necrosis and microabscesses in the middle cerebral artery territory.

In candidal infection, CSF usually shows lymphocytic pleocytosis or decreased CSF glucose in 50% of culture positive patients. The diagnosis is established by microscopic detection of the spores / yeast cells and confirmed by recovery of the fungus in culture of CSF, blood or neural tissue.[1] Catheter tips and urine also should be cultured. Identification of the species helps to give appropriate antifungal therapy.

Though there are no pediatric guidelines, there are Infectious Disease Society of America (IDSA) guidelines for treating adults with Candida albicans CNS infection with Liposomal Amphotericin (3-5 mg/kg/day) with or without oral 5 Flucytosine (100 mg/kg/day in 4 divided doses) followed by oral Fluconazol (6-12 mg/kg/day in 2 divided doses).[6] As an alternative treatment, IV Fluconazole (6-12 mg/kg/day) or IV Voriconazole (6 mg/kg/day in 2 divided doses followed by 3 mg/kg/day) may be used.

In neonates, Amphotericin B is the treatment of choice in a dose of 0.5-1 mg/kg/day; duration of therapy depends on severity and clinical response and should be continued till all signs and symptoms have disappeared and there is resolution of CSF and radiological abnormalities.[5] Monitoring for side effects of the drug, specially renal, is essential during therapy. Meningitis, in the presence of a shunt, resolves only by removing the shunt and placing an external drain and treating for 4-6 weeks. Candida meningitis has a mortality of 10-20% with neurologic sequelae in the survivors.

Cryptococcal Infections

Cryptococcal CNS infections are due to monomorphic encapsulated yeast Cryptococcus neoformans found particularly in bird feces and soil visited by birds, or Cryptococcus gatti. The mode of infection is by inhalation or ingestion. Dissemination to the CNS usually occurs from primary lung disease. Cryptococcus causes meningoencephalitis, but sometimes can cause brain abscess or cryptococcomas or partially cystic and solid lesions involving the basal ganglia and cortical grey matter.[7] The cystic lesions contain a gelatinous polysaccharide detectable on CSF examination and can be used for diagnosis.

The clinical presentation ranges from typical meningitis to no symptoms in healthy children and from acute to subacute in children infected with HIV. In AIDS patients, CNS cryptococcosis presents with an acute febrile illness with headache in 70% and meningismus, photophobia and altered sensorium in 25%.The symptoms are severe with underlying HIV infection or when the child is on high-dose corticosteroids. In a few patients, CSF findings are normal, in the initial stages. Mass lesions seen in Cryptococcus neoformans can cause cranial neuropathies, papilledema, hemiparesis or hydrocephalus, which requires shunting. If the hydrocephalus is not treated, it can be fatal.

Diagnosis is established by culture of CSF on Sabouraud's agar. India ink preparation is useful for detection of the fungus. A latex agglutination test for rapid detection of cryptococcal antigen in serum and CSF is also available. The sensitivity is 90% for antigen detection in the cerebrospinal fluid. A recently developed affordable, lateral-flow immunoassay for detection of cryptococcal antigen (LFA Cr Ag) gives reliable results in 15 minutes.[8] Titres of antigen in CSF and Serum less than 1:32 indicate good prognosis. CT and MRI brain scans may reveal cryptococcomas, abscesses as well as hydrocephalus and assist in diagnosis.[9-11]

The treatment of choice has been amphotericin B. Although there are no pediatric guidelines, the recent IDSA treatment guidelines recommend a combination of amphotericin B and flucytosine initially for 2 weeks, for all CNS cryptococcal disease in all age groups, irrespective of HIV status.[12] This should be followed by oral fluconazole for 8-10 weeks for consolidation and for 6-12 months for long-term suppression. A CSF examination may be essential in HIV patients at the end of 2 weeks of amphotericin, before starting fluconazole. In HIV patients, sometimes sudden deterioration with raised intracranial pressure, sudden loss of vision and death may occur in the first 2 weeks of treatment and requires immediate management of raised intracranial pressure.[13]

Alternative treatment used successfully is intraventricular amphotericin B and where amphotericin and flucytosine is not available, high dose oral fluconazole has been tried. In HIV patients, with CNS cryptococcal infections, corticosteroid administration should first be discontinued or reduced. Then antifungals should be started and after response is obtained, antiretroviral therapy should be introduced. In cryptococcomas, usually antifungal therapy suffices, but in large lesions, surgical removal may be required. Fluconazole and itraconazole can prevent cryptococcal meningitis in HIV infected patients. The outcome of cryptogenic meningitis is better than other fungal meningitis.

Coccidioidomycosis is caused by soil dwelling dimorphic fungi Coccidioides immitis, that exist in mycelial form or as a spherule. Coccidioidomycosis is acquired by inhalation or spore laden dust or through broken skin but not from person to person. Coccidiodes CNS infection in children is very rare. The most common manifestation is basilar meningitis. Ventriculitis, cerebral vasculitis and abscess may be seen. The clinical picture is similar to tuberculous meningitis with headache, vomiting, meningismus and cranial nerve palsies.[14-16]

CSF findings are similar to those seen in tuberculous meningitis. Eosinphilic pleocytosis may be seen in the CSF. X-ray chest may show sharply circumscribed lesions, hilar lymphadenopathy and even military mottling. Raised ESR, peripheral eosinophilia and increased alkaline phosphatase are common. Diagnosis can be confirmed by culture but often culture is negative. DNA probe, exoantigen test and animal inoculation are also confirmatory. C. immitis antibodies in CSF are also detectable in about 90% of cases are of great use in diagnosis. A quantitative enzyme immunoassay that detects coccidioidal galactomannan in the urine has excellent specificity and is found to be positive in 70% of severe infections. Complement fixating antibody (CFA) titre of 1:32 or more is found in CSF of more than 90% patients with coccidioidomycosis meningitis.

Oral fluconazole or itraconazole are currently used in isolated coccidioidal meningitis.[16] Earlier Amphotericin B was the treatment of choice. In disseminated disease, a combination of amphotericin B and fluconazole is used and as an alternative intrathecal amphotericin B injection followed by a lumbar, cisternal or ventricular reservoir has been tried. This infection is difficult to cure. Morbidity and mortality are very high.

Histoplasmosis, caused by Histoplasma capsulatum, a fungus occurring in mycelial form rarely causes meningitis. The disease usually follows primary infection in the lungs and common associations are anemia, lymphadenopathy, hepatosplenomegaly, pneumonia, thrombocytopenia.[17] Diagnosis is by culture. The fungus may also be recovered from blood and bone marrow in disseminated histoplasmosis. Histoplasma associated antigen can be detected in disseminated disease by radioimmunoassay. Amphotericin B is the drug of choice for treatment.[17] Histoplasma meningitis has a mortality of 20-40% with a high relapse of 50%.[18]

Blastomycosis caused by Blastomycosis dermatiditis occurring in mycelial form is again a rare cause of meningitis. The three major CNS manifestations are meningitis, intracranial mass and spinal mass. Diagnosis is confirmed by culture. An ELISA test is also available that has good sensitivity and specificity. Liposomal Amphotericin B for 4-6 weeks followed by prolonged treatment with oral fluconazole, itraconzole or voriconazole is the recommendation.[19,20]

Aspergillosis is caused by the fungus Aspergillus which enters the lungs by inhalation. CNS aspergillosis was rare before the immunocompromised host population increased and now accounts for 10-20% of invasive disease. CNS aspergillosis has three distinct types of clinical presentation: as an intracranial space occupying lesion, a rhinocerebral form and a vascular form with stroke like symptoms. Occasionally, meningitis, meningoencephalitis and other CNS involvement may be seen. Definitive diagnosis of invasive Aspergillosis is made by smear and culture of biopsy material. Serum galactomannan is a non-invasive test for invasive aspergillosis.

Amphotericin B was the drug of choice. Now the drug of first choice for treatment of CNS Aspergillosis, in children 2-11 years of age, is voriconazole.[21] Itraconazole, posaconazole and liposomal formulation of Amphotericin B are alternatives in this age group, while capsofungin and micafungin are alternatives in younger children.[22] CNS aspergillosis has a very poor prognosis and although case fatality rate has halved to 40% now, but disseminated aspergillosis including CNS involvement is 100% fatal.

Zygomycosis (Mucormycosis)

These fungi do not cause meningitis but account for important CNS infections. Mucormycosis can cause sudden onset stroke, seizures or focal neurological deficit, due to vasculitis or occasionally hemorrhage secondary to rupture of mycotic aneurysms. Rhinocerebral syndrome characterized by orbital pain, blackish nasal discharge and facial edema can occur with zygomycosis in patients suffering from renal failure, diabetes mellitus or neutropenia. Proptosis, visual loss, trigeminal nerve involvement and blackish necrotic areas on palate can be seen in mucormycosis. Involvement of carotid arteries can lead to infantile hemiplegia.

Diagnosis is made on the basis of the classical presentation, examination and investigations. CSF analysis reveals high proteins, decreased glucose and polymorphonuclear leucocytosis and culture may identify the species. Methamine Silver stain of direct aspirate or biopsy is useful for identification of Zycomycetes. CT or MRI scan helps in diagnosis and in excluding a mass lesion. Liposomal Amphotericin B is the treatment of choice.[23] Prognosis is usually poor.

Scedosporium spp are seen in survivors of near drowning in polluted water and immunocompromised hosts.[24] The CNS manifestations are usually brain abscess and occasionally meningitis. There are no noninvasive or antigen detection tests. On microscopy, the organism can be confused with Aspergillus or Fusarium spp. but can be distinguished after culture. The drug of choice is Voriconazole.[24] Prognosis is poor and most patients with CNS disease succumb.

MYCOPLASMAL MENINGITIS

Mycoplasma pneumoniae, a primary respiratory pathogen, member of the class Mollicutes, the smallest self replicating organisms capable of free existence, has been shown to cause meningitis. Mycoplasma meningitis may be associated with features of mycoplasma pneumonia that is characterized by gradual onset of headache, malaise, sore throat, hoarseness, cough and pneumonia. Characteristically, coryza is absent. Cough is usually non-productive and symptoms worsen during the first 2 weeks, gradually subsiding over 3-4 weeks. The disease usually occurs in school going children and adolescence and spreads through contact. Diagnosis can be established by culture, high titer of cold agglutinins in blood, four-fold rise in IgM antibody titre and also PCR.

Neurological manifestations or complications are varied and include meningoencephalitis, aseptic meningitis (direct infection), cerebellar ataxia, brainstem syndrome, transverse myelitis, Bell's palsy, deafness, acute demyelinating encephalitis and Guillian-Barré syndrome (immune mediated) and stroke (vascular occlusion). These complications can occur 3-28 days after the respiratory illness, but in about 20% of patients, may occur in the absence of respiratory illness. Encephalitis occurring within 5 days of prodromal symptoms is due to direct infection of the CNS by M. pneumoniae while after 7 days of prodrome is attributable to autoimmune response.

M. pneumonia has been found to be the etiologic agent in 5-15% of all encephalitis. The typical presentation is fever, lethargy and impaired consciousness while seizures, focal motor deficit, ataxia or meningeal signs are less common. Concurrent viral infection is present in one third of patients. Brainstem involvement results in severe dystonia and movement disorders.

CSF is normal or shows mild mononuclear pleocytosis. Positive CSF PCR confirms the diagnosis supported by PCR from throat swab or definitive serum antibody titers. MRI changes reflect the spectrum of neurological involvement–focal ischemic changes, ventriculomegaly diffuse edema or multifocal white matter inflammatory lesions consistent with postinfectious demyelinating encephalomyelitis.

Mycoplasma pneumoniae infection of the CNS is effectively treated with azithromycin.[25-26] For improved CSF penetration, addition of a fluoroquinolone or chloramphenicol may be required. Corticosteroids, intravenous immunoglobin and plasmapheresis play a role in resolution of immune mediated mycoplasma associated CNS disease.

PARASITIC MENINGITIS

Protozoa-Amoeba

A few protozoa are responsible for CNS infection. Naegleria fowleri causes acute primary amebic meningoencephalitis (PAM). Acanthamoeba spp. and Balamuthia mandrillaris produce chronic and opportunistic granulomatous amebic (meningo) encephalitis (GAE). Very recently, Sappinia diploidea has been identified as an agent that causes comparatively acute type of encephalitis.

Primary amoebic meningitis/meningoencephalitis is caused by the ameba Naegleria fowleri. The portal of entry is the nasal cavity when air or water contaminated with trophozoite or cysts of the ameba enters it.[27] The ameba then infects the olfactory nerve and bulb and subsequently spreads to the meninges causing meningitis with fibrinopurulant exudates. It occurs in previously healthy children. The clinical presentation is similar to bacterial and viral meningitis. The disease usually terminates fatally.

Diagnosis is by demonstration of the motile ameba in wet mount of CSF, preferably hanging drop preparation.[28] Naegleria fowleri could be identified by PCR with specific primers on DNA extracted from frozen cerebrospinal fluid samples. As the internal transcribed spacer (ITS1) region of DNA is variable in length, sequencing of the amplified ITS1helps to identify the strain.[29]

Treatment is not very clear. Amphotericin B, rifampicin, chloramphenicol, fluconazole or ketoconazole for 4 weeks were found to be successful. Ventriculoperitoneal shunt may be required for obstructive hydrocephalus.[28]

Granulomatous amebic meningoencephalitis is caused by the amebae acanthamoeba spp. and balamuthia spp. It usually occurs in immunocompromised children. There is widespread meningoencephalitis with clinical features of diffuse parenchymal involvement. Fever, headache, vomiting, ataxia, seizures, hemiparesis, cranial nerve palsies following otitis media is the presentation. Diagnosis is by culture of the protozoa. There is no satisfactory treatment. Flucytosine, sulfadiazine and intravenous pentamidine, fluconazole, ketoconazole, miltefosine and macrolide antibiotics have been shown to be effective in an occasional patient.[30]

Neurocysticercosis is also known to cause meningeal inflammation when it infects the subaracnoid space (subarachnoid cysticerosis) and the ventricles (intraventricular NCC). It is characterised by features of intracranial hypertension, seizures and CSF showing increased protein and pleocytosis, often usually lymphocytic and at times eosinophilic.[31-33]

EOSINOPHILIC MENINGITIS

Eosinophilic meningitis is characterized by 10 or more eosinophils/mm^3 of CSF. The common causes of eosinophilic meningitis are tissue migrating helminthic infections like Angiostrongylus cantonensis, Ascaris lumbricoides, Trichinella spiralis, Toxocara canis, Toxoplasma gondii, Paragonimus westermani, Echinococcus granulosus, Schistosoma japonicum, Onchocerca volvus, and T. Solium. Angiostrongylus cantonensis is the primary cause of human eosinophilic meningitis worldwide. Rarely fungal, viral and bacterial meningitis can have CSF eosiniphilia.

In eosinophilic meningitis due to helminthic infestation, the child becomes unwell about 1-3 weeks after exposure, the time required for parasites to migrate from the GI tract to the CNS. The child can present with fever, vomiting, abdominal pain, creeping skin eruptions or pleurisy. Neurological symptoms include headache, meningismus, paraesthesias, ataxia, cranial nerve palsy and sometimes even paraparesis or incontinence.[34-38] Peripheral and CSF eosinophilia is seen.

Treatment is supportive because the infection is self limited. Antihelminthic drugs do not help but analgesics are useful for headaches. Shunting may be required if hydrocephalus occurs. Prognosis is good with 70% recovering in 2 weeks.

Certain non-infectious disorders also can cause eosinophilic meningitis: malignancy, hypereosinophilic syndrome, reaction to a medication or ventriculoperitoneal shunt, SLE, multiple sclerosis and sarcoidosis.[36] Clinically, these patients may have features related to the primary disorders besides features of meningitis. Peripheral eosiniphilia is common. Investigations will depend on the suspected etiology. Treatment of the meningitis is supportive. Prognosis is good although it depends on the etiology.[34-38]

Summary

Unusual meningitis and other CNS infections are on the rise and a high index of suspicion must be kept while treating children with uncommon, prolonged or difficult-to-treat neurological symptoms.

References

1. Fegin RD, Cherry JD, Demmler GJ, Kaplan SL. Textbook of Pediatric Infectious Disease. Vol 11. 5th Edition. Saunders, Philadelphia 2004;2548-50.
2. Dreizen S. Oral Candidiasis. Am J Med 1984;77:28.
3. Bayer AS, Edweards JE, Jr., Seidel JS, Guze LB. Candida Meningitis. Medicine (Baltimore) 1976:55:477.
4. Johnson DE, Thompson TR, Green TP *et al.* Systemic Candidiasis in Very Low Birth Weight (1500 gms). Pediatrics 1984;73:138.
5. Ericson J, Smith BP, Benjamin DK Jr. Candida. In: Nelson Textbook of Pediatrics 20th Edition. Kliegman RM, Stanton BF, St Geme JW, Schor NF (eds.) New Delhi, Reed Elsevier India 2016:1515-18.
6. Pappas PG, Kauffman CA, Andes D *et al.* Clinical Practice Guidelines for the Management of Candidiasis: 2009 Update by the Infectious Diseases Society of America. Clin Infect Dis 2009;48:503-35.
7. Hong XY, Chou YC, Lazareff JA. Brain Stem Candidiasis Mimicking Cerebellopontine Angle Tumor. Surg Neurol 2008;70:87-91.

8. Lindsley MD, Mekha N, Bagget HC, *et al.* Evaluation of a Newly Developed Lateral Flow Immunoassay for the Diagnosis of Cryptococcosis. Clin Infect Dis 2011:53:321-25.

9. Gould JM, Arnoff SC. Cryptococcus Neoformans. In: Nelson Textbook of Pediatrics, 20th Edition, Kliegman RM, Stanton BF, St Geme JW, Schor NF (eds.) New Delhi, Reed Elsevier India 2016:1518-20.

10. Leggiadro RJ, Barret FF, Hughes WT. Extrapulmonary Cryptococcosis in Immunocompromised Infants and Children. Pediatr Infect J 1992;11:43-47.

11. Abadi J, Nachman S, Kressel AB, Pirofski LA. Cryptococcosis in Children with AIDS. Clin Infec Dis 1999:28:309-13.

12. Perfect JR, Dismukes WF, Dromer F, *et al.* Clinical Practice Guidelines for the Management of Cryptococcal Disease: 2010 Update by the Infectious Diseases Society of America. Clin Infect Dis 2010:50:291-322.

13. Graybill JR, Sobel J, Saag M, *et al.* Diagnosis and Management of Increased Intracranial Pressure in Patients with AIDS and Cryptococcal Meningitis. Clin Infect Dis 2000:30:47-54.

14. Galgiani JN. Coccodioidomycosis. West Med J 1993:159: 153-17.

15. Kleigman MB. Coccodioides immitis (Coccodioidomycosis). In: Principles and Practice of Pediatric Infectious Disease, 2nd Edition, Long SS, Pickering LK, Prober CG (Eds). Churchill Livingstone 2003:1246-52.

16. Kleiman MB. Coccidioidomycosis. In: Nelson Textbook of Pediatrics 20th Edition, Kliegman RM, Stanton BF, St Geme JW, Schor NF (eds.) New Delhi, Reed Elsevier India 2016;1529-32.

17. Odio CM, Navarrete M, Carrilo JM *et al.* Disseminated Histoplasmosis in Infants. Pediatrics Infect Dis J 1999;18: 1065-68.

18. Pereira GH, Padua SS, Park MV, *et al.* Chronic Meningitis by Histoplasmosis: Report of a Child with Acute Myeloid Leukemia. Braz J Infect Dis 2008:12:555-57.

19. Bariola JR, Perry P, Pappas PG, *et al.* Blastomycosis of the Central Nervous System: A Multicenter Review of Diagnosis and Treatment in the Modern Era. Clin Infect Dis 2010;50: 797-804.

20. Yogev R, Davis T. Blastomycosis in Children: A Review of Literature. Mycopathologica 1999;28:139-43.

21. Traunmuller F, Popovic M, Konz KH, *et al.* Efficacy and Safety of Current Drug Therapies for Invasive Aspergillosis. Pharmacology 2011;88:213-24.

22. Amador JT, Guillen Martin S, Prieto Tato L. Why Might Micafungin be the Drug of Choice in Paediatric Patients? Enferm Infec Microbiol Clin 2011:29 (Suppl 2):23-28.

23. Spellberg B, Walsh TJ, Kontoyiannis DP, *et al.* Recent Advances in the Management of Mucormycosis: From Bench to Bedside. Clin Infect Dis 2009;48:1743-51.

24. Katragkou A, Dotis J, Kotsiou M, *et al.* Scedosporium Apiospermum Infection After Near Drowning. Mycoses 2007; 50:412-21.

25. Mejias A, Ramilo O. Mycoplasma Pneumoniae. In: Nelson Textbook of Pediatrics, 20th Edition, Kliegman RM, Stanton BF, St Geme JW, Schor NF (eds.), New Delhi, Reed Elsevier India 2016:1487-90.

26. Lind K, Zoffmann H, Larsen SO, Jessen O. Mycoplasma Pneumoniae Infection Associated with Infection of the Central Nervous System. Acta Med Scand 1979:205:325-32.

27. Eberly MD, Weisse ME. Primary Amebic Meningoencephalitis. In: Nelson Textbook of Pediatrics, 20th Edition, Kliegman RM, Stanton BF, St Geme JW, Schor NF (eds.), New Delhi, Reed Elsevier India 2016;1688-92.

28. Yadav D, Aneja S, Dutta R, Maheshwari A, Seth A. Youngest Survivor of Naegleria Meningitis. Indian J Pediatr 2013 March:80(3):253-54. doi: 10.1007/s12098-012-0756-2.Epub 2012 April 28.

29. Nicolas M, De Jonckheere JF, Pernin P, *et al.* Molecular Diagnosis of a Fatal Primary Amoebic Meningoencephalitis in Guadeloupe (French West Indies). Bull Soc Pathol Exot 2010 February;103(1):14-18. doi: 10.1007/s13149-009-0028-1. Epub 2010 January 22.

30. Cuevas PM, Smoje PG, Jofré ML, *et al.* Granulomatous Amoebic Meningoencephalitis by Balamuthia Mandrillaris: Case Report and Literature Review. Rev Chilena Infectol 2006 September;23(3):237-42. Epub 2006 August 4.

31. Flisser A. Larval Cestodes. In: Topley & Wilson's Microbiology and Microbial Infections, Vol. V (Parasitology), 9th Edition, 1998, Cox FEG, Krier JP, Wakelin D (Eds.), Arnold, London 539-60.

32. Garcia LS. Intestinal Cestodes 363-385, T. solium 368-377, Diagnostic Medical Parasitology, 4th Edition, ASM Press, Washington DC, 2001.

33. Lopez-Hernandez A, Garazier C. Manifestations of Infantile Cerebral Cysticercosis. In: Palacios E, Rodriguez-Carbazal J, Taveras JM, eds. Cysticercois of the Central Nervous System. Springfield, 111, Charles C Thomas 1983:69-83.

34. Hollister D, Clements M, Coleman M, Petilo F. Eosiniphilic Meningitis in Hodgkin's Disease. Ann Int Med 1983;143: 590-92.

35. Wiengarten JS, O'Sheal SF, Margolis WS. Eosinophilic Meningitis and Hypereosinophilic Syndrome. Am J Med 1985;78:674-76.

36. Vinchon M, Vallee L, Prin L, *et al.* Cerebrospinal Fluid Eosinophilia in Shunt Infection. Neuripaediatrics 1992;23: 235-40.

37. Weller PF. Eosinophilic Meningitis. Am J Med 1993;95: 250-53.

38. Prober CG, Srinivas NS. Eosinophilic Meningitis. In: Nelson Textbook of Pediatrics, 20th Edition, Kliegman RM, Stanton BF, St Geme JW, Schor NF (eds.) New Delhi, Reed Elsevier India 2016:2948.

39 Chapter

ACUTE VIRAL ENCEPHALITIS

Bibek Talukdar, Medha Mittal

Acute viral encephalitis, inflammation of the brain parenchyma due to invasion by viruses, is one of the most serious CNS infections of childhood. Difficulty in establishing the etiologic diagnosis specially in developing countries, unpredictable course, significant mortality and sequelae and virtual absence of specific treatment have made it a disease of serious nature. The overall outcome remains poor in developing countries, mostly related to management issues. Viral encephalitis can be acute, subacute and chronic. Acute viral encephalitis is the most common form encountered in clinical practice in India.

EPIDEMIOLOGY, ETIOPATHOGENESIS AND PATHOLOGY

Viruses causing acute encephalitis shows wide *regional variation* probably depending upon type of vector and climate. Based on western literature, the incidence seems to be approximately 10.5-13.8 per 100000 children; this may however be quite an underestimation mainly due to difficulty in confirming the etiology. *Seasonal variation* is seen with some viruses like adenovirus and arbovirus occurring more commonly in summer (when insect vectors are most active), enterovirus in summer and fall, mumps in late winter and spring and lymphocytic choriomeningitis virus in winter. Herpes virus group on the other hand does not show significant seasonal variation. Host's *immune status* is also an important factor in the occurrence of viral infections, maximum susceptibility is shown by infants and young children between the age group of 6 months and 5 years.[1-4]

Large number of viruses causes acute encephalitis.[1-6] The viruses that have *been well documented* to cause acute encephalitis in children worldwide are shown in the Inset 39.1.

Inset 39.1: Viruses Causing Encephalitis in Children

**Arboviruses* namely eastern, western and Venezuelan equine encephalitis viruses, St. Louis encephalitis virus, California encephalitis virus, west nile virus, Colorado tick fever virus, Powassan encephalitis, Japanese encephalitis virus (JE) and dengue virus, **Herpesviruses* namely herpes simplex virus (HSV), type I and type II, human herpesvirus type 6 (HSV 6), human herpesvirus type 7 (HSV type 7), varicella zoster virus (VZV), **cytomegalovirus* and **Epstein Bar virus*, **Enteroviruses* namely polio, coxsakie, echo, enterovirus 70, enterovirus 71, **Mixoviruses* namely influenza, parainfluenza, measles, mumps, **Adenoviruses*, *Rubella*, *Rhabdoviruses* like Chandipura and other less common ones, i.e., **Nipah*, **Lymphocytic choriomeningitis* virus and *Polyomavirus.

Because of technical difficulties in confirming the diagnosis, only a few viruses causing encephalitis in children in India have been documented, mostly in hospital-based studies. These are Herpes simplex virus (HSV 1), varicella zoster virus, Japanese encephalitis virus (JE), Adenoviruses, Enteroviruses, ECHO viruses, Coxsackie, Mumps, Ebstein Bar virus, Chandipura, Papovirus, Dengue and Nipah.[7-32] Viral etiology in these cases has been established based on isolation of viruses in some and PCR and other serologic methods in others. HSV1 seems to be the most commonly occurring one, followed by adenovirus and JE. These viruses have been causing sporadic outbreaks in different parts of the country. Such outbreaks have been common with JE,[16,21,22,26,27] enteroviruses,[10,13] Chandipura,[12,13] ECHO[28] and measles.[19] Viruses commonly reported in non-endemic times in hospital-based studies are HSV, JE, Enterovirus, Coxsackie, ECHO, measles and mumps.

Viruses are obligate intracellular parasite. Infection of the body by a virus involves adsorption/attachment to the host's cell membrane, penetration into the cell, virus uncoating, replication of viral nucleic acid and production of viral protein, virus assembly, production of virion or mature virus particle and finally the spread. Initial attachment and replication of the virus occurs at the mucosal surfaces of the skin, conjunctiva, gut, respiratory tract and urinary tract from where they spread to the regional lymph nodes. The initial or primary replication of the virus depends on permissiveness of the host's cell.[1,2,3,4]

The usual mode of spread is through the hematogenous route. After the primary replication, viraemia occurs in the susceptible host resulting in dissemination of the virus to other organs and tissues. Secondary replication occurs in these tissues that intensifies the infection. Spread through neural route (retrograde axonal transport) occurs in cases of herpes (HSV and VZV) and rabies viruses; it starts with infection of the peripheral nerve endings that spreads, along the nerve, to the spinal cord and finally reaching the brain through infection of the spinal neurons. Once neurons are affected antegrade transmission also can occur. Viruses exhibit variable neurotropism and neurovirulence that have important role in pathogenesis. Host factors like age, sex and genetic differences are also important in pathogenesis.[1,2,3,4]

Infection of the body by a virus is associated with marked immune response. IgM antibodies usually appear within 2 weeks of infection. IgG antibodies usually appear within 2-6 weeks of infection peaking around 8 weeks.[2] Cell mediated immunity also becomes active soon after the infection and parallels the humoral response. The salient features of cell mediated immunity are activation of cytotoxic T lymphocytes (CTLs), natural killer cells (NK) and macrophages. The alternate complement pathway is also activated in certain viral infections. These immune responses are ultimately aimed at neutralization of the virus particles. Viral infection is also associated with the production of interferon which inhibits virus multiplication. Numerous other complex immune responses take place, all aimed at virus elimination. Sometimes these immune responses result in adverse consequences; the intense reaction may result in destruction of the host's own cells.[1,2,3,4]

The pathology in viral encephalitis depends upon neurotropism and neurovirulence of the viruses that are extremely variable, and some features are unique to certain virus; however, many of features are common like cellular infiltration especially mononuclear, cell lysis and phagocytosis by macrophages and occasional cellular inclusions in neurons and glial cells. Pathologically, the brain often becomes edematous, although can be normal at times, on macroscopic examination. Important microscopic features are lymphocytic infiltration of the leptomeninges, mononuclear cell infiltration of the brain parenchyma, perivascular cuffing, infarcts, necrosis, and microglial nodule formation. Punctate hemorrhage can also be seen. These changes may be focal or diffuse. Electron microscopic examination may show virus particles. Severity of the pathology depends on the virulence of the virus, host response and the intensity of the immunologic reactions. Viruses at times show predilection for specific areas of brain, i.e., arboviruses tend to affect the whole brain while HSV frequently affects the temporal lobe. Marked demyelination involving the oligodendrocytes with preservation of the neurons and axons is frequently seen in post and parainfectious encephalitides. There may be involvement of the meninges and also the spinal cord with or without involvement of the peripheral nerves.[1,2,3,4]

CLINICAL FEATURES

The most common presenting features of acute viral encephalitis are *fever, altered sensorium and seizures*. The clinical picture is very similar practically in all cases irrespective of the viral etiology. The disease is often preceded by a prodrome of varying severity that is followed by the florid symptomatology.[5,6]

Prodrome or Antecedent Illness

Encephalitis usually occurs during the course of a systemic viral infection. The prodrome consists of certain features suggestive of a systemic viral illness like fever, cough, coryza, sleepiness, headache, myalgia, vomiting, loose motions, decreased appetite, conjunctivitis, rash photophobia and mumps. After an interval of 3-7 days (maximum of 4 weeks) in most cases, the encephalitic symptoms start manifesting. About 2% of cases do not have such antecedent illness, but present straight away with symptoms of encephalitis.[4,5]

SYMPTOM AND SIGNS

The mode of presentation is acute in the majority of cases. It can however be insidious in some.

Fever is common and is present in almost all the cases. The fever is often intermittent and irregular. It may be associated with chills; hyperpyrexia may occur.

Cerebral parenchymal involvement: Fever is soon followed by a wide variety of symptoms and signs pointing towards *cerebral parenchymal involvement* that may be *diffuse* or *focal*. The features of cerebral parenchymal involvement are the hallmarks of acute viral encephalitis.

Diffuse cerebral involvement is usually manifested by altered sensorium, convulsion, vomiting, headache, photophobia, abnormal movements, abnormal respiration, behaviour disturbances, signs of raised intracranial pressure, neck stiffness and altered tone and reflexes.[1-6] *Altered sensorium*, the most important feature of encephalitis, indicates inflammation of brain parenchyma with or without raised intracranial pressure; it is characterized by irritability, agitation, confusion, screaming spells, drowsiness, delirium, stupor and/or coma. Infants usually show excessive and/or intermittent crying. *Seizures and convulsions* are usually generalized; status can occur in about 50% of case. *Abnormal movements* may take the form of bizarre movement of the body, ataxia, tremor and decerebrate and dystonic postures. Respiration may be irregular, and hyperventilation can occur. *Altered behaviour* occurs in the form of changes in mood, hallucinations, apathy, aggressiveness, shrill cry, emotional outbursts and staring spells. *Raised intracranial* pressure is suggested by rapid deterioration in consciousness, frequent seizures, bulging fontanelle in infants, decerebration, respiratory abnormality, pupillary abnormalities and sometimes papilledema in older children. Headache is often complained of by older children. *Neck stiffness* is observed in a small proportion of children because of associated meningeal reaction. *Tone and reflexes* are variable, plantar reflex is mostly extensor. There may be loss of *bladder and bowel* control.

Focal cerebral involvement is manifested commonly by *cranial nerve palsies*, hemiplegia, monoplegia and aphasia. HSV encephalitis, that has a predilection for the temporal lobe, is often associated with focal neurological signs and features of *temporal lobe involvement* like visual and auditory hallucination, abnormal behaviour and aphasia. *Brainstem involvement*, commonly associated with entro-flavi-alpha viruses, results in 'brainstem encephalitis' manifested by respiratory irregularity, vasomotor instability, autonomic dysfunction, lower cranial nerve palsies, myoclonus, bulbar and pseudobulbar palsies and locked-in syndrome. *Cerebellar involvement*, manifested primarily by ataxia, nystagmus and incoordination, is often associated with coxsackie virus infection. *Hypothalamic disturbances* can occur resulting in abnormal temperature control and fluid and electrolyte disturbance.

Non-CNS features like vomiting, diarrhea, respiratory difficulty, are also commonly seen. *Exanthems* are common with several viruses like coxsackie, echo, varicella-zoster, measles and rubella.

The ***severity of illness and subsequent course*** varies widely and often unpredictable. Some cases present as mild encephalitis and progress rapidly to coma and death; others presenting apparently as severe encephalitis with marked sensorial changes and decerebration recover within a short time with minimal sequelae. Some patients continue to remain in coma for prolonged period and ultimately show remarkable recovery or develop severe sequelae. Majority however continue to be ill for quite some time showing diffuse and/or focal cerebral features that keep fluctuating finally recovering with or without sequelae.

In a study of confirmed acute viral encephalitis in children by Wong *et al.*,[5] the important clinical features observed were signs of cerebral involvement (100%), convulsions (30%), focal neurological deficit (33%), headache (5%), drowsiness (18%), neck rigidity (10%), behavioural changes (9%), coma (9%) and hallucination (1%).

DIAGNOSIS

Once the acute viral encephalitis is suspected in a case after detailed history and physical examination, a careful **plane of work up** should be made with the objectives of confirming the diagnosis and picking up problems that may help in management. This should include:

1. Establishing cerebral parenchymal infection – CSF examination, routine (macroscopy, smear, cell counts, sugar and protein, chloride and culture).
2. Establishing the viral etiology – Appropriate virologic study in CSF, blood and other tissue; discussion with microbiologist / virologist wherever possible is useful.
3. Investigations useful as an adjunct to diagnosis acute viral infection – Hemogram with CBC and PS. Inflammatory markers like ESR, CRP, procalcitonin should be done whenever possible (in acute viral encephalitis values are usually normal).
4. Investigations useful in maintaining body homeostasis and management of complications – Blood sugar, electrolytes, blood osmolality, LFT, KFT and coagulogram.
5. Investigations aiding in diagnosis of cerebral parenchymal involvement – Imaging studies, EEG.
6. Investigations needed to exclude conditions mimicking acute viral encephalitis, guided by clinical suspicion (differential diagnosis), i.e., PS and/or serology for malaria.

Clinical Evaluation

Detailed history and good clinical examination remain the mainstay of diagnosis of acute viral encephalitis. As detailed above, the important features should be looked for in each and every case. The most important clinical pointers to diagnosis are fever and features of encephalopathy. The most important features of encephalopathy are altered sensorium of varying grade and seizures. In some cases, however, even detailed investigation may remain non-contributory, and diagnosis basically remains clinical.

Certain clinical features can give *clue to the etiology* and should be looked for in every case, these are shown in Inset 39.2.

Inset 39.2: Clinical Clues to Viral Etiology in Acute Viral Encephalitis
*History of travel (encephalitis prevalent in the area), *Travel and exposure to ticks, insects and mosquitoes (arbovirus, tickborne encephalitis), *Preceding rash (measles, mumps, rubella, varicella), *Accompanying rash (coxsackie, echo, varicella, enterovirus), *Kerato-conjunctivitis (adenovirus, enterovirus 71), cold and cough (respiratory viruses), *Gastroenteritis (enterovirus), *Parotitis and orchitis (mumps), *Dog bite (rabies), *History of measles, mumps, influenza in the family and/or around (encephalitis due to these viruses), *Fever and rash in the family and around (varicella, roseola, enterovirus), *Retinitis (toxoplasma, rubella, CMV), *Hemorrhage (enterovirus 70), *Features of hand-foot-mouth disease (enterovirus 70), *Flaccid paralysis (tickborne encephalitis)

CSF Examination

The CSF in viral encephalitis usually shows predominantly lymphocytic pleocytosis, moderately increased protein and normal sugar. Smear examination is negative for bacteria and routine culture is sterile. Sugar may however be low, on occasion, in mumps encephalitis and also in HSV encephalitis. Early in the course of illness in viral encephalitis, the CSF sometimes may show predominantly polymorphonuclear response. In such a situation a repeat CSF after 24-48 hours usually shows reversal of the cellular response to predominantly lymphocytic. CSF abnormalities are diagnostic of inflammation of brain parenchyma and meninges; it helps in excluding a wide variety of encephalopathies where CSF is usually normal. *CSF examination is thus vital for diagnosis of acute viral encephalitis.* CSF however can be normal early in the course of the illness; a repeat examination after 24-48 hours usually shows the usual findings of viral encephalitis.

Before doing LP, the time-tested precautions must be taken. Contraindications to LP are raised ICP (suggested by papilledema, increasing stupor progressing to coma, deteriorating consciousness, neurogenic shock), too sick child with cardio-respiratory embarrassment/compromise, shock, bleeding disorder, local infection at LP site etc. If raised ICP is suspected, imaging should be done before LP. It is extremely important to keep in mind that LP in a child with raised ICP may precipitate herniation sudden death. Imaging however may not always detect raised ICP accurately, clinical signs must also be considered for the diagnosis. Imaging features of raised ICP are: cerebral edema, chinked ventricles, tight basal cisterns and midline shift. If LP cannot be done due to poor general condition of the child, it should be done at the earliest possible time once the child is stabilized.[33-35]

Routine examination of CSF should be done as quickly as possible after collection of the sample. CSF samples should be preserved for virologic study.

Virological Studies

Confirmed etiologic diagnosis of acute viral encephalitis is possible only by *isolation of virus* through tissue culture of brain tissue obtained by brain biopsy that is however not always possible and also not needed in most cases now-a-days as there are good newer diagnostic techniques. Virus isolation is commonly done using CSF in mouse model. Molecular diagnosis is the mainstay for finding the etiology.[36] Molecular diagnostic tests are based primarily on (a) *antigen detection* like PCR, RTPCR and DNA probe and (b) *antibody detection* like variety of serologic tests for detection of IgM and IgG antibodies. Properly done, these tests have virtually replaced brain biopsy. These tests that can give the diagnosis relatively early, are of extreme clinical importance since it can lend great help in acute management as in cases of HSV encephalitis for which there is a specific treatment the early institution of which is related to improved outcome. *Demonstration of virus particles* using electron microscopy in appropriate body tissue or fluid is also useful. Virologic studies thus usually involve viral culture, electron microscopy, histology, antigen detection tests and antibody detection tests.[1-4] The antigen detection tests are commonly done in CSF and blood and can be done in other appropriate tissues.

Polymerase chain reaction (PCR) that detects the viral genome has revolutionized the etiologic diagnosis of acute viral encephalitis. PCR has been shown to be extremely useful in diagnose of HSV and enterovirus infections, two very common causes of encephalitis in children. PCR has also been useful in the diagnosis of certain other viruses like VZV, EBV, CMV and some arboviruses. The spectrum is growing. Currently PCR/RTPCR are most widely used diagnostic tests in acute viral encephalitis.[1-4]

With PCR diagnosis can be obtained within about 48 hours depending on the viral load in the sample.

The high sensitivity (75-95%) and specificity (100%) of PCR for detection of HSV infection has virtually eliminated the need for brain biopsy to confirm the diagnosis of HSV encephalitis. CSF PCR has High sensitivity and specificity for HSV > 95% in adult.[35] It can however be negative in the first few days of illness.[35] Negative results thus need to be interpreted carefully in the context of the patient's clinical presentation and the timing of the CSF sampling.

Antibody detection like IgM and IgG, are commonly done using different tests like ELIZA, compliment fixation, hemagglutination inhibition, immunofluorescence, radio-immunoassay, latex agglutination, and immunoperoxidase. IgM has been extremely useful in diagnosis of encephalitis due to HSV, JE, Nipah and measles viruses.

Serologic methods provide a relatively easy alternative for diagnosis of viral infection, although the evidence obtained is indirect and often retrospective. IgM antibody appears within 2 weeks of infection and IgG antibody appears later, peaking around 8 weeks. Detection of IgM antibody is more important for early and specific diagnosis. Recent infection with a viral pathogen is strongly supported by detection of virus specific IgM, seroconversion or a fourfold rise in IgG antibody titre.[1-4]

Tests in other body tissues and fluid: PCR in throat swab, nasopharyngeal aspirate, rectal swab, feces, urine samples are done for certain viruses like enterovirus, adenovirus, influenza, measles. Tissue smear and EM is useful in varicella infection. Isolation of virus or positive serologic tests in tissues other than brain tissue or CSF are also considered to be the etiology of the encephalitis, in presence of clinical symptoms, signs and other positive investigative findings.[1-4]

Specimen for virologic studies: For virologic studies specimens of body tissues, body fluids and other tissue fluids and/or whole blood is needed. Sampling of specimens may be determined according to clinical suspicion, i.e., *for HSV* (scrapings of mucocutaneous lesions, blood, CSF, brain tissue obtained by biopsy), *for adenovirus* (respiratory secretions, urine, feces), *for enterovirus* (oral secretions, CSF, feces), *for influenza virus* (oral secretions), *for arbovirus* (blood and brain tissue), *for measles* (oral secretions), *for rubella* (CSF, urine, oral secretions), and *for varicella* (scrapings of cutaneous lesion, CSF). When etiology is uncertain, specimens of whole blood, CSF, urine, feces, and throat washings should be sent. Proper collection, storage and transport of specimens are extremely important and should be carried out in consultation with the reference laboratory. Tissues are usually collected without preservative. Specimens obtained within the first 72 hours of illness are more likely to yield a viral pathogen than specimens obtained later. For serologic studies two serum samples are needed, acute serum (at the beginning of illness/hospitalization) and convalescent serum (after at least 2-3 weeks).[1-4]

Other Laboratory Investigations

Several other investigations are useful in diagnosis and in basic supportive management.

Routine examination blood: Blood counts in acute viral encephalitis usually show lymphocytic pleocytosis. Routine blood culture also should be taken for any unidentified system in bacterial infection.

Blood glucose, serum electrolytes, blood osmolality, blood urea and creatinine, liver function tests: These are essential in initial stabilization and management of complications.

Inflammatory markers: Acute inflammatory markers like ESR, CRP, procalcitonin, whatever is possible should also be done to rule out bacterial infections. Whenever possible, CSF lactate may be done; CSF lactate has been shown to be useful in excluding bacterial meningitis where it is high. CSF lactate < 2 mmol/l is said to exclude bacterial meningitis.[35]

Neuroimaging

Neuroimaging modalities like CT scan and MRI has been shown to provide information about infection induced damages and changes in the brain parenchyma that is helpful in management.[37-42] Imaging is also extremely useful in detecting raised intracranial pressure (ICP). Diffuse cerebral edema is a frequent finding. Focal abnormalities involving the temporal lobe and sometimes the inferior frontal lobe and insula have been found to be common in HSV encephalitis and are considered as good supportive evidence of HSV encephalitis. The usual abnormalities found on imaging are low attenuating lesions with or without contrast enhancement in temporal lobe and areas of increased signal in mesial temporal lobe. On radionuclide brain scan areas of increased uptake in temporal lobe commonly seen in patients with HSV encephalitis.[43] FLAIR sequence of MRI has been shown to be better for localizing the infection in HSV encephalitis. Involvement of basal ganglia, brainstem and thalamus has been reported in JE and also in Eastern equine encephalitis. Generalized parenchymal involvement can be seen in enteroviral infection. Compared to CT scan MRI is more advantageous as it is more sensitive to changes in brain water content alterations, detects the changes earlier, detects the extent of changes better, is more sensitive to demyelination and does not produce confusing bony artefacts. CT however is quite useful in emergency because of easy availability. Imaging findings can however be non-specific in many cases.

Imaging modalities also are valuable in differential diagnosis of viral encephalitis. It is helpful in differentiating acute viral encephalitis from conditions having similarity in clinical picture like bacterial and tuberculous meningitis. These techniques also help in excluding unexpected focal or other structural lesions that may have encephalitis like presentation like brain abscess, brain tumour, stroke, intracranial hemorrhage, acute demyelinating encephalomyelitis (ADEM), acute hemorrhagic leukoencephalopathy. In cases presenting with coma at emergency, where acute viral encephalitis is suspected, imaging can give useful clues to diagnosis of conditions mentioned above. Thus, we feel, imaging, specially MRI, is indicated in all cases of clinically suspected acute viral encephalitis.

EEG

EEG usually shows diffuse/generalized slowing with or without discharges suggestive of diffuse parenchymal disease and although non-specific this may be helpful in differentiating other conditions mentioned above. Focal slowing, with or without epileptiform discharges, over the temporal lobe, periodic lateralized discharges (PLDs) in the temporal lobe, sometimes over the frontal lobe is highly suggestive of HSV encephalitis.[44] Sensitivity and specificity of EEG in diagnosis of HSV encephalitis is modest. EEG is also helpful in diagnosis and management of seizure in these cases. EEG is also the only tool to diagnose non-convulsive status epilepticus that can be present during the illness that needs proper management.[35]

DIFFERENTIAL DIAGNOSIS

Some diseases may mimic viral encephalitis closely; common ones that we see in our setup are *acute bacterial meningitis* (ABM), *tuberculous meningitis*, and *fungal meningitis (in infants and immunocompromised cases), cerebral malaria, brain abscess, occasional case of dengue, occasional case of stroke, acute demyelinating encephalomyelitis* (ADEM), *complex febrile seizure, status epilepticus precipitated by fever, autoimmune antibody mediated encephalitis, certain neurometabolic disorders and occasional toxic disorders*. These disorders, if associated with coma besides fever as is seen quite often, can be confounding and needs to be excluded carefully. All these disorders have typical clinical picture and most of these disorders can be easily differentiated through good history, physical examination and appropriate investigation.

TREATMENT

Except acyclovir for herpesvirus, treatment is basically supportive. Some cases of viral encephalitis are relatively mild and can be treated well with antipyretics, analgesics, and maintenance of hydration. Others, especially the severe cases, are a challenge to our health care system; they can present with variety of homeostatic disturbances and complications, some of which can be life threatening. Treatment is primarily directed at supporting the vital functions and treating the acute complications. Circulatory and respiratory functions need utmost attention. The acute complications that are frequently seen and need urgent attention are cerebral edema, seizures, airway obstruction, hyperpyrexia, fluid, electrolyte, and acid-base disturbances, DIC and cardio-respiratory arrest.

Initial Empirical Therapy

Acute viral encephalitis is an emergency condition and bacterial infection of the CNS, specially ABM, is often difficult to rule out at presentation in the hospital, missing the diagnosis of which may seriously compromise the outcome. That is why antibiotic for ABM, usually ceftriaxone is started in all cases till it is ruled out. Cerebral malaria is another similar condition; we start its treatment if strongly suspected pending confirmation. We feel, in areas with high incidence of malaria antimalarial drugs should be started.

Specific Therapy

Specific therapy is available only for HSV encephalitis and the drug is acyclovir.[35,45,46] Acyclovir is a purine analogue that inhibits virus replication by inhibiting viral DNA polymerase. Patients showing features suggestive of HSV encephalitis, i.e., focal neurological signs, focal abnormalities on neuroimaging and EEG as mentioned already, are put on acyclovir while waiting for the confirmed diagnosis as HSV encephalitis is a life-threatening form of encephalitis, is the only form of viral encephalitis having specific drug therapy and is a very common form of viral encephalitis. The drug has proved to be reasonably safe and effective over time.

HSV being the most common and treatable form of acute viral encephalitis, currently it is recommended that acyclovir should be started in all cases of viral encephalitis[35] irrespective of the cause pending confirmation.

Children with proven or strongly suspected HSV encephalitis should be treated with acyclovir, 10 mg/kg/8 hourly, each dose infused intravenously over a period of one hour. The recommended dose for children 3 months 12 years is 500 mg/sqm 8 hourly. Acyclovir should be continued for 14-21 days,[35] as a high rate of relapse, upto about 29% has been shown to occur if used for a duration of < 14 days.

Treatment with acyclovir should be started as early as possible, preferably > 6 hours. It is most effective when started early. *The outcome has been shown to be influenced by age, level of consciousness at presentation and duration of illness before presentation, it is poor with younger age, Glasgow coma score less than 6, and duration of illness more than 4 days.*[47,48] After completion of therapy, repeat CSF PCR can confirm the elimination of replicating virus, aiding further in management.

HSV PCR has been used to monitor the treatment. If HSV PCR/antigen detection test is positive treatment is continued for 14-21 days guided by the clinical course. Many like to continue acyclovir till HSV PCR is negative. If initial test is negative but HSV is strongly suspected, test is repeated. Duration of treatment also can be guided by PCR.[35]

While on acyclovir, the patient should be monitored for side effects. The drug is excreted through kidney and can cause crystalluria and obstructive nephropathy leading to renal impairment. The dose of acyclovir should be reduced in patients with pre-existing renal impairment. Other rare adverse events include hepatitis, bone marrow failure and encephalopathy.

Acyclovir has also been used for VZV encephalitis although it is less sensitive compared to HSV encephalitis. The dose suggested is 15 mg/kg/dose 8 hourly for children >12 years of age and 500 mg/sq m 8 hourly for 10 days.

Few other drugs are undergoing trials in other forms of viral encephalitis, but their efficacy is yet to be proved beyond doubt although they appear to be promising; these are pleconaril for enteroviruses, amantadine or rimantadine for influenza A virus, and oseltamivir for influenza B virus.

Supportive Treatment

Baseline Data and Monitoring: Intensive monitoring is vital for proper management of acute viral encephalitis that is frequently beset with complications. After admission, intravenous line should be started and blood samples collected for hemogram and CBC, PS, electrolytes, sugar, calcium and blood gas and also blood culture. A monitoring chart should be made incorporating important clinical and biochemical data. The clinical parameters for monitoring should include vital signs (pulse, BP, temperature and respiration), sensorium, tone, reflexes, any focal deficit, appearance of new signs, intake and output. Biochemical parameters for monitoring should include reports of serum electrolyte, serum calcium, blood sugar, and acid-base status. Clinical parameters should be monitored everyday and frequently according to the condition of the patient. Biochemical parameters also need to be monitored frequently in the early stage. Such monitoring helps in early detection of complications and prompt treatment that should influence the outcome.

Fluid and Electrolyte Balance: All cases should be put on intravenous fluid therapy at the initial stage. Any dehydration present should be corrected. The 24 hours maintenance fluid is usually reduced to 2/3rd of the normal in presence of cerebral oedema. In children it is often difficult to exclude the presence of cerebral oedema in the acute stage and restricted fluid is usually prescribed for all such cases in this stage. Dextrose saline with supplemental potassium is commonly used for the maintenance fluid therapy. So long the child is on I.V. fluid, daily electrolyte estimations is essential for detection of abnormalities of sodium and potassium. The status of hydration should be checked frequently besides the intake and output. It is important to keep in mind that overloading the circulation will aggravate cerebral oedema and dehydration will compromise cerebral perfusion. The amount of fluid and electrolyte administered daily should thus be guided by the status of hydration, cerebral oedema, and disturbance in electrolytes. SIADH can occur and should be treated promptly.

Acid Base Disturbance: Acidosis can aggravate cerebral edema by causing cerebral vasodilation. Cerebral edema can itself lead to acid-base disturbance by compromising the function of the vital centers; alkalosis from hyperventilation is common. Effort should be made to maintain a normal acid-base status. Blood gas should be repeated in the acute stage at least once a day or as warranted by cardio-respiratory status or special circumstances like treatment of cerebral edema.

Cerebral Edema and Intracranial Hypertension: Cerebral edema is the most important cause of raised intracranial pressure (ICP) and is probably the most important and serious complication of viral encephalitis that demands urgent treatment.[34-36] Many cases in acute stage do have cerebral edema. Monitoring for raised ICP is extremely important, and it should be done using the clinical signs mentioned under clinical features. Common measures used to treat cerebral edema and raised ICP are: (i) raising the head approximately to 30° or above the level of the heart; (ii) restriction of I.V. fluid to 2/3rd of maintenance, this however should be for a short period; (iii) intravenous infusion of 20% mannitol, 0.25-0.5 g/kg over 20-30 mins; (iv) administration of furosemide, 1-3 mg/kg/dose I.V.; and (v) mild hyperventilation, manually by bag and mask or through endotracheal intubation, to maintain the PaCO between 25-30 mm of Hg. and (vi) mechanical ventilation if needed to keep the PaO_2 at 30-35 mm Hg.

Hyperventilation is a quick and effective way of reducing raised ICP in bed side, however, it should not be too aggressive as it may result in cerebral ischemia. Mannitol, the commonly used agent for reducing ICP, can be repeated 2-3 times if the situation demands. After about 72 hours, its effects start waning because of rebound phenomena and the drug should not be continued further. If some cerebral edema persists oral administration of glycerol 0.5-1 ml/kg/dose 8 hourly and/or acetazolamide 50 mg/kg/day is often started although their efficacy is unclear. Presently hypertonic saline, i.e., 3% sodium chloride, has been shown to be beneficial in managing intracranial hypertension. Complications can however occur and needs constant monitoring of electrolytes and ICP.

The various measures to reduce ICP can give rise to several complications. Mannitol and furosemide use can lead to fluid and electrolyte disturbances like dehydration, hyponatremia and hypokalemia; vigorous hyperventilation can cause depressed cardiac output and acetazolamide use can cause acidosis. Close monitoring of fluid, electrolyte and acid-base status are therefore essential during treatment of raised ICP.

In difficult cases not responding to treatment, invasive intracranial pressure monitoring is indicated that needs ICU setup and neurosurgical facilities. Here more aggressive measures for monitoring and reduction of raised ICP can be initiated like ventricular drainage of CSF, ICP monitoring using different techniques like subdural screw; these measures have been shown to improve the outcome of treatment of raised ICP.[47,48] The result is likely to be best if cerebral perfusion pressure is kept above 50 mm of Hg and ICP at or below 15 mm of Hg.

Treatment of Seizures: Seizures probably result from several factors like raised ICP, toxic encephalitis, hypothermia/hyperthermia, vasculitis, dyselectrolytemia, hypocalcemia and hypoglycemia. Seizures increase the metabolic demand of the brain, increase the risks of aspiration and asphyxia and neuronal damage and should therefore be treated vigorously. An occasional seizure is best treated with intravenous diazepam in a dosage of 0.3 mg/kg/dose or lorazepam in a dose of 0.05-0.1 mg/kg/dose. In case of further recurrence, it should be treated with other long acting anti-convulsant; we usually use phenytoin, 5-6 mg/kg/day after an initial loading dose of 15-20 mg/kg. Seizures can, at times, take the form of status epilepticus that must be managed aggressively. Biochemical imbalances like hypocalcemia, hypoglycemia and dyselectrolytemia should be corrected promptly.

Cardio-respiratory Complications: Airway obstruction of varying severity due to accumulation of secretions and/or vomitus in the throat is often seen in encephalitis specially in the comatose cases. Such obstructions can lead to episodes of hypoxia, cyanosis or even respiratory arrest. Aspiration of secretions often lead to pneumonia. Frequent suction of the throat should therefore be done in the acute stage, specially in the comatose cases. Frequent change of posture is also important.

Circulatory failure, central and/or peripheral, and also cardio-respiratory arrests often occurs unpredictably in the acute stage of the illness; it is therefore important to remain alert for the need of intubation and resuscitation. Patients with respiratory failure will need mechanical ventilatory support.

Other Complications: Hyperpyrexia, that increases the metabolic demand of the brain and also the chances of seizures, should be treated with conventional measures like antipyretics and tepid sponging. Prophylactic antibiotic is indicated in view of initial difficulty/dilemma in excluding serious bacterial CNS infections and also life-threatening nature of the disease. Bleeding may need FFP/blood transfusion.

Convalescent Phase: Care of the nutrition and prevention of infection in bedridden patients is important. Some patients may require prolonged nasogastric feeds. Neurologic handicaps, which may gradually start manifesting as the patient recovers, need appropriate management.

OUTCOME

The outcome of viral encephalitis is guarded. Because of the diverse etiopathogenesis and epidemiologic factors generalization of outcome is not possible. Mortality and sequelae may vary according to causative agent, the severity of infection and host defense mechanism and also availability of quality health care. HSV and JE are well known to be associated with high mortality. Mortality in general has been shown to be high in infants, in cases who had altered sensorium and/or coma before admission into hospital.[49] High risk for death and brain damage was seen with HSV encephalitis and JE in our country.

Viral encephalitis is frequently followed by many sequelae in the survivors, mostly neuromotor and neurodevelopmental like behavior disorders, intellectual impairment, visual, hearing and speech defects, epilepsy, spasticity, rigidity, dystonia and various palsies.[49-52] Severe, cases, although few, may continue to remain in a vegetative state. About 50% of viral encephalitis especially due to HSV, has been reported to be left with cognitive, motor, behavioral problems and epilepsy.[50] In presumed viral encephalitis (in cases without prior neurologic condition) almost half of the cases have been observed to develop some sequelae,[51] the disabilities observed being developmental delay, learning difficulties, behavioral problems, or focal neurological findings. Younger age and presence of seizure at admission were found to have significant association with neurological sequelae. In another report almost half of childhood infective encephalitis survivors had incomplete recovery in the long-term, most commonly having developmental delay, behavioral abnormality, and neurological impairments primarily seizure.[52]

PREVENTION

Vaccines are the best way of preventing viral encephalitis. This has been well exemplified by reduction in incidence of encephalitis due to measles, mumps and rubella. Effective vaccine for Japanese encephalitis is also now available. The multiplicity of viruses and difficulty in making vaccines for every virus however make prevention of all types of encephalitis by vaccines impossible.

Vector control, which should be useful in preventing infections due to arboviruses, is difficult to achieve in practice. However, measures to minimize individual exposure to vectors is possible and should be encouraged.

References

1. Green RJ, Smuts I, Lamb GV. Viral infections of the central nervous system; vol II, 83-123, Published online 2017 May 5.
2. Pallansch M, Roos R. Enteroviruses: Polioviruses, Coxsackie viruses, Echoviruses and Newer Enteroviruses. In: Field's Virology, Knipe M, Howley PM (Eds), Lippincott Williams and Wilkins, Philadelphia 2007:839-91.
3. Koskiniemi M, Rautonen J, Lehtokoski-Lehtiniemi E, Vaheri A. Epidemiology of Encephalitis in Children: A 20-year Survey. Ann Neurol 1991;29:492-97.
4. Johnson RT. The Pathogenesis of Acute Viral Encephalitis and Postinfectious Encephalomyelitis. J Infect Dis 1987;155: 359-64.
5. Wong V, Yeung CY. Acute viral encephalitis in children. Aust Pediatr J 1987;23:339-42.
6. Wang D, Bortolussi R. Acute Viral Infection of the Central Nervous System in Children: An 8-Year Review. Can Med Assoc J 1981:125:585-89.
7. Kumar R, Kumar P, Singh MK, Agarwal D, Jamir B, Khare S, Narayan S. Epidemiological Profile of Acute Viral Encephalitis; Indian J Pediatr 2018;85(5):358-63.
8. Sharma S, Mishra D, Aneja S, Kumar R, Jain A and Vashishtha VM. Consensus Guidelines on Evaluation and Management of Suspected Acute Viral Encephalitis in Children in India. Indian Pediatr 2012;49:897-910.
9. Joshi R, Kalantri SP, Reingold A, Colford JM. Changing Landscape of Acute Encephalitis Syndrome in India: A Systematic Review. The Natl Med J India 2012;25:212-20.
10. Kumar A, Shukla D, Kumar R, Idris MZ, Misra UK, Dhole TN. An Epidemic of Encephalitis Associated with Human Enterovirus B in Uttar Pradesh, India, 2008. J Clin Virol 2011;51:142-45.
11. Beig FK, Malik A, Rizvi M, Acharya D, Khare S. Etiology and Clinico-Epidemiological Profile of Acute Viral Encephalitis in Children of Western Uttar Pradesh, India. Int J Infect Dis 2010:14:e141-46.
12. Gurav YK, Tandale BV, Jadi RS, Gunjikar RS, Tikute SS, Jamgaonkar AV *et al.* Chandipura Virus Encephalitis Outbreak Among Children in Nagpur Division, Maharashtra, 2007. Indian J Med Res 2010;132:395-99.
13. Sapkal GN, Bondre VP, Fulmali PV, Patil P, Gopalkrishna V, Dadhania V *et al.* Enteroviruses in Patients with Acute Encephalitis, Uttar Pradesh, India. Emerg Infect Dis 2009;15: 295-98.
14. Karmarkar SA, Aneja S, Khare S, Saini A, Seth A, Chauhan BK. A Study of Acute Febrile Encephalopathy with Special Reference to Viral Etiology. Indian J Pediatr 2008;75:801-05.
15. Chadha MS, Comer JA, Lowe L, Rota PA, Rollin PE, Bellini WJ *et al.* Nipah Virus-associated Encephalitis Outbreak, Siliguri, India. Emerg Infect Dis 2006;12:235-40.
16. Kumar R, Tripathi P, Singh S, Banerjee G. Clinical Features in Children Hospitalized During the 2005 Epidemic of Japanese Encephalitis in Uttar Pradesh, India. Clin Infect Dis 2006; 43:123-31.
17. Rao BL, Basu A, Wairagkar NS, Gore MM, Arankalle VA, Thakare JP, Jadi RS, Rao KA, Mishra AC. A Large Outbreak of Acute Encephalitis with High Fatality Rate in Children in Andhra Pradesh, India, in 2003, Associated with Chandipura Virus. Lancet 2004;364:821-22.

18. Potula R, Badrinath S, Srinivasan S. Japanese Encephalitis in and Around Pondicherry, South India: A Clinical Appraisal and Prognostic Indicators for the Outcome. J Trop Pediatr 2003; 49:48-53.

19. Wairagkar NS, Shaikh NJ, Ratho RK, Ghosh D, Mahajan RC, Singhi S, *et al.* Isolation of Measles Virus from Cerebrospinal Fluid of Children with Acute Encephalopathy Without Rash. Indian Pediatr 2001;38:589-95.

20. Kabilan L, Edwin N, Balashankar S, Meikandan D, Thenmozhi V, Gajanana A. Japanese Encephalitis Among Paediatric Patients with Acute Encephalitis Syndrome in Tamil Nadu, India. Trans R Soc Trop Med Hyg 2000;94:157-58.

21. Devi PS, Behera PL, Swain A. Japanese Encephalitis in Orissa. Indian Pediatr 1996;33:702-03.

22. Rathi AK, Kushwaha KP, Singh YD, Singh J, Sirohi R, Singh RK, Singh UK. JE virus encephalitis: 1988 Epidemic at Gorakhpur Indian Pediatr 1993;30:325-33.

23. Kumar R, Mathur A, Kumar A, Sethi GD, Sharma S, Chaturvedi UC. Virological Investigations of Acute Encephalopathy in India. Arch Dis Child 1990;65:1227-30.

24. John TJ, Feldman RA, Patoria NK, Christopher S, George S. Enteroviruses and Acute Encephalopathy Syndrome in Nagpur Indian J Pediatr 1984;51:621-31.

25. Benakappa DG, Prasad SR, Sastry NS, George S. Acute Encephalopathy Syndrome in Bangalore. Indian J Pediatr 1983;50:121-27.

26. Mathur A, Chaturvedi UC, Tandon HO, Agarwal AK, Mathur GP, Nag D, *et al.* Japanese Encephalitis Epidemic in Uttar Pradesh, India During 1978. Indian J Med Res 1982;75: 161-69.

27. Mathur KK, Bagchi SK, Sehgal CL, Bhardwaj M. Investigation on An Outbreak of Japanese Encephalitis in Raipur, Madhya Pradesh. J Commun Dis 1981;13:257-65.

28. Balakrishan S, John E, Madhavan HN. Echovirus Encephalitis in Pondicherry. Indian Pediatr 1970;7:212-18.

29. Athavale VB, Desai NN, Kadoth WK, Aiyer RR. Acute Viral Meningoencephalitis. Indian Pediatr 1970 Oct;7(10):547-56.

30. Hardas UD, Pathak AA, Jahagirdar VL. Virological Studies in Encephalitis. Indian J Pediatr 1976;43:270-71.

31. Nair E, Kalra SL. Cytopathic Enteroviruses in Delhi Area. II. From Cases of Febrile Illnesses with Neurological Involvements. Indian J Med Res 1969;57:272-76.

32. Madhavan HN, Sharma KB. Enteroviruses from Cases of Encephalitis in Pondicherry. Indian J Med Res 1969;57: 1607-10.

33. Gutierrez K, Pinsky B, Arvin MM. Herpes Simplex Viruses 1 and 2. In: Cherry JD, Harrison GJ, Kaplan SL, Steinbach WJ, Hotez PJ (Eds). Fegin and Cherry's Textbook of Pediatric Infectious Disease, 7th edition, Elsevier, Saunders, Philadelphia 2019:1933.

34. Janowski AB, Hunstad DA. Viral Meningoencephalitis. In: Nelson Textbook of Pediatrics, Kleigman RM, Blum NJ, Shah SS, St Geme JW, Tasker RC, Wilson KM, Behrman RE (Eds), 21st edn, 2020, Elsevier, 32 Philadelphia 3232-34.

35. Kneen R, Michael BD, Manson E, Mehta B, Easton A, Hemingway C, *et al.* Management of Suspected Viral Encephalitis in Children–Association of British Neurologists and British Pediatric Allergy Immunology and Infection Group National Guidelines. J Infect 2012;64:449-77.

36. Lakeman FD, Whitley RJ. Diagnosis of Herpes Simplex Encephalitis: Application of Polymerase Chain Reaction to Cerebrospinal Fluid from Brain-biopsied Patients and Correlation with Disease. National Institute of Allergy and Infectious Diseases Collaborative Antiviral Study Group. J Infect Dis 1995;171:857-63.

37. Jayaraman K, Rangasami R, Chandrasekharan A. Magnetic Resonance Imaging Findings in Viral Encephalitis: A Pictorial Essay. J Neurosci Rural Pract 2018;9:556-60.

38. Granerod J, Davies NW, Mukonoweshuro W, Mehta A, Das K, Lim M, Solomon T, Biswas S, Rosella L, Brown DW, Crowcroft NS. UK Public Health England Aetiology of Encephalitis Study Group. Neuroimaging in Encephalitis: Analysis of Imaging Findings and Interobserver Agreement. Clin Radiol 2016;71:1050-58.

39. Gupta RK, Soni N, Kumar S, Khandelwal N. Imaging of Central Nervous System Viral Diseases. J Magn Reson Imaging 2012;35:477-91.

40. Polllock AN, Henesch SM, Rorke-Adams LB. Brain infections. In Caffey's Pediatric Diagnostic Imaging, 11th edn, Morley Elsevier, Philadelphia 2008:751-89.

41. Kumar S, Misra UK, Kalita J, Salwani V, Gupta RK, Gujral R. MRI in Japanese Encephalitis. Neuroradiology 1997;39: 180-84.

42. Zimmerman RA, Russell EJ, Leeds NE, Kaufman D. CT in the Early Diagnosis of Herpes Simplex Encephalitis. AJR Am J Roentgenol 1980;134:61-66.

43. Karlin CA, Robinson RG, Hinthorn DR, Liu C. Radionuclide Imaging in Herpes Simplex Encephalitis. Radiology 1978; 126:181-84.

44. Ch'ien LT, Boehm RM, Robinson H, Liu C, Frenkel LD. Characteristic Early Electroencephalographic Changes in Herpes Simplex Encephalitis. Arch Neurol 1977 Jun;34(6): 361-64.

45. Whitley RJ, Alford CA, Hirsch MS, Schooley RT, Luby JP, Aoki FY, Hanley D, Nahmias AJ, Soong SJ. Vidarabine Versus Acyclovir Therapy in Herpes Simplex Encephalitis. N Engl J Med 1986 Jan 16;314(3):144-49.

46. Whitley RJ, Alford CA, Hirsch MS, Schooley RT, Luby JP, Aoki FY, Hanley D, Nahmias AJ, Soong SJ. Factors Indicative of Outcome in a Comparative Trial of Acyclovir and Vidarabine for Biopsy-proven Herpes Simplex Encephalitis. Infection 1987;15 Suppl 1:S3-8.

47. Dean JM, Moss JD. Intracranial Hypertension. In: Pediatric Critical Care. Fuhrman BP, Zimmerman JJ (Ed) St. Louis, Mosby Year Book 1992;557-87.

48. Tasker RC, Matthew DJ, Helms P, Dinwiddie R, Boyd S. Monitoring in Non-traumatic Coma. Part I: Invasive Intracranial Measurements. Arch Dis Child 1988 Aug;63(8):888-94.

49. Rautonen J. Koskiniemi M. Vaheri A. Prognostic Factors in Childhood Acute Encephalitis. Pediatr Infect Dis J 1991 Jun:10(6):441-46.

50. Schmutzhard E. Viral Infections of the CNS with Special Emphasis on Herpes Simplex Infections. J Neurol 2001 Jun:248(6):469-77.

51. Rismanchi N, Gold JJ. Sattar S. Glaser C. Sheriff H. Proudfoot J. Mower A. Nespeca M. Crawford JR. Wang SG. Neurological Outcomes After Presumed Childhood Encephalitis. Pediatr Neurol 2015 Sep:53(3):200-06.

52. Khandaker G. Jung J. Britton PN. King C. Yin JK Jones CA. Long-term Outcomes of Infective Encephalitis in Children: A Systematic Review and Meta-analysis. Dev Med Child Neurol 2016 Nov:58(11):1108-15.

40 Chapter

JAPANESE ENCEPHALITIS

Arvind K Rathi, Mahima Mittal

Japanese Virus Encephalitis (JE) is the most important cause of encephalitis worldwide with approximately 67,900 cases of clinical JE are estimated to occur every year, about 75% them being under 15 years of age.[1] The disease is fatal in 20-25% of symptomatic subjects and nearly 40-45% of the children who recover suffer from neuropsychiatric sequelae.[2] Though JE is an uncommon event in most of the Western Hemisphere, in the East particularly in South Asia, it poses enormous problems.[3] Not only epidemic outbreaks of JE have occurred in different countries of Asia for the last several decades, the disease is endemic in many countries of eastern globe and for long has become an important public health problem.

The first epidemic of JE was recorded in Japan in 1871 and since then it has been occurring there frequently. However, the illness was recognized as viral encephalitis in 1924 and the JE virus was isolated in 1925. The disease was named Japanese B Encephalitis to differentiate it from Von Economo's disease, which that time was referred to as Japanese A encephalitis. Following change in taxonomy the letter 'B' was dropped. Infections with Japanese Encephalitis Virus (JEV) have been occurring in all islands of Japan as well as in Okinawa, Korea, China, Philippines, Taiwan, Thailand, Cambodia, Lao Pupil Democratic Republic, South Eastern Soviet Union, Indonesia, Jawa, Sumatra, Malaya, Burma, India, Pakistan, Bangladesh, Nepal and Srilanka. Most of these countries have a similar environmental, ecological and agricultural background which favors JEV transmission. During the last decade of 20th century, JE emerged in new geographic regions of Asia.[4] Effective immunization program against JE has drastically brought down the incidence of disease in China, Japan, Malaysia, South Korea,Taiwan, and Thailand and Indian subcontinent.[5] Significant decrease in the occurrence of JE has also been observed in India after large scale anti JE immunization since 2006 adopting various strategies.

In India, the first patient of JE was reported in 1954 from Jamshedpur. It was identified as a disease entity in 1955 when cases were reported from North Arcot district of Tamil Nadu and Pondicherry. Till 1973, the disease was not commonly identified and was restricted to southern states of Andhra Pradesh, Tamil Nadu and Karnataka.[6,7] In 1973, a large outbreak of JE occurred in Burdwan and Bankura district of West Bengal.[8,9] In subsequent years, cases of JE were diagnosed in West Bengal with serological evidence of infection in healthy population. During 1978, outbreaks of JE occurred in several parts of India including Gorakhpur region of Eastern Uttar Pradesh.[10] Since then the virus had rapidly spread in India in as much it was present in 24 states and Union territories. A total of 745 cases and140 deaths in 2012 and nearly 1000 cases and 200 deaths in 2013 have been reported from India.[11] Presently, JE encephalitis cases are reported from the states of Andhra, Assam, Bihar, Delhi, Goa, Haryana, Jharkhand, Kerala, Karnataka, Maharashtra, Manipur, Nagaland, Punjab, Tamil Nadu, Uttar Pradesh, Uttarakhand, West Bengal and Pondicherry. There are 171 JE epidemic Districts with a population of 375 millions. Assam, West Bengal, Bihar and U.P. remain the worst affected states.[12] Longest and most severe epidemic of Japanese Encephalitis was seen in Eastern U.P. with Gorakhpur as the centre during summer–rainy season of 2005, a total of 5737 persons were affected and 1344 died. Besides, disease spread to several other districts of Eastern UP for the first time during this year.[13]

To contain JE, Government of India has carried out extensive immunization against the disease from 2006 to 2009 in which high risk districts of the country (11 districts in Assam, Karnataka and Uttar Pradesh) were covered. Children between the age group of 1 to 15 years were vaccinated with a single dose of Chinese live attenuated SA-14-14-2 JE vaccine. In 2011, the same SA-14-14-2 JE vaccine was introduced in the routine immunization under

Universal Immunization Program (UIP) in 181 endemic districts as a single dose at 16 to 18 months, at the time of the 1st booster of DTP vaccine. In 2013, another dose of SA-14-14-2 vaccine was added at 9 months of age along with measles vaccine.[14] After such a large vaccination coverage the incidence of JE has come down,[15] however both in its endemic and epidemic form, the illness still remains an important public health problem in many states of India.

JAPANESE ENCEPHALITIS VIRUS (JEV)

The JEV is an arbovirus and belongs to the family Toga-viridae, genus Flavivirus and is closely related immunologically to Yellow fever, Dengue, West Nile virus and St. Louis Encephalitis virus. It has a 40-50 nm lipoprotein envelope surrounding a nucleocapsid comprising core protein and single stranded RNA. The lipid envelope is derived from host and is soluble in lipid solvents. Lipases, organic solvents and detergents disrupt the virus envelope and inactivate JEV. Embedded in the lipid envelope is the envelope (E) protein, which projects from the surface and is responsible for all the biological properties of the virus such as attachment to host cell, haemagglutination (HA) and neutralization (Nt). The other structural proteins present are matrix (M) and capsid (C) proteins. Besides, there are seven non-structural proteins.

Four genotypes, I to IV of JEV are presently recognized.[16] Genotype I from North Thailand, Korea and Cambodia, Genotype II from South Thailand, Malaysia, Indonesia and Northern Australia, Genotype III from Japan, China, India, Nepal and Sri Lanka and Genotype IV from Indonesia. In addition a fifth Genotype has also been isolated. Genotype III and I occur in epidemic regions and Genotype II and IV are said to be associated with endemic disease. However, strains are being isolated which do not fit this paradigm. Genotype III is the most common genotype found in India in all the geographical locations so far. JEV isolates responsible for 2005 epidemic of Gorakhpur have been shown to belong to this group (G III) but it form a cluster separate from earlier Indian isolates.[17] The prevalence of genotypes III and I among the JE cases of West Bengal[18] was reported in 2012. Newer studies from Gorakhpur also indicate the presence of genotypes I and III[19] in this area.

Epidemiology

JE is a zoonotic disease. The mode of dissemination and maintenance of JEV in the nature is not precisely known. JEV has been isolated from 12 species of mosquitoes in India of which three belong to genus Anopheles, eight to Culex and one to Mansoni.[20] Culextritaeniorhynchus, Culexvishnui and Culexpseudovishnui appear to be competent vectors. These mosquitoes breed in irrigated rice fields, shallow ditches and pools where the decomposition takes place. C. Vishnui has more attraction to children, birds and pigs. NIV Pune has suggested that C. whitomores and C. epidesmus may also be responsible for the transmission of the disease to some extent.[21]

Arboviruses are maintained in nature by vertebrate hosts. Birds belonging to the family of Ardeidae have been incriminated both for dissemination and maintenance of JEV in Japan. There has been considerable controversy with regard to vertebrate host for JEV in India. In the studies carried out in Andhra Pradesh, Ardeolagrayii (pond heron) and Bubulcusibis (cattle egret), both belonging to Ardeidae have been found having antibodies against JEV in nearly 85% of samples and also have been shown to develop viraemia in sufficiently high titers to infect mosquitoes. The possible role of ducks is yet to be determined. However, ducks have been shown to develop adequate level of viraemia as mosquitoes fed on them get infected and effectively transmit the disease.

It seems reasonably clear that the normal enzootic cycle of JEV is a bird-mosquito-bird cycle. However, evidences suggest that the pigs act as amplifying hosts. Pigs bitten by infected C. tritaeniorhynchus have been shown to develop sufficient viraemia to infect mosquitoes. Mosquito-pig-mosquito cycle appears to be temporary and epizootic, the epidemics in man appear to follow pig epizootics. Pigs have been incriminated as major vertebrate host for JE virus in Malaysia, Singapore, Taiwan, Korea and Japan.[22] The pig to man population in India is comparatively small and serological evidence suggests that buffaloes and cattle also possess neutralizing antibodies and may play a role like pigs. Cattle and buffaloes may, however, have a dampening effect in causation of the disease in man as C. tritaeniorhynchus has predilection for cattle, which are found in large numbers in India. Cattle and buffaloes also support mosquito population by providing them the blood meal. Other vertebrate hosts viz. horse, bats, snakes and other reptiles have been suspected to be having some role in survival of virus in nature specially in winter months.

Man is the dead end host and JEV is rarely isolated from human blood suggesting that man is not a suitable host to infect C. tritaeniorhynchus, the major vector which is mainly zoophilic and bites man only in absence of usual host or when its population is high.

JE is predominantly reported from rural area, particularly among low socioeconomic group. Flooded rice fields provide ideal conditions for mosquito breeding. It is often seen that only few cases are reported from a village. This is because most of the infections by JEV in man are asymptomatic and the ratio of symptomatic to asymptomatic cases may be as high as 1:1000 in Japan to 1:200 to 1:6300 in other parts of Asia. In India, though this figure is not precisely known, it is believed to be very high as demonstrated by large percentage of population possessing antibodies in endemic areas without any symptoms.

Seasonal Incidence

Patterns of JEV transmission vary regionally as per climatic conditions, year to year variations also occur within the same region. Two epidemiological patterns have been recognized in temperate zone (northern Thailand, northern Vietnam, Korea, Japan, Taiwan, China, Nepal and northern India) the disease occurs in epidemics during summer and rainy months; in tropical areas (southern Thailand, southern Vietnam, Indonesia, Malaysia, Philippines, Sri Lanka and southern India) the JE is endemic at low rates throughout the year. However, in India, the disease has not always followed the above pattern. In south, illness occurs during later half of the year, coinciding with the rainy season and the period of high mosquito prevalence. In eastern states of India, the disease occurs between May and October, related to summer monsoon.[20] In eastern Uttar Pradesh, the outbreaks which have followed end of rainy season and floods (starting in the September and ending sometimes in November) have now started occurring early, large number of cases of JE are being reported in the month of July.[9] Moreover, sporadic cases of JE occur round the year.

Age and Sex Incidence

JE mostly is a disease of children and young adults[20] and the incidence is 1.5 to 2 times higher in males over females. The disease commonly affects families of poor field workers having unsatisfactory living conditions with abundance of mosquitoes. The prevalence of antibody to virus rises with increasing age in inhabitants of the endemic areas. However, when epidemics occur at new location, both adults as well as children are affected. The disease mainly affects children of 2-5 years in China and school going children in Republic of Korea. In Japan, since children are vaccinated, disease mainly affects elderly persons. Recent data from Thailand has shown that after vaccination incidence of JE in children has come down to 15-16% from 46% occurring before vaccination.[23] In India and Nepal, though JE affects people of all ages, school going children between 5 and 12 years of age are mainly affected, both during epidemics as well as in sporadic occurrence throughout the year. Though the effect of vaccination on age of occurrence of JE in these two countries is not clear, as there is no data available on this, it is logical to presume that in line with the age shift seen in Japan and Thailand,[23] the age of occurrence of JE may shift to older children and adults.

Pathogenesis

JEV gets into lymphatic system from the site of mosquito bite, multiplication begins and the seeding of blood stream leads to infection of several organs.[15] At this extra-neural stage non specific febrile illness is commonly present. With further viral multiplication secondary viraemia takes place and central nervous system along with lungs, liver, kidneys, GIT are invaded. The means of crossing the blood-brain barrier is unknown, passage through the vascular endothelium is now thought to be more likely than via olfactory nerves.[24]

The virus involves whole of the brain tissue including cortex and spinal cord. Neurological damage is caused by direct invasion and destruction of neural tissue by JE virus and also by reaction of the nervous tissue to viral antigens. Multiple factors lead to cerebral edema, most important being inflammation of brain leading to exudation. Central respiratory depression along with peripheral ventilatory insufficiency and decreased cerebral perfusion leads to tissue hypoxia and edema. Finally, increased secretion of ADH leads to transfer of fluids to intracellular compartment as an osmotic effect to hyponatremia and water retention.

The course and outcome of the disease depends upon the dose and virulence of the virus, age and nutritional status of the host, immune status by earlier infections by JEV or other viruses of the group. The immature brain is generally more susceptible to infection explaining higher morbidity and mortality in children due to JEV infection. The neurological permissiveness to Flava virus replication decreases with age and slower replication in older people allows clearance of virus by host defense before clinical signs manifest.

Pathology

Invasion of brain by JEV is followed by perivascular cuffing, infiltration of inflammatory cells (T cells and macrophages) into the parenchyma and phagocytosis of the infected cells.[25-26] These changes are most marked in the thalamus and brainstem. Pathological lesion in fatal cases of JE is polymorphic and diffuse in various parts of the nervous system. Meningeal blood vessels are congested with very little overlying cellular exudate.

The brain substance becomes edematous leading to uncal and cerebellar tonsillar herniation. Cut sections through various regions show punctate hemorrhages. On closer examination, small, circular necrotic zones can be seen in superficial cortical and deep grey matter.

Microscopic evidence of leptomeningitis is seen in all the cases with minimal mononuclear infiltration extending into deep parenchyma. Brain parenchyma becomes moderately congested with neuronophagia and perivascular cuffing and occasional focal hemorrhages in many cases. Degenerative changes in the Purkinje cells is an interesting feature in most cases. Focal areas of cellular encephalomalacia and presence of numerous cellular inflammatory nodules mostly consisting of glial cell, often including red cells, have been observed in many cases. Focal, small rounded to oval areas of cystic necrosis are seen in grey matter, thalamic nuclei, midbrain, pons, corpus striatum and less frequently in medulla oblongata. These areas may remain discrete or may become confluent. In spinal cord, anterior horns are damaged causing changes similar to poliomyelitis.[27] However, the astroglial reaction in JE is negligible.

In patients who die rapidly, there may be no histological signs of inflammation but immunohistochemical studies demonstrate viral antigen in histologically normal neurons. This explains the normal CSF findings in some patients of JE. Lungs, liver and kidneys are the other important organs affected by JEV. Lungs show interstitial pneumonitis and interalveolitis together with the areas of hemorrhage. Hydropic degeneration and fatty changes of perilobular distribution have been demonstrated in liver in JE patients. Areas of focal hemorrhages are seen in kidneys and interstitial myocarditis has been reported in some cases.

Clinical Presentation

Infections with JEV range in severity from asymptomatic, through mild febrile illness, to aseptic meningitis and lethal meningoencephalitis. The incubation period in man is not precisely known, but it is believed to be from 5 to 15 days. Extrinsic incubation period in vector mosquito is 9 to 12 days. Clinically the disease may be divided into three stages, prodromal stage, stage of acute encephalitis and stage of late convalescence and sequelae.[28,29]

Prodromal stage is characterized by general malaise, headache and fever, resembles any acute febrile illness and is difficult to be diagnosed except during epidemics. Headache and fever are often accompanied by nausea, vomiting and rigors. Duration of prodromal stage is usually 1 to 6 days, it can be less than 24 hours or sometimes as long as two weeks. Most of the patients are brought to the hospital during acute encephalitic stage. Fever becomes moderate to high; child, who may be confused initially, rapidly passes into coma, develops nuchal rigidity, seizures and may have focal neurological signs. The convalescent stage begins with the fever returning to normal, improvement of neurological signs or persistence of neurological deficits of irreversible brain damage.

Encephalitic stage usually starts acutely. Moderate to severe fever occurs in nearly all patients and may continue from 3 days to several weeks; however, it commonly lasts for 5 to 7 days. Headache and vomiting are associated with fever in more than half of the cases, a good number of children rapidly pass to coma without having noticed headache. Sensorium of varying degree is altered in all cases, appearing in the form of confusion, disorientation, delirium and finally coma. Recovery from unconsciousness varies, depends upon overall recovery of the patients and has no relation to the degree of coma in acute stage. With the subsidence of fever, recovery from unconsciousness is rapid in some patients, while in others it may be slow and associated with mental and physical sluggishness. Patients may develop vacant expression often accompanied by akineticmutism. Seizures in acute stage are seen in more than ninety percent of cases, they are tonic or tonic-clonic with typical twisting movement of the upper limbs and are commonly associated with hypertonia of the extremities and retraction of the neck backwards. Generalized clonic and focal seizures have also been reported. Gastric hemorrhage due to erosion of gastric mucosa, lasting for initial 3 to 4 days and sometimes leading to fatality, occurs in about one fifth of the patients. Nearly similar number of patients also develop peripheral vascular failure (PVF) in acute stage, half of the patients developing PVF also develop gastric bleeding. Neurological deficits viz. cranial nerve palsies, monoparesis and hemiplegia are seen in acute stage of JE in less than ten percent of cases. Neck rigidity and positive Kernig's sign are present in one third of the patients and planter reflex is usually extensor. Some patients have respiratory irregularities of central origin due to involvement of the brainstem and a few develop pneumonitis leading to respiratory difficulties. Pulmonary edema, especially after use of mannitol to reduce intracranial tension, occurs occasionally. Constipation with poor bowel sounds is seen in fairly good number of patients, it may become severe in some patients leading to marked gastric distention. Loose motions have been reported in a few patients.

In some conscious patients, acute flaccid paralysis of the limbs reflecting the disease of the spinal cord may be the only feature.[30] Muscle wasting seen in few cases of JE has also been attributed due to the same reason. Occasionally, particularly during epidemics, altered behavior may be the predominant presenting feature and the illness may resemble hysteria or neurosis.

Course of the disease usually becomes clear within first few days. Majority of patients who succumb to illness do so within 3 to 4 days.[28,31] Patients with good recovery fully recover in 7 to 10 days, fever and seizures subside and child becomes conscious. Most of the children with smart recovery go home within 10 days. Children of JE not showing recovery within first 7 to 10 days have higher chances of developing neurological deficits, brain damage and have poorer outcome. Deterioration of mental faculties, aphasia, choreoathetoid and dystonic movements, seizures, cranial nerve palsies and hemiparesis, irrelevant talk and behavior are some of the commonly seen problems in these children. Some of the children of this group eventually show good recovery, however, a fair number pass to the so called subacute stage, take a long course to recovery and show features of marked permanent brain damage. Recurrence of the disease has also been reported. Children who clinically seem to have come out of the acute illness fully in 7-10 days, after a gap of few days develop recurrence of symptoms and may pass to subacute stage with permanent brain damage.

Diagnosis

Clinical manifestations of acute encephalitis similar to JE can be caused by numerous agents viz. viruses, bacteria, fungi, parasite, spirochetes, chemicals, toxins etc. and the outbreaks of several viral infections coincide with outbreak of JE in monsoon and post monsoon season. Moreover, facilities of making definitive virological diagnosis are limited in India and initial management of all acute encephalitis remains the same. Taking this into consideration, National Vector Born Disease Control Program, Ministry of Health, Government of India in consultation and advise of WHO has recommended that all encephalitis patients should be labeled as Acute Encephalitis Syndrome (AES)[32] and treated on the line of acute encephalitis as per guidelines issued by them till the etiological diagnosis is made. In endemic areas and during epidemics however, JE may be diagnosed on the basis of epidemiology, clinical presentation and by excluding other related illnesses clinically and by simpler and less time consuming investigations, keeping in mind the possibility of other conditions viz. other flavivirus encephalitis (West Nile, Dengue), Reye syndrome, heat stroke, toxic encephalopathies, cerebral malaria, intracranial infections including bacterial infections etc.

Blood of these patients show moderate to marked polymorphonuclear leukocytosis. CSF pressure is raised, fluid is clear with mild mononuclear pleocytosis, cell count is seldom above 100/cmm.[23] Levels of CSF proteins range between 40 and 100 mgs percent while sugar and chloride stay normal. Electroencephalographic recordings show diminution of electrical activity, dysrhythmia and slowing.

The specific etiological diagnosis of JE may be made by isolation of virus, detecting virus genome, demonstration of viral antigens in brain tissue or by detection of antibodies against JEV.[33,34] Isolation of virus can be made from autopsied brain tissue, CSF of patients and occasionally from blood collected in very early stage of illness using infant mice model, insect tissue culture or cell lines of fibroblast origin. The virus so grown is identified by neutralization (Nt), haemagglutination inhibition (HI) or complement fixation (CF) tests. Isolation of JE virus from clinical specimens is usually unsuccessful, probably because of low viral load and the rapid production of neutralizing antibodies. Currently virus genomes are detected in CSF of the patients by Reverse transcriptase polymerase chain reaction (RTPCR) or by using quantitative PCR. Viral antigens can also be demonstrated in the brain tissue and in CSF using immunofluorescent techniques.

However, for most practical purposes Japanese encephalitis is diagnosed serologically. In the primary response to JEV infection, monotypic rise of CF and HI antibodies takes place, and a four-fold or more rise in antibodies to JE is diagnostic. Difficulties in diagnosis arise because of cross reactivity to closely related Dengue-2 and West Nile viruses, which are also widely prevalent in India. However, the titers of cross-reacting antibodies are lower. A single high titer (HI > 80, CF > 32) in convalescent sera is also quite suggestive of JE infection. The serological diagnosis of JE may be difficult in the secondary response where the rise in antibody titers to flavivirus may already be present. Usually a four-fold or more rise in antibodies in paired sera along with the presence of IgM antibodies in such patients helps in reaching a diagnosis. Presence of anti-Japanese encephalitis virus IgM in the CSF has a sensitivity and specificity of > 95% for CNS infection with the virus. In the 1980s IgM and IgG capture enzyme linked immunosorbent assays (ELISAs) were developed which have become the accepted standards for diagnosis of Japanese encephalitis.[35] CurrentlyJapanese Encephalitis IgM capture MAC ELISA qualitative kit developed by National Institute of Virology, Pune, is being used for presumptive diagnosis of JE all over India.

Imaging techniques have provided valuable insights into the topographic distribution of lesions. Abnormalities seen on CT/MRI are diffuse white matter hypo densities suggestive of cerebral edema and low-density areas in the cerebral cortex in frontal, parietal, and temporal areas. Bilateral low-density areas and abnormal signal intensities in the thalamus and basal ganglia including putamen are considered to be characteristic features of JE.[36]

Management

There is no specific drug available against JEV. Symptomatic and supportive treatment plays an important role in reducing mortality and morbidity.[28,34] Pending etiological diagnosis, treatment of all patients of AES including JE should be started as soon as possible on similar lines, necessary changes be made once the offending agent is identified.

Patients are usually brought in coma with high fever and seizures. Airways are kept patent by proper positioning and using advanced airway adjusts as per requirement. Oxygen inhalation, specially in patients with central and peripheral respiratory insufficiency, helps in reducing cerebral edema and hypoxic brain injury. Temperature should be brought down immediately and kept under control by tepid sponging and antipyretics as persistent fever not only increases the extent of brain injury but also makes the control of seizures very difficult. Stomach should be kept empty using gastric tube to prevent aspiration of the gastric contents which also helps in early diagnosis of gastric bleeding.

Seizures should be brought under control by intravenous (IV) diazepam 0.1-0.3 mg/kg or lorazepam 0.05 to 0.1 mg/kg or midazolam 0.2 mg/kg administered over 3 to 5 minutes. To prevent recurrence of seizures phenobarbitone (5-8 mg/kg in three divided doses) or hydantoins (5-10 mg/kg in two divided doses) are also started simultaneously. Alternatively, phenobarbitone in dosage of 20-25 mg/kg or fosphenytoin in dosage of 30 mg/kg given intravenously over a period of 15-20 minutes under respiratory and cardiac monitoring can also be used to control seizures in acute stage. Anticonvulsants should be continued for twelve weeks or longer depending upon neurological recovery. Reduction of cerebral edema and raised intracranial pressure is of prime importance in reducing mortality and morbidity from JE. Mannitol is administered IV in dose of 1.5 to 2.0 mg/kg as 20 percent solution over a period of half to one hour, two to three times a day for initial three to four days. Frequent use of mannitol may lead to heart failure and pulmonary edema and patients on mannitol need to be supervised closely. However, 3% hypertonic saline (HS) is gaining favour over mannitol to bring down intracranial pressure, its use has been shown to decrease ICP and improve outcome.[37] Unlike mannitol 3% saline preserves intravascular status and can be administered in a hemodynamically unstable patient. Additional benefits include restoration of normal cellular resting membrane potential and cell volume, stimulation of atrial natriuretic peptide release, inhibition of inflammation, and enhancement of cardiac output. It is contraindicated if serum sodium is >150 mEq/l, and/or osmolality > 320 mOs mol/l. Glycerol, 0.5-1.0 mg/kg diluted with equal amount of fruit juices helps in reducing cerebral edema and can be given 8 hourly by gastric tube in acute stage. It is an agent of choice on discontinuation of mannitol, is non-toxic and can be used for extended period in patients with slow recovery. Fever should be treated and repeated suctioning should be avoided. Hyperventilation, artificial hypothermia, barbiturate coma and surgical decompression if available are other modalities during impending herniation.

Patients when first seen are hypoglycemic and have some degree of dehydration due to vomiting, fever and inadequate intake. IV infusion should include 5% glucose with half strength saline. Keeping in mind the inappropriate release of ADH, fluid intake should be restricted to less than normal and needs close monitoring. A slight excess of IV fluids and mannitol in JE may cause pulmonary edema. Blood transfusion may be required for the patients having excessive gastric bleeding, dopamine and dobutamine are used to control PVF.

IV fluids should be stopped and tube feeding initiated as soon as the critical stage is over, which generally takes 3-5 days. Adequate intake of fluids, calories, proteins and vitamins should be ensured at this stage as most of the patients of JE in India are malnourished. Antibiotics have no role in acute stage and should be reserved for secondary bacterial infections which are particularly common in lungs. Corticosteroids used routinely have not been found beneficial.

Recombinant interferon alpha has been given in open trials to small number of patients with promising results, however, this needs to be assessed further by large double-blind trials.[38] Intravenous immunoglobulin (IVIG) in children showed no difference in outcome in those who received IVIG or placebo.[39] Suramin,[40] diethyldithiocarbamate,[41] plant lignan called arctigenin[42] are still in the experimental stage.

Some studies have shown that tetracyclines and aminoglycoside-derivative compounds have been beneficial against reovirus, West Nile virus, and dengue virus.[43] Minocycline was investigated for its role in protecting against encephalitis and neurodegeneration. Proposed protective effects may result from direct inhibition of viral replication and its anti-inflammatory and immunomodulatory properties.[44]

Physiotherapy and drugs are used in sub-acute stage to control abnormal posture and behavior. Multidisciplinary approach including pediatrician, child psychologist, psychiatrist, physiotherapist, neurologist and social worker is required in managing such patients. Families of these patients needs to be supported.

Outcome

In general, outcome is better during epidemics than in the patients coming sporadically round the year. It is better in the second half of the epidemics compared to first half. On the whole about 25-30 percent of the patients die in acute stage, nearly 40 percent recover completely and the remaining pass to the sub-acute stage and land up in prolonged convalescence.[28,34] Many of these children develop flexion of upper limbs and extension of lower limbs with pes cavus. Neurological deficits viz. hemiparesis, cranial nerve palsies, monoparesis are common at this stage as are seizures, tremors, dystonia and choreoathetoid movements.[45,46] Abnormal behavior, irrelevant talk, weeping, laughing, excitement, aggression and lack of sleep are other problems commonly seen. Children once conscious appear mentally sluggish, subnormal and many of them remain aphasic for long. Peculiar protrusion of tongue has been observed in fair number of cases.[28,45] Prolonged follow-up of these children has shown that many of them recover completely after a variable period, others develop permanent brain damage and continue with above difficulties, few of them lead a vegetative life.[46,47] Mental retardation and learning disabilities are the major problems even in children who otherwise are found doing well.

Prevention

Preventive measures need to be directed to control mosquitoes and preventing them from biting humans. While protective measures against reservoirs and control of mosquitoes may help, vaccination of population at risk remains the mainstay in prevention of JEV disease.[20]

Varying in the geographical conditions, several species of mosquitoes seem to be involved in transmission of JEV in India. Physical, chemical, biological, ecological and genetic methods to control mosquitoes have not brought desired results, vector control does not seem to be in sight. People, however, can be motivated and educated to avoid exposure to mosquitoes and to prevent mosquito bite in the affected areas. Pictures, posters, radio, television may be used to show how mosquito nets, mosquito repellents etc. may be effectively used to prevent mosquito bite. Pigs seem to be the most important amplifying host. Though the population of the pigs in India is relatively low, piggeries are in bad shape. Pigs reared for consumption are used as scavengers till they are consumed. Piggeries should be away from human dwellings, their condition needs to be improved and should be mosquito proof. Vaccination of pigs in Japan has also given encouraging results.

Vaccination

Japanese encephalitis vaccines used worldwide fall into 4 classes.[48] They are based on Japanese encephalitis virus genotype III but are cross-protective against the other genotypes. Each of the vaccines incorporates a different vaccination schedule and booster dose requirement:

(1) Inactivated mouse brain-derived vaccine (JE-MB) manufactured in countries other than Japan.

(2) A cell-culture-derived (primary hamster kidney) live attenuated vaccine based on the SA 14-14-2 strain manufactured in China.

(3) Inactivated Vero cell culture vaccine (JE-VC); and

(4) A live attenuated chimeric vaccine based on the genes of yellow fever 17D backbone combined with Vero cell propagated SA 14-14-2 strain.

1. The mouse brain inactivated vaccine being produced in Kasauli (Himachal) with Japanese assistance was the only vaccine available in India, since 1960. This vaccine has been abandoned as there has been a rapid development of more effective vaccines during last couple of years.

2. Live Attenuated SA-14-14-2 Vaccine (cell culture derived)[49] is imported from China and has been extensively used for prevention of JE in endemic areas since 2006. In 2011, SA-14-14-2 JE vaccine was introduced in the routine immunization under Universal Immunization Program (UIP) in the 181 endemic districts as a single dose at 16 to 18 months at the time of 1st booster of DTP vaccine. In 2013, another dose of SA-14-14-2 vaccine was added at 9 months of age along with measles vaccine.Though there is no conclusive data on the precise efficacy/effectiveness of this vaccine in India, it appears quite effective, its efficacy has been shown to be from 60%-94.5%

in various studies.[14] Vaccine may have occasional side effects in the form of mild JE like illness (fever, headache, vomiting, delirium etc).

3. Inactivated Vero cell culture-derived SA 14-14-2 Vaccine (JE-VC) was developed by Intercell AG[50] and has been approved by US FDA and EU for use in children beyond 2 months of age. In India, a variant of Intercell AG SA 14-14-2 Vaccine has been launched by Biological E. Ltd. with the trade name JEEV. The vaccine is WHO prequalified and studies show a seroconversion rate of 57% on 28th day and 96% on 56th day following vaccination. The vaccine has been licensed by Drug Controller General of India for prevention of JE in children and adults. Two doses of inactivated SA 14-14-2 vaccine are recommended for primary immunization, 0.25 ml in children between 1-3 years and 0.5 ml after 3 years. The first dose of vaccine may be given with measles vaccine and the second with booster of DPT in endemic area for JE. An interval of four weeks between the two doses is required if the vaccine is used in older children and adults.

   Another Vero Cell cultured derived inactivated vaccine has been developed by Bharat Biotech International Limited (BBIL) using original Kolar (Karnataka) strain[51] of JE isolated by NIV Pune and transferred to BBIL for vaccine development. The vaccine uses Indian strain and has been licensed for use in India by the name JENVAC. Similar to the other inactivated vaccines, two doses of vaccine (0.5 each) are required to be administered for primary immunization and for immunization of older children and adults. The safety profile of all the inactivated vaccines is good. There appears a need for booster dose of inactivated vaccines in endemic areas after primary immunization in view of the fact that JE occurs in older children and adults in areas where only young children are immunized; timing of the booster dose need to be worked out after studying epidemiology and waning of seroprotection following initial vaccination. Due to its high cost this vaccine is still not included in the National Programmes.

4. Live Chimeric Virus Vaccine (genetically engineered licensed vaccine)[52] is prepared by using JE/Yellow fever chimera is undergoing extensive field trials and the reports suggest that a single dose achieves seroprotective antibodies after 28th day of administration lasting over 60 months. The vaccine has no unexpected adverse events (AEs) and may turn out to be most effective vaccine in JE prevention. Vaccine still not available in India.

In addition to above vaccines novel non-parentral vaccination approaches such as intranasal inoculation using mouse brain-derived inactivated Japanese encephalitis virus appear to have some potential but still is in the developmental stage.[53]

Since immunization against JE has a major role in decreasing JE all over the world, the World Health Organization (WHO) recommends that the JE vaccine be incorporated into immunization programs in all areas where the disease is a public health problem.[11]

References

1. Campbell GL, Hills SL, Fischer M, Jacobson JA, Hoke CH, Hombach JM, Marfin AA, Solomon T, Tsai TF, Tsu VD, *et al.* Estimated Global Incidence of Japanese Encephalitis: A Systematic Review. Bull World Health Organ 2011:89:766-74; PMID:22084515; https://doi. org/10.2471/BLT.10.085233.
2. Solomon T, Vaughn DW. Pathogenesis and Clinical Features of Japanese Encephalitis and West Nile Virus Infections. Curr Top Microbiol Immunol 2002;267:171-94. PMID:12082989.
3. Umenai T, Krzysko R, Bektimirov TA, Asaad FA, Japanese Encephalitis: Current Worldwide Status, Bull World Hlth Org 1985:63:625-31.
4. Igarashi A, Tanaka M, Morita K *et al.* Detection of West Nile and Japanese Encephalitis Viral Genome Sequences in Cerebrospinal Fluid from Acute Encephalitis Cases in Karachi, Pakistan, Microbiol, Immunol 1994;38:827-30.
5. Nagendra R Hegde and Milind M Gore. Japanese Encephalitis Vaccines: Immunogenicity, Protective Efficacy, Effectiveness and Impact on the Burden of Disease. Human Vaccines and Immunotherapeutics 2017, Vol. 13, No. 6, 1320-37 https://doi. org/10.1080/21645515.2017.1285472.
6. Nihal A. Global Scenario of JE/AES, Prevention and Control. WHO Workshop at Gurgaon, Haryana (India) 2013 March:5-6.
7. Banerjee K. Japanese Encephalitis in India. Ann Indian Acad Med Sci 1975;11:51-76.
8. Medappe N. Japanese Encephalitis in India. Bull ICMR 1980; 10:29-38.
9. Biswas SK, Bose SN, *et al.* Epidemic of Japanese Encephalitis in Bankura1973: Clinicopathological Findings, Ind J Med Res 1976;64:801-07.
10. Chakraborty MS, Chakraborty SK, *et al.* Recurrent Japanese Encephalitis Epidemics in West Bengal. Ind J Med Res 1980;72:1-6.
11. World Health Organization, Outbreak Encephalitis 2005: Cases of Japanese Encephalitis in Gorakhpur, Uttar Pradesh, India

2005 Core Programme Clusters Communicable Disease and Disease Surveillance. 2005 October 21:(cited 2006 July 11).

12. Details of AES/JE Cases and Deaths 2008-2013. Information Bulletin. National Vector Borne Disease Control Programme. Ministry of Health. Government of India. October 2013.
13. Mathur A. Chaturvedi UC. *et al.* JE Epidemic in Uttar Pradesh. India During 1978. Ind J Med Res 1982;75:161-64.
14. Vashishtha VM and RamachandranVG. Vaccination Policy for Japanese Encephalitis in India: Tread with Caution!. Indian Pediatrics 2015: Vol. 52. October 15.
15. PK Sen. AC Dhariwal. RK Jaiswal. Shiv Lal. VK Raina. A Rastogi. Epidemiology of Acute Encephalitis Syndrome in India: Changing Paradigm and Implication for Control. J Commun Dis 2014;46(1):4-11.
16. Jaiswal RK National Vector Borne Disease Control Workshop on Disease Surveillance. Lab Networking and Other Related Aspects of JE. Gurgaon. Haryana (India) 2013: March 5-6.
17. Fulmali PV. Sapkal GN. Athawale S. Gore MM. Mishra AC. Bondre VP. Introduction of Japanese Encephalitis Virus Genotype I. India Emerg Infect Dis 2011;17(2):319-21.
18. Sarkar A. Taraphdar D. Mukhopadhyay SK. Chakrabarti S. Chatterjee S. Molecular Evidence for the Occurrence of Japanese Encephalitis Virus Genotype I and III Infection Associated with Acute Encephalitis in Patients of West Bengal. India 2010. Virol J 2012;9:271.
19. Solomon T. Haolin Ni. *et al.* Origin and Evolution of Japanese Encephalitis Virus in Southeast Asia. J of Virology 2003;5:3091-98.
20. Manmohan M Parida. Paban K Dash. Nagesh K Tripathi. Ambuj. Santosh R Santosh. Parag Saxena. Surekha Agarwal. Ajay K Sahni. Sanjay P Singh. Arvind K Rathi. Rakesh Bhargava. Ajay Abhayankar. Shailendra K Verma. Putcha V Lakshmana Rao and Krishnamurthy Sekhar. Japanese Encephalitis Outbreak. India. 2005. Emerging Infectious Disease. www.cdc.gov/eid. Vol. 12. No. 9. September 2006.
21. Japanese Encephalitis in India–Information Document. National Institute of Virology. Pune. ICMR Offset Press 1998. New Delhi.
22. Rodrigues FM. Epidemiology of Japanese Encephalitis in India: A Brief Overview. In: Proceedings of the National Conference on Japanese Encephalitis. New Delhi: Indian Council of Medical Research 1984;1-9.
23. Innis BL. Japanese Encephalitis. In: Exotic Viral Infections Porterfield JS. ed. Chapman and Hall. London 1996:147-74.
24. Daniel ET. *et al.* Effect of Vaccination Coverage and Climate on Japanese Encephalitis in Sarawak. Malaysia. Plos Neglected Tropical Diseases 7.8.1-9.
25. Johnson RT. The Pathogenesis of Acute Viral Encephalitis and Postinfectious Encephalomyelitis. J Infect Dis 1987;155:359-64. Zimmerman HM. The Pathology of Japanese B Encephalitis. Am J Pathol 1946;22:965-91.
26. Miyake M. The Pathology of Japanese Encephalitis. Bull WHO 1964;30:153-60.
27. Misra UK. Kalita J. Anterior Horn Cells are also Involved in Japanese. Acta NeurolScand 1997;96:114.
28. Rathi AK. Kushwaha KP. *et al.* JE Virus Encephalitis: 1988 Epidemic at Gorakhpur. Indian Pediatr 1993;30:325-33.
29. Kharya G. Rathi AK. Kushwaha KP. *et al.* Clinical Features of Immunologically Proven Cases of JE–Epidemic 2003. Personal Communication.
30. Solomon T. Kneen R. Dung NM. *et al.* Poliomyelitis-like Illness Due to Japanese Encephalitis Virus. Lancet 1998;351: 1094-97.
31. Kumar R. Misra PK. Japanese Encephalitis in India. Indian Pediatr 1988;25:354-58.
32. Guidelines on Clinical Management of AES. Including JE. Guidelines Issued by National Vector. Borne Disease Control Programme. Ministry if Health. Government of India.
33. Leake CJ. Burke DS. Nisalak A. *et al.* Isolation of Japanese Encephalitis Virus from Clinical Specimens Using a Continuous Cell Line. Am J Trop Med Hyg 1986;35:1045-50.
34. Ravi V. Vanajakshi S. Gowda A. Chandramukhi A. Laboratory Diagnosis of Japanese Encephalitis Using Monoclonal Antibodies and Correlation of Findings with Outcome. J Med Virol 1989;29:221-23.
35. Japanese Encephalitis Surveillance Standards (2007) from WHO-Recommended Standards for Surveillance of Selected Vaccine-Preventable Diseases.
36. Misra UK. Kalita J. Jain SK. *et al.* Radiological and Neurophysiological Changes in Japanese Encephalitis. J Neurol Neurosurg Psychiatry 1994;57:1484-87.
37. Peterson B. Khanna S. Fisher B. Marshall L. Prolonged Hypernatremia Controls Elevated Intracranial Pressure in Head-Injured Pediatric Patients. Crit Care Med 2000 April; 28(4):1136-43.
38. Harinasuta C. Nimmanitya S. Titsyakorn U. The Effect of Interferon Alpha on Cases of Japanese Encephalitis in Thailand. Southeast Asian J Trop Med Pub Health 1985;16:332-36.
39. Rayamajhi A. Nightingale S. Bhatta NK. Singh R. Kneen R *et al.* A Preliminary Randomized Double Blind Placebo-Controlled Trial of Intravenous Immunoglobulin for Japanese Encephalitis in Nepal. PLoS One 2015;10(4):e0122608.
40. Lee E. Pavy M. Young N. Freeman C. Lobigs M. Antiviral Effect of the Heparan Sulfate Mimetic. PI-88. Against Dengue and Encephalitic Flaviviruses. Antiviral Res 2006;69(1):31-38.
41. Saxena SK. Mathur A. Srivastava RC. Inhibition of Japanese Encephalitis Virus Infection by Diethyldithiocarbamate is Independent of Its Antioxidant Potential. Antivir Chem Chemother 2003;14(2):91-98.
42. Swarup V. Ghosh J. Mishra MK. Basu A. Novel Strategy for Treatment of Japanese Encephalitis Using Arctigenin. a Plant Lignan. J Antimicrob Chemother 2008;61(3):679-88.
43. Topno R. Khan SA. Chowdhury P. Mahanta J. Pharmacodynamics of Aminoglycosides and Tetracycline Derivatives Against Japanese Encephalitis Virus. Asian Pac J Trop Med 2016;9(3):241-46.

44. Kumar R, Basu A, Sinha S, Das M, Tripathi P *et al.* Role of Oral Minocycline in Acute Encephalitis Syndrome in India – A Randomized Controlled Trial. BMC Infect Dis 2016;16:67.

45. Rathi AK, Kushwaha KP, *et al.* Neurological Deficits and Behaviour Disorders in Children of Japanese Encephalitis. The Vivekananda Institute of Sciences 1993;16:34-37.

46. Misra UK, Kalita J. Movement Disorders in Japanese Encephalitis. J Neurol 1997;234-99.

47. Schneider RJ, Firestone MH, *et al.* Clinical Sequelae After Japanese Encephalitis. One Year Follow-up Study in Thailand. Southeast Asian J Trop Med Public Health 1977;8:113-20.

48. Hui-LanChen, Jia-Kan Chang B, Ren-Bin Tang B. Current Recommendations for the Japanese Encephalitis Vaccine. Journal of the Chinese Medical Association 2015;78:271-75.

49. VM Vashishtha *et al.* I.A.P. Recommended Immunization Schedule for Children Aged 0 through 18 Years–India. Indian Pediatrics 2013;50,12:1095-110.

50. Intercell Announces Pediatric Approval of Its Japanese Encephalitis Vaccine in the U.S. Available from http://www.vaccines.mil/documents/1624_2013A21_JEVpediatric_US_ENG_Final.pdf. Accessed on October 3, 2013.

51. JENVAC Available from http://www.cdsco.nic.in/SMPC/Bharat%Biotech%20JE.pdf.

52. Nasveld PE *et al.* Long-term Immunity to Live Attenuated Japanese Enceohalitis Chimeric Virus Vaccine. Human Vaccines 2010; 6,12:1-9.

53. Harakuni T, Kohama H, Tadano M, Uechi G, Tsuji N, Matsumoto Y, Miyata T, Tsuboi T, Oku H, Arakawa T. Mucosal Vaccination Approach Against Mosquito-borne Japanese Encephalitis Virus. Japan J Infect Dis 2009;62(1):37-45 (ISSN: 1344-6304).

41 Chapter

POLIOMYELITIS

Satinder Aneja, Bina Ahuja

Acute anterior poliomyelitis (polio) is a disease that gives rise to localized or widespread destruction of motor neurons in the spinal cord or brainstem. It is characterized by the appearance of acute flaccid paralysis (AFP) of the muscles supplied by the affected motor neurons.[1] This disease was most commonly caused by infection with poliovirus before the global efforts to eradicate poliovirus was launched. Currently the AFP rates have declined and most cases of so called poliomyelitis are due to other viruses.

Etiopathogeneis

Poliovirus is a member of the enterovirus subgroup, family Picornaviridae. Picornaviruses are small viruses with an RNA genome. The poliovirus consists of four polypeptide chains that form a very highly structured shell. Located inside this shell, the viral genome consists of a single molecule of ribonucleic acid (RNA), which is about 7500 nucleotides long. The four capsid polypeptides are produced by the proteolytic cleavage of a single polyprotein precursor, and are designated VP1 through VP4.

The poliovirus is rapidly inactivated by heat, formaldehyde, chlorine and ultraviolet light. There are three antigenically distinct poliovirus serotypes (P1, P2 and P3) which have minimal heterotypic immunity. Studies with monoclonal neutralizing antibodies and mutant viruses resistant to them have revealed four main antigenic sites on the virus. The relative importance of individual sites is different for each of the three serotypes of poliovirus. Thus immunity to one serotype does not produce significant immunity to the other serotypes. Type 1 poliovirus accounted for most of cases when vaccination coverage was low.[2] Type 2 and 3 are responsible for most of cases reported in well immunized population.[3]

The virus enters through the mouth, and primary multiplication of the virus occurs at the site of implantation in the pharynx and gastrointestinal tract. The virus is usually present in the throat and in the stool before the onset of illness. The virus invades local lymphoid tissue, enters the bloodstream, and then may infect cells of the central nervous system. Replication of poliovirus in motor neurons of the anterior horn and brainstem results in cell destruction and causes the typical manifestations of poliomyelitis.

Other Neurotropic Viruses

Infection due to a variety of viruses other than poliovirus can cause flaccid paralysis. These include enterovirus 70 and 71, echovirus, coxsackie virus and West Nile fever virus. The proportion of cases of AFP due to non-polioviruses has increased due to increased vaccination coverage.[4]

Epidemiology

Humans are the only known reservoir of poliovirus, which is transmitted most frequently by persons with inapparent infections. There is no asymptomatic carrier state except in immune deficient persons.

Person-to-person spread of poliovirus via the fecal-oral route is the most important route of transmission, although the oral-oral route may account for some cases. In countries with good sanitation the main route is droplet infection from nasopharynx. Direct involvement of CNS can occur after tonsillectomy through severed cranial nerve filaments. There are a large number of subclinical infections and such cases are capable of spreading infection to others. Unimmunized contacts of infants immunized by OPV are also at risk of getting the infection.

With increase in standard of hygiene coupled with immunization programme polio has ceased to be a problem in developed countries. Wild virus infection has been eliminated from many countries. However asymptomatic carrier from an endemic area can import wild virus. Antigenic drift of the virus resulting in the strain not fully covered by vaccine can also lower the herd immunity to wild virus as was seen in outbreaks in Finland.[5] There has been a steady decline in the number of cases of poliomyelitis. Four countries namely India, Nigeria, Pakistan and Afghanistan have never been free of polio. In 2006, addition to these four, 12 countries have reported cases which is due to importation – Saudi Arabia, Yemen, Indonesia, Bangladesh, Ethopia, Kenya, Angila, Cameron, Namibia, Nigeria, Nepal and D R Congo.[6]

Pathology

It is primarily an intestinal infection. The virus multiplies in the gut and the associated lymph nodes from which it may spread and cause viremia. In some patients the CNS is invaded producing a variable spectrum of neurological manifestations. There is extensive non-specific infiltration of anterior horn cells. This is followed by wallerian degeneration of axons and atrophic changes in muscles. Besides the anterior horn cells in the spinal cord, cranial nerve nuclei, nuclei in the roof of cerebellum and vermis may be involved. The cerebral cortex is generally spared.

Clinical Features

The **incubation period** for poliomyelitis is commonly 7-20 days with a range of 3-35 days. The response to poliovirus infection is highly variable and has been categorized on the basis of the severity of clinical presentation. If the infection is not massive and antibody production is adequate, no clinical disease is seen. Upto 95% of all polio infections are *inapparent or asymptomatic*. Estimates of the ratio of inapparent to paralytic illness vary from 50:1 to 1,000:1 (usually 200:1). Infected persons without symptoms shed virus in the stool and are able to transmit the virus to others.

Approximately 4%-8% of polio infections consist of a minor, nonspecific illness without clinical evidence of central nervous system invasion. This clinical presentation is known as *abortive poliomyelitis*, and is characterized by complete recovery in less than a week. Three syndromes observed with this form of poliovirus infection are upper respiratory tract infection (sore throat and fever), gastrointestinal disturbances (nausea, vomiting, abdominal pain, constipation or, rarely, diarrhea), and influenza-like illness. These syndromes are indistinguishable from other viral illnesses.

Nonparalytic aseptic meningitis occurs in 1% of polio infections and is indistinguishable from other aseptic meningitis. Typically these symptoms will last from 2 to 10 days, followed by complete recovery.

Fewer than 1% of all polio infections in susceptible persons result in *flaccid paralysis*. Paralytic symptoms generally begin within a week after prodromal symptoms and progress for 2 to 3 days. The prodrome may be biphasic, especially in children, with initial minor symptoms separated by a 1- to 7-day period from more major symptoms. Additional prodromal signs and symptoms can include a loss of superficial reflexes, initially increased deep tendon reflexes and severe muscle aches and spasms in the limbs or back. The illness progresses to flaccid paralysis with diminished deep tendon reflexes, reaches a plateau without change for days to weeks, and is usually asymmetrical. Strength then begins to return. There is no sensory loss or changes in cognition. Weakness or paralysis still present 12 months after onset is usually permanent.

Paralytic polio is conventionally classified into spinal, bulbar and bulbo-spinal depending upon the involvement.

Spinal polio is most common, and is characterized by asymmetric and patchy paralysis that most often involves the legs.

Single limb involvement (generally of lower limb) is the most common presentation. Large group of muscles are more often involved because of selective destruction of motor neurons with fibres of large diameter and heavy myelination. Paralysis of respiratory muscles may occur if there is damage to cervical or thoracic segments of spinal cord. Diaphragmatic involvement is more serious than intercostals muscles as diaphragm is a more powerful muscle, urinary retention and constipation is common but a temporary phenomenon.

Bulbar polio leads to weakness of muscles innervated by cranial nerves. It is the most life threatening form of polio. 7th and 10th cranial nerves are the most commonly involved. Involvement of 10th nerve results in difficulty in swallowing, regurgitation of feeds and nasal twang to voice. There may be involvement of vasomotor and respiratory center which can result in respiratory/circulatory failure. **Bulbospinal polio**, is a combination of bulbar and spinal paralysis was seen in 3-8.16% of cases in our center. Uncommon presentations of poliomyelitis include polyneuritic form simulating GBS,[7] myelitic form, isolated Bell's palsy[8] and acute cerebellar syndrome.[9]

Poliomyelitis

Diagnosis of poliomyelitis can be made on the basis of 2 parameters – Clinical and Laboratory.

(i) *Clinical:* In paralytic stage the diagnosis is made by typical clinical presentation of patchy asymmetric motor paralysis in an unimmunized child. The major signs and symptoms of paralytic poliomyelitis in acute phase are: (i) Acute onset, (ii) Fever prior to paralysis, (iii) Muscle pain, (iv) Asymmetric paralysis, (v) Absent or diminished deep tendon reflexes with (vi) No sensory loss. Clinical diagnosis of abortive polio is possible only in epidemics.

Lab Diagnosis

Diagnosis is confirmed by isolation of wild virus. Serological tests such as complement Fixation and Neutralising Antibody titres show 4-fold rise in titres but are not widely used. EMG and Nerve Conduction Velocity studies show the involvement of anterior horn cells and are thus helpful to differentiate polio from other causes of AFP.

Polio virus isolation in stool is mandatory to make a definite diagnosis of poliomyelitis in child with acute flaccid paralysis. This is also required during suspected polio outbreak investigation for confirmation of the diagnosis.

Viral Isolation

The likelihood of poliovirus isolation is highest from stool specimens, intermediate from pharyngeal swabs, and very low from blood or spinal fluid. The isolation of poliovirus from stool specimens contributes to the diagnostic evaluation but does not constitute proof of a causal association of such viruses with paralytic poliomyelitis. Isolation of virus from the cerebrospinal fluid (CSF) is diagnostic but is rarely accomplished. To increase the probability of poliovirus isolation, at least two stool specimens and two throat swabs should be obtained 24 hours apart from patients with suspected poliomyelitis as early in the course of the disease as possible but ideally within the first 14 days after onset of paralytic disease. A rectal swab is dipped into the stool and then immersed into test tubes containing VTM (Viral transport medium) or Buffered saline. If no media is available, 4-8 gm stool sample should be sent to the nearest laboratory immediately while maintaining cold chain technique during transport and storage.

Poliovirus may be recovered from the stool or pharynx of a person with poliomyelitis. Isolation of virus from the cerebrospinal fluid (CSF) is diagnostic, but is rarely done. The next step in the poliomyelitis eradication initiative is to identify polioviruses isolated from clinical specimens. A polyclonal is first used to identify poliovirus antisera to types 1, 2 and 3 combined as antiserum pools. Monospecific antisera is then used for confirmation of serotype.

If poliovirus is isolated from a person with acute flaccid paralysis, it must be tested further, using oligonucleotide mapping or genomic sequencing, to determine if the virus is "wild type" or vaccine type. All poliovirus isolates are subjected to two methods of intratypic differentiation (ITD): one antigenic and one molecular. Concordant non-Sabin-like ITD results are classified as wild polioviruses, concordant Sabin-like results are classified as Sabin-like (vaccine virus), and any discordant results or Sabin-like isolates lacking two ITD tests are forwarded immediately for sequence analysis of the major viral capsid surface protein (VP1). These isolates are then classified based on the sequencing results: <1% difference from Sabin vaccine virus is classified as Sabin-like, 1%-15% difference is classified as VDPV, and >15% difference is classified as wild virus.[10]

Reverse transcriptase and PCR has been used for detection and identification of poliovirus based upon the nucleotide sequence characteristic of their genome. The specificity and sensitivity of PCR is well established and it is now being routinely used to identify cell culture isolates from polio cases. Antigen capture PCR further increase the sensitivity in analyzing the clinical specimens directly.[11] The full-length viral cDNA can be PCR amplified directly from stool samples and immediately subjected to genomic analysis by oligonucleotide microarray hybridization and nucleotide sequencing.[12]

Detection of poliovirus antibodies: Serum can be tested for neutralizing antibodies and complement fixing antibodies. Paired samples carried 4-6 weeks apart after the onset showing four-fold or greater rise is significant and confirmatory of polio infection. Non-detectable antibody titers in both specimens may help rule out poliomyelitis but may be falsely negative in immunocompromised persons.

Demonstration of polio specific IgM antibodies in cerebrospinal fluid is a specific test for poliomyelitis and indicates a true causal relationship between disease and infection. Isotype-specific capture ELISA tests have been developed for detection of IgM antibodies specific for the three strains of poliovirus which is easy to perform and gives result in less than 2 days. Since the virus isolation rate is maximal during the first 2 weeks after the onset of paralysis and then drops sharply the serology is useful in diagnosis of the cases who are detected at a later stage. A high percentage of patients test positive for poliovirus-specific IgM in the early phase of the infection and remain positive for upto 8 weeks.[13]

Neuroradiology: Neuroradiology has not been used as a diagnostic modality as it shows non-specific hyperintensity of anterior horn cells on MRI of spinal cord.

Electrodiagnostic changes: During the acute phase the affected muscles may be electromyographically silent or may show increase in polyphasic pattern. Evidence of denervation appears after about 3 weeks. Numerous fasciculation may be seen at this time. Giant action potentials signify the reinervation of muscle fibres by healthy neurons in recovery phase. However polyphasic pattern and neuropathic potentials can be found even after a good clinical recovery and in many cases fibrillation may persist for many years. Nerve conduction velocity is normal in acute poliomyelitis in the first 2-3 weeks. The response to peripheral nerve stimulation depends upon the extent of axonal damage. When the axonal damage is severe there may be no response to stimulation. In the presence of intact residual motor neurons the conduction speed is normal. Sensory latencies are always normal.

Differential Diagnosis

Non-paralytic form of polio should be distinguished from aseptic meningitis due to other viruses and meningismus associated with systemic illnesses. Paralytic form should be distinguished other causes of lower motor neuron paralysis and pseudoparalysis.

Table 41.1 shows the points of differentiation between poliomyelitis and other common causes of AFP which include GBS, transverse myelitis and injection neuritis.

Table 41.1: Differential Diagnosis of Poliomyelitis[14]

Signs and Symptoms	**Polio**	**GBS***	**TM****	**TN*****
Progression of paralysis	24-48 hours	Hour-10 days	Hours - 4 days	Hours-days
Fever	High, always present at onset of FP	Not common	Rarely present	Often present before, during and after FP
Flaccid paralysis (FP)	Acute asymmetrical mainly proximal	Acute symmetric distal	Acute lower limbs symmetrical	Acute asymmetrical, only one limb
Tone	Decreased or absent in affected limb	Diminished	Hypotonia of lower limbs	Decreased or absent in affected limb
Deep tendon reflexes	Decreased to absent	Global areflexia	Absent in acute phase later exaggerated	Decreased to absent
Sensation	Severe myalgia No sensory changes	Cramps, Tingling Hypo/ anaesthesia palms and soles	Anaesthesia LL and sensory level	Pain in gluteus hypothermia
Cranial nerve involvement	Only in bulbar form	Often present	Absent	Absent
Respiratory insufficiency	Mainly in cases with respiratory paralysis	In severe cases	If lesion is cervical or thoracic	Not present
CSF: WBC: Protein:	Increased normal	< 10 WBC high	Normal N or mild ↑	Normal
Bladder dysfunction	Generally absent	Sometimes transient	Present	Never
Nerve conduction velocity: 3rd week	Abnormal : Ant. horn cell disease normal in 1st 2 weeks	Abnormal: Demyelination	No diagnostic value	Abnormal in sciatic nerve
EMG –3 weeks	Abnormal denervation	Normal	Normal	Normal
Sequel at 3 months	Severe asymmetric atrophy, skeletal deformities later	Mild, symmetric atrophy of distal muscles	Flaccid diplegia	Moderate atrophy only in affected limb

*GBS: Guillain-Barré Syndrome

*TM: Transverse Myelitis

*TN: Traumatic Neuritis

Adapted from Reference No. 14.

Guillain-Barré Syndrome (GBS): An acquired demyelinating disease of peripheral nervous system is a common cause of AFP in childhood. Children with GBS may have sensory complaints in form of hypoanesthesia in a glove stocking distribution or tingling and burning sensation. GBS is differentiated from polio by the following features.

GBS is common in children >2 years while polio is common in children < 3 years. Fever is present in polio just before onset of paralysis, in GBS there may be history of fever 2-3 weeks prior to paralysis. Symmetric ascending paralysis involving distal muscles is seen in GBS while in polio paresis is patchy involving proximal muscles. CSF shows albumino-cytological disassociation in GBS.

Traumatic neuritis and **transverse myelitis** are other common causes of AFP which are differentiated by clinical features (Table 41.1). Symptoms of Infantile botulism may simulate bulbar poliomyelitis.

Other conditions which can cause confusion are peripheral neuropathies due to toxins such as lead and organophosphorous compounds and post diphtheria paralysis. The clinical picture of post diphtheretic paralysis is similar to GBS but there is a history of sore throat, nasal twang and nasal regurgitation of fluids 2-5 weeks prior to paralysis.

Pseudoparalysis: Certain conditions may present with pseudoparalysis due to local inflammatory conditions of hip or knee and can be confused with other causes of AFP. These are not to reported as AFP. Common causes of pseudoparalysis are hypokalaemia, inflammatory condition of femur, hip and knee such as toxic synovitis, arthritis, osteomyelitis; scurvy and congenital syphilitic. Rarely dengue virus infection can also result in acute pure motor quadriplegia due to myositis.[15]

Other Non-Polio Enteroviruses: A number of other non-polioenteroviruses (NPEV) are known to cause AFP.[16] Coxsackie A, coxsackie B, echovirus, enteroviruses types 70 and 71 have been associated with polio like illness. Most of cases of infection with NPEV show complete recovery within 60 days of onset. The paralytic sequelae of polio are more severe and permanent leading to atrophy of muscles and shortening of limb. Infection with West Nile virus causes an overlapping spectrum of aseptic meningitis, encephalitis, and myeloradiculitis causing asymmetric flaccid weakness, and with pathologic changes in the CNS which resemble poliomyelitis.[17]

Treatment

Management is primarily symptomatic as there is no specific treatment for poliomyelitis. In abortive and preparalytic stage complete bed rest is advised. Breast-feeding is continued in infants. Parents are advised not to give massage and intramuscular injections. Patient should be given analgesics for pain. The patient is closely observed for any weakness.

Patients with paralytic polio should be kept in close observation and may require hospitalization if there is rapid progression, bulbar involvement, respiratory insufficiency, bladder and bowel involvement or alteration of sensorium. The patient is given complete bed rest and kept on a firm bed with foot in a neutral position. The limbs are put in optimum position for relaxation of paralysed muscles. The affected limb can be positioned with pillows or rolled towels. The affected joints should be moved passively and gently through full range of movements to prevent contractures. Such movements are done 2-3 times a day. Symptomatic treatment for fever and pain is given as required. Warm water fomentation can be started in acute phase and continued for upto 6 weeks. Massage and intramuscular injections are contraindicated.

After the acute phase is over, active movements should be started and patient referred to centre equipped with physiotherapy services. Continued physiotherapy is required to prevent deformities and improve function.

Post-Polio Syndrome

After an interval of 25-40 years, 25%-40% of persons who contract paralytic poliomyelitis in childhood may experience muscle pain and exacerbation of existing weakness or develop new weakness or paralysis. The pathogenesis of this disease entity, which is referred to as post-polio syndrome, is not clear though premature ageing of motor neurons has been suggested to cause it. The most common symptoms are excessive fatigue and deterioration of functional capacity. Muscle weakness usually involves the same group of muscles which had residual paresis although in some cases muscles which were not involved earlier may show weakness. Risk factors for post-polio syndrome include (a) increasing length of time since acute poliovirus infection, (b) presence of permanent residual impairment after recovery from the acute illness; and (c) female sex. The treatment consists of reducing fatigue, use of assistive devices and bracing of weak muscles and joints. The exact magnitude of problem in India is not known.

Prevention

Poliovirus Vaccines: Currently three types of polio-vaccines are available, i.e., oral poliovaccine (OPV); inactivated polio vaccine (IPV) of Salk which has been largely replaced by enhanced potency inactivated vaccine (IPV-EP). All these are trivalent with mixture of 3 strains of polioviruses.

OPV: Trivalent OPV contains live attenuated strains of all three serotypes of poliovirus. The viruses are propagated in monkey kidney cell culture. After complete primary vaccination with three doses of OPV, greater than or equal to 95% of recipients develop long-lasting (probably life-long) immunity to all three poliovirus types. OPV consistently induces immunity of the gastrointestinal tract that provides a substantial degree of resistance to reinfection with poliovirus. Because of continued excretion it also gives rise to herd immunity. Administration of OPV interferes with subsequent infection by wild poliovirus, a property that is important in vaccination campaigns to control polio epidemics.

The major concern with OPV is vaccine associated poliomyelitis. The overall risk for VAPP is approximately one case in 2.4 million doses distributed. Immunodeficient persons, particularly those who have B-lymphocyte disorders that inhibit synthesis of immune globulins are at greatest risk for VAPP (3,200-fold to 6,800-fold greater than the risk for immunocompetent OPV recipients).[18] VAPP is more likely to occur in persons 18 years of age and older than in children. The mechanism of VAPP is believed to be a mutation or reversion, of the vaccine virus to a more neurotropic form. These mutated viruses are called revertants. The paralysis that results are similar to that caused by wild virus, and may be permanent.

IPV

The original salk strain was grown in tissue culture of human diploid cell line or vero cell and inactivated by formalin. This has been replaced by IPV-EP which is manufactured by means of microcarrier culture technique and has a high antigenic content. Inactivated vaccines are not associated with VAPP and can be given to immunodeficient individuals. Whereas the systemic antibody response of OPV and IPV/ IPV-EP is comparable, the mucosal immune response is virtually absent in case of IPV and weak in case of IPV-EP. Besides high cost, absence of herd effect and shorted duration of immunity are the drawbacks of inactivated vaccines.

Vaccination Schedules

Vaccination schedules followed by various countries depends on the circulation of wild virus in that country. In country like India 0 dose is given at birth followed by 3 primary doses of OPV at 6, 10 and 14 weeks. Subsequently 2 booster doses at 18 months and 41/2 years are recommended. In countries where wild poliovirus is not reported, inapparent infection with wild poliovirus no longer contributes to establishing or maintaining poliovirus immunity because these viruses no longer circulate in the population. However universal vaccination of infants and children is required to maintain population immunity against poliomyelitis until the wild virus is totally eradicated from the world. In such countries the risk of OPV associated VAPP is considered significant, immunization with IPV or alone sequelae of IPV+ OPV is recommended. The primary series of sequential use is administered at age 2 months and 4 months with IPV followed by 2 doses of OPV at 16-18 months and 4-6 years.[19] Pentavalent (5-component) combination vaccine containing IPV is also available. The vaccine contains IPV, DTaP and a pediatric dose of hepatitis B vaccine.

Poliomyelitis Eradication

In May 1988, members of the 41st World Health Assembly (WHA) passed a resolution calling for the above global eradication of poliomyelitis by the year 2000.[20]

The Government of India also committed to the goal. Specific targets to achieve this included:

(a) No case of clinical poliomyelitis caused by wild polio virus.

(b) No wild polio virus found world wide despite intensive efforts to do so.

The polio eradication initiative (PEI) is global collaborative effort of WHO, UNICEF, US Centre for Disease Control and Prevention (CDC) and number of national governments and NGOs who are strongly committed to the initiative. The primary strategies for achieving the goal are:

(1) **Routine Immunization:** Attaining high routine immunization coverage, every child <1 year should get at least 3 doses of OPV. The EPI schedule comprises zero dose at birth and three doses of OPV3 at 6, 10 and 14 weeks of age.

(2) **Supplementary Immunization Activities (SIA)** which provide additional OPV doses to every child

in age group of 0-5 years to interrupt wild virus transmission. The aim of SIA is to flood the community with OPV within a very short period of time thereby interrupting transmission of wild polio virus and to increase immunity amongst children. SIAs include:

(a) National Immunization Days (NIDs) when entire country is covered.

(b) Sub National Immunization Days (SNID) when some states or parts of state are covered.

(c) Mop-ups are conducted as soon as possible after identification of virus as an end stage strategy, when virus transmission is focalized and polio case are found in specific areas.

The basic aim of conducting SIA is to reach all under five children with potent vaccine in each round. This is achieved by offering:

- Immunization to all children at booths on the first day of round.
- Follow up of missed children through house-to-house search and vaccinate component by vaccination teams.
- Immunize children in transit by transit teams.

The number of PPI rounds conducted during a particular year is determined by extent of polio virus transmission. The first PPI round in India was held on 9th December 1995 and 20th January 1996 only as booth days and reached 87 million children aged 0-3 years with OPV doses. In subsequent years the target age group was expanded to include children aged 0-5 years. Later the programme was intensified to include house to house and transit teams activity. Intensification of PPI required meticulous micro planning, intensive supervision monitoring and extensive social mobilization.

(3) **Surveillance of Acute Flaccid Paralysis (AFP):** This is to identify all reservoirs of wild polio virus transmission, it includes AFP case notification investigation and laboratory investigation of stool specimens collected from AFP cases. In 1997 National Polio Surveillance Project (NPSP) was established as joint collaboration between World Health Organization and Ministry of Health and Family Welfare Government of India with primary objective to intensify and assist states and Government of India in polio surveillance.[21]

For surveillance purposes AFP is defined as in **Sudden onset of weakness and floppines in any part of body in a child. < 15 years of age or paralysis in a person of any age in whom polio is suspected.**

In India the AFP surveillance system is based on comprehensive network of surveillance medical officers (SMO) in each districts and reporting sites which include all health facilities right from medical colleges, private nursing homes, practitioners, popular quacks or polio doctors even religious places visited by AFP cases.

As of 2005, 9500 reporting units and 12,300 informers units have been enrolled under AFP Surveillance network throughout the country. Each reporting unit has been designated a nodal officer to report an AFP case immediately and also send weekly report on an assigned format even if it is a nil report.

Two stool samples must be collected from each AFP case upto 60 days of paralysis onset. A stool specimen is **adequate** "when two stool specimen are collected within 14 days of paralysis onset and at least 24 hours apart in adequate volume (8-10 gms) and arrive in a WHO accredited laboratory in good condition (no desiccation, no leakage with adequate documentation and evidence that cold chain was maintained)".

Polio virus laboratory network: Eight national laboratories accredited by WHO constitute the India polio virus lab network, ERC Mumbai is one of the seven global specialized lab to perform intra typic differentiation (ITD) and genetic sequencing all wild polio virus isolates to guide the programme. This information is powerful tool to determine reservoir areas of transmission and sources of outbreaks; it helps to determine if a case that appears in previously polio free area is due to re-establishment of indigenous circulation or an importation of virus from elsewhere.

India is closer to eradication of wild polio virus transmission than any time in its history. Only 66 cases of confirmed polio cases were identified in 2005. The disease is confined to the smallest geographic area, only in few districts of western UP and North Bihar. Most of the genetic families of virus circulating in 2002 are now extinct. This has resulted from intensified and focused Supplementary Immunization Activities (SIA). Enhanced AFP surveillance and introduction of monovalent oral polio vaccine (MOPV) targeted to those areas, which continue to report wild virus cases.[21]

There was increase in cases of paralytic polio due to wildpoliovirus in 2006. The main concern is that longer it takes to interrupt WPV transmission in the endemic region. The greater the danger of WPV being exported to polio-free countries. Currently Nigeria, Uttar Pradesh and Indonesia pose a constant threat to polio-free areas within the country as well as neighbouring countries.[22]

An outbreak of circulating vaccine derived poliovirus (cVDPV), which was reported for Indonesia in 2005 is another area of concern which illustrate the risk of emergence of cVDPV in areas with low level of population immunization. This emphasizes the need to eventually stop all route use of OPV once wild poliovirus is eradicated.[23]

References

1. World Health Organization. Acute onset flaccid paralysis. WHO: Geneva 1993 WHO/MNH/EPI.
2. Sharma M, Sen S, Ahuja B, Dhamija K. Paralytic Poliomyelitis 1975-1988. Report from a Sentinel Center. Indian Pediatr 1990;27:143-50.
3. Sen S, Sharma D, Santhanam S. Clinical and Serological Study of Acute Paralytic Poliomyelitis in Immunized and Non-Immunized Children. Indian J Pediatricsn 1985;22:891-97.
4. Deivanayagam N, Nedunchelian K, *et al.* Etiological Agents of Acute Poliomyelitis in South India. Indian J Pediatr 1994;61:257-62.
5. Hovi T, Huovilacnem A, Kurouen T, *et al.* Outbreak of Paralytic Poliomyelitis in Finland: Widespread Circulation of Antigenically Altered Poliovirus Type 3 in a Vaccinated Population. Lancet 1986:1427.
6. CDC – Progress Towards Interruption of Wild Poliovirus Transmission – Worldwide, January 2005 – March 2006. MMWR 2006;55:458-62.
7. Yohannan MD, Ramia S, Al Frayh AR. Acute Paralytic Poliomyelitis Presenting as Guillian Barré Syndrome. J Infect 1991;22:129-33.
8. Vijayan P, Mukundan P, Shukoor AA, Panicker CKJ, John TJ. Epidemic Poliomyelitis. Indian J Pediatr 1985:22:569-73.
9. Gupta PC, Gathwala G, Aneja S, Arora SK. Acute Cerebellar Ataxia–An Unusual Presentation of Poliomyelitis.
10. CDC Laboratory Surveillance for Wild and Vaccine Derived Poliovirus 2000-2001. MMWR 2002;51:369-71.
11. Boot HJ, Schepp RM, van Nunen FJ, Kimman TG. Rapid RT-PCR Amplification of Full-length Poliovirus Genomes Allows Rapid Discrimination Between Wild-type and Recombinant Vaccine-derived Polioviruses. J Virol Methods 2004:1:116(1):35-43.
12. Laassri M, Dragunsky E, Enterline J, Eremeeva T, Ivanova O, Lottenbach K, Belshe R, Chumakov K. Genomic Analysis of Vaccine-derived Poliovirus Strains in Stool Specimens by Combination of Full-length PCR and Oligonucleotide Microarray Hybridization. J Clin Microbiol 2005;43(6): 2886-94.
13. Herremans T, Koopmans MP, van der Avoort HG, van Loon AM. Lessons from Diagnostic Investigations of Patients with Poliomyelitis and Their Direct Contacts for the Present Surveillance of Acute Flaccid Paralysis. Clin Infect Dis 1999;29(4):849-54.
14. Alcala H, Olive JM, de Quadros C. The Diagnosis of Polio and Other Acute Flaccid Paralysis–A Neurological Approach. Draft of EPI Research and Development Group Meeting 1990. Expanded Program on Immunization Pan American Health Organization, Washington DC.
15. Kalita J, Misra UK, Mahadevan A, Shankar SK. Acute Pure Motor Quadriplegia: Is It Dengue Myositis? Electromyogr Clin Neurophysiol 2005;45:357-61.
16. Soloman T, Willison H. Infectious of Acute Flaccid Paralysis. Curr Opin Infect Dis 2003;16:275-81.
17. Jeha LE, Sila CA, Lederman RJ, Prayson RA, Isada CM, Gordon SM. West Nile Virus Infection: A New Acute Paralytic Illness. Neurology 2003;61:55-59.
18. Sutter RW, Prevots DR. Vaccine-associated Paralytic Poliomyelitis Among Immunodeficient Persons. Infect Med 1994; 11:426,429-30,435-58.
19. Poliomyelitis Prevention in United States: Introduction of a Sequential Vaccination Schedule of Inactivated Polio-virus Vaccine Followed by Oral Poliovirus Vaccines: Recommendation of the Advisory Committee in Immunization Practices (ACIP). MMWR 1997;46:1-25.
20. World Health Assembly. Global Eradication of Poliomyelitis by the Year 2000: Resolution of the 41st World Health Assembly Geneva Switzerland. WHO 1988.
21. National Polio Surveillance Project India Field Guide. Surveillance of Acute Flaccid Paralysis. Department of Family Welfare. MOHFW, New Delhi 2005.
22. CDC–Progress Towards Interruption of Wild Poliovirus Transmission–Worldwide, January 2005–March 2006.MMWR 2006;55:458-62.
23. Kew OM, Sutter RW, de Gourville EM, Dowdle WR. Vaccine Derived Poliovirus in the Endogenic Strategy of Global Polio Eradication. Ann Rev Microbiol 2005;69:587-639.

42 Chapter

CEREBRAL MALARIA

Medha Mittal

BURDEN OF DISEASE

Malaria is caused by Plasmodium species with life cycle stages alternating between the mosquito and a variety of mammals and birds. It persists as a major public health problem throughout the world primarily in developing tropical and subtropical regions. In the recently published global burden of disease study, malaria accounted for 25,652 deaths among children and adolescents in India in the year 2013.[1]

Cerebral malaria is defined as coma without apparent etiology in presence of Plasmodium falciparum (P. falciparum) (asexual stage) parasitemia.[2] However, with the increasing number of cases of cerebral malaria due to Plasmodium vivax (P. vivax) being reported from across the globe this definition would need to be revised. The earliest known such case was reported in the year 1921.[3] Most of the reports are of isolated cases with only a few case series. In the author's own study of 198 admitted cases of malaria, 128 (64.6%) were due to P. vivax, 66 (34.3%) due to P. falciparum and 4 (2.0%) had evidence of mixed infection. Sixty-four (50%) patients with *vivax* infection had one or more complications, with severe anemia in 33 (26%), cerebral malaria in 16 (12.5%), and death in 6 (4.7%) cases. In the falciparum group, 52 (78.8%) had one or more complications with severe anemia in 37 (56.1%), cerebral malaria in 24 (36.4%) and death in 4 (6.1%) cases. Overall, because of their larger numbers, *vivax* infection comprised the major bulk of the burden of severe complications and death.[4] In studies from Bikaner and New Delhi, cerebral malaria was reported in 21.5% and 16.8% children with severe vivax malaria.[5,6] P. vivax monoinfection has been reported in 21-27% cases of severe malaria from Papua New Guinea, Indonesia and Thailand.[7]

Etiology and Pathogenesis

Hippocrates first described the clinical presentation and complications of malaria in the fifth century BCE. The term malaria was coined much later in the eighteenth century. It was believed that the disease was transmitted through the foul air of swampy areas (and hence malaria or bad air). The first description of malaria parasites in the blood was given by a French physician, Laveran, in 1880, while working in Algeria. Transmission of malaria by Anopheles mosquito was discovered in 1897 by Ross, a British military physician, working in India.[8] Thereafter scientists elucidated the life cycle of the parasite which led to the initiation of control efforts.

The definitive host and vector, the female anopheles mosquito, is the site of sexual reproduction of plasmodia. Anopheles culicifacies is the principal vector in rural areas while An. Stephensi is the primary urban vector.[9] When the mosquito bites a human being it releases an average of 100-500 sporozoites into the blood stream. They travel to the hepatic sinusoids, invade hepatic cells where the sporozoite develops to a mature liver stage schizont, inside which develop about 30,000 uninucleated merozoites (asexual reproduction).[10] The hepatic cell dies or ruptures and the released merozoites invade the erythrocytes. Here the merozoites consume red cell hemoglobin and develop into trophozoites. When fully mature, the infected erythrocyte ruptures, releasing the merozoites which then invade normal erythrocytes initiating the cycle again. This increases the number of parasites manifold and leads to all the manifestations of the illness. This erythrocytic phase lasts for 1-3 weeks. In its early stages of schizogony, the parasite appears as a ring like structure within the parasitized erythrocyte. The hemoglobin degraded by the parasite accumulates as hemozoin inside the erythrocyte. Some merozoites differentiate into gamete precursors. When the human host is bitten, the infected erythrocytes enter the mosquito where sexual reproduction takes place.[10]

Inside the human host the parasite lodged in the erythrocyte influences and changes the properties of the erythrocyte membrane. An increased red blood cell (RBC) membrane rigidity, reduced plasticity, greater adhesiveness of the cell membrane lead to microvascular slugging and capillary clogging.[11-14] This depletes the local oxygen level providing an optimum environment for parasite replication.[14] Thrombi may form followed by DIC. The theories also attribute pathogenic role to proinflammatory cytokines and interleukins in causing endothelial damage. The most serious consequence develops when the parasitized RBCs bind to the microvascular endothelium in the brain vasculature impairing the blood flow and depleting oxygen levels. The blood brain barrier too gets disrupted due to the changes in endothelial cell junctional permeability causing cerebral edema. This is more commonly seen in children than adults.[15]

Elevated levels of TNF (tumor necrosis factor), inerleukin (IL)-6 and anti-inflammatory IL-10 are observed in patients with cerebral malaria compared with those without malaria.[16] Several polymorphisms in the TNF gene promoter are associated with an increased risk of cerebral malaria, neurological sequelae and death.[17] Nitric oxide has been suggested as a key effector for TNF in the pathogenesis of malaria. This influences cerebral blood flow and reduces level of consciousness rapidly and reversibly because of its easy diffusibility across the blood brain barrier.[17,18]

Clinical Features

Classically there *is high fever with chills, rigors, sweats* and headache but symptoms can be notoriously nonspecific and include vomiting, diarrhea, abdominal pain, respiratory distress. Cerebral malaria is most often heralded by mental deterioration and often has a rapid onset (mean duration of symptoms prior to admission being 47 hours) followed by progression to stupor or coma.[19] Hypoglycemia should always be suspected in any patient with altered sensorium. Patients with cerebral malaria fail to arouse even after dextrose correction.

Physical findings include *high fever, pallor, hepatosplenomegaly*, seizures (may be repeated), abnormal movements, upper motor neuron dysfunction, extensor plantar, cerebellar involvement and even psychosis. Decorticate or decerebrate posturing may be seen. Seizures are seen in 80% of children with cerebral malaria compared with only 15-20% of adults. Seizures are mostly generalized though EEG identifies a focal origin in many patients. Focal deficits such as hemiparesis and isolated cranial nerve lesions may occur. Tendon jerks though usually increased may be normal or even depressed. Neck stiffness is only occasionally seen. Disorders of conjugate gaze are typically present and pupillary abnormalities are also often seen.[18,19] Papilledema, extramacular retinal edema, prolonged seizure activity, deep and prolonged coma, hypoglycemia, metabolic acidosis and respiratory distress identify those with poor prognosis (mortality or sequelae).[20,21] Patients may have other features of severe malaria that include metabolic acidosis, severe anemia, acute renal failure, acute pulmonary edema, jaundice, significant bleeding or shock.[20] Neurologic sequelae may occur in those recovering, in about 10-30%, the most commonly seen being ataxia and paresis.[2,20] Others include epilepsy, hemiparesis, cortical blindness, impaired hearing, behavioral abnormalities and cognitive deficits.[2,21-25] Cerebellar atrophy and acute disseminated encephalomyelitis have also been reported.[26,27]

According to a study published in 2004, about a quarter of the pediatric patients diagnosed with CM using the WHO criteria were shown at autopsy to have died of non-CM causes[28] (which highlights the importance of accurate and reliable diagnostic tools while emphasizing careful clinical judgement). In pediatric patients, retinal microvessels have been shown to sustain damage comparable to the ones occurring in the brain, making them an easily observable surrogate marker to assess the severity of cerebral pathology during CM.[29,30] Retinal changes include vessel color changes, white-centered hemorrhages, and peri- and extramacular whitening.[31] The severity of these changes during P.falciparum infection correlates strongly with patient mortality, and their early detection may help identify the at-risk patient.[32,33] The modalities to pick up such changes include fundoscopy and the newer methods such as Optical Coherence Tomography (OCT), use of retinal cameras and automated analysis of the retinal vasculature as seen on fluorescein angiogram.[31]

Investigations

Prompt and accurate diagnosis remain the key to effective management. All patients should undergo examination of a blood smear and rapid diagnostic test. While thick smear remains the gold standard being more sensitive in detecting the parasite at density of <10 per μL of blood, thin smears aid in parasite species identification and quantification. They can also determine parasite density and presence of gametocytes besides being cost effective. They also allow monitoring of response to therapy. Both microscopy and rapid diagnostic tests (RDT) must be supported by a quality assurance programme.[20] Examination of quantitative buffy coat and detection of parasites in smears stained with acridine orange can improve the yield of microscopy.[9] Unavailability or delay of the test results should not delay the antimalarial treatment which should be initiated promptly.

The RDTs are immunochromatographic tests based on detection of pLDH (plasmodium lactate dehydrogenase) antigen from P. vivax or pan-malarial antigens pan-pLDH and HRP2 (histidine rich protein 2) that detects P. falciparum. RDTs are simple to perform and interpret. The sensitivity and specificity of HRP2 was 95% and 95.2% respectively in one report.[34] It can persist in blood stream for several weeks and so cannot be used to detect parasite clearance. The pLDH on the other hand gets rapidly cleared (though sexual stages may give some positivity) and along with smear examination can be used to see for clearance.

Polymerase chain reaction based tests are highly sensitive but are not generally available and are not appropriate for routine diagnosis in endemic areas where a large proportion of the population may have low-density parasitemia.[20]

CT findings correlate well with level of consciousness and severity of disease[35] and are helpful in determination of cerebral volume variation and the detection of infarctions in large vessels.[36] In children with retinopathy-confirmed CM, acute head CTs revealed findings consistent with autopsy studies and showed abnormality in basal ganglia, white matter and corpus callosum.[35]

Other tests may be required as per the clinical condition of the patient–such as PT, aPTT to assess coagulation, liver function and renal function tests, screen for any bacterial infection etc.

In addition to prevention strategies and effective treatment, one of the most important factors influencing the outcome of CM is its early diagnosis. Early screening biomarkers allow the identification of individuals destined to become affected or who are in the "preclinical" stages of the illness. The role of endothelial intracellular adhesion molecule-1 (ICAM-1) in the sequestration of PRBC is well-understood, and specific binding of PRBC to ICAM-1 has been implicated in the development of CM[37] Angiopoetin-1 and -2 (ANG-1 and -2) are critical regulators of endothelial activation and integrity, and their levels have also been described as reliable biomarkers of CM. Indeed, ANG-1 and -2 levels profiled from serum or whole blood were shown to discriminate accurately between cerebral and uncomplicated malaria in African patients[38] and between cerebral, severe non-cerebral malaria, and uncomplicated malaria in a cohort of Thai patients.[39] Compared to uncomplicated malaria, CM patients presented significant decreases in ANG-1 and increases in ANG-2 levels and the ratio of ANG-2: ANG-1. This is consistent with the pathophysiology of CM, which involves endothelial activation and dysfunction. Indeed, ANG-1 maintains vascular quiescence, while ANG-2 displaces ANG-1 upon endothelial activation and sensitizes the cells to become responsive to sub-threshold concentrations of tumor necrosis factor (TNF).[40] These tests hold promise for the future.

Treatment

Cerebral malaria should be treated as a medical emergency with emphasis on management of fluid and electrolyte balance, hypoglycemia, metabolic acidosis and renal failure. Any suspicion of coexisting bacterial infection or meningitis should be treated with parenteral antibiotics. Mechanical ventilation may be required to protect the airway. Data do not support the use of mannitol for control of raised intracranial pressure in cerebral malaria and dexamethasone use prolongs coma and is contraindicated.[2]

Parenteral artesunate (or artemether) should be started for at least 24 hours and until patients can tolerate oral medication. Children weighing < 20 kg should receive a higher dose of artesunate (3 mg/kg body weight per dose) than larger children and adults (2.4 mg/kg per dose). Artesunate has been shown to decrease mortality by about 25% as compared to quinine whereas, artemether reduced mortality similar to quinine. There may be a phase of post treatment hemolysis especially in those with hyperparasitemia. This is because the drug acts on the intraerythrocytic ring stage of the parasite which are then removed from the red cells by the spleen. These erythrocytes return to the circulation but with a reduced life span. Post artesunate anemia has to be watched for. Quinine may be required for those not resistant to artesunate to be given as slow controlled infusion in 5% dextrose solution.

Supportive treatment to manage complications is also essential. Hypoglycemia should be managed as per standard treatment though hyperinsulinemic hypoglycemia may require somatostatin analogue. Seizures can be terminated with benzodiazepines although they may be less effective as malaria seems to downregulate amunobutyric acid receptors. Co-existent bacterial infection would need antibacterial therapy. Blood transfusions would be required for severe anemia; exchange transfusion to manage hyperparasitemia remains controversial. Cerebral perfusion pressure must be optimized and raised intracranial pressure managed cautiously. Primaquine should be given for radical cure.

Artesunate: Two 2.4 mg/kg doses given intravenously 12 h apart on day 1, then 2.4 mg/kg daily for 6 days, given orally if patient can swallow. Side effects include hypersensitivity reactions (risk estimate, 1 in 3000), gastrointestinal disturbances, cough, rash, arthralgia, dizziness and delayed haemolysis.

Artemether: 3.2 mg/kg intramuscular loading dose, then 1.6 mg/kg per day for 6 days, given orally if patient can swallow. Absorption might be erratic in patients in shock. It has similar side-effects to other artemisinin derivatives, including hypersensitivity reactions (risk estimate, 1 in 3000), mild gastrointestinal disturbance, dizziness, reticulocytopenia, neutropenia and elevated liver enzyme activity. Bradycardia may also occur.

Quinine: Dilute quinine dihydrochloride with normal or dextrose saline and infused over 4 h (preferably via syringe or infusion pump); Loading dose: 20 mg/kg body weight (salt) infused over 4 h; Maintenance dose: 10 mg/kg body weight infused every 8 h until oral administration possible. Side-effects are seen commonly. "Cinchonism" includes tinnitus, slight impairment of hearing, headache, nausea, dizziness, dysphoria and sometimes disturbed vision. When severe, there can be vertigo, vomiting, abdominal pain, diarrhea, marked auditory loss and visual symptoms, including loss of vision. Hypoglycemia (due to hyperinsulinemia), cardiotoxicity (prolongation of QTc interval, hypotension and even cardiac arrest), venous thrombosis and hypersensitivity reactions are other important side effects. Hepatic injury and psychosis occur very rarely.

Primaquine: 0.25 mg base/kg bw per day for 14 days for P. vivax and 0.5 mg/kg bw base upto maximum oral dose of 30 mg daily for P. falciparum. While primaquine is generally well tolerated, it may cause dose-related gastrointestinal discomfort, including abdominal pain, nausea and vomiting. Administration with food improves tolerability. Hypertension and cardiac arrhythmia have been reported rarely. The most important adverse effect is haemolysis in patients with glucose-6-phosphate dehydrogenase (G6PD) deficiency. Leukopenia, methaemoglobinaemia with cyanosis and granulocytopenia may also occur.

References

1. Global Burden of Disease Pediatrics Collaboration, Kyu HH, Pinho C, Wagner JA, Brown JC, Bertozzi-Villa A, Charlson FJ, *et al.*, Global and National Burden of Diseases and Injuries Among Children and Adolescents Between 1990 and 2013: Findings From the Global Burden of Disease 2013 Study. JAMA Pediatr 2016 January 25.
2. Chandy C John. Malaria. In: Kliegman RM, Stanton BF, Schor NF, St Geme III JW, Behrman RE eds. Nelson Textbook of Pediatrics, 20th Edition, Philadelphia: Elsiever 2016:1709-21.
3. Vietze G. Malaria and Other Protozoal Disease, Vinken PG, Bruyn GW eds. Handbook of Clinical Neurology, Infections of the Nervous System. Amsterdam: North Holland Publishing Company 1978;143-60.
4. M Mittal M, Jain R, Talukdar B, Kumar M, Kapoor K. Emerging New Trends of Malaria in Children: A Study from A Tertiary Care Centre in Northern India. J Vector Borne Dis 2014 June;51(2):115-18.
5. Kochar DK, Tanwar GS, Khatri PC, Kochar SK, Sengar GS, Gupta A *et al.* Clinical Features of Children Hospitalized with Malaria–A Study from Bikaner, Northwest India. Am J Trop Med Hyg 2010;83:981-89.
6. Yadav D, Chandra J, Aneja S, Kumar V, Kumar P, Dutta AK. Changing Profile of Severe Malaria in North Indian Children. Indian J Pediatr 2012;79(4):483-87.
7. Price RN, Douglas NM, Anstey NM. New Developments in Plasmodium Vivax Malaria: Severe Disease and The Rise of Chloroquine Resistance. Curr Opin Infect Dis 2009 Oct; 22(5):430-5. doi: 10.1097/QCO.0b013e32832f14c1. Review. PubMed PMID:19571748.
8. The History of Malaria: An Ancient Disease at www.cdc.gov/malaria accessed on 18.02.2016.
9. Mengi S, Singh VA, Vohra P, Sawhney N. Malaria: Mini Review on Disease and Diagnostic Challenges Int. J. Pharm. Med. and Bio. Sc 2014 Vol. 3.(2)2014:53-60.
10. Hoffman SL, Campbell CC, White NJ Chapter 96 Malaria In: Tropical Infectious Diseases Principles, Pathogenesis and Practice, 3rd Edition. Eds Guerrant RL, Walker DH, Weller PF, Saunders Elsevier.
11. Krogstad DJ. In: Principles and Practice of Infectious Diseases, Mandell GL, Bennett JE, Dolin R, Editors, New York: Churchill Livingstone 1995;2415-27.
12. McQueen PG, McKenzie FE. Age-Structured Red Blood Cell Susceptibility and the Dynamics of Malaria Infections, Proc NatlAcadSci USA 2004;101:9161-66.
13. Newton CR, Krishna S. Severe Falciparum Malaria in Children: Current Understanding of Pathophysiology and Supportive Treatment, Pharmacol Ther 1998;79:1-53.
14. Cooke BM, Mohandas N, Coppel RL. Malaria and the Red Blood Cell Membrane. Semin Hematol 2004:41(2):173-78.
15. Adams S, Brown H, Turner G. Breaking Down the Blood Brain Barrier: Signaling a Path to Cerebral Malaria? Trends in Parasitol 2002;18:360-66.
16. Day NP, *et al.* The Prognostic and Pathophysiologic Role of Pro- and Antiinflammatory Cytokines in Severe Malaria. J. Infect. Dis 1999;180:1288-97.
17. Gimenez F, de Lagerie S. Barraud, Fernandez C, Pino P, Mazier D. Tumor Necrosis Factor α in the Pathogenesis of Cerebral Malaria. Cell. Mol. Life Sci 2003;60:1623-35.
18. Mishra SK, Newton CR. Diagnosis and Management of the Neurological Complications of Falciparum Malaria. Nat Rev Neurol 2009 Apr;5(4):189-98.
19. Molyneux ME. Malaria–Clinical Features in Children. J R Soc Med 1989:82Suppl17:35-38Review.
20. Guidelines for the Treatment of Malaria, 3rd edn. Geneva: World Health Organization 2015, Available from: http://apps.who.int/iris/bitstream/10665/162441/1/9789241549127_eng.pdf (accessed on October 25, 2017).
21. Idro R, Kakooza-Mwesige A, Balyejjussa S, Mirembe G, Mugasha C, Tugumisirize J *et al.* Severe Neurological Sequelae and Behaviour Problems After Cerebral Malaria in Ugandan Children, BMC Res Notes 2010April16:3:104.
22. Molyneux ME, Taylor TE, Wirima JJ, Borgstein A. Clinical Features and Prognostic Indicators in Paediatric Cerebral

Malaria: A Study of 131 Comatose Malawian Children. Q J Med 1989:71:441-59.

23. vanHensbroek MB, Palmer A, Jaffar S, Schneider G, Kwiatkowski D. Residual Neurologic Sequelae After Childhood Cerebral Malaria. J Pediatr 1997:131:125-29.

24. Idro R, Carter JA, Fegan G, Neville BG, Newton CR. Risk Factors for Persisting Neurological and Cognitive Impairments following Cerebral Malaria. Arch Dis Child 2006:91:142-48.

25. Idro R, Karamagi C, Tumwine J. Immediate Outcome and Prognostic Factors for Cerebral Malaria Among Children Admitted to Mulago Hospital, Uganda. Ann Trop Paediatr 2004:24:17-24.

26. Sriram P, Balachandar BV, Raja AJ. Cerebellar Atrophy in Falciparum Malaria. Indian Pediatr 2013:50:505-06.

27. Agrawal A, Goyal S. Acute Demyelinating Encephalomyelitis in a Child Following Malaria. Indian Pediatr 2012:49:922-23.

28. Taylor TE, Fu WJ, Carr RA,Whitten RO, Mueller JG, Fosiko NG, *et al.* Differentiating the Pathologies of Cerebral Malaria by Postmortem Parasite Counts. Nat. Med 2004:10:143-45.

29. Beare NA, Taylor TE, Harding SP, Lewallen S and Molyneux ME. Malarial Retinopathy: A Newly Established Diagnostic Sign in Severe Malaria. Am. J. Trop. Med. Hyg 2006:75:790-97.

30. Maude RJ, Dondorp AM, Sayeed AA, Day NP, White NJ and Beare NA. The Eye in Cerebral Malaria: What Can it Teach Us? Trans R. Soc. Trop. Med. Hyg 2009:103:661-64.

31. Sahu PK, Satpathi S, Behera PK, Mishra SK, Mohanty S, Wassmer SC. Pathogenesis of Cerebral Malaria: New Diagnostic Tools, Biomarkers and Therapeutic Approaches. Front Cell Infect Microbiol 2015Oct 27:5:75.

32. Maccormick IJ, Beare NA, Taylor TE, Barrera V, White VA, Hiscott P, *et al.* Cerebral Malaria in Children: Using the Retina to Study the Brain. Brain 2014:137(Pt8):2119-42.

33. Kariuki SM, Gitau E, Gwer S, Karanja HK, Chengo E, Kazungu M, *et al.* Value of Plasmodium Falciparum Histidine-Richprotein 2 Level and Malaria Retinopathy Indistinguishing Cerebral Malaria from Other Acute Encephalopathies in Kenyan Children. J. Infect. Dis 2014:209: 600-09.

34. Abba K, Deeks JJ, Olliaro P, Naing CM, Jackson SM, Takwoingi Y, Donegan S, Garner P. Rapid Diagnostic Tests for Diagnosing Uncomplicated P. Falciparum Malaria in Endemic Countries. Cochrane Database Syst Rev 2011July6:(7).

35. Patankar TF, Karnad DR, Shetty PG, Desai AP and Prasad SR. Adult Cerebral Malaria: Prognostic Importance of Imaging Findings and Correlation with Postmortem Findings. Radiology 2002:224:811-16.

36. Taylor TE. Neuroimaging Findings in Children with Retinopathy-confirmed Cerebral Malaria. Eur J Radiol 2010 April: 74(1):262-68.

37. Smith JD, Craig AG, Kriek N, Hudson-Taylor D, Kyes S, Fagan T, *et al.* Identification of a Plasmodium Falciparum Intercellular Adhesion Molecule-Binding Domain: A Parasite Adhesion Trait Implicated in Cerebral Malaria. Proc. Natl. Acad. Sci. USA 2000:97:1766-71.

38. Lovegrove FE, Tangpukdee N, Opoka RO, Lafferty EI, Rajwans N, Hawkes M, *et al.* Serum Angiopoietin-1 and -2 Levels Discriminate Cerebral Malaria from Uncomplicated Malaria and Predict Clinical Outcome in African Children. PLoSONE 2009;4:e4912.

39. Conroy AL, Lafferty EI, Lovegrove FE, Krudsood S, Tangpukdee N, Liles WC, *et al.* Whole Blood Angiopoietin-1 and - 2 Levels Discriminate Cerebra and Severe (Non-Cerebral) Malaria from Uncomplicated Malaria. Malar J 2009:8:295.

40. Kim H, Higgins S, Liles WC and Kain KC. Endothelial Activation and Dysregulation in Malaria: A Potential Target for Novel Therapeutics. Curr. Opin. Hematol 2011:18:177-85.

43 Chapter

NEUROCYSTICERCOSIS

Bibek Talukdar

Neurocysticercosis (NCC), resulting from infection of the brain and spinal cord by pork tape worm taenia solium and characterized primarily by seizure, is a common neurological disorder worldwide. The disease is endemic in many developing countries including India probably because of poor sanitation and hygiene. The exact prevalence of the disease in India is not known there being no systematic epidemiologic study; it is likely to be high as can be gauzed from the large number of cases being reported every year.

Pathophysiology

Human gets cysticercosis from accidental ingestion of taenia solium egg. Such ingestion can occur through (a) Consumption of water, vegetables, and other food contaminated by eggs; (b) Oro-fecal route if his immediate environment was contaminated by ova of T. solium because of some close contact harboring a tapeworm who keeps excreting eggs off and on; and (c) Due to reverse peristalsis if the man himself has harbored the worm in his own intestine. The oncospheres liberated from the eggs in his intestine by the action of gastric juice invade the intestinal mucosa, enters the circulation and gets lodged in different tissues where they mature into larva that soon transforms into a cystic metacystode termed the cysticercus. The cysticercus contains the scolex or the mature larva. The man thus acts as the intermediate host in the life cycle of the tapeworm. The parasite has special predilection for skeletal muscles, subcutaneous tissues, brain and eye.

Cysts *can be located anywhere in the brain* and in any number. Location and number often have important bearing on clinicopathologic diversity of the disease. *Parenchymal* cysts are more frequently seen in the highly vascular areas and can be single, multiple or be scattered throughout the brain or may occur in clumps. *Subarachnoid* cysts can be small or large, may occur in clumps or may be scattered around; these are usually associated with leptomeningeal inflammation and thickening. *Ventricular* cysts are usually large, commonly seen in forth ventricle and are often associated with granular ependymitis. *Spinal* cysticercosis are often intramedullary or leptomeningeal that may be associated with severe inflammation. *Ocular* cyst occurs more commonly in posterior chamber than anterior and common locations are retinal, subretinal, vitreous and infratemporal subretinal. In children parenchymal cerebral cysts are most common, subarachnoid and ventricular cysts are uncommon and spinal cysts are rare. Ocular cysts are also uncommon. Single parenchymal cysts are the most commonly seen form of NCC in children. Uncommonly the whole brain parenchyma can be studded with cysts giving rise to a serious form of the disease with poor outcome commonly known as the *encephalitic NCC*.

The cysts have been observed to grow in *two different forms* probably related to the surrounding environment, the cellular cyst and the recemose cyst. The *cellular cyst*, cysticercus cellulose, is the classic cyst that is usually small, spherical, often yellowish, fluid filled vesicle having a thin translucent wall through which the scolex can be seen as a small eccentric granule. These are common in brain parenchyma. The *recemose* cyst is a large rounded fluid filled bladder having a delicate wall and is lobulated resembling cluster of grapes. These occur commonly in subarachnoid space and the ventricular system where they may grow into enormous size; scolex is usually not visible in these as they disappear, may be because of hydropic changes.

The parasite remains alive and *grows* in the brain for variable period of time, even many years, often without producing any symptom (host showing immune tolerance to the parasite) and subsequently it dies, *degenerates*, gets absorbed and disappears. How the parasite evades destruction for long time remains unclear; this has been hypothesized to be due to modulation of host immunity by the parasite through mechanisms like sequestration within immunologically privileged sites, production of distractive antigens, complement blockage, release of anti-inflammatory cytokines and masking of cysticercal antigens by host immunoglobulins. The symptoms appearing after the cysts have stayed for variable period of time, have been related to onset of degeneration / death of the cyst, antigen release and subsequent *inflammatory reaction.* The degenerating cyst subsequently disappears after variable period of time that may extend for a month or so to several years. Before disappearing they often get calcified.

While growing, the live cysts act as a *space occupying lesion* resulting in symptoms, commonly headache and sometimes intracranial hypertension. The growing cyst can also cause obstruction of the CSF pathway and *hydrocephalus* and in the spinal cord it can cause symptoms of mass effect and *cord compression.* Subsequent degeneration of the cysts may be quite or it may be associated with varying degree of inflammatory reaction, severe at times, in the surrounding neural tissue of the host, as the cyst is highly antigenic. The most common manifestations of this reaction in brain parenchyma are *seizure and cerebral edema.* Most of the symptoms of NCC are thus results of acute inflammation occurring around the dying/degenerating cysticercus. The inflammatory reaction often results in leptomeningitis in brain and arachnoditis and myelitis in spinal cord and adds to complications like development of *hydrocephalus, infarct,* spinal *cord* symptoms. The *degenerating cysts usually courses through different stages like nodular, granular and calcific,* and subsequently get absorbed and disappear (healed). The whole process of healing may be quiet or may be associated with symptoms till the cyst disappears. Recurrence of symptoms in presence of different stages of resolution may be due to persistence of some immunogenic cyst components within them. At times cyst heals but leaves behind scars resulting from the inflammation, exudation and subsequent gliosis occurring during the process of healing. Scars in the brain parenchyma often act as focus for subsequent *seizures* and *epilepsy* and those in the CSF pathway often result in development of hydrocephalus.

The important manifestations of these pathologies are thus seizures, intracranial hypertension and spinal cord dysfunction. These result from (a) Mass effect exerted by the growing cyst or (b) Inflammatory phenomena, probably immune mediated, associated with the innnunogenic cyst or (c) Damaged brain tissues/scars resulting from the inflammation that act as epileptogenic foci.

NCC however may not always be associated with symptoms and remain *asymptomatic* for a long time. This is demonstrated by the observation of accidental finding of cysts of T. solium at autopsy of accident victims.[9] We also see NCC in CT/ MRI done for some other reason like intracranial hypertension in bacterial meningitis, mental retardation, cerebral palsy and dysmorphism. The cyst may live, grow, die, degenerate and disappear without producing any symptoms. Cysts can remain in the brain for a long time in any particular stage of degeneration. Also symptoms may be associated with all or any one stage of degeneration like the calcific one. The exact mechanism of many of the symptoms however, remains unclear obviously due to lack of pathological correlation.

NCC is associated development of *immunity* in the host. Anti-cysticercous antibodies of several immunoglobulin isotypes have been detected. IgG is most commonly found in blood, CSF and saliva. It usually indicates past or long-term infection. IgM is not found regularly.[5] Uncommonly IgA and also IgE has been detected. Development of antibodies is however inconsistent, unpredictable and of varying degree and intensity.

Pathology and Imaging Findings of NCC

Imaging studies like MRI and CT gives virtual anatomy and pathology of the disease. Imaging shows the cyst / cysts in the brain in different forms and stages till its death and disappearance.

The evolution and subsequent resolution of the cyst in imaging studies have been shown to pass through different phases namely *vesicular, colloidal, nodular-granular and calcified* (Fig. 43.1 to 43.5) based on clinical- pathological-radiological correlations. Each of these phases has characteristic imaging findings. In the vesicular phase, the cyst is filled with a thin translucent fluid and is believed

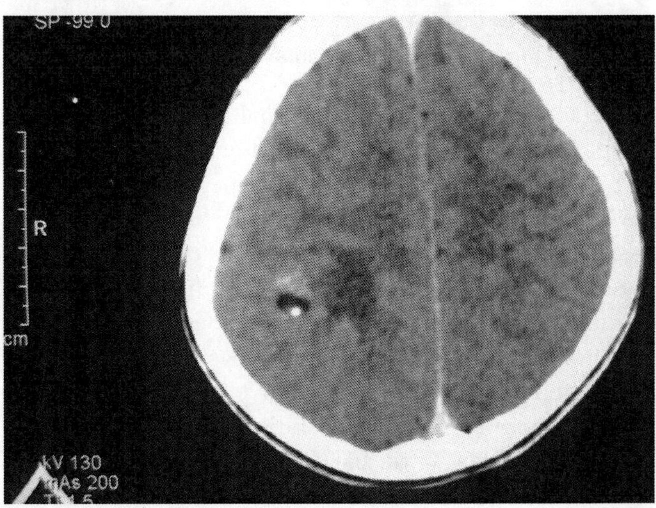

Fig. 43.1: NCC–showing the scolex

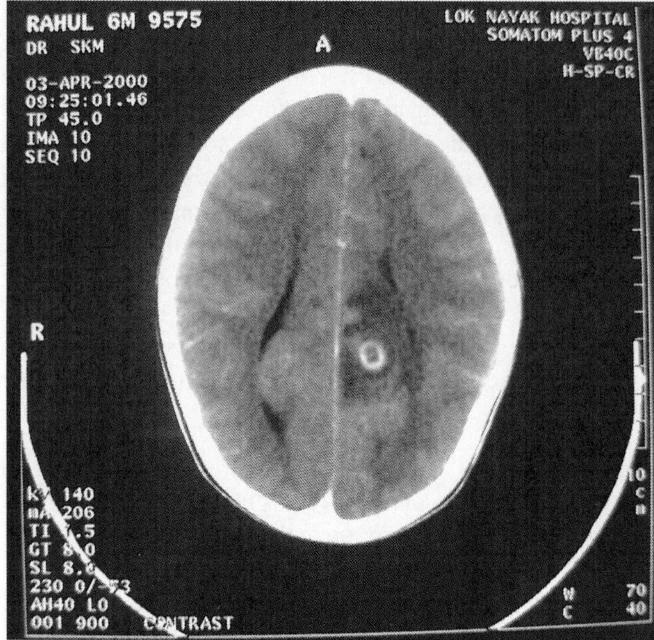

Fig. 43.2: Degenerating NCC – colloidal stage showing

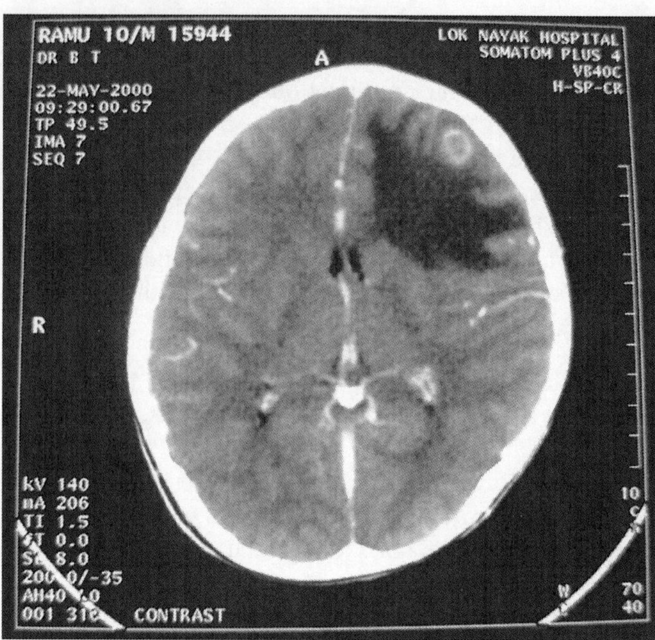

Fig. 43.3: NCC – advanced colloidal stage

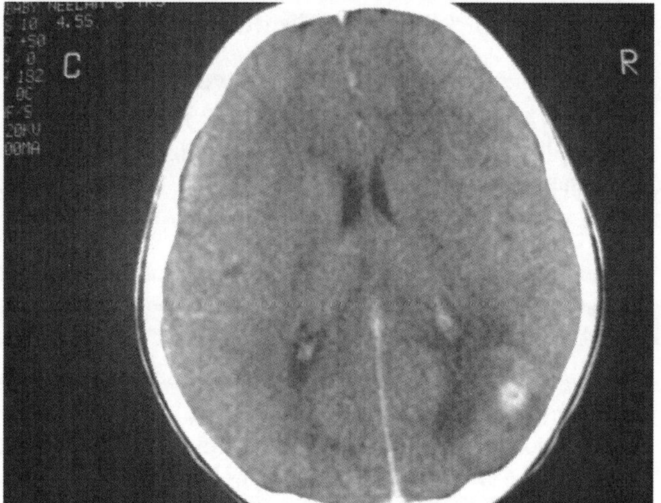

Fig. 43.4: NCC in nodular granular stage

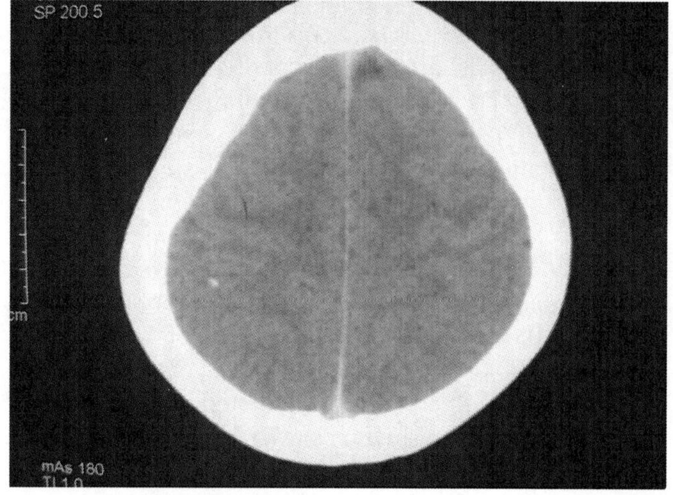

Fig. 43.5: Calcified NCC

to be active or live. In the colloidal phase, the cyst fluid becomes gelatinous and the wall thickens; this phase is believed to represent the onset of degeneration. In the nodular-granular phase, the contents become semisolid because of being progressively replaced by granulomatous tissue followed by hyalinization and the cyst tends to shrink. In the calcified phase the dead parasite gets mineralized while resorption also goes on. The vesicular phase represents the active or live cyst and the other subsequent phases the degenerating cyst, dying or dead. Imaging studies give virtual depiction of the pathology of the disease and its course. This has obviated the need of diagnostic brain biopsy in the cases.

MRI/CT findings in the *vesicular phase* – CT shows a round hypodense lesion, of size varying from about 4-20 mm, with or without a mural nodule (scolex) within, of size varying from 2-4 mm. They look like punched out lesions in the brain parenchyma. The surrounding brain parenchyma is more or less normal. MRI shows CSF signal intensity in all sequences, besides showing the scolex. This imaging picture has been given names like 'hole with eccentric dot on imaging', 'starry night effect'.

MRI/CT findings in the *colloidal phase*–CT characteristically shows the cyst as a round hypodense lesion with enhancement of the margin (ring enhancing lesion) with contrast surrounded by perilesional edema of varying intensity appearing hypodense and with or without the calcified mural nodule (scolex), usually eccentric. MRI findings vary in different sequences. In T1 weighted MRI, the signal intensity of the contents of the cyst (cyst fluid) is hypointense, that of the margin (capsule) is isointense with thick ring enhancement and that of the surrounding oedema fluid is hypointense. In T2 weighted MRI the signal intensity of the cyst fluid is hyperintense, that of the capsule hypointense and that of the surrounding oedema fluid hyperintense. Eccetntric nodule also may be seen. Effacement of the ventricles and midline shift are seen at times resulting from the edema. These findings often coincide with development of symptoms specially seizures and are considered to be the beginning of degeneration of the cyst.

MRI/CT findings in the *nodular-granular phase*–non contrast CT shows diffuse hypodensity with irregular margin of the cyst; with contrast, small hyperdense, rounded nodular image surrounded by edema is seen. T2 weighted MRI images often show isointense or low intensity signals signifying probably early mineralization associated with hyalinization.

MRI/CT findings in the *calcified phase*–non contrast CT shows rounded homogeneous hyperdense lesion with no enhancement on contrast. MRI shows low intensity lesion.

Classification of NCC

Based on CT findings, clinical findings and the course, a few classifications of the disease have been proposed. Sotello *et al.* ('85) classified NCC as (a) *Active* that includes cysts, parenchymal, intraventricular and spinal, and also arachnoditis, hydrocephalus secondary to meningeal inflammation, brain infarcts secondary to vasculitis and mass effects secondary to large cysts and clumps of cysts and (b) *Inactive* that includes the calcified lesion and hydrocephalus secondary to meningeal fibrosis. Carpio *et al.* ('94), who felt that the degenerating parasite cannot be considered active or inactive because of the surrounding inflammatory changes and put forward a classification based on viability and location of the parasite as (a) *Active* when the parasite is alive, (b) *Transitional* if it is in the degenerating phase and (c) *Inactive* if there is evidence of death. Each category is further subdivided according to location, parenchymal or extraparenchymal.

CLINICAL FEATURES

Cerebral Parenchymal NCC

The disease can affect any *age group* from infancy onwards as can be seen from studies that have included cysts in different stages based on CT findings. The mean/median age at presentation however vary between 7.5-9 years (Baranwal *et al.*,'98, Singhi *et al.*, 2000, Talukdar *et al.*,'02, Gogia *et al.*,'03, Kalra *et al.*,'03, Thomson *et al.*, '84, Dawood *et al.*,'84, Mitchell *et al.*,'88, Puri *et al.*,'91, Rosenfield *et al.*,'96, Morales *et al.*, 2000). Clinical manifestations are however less common before 5 years of age and is extremely uncommon in infancy; this is likely to be due protective food habits in early years of life. The youngest patients observed in reported Indian studies have been aged 1.5 years (Singhi *et al.*, 2000, Gogia *et al.* '03). *Sex* difference does not seem to be significant although slight male preponderance is common. *Dietary habit* does not seem to be important in presence of poor hygiene and pigs around; the disease is seen in non-vegetarians as well as vegetarians, although it is more common in pork eaters (Table 43.1).

The clinical findings of NCC closely relate to number, location and evolution the cysts and the degree of host immune response they induce during the process of degeneration. The location of the cysts in Indian children with NCC based mostly on CT scan findings reported in a few systematic studies from India is shown in Table 43.2.

The most common symptom of parenchymal NCC is *seizure* (Baranwal *et al.*,'98, Singhi *et al.*, 2000, Talukdar *et al.*, '02, Gogia *et al.*,'03, Kalra *et al.*,'03, Thomson *et*

Table 43.1: Certain Case Characteristics in Neurocysticercosis in Children

Symptoms and signs	Baranwal *et al.*, 1998	Singhi *et al.*, 2000	Talukdar *et al.*, 2002	Gogia *et al.*, 2003	Kalra *et al.*, 2003
Age range (years)	2-12	1.5-12.5	3-14	1.5-12	1-14
Mean age (years)	7.44	8.02	8.5	8.05	7.7
Vegetarian	-	-	-	52.8%	-
Non-vegetarian but non pork-eater	-	-	-	33.3%	-
Non-vegetarian and pork-eater	-	-	-	13.9%	-
Pork-eater	-	-	-	-	14%

Table 43.2: Location of CT Lesions in Neurocysticercosis in Children

Study and Type of Lesions Included	Parietal	Frontal	Temporal	Occipital	Others
Baranwal *et al.*, 1998 (n=63) SSECTL	41%	27%		9.5%	Frontoparietal 9.5%, parieto occipital 6.4%
Singhi *et al.*, 2000 (n=500) All types of lesions	46%	19.8%	18.2%	8.2%	57.4%
Talukdar *et al.*, 2002 (n= 176) RELs, single or multiple	81%	11%	0.6%	7.2%	-
Gogia *et al.*, 2003 (n=72) RELs, consecutive cases, single or multiple	65.3%	9.7%	6.9%	8.3%	Frontoparietal-5.6%, parietooccipital - 4.2%, parafalcine - 2.8, periventricular 1.4, basal ganglia-1.4, thalamus 1.4
Kalra *et al.*, 2003 (n=123) RELs – one or two	58.5%	31.7%	5.7%	4.1%	

Note: SSECTL (Single Small Enhancing CT Lesions), REL (Ring Enhancing Lesions)

al., Dawood *et al.*,'84, Mitchell *et al.*,'88, Puri *et al.*,'91, Rosenfield *et al.*,'96, Morales *et al.*, 2000). Seizures are commonly focal motor, focal motor evolving into generalized and generalized. Types of seizures seen in Indian children with NCC reported in a few systematic studies from India are shown in Table 43.3. Seizure type is usually determined by location of the cyst. Cyst or cysts located in one hemisphere usually results in focal seizure. Multiple cysts located in both the hemispheres are usually associated with generalized or at times, focal seizure. Some of the apparently generalized seizures are actually focal motor, focal motor evolving into generalized seizure that can be demonstrated by EEG.

Sometimes the same child can have mixed type / more than one type of seizures, i.e., sometimes right focal sometimes left focal and sometimes generalized. Associated or preceding sensory symptoms are also not uncommon. Common sensory symptoms as described by our patients / parents are sensations of tingling, pins and needles, numbness and feeling of passage of an electric current the extremities. Uncommon types of seizures like myoclonic and akinetic have also been reported.

Seizures are brief (lasting for <5 minutes) in about 25-33% although status epilepticus (seizures lasting > 5 mins) is not uncommon. Majority of cases have single seizures at presentation, some however have seizures in cluster within the first 48-72 hours or so (Branwal *et al.*,'98, Gogia *et al.*,'03) while some have multiple recurrences occurring over a few days that gradually subside (Singhi *et al.*, 2000, Gogia *et al.*,'03, Kalra *et al.*,'03). Recurrent seizures in a child are usually stereotyped.

Table 43.3: Seizure Types in Neurocysticecosis in Children

Study and type of lesions included	Total partial	SPS	CPS	PS-G	Total generalised	Gen tonic	g-tonic-clonic	Others
Baranwal *et al.*, 1998 (n=63), SSECTL	-	25.4%	49.2%	25.4%	-	-	-	SE 38.8%
Singhi *et al.*, 2000 (n=500), All types of lesions	83.7%	-	-	70%	-	-	8.7%	TLE 2.4%, others 5.2%
Talukdar *et al.*, 2002, (n= 176), RELs, single or multiple	86.9%	21%	61.9%	4%	10.8%	2.3%	8.5%	Mixed-2.3%, prls 1.7%
Gogia *et al.*, 2003 (n=72), RELs, consecutive cases, single and multiple	79.2%	23.6%	47.2%	8.3%	20.8%	4.2%	16.7%	prls 27.8%
Kalra *et al.*, 2003 (n=123), RELs – single or two lesions	70.7%	-	-	-	24.4%	-	-	-

Note: SPS (Simple Partial Seizure), CPS (Complex Partial Seizure), PS-G (Complex Partial Seizure Secondarily Generalised), SE (Status Epilepticus), prls (prolonged seizures > 15 mins).

A number of other *pre and peri-ictal symptoms* (symptoms seen at or around the time of seizures) are observed in some cases most common being headache and nausea / vomiting (Table 43.4); these however resolve quickly. Aura is not commonly seen, may be due to inability of the child to describe it.

At times a case can present with features of acute *encephalopathy* (Thompson *et al.*,'84, Dawood *et al.*,'88, Puri *et al.*,'91, Thakur *et al.*,'91). Intracranial hypertension is commonly associated with these cases. Encephalopathic features are common with multiple parenchymal NCC. Rarely a child can have *only headache* that is persistent and nagging.

Clinical examination is usually non-contributory, most of the children being normal except features of unrelated problems in some. Transient focal neurological deficits and Todd's palsy are seen in some cases, while papilledema is seen infrequently. Subcutaneous nodules are not common but has been reported. Simultaneous presence of ocular cyst is rare.

Encephalitic NCC, a distinctive type of NCC seen rarely in children, is due to extensive infection of the brain (Fig. 43.6) and commonly presents as acute to subacute encephalopathy with features of intracranial hypertension, altered sensorium, behaviour, papilledema, and frequent / off and on seizures.

Recurrence of symptoms, specially seizure, is common in NCC. These recurrences however die down in most cases, in time with healing and disappearance of the lesions.

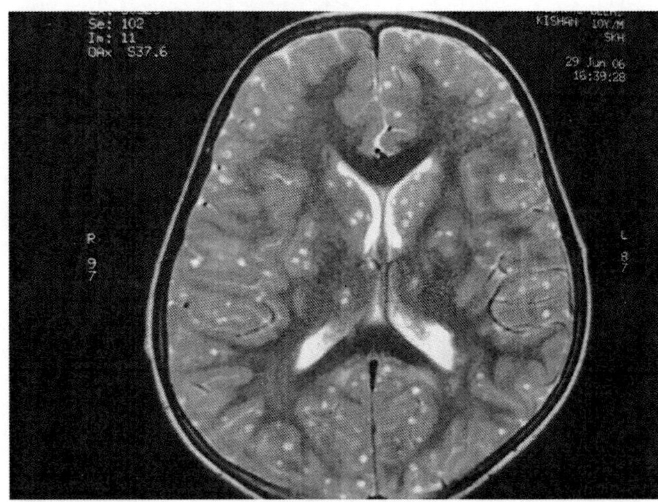

Fig. 43.6: Encephalitic NCC; the brain is studded with NCC

Subarachnoid, Intraventricular, Spinal and Ocular NCC

Intraventricular and subarachnoid NCC are uncommon/ rare in children. These cases are usually associated with hydrocephalus and manifest mostly with features of raised intracranial pressure and at times seizures (Lopez-Hernandez,'82, Puri *et al.*,'91, Rosenfield *et al.*'96, Thakur *et al.*,'91). Spinal NCC, rare in children, manifests with features of cord compression and paraplegia (Thomson *et al.*,'84, Dawood *et al.*,'84). Ocular NCC is associated with visual problems.

Table 43.4: Important Clinical Findings at Presentation in Neurocysticercosis in Children

Symptoms and signs	Baranwal *et al.*, 1998	Singhi *et al.*, 2000	Talukdar *et al.*, 2002	Gogia *et al.*, 2003	Kalra *et al.*, 2003
Headache	y	28.2%	2.8%	18.1%	26.8%
Vomiting / nausea	y	31.4%	3.4%	15.3%	5.7%
Blackening-visual	-	-	-	2.8%	-
Sensory symptoms (mostly tingling sensation, extremities)	y- 20.6%	15%	-	1.4%	-
Focal deficit, mono-hemiparesis	-	4%	-	8.3%	2.4%
Todd's palsy	y-28.6%	28%	-	8.3%	-
Extensor plantars	-		-	4.2%	-
Gen hyporeflexia	-		-	2.8%	-
Cranial n palsy (6th)	-	1.2%	-	1.4%	2.5%
Cerebellar ataxia	-	0.2%	-	-	-
Papilledema	None	6.6%	1.7%	4.2%	-
Skin nodule	-	-	None	None	-

INVESTIGATIONS

Imaging Studies

Neuroimaging studies like MRI/CT are essential for diagnosis of NCC, in fact it is neuroimaging that gives the diagnosis. These studies show the cysts in different stages of evolution, number of cysts, location, and also complications like intracranial hypertension. Many such CT lesions have been histopathologically demonstrated to be due to NCC time and again in parenchymal brain biopsy specimens done for confirmation, in cysts removed at surgery for ventricular disease, at autopsy of cases having such CT lesions who died (Lopez-Hernandez,'82, Percy *et al.*,'90,) and also in diagnostic brain biopsy studies done prospectively in India (Chandy *et al.*,'91, Rajsekhar,'91, Sethi *et al.*,'94). It is worth remembering that these lesions were earlier thought to be mostly due to tuberculosis, so common in India. The pioneering work of Chandy ('91) and Rajsekhar ('94) using stereotactic brain biopsy and histopathology showed that most of these lesions are due to NCC.

MRI and CT both are useful in diagnosis. CT is better for calcified lesions and MRI is better for detailed delineation of the cyst anatomy including the different stages. In live cyst the fluid is of same density as CSF and with onset of degeneration (usually hyaline) the density increases. MRI is more sensitive for detection of the scolex. Edema is also better defined by MRI and also subarachnoid cyst that is sometimes missed by CT.

Other imaging technique like magnetic resonance spectroscopy (MRS) and magnetic transfer spectroscopy (MTS) that characterizes the content of the cyst, have been shown to be useful in diagnosis of NCC. Tuberculomas have been reported to show high lipid peak and neurocysticercosis high choline peak and also a choline/creatine ratio greater than 1.

In Indian children degenerating single parenchymal cysts appearing in imaging studies as ring enhancing lesions (REL) are the most common type of NCC. Most of such lesions are small, usually less than 20 mm (Baranwal, *et al.*,'98, Singhi *et al.*, 2000, Talukdar *et al.*,'02). Single lesions have been reported in 76-86.9% of cases and multiple lesions in 13.1-29.2% cases (Baranwal,'98, Singhi *et al.*, 2000, Talukdar *et al.*,'02) of NCC in Indian children. Other important and clinically relevant imaging findings reported in Indian children are: peri-lesional edema (suggestive of inflammatory reaction) in 57.4-100% of cases, mural nodule (larva/scolex, appearing as eccentric dot) in 10.8-44% of cases, mass effects in the form of effacement of lateral ventricle in 11.1%, midline shift in 4.2%[28] and unspecified in 9.5%.[26] Basal subarachnoid NCC at times associated is with spinal NCC. In such situation MRI of the spine also should be done.

Immunodiagnosis

As indicated already NCC is associated with development of antibodies and immunologic tests have been developed for serologic diagnosis. The earlier hemagglutination inhibition (HI) and complement fixation (CF), has now been replaced by newer tests like Enzyme-Linked immunosorbent Assay (EITB) and Enzyme-Linked Immunoelectrotransfer Blot Assay (EITB). Intense research is going on at present for sero-diagnostic methods having better sensitivity and specificity.

Enzyme-Linked Immunosorbent Assay (ELISA) using purified extract of cysticerus detects IgG and IgM antibodies. IgM antibody is usually used for diagnosis of NCC. In active or viable NCC, its sensitivity and specificity has been found to be 50% and 70% in serum and 87% and 97% in CSF. Frequency of positive tests are more when there are multiple cysts and cysts in or closer to the CSF space (as in intraventricular and subarachnoid cysts) and it is less when there are single parenchymal cysts and it is least with calcified cysts. Development of antibody is also believed to be more local.

Many false positive and false negative results with ELISA has been reported in the literature. Cross reactivity to antibodies due to infection with other helminthes parasites specially hydatid disease and also host's immune tolerance to the parasite has been believed to be the causes of such reactions. Negative ELISA thus does not rule out the diagnosis of NCC. Poor sensitivity in cases with single lesions, calcified lesions and other stages during degeneration of the cysts reduces significantly the usefulness of this test in initial diagnosis of NCC in India where such lesions are the predominating ones.

Enzyme-Linked Immunoelectrotransfer Blot (EITB) assay using enriched fraction of parasite glycoprotein has good sensitivity and specificity, 98% and 100% respectively.[52] Sensitivity and specificity have been shown to be 72% and 96% respectively in a study in children. Sensitivity of the test in serum is similar to better than in CSF so that only serum is needed to be used which is an advantage over ELISA. Sensitivity is also high with multiple lesions at multiple sites and in parenchymal lesions.

However, EITB also has limitations. Sensitivity and specificity are poor in cases with single lesions and calcified lesions besides false positivity in presence of extracranial cysticercosis and even recent infections. Discrepancy between CT dignosis and EITB diagnosis has also been significant. Negative EITB also thus does not rule out NCC. In Indian children most common lesions of NCC on imaging are single ring enhancing ones followed by other stages of degeneration including calcifications as already mentioned and EITB like ELISA, also does not seem to be of significant help in initial diagnosis of NCC in India. Few studies from India in adult subjects have shown low positivity of this test. The test is also costly and is not available everywhere.

Thus both ELISA and EITB have their limitations and may be used judiciously. ELISA is likely to be fruitful in cases with non-enhancing lesions (active cysts), with multiple lesions and lesions in subarachnoid space or ventricles. EITB is also likely to be fruitful in similar situations. In both cases gastrointestinal infestation with tapeworm and other parasitic disease like helminthiasis and hydatid disease and also extracranial cysticecosis should be excluded. Because of relative ease of doing the test (as testing only in serum is needed) and better sensitivity and specificity, EITB is currently the sero-diagnostic method of choice.

Newer diagnostic tests like antigen detection test is in the offing. The antigen can be detected in serum, CSF and even urine.

Other Aids in Diagnosis

Eosinophilia in peripheral blood is sometimes observed. CSF changes like raised protein and pleocytosis, usually lymphocytic and at times presence of eosinophils have been reported; these changes seem to be more common in hydrocephalus and meningo-ephalitic features. These may provide indirect support to the diagnosis.

FNAC or biopsy of any subcutaneous nodule may show the parasite. *Stool examination* of the patient may rarely show T. solium ova or proglotids.[28] *X-ray of the thigh* may show ciger-shaped calcification, rarely observed in children. These findings may give corroborative evidence that the cyst in the brain is probably that of T. solium.

EEG is useful in establishing the exact seizure type. Focal abnormality, a frequent finding in NCC (Gogia *et al.*, '03, Puri *et al.*,'91) corroborates a focal pathology as in cases with single cysts. It is also quite helpful in management of encephalitic form of NCC.

Diagnosis of NCC

In the absence of brain biopsy and histology the diagnosis of NCC remains unconfirmed. Brain biopsy however is not always possible and may not be warranted for a disease that is relatively benign, self-healing and almost accurate diagnosis can be arrived at by clinical evaluation, imaging studies and serology.

As discussed already, *imaging* remains the mainstay of diagnosis of NCC. All cases of suspected NCC should be subjected to imaging studies. Seizures being the most common manifestation of NCC in children in India, imaging should be advised in all such cases. MRI/CT showing ring lesion with mural nodule (scolex) is considered to be the most useful finding and almost diagnostic of NCC.[2] **Serology,** being a biologic tool, is of great diagnostic value if positive and hence should be done whenever possible; currently immunoblot assay is recommended diagnostic purpose.

An initial *blood count* with ESR also should be done as it may be helpful more in excluding other diagnostic confounders specially tuberculomas, so common in developing countries like India. Tuberculosis, so common in India, should be ruled out in all cases of suspected NCC. *Biopsy of subcutaneous nodule,* if present, should be done. Examining of *stool* that is simple, should also be done, besides diagnostic corroboration, it has preventive implications as well.

Early / spontaneous regression or disappearance of the MRI/CT lesion, i.e., the cyst, also gives a good support to the diagnosis.[2] Imaging studies therefore may be repeated after some time to detect this, first repetition preferably being done after 6 months of initial diagnosis (Talukdar *et al.*,'02).

Because of the difficulty in having histologic diagnosis in all cases, efforts have been made to evolve diagnostic criteria for diagnosis of NCC taking into consideration imaging, clinical, investigational and epidemiological findings (Del Bruto *et al.*,'01, Carpio *et al.*,'16); however, the essence of these criteria are primarily imaging findings without which diagnosis of NCC is not possible at present.

Differential Diagnosis

In cases of NCC presenting with acute seizures, common *causes of acute seizures* like trauma, CNS infections, static and developmental lesions of the brain, ICSOL, genetic and metabolic conditions, stroke and recurrence of an attack in known epileptic. In cases primarily having features of raised ICP, all conditions leading to *intracranial hypertension* in children commonly meningoencephalitis, hydrocephalus and ICSOL should be excluded. In cases with *focal neurological deficit* stroke, mass lesion and other structural lesion should be kept in mind. Thus all cases of NCC, even if they look benign, should be evaluated carefully worked up as required. Most of these conditions, however, can be ruled out by good clinical evaluation and need for extensive investigation remains in only in a few cases. NCC should be considered in any child with seizures especially focal, even if he is normal otherwise.

Imaging findings also should be considered in making a diagnosis. The ring lesions, enhancing or unenhancing, should be differentiated from tuberculoma, hydatid cyst, small brain abscess, focal encephalitis, lymphomas, metastatic lesions, fungal infections like sarcoidosis, histoplasmosis, toxoplasmosis. Degenerating lesions like nodular-granular and calcific lesion can also result from the same conditions. Tuberculoma, so common in India, have certain distinctive imaging features (Fig. 43.7) like being bigger in size, usually >20 mm, irregular in outline and also more associated with midline shift compared to NCC as observed in some histologically proved cases in adults (Rajsekhar,'93, Rajsekhar,'97) .

TREATMENT

Parenchymal NCC

The treatment neurocysticercosis is primarily treatment of (a) Symptoms commonly the seizures and (b) Cysticidal drugs.

Treatment of Acute Seizures

The acute episodes of seizures have to be managed as usual. Many cases of NCC do have status convulsive status epilepticus and needs appropriate management. These apply to NCC in any location.

Treatment of Other Acute Symptoms

Headache and vomiting due to intracranial hypertension

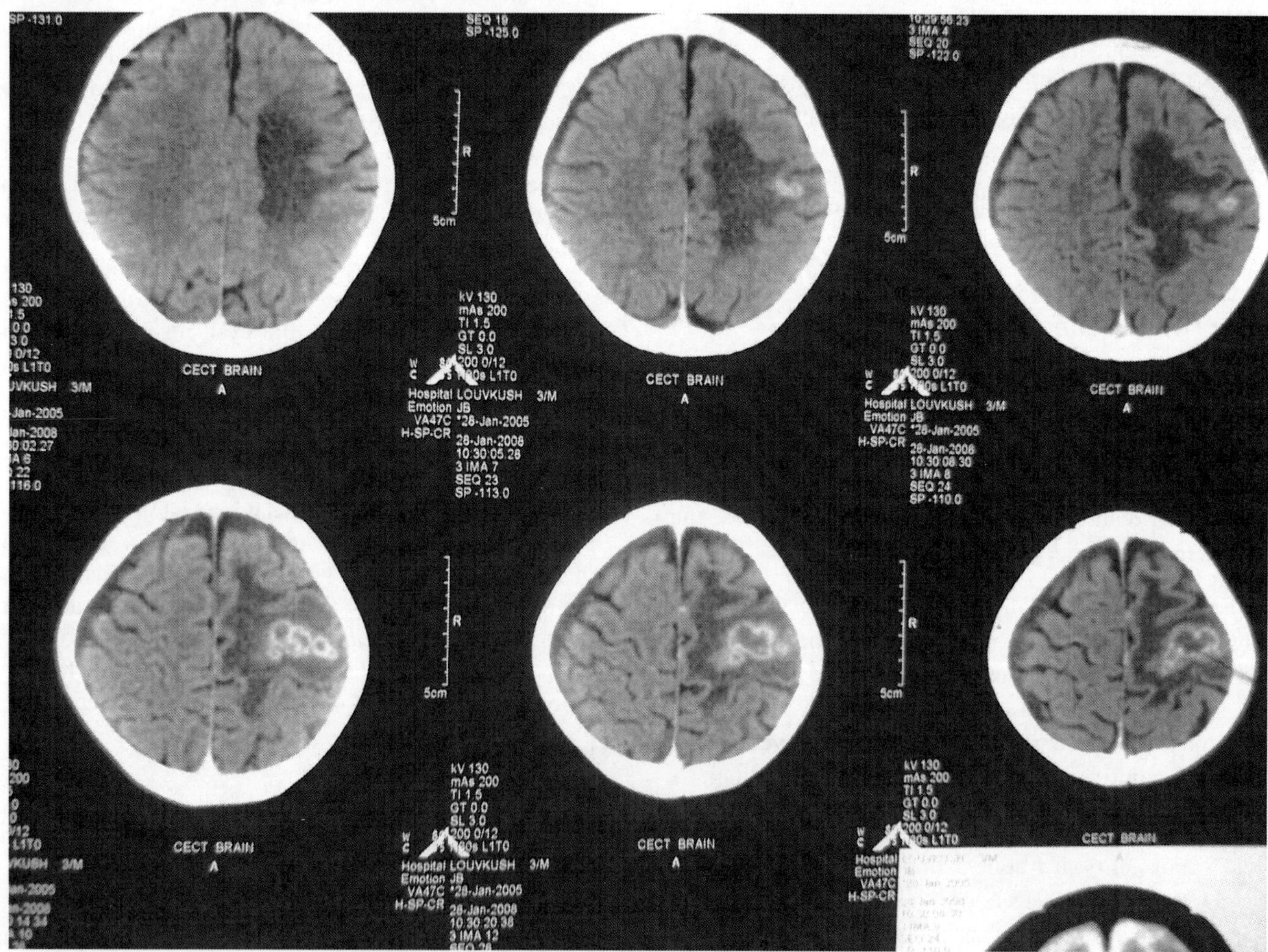

Fig. 43.7: Tuberculomas, the case had tuberculous meningitis

(once established) should be managed as usual, i.e., fluid balance, posture (raised head end), decompressive therapy using mannitol / 3% sodium chloride and dexamethasone to reduce inflammation if needed. The same applies for associated hydrocephalus if there is. The IH is usually due to cerebral edema mostly around the cyst with or without hydrocephalus.

Use of Cysticidal Drugs

Cysticidal drugs specially albendazole and praziquantel have been used in NCC. Albendazole is weakly absorbed from the gut. Albendazole has been used in a dose of 15 mg/kg/d divided into 2 doses orally varying from 3-28 days. The drug is poorly absorbed from the gut, it should be taken with meal to improve availability. The reported side effects are: abdominal pain, nausea, vomiting, headache, hair loss, leukopenia, agranulocytosis, hepatotoxicity, aggravation of seizure and suspected teratogenicity. If it is prescribed for more than 14 days, monitoring for blood counts and liver functions is indicated. In case of absolute neutropenia and liver enzymes high for more than five times the normal it should be withheld until normalization of these parameters and/or alternative approach considered, i.e., praziquantel or no cysticidal drug (ASTMH, '18). Praziquantel is used in a dose of 50 mg/kg/day orally for 14 days. The side reported effects are abdominal pain, allergic reactions commonly urticaria and rash, diarrhoea, dizziness, drowsiness, malaise, fever. Because of easy availability and ease of administration albendazole is commonly used in India. Praziquantel on the whole is less effective than albendazole.

Most of the experience in the use of these drugs in NCC have originated from the Latin American countries. The use of cysticidal drugs however has controversies in many areas like efficacy in different situations, dose, duration of treatment since the first reported trial was in 1979. It is well-known fact that NCC is a self-limiting disease and lesions disappear on its own, symptoms commonly disappear with disappearance of the lesion, persistence of the lesion is not always associated with recurrence of symptoms and lesions, often calcific, may remain in the brain for many years. Occurrence of lesions in different stages at the same time and also spontaneous degeneration of the lesions in some complicates the issue. Some earlier studies have showed cysticidal drugs to be useful in hastening the resolution of lesions and reduction in severity seizures, whether some not. Studies from India on neurocysticercosis have shown variable findings as already indicated, however, overall benefit has been observed in resolution of lesions (although not always significant) in most of them (Table 43.5).

Several reviews and meta-analysis have tried to resolve these issues. Abba *et al.* (2010) in an analysis of data of RCTs, observed that in viable lesions in adults albendazole may reduce the number of lesions, but no difference was seen in recurrence of seizure. Trials on non-viable lesions in adults are few. It is interesting to find that there is hardly any study on viable lesions in children. For non-viable lesions in children, seizures recurrence was less common with albendazole compared with no treatment. However no difference was detected in the persistence of lesions at follow-up. A Guideline Development Subcommittee of the American Academy of Neurology (Baird *et al.*, 2013) on neurocysticercosis has observed that albendazole therapy, administered with or without corticosteroids, is probably effective in decreasing both long-term seizure frequency and the number of cysts demonstrable radiologically in adults and children with neurocysticercosis. They have recommended that Albendazole plus either dexamethasone or prednisolone should be considered for adults and children with neurocysticercosis, both to decrease the number of active lesions on brain imaging studies (Level B) and to reduce long-term seizure frequency (Level B). There is insufficient data to recommend the use of praziquantel. In another observation Romo *et al.* (2015) concluded that albendazole treatment may be associated with some symptomatic improvement; however, this association seems to be specific to generalized seizures. Otte *et al.* (2013) have observed that anthelminthic treatment in neurocysticercosis was associated with significantly increased rates of seizure freedom, and significantly higher rates of granuloma resolution, but did not alter the risk of residual calcification. Corticosteroid treatment was not significantly associated with any outcome.

These differences and controversies have led to formulation of guidelines off and on regarding management of NCC. A guideline formulated recently by the American Society of Tropical Medicine and Hygiene (ASTMH) (2018) is useful in day-to-day management of NCC. This guideline, an update on existing knowledge, has brought about some clarity in a better way in management of different types of lesions in different locations and also in duration of treatment in different situations; the use of cysticidal drug has also been better clarified.

Viable (Active) Cysts of Parenchymal NCC

If there are 1-2 viable cysts: The ASTMH guideline proposes albendazole monotherapy in all such cases for 14 days (evidence-strong to high), as against no antiparasitic therapy (evidence strong-high) or combination therapy

Table 43.5: Albendazole Trials in Neurocysticercosis

Study and year	Sample size and type	Type of study	Type of CT lesions	Duration of albendazole therapy	Results analysed at	Statistical significance–albendazole vs control
Padma *et al.*, 1994	n=75 Adults	Randomized double blind placebo controlled trial	SSECTL	7 days	3 months	Resolution of lesions not significant
Padma *et al.*, 1995	n=29 Adults	Randomized double blind placebo controlled trial	Multiple cystic lesions	7 days	3 months	Resolution of lesions not significant
Carpio *et al.*, 1995	n=138 Adults	Randomised controlled trial (prednisolone orally for 15 days to all)	Non-enhancing	8 days	6 months, 1year and 2 years	Resolution and disappearance of lesions and also seizure control not significant
Garcia *et al.*, 2004	n=120 Adults	Randomized double blind placebo controlled trial		10 days	30 months or 6 months of seizure free state	Resolution of lesions during therapy significant; seizure control not significant
Baranwal *et al.*, 1998	n=63 Children	Randomized double blind placebo controlled trial (prednisolone orally for 5 days to all)	SSECTL	28 days	3 months	Disappearance of lesions significant, seizure control not significant
Gogia *et al.*, 2003	n=72 Children	Randomized double blind placebo controlled trial (prednisolone orally for 3 days to all as pretreatment)	RELs single and multiple	28 days	6 months	Disappearance of lesions and also seizure control not significant
Kalra *et al.*, 2003	n=123 Children	Randomized controlled trial, one or two CT lesions included, dexamethasone given orally for 5 days to the albz group	RELs one and two lesions	28 days	3 months and 6 months	Disappearance of lesions alone not significant; disappearance, size-reduction and calcification taken together is significant and seizure control significant
Das *et al.*, 2007	n=250 Adult	Randomized controlled trial, one group received dexamethasone, albendazole, and AED and the other only AED and placebo	RELs 2 or more		6 months	Significant increase seen in seizure frequency, hospital readmission and encephalopathy in the group receiving albendazole, dexamethasone and AED; albendazole did not have greater beneficial effect
Singhi *et al.*, 2004	N=110, Children	Randomized controlled trial: one group received corticosteroid, 2nd albendazole and 3rd corticosteroid+albendazole	REL, single, small	28 days	6 months	No significant difference in resolution of CT lesions in 3 groups. Corticosteroid group had significantly more seizure recurrence

(weak to moderate). Before starting it a short course of steroid should be given to the patient to counteract any inflammatory reaction resulting from antiparasitic drug; we have been using prednisolone in a dose of 2 mg/kg/day for 3 days. Albendazole should be started after managing the acute problems like seizure, intracranial hypertension etc.

If there are more than 2 viable cysts: The ASMTH guideline suggests using albendazole combined with praziquantel rather than albendazole monotherapy for 10-14 days (evidence strong to moderate). We however have very little experience on using such a combination in our children and will need evaluation in Indian children.

If cysts continue to persist despite using cysticidal drug: If parenchymal cysts/cysts persist for more than 6 months after the initial course of treatment, ASMTH guideline has suggested retreatment as the initial course (evidence weak to low).

Degenerating (Transitional) Parenchymal NCC

These are the most common form of NCC that we see in Indian children presenting as ring enhancing lesion (REL) on imaging. The larva of the parasite larva is already dead.

If there is single lesion: AAMTH guideline recommends use of cysticidal drug, rather than no antiparasitic therapy, for all cases of single REL (evidence weak to moderate). They also have suggested MRI every 6 months till resolution of the cystic lesions.

If there are multiple lesions: AAMTH guideline recommends use of antiparasitic drug in this situation, similar to single lesion, as well (evidence weak to moderate).

Calcified Parenchymal NCC

Cysticidal drug is not used in calcified parenchymal lesions and the treatment is symptomatic; this has also been suggested in ASTMH guideline.

Encephalitic NCC

Cysticidal drug is not indicated here. It can precipitate severe inflammatory reaction as already there is inflammatory reaction and edema in most cases.

TREATMENT OF NCC IN OTHER LOCATIONS

NCC in other locations, i.e., ventricular, subarachnoid space, spinal cord and eye are uncommon, rather rare in children in India. Occasionally we come across a lesion in ventricles / subarachnoid space in cases of multiple NCC. These types of NCC are relatively common in adults. NCC leading to development of hydrocephalus needing shunting is also rare in Pediatric NCC. All the related guidelines are practically based on adult experience.

Treatment of Intraventricular NCC

Removal of cyst is recommended, whenever possible (ASTMH). Cysticidal drug is not indicated pre-operatively as the inflammatory reaction following its use may make removal difficult /complicated. Shunt surgery is indicated for hydrocephalus after removal of cyst. When surgical removal of cyst is technically difficult shunt surgery is indicated for hydrocephalus as inflamed ventricular cysts may result in complications. Antiparasitic drug and corticosteroid are indicated after shunt insertion to decrease subsequent shunt failure (ASTMH)

Treatment of Subarachnoid NCC

Cysticidal drug has been recommended here (ASTMH) (evidence strong to weak). It may have to be used for prolonged period till radiological clearance of cysts (ASTMH). Associated hydrocephalus has to be managed with shunting.

Treatment of Spinal NCC

Both medical and surgical management is indicated (ASTMH). In cases with spinal cord dysfunction, corticosteroid is recommended, or as an adjunct to cysticidal drug (ASTMH). Treatment should be invidualized depending on symptoms, location of cysts and degree of arachnoiditis (ASTMH). Follow-up reimaging is needed.

Treatment of Ocular NCC

Surgical removal, rather than antiparasitic drug, is recommended (ASTMH) (weak to low).

COURSE AND OUTCOME

Most of the cases of NCC continue to have problems specially recurrent seizures. They need regular follow-up for proper management. Most of the cases with seizures need prolonged antiepileptic drug (AED) for variable duration that is difficult to define. Most cases need AED for 2 or more years. Long-term outcome on the whole is good.

We commonly find recurrences to be associated with calcified lesions and also persistence of the degenerating lesion. We also find recurrence in some cases where AED was stopped after remaining seizure free for 2 years or more and also in some cases where AED was stopped after disappearance of lesions on imaging. AED use in every case has to be individualized. Disadvantages of prolonged AED therapy in children should always be kept in mind and it should be withdrawn whenever possible. Majority of the cases can be controlled with AED monotherapy. Some cases turn difficult to treat / intractable and need polytherapy and also need for prolonged AED prophylaxis beyond 2 years.

If at any point cysts has been found to be resolved, AED should be stopped after tapering it off gradually. In cases of single lesion if there is no recurrence of seizure for 6 months, we give a trial of tapering off and withdrawing AEDs, irrespective of the lesion being resolved or not, as in our experience lesions can persist. Most cases remain well. We also find that many cases remain seizure free even if the lesions continue to persist. The ASTMH guidelines has suggested that in patients who have been seizure free for 6 months, antiepileptic drugs be tapered off and stopped after resolution of the lesion in patients with SEL without risk factors for recurrent seizures (weak, moderate).

In cases having recurrences off and on we continue AED till the child is seizure free for at least 2 years. We do repeat imaging guided by recurrence and severity of seizure. The ASTMH guideline suggests tapering off and stopping AED in cases with few seizures before starting antiparasitic therapy, resolution of cystic lesions on imaging studies and no seizure for 24 consecutive months. They also suggest repetition of MRI every 6 months, until resolution of cystic component. Risk of recurrence are residual cystic lesions or calcifications on repeat imaging studies, breakthrough seizures or more than 2 seizures. We also find appearance of new viable lesions in MRI/CT, repeated in cases who had recurrence of seizure. It is unclear whether cysticidal drug should be used in such cases or not, we have used another course in some depending on frequency of recurrence. Cases with recurrence can have problems of intracranial hypertension and have to be managed accordingly. This is commonly seen in cases of encephalitic NCC. Few cases develop intractable epilepsy; they may be candidate for surgery.

PREVENTION

The most important mode if infection in NCC in India appears to be through food items contaminated by taenia solium eggs like, vegetables, fruits, water, milk etc mostly due to unhygienic environment. Through washing of vegetables, fruits and other raw eatables is extremely important. Appropriate purification/sterilization of water and milk needs to be ensured. Proper boiling of milk before use is essential. Raw food outside like salads, fruit juices, drinks and even water, if appears to be unhygienically prepared, stored and dispensed, should be avoided. Washing hands well after visiting the toilet is important to prevent oro-fecal contamination. Thus good hygiene, environmental and personal is of utmost need for curbing this preventable menace.

Pigs are the most important reservoir. It is interesting to find that countries where pork is not eaten, incidence of NCC is low or nil. Avoiding taking pork infected with cyst is important. Pork eaters should be careful that the meat is not infected with taenia solium cysts and this can be ensured to some extent by careful inspection. Prolonged boiling of pork before cooking is essential to kill the cysts. Inspecting the meat at the slaughter houses is compulsory in many endemic countries in Latin America. Prompt treatment of intestinal infection with taenia solium, if detected by examination of stool or if found from history of passage of tapeworms, is also important. Pork eaters should get his stool examined off and on for evidence of taenia solium infestation. Vaccination of pigs is also being explored as an option. Restricted trials seem to have shown some promise.

Suggested Reading

- Aguilar-Rebolledo F, Meza-Lucas A, Torres J, Cedillo-Rivera R, Enciso A, Garcia RC, Munoz O, Correa D. Evaluation of Enzyme Linked Immunotransfer Blot Assay for Diagnosis of Neurocysticercosis in Children. J Child Neurol 2002;17:416-20.
- Alarcon F, Escalante L, Duenas G, Montalvo M and Roman M. Neurocysticercosis Short Course of Treatment with Albendazole. Archives of Neurology 1989;46:1231-36.
- Baird RA1, Wiebe S, Zunt JR, Halperin JJ, Gronseth G, Roos KL. Evidence-based Guideline: Treatment of Parenchymal Neurocysticercosis: Report of the Guideline Development Subcommittee of the American Academy of Neurology. Neurology 2013 Apr 9;80(15):1424-29. doi: 10.1212/WNL.0b013e31828c2f3e.
- Baranwal AK, Singhi PD, Singhi SC. Seizure Recurrence in Children with Focal Seizures and Single Small Enhancing Computed Tomographic Lesions: Prognostic Factors on Long-Term Follow-up. J Child Neurol 2001;16:443-45.
- Baranwal NK, Singhi PD, Khandelwal N, Singhi SC. Albendazole Therapy in Children with Foal Seizures and Single Small Enhancing Computed Tomographic Lesions: A Randomised, Placebo-controlled, Double Blind Trial. Pediatr Infect Dis J 1998;17:696-700.
- Carpio A, Placencia M, Santillan F, Escober A. Proposal for A New Classification of Neurocysticercosis. Can J. Neurosc Neurol sc. 1994:21:43-47.
- Carpio A, Santillan F, Leon P, Flores C and Hauser WA. Is the Course of Neurocysticercosis Modified by Treatment with Antihelminthic Agents? Archives of Internal Medicine, 1995:155:1982-88.
- Carpio A1,2, Fleury A3,4, Romo ML5,6, Abraham R7, Fandiño J8, Durán JC9, Cárdenas G3, Moncayo J10, Leite Rodrigues C11, San-Juan D3, Serrano-Dueñas M12, Takayanagui O13, Sander JW14,15. New Diagnostic Criteria for Neurocysticercosis: Reliability and Validity. Ann Neurol 2016 Sep;80(3):434-42. doi: 10.1002/ana.24732. Epub 2016 Aug 13.
- Chandy MJ, Rajsekhar V, Ghosh S et al. Single Small Enhancing CT Lesions in Indian Patients with Epilepsy: Clinical, Radiological and Pathological Considerations. J Neurol Neurosurg Psychiatry 1991;54:702-05.
- Correa D, Medina E. Host-Parasite-Immune Relationship in Taenia Solium Taeniasis and Cysticercosis. In: Garcia HH, Martinez SM (Eds), Taenia Solium Taeniasis and Cysticercosis, 2nd edn, Universo, Lima 1999;15-24.
- Das K, Mondal GP, Banerjee M, Mukherjee BB, Singh OP. Role of Antiparasitic Therapy for Seizures and Resolution of Lesions in Neurocysticercosis Patients: An 8-Year Randomised Study. J Clin Neurosci 2007 Dec;14(12):1172-77.

- Dawood AA, Moosa A. Cerebral Cysticercosis in Children. J Trop Ped 1984:30:136-39.
- Del Brutto OH, Roos KL, Coffey CS, García HH. Meta-analysis: Cysticidal Drugs for Neurocysticercosis: Albendazole and Praziquantel. Ann Intern Med 2006;145: 43-51.
- Del Brutto, Rajshekhar V, White AC Jr.,Tsang VCW, Nash TE, Takayanagui OM, Schantz PM, Evans CAW, Flisser A, Correa D, Botero D, Allan JC, Sarti E, Gonzalez AE, Gilman RH and García HH. Proposed Diagnostic Criteria for Neurocysticercosis. Neurology 2001;57:177-83.
- Diagnostic Imaging. Adam A, Dixon AK, Gillard JH, Schaefer-Prekop CM (Eds).Vol II, 6th Edition, 2015. Churchill Livingstone, Vol II, 2015.
- Dixon HBF, Lipscomb FM. Cysticercosis: An Analysis and Follow-up of 450 Cases. Med Res Council Spec Rep Ser No. 299. London: Her Majesty's Stationery Office 1961:1-58.
- Escobar A. The Pathology of Neurocysticercosis. In: Palacios E, Rodriguez-Carbazal J, Taveras JM, eds, Cysticercosis of the Central Nervous System. Springfield, Charles C Thomas 1983:27-54.
- Escobedo F, Penagos P, Rodriguez J, Sotelo J. Albendazole Therapy for Neurocysticercosis. Arch Intern Med 1987;147: 738-41.
- Espinoza B, Ruiz-Palacio G, Tovar A, Sandoval MA, Plncarte A, Flisser A. Characterization by Enzyme-Linked Immunosorbent Assay of the Humoral Immune Response in Patients with Neurocysticercosis and Its Application in Immunodiagnosis. J Clin Microbiol 1986;24:536-41.
- Garcia HH, *et al.* Cysticidal Efficacy of Combined Treatment with Praziquantel and Albendazole for Parenchymal Brain Cysticercosis. Clin Infect Dis 2016;62:1375-79. [PMC free article] [PubMed] [Google Scholar].
- Garcia HH, *et al.* Efficacy of Combined Antiparasitic Therapy with Praziquantel and Albendazole for Neurocysticercosis: A Double-blind, Randomised Controlled Trial. Lancet Infect Dis 2014;14:687-95. [PMC free article] [PubMed] [Google Scholar].
- Garcia HH, Evans CAW, Nash TE, Takayanagui OM, White AC Jr, Botero R, Rajshekhar V, Tsang VCW, Schantz PM, Allan JC, Flisher A, Correa D, Sarti E, Friedland JS, Martinez SM, Gonzalez AE, Gilman RH, Del Brutto OH. Current Consensus Guidelines for Treatment of Neurocysticercosis. Clin Microboil Rev 2002;15:747-56.
- Garg RK and Nag D. Single Enhancing CT Lesions in Indian Patients with Seizure: Clinical and Radiological Evaluation and Follow-up. Journal of Tropical Pediatrics, 1998:44:204-10.
- Gogia S, Talukdar B, Aurora BS, Choudhury V. Neuro-cysticercosis in Children: Clinical Findings in Newly Diagnosed Cases and Response to Albendazole Therapy in A Randomized Double Blind Placebo Controlled Trial. Trans R Soc Trop Med Hyg 2003;97:416-21.
- Gonzalez AE, Gauci CG, Barber D, Gilman RH, Tsang VC, Garcia HH, Verastegui M, Lightowlers MW. Vaccination of Pigs to Control Human Neurocysticercosis. Am J Trop Med Hyg 2006;72:837-39.
- Kalra V, Dua T, Kumar V. Efficacy of Albendazole and Short-course Dexamethasone Treatment in Children with 1 or 2 Ring-enhancing Lesions of Neurocysticercosis: A Randomized Controlled Trial. J Pediatr 2003 July;143(1):111-14.
- Lopez-Hernandez A, Garazier C. Childhood Cerebral Cysticercosis: Clinical Features and Computed Tomographic Findings in 89 Meixcan Children. Can J Neurol Sci 1982;9: 401-07.
- Lopez-Hernandez A, Garazier C. Manifestations of Infantile Cerebral Cysticercosis. In: Palacios E, Rodriguez-Carbazal J, Taveras JM, eds, Cysticercois of the Central Nervous System. Springfield, 111, Charles C Thomas 1983:69-83.
- Mandal J, Singhi PD, Khandelwal N, Malla N. Evaluation of ELISA and Dot Blots for the Serodiagnosis of Neurocysticercosis in Children Found to Have Single or Multiple Enhancing Lesions in Computerized Tomographic Scans of the Brain. Ann Trop Med Parasitol 2006 Jan;100(1):39-48.
- Mitchell WG, Crawford TO. Intraparenchymal Cerebral Cysticercosis in Children: Diagnosis and Treatment. Pediatrics 1988:82:76-82.
- Morales NMO, Agapejev S, Morales RR, Padula NAMR, Lima MMF. Clinical Aspects of Neurocysticercosis in Children. Pediatric Neurology 2000:22:287-91.
- Otte WM, Singal M, Sander JW, Singh G. Drug Therapy for Solitary Cysticercus Granuloma: A Systematic Review and Meta-analysis, Neurology, Jan 8, 2013;80(2):152-62. doi: 10.1212/WNL.0b013e31827b90a8 PMCID: PMC3589189.
- Padma MV, Behari M, Misra NK, Ahuja GK. Albendazole in Neurocysticercosis. Natl Med J India 1995;8(6):255-58.
- Padma MV, Behari M, Misra NK, Albendazole in Single CT Ring Lesions in Epilepsy. Neurology 1994;44:1344-46.
- Pandit S, Lin A, Gahbauer H, Libertin CR, Erdogan B. MR Spectroscopy in Neurocysticercosis. J Comput Assist Tomogr. 2001 Nov-Dec;25(6):950-52.
- Percy AK, Byrd SE, Locke GE. Cerebral Cysticercosis. Pediatrics 1980;66:967-71.
- Pretell EJ, Garcia HH, Gilman RH, Saavedra H, Martinez M. Failure of One-day Praziquantel Treatment in Patients with Multiple Neurocysticercosis Lesions. Clin Neurol Neurosurg 2001;103:175-77.
- Principles and Practice of Infectious Diseases; Bannett JE, Dolin R, Blaser MJ (Eds); Vol II, 8th Edition, 2015.
- Proano-Narvaez JV, Meza-Lucus A, Mata-Ruiz O, Garcia-Jeronimo RC, Correa D. Laboratory Diagnosis of Human Neurocysticercosis: Double-blind Comparision of Enzyme-Linked Immunosorbent Assay and Electroimmunotransfer Blot Assay. J Clin Microbiol 2002;40:2115-18.
- Puri V, Sharma DK, Kumar S, Choudhuy V, Gupta RK, Khalil A. Neurocysticercosis in Children 1991;28:1309-17.
- Rajsekhar V, Haran RP, Prakash GS, Chandy MJ. Differentiating Solitary Small Cysticercous Granulomas and Small Tuberculomas in Patients with Epilepsy. Clinical and Computerized Tomographic Criteria. J Neurosurg 1993;78:402-07.

- Rajsekhar V. Etiology and Management of Single Small CT Lesions in Patients with Seizures: Understanding a Controversy. Acta Neurol Scand 1991;84:465-70.
- Rajshekhar V. Oommen A: Serological Studies Using ELISA and EITB in Patients with Solitary Cysticercus Granuloma and Seizures. Neurological Infections and Epidemiology 1997;2: 177-80.
- Ramos-Kui M. Montoya RM. Padilla A et al. Immunodiagnosis of Neurocysticrcosis: Disappointing Performance of Serology (Enzyme-linked Immunosorbent Assay) in an Uniased Sample of Neurological Patients. Arch Neurol 1992;49:633-36.
- Romo ML1. Wyka K2. Carpio A3. Leslie D4. Andrews H5. Bagiella E5. Hauser WA6. Kelvin EA7. Ecuadorian Neurocysticercosis Group. The Effect of Albendazole Treatment on Seizure Outcomes in Patients with Symptomatic Neurocysticercosis. Trans R Soc Trop Med Hyg. 2015 Nov;109(11):738-46. doi: 10.1093/trstmh/trv078. Epub 2015 Oct 3.
- Rosas N. Sotelo J. Nieto D. ELISA in the Diagnosis of Neurocysticercosis. Arch Neurol 1986;43:353-56.
- Rosenfeld EA. Byrd SE. Shulman ST. Neurocysticercosis Among Children in Chicago. Clin Infect Dis 1996;23:262-68.
- Sethi PP. Wadia RS. Kiyawat DP. Ichaporia NR. Kothari SS. Sangle SA and Wadhwa P. Ring or Disc Enhancing Lesions in Epilepsy in India. Journal of Tropical Medicine and Hygiene 1994;97:347-53. Sotelo J. Guerrero V. Sotelo J. Guerrero V. Rubio F. Neurocysticercosis: A New Classification Based on Active and Inactive Form: A Study of 753 Cases. Arch Intern Med 1985;145:442-45.
- Singh G. Kaushal V. Ram S et al. Cysticercus Immunoblot Assay in Patients with Single. Small Enhancing Lesions and Multilesional Neurocysticercosis. JAPI 1999;47:476-79.
- Singhi P. Jain V. Khandelwal N. Corticosteroids Versus Albendazole for Treatment of Single Small Enhancing Computed Tomographic Lesions in Children with Neurocysticercosis. J Child Neurol 2004;19:323-27.
- Singhi P. Ray M. Singhi S and Khandelwal N. Clinical Spectrum of 500 Children with Neurocysticercosis and Response to Albendazole Therapy. Journal of Child Neurology 2000;15:207-13.
- Singhi PD. Dinakaran J. Khandelwal N. Singhi SC. One vs Two Years of Anti-epileptic Therapy in Children with Single Small Enhancing CT Lesions. J Trop Pediatr 2003;49:274-78.
- Sotelo J. Del Brutto OH. Penagos P et al. Comparison of Therapeutic Regimen of Anticysticercal Drugs for Parenchymal Brain Cysticercosis. J Neurol 1990;237:69-72.
- Sotelo J. Penagos P. Escobedo F and Del Brutto OH. Short Course of Albendazole Therapy for Neurocysticercois. Archives of Neurology 1988;45.1130-33.
- Talukdar B. Saxena A. Popli VK and Choudhury V. Neurocysticercosis in Children: Clinical Characteristics and Outcome. Annals of Tropical Paediatrics 2002;22:333-39.
- Thakur LC. Anand KS. Childhood Neurocysticercosis in South India. Indian J Pediatr 1991;58:815-19.
- Thomson AJ. De Villiers JC. Moosa A. Van Dellen J. Cerebral Cysticercosis in Souh Africa. Ann Trop Paediatr 1984;4:67-77.
- Tsang-Tsang VCW. Brand JA. Boyer AE. An Enzyme-linked Immunoelectrotransfer Blot Assay and Glycoprotein Antigens for Diagnosis of Human Cysticercosis (Taenia solium). J Infect Dis 1989;159:50-59.
- Verma A. Misra S. Outcome of Short-term Antiepileptic Treatment in Patients with Solitary Cerebral Cysticercus Granuloma. Acta Neurol Scand 2006 Mar;113(3):174-77.
- White C Jr., Coyle CM. Rajshekhar V. Singh G. Hauser WA. Mohanty A. Garcia HH and Nash TE. Diagnosis and Treatment of Neurocysticercosis: 2017 Clinical Practice Guidelines by the Infectious Diseases Society of America (IDSA) and the American Society of Tropical Medicine and Hygiene (ASTMH). Am J Trop Med Hyg 2018 Apr; 98(4): 945-66.doi: 10.4269/ajtmh.18-88751.
- Wilson M. Bryan R. Fried J. Ware D. Schantz P. Pilcher JB. Tsang VCW. Clinical Evaluation of the Cysticercosis Enzyme-linked Immunoelctrotransfer Blot in Patients with Neurocysticecosis. J Infect Dis 1991;164:1007-09.

44 Chapter

HEADACHE IN CHILDREN AND ADOLESCENTS

Devendra Mishra, Prarthana Kharod

INTRODUCTION

Headache is the most common neurological symptom in children. It causes significant morbidity for a significant number of children, most notably in days lost and days affected at school. Headache impact is directly related to headache frequency and severity. Childhood headache has a high risk of developing into a chronic condition and persisting into adulthood in the form of physical and/or psychiatric morbidity. Despite its public health and medical importance, many barriers to care exist for patients suffering from headache disorders, especially children.

EPIDEMIOLOGY

Headache is a common complaint in childhood with upto 75% of children reporting a notable headache by the age of 15 years. It is common across the age range and across the world. In a recent systematic review of population based studies on headache in children and adolescents, it was found that about 60% of children and adolescents were prone to headache over at least a 3-month period. In this analysis of 50 population-based studies, estimated prevalence of headache over periods between 1 month and lifetime in children and adolescents was found to be 58.4% (95% confidence interval [CI] 58.1-58.8%). It was found significantly more commonly in females (67%) than in males (58%).

Migraine is a common disorder in children and adolescents: approximately 8% of children and adolescents are prone to it over at least a 3-month period. The overall prevalence of migraine in children and adolescents is 7.7% (95% CI 7.6-7.8). There is lower prevalence of migraine in children under the age of 14 years than in the general childhood population. The study showed that migraine affects males and females equally at a young age (< 14 years), and more females than males in adolescence and young adulthood. The overall prevalence of migraine in female children and adolescents is 9.7% (95% CI 9.4-9.9) and in males 6.0% (95% CI 5.8-6.2); the difference is 3.7% (95% CI 3.4-3.9, $p < 0.001$). Statistically significant differences in prevalence of migraine among different regions are observed– between Europe and the Middle East on the one hand and the USA and the Far East on the other, probably due to a combination of genetic predisposition as well as environmental factors.[1]

Data on pediatric headache in India is limited. In a study done to analyze the pattern of headache at a tertiary referral center in India, out of 1000 patients (of all ages) who presented with headache, 86% had primary headaches that were classifiable, 11% were unclassifiable and 3% had secondary headaches. Of the primary headaches, 55% had migraine, 28.3% had tension-type headache, 22.2% had cluster headache and 0.5% had miscellaneous primary headaches.[2,3] Our recent data on recurrent headache among pediatric patients presenting to a public hospital evaluated 43 new patients with recurrent headache over an 8-month period. 60.2% were suffering from migraine with majority having significant disability.[4,5]

CLASSIFICATION

International Classification of Headache disorders is a hierarchical classification of headache disorders, with the third edition currently in use (Table 44.1). Using this classification, the diagnosis given is according to the current headache pattern or that experienced in last one year. In case patient receives more than one diagnosis, they are listed in order of importance to the patient. When a new headache occurs for the first time in close temporal relation to another disorder that is known to cause headache, or fulfils other criteria for causation by that disorder, the new headache is coded as a secondary headache attributed to the causative disorder. This remains true even when the headache has the characteristics of a primary headache (migraine, tension-type headache, cluster headache or one of the other trigeminal autonomic

Table 44.1: International Classification of Headache Disorders, III Edition

1. Migraine
2. Tension-type headache
3. Trigeminal autonomic cephalgias (TACs)
4. Other primary headache disorders
5. Headache attributed to trauma or injury to the head and/or neck
6. Headache attributed to cranial or cervical vascular disorder
7. Headache attributed to non-vascular intracranial disorder
8. Headache attributed to a substance or its withdrawal
9. Headache attributed to infections
10. Headache attributed to disorder of homeostasis
11. Headache or facial pain attributed to disorder of the cranium, neck, eyes, ears, nose, sinuses, teeth mouth or other facial or cervical structure
12. Headache attributed to psychiatric disorder
13. Painful cranial neuropathies and other facial pains
14. Other headache disorders

cephalalgias). When a pre-existing primary headache becomes chronic in close temporal relation to such a causative disorder, both the primary and the secondary diagnoses should be given. When a pre-existing primary headache is made significantly worse (usually meaning a two-fold or greater increase in frequency and/or severity) in close temporal relation to such a causative disorder, both the primary and the secondary headache diagnoses should be given, provided that there is good evidence that the disorder can cause headache.

APPROACH TO A CHILD WITH HEADACHE

Clinical approach to a childhood headache is similar to that in adults, although the differences exist. Certain diagnoses are less common in children. Also, there are differences in clinical presentation and treatment in adult and pediatric migraine. It is more difficult to interpret the nature of headache in children as the description is often difficult especially in young children. Child's behaviour during the episode gives crucial clues to nature, onset and severity of the symptoms. Parents' observation and description are of key importance.

Evaluation of a child with headache begins with detailed history and thorough physical examination. History may have to be taken on repeated visits to know the exact nature of illness. Children and parents can be taught to maintain a headache diary for detailed description of each episode. One of the examples of a headache diary is given below (Fig. 44.1).

Date:	**Date:**	**Date:**
Warning Signs:	**Warning Signs:**	**Warning Signs:**
Time Begun:	**Time Begun:**	**Time Begun:**
Time Ended:	**Time Ended:**	**Time Ended:**
Type of Pain: e.g., piercing, throbbing, etc.	**Type of Pain:** e.g., piercing, throbbing, etc.	**Type of Pain:** e.g., piercing, throbbing, etc.
Intensity of Pain: Circle one **Low** 1 2 3 4 5 6 7 8 9 10 **high**	**Intensity of Pain:** Circle one **Low** 1 2 3 4 5 6 7 8 9 10 **high**	**Intensity of Pain:** Circle one **Low** 1 2 3 4 5 6 7 8 9 10 **high**
Location: e.g., between the eyes, back of head, etc.	**Location:** e.g., between the eyes, back of head, etc.	**Location:** e.g., between the eyes, back of head, etc.
Treatment or Medication Taken:	**Treatment or Medication Taken:**	**Treatment or Medication Taken:**
Effect of Treatment:	**Effect of Treatment:**	**Effect of Treatment:**
Hours of Sleep Previous Night:	**Hours of Sleep Previous Night:**	**Hours of Sleep Previous Night:**
Foods/Beverages:	**Foods/Beverages:**	**Foods/Beverages:**
Events Prior to Headache: e.g., strenuous activities, elevated stress etc	**Events Prior to Headache:** e.g., strenuous activities, elevated stress, etc.	**Events Prior to Headache:** e.g., strenuous activities, elevated stress etc.
Comments:	**Comments:**	**Comments:**

Fig. 44.1: Headache diary

There are five temporal patterns of headache described by Rothner:[6] Acute, acute recurrent, chronic progressive, chronic non-progressive and mixed. These are suggestive of differing pathophysiologic processes. Each of these patterns has distinctive differential diagnosis (Table 44.2).

Table 44.2: Differential Diagnosis of the Five Temporal Patterns[5]

Temporal pattern	Etiology
Acute: Generalized	– Fever – Systemic infection – CNS infection – Toxins: lead, CO – After seizure – Electrolyte imbalance – Hypertension – Hypoglycemia – Post lumbar puncture – Trauma – Embolic – Vascular thrombosis

Contd.

Contd.

	– Hemorrhage – Autoimmune/Collagen vascular disease – Exertional
Acute-Localised	– Sinusitis – Otitis – Ocular abnormality (glaucoma) – Dental disease – Trauma – Cranial neuralgia (occipital) – Temporomandibular joint dysfunction
Acute-Recurrent	– Migraine – Complex migraine – Migraine variants – Cluster – Paroxysmal hemicrania – After seizure – Tic douleureux – Exertional
Chronic Progressive	– Brain tumor – Idiopathic intracranial hypertension – Brain abscess – Subdural hematoma – Hydrocephalus – Hemorrhage – Hypertension – Vasculitis
Chronic Nonprogressive and Mixed*	– Chronic daily headache (chronic migraine) – Chronic tension-type – Chronic hemicrania continuum – Conversion disorder – Malingering – After concussion – Depression – Anxiety – Adjustment reaction

*With superimposed migraine.

Figure 44.2 graphically explains the presentation in different temporal patterns of headache. The acute, sudden onset of headache in an otherwise healthy child is usually due to intercurrent viral infection. Presence of focal neurological signs or fever should raise the suspicion of intracranial haemorrhage or meningitis, respectively. These patients should undergo relevant investigations to rule out serious pathology. An acute-recurrent pattern implies episodes or attacks of headache, separated by symptom-free intervals. Most common causes are primary headache disorders like migraine and tension type, although complex partial seizures, cluster headache and recurrent trauma are important differentials. Chronic progressive headache is the most ominous of the five patterns as it implies gradually increasing frequency and severity of headache, mostly suggestive of increasing intracranial pressure. Chronic non-progressive or chronic daily headache represents a pattern of frequent or near-constant headache, the most common form being chronic migraine. These patients usually have normal neurological examination and there are usually interwoven psychological factors and heightened anxiety about unrecognized, underlying organic causes.

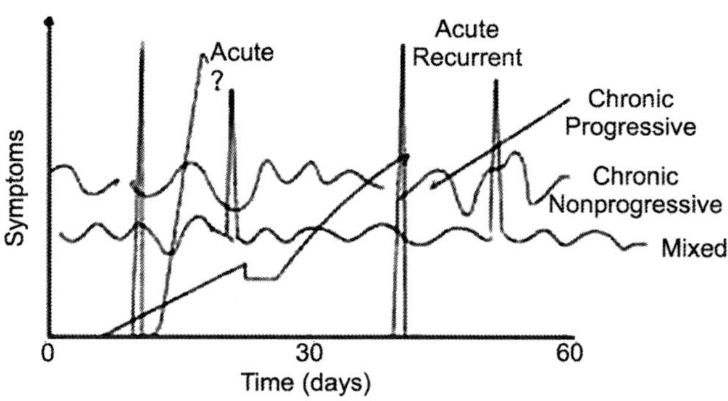

Fig. 44.2: Five temporal patterns of pediatric headache

History-taking should preferably involve both the child and the parent; though for older children it's the latter's version that takes precedence. Similar to any other disorder, history involves asking the characteristic features of a typical episode, frequency, onset, progression and disability. However, there are some important differences need to be kept in mind:

1. When did the headache begin?

Chronic headaches are unlikely to reflect intracranial pathology. New onset worsening headaches are more likely to be due to a space-occupying lesion and require neuroimaging.

2. How did the headache begin?

Look for precipitants, such as head injury or social stresses.

3. What is the temporal pattern of the headaches?

Intermittent headaches separated by intervals of well-being are most likely to be migraines. Progressively more severe headaches are more likely to reflect pathology and require further investigations. Tension-type headaches (TTH) are usually chronic and non-progressive.

4. What is the headache frequency?

Migraines typically occur weekly or less often. TTH occur daily or several times per week. Headache syndromes in childhood, such as cluster headache, may have their own unique pattern, occurring in clusters of two to three per week over a few weeks or months, followed by long periods of headache freedom. Headaches due to increased intracranial pressure (ICP) often occur nightly.

5. How long does the headache typically last?

Migraines are often brief, lasting 30 min to 120 min. Although the International Headache Society criteria define paediatric migraine as lasting upto 72 hours, few paediatric patients have regular migraines that last this long. TTH often lasts 'all day'. Cluster headaches are brief.

6. Do the headaches happen at any particular time or circumstance?

Headaches that occur at night or in the early morning are more likely to reflect increased ICP, although as many as 25% of migraine episodes occur at night. Children with TTH may describe waking with their headache, although this is typically after the child arises in contrast with increased ICP, which may weaken the child. Occasionally, headaches occur exclusively in one situation or circumstance (e.g., school, when hungry or with changes in weather). Children with chronic morning headaches and a history of bruxism should be examined for temporomandibular joint dysfunction.

7. Is there an aura or prodrome?

Children with migraines may be able to describe or draw their aura. If the aura is persistently on the same side, a structural lesion should be excluded. Parents may predict a migraine hours before it occurs because their child may show a prodrome of lethargy, mood change, thirst or food cravings, yawning or pallor.

8. Where is the pain?

Migraine is bifrontal in more than 55%. TTH is usually more diffusely located. The severity of pain is not helpful in identifying serious causes of headaches. An inability to describe the quality of the headache is much more likely to distinguish those with brain tumours or ventriculoperitoneal shunt malfunctions; occipital headaches are more likely to occur in children with brain tumours. Persistently unilateral headaches should be considered to be suspicious.

9. What is the pain like?

Offering choices helps to determine the quality of the pain. Migraines are typically throbbing, but may be described as heavy or pressing. An inability to describe the pain is more significant than the actual choice of adjective. Historical concepts of throbbing equating to migraine and band-like to TTH are probably inaccurate.

10. Are there associated symptoms?

Migraines are usually accompanied by nausea, vomiting, anorexia, photophobia, phonophobia or osmophobia. Vomiting without accompanying nausea is suspicious. Migraine with aura may be associated with aphasia, vertigo, visual, sensory or other associated symptoms. If symptoms persist beyond the headache or if the associated phenomenon is persistent from one headache to the next, thought should be given to possible underlying pathology.

11. What do you do during the headache?

What a child does if a headache begins during play is often more informative than asking what they do if a headache begins at school. Those with migraines will usually interrupt their activity to return home. Children with TTH will often watch television or play video games. In comparison, those with migraines usually seek refuge in a quiet and darkened bedroom.

12. Would I know you had a headache if I saw you?

The child with migraines usually looks ill. Those with TTH usually appear normal.

13. What makes the headache better and worse?

Details on medication use can provide insight into both the headache and the patient/family's preferences for headache management. Many report using large doses of medication despite its lack of benefit. Migraineurs often describe benefit from sleep or simple analgesics taken early in the headache course. Aggravating factors in migraine include activity, light, noise and smells. Those with increased ICP will often find increased discomfort on lying down. Headaches due to low ICP are usually worse on sitting or standing up.

14. Are there symptoms between headaches?

Patients with migraines or TTH are asymptomatic between headaches. Ongoing symptoms, such as forgetfulness, confusion or localizing neurological symptoms suggest a structural lesion. Brain tumours may manifest as lethargy, personality changes or recent school failure.

Difficulties with concentration may persist beyond the headaches in those who have suffered a concussion. In the setting of chronic daily headache, comorbid symptoms of depression may be present. Underlying psychosocial factors are common and may relate to learning difficulties, bullying, parental conflict, grieving reactions, and drug or alcohol abuse.

15. Are there any other health problems?

Children with chronic illnesses often feel stressed by their prognosis, they need to attend hospital visits and take medications. Those with hypertension may have 'migraine-like' headaches.

16. Are you taking medications?

Headaches may occur as an adverse effect to medications used to treat other conditions or to treat the headaches themselves. It is important to understand the attitudes of the patient and parents toward medication. Quantifying the child's use of nonprescription analgesics will identify those at risk for rebound analgesic headaches. A medication history may also reveal exposure to medications associated with idiopathic intracranial hypertension, such as oral contraceptives, vitamin A, isotretinoin, tetracycline and corticosteroids.

17. Is there a family history of headaches?

Many children with migraine or TTH have first-degree family members with similar headaches. In these families, educational efforts should be directed toward all those in the family with headaches.

18. What do you think is causing the headaches?

This is usually a very valuable question. Some children will identify a particular stressor of which the parents are often unaware. Both children and parents are also afforded the opportunity to discuss their fears of underlying pathology. A number of families will demonstrate a remarkable misunderstanding of the potential causes of their child's headaches. Many believe the headaches are caused by chronic sinusitis. There is no evidence to support chronic headaches as a result of chronic sinusitis.

(Adapted from Rothner AD. Evaluation of headache. In: Winner P, Rothner AD, eds. Headache in Children and Adolescents. Hamilton: BC Decker Inc, 2001:20-32)

Severity of pain can also be judged by adopting a pain-scoring system like 'pain-faces' scoring method for children to help tell mild from severe headaches, as well as to monitor the response to therapy.

The physician should always look for 'Red flags' in the headache history, presence of which is suggestive of possible serious pathology. Presence of any of the red flags lowers the threshold for neuroimaging/other investigations. These 'Red flags' are as follows:

- A short history ('First' or 'worst'), or recent recurrent severe headache for few weeks.
- Accelerated course, change in character over weeks or days.
- Headache suggesting raised intracranial pressure (early morning headache, vomiting in morning, pain disturbing sleep, headache worse with cough or valsalva).
- Associated symptoms of personality changes, weakness, visual disturbances, confusion, focal weakness, seizures or fever.
- Underlying history of neurocutaneous syndrome, history of systemic illnesses, e.g., known malignancy with possible metastases, hypercoagulopathy.
- Young age of child (< three years old).

Physical Examination[7]

Physical examination in case of headache should focus on secondary causes. Linder[8] pioneered formalised headache specific examination.

Vital Signs

Measurement of temperature is important as fever per se can cause acute headache. Fever can also be one of the signs of underlying central nervous system infection. Blood pressure should be measured as hypertension is an important cause of long standing headache. Moreover, acute, severe hypertension can lead to subarachnoid haemorrhage leading to headache.

Growth Parameters

Anthropometry should be done in all patients. Growth failure is associated with chronic disorders and tumours. Head circumference should be measured and monitored to look for macrocephaly, which may be due to hydrocephalus or associated with neurocutaneous disorders, e.g., neurofibromatosis type I.

Infections

One should always look for signs of meningeal irritation with passive neck flexion, Kernig's sign and Brudzinski's sign. However, the physician should be aware that even where meningeal infection is present, neck stiffness or positive Kernig's sign can be absent, especially in young children. Hence, if the suspicion of meningitis is high, the child should be carefully evaluated and observed, with appropriate investigations where necessary.

Acute sinusitis is one of the common secondary causes of headache. Chronic sinusitis usually does not cause headache. One should keep in mind that many 'sinus headaches' eventually turn out to be migraines. Mueller's manoeuvre can be used to detect increased pressure in the sinuses. It is performed by getting the child to hold their nose while counting to three. The child then coughs, and the transient increase in sinus pressure aggravates a headache caused by sinusitis. However, this manoeuvre should not be attempted if there is evidence of raised intracranial pressure (ICP) or during an acute migraine.

Mouth should be examined for dental caries, although most children can identify dental pain. One should also look for focus of infection in oropharynx (e.g., acute tonsillitis) and ear (e.g., acute otitis media) which can lead to referred pain.

Eyes

Careful evaluation by ophthalmologist should be done especially in children with headache associated with eye strain, watering from eyes, difficulty in distant/near vision, ocular pain. One should look for uncorrected refractive errors, raised intraocular pressure or latent squint.

Increased ICP

Children with headaches secondary to raised ICP may have evidence of papilledema or optic nerve pallor, especially with long-standing increased pressure.

Trauma

Signs of head trauma suggest a possible concussion. Some children with concussion may have very mild ataxia and subtle coordination deficits as the only findings. Mild ataxia can be demonstrated by having the child pirouette three times. This will detect ataxia, which is not evident on tandem gait testing.

Skin and Musculoskeletal

The child with headache should also be examined for neurocutaneous stigmata and systemic signs of connective tissue disorders/vasculitis.

Cervical spine involvement can lead to headache, which may be perceived beyond the expected dermatomal distribution. The discomfort is usually elicited by having the child push the head forward against examiner's hand and by checking the range of lateral movement. When the head is tilted 15°, one can test C1-C2 at 45° one tests C3-C6 and with neck fully flexed to place the chin on the chest, one can test C7-T1.

Examine the temporomandibular joint for tenderness. The joint should be palpated with the mouth open and then closed. Lateral meniscus palpation is done by applying pressure in front of the tragus of the ear, while the medial meniscus is most easily felt with examiner's finger in the child's ear. The normal adolescent should be able to open the mouth at least 4.5-5 cm.

Investigations

The role of ancillary diagnostic studies, such as laboratory testing, electroencephalography (EEG), and neuroimaging, has been extensively reviewed. The American Academy of Neurology (AAN) Practice Parameter determined that there is inadequate documentation in the literature to support any recommendation as to the appropriateness of routine laboratory studies, e.g., hematology or chemistry panels or performance of lumbar puncture. Routine EEG is not recommended as part of the headache evaluation. The role of neuroimaging is better defined. The recommendations for neuroimaging in pediatric headache are as mentioned below:

1. Obtaining neuroimaging study on a routine basis is not indicated in children with recurrent headaches and a normal neurologic examination.
2. Neuroimaging should be considered in children in whom there are historic features to suggest:
   - Recent onset of severe headache.
   - Change in the type of headache.
   - Neurologic dysfunction.
3. Neuroimaging should be considered in children with an abnormal neurologic examination (e.g., focal findings, signs of increased intracranial pressure, significant alteration of consciousness), and/or the coexistence of seizures.

Care must be taken not to over- or under-interpret these recommendations. Neuroimaging may be considered in children with recurrent headache based upon clues extracted from the medical history or based upon the findings on neurologic examination. The findings of the AAN Practice Parameter support the medical decision to perform scans, or to withhold scans, based upon clinical determinants for the individual patient.[5]

PRIMARY HEADACHE DISORDERS

Migraine

Migraine is a common disabling primary headache disorder. Epidemiological studies have documented its high prevalence and high socio-economic and personal impacts. In the Global Burden of Disease Survey 2010, it was ranked as the third most prevalent disorder and seventh highest specific cause of disability worldwide.[4] Pediatric migraine is the most frequent recurrent headache, occurring in upto 28% of older teenagers. Migraine can have a substantial effect on the life of the child, as well as their family, leading to lost school days and withdrawal from social interactions.[9]

Diagnostic Criteria[4]

There two major subtypes of migraine–migraine without aura and migraine with aura.

The International Classification of Headache Disorders, 3rd edition classifies migraine into following categories:

- Migraine without aura.
- Migraine with aura.
- Chronic migraine.
- Complications of migraine (status migrainosus, persistent aura without infarction, migrainous infarction, migraine aura-triggered seizure).
- Probable migraine.
- Episodic syndromes that may be associated with migraine (cyclical vomiting syndrome, abdominal migraine, benign paroxysmal vertigo, benign paroxysmal torticollis).

Migraine without aura (previously known as common migraine/hemicranias simplex) is a clinical syndrome characterized by headache with specific features and associated symptoms. The diagnostic criteria are given in Box 44.1. Migraine with aura (previously known as classic or classical migraine/ophthalmic, hemiparaesthetic, hemiplegic, aphasic migraine/migraine accompagnee/ complicated migraine) is primarily characterized by the transient focal neurological symptoms that usually precede or sometimes accompany the headache. The diagnostic criteria are given in Box 44.2.

Box 44.1: The Diagnostic Criteria for Migraine Without Aura

A. At least five attacks fulfilling criteria B-D

B. Headache attacks lasting 2-72 hours (untreated or unsuccessfully treated)

C. Headache has at least two of the following four characteristics:
   i. Unilateral location
   ii. Pulsating quality
   iii. Moderate or severe pain intensity
   iv. Aggravation by or causing avoidance of routine physical activity (e.g., walking or climbing stairs)

D. During headache at least one of the following:
   i. Nausea and/or vomiting
   ii. Photophobia and phonophobia

E. Not better accounted for by another ICHD-3 diagnosis

Box 44.2: The Diagnostic Criteria of Migraine With Aura

A. At least two attacks fulfilling criteria B and C

B. One or more of the following fully reversible aura symptoms:
   i. Visual
   ii. Sensory
   iii. Speech and/or language
   iv. Motor
   v. Brainstem
   vi. Retinal

C. At least two of the following four characteristics:
   i. At least one aura symptom spreads gradually over ≥ 5 minutes, and/or two or more symptoms occur in succession
   ii. Each individual aura symptom lasts 5-60 minutes
   iii. At least one aura symptom is unilateral
   iv. The aura is accompanied, or followed within 60 minutes, by headache

D. Not better accounted for by another ICHD-3 diagnosis and transient ischaemic attack has been excluded.

Pathophysiology

The pathophysiology of migraine in children and adolescents is presumed to be the same as in adults. The principal underlying phenomenon of migraine is hyperexcitable neurons. Polygenic influences produce disturbances of neuronal ion channels, leading to episodes of cortical spreading depression and trigeminal vascular activation with transmission through the thalamus to higher cortical structures. Cortical spreading depression is now viewed as cause of migraine aura. As only about 30% of patients experience aura, occurrence of pain is possibly due to other cerebral circuits. Various factors involved in complex pathogenesis of migraine headaches are described below:

Genetics

The risk of developing migraine depends upon a balance between the genetic inheritance and the environmental effects that contribute to the phenotypic expression. The environmental influences could be shared and non-shared ones.[10-17]

The roles of individual genes in migraine are beginning to be understood. Mutations in a calcium channel gene, CACNA1A, a sodium/potassium pump gene, ATP1A2, and a sodium channel gene, SCN1A, directly cause a rare subtype of migraine, familial hemiplegic migraine.[18-22] This highlights the importance of neurotransmission between neurons that might contribute to the hypersensitivity in some patients with migraine (cases of allodynia). Also, as astrocytes provide a connection between the neurons and blood vessels and regulate the extracellular milieu in which neurons exist, involvement of the ATP1A2 gene suggests that this connection is important in migraine expression.[9]

There are potential genetic biomarkers, which are being studied in patients with migraine. The candidate genes which are under study are the ones which encode serotonin transporters, a potassium channel (KCNN3), 5'10'-methylenetetrahydrofolate reductase (MTHFR), and angiotensin-converting enzyme and matrix metalloproteinase 3. This suggests a possible complex interaction between neurotransmitters, channels and metabolism.[23-27]

Biological Changes

Studies have shown immunological and inflammatory changes in children with migraine. Children with a history of migraine have been found to have detectable levels of interleukin 1α that are not seen in children with a history of TTH. The concentrations of both soluble tumour necrosis factor receptor 1 and tumour necrosis factor are also found to be increased in children with migraine.[28] Potential biological markers have been identified for some groups of patients with migraine, which include increased levels of calcitonin gene-related peptide and decreased levels of coenzyme Q10.[29-30]

Hormonal changes possibly explain the predominance of migraine in girls during adolescence. Menstrual migraine has also possibly hormonal basis.

Neurophysiological Changes

The neurophysiological changes specific to migraine suggest that migraine is not just a vascular disease. Adult migraine patients have been found to have interictal trigeminal sensitisation as evidenced by an altered blink reflex, altered visual-evoked responses during the oddball paradigm, and altered auditory responses.[31-39] The changes are similar in children. Additionally, there are changes in somatosensory-evoked potentials with treatment of pediatric migraine.[40] These neurophysiological changes indicate that the altered sensitivity in the migraine brain might be involved in the initiation and propagation of migraine.

Children with migraine have also been found to have altered occipital response (but not motor cortex response) at the time of migraine as shown in a study which used transcranial magnetic stimulation to examine cortical excitability in children.[41] This suggests a neurophysiological sensitivity in adolescent migraine that can change during the migraine cycle, which has implications for treatment.

CLINICAL FEATURES

Migraine Without Aura

It is the more common form of migraine in pediatric population, seen in 60-85% of the patients. Patients often recognize prodromal features: mood changes, irritability, lethargy, yawning, food cravings, or increased thirst. Perhaps the most frequent heralding feature is a change in behavioral patterns or withdrawal from activities.

A migraine headache begins gradually and is usually localized to the frontal or temporal region. The pain may be unilateral. The quality is generally described as pounding, pulsing and throbbing, but the key feature is intensity. Routine activities will be interrupted. Photophobia and/or phonophobia are common, and may be inferred by the child's desire to seek a quiet, dark place to rest or even to sleep, since sleep often produces significant relief.

Migraine headaches typically last for hours, even days, but do not generally, occur more frequently than 6-8 times per month.

The time of the day when the headache occurs tends to shift through childhood. Younger children will complain in the afternoon, after school. The early teenagers will frequently begin to report their headaches about lunchtime. Older teens will acquire a cause for concern since morning occurrence frequently raises suspicion of space-occupying lesions.

In case of developmentally challenged or pre-verbal child, the symptoms can be inferred by caregiver's report of repeated, cycling, events of quiet, withdrawn behaviour with pallor, regurgitation, vomiting and desire to rest.

Migraine With Aura

The aura is an inconsistent feature in children and adolescents with migraine. It is seen in 14-30 percent of children. Children usually report visual disturbances, distortions, or obscuration before or as the headache begins. Typically, the aura is a visual phenomenon, but the cortical spreading depression responsible for aura may disturb virtually any cortical region, including language, motor, or sensory areas.

Episodic Syndromes Associated With Migraine[4]

These were previously known as childhood periodic syndromes/periodic syndromes of childhood. This group of disorders occurs in patients who also have migraine without aura or migraine with aura or who have an increased likelihood to develop either of these disorders. Although historically noted to occur in childhood, they may also occur in adults. Additional conditions that may also occur in these patients include episodes of motion sickness and periodic sleep disorders including sleep walking, sleep talking, night terrors and bruxism.

Recurrent gastrointestinal disturbance was previously known as chronic abdominal pain/functional abdominal pain/irritable bowel syndrome. It is characterised by recurrent episodic attacks of abdominal pain and/or discomfort, nausea and/or vomiting, occurring infrequently, chronically or at predictable intervals, that may be associated with migraine.

Cyclic vomiting syndrome is characterized by recurrent episodic attacks of intense nausea and vomiting, usually stereotypical in the individual and with predictable timing of episodes. Attacks may be associated with pallor and lethargy. There is complete resolution of symptoms between attacks.

Abdominal migraine is an idiopathic disorder seen mainly I children as recurrent attacks of moderate to severe midline abdominal pain, associated with vasomotor symptoms, nausea and vomiting, lasting 2-72 hours and with normality between episodes. Headache does not occur during these episodes.

Benign paroxysmal vertigo is characterised by recurrent brief attacks of vertigo, occurring without warning and resolving spontaneously, in otherwise healthy children.

Benign paroxysmal torticollis leads to recurrent episodes of head tilt to one side, perhaps with slight rotation, which remit spontaneously. The condition occurs in infants and small children, with onset in the first year.

TREATMENT

The treatment of paediatric migraine can be divided into pharmacological (both acute and preventive strategies) and biobehavioural interventions to minimise the effects of the attacks. The goals of treatment need to be determined at the initial visit, and should include a rapid return to normal function with acute treatment, and a reduction in the frequency and effect of the migraine with preventive and biobehavioural treatment. A crucial component of management of paediatric headache is education of the patients and parents on the incorporation of all these strategies.

Acute pharmacological treatment is done with the goals of consistent response with minimal side effects and rapid return to normal function. There are various drugs available for management of acute attack (Table 44.3). NSAIDs (particularly ibuprofen) are effective when used early in the attacks at an adequate dose (7.5-10.0 mg/kg per dose) and that triptans are effective when NSAIDs do not completely relieve symptoms, particularly during more severe attacks.

One aspect of acute treatment that needs to be included in any treatment plan is the avoidance of medication overuse. This is a common component of chronic daily headache that can be avoided by limiting the number of headaches treated with acute medications. Clinical experience suggests that non-specific analgesics should be used fewer than 2-3 times per week, and migraine-specific drugs should be used fewer than 6 times per month. On the basis of controlled studies of acute treatment to date, the general conclusions that can be drawn are that NSAIDs (particularly ibuprofen) are effective at appropriate doses (7.5-10 mg/kg) when taken early and when these drugs are used fewer than 2-3 times per week to minimise the risk of medication overuse. When this approach is not consistently effective, triptans can be a well-tolerated and successful addition to the acute treatment. When treatment

Table 44.3: Drugs Used in Treatment of Acute Attack of Migraine in Children and Adolescents[42]					
Drug	**Licensed for**	**Single dose**	**Maximum dose**	**Minimum interval**	**Dose form**
Ibuprofen	All ages	10-20 mg/kg	40 mg/kg/day	2 hours	Oral suspension: Effervescent tablet
Paracetamol	All ages	10-15 mg/kg	60 mg/kg/day	2 hours	Rapid tablet: Oral suspension
Sumatriptan	>12 years	10 mg (20-39 kg) 20 mg (>39 kg)	10 mg/day 20 mg/day	2 hours	Nasal spray
Rizatriptan	>18 years	5 mg (20-39 kg) 10 mg (>39 kg)	10 mg/day 20 mg/day	2 hours	Tablet
Zolmitriptan	>18 years	2.5 mg, 5 mg	5 mg/day, 10 mg/day	2 hours	Nasal spray, Tablet
Prochlor-perazine	Weight >10 kg	0.10-0.30 mg/kg 0.1-0.15 mg/kg	0.4-0.5 mg/kg/day Max single dose 10 mg	4 hours	Tablet Injection solution

with NSAIDs or triptans at home is ineffective, the use of dopamine antagonists with intravenous NSAIDs in the emergency department and infusion centres seems to be effective, but larger studies are needed to confirm this result. Intravenous dihydroergotamine remains one of the few options with supporting evidence for inpatient management of migraine in children.[9]

Preventative treatment of migraine is indicated if attacks occur on at least four occasions per month and are severe and long enough to stop activities. Various drugs which are available and used for prophylaxis against migraine are shown in Table 44.4. There are no reliable medications to prevent headache in all children all of the time. Medications should be taken regularly for at least two months in appropriate dosages before their success or failure can be confidently decided.

Table 44.4: Drugs Used for the Prevention of Migraine in Children			
Drug	**Total daily dose**	**Dose frequency**	**Evidence**
Flunarizine	5-10 mg	Once per day	DB, PC, RTs
Topiramate	1-2 mg/kg	Once per day	DB, PC trials
Pizotifen	0.5-1.0 mg	Once per day	DB, open trials
Propranolol	1-3 mg/kg	Twice per day	DB, open trials
Amitriptylline	0.25-1 mg/kg	Once per day	Open trials
Sodium valproate	500-1000 mg	Twice per day	DB, open trials
Cyproheptadine	2-8 mg	One or two doses per day	Open trials
DB: double blind; PC: placebo controlled; RT: randomised trials			

Status migrainosus is one of the complications of migraine. It is defined as attack of migraine (the) headache phase lasting for >72 hours despite of treatment. Headache free intervals of not more than 4 hours (excluding sleep) may occur. Approach to a patient with status migrainosus is shown in Figure 44.3. The treatment options for the management of status migrainosus are given in Table 44.5.

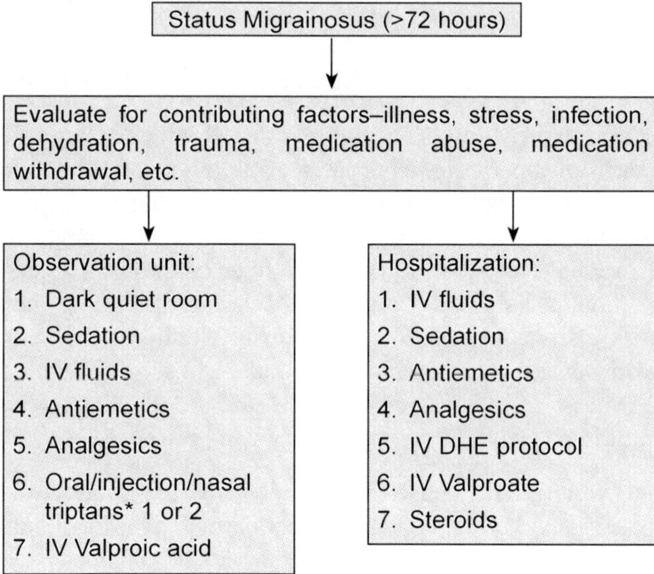

Fig. 44.3: Status migrainosus management approach[42]

Table 44.5: Treatments of Status Migrainosus[43]	
1.	Subcutaneous sumatriptan (2-6 mg)
2.	IM or IV Ketorolac (10-30 mg)
3.	IV Neuroleptics/Antiemetics
	Prochlorperazine (2.5-10 mg)
	Metoclopramide (1-2 mg/kg/dose)
	Chlorpromazine (0.5-1 mg/kg/dose)
4.	IM or IV DHE
	Pretreatment with antiemetic
	Test dose 0.1 mg
	Treatment dose (0.1-0.2 mg/dose Q8 hours)

Contd.

Contd.

5.	IV Steroids Hydrocortisone 1-2 mg/kg/dose Methylprednisolone 1 mg/kg/dose Dexamethasone 0.25-0.5 mg/kg/dose
6.	IV Opioids

TENSION-TYPE HEADACHE

TTH is atleast as common as migraine headache in school aged children and adolescents. It is characterised by mild (no interference with normal activities) to moderate (interferes with some but not all activities) intensity of headache (Box 44.3). The pain is dull or pressure around the head, and is not associated with other symptoms such as nausea, vomiting or intolerance to light and noise.

Box 44.3: The ICHD Criteria for Diagnosis of Tension-Type Headache

A. At least 10 episodes of headache occurring on fulfilling criteria B–D

B. Lasting from 30 minutes to 7 days

C. At least 2 of the following 4 characteristics:
   1. Bilateral location
   2. Pressing or tightening (non-pulsating) quality
   3. Mild or moderate intensity
   4. Not aggravated by routine physical activity such as walking or climbing stairs

D. Both of the following:
   1. No nausea or vomiting
   2. No more than one of photophobia or phonophobia

E. Not better accounted for by another ICHD-3

Infrequent TTH Frequent TTH Chronic TTH

< 1 day/month 1–15 days/month >15 days/month

The exact mechanisms of tension-type headache are not known. Peripheral pain mechanisms are most likely to play a role in infrequent episodic tension-type headache and frequent episodic tension-type headache, whereas central pain mechanisms play a more important role in chronic tension-type headache.

Increased pericranial tenderness recorded by manual palpation is the most significant abnormal finding in patients with tension-type headache. The tenderness is typically present interictally, is further increased during actual headache and increases with the intensity and frequency of headaches. Pericranial tenderness is easily recorded by manual palpation by small rotating movements and a firm pressure (preferably aided by use of a palpometer) with the second and third fingers on the frontal, temporal, masseter, pterygoid, sternocleidomastoid, splenius and trapezius muscles. Local tenderness scores of 0-3 for each muscle can be summed to yield a total tenderness score for each individual. Palpation is a useful guide for treatment strategy. It also adds value and credibility to the explanations given to the patient. Increased tenderness is most likely of pathophysiological importance.

Most tension-type headache is best managed by primary care. Episodic tension-type headache is self-limiting, but children and their parents generally consult doctors when headaches become frequent and are no longer responsive to analgesics. For acute treatment of episodic tension-type headache, paracetamol and aspirin are effective and inexpensive drugs for those age 16-65 years. Together with aspirin and paracetamol, non-steroidal anti-inflammatory drugs are effective first-line therapy for episodic tension-type headache in adults. In children younger than 15 years, aspirin is not recommended because of the concern of Reye's syndrome. However, paracetamol is safe even in young children. Prophylactic pharmacological treatment should be considered in chronic tension-type headache if non-pharmacological management is inadequate. For children with frequent headache, amitriptyline might be beneficial for the prophylaxis, although no placebo-controlled studies have been done.

Behavioural headache treatments include relaxation training, biofeedback training, cognitive-behavioural therapy, or combinations of these treatments. Relaxation techniques are often used in combination with biofeedback and stress management. Relaxation and cognitive behavioural therapy might reduce the severity and frequency of chronic headache in childhood and adolescence.[44]

References

1. Abu-Arafeh I, Razak S, Sivaraman B, Graham C. Prevalence of Headache and Migraine in Children and Adolescents: A Systematic Review of Population-based Studies. Dev Med Child Neurol 2010;52:1088-97.
2. Ravishankar K. Headache Pattern in India: A Headache Clinic Analysis of 1000 Patients. Cephalalgia 1997;17:316-17.
3. Shah PA, Nafee A. Clinical Profile of Headache and Cranial Neuralgias. J Assoc Physicians India 1999 November; 47(11):1072-75.
4. The International Classification of Headache Disorders, 3rd Edition (Beta version), Cephalalgia 2013;33(9):629-808.

5. Lewis DW. Headaches in Infants and Children. In: Swaiman's Pediatric Neurology: Principles and Practice. 5th Edition. Elsevier Saunders 880-99.

6. Rothner AD. Evaluation of Headache. In: Winner P, Rothner AD, eds. Headache in Children and Adolescents. Hamilton: BC Decker Inc 2001;20-32.

7. Dooley JM. The Evaluation and Management of Paediatric Headaches. Paediatr Child Health 2009:14(1):24-30.

8. Linder S. Understanding the Comprehensive Pediatric Headache Examination. Peditric Annals 2005:34:442-47.

9. Hershey AD. Current Approaches to the Diagnosis and Management of Paediatric Migraine. Lancet Neurol 2010: 9:190-204.

10. Honkasalo ML, Kaprio J, Winter T, Heikkila K, Sillanpaa M, Koskenvuo M. Migraine and Concomitant Symptoms Among 8167 Adult Twin Pairs. Headache 1995:35:70-78.

11. Gervil M, Ulrich V, Kyvik KO, Olesen J, Russell MB. Migraine Without Aura: A Population-based Twin Study. Ann Neurol 1999:46:606-11.

12. Svensson DA, Larsson B, Bille B, Lichtenstein P. Genetic and Environmental Influences on Recurrent Headaches in Eight to Nine-year-old Twins. Cephalalgia 1999;19:866-72.

13. Ulrich V, Gervil M, Fenger K, Olesen J, Russell MB. The Prevalence and Characteristics of Migraine in Twins from the General Population. Headache 1999;39:173-80.

14. Ulrich V, Gervil M, Kyvik KO, Olesen J, Russell MB., Evidence of a Genetic Factor in Migraine with Aura: A Population-based Danish Twin Study. Ann Neurol 1999;45:242-46.

15. Ulrich V, Olesen J, Gervil M, Russell MB. Possible Risk Factors and Precipitants for Migraine with Aura in Discordant Twin-pairs: A Population-based Study. Cephalalgia 2000;20: 821-25.

16. Ulrich V, Gervil M, Olesen J. The Relative Influence of Environment and Genes in Episodic Tension-type Headache. Neurology 2004;62:2065-69.

17. Gervil M, Ulrich V, Kaprio J, Olesen J, Russell MB. The Relative Role of Genetic and Environmental Factors in Migraine without Aura. Neurology 1999:53:995-99.

18. Ophoff RA, Terwindt GM, Vergouwe MN, *et al.* Familial Hemiplegic Migraine and Episodic Ataxia type-2 are Caused by Mutations in the Ca2+ Channel Gene CACNL1A4. Cell 1996:87:544-52.

19. Terwindt GM, Ophoff RA, Haan J, *et al.* Variable Clinical Expression of Mutations in the P/Q-type Calcium Channel Gene in Familial Hemiplegic Migraine. Neurology 1998:50: 1105-10.

20. De Fusco M, Marconi R, Silvestri L, *et al.* Haploinsufficiency of ATP1A2 Encoding the Na+/K+ Pump Alpha2 Subunit Associated with Familial Hemiplegic Migraine Type 2. Nat Genet 2003;33:192-96.

21. Vanmolkot KR, Kors EE, Hottenga JJ, *et al.* Novel Mutations in the Na+, K+-ATPase Pump Gene ATP1A2 Associated with Familial Hemiplegic Migraine and Benign Familial Infantile Convulsions. Ann Neurol 2003:54:360-66.

22. Dichgans M, Freilinger T, Eckstein G, *et al.* Mutation in the Neuronal Voltage-gated Sodium Channel SCN1A in Familial Hemiplegic Migraine. Lancet 2005:366:371-77.

23. Mossner R, Weichselbaum A, Marziniak M, *et al.* A Highly Polymorphic Poly-glutamine Stretch in the Potassium Channel KCNN3 in Migraine. Headache 2005;45:132-36.

24. Scher AI, Terwindt GM, Verschuren WM, *et al.* Migraine and MTHFR C677T Genotype in a Population-based Sample. Ann Neurol 2006;59:372-75.

25. Kaunisto MA, Kallela M, Hamalainen E, *et al.* Testing of Variants of the MTHFR and ESR1 Genes in 1798 Finnish Individuals Fails to Confirm the Association with Migraine with Aura. Cephalalgia 2006;26:1462-72.

26. Kara I, Ozkok E, Aydin M, *et al.* Combined Effects of ACE and MMP-3 Polymorphisms on Migraine Development. Cephalalgia 2007;27:235-43.

27. Kowa H, Fusayasu E, Ijiri T, *et al.* Association of the Insertion/ Deletion Polymorphism of the Angiotensin I-converting Enzyme Gene in Patients of Migraine with Aura. Neurosci Lett 2005:374:129-31.

28. Bockowski L, Sobaniec W, Zelazowska-Rutkowska B. Proinflammatory Plasma Cytokines in Children with Migraine. Pediatr Neurol 2009;41:17-21.

29. Fan PC, Kuo PH, Chang SH, Lee WT, Wu RM, Chiou LC. Plasma Calcitonin Gene-related Peptide in Diagnosing and Predicting Paediatric Migraine. Cephalalgia 2009;29:883-90.

30. Hershey AD, Powers SW, Vockell AL, *et al.* Coenzyme Q10 Deficiency and Response to Supplementation in Pediatric and Adolescent Migraine. Headache 2007;47:73-80.

31. Katsarava Z, Lehnerdt G, Duda B, Ellrich J, Diener HC, Kaube H. Sensitization of Trigeminal Nociception Specific for Migraine but not Pain of Sinusitis. Neurology 2002;59: 1450-53.

32. Kaube H, Katsarava Z, Przywara S, Drepper J, Ellrich J, Diener HC. Acute Migraine Headache: Possible Sensitization of Neurons in the Spinal Trigeminal Nucleus? Neurology 2002:58:1234-38.

33. De Marinis M, Pujia A, Natale L, D'Arcangelo E, Accornero N. Decreased Habituation of the R2 Component of the Blink Reflex in Migraine Patients. Clin Neurophysiol 2003;114: 889-93.

34. Katsarava Z, Giffin N, Diener HC, Kaube H. Abnormal Habituation of 'Nociceptive' Blink Reflex in Migraine–Evidence for Increased Excitability of Trigeminal Nociception. Cephalalgia 2003:23:814-19.

35. Burstein R, Levy D, Jakubowski M. Effects of Sensitization of Trigeminovascular Neurons to Triptan Therapy During Migraine. Rev Neurol 2005;161:658-60.

36. Evers S, Bauer B, Grotemeyer KH, Kurlemann G, Husstedt IW. Event-related Potentials (P300) in Primary Headache in Childhood and Adolescence. J Child Neurol 1998;13:322-26.

37. Wang W. Schoenen J. Interictal Potentiation of Passive "Oddball" Auditory Event-related Potentials in Migraine. Cephalalgia 1998:18:261-65.

38. Siniatchkin M. Kropp P. Gerber WD. What Kind of Habituation is Impaired in Migraine Patients? Cephalalgia 2003:23:511-18.

39. Buodo G. Palomba D. Sarlo M. Naccarella C. Battistella PA. Auditory Event-related Potentials and Reaction Times in Migraine Children. Cephalalgia 2004:24:554-63.

40. Vollono C. Ferraro D. Miliucci R. Vigevano F. Valeriani M. The Abnormal Recovery Cycle of Somatosensory Evoked Potential Components in Children with Migraine Can be Reversed by Topiramate. Cephalalgia 2009; Published online June 1. DOI:10.1111/j.1468-2982.2009.01892.x.

41. Siniatchkin M. Reich AL. Shepherd AJ. van Baalen A. Siebner HR. Stephani U. Peri-ictal Changes of Cortical Excitability in Children Suffering from Migraine Without Aura. Pain 2009; 147:132-40.

42. Diagnosis and Management of Headache in Children and Adolescents. Arafeh IA. Prgoress in Neurology and Psychiatry; July/August 2014:16-20.

43. Lewis DL. Headache in the Pediatric Emergency Department. Semin Pediatr Neurol 2001;8:46-51.

44. Anttila P. Tension-type Headache in Childhood and Adolescence. Lancet Neurol 2006;5:268-74.

45. Mishra D. Sharma A. Juneja M. Singh K. Profile of Pediatric Headache at a Public Hospital in India. Indian Pediatr 2013: 50:775-78.

45 Chapter

CEREBROVASCULAR DISEASES

Devendra Mishra, Richa Mittal

INTRODUCTION

Cerebrovascular diseases (CVD) are an important cause of mortality and morbidity in children. They are already amongst the top 10 causes of childhood death and are increasing in prevalence. These disorders may exhibit an entire spectrum of neurological presentations. Also, the diagnosis and management of CVD in children can be difficult because of diversity of underlying risk factors and the absence of a uniform treatment approach. Children and adolescents with stroke have remarkable differences in presentation as compared to older children. Stroke has been defined as the sudden occlusion or rupture of cerebral arteries or veins resulting in focal cerebral damage and clinical neurologic deficits.[1] Stroke can be ischaemic, haemorrhagic or both. Ischaemic stroke is more frequently caused by arterial occlusion, but it may also be caused by venous occlusion of cerebral veins or sinuses. Haemorrhagic stroke is the result of bleeding from a ruptured cerebral artery or from bleeding into the site of an acute ischemic stroke (AIS). AIS accounts for about half of all strokes in children, in contrast to adults in whom 80-85% of all strokes are ischemic.[2,3] Children also have a more diverse and larger number of risk factors for stroke that differ significantly from adults which are predominated by hypertension, diabetes and atherosclerosis[4,5] (Box 45.1). Roughly 10-25% of children with a stroke will die, upto 25% of children will have a recurrence, and upto 66% will have persistent neurological deficits or develop subsequent seizure disorders, learning, or developmental problems.[4,6,7] Given the onset of impairment during childhood and the effect on quality of life for the child and family, the economic and emotional costs to society are amplified. Early recognition of pediatric stroke should lead to more rapid neurological consultation, imaging, treatment and improved outcomes.

Box 45.1: Common Disorders Causing Cerebrovascular Disease in Children

Ischemic Stroke	Hemorrhagic Stroke
Intravascular	
Sickle cell anemia Antithrombin III deficiency Protein C and S deficiency Hyperhomocysteinemia Lupus anticoagulant Anticardiolipin antibodies Lipoprotein (a) elevation Factor V Leiden gene defect MTHFR mutations	Immune thrombocytopenic purpura Clotting factor deficiencies • Congenital • Liver dysfunction • Vitamin K deficiency Systemic conditions Hypertension Hemolytic-uremic syndrome Trauma • Accidental • Child abuse
Vascular	
Meningitis Intra-oral trauma Post-traumatic arterial dissection Primary angiitis of the CNS Homocystinuria Post-Varicella angiopathy Transient cerebral arteriopathy Moyamoya disease and syndrome Post-radiation vasculopathy	Arteriovenous malformations Aneurysms Cavernous malformation Venous angioma Hereditary hemorrhagic telangiectasia Moyamoya syndrome Sickle cell disease Ehlers-Danlos syndrome-IV
Embolic Congenital heart disease Acquired heart disease Cardiac procedures Fat/air embolism	

EPIDEMIOLOGY

There is no population-based published data on the incidence or prevalence of pediatric stroke in India. The reported incidence of combined ischemic and hemorrhagic pediatric stroke ranges from 1.2 to 13 cases per 100,000 children under 18 years of age.[3,8-16] However, pediatric stroke is likely more common than we may realize since it is thought to be frequently undiagnosed or misdiagnosed. In one report, 19 out of 45 children with a stroke did not receive a correct diagnosis until 15 hours to 3 months after initial presentation.[17] Another study demonstrated upto a 28-hour delay in seeking medical attention from the onset of symptoms and a 7.2-hour average delay after presentation before any brain imaging was done.[18] However, the reported incidence of pediatric stroke has more than doubled from prior decade estimates.[19] This may be due to a combination of increased survival in children with risk factors for stroke, such as congenital heart disease, sickle cell disease, and leukemia, and increased awareness.[19] Stroke is more common in boys than girls, even after controlling for differences in frequency of causes such as trauma. There appears to be a predominance of stroke in black children.[10] This difference remains true even after accounting for sickle cell disease patients with stroke.[16] In hospital-based studies, pediatric stroke constitutes <1% of all pediatric admissions. Incidence rates of 10.7 per 100,000 children per year (2.9 for ischemic stroke and 7.8 for hemorrhagic stroke) have been reported.[12] A population-based study estimated the relative proportion of AIS and CVT as 2:1 among an incidence of 1.8/100,000 for ischemic stroke.[20]

CLINICAL MANIFESTATIONS

Few presentations of stroke in children can be generalized. AIS most often presents as a focal neurologic deficit. Hemiplegia is the most common focal manifestation, occurring in upto 94% of cases.[2,11,21-23] Hemorrhagic strokes most commonly present as headaches or altered level of consciousness, and are more likely to cause vomiting than in AIS.[2,11,24] Seizures are common in both ischemic and hemorrhagic strokes. They occur in upto 50% of children with strokes, are not restricted to any age group, and are not limited to any specific seizure type. based on the child's age. The younger the child, the more nonspecific their symptoms may be. Perinatal strokes are more likely to initially present with focal seizures or lethargy in the first few days after birth.[26] Although focal neurological deficits from these events may not develop until weeks or months later, infants within the first year of life can still present acutely with lethargy, apnea spells, or hypotonia.[27] Toddlers can also present with protean symptoms such as deterioration of their general condition, increased crying and sleepiness, irritability, feeding difficulty, vomiting, and sepsis-like symptoms with cold extremities.[28] Older children demonstrate more specific neurological defects similar to adults. These include hemiparesis, language (e.g., aphasia) and speech difficulties, visual deficits, and headache.[29-31] If symptoms last less than 24 hours, they are defined as a transient ischemic attack (TIA).[32] Deficits are frequently brief and may resolve as quickly as within one hour. However, it is increasingly being recognized that neuroimaging evidence of an infarct is present in up to 50% of adults with a neurological deficit lasting less than 24 hours. TIA is therefore now defined as "a brief episode of neurologic dysfunction caused by focal brain or retinal ischemia, with clinical symptoms typically lasting less than one hour, and without evidence of acute infarction". Recent data suggests that 33% of children with arterial strokes had preceding TIAs that were undiagnosed at that time.[19] Venous sinus thrombosis can present in all ages with fever and lethargy, but young infants can present with a history of decreased oral intake or respiratory distress.[33-36] Physical examination may reveal dilated scalp veins, eyelid swelling, or a large anterior fontanelle whereas an older child would likely present with more slowly progressing signs, such as vomiting, headache, or any other signs of increased intracranial pressure.[33-36] A subarachnoid hemorrhage can also present as irritability and a bulging fontanelle in infants, but should be suspected in older children complaining of sudden acute onset headache, neck pain, meningismus, or photophobia.[37] The clinical presentation is also useful for localizing the lesion. The majority of pediatric ischemic strokes occur in the distribution of the middle cerebral artery, which results in hemiplegia with upper limb predominance, hemianopsia, or dysphasia. Primarily lower extremity weakness would suggest anterior cerebral artery involvement whereas vertigo, ataxia, and nystagmus are consistent with an ischemic event in the posterior circulation.[38] Bulbar dysfunction and dysarthria points towards lower brainstem involvement whereas aphasia suggests involvement of the basal ganglia, thalamus, or cerebral hemispheres. If the hemispheres are involved, then the eyes will look towards the lesion, rather than away as if the brainstem were involved. Neurodeficit due to thrombosis is slow to develop whereas embolism produces a rapidly evolving clinical picture with maximum deficit within minutes. Shedding of emboli from a thrombus may lead to cerebral symptoms in a typical 'stuttering presentation'. CVD associated with congenital heart disease is most frequently observed among infants whereas trauma and bacterial infection are more common in preschoolers.

Arterial Ischaemic Stroke

Clinical manifestations of AIS in childhood are age-related with the presentations being similar to many common childhood illnesses like focal seizure, focal encephalitis, migraine, or demyelination.[25] In late infancy or childhood, an acute onset hemiparesis with or without seizures is the most common manifestation. In addition to seizure, fever, headache, and lethargy may occur specially in younger children.[39] Children with arterial dissection or other physical injuries may frequently present with headache. Dystonia is commonly present in those with basal ganglia infarction.

Sinovenous Thrombosis

In *septic* sinovenous thrombosis (SVT), spread of infection from an adjacent structure leads to thrombophlebitis whereas the pathological mechanism for *nonseptic* SVT is still unclear. In contrast to AIS, there is a zone of prolonged increased pressure in the brain of patients with SVT. Thus delayed recanalisation of the obstruction to venous drainage days after the initial occlusion can potentially relieve circulatory congestion.[1] Moreover, in contrast to AIS, the location of the cerebral venous infarct and the resulting clinical presentation do not correlate highly with the site of cerebral sinovenous thrombosis.

Seizures are more common in neonates (~75%) than in infants and children with SVT. The relative proportion of various clinical features in post-neonatal patients with SVT is headache in 54%, focal neurological signs in 53%, altered consciousness in 49%, seizures in 45%, and papilledema in 22%.[20] Older children can present with sign and symptoms suggestive of 'idiopathic intracranial hypertension', including headache, papilledema, abducens palsy and altered level of consciousness, especially when the superior sagittal sinus is the site of thrombosis.[1]

Hemorrhagic Stroke

The term signifies bleeding either into the brain parenchyma *(intracerebral hemorrhage)* or the subarachnoid space (*subarachnoid hemorrhage,* SAH). Amongst children with HS, 68% have intracerebral hemorrhage and SAH is found in 25%.[40] *Intraventricular hemorrhage* is rare beyond the neonatal period and usually occurs due to rupture of vascular malformation and aneurysm or with a sinus thrombosis and bleeding diathesis. Intracerebral hemorrhage typically presents with severe headache with focal signs, rapid decrease in consciousness and seizures. Smaller bleeds may lead to isolated focal signs correlating with the area involved. If posterior fossa is involved, gaze palsies, ataxia and rapidly deteriorating coma occur. SAH typically presents with a severe headache associated with meningeal signs and features of raised intracranial pressure. Occasionally, low-grade fever, leukocytosis, and subhyaloid retinal hemorrhage[1] may also be present.

Hemorrhage in Infants and Term Neonates

The signs and symptoms of an ICH can be more subtle and less specific in infants and neonates than in older children, especially with smaller hemorrhages which may go unrecognized.[41] A term newborn with an intraparenchymal hemorrhage is less likely to have an identifiable cause for the hemorrhage than older children. Additionally, a few clinical situations are distinct to infants and neonates. Some infants whose mothers took warfarin, phenytoin, or barbiturates during pregnancy bleed excessively owing to a reduction in vitamin K-dependent coagulation factors. These babies require a higher dose of vitamin K after birth to prevent bleeding; vitamins during the last trimester of pregnancy may also be of value. The clinical presentation of an AVM or arteriovenous fistula varies with age. Symptomatic neonates, for example, frequently present with unexplained high-output cardiac failure, and these neonates tend to fare much worse than individuals presenting later.[42] Older children and adolescents present much like adults, with seizures or ICH, whereas some infants develop hydrocephalus, particularly when a posterio fossa lesion results in aneurysmal dilatation of the vein of Galen and aqueductal compression.

RISK FACTORS

I. Arterial Ischaemic Stroke

Majority of children with AIS have an underlying infectious or inflammatory disorder,[43] with meningitis being the most frequent. In a population based study 72% of children with AIS had an identifiable primary risk factor[44] with quite a few having multiple risk factors. Cardiac disease was found in 24% patients, with stroke occurring spontaneously in 63% of these children.[44] Anemia in 40% and elevated homocysteine levels or homozygosity for t-MTHFR mutation in 21% children has been reported in a more recent study.[45] In another study mechanism of stroke was arteriopathy in 53%, cardioembolic in 12% and systemic disease in 14%.[46] Children with genetic disorders like sickle cell disease, homocystinuria, Menke disease and neurofibromatosis have significant predisposition to stroke. Air embolism during surgery and fat emboli occurring with fracture long bones are other causes of embolism leading to stroke.

A. **Cardiac Disorders:** Cardiac disease is the most common cause of stroke in childhood, accounting for upto a third of all AIS.[5] In children with a cardiac repair or catheterization, nearly 50% of strokes occur within 72 hours. Long-standing cyanotic lesions cause polycythemia and anemia, which both increase the risk of thromboembolism and cerebral infarction.[3] Embolic clots can arise in children with cardiomyopathies, rheumatic heart disease, prosthetic valves, or valvular vegetation from endocarditis.[2,26] A patent foramen ovale (PFO) can occur in as many as 35% of people between ages 1 and 29 years, and may serve as a portal for venous embolic events to pass from the right to left side of the heart. These are reported to be present in 12-28% of infants and children with AIS.[44-46] AIS may be associated with congenital cardiac problems (specially complex CHD, arrhythmias, myxoma), acquired conditions (like rheumatic heart disease, infective endocarditis) or may even occur in children with prosthetic heart valves or those undergoing cardiac procedures. The pathophysiologic mechanism involves the emboli from a thrombus formed in the heart, reaching the cerebral circulation. This occurs with prosthetic heart valves, or right to left shunt in those with septal defects, which allows systemic venous clots to reach the cerebral circulation. Although small insignificant intracardiac septal defects have been shown to be risk factors for stroke, they are associated with low risk of recurrence with aspirin therapy.[47] In approximately half the children with CHD and stroke, the stroke occurs in relation to a cardiac intervention, either surgery or cathetarisation. The frequency of stroke following cardiac procedures in children is 1 in 250-400 cardiac surgeries, 1 in 600-700 cardiac cathetarisations and in 3-19% of Fontan procedures. Rheumatic valve disease (mitral, aortic) is an important cause of embolic stroke in India. Infected valves in bacterial endocarditis pose considerable risk for the occurrence of embolic stroke, which may even occur after successful sterilization of vegetations.

B. **Infection:** Besides the established stroke risk factors (e.g., hypertension, diabetes, hypercholesterolemia, atrial fibrillation) both acute and chronic infectious diseases have emerged as risk factors for stroke A variety of infective illnesses have been reported to be associated with pediatric stroke. In an International Pediatric Stroke Children (29 days–18 years) were analyzed, upto 50% of children with cerebral infarcts had infections including acute systemic conditions and acute head and neck infections.[45] Mainly acute respiratory tract infection but also urinary tract infections independently increase the risk of ischemic stroke. The risk was shown to be highest for infection within 3 days before ischemia and the risk steadily declines with increasing time intervals between infection and stroke.[48] Also associations between stroke incidence and mortality and influenza epidemics have been demonstrated. Chronic infection including periodontitis and infections with Helicobacter pylori (Hp) and Chlamydia pneumoniae (Cp) have found to be associated with stroke recurrence.[48] Inflammation of the vessel intima is the pathophysiological mechanism associated with stroke following retropharyngeal abscess or other nasopharyngeal infections. A high incidence of multiple infarcts and cerebral aneurysms, frequently asymptomatic is increasingly being recognized with HIV infection in children. However, the most common cause is bacterial meningitis with 5-12% of these children having arterial or venous stroke.[1] In infants under one year, upto 75% with acute bacterial meningitis may have stroke. Local inflammation of meninges with thrombophlebitis of cerebral vessels is the principal mechanism.

Several traditional vascular risk factors are associated with proinflammatory alterations, including leukocyte activation, and predispose cerebral vasculature to thrombogenesis on inflammatory stimulation. Further-more, accumulation of inflammatory cells, mainly monocytes/macrophages, within the vascular wall starts early during atherogenesis. During later disease stages, their activation can lead to plaque rupture and thrombus formation, increasing stroke risk. Inflammatory markers (e.g., leukocytes, fibrinogen, C-reactive protein) are independent predictors of ischemic stroke. Chronic infections (e.g., infection with Chlamydia pneumoniae or Helicobacter pylori) were found to increase the risk of stroke. Acute infection within the preceding week has been seen as trigger factor for ischemic stroke. Acute and exacerbating chronic infection may act by activating coagulation and chronic infections and may contribute to atherogenesis. Also, genetic predisposition of the inflammatory host response may be an important codeterminant for atherogenesis and stroke risk.[49] In tubercular meningitis, infarcts due to basal arteritis are an important and not an uncommon finding. There are four changes in intracranial vessels associated with tubercular meningitis viz.:

(i) Inflammatory changes in the vessel wall leading to endarteritis.

(ii) Thrombus formation in the vessel leading to vessel occlusion or narrowing.

(iii) Fibrinoid degeneration leading to aneurysm formation; and

(iv) Focal hemorrhages occasionally. Cerebral infarction occurs most commonly around the sylvian fissure and in basal ganglia in the distribution of medial striate and thalamic perforating arteries.[50]

C. **Prothrombotic Disorders:** These are inherited or acquired disorders of the coagulation system, fibrinolytic system, endothelial cells or platelets, which lead to a reduced threshold for pathologic thrombus formation. Prothrombotic disorders may contribute to the etiology of childhood stroke, and include deficiencies of antithrombin, protein C, protein S, plasminogen, and presence of Factor V Leiden, Prothrombin gene G20210A, dysfibrinogenemia, antiphospholipid antibodies, hyperhomocysteinemia, and elevated lipoprotein (a). The overall incidence of prothrombotic disorders in childhood AIS is estimated to be 20% to 50% in most studies and, in childhood SVT, to be 33% to 99%. Also, hyperlipidemia, polycythemia, iron deficiency anemia, and platelet disorders may result in a prothrombotic state associated with ischemic stroke.[51] One or more prethrombotic disorders were present in around 30% with AIS and 50% with SVT,[52] with acquired disorders being more common than congenital ones. There is also evidence that activated protein C resistance or its underlying genetic defect, the factor V (FV) G1691A mutation, plays a role in the early onset of childhood ischemic stroke, which is in contrast to data obtained in adult populations. The 20210A allele within the 3'-untranslated region of the prothrombin (PT) gene, which is a common but mild risk factor of venous thrombosis in the CNS has also been controversially discussed as a risk factor for arterial thrombosis, i.e., myocardial infarction or stroke.[53] The most frequently reported abnormalities include factor V Leiden deficiency, prothrombin G20210A mutation, elevated lipoprotein (a) and homocysteine levels, protein C deficiency, and antiphospholipid antibodies. In children, the prothrombin G20210A mutation is more frequently seen with arterial thrombosis as compared to the other conditions, which promote venous thrombosis. Some studies have shown that stroke recurrence risk is significantly increased in children with familial protein C deficiency or increased Lipoprotein (a) levels though it has been shown that children with prothrombotic disorders usually have additional "triggering" risk factors at the time of AIS.[54,55]

D. **Hematologic Disorders:** Around a quarter of patients with sickle cell disease develop cerebrovascular complications that include overt AIS (as part of a thrombotic crisis), subclinical small-vessel occlusive AIS (due to a progressive cerebral vasculopathy), and subarachnoid or intracranial hemorrhage.[56] Sickle cell disease (SCD) is a very common cause of pediatric stroke, occurring in 285 cases per 100,000 affected children.[2] Children less than 2 years of age with sickle cell disease had the lowest CVA incidence, suggesting that there may be a protective mechanism operative in early life or that, in SCD, the pathology responsible for CVA develops over time. However, studies have shown risk of CVA to be higher in the 1 to 9 years of age group than in the 10 to 19 years of age group.[57] This finding suggests that a subset of patients may have additional risk factors for early stroke. Stroke can be ischemic in 15% and hemorrhagic in 25% cases but hemorrhage is rare until teenage years. Stroke is the cause of death in 10% children with sickle cell disease. Anemias, including iron-deficiency anemia[58] may be associated with AIS and was observed in more than 25% children with AIS in one study.[45] Strokes may occur in the absence of pain or aplastic crises.[60] Two-thirds of children with SCD who have had previous strokes but remain untreated will have a recurrence.[61] The exact pathophysiology is not entirely clear, although it likely involves elements of anemia, microvascular occlusion, stasis causing reperfusion injury physiology and endothelial dysfunction.[62]

E. **Moyamoya Disease:** Moyamoya is a chronic, noninflammatory occlusive intracranial vasculopathy of unknown cause and accounts for 10% to 20% of arterial infarcts in children.[59,63] Moyamoya is seen primarily in the Japanese but has been reported in all ethnic groups. Ten percent of cases are familial and a concordance rate of 80% has been reported in monozygotic twins. Moyamoya causes symptoms of transient ischemic attack (TIA), seizures, involuntary movements, and in teenagers and adults, intracranial and subarachnoid hemorrhage. The diagnosis is based on an angiographic finding of bilateral stenosis of the internal carotid and the development of an extensive collateral network with the appearance of a "puff of smoke". It is characterized by progressive idiopathic stenosis and eventual occlusion of the large cerebral arteries involving the circle of Willis. Similar angiographic findings may also be found in a variety of conditions causing slowly progressive occlusive cerebral vasculopathies – the *Moyamoya Syndrome*, e.g., sickle cell disease, post-radiation vasculopathy, Down syndrome, neurofibromatosis, Williams syndrome etc.[1] Moyamoya disease is characterized by recurrent TIAs and strokes, and progressive cognitive decline and motor impairment. The disease usually follows a progressive course though may occasionally remain stable.

F. **Vasculopathies:** Head and neck trauma are at risk of developing an ischemic event subsequent to dissection of the carotid or vertebral arteries. Dissection and other physical injuries are responsible for 8-20% of children with AIS.[64,65] This can result from direct intraoral trauma delivered by a foreign object such as a pencil in the mouth or after tonsillectomy, and can also occur spontaneously.[66] Hyperextension or rotational injuries experienced during minor head trauma, motor vehicle collisions, sports such as wrestling, can also result in strokes. Symptoms of traumatic arterial dissection can be delayed by 24 hours, and the risk is greatest within a few days of the vascular injury. Intraoral trauma (blunt trauma to posterior pharynx specially by fall with popsickle stick or pencil in mouth) and mechanical injuries to neck, may cause a tear in the intima of the vessel wall which may lead to dissection of the carotid or vertebral arteries in the neck or formation of a thrombus at the site.[64] Headache is a common feature seen in upto 75% of the patients. Recurrent TIA or strokes are documented in 8-19% of children with large-vessel dissection and recurrent dissection in other arteries occurs in upto 20% of children with dissection involving the anterior circulation.[64,65]

Postvaricella angiopathy occurs weeks or months after uncomplicated varicella and characteristically manifests as basal ganglia infarction and self-resolving unilateral stenosis of the distal ICA or proximal anterior or middle cerebral arteries. It is reported to account for nearly 1/3rd of childhood AIS.[67] Varicella infection within the past year can result in basal ganglia infarction. HIV infection can cause stroke secondary to HIV-induced vasculitis, vasculopathy with subsequent aneurysms, or hemorrhage due to immune thrombocytopenia.[68,69] More commonly associated organisms include mycoplasma and chlamydia, as well as enterovirus, parvovirus 19, influenza. A, coxsackie, Rocky Mountain spotted fever, or cat scratch disease.[68,70] Five to twelve percent of children with bacterial meningitis, TB meningitis, and viral encephalitis will have a stroke due to local vasculitis and thrombosis. A history of drinking raw milk or visiting a farm may point to a diagnosis of neurobrucellosis.[71] Head and neck infections, such as mastoiditis or periorbital infections, remain important causes of CVT.[3] Post-radiation vasculopathy presents with TIA or strokes several years after irradiation of cerebral tumours in children because of progressive large vessel stenosis, visible on MRI as arterial wall thickening and contrast enhancement. In children with *raised intracranial pressure* due to whatever cause, cerebral arteries at the base of brain, especially posterior cerebral arteries are susceptible to extrinsic mechanical compression and occlusion.

Cerebral vasculitis is a less common cause of stroke in children, and is more common in children older than 14 years of age.[9] Although idiopathic vasculitis is most often diagnosed, signs and symptoms of systemic vasculitides with Kawasaki disease, Henoch-Schönlein Purpura (HSP), polyarteritis nodosa, Takayasu's arteritis, juvenile rheumatoid arthritis, systemic lupus erythematosus, inflammatory bowel disease, sarcoidosis, Sjögren syndrome, or Behcet disease should be considered. Vasculitis involving the CNS vessels in children may be secondary to a variety of disorders (more common) or primary (also called as *isolated angiitis of the CNS – IACNS)*. Stroke is common in children with SLE but vasculitis as the etiology is rare. IACNS is a condition involving any of the large, medium-sized and small vessels with a granulomatous to non-granulomatous, primary lymphocytic process leading to progressive irregular arterial narrowing.[72] The disease is milder in children as compared to adults and is a diagnosis of exclusion. A brain or leptomeningeal biopsy is required for definitive diagnosis. *Transient cerebral arteriopathy* is likely the most common type of arteriopathy in children with AIS and presents angiographically as unilateral irregular stenosis involving the distal part of anterior cerebral artery, the middle cerebral artery, or the posterior cerebral artery. It is likely a focal self-limited vasculitis with average age of onset at 5 years with unilateral infarcts located in the basal ganglia and internal capsule being the typical feature.[1] The lesion stabilizes or regresses within 3-6 months of presentation. The likely pathophysiological mechanism is a transient acute vasculitis induced by a viral infection. If the lesion is preceded by varicella within the last one year, then the condition is labeled as post-varicella angiopathy.

G. **Others:** Although rare, children with Marfan syndrome are at risk of ischemic neurovascular complications.[73] Children with tuberous sclerosis have a higher risk of embolic events, and may also have hemorrhagic strokes secondary to hypertension, hemorrhage into a tumor, or rupture of an abnormal vessel.[41] Homocysteinuria can cause AIS and should be suspected in the presence of mental retardation associated with lens dislocation and occasionally pectus excavatum. Nutritional deficiencies of folic acid or vitamin B_{12} may also cause hyperhomocysteinemia, leading to stroke.[3]

There is an elevated risk for AIS secondary to thrombosis and premature arteriosclerosis, the latter of which is also caused by familial lipoprotein disorders. Stroke due to migraine has been reported commonly in adults but is rare in children. The distribution is usually in the posterior circulation. The diagnosis needs to fulfill strict diagnostic criteria.[74] Thromboembolic manifestations are inherent part of the clinical features of homozygous *homocystinuria,* which includes arterial and venous thrombosis, and these may even be the first manifestation of the disease. However, upto 1/5th of children with AIS have been found to have more subtle forms of hyperhomocysteinemia[26] and may play an important pathogenic role.[1] Hyperhomocystinemia therefore must be considered as a possible risk factor for AIS even in the absence of a vasculopathy.[1] *Fabry's disease,* is a rare X-linked disorder of lipid storage attributable to ceramide trihexosidase deficiency. Endothelial accumulation of sphingoloipid in vessel wall is responsible for cerebrovascular occlusion. *Mitochondrial disorders* include in their phenotype, recurrent and sometimes catastrophic stroke. MELAS (mitochondrial encephalomyopathy, lactic acidosis and stroke) presents in childhood with acute onset neurologic deficit and an elevated serum and/or CSF lactate helps in suspecting the condition.

II. Sinovenous Thrombosis

Septic SVT is the thrombosis of venous sinuses associated with head and neck infections (otitis media, mastoiditis and sinusitis) and is reported to account for only 18% of cases pediatric SVT in Western studies.[5] Data reveal that the incidence of SVT in children is 0.6/100000 children per year and is highest in the first year of life.[75] The clinical presentation of SVT in children is often subtle and approximately 50% present with focal abnormalities or seizures. The majority of thromboses are located within the superior sagittal sinus with or without associated lateral sinus thrombosis. A number of risk factors are linked to the development of SVT, including head and neck infections, dehydration, perinatal complications, and coagulation disorders. In one study, prothrombotic abnormalities were present in half of children with SVT and many of these children had multiple risk factors. Among Indian children it is still an important cause. Risk factors are age-related and in contrast to AIS, risk factors are definable in most of the children. Nearly two-thirds of the children studied in a population-based sample had more than one risk factor. The various factors reported are prothrombotic disorders in 41%, dehydration in 25%, head and neck infections in 18%, other head and neck disorders in 12%, hematologic disorders in 12%; systemic infections, malignancies and cardiac disorders in <10% each.[5] Dehydration is more common as a risk factor in neonates and younger infants, with anemia and cardiac disorders in older infants. Iron deficiency anemia has also been reported as an important cause.[2] In preschoolers with SVT, upto a third may have infection of head and neck whereas in older group chronic systemic diseases (SLE, nephrotic syndrome, inflammatory bowel disease, underlying cardiac disease) are commonly found. In addition, acute illnesses like sepsis and dehydration, and head trauma may be found in many patients. Although nearly half of the infants and children will have involvement of multiple sinuses and veins, thrombosis of the superficial system (superior sagittal sinus and lateral sinus) is present in the majority (86%).[5] In addition to the thrombosis, either bland (in 1/3rd) or hemorrhagic (2/3rd) venous infarcts are present in 41% of these children. *Prothrombotic disorders* have been reported in 20-80% of pediatric patients with SVT, with acquired states being more common. The commonly reported abnormalities are Factor V Leiden, anticardiolipin antibody, elevated lipoprotein (a), activated protein C resistance, and protein C and protein S and antithrombin deficiency.[5]

III. Hemorrhagic Stroke

Hemorrhagic stroke is less common than ischemic stroke in children. Several risk factors for hemorrhagic stroke have been identified in children, including vascular malformations, malignancy and trauma. Hemorrhagic stroke in children is also associated with primary and secondary coagulation disorders including hemophilia, thrombocytopenia, liver failure, leukemia and warfarin therapy.

Arteriovenous malformations (AVM) are the most common cause of hemorrhagic stroke in children. The development of an AVM results from failure in the formation of the capillary bed between primitive arteries and veins in the brain during the first trimester of fetal life. The incidence of AVM in children is 1/100000 and approximately 10% to 20% of all AVMs will become symptomatic during childhood.[76] The average probability of a first hemorrhage is 2% to 4% per year, with a recurrence risk as high as 25% by 5 years.[77] Magnetic resonance (MR) imaging and MRA confirm the diagnosis of AVM. Approximately 1% to 2% of aneurysms become symptomatic during childhood. Aneurysms in children are typically associated with other vascular lesions or chronic disorders. Cavernous malformations can also lead to hemorrhagic stroke in children. One third of cavernous malformations are familial. Cavernous malformations have recently been linked to abnormalities in the long arm of chromosome 7.[78] In a study of 56 children with HS, the underlying causes included arteriovenous malformations in 23, hematologic disorders in 9 and aneurysms in 5. Long-term follow-up showed death directly due to hemorrhage in 25% and 25% having no physical or cognitive deficits at a mean follow-up of ten years.[50] However, amongst Indian children with HS, coagulation abnormalities are responsible for the majority.

Intracerebral hemorrhage: Congenital vascular anomalies are the most common cause and present in 43-62% of patients whereas bleeding diathesis due to inherited or acquired disorders is found in 32% of children.[79] Bleeding from cerebral lesions like brain tumour and arterial or venous infarcts is also an important cause.

Subarachnoid hemorrhage: The principal cause is rupture of an arteriovenous malformation or more commonly an aneurysm. *Head trauma*, accidental or intentional, is the most common cause of intracranial hemorrage in childhood. In infants, unexplained subdural and other intracranial hemorrhage, particularly when bilateral, should raise suspicion of inflicted trauma. An important diagnostic clue is the presence of retinal hemorrhage in upto 75% of children with "shaken baby syndrome".

Vascular malformations are of four types namely arteriovenous malformation, cavernous malformation, venous angiomas and capillary telangiectasias. The last two are very common but rarely cause hemorrhage. Cavernous malformations are dense collection of thin-walled blood vessels and usually remain asymptomatic. Hemorrhage, if it occurs, is rarely life threatening. Arteriovenous malformation results due to failure of formation of the capillary bed between primitive arteries and veins in brain during development and its incidence in children is 1 in 100,000 with approximately 10-20% becoming symptomatic during childhood.[80] Around 80% of patients present with hemorrhage and the recurrence risk is as high as 25% by five years. *Aneurysms* likely arise from a focal congenital weakness of the elastic and muscular layers of the cerebral artery. Rupture commonly occurs in those less than 2 years or above 10 year of age. Aneurysms usually present with acute SAH, frequently associated with intracranial and intraventricular hemorrhage. Acquired aneurysms commonly are due to bacterial endocarditis because of release of infected emboli into cerebral arteries, which seed the adventitia of the cerebral vessel, and the resultant infection and inflammation results in the weakening of the vessel and development of a 'mycotic aneurysm'. Post-traumatic aneurysms are also an important cause said to be under-recognized in children. HS may also occur with tubercular meningitis.

EVALUATION

The evaluation should rule out other nonvascular causes and identify the cause of the stroke (Box 45.2). All conditions presenting with an acute onset neurologic deficit need to be considered in the differential diagnosis of stroke. These include postictal hemiparesis (Todd's paresis), intracranial space occupying lesions that may be infective (abscess, inflammatory granuloma) or non-infective (malignancy) and ADEM. Rare causes are hemiplegic migraine and alternating hemiplegia of childhood.

Box 45.2: Investigations to be Carried Out for Determining Etiology of Stroke*

Neuroimaging

- Computed tomography
- MRI and MRA
- Conventional angiography

Investigations in Ischemic Stroke (in all)

- Full blood counts with ESR
- Hb electrophoresis for sickle cell anemia
- Workup for iron-deficiency anemia
- Protein C and S, Antithrombin III
- Infection screen (if suggestive features)

Ischemic Stroke (Selectively)

- Factor VIII, Factor XII
- Lupus anticoagulant, anticardiolipin antibody
- Factor V Leiden
- Total Homocysteine
- Lipoprotein (a) levels

Contd.

Contd.

Hemorrhagic Stroke
• Platelet counts • Coagulation studies • Angiography
Echocardiography
• Precordial • Transesophageal and bubble contrast
Infarct not Correlating with Typical Vascular Distribution
• Blood and CSF lactate • Plasma ammonia and aminoacids • Urine organic acids
Further Tests – If resources permit
• Serum and CSF antibodies to Varicella Zoster virus • Sleep studies • EEG (unihemispheric slowing in hemiplegic migraine)

*Many other investigations are available and may be carried out depending on the resources available.

The evaluation of stroke in children should also include hematologic, metabolic, and angiographic studies, as recent evidence suggests that the identification of multiple risk factors predicts worse long-term outcome. Risk factors may not be identified in about one third of patients with stroke. Stroke may also be the first presentation of serious underlying disease like congenital heart disease, inherited coagulation abnormalities, SLE etc.

The evaluation should include questions about any history of head or neck trauma, unexplained fever or recent infection, drug ingestion, developmental delay, family history of bleeding problems, and associated headache. A careful family and birth history should also be taken, with special attention to premature vascular disease hematologic disease and mental retardation.

Imaging studies like CT, MRI, MR angiography, that delineates the anatomy of the process, remains the most important tool in the evaluation of stroke. Computed tomography scanning is sreadily available and useful for identifying acute hemorrhage.

CT: Non contrast CT is a sensitive means of detecting ICH, and abnormal CT findings have been identified 6 hours after onset of symptoms from AIS, although CT findings also may be absent at this early stage. Although CVST is sometimes evident on CT, these lesions are more reliably identified with MRI and MRV. In the neonate, the normally occurring high hematocrit can result in increased attenuation of normal cerebral vessels, and this finding can be misinterpreted as a vessel thrombosis. CT of the brain is often normal within the first 12 hours after ischaemic stroke. Bland infarcts are hypodense lesions corresponding to the vascular territory of the affected artery whereas hemorrhagic infarcts have additional hyperdense components. CT is helpful in making the diagnosis of SVT but diagnosis may be missed in 16% of scans[44] in addition to yielding false positive results especially in neonates. Newer CT techniques and CT venography have improved its sensitivity. There is a small but finite incidence of adverse reaction to intravenous administration of contrast agents, and compromised renal function can limit the volume of contrast that can be administered safely.

Several new MR techniques have been used for the evaluation of ischemic stroke in children, including diffusion, perfusion, gradient echo, and FLAIR imaging. MRA is also useful in the evaluation of arteriopathies and computed tomography and MR venography for SVT. MRI is the most versatile and sensitive imaging technique for identifying ischemic brain lesions. MRI is better than CT for evaluation of acute arterial ischemic stroke. This is so because of its sensitivity for detecting early, small, and multiple infarcts,[1] especially in the posterior fossa (where it avoids bone artifacts) and higher sensitivity for detecting hemorrhagic conversion of infarct, that has important treatment implications. Modifications like diffusion-weighted imaging have improved the sensitivity of MRI. Prediction of ischemic tissue that will progress to infarction and detection of microbleeds before intracranial hemorrhage are recently reported features of MRI.[81] *Magnetic resonance angiography* can be performed at the same time as MRI and adequately visualizes the flow in major cerebral arteries at the circle of Willis and extracranial carotid and vertebral arteries at sites prone to dissection. MR spectroscopy uses MR pulse sequences to generate a linear spectrum of metabolite resonances that reflect tissue physiology. Contrast enhanced MRA and higher field (3 Tesla) machines have improved the sensitivity of the technique. Typical MRI sequences require 3 to 5 minutes each to acquire, and assessment for cerebrovascular disease takes from 15 to 35 minutes. The absence of radiation and the ability to visualize both absent flow and the presence of thrombus, clot progression and resolution over time, and associated parenchymal lesions have made MRI the diagnostic study of choice in SVT.[1] Determining the age of the thrombus may also be possible in some cases. MR venography and contrast enhanced MR venography are used to study the cerebral sinovenous system. MR imaging should be considered in the evaluation of children. Ultrasonography may also be useful, as ultrasound can detect abnormal flow patterns in greater than 90% of patients with extracranial arterial dissection. Intracranial MRA or MRV can confirm vessel patency and define the vascular anatomy. Degradation of the MRA signal by turbulent flow may lead to overestimation of pathology; further evaluation with CTA may obviate the need for CA. Functional MR evaluates changes in blood flow with motor or language function, and is useful in monitoring changes in the localization of function over time related to recovery. Recent work with MR spectroscopy demonstrates lactate changes in children with hypoxic ischemia at birth that may be related to prognosis.

Conventional angiography is recommended when MR scanning has failed to identify a cause. Conventional angiography is still the definitive method of visualizing the extra and intracranial vasculature.[1] This is either because MRA does not visualize small or medium sized cerebral arteries reliably and also because specific signs of various CVD may be well defined only with conventional arteriography. Conventional arteriography should therefore be performed in all children with AIS in whom a specific etiology has not been determined; and the rate of major complications with this procedure in children with AIS is rare. For diagnosing SVT, conventional angiography is rarely needed and is used only when other techniques cannot confirm the diagnosis.[1] Lack of filling of cerebral veins or sinuses (either partial or complete) suggests SVT. Conventional angiography should be performed in all older infants and children with intracerebral hemorrhage of unclear origin because >50% will have a definable etiology. Although CA is superior to MRA and CTA for the visualization of tertiary branches and small cerebral arteries, the likelihood of identifying a larger vessel abnormality with CA in the face of a negative MRA is relatively low.

Doppler studies of carotid vessels and transcranial Doppler can assist in detection of large vessel vasculopathy. The risk of future stroke in children with SCD can be predicted based on transcranial Doppler imaging.[82] MR perfusion and SPECT provide information about perfusion of cerebral areas and can be helpful in assessing cerebrovascular reserve in children with severe arterial vasculopathy. In neonates and young infants with an open fontanel, US is helpful in identifying and monitoring the course of SVT. Its short scan time, non-invasiveness and portability may be additional advantages in unstable patients. Recent improvements like "power Doppler" (that measures the energy of moving RBCs instead of velocity and direction of flow) are more sensitive. Echocardiography should be performed in all children with AIS of undetermined cause and use of agitated saline (to establish the presence of PFO) and/or transesophageal echocardiography to increase the sensitivity of testing should be considered.

Ultrasound: Transcranial Doppler can be performed at the bedside and is useful in sickle cell-related stroke. Children with SCD that have a peak mean velocity of greater than 200 cm within the terminal ICA or proximal MCA are at an increased risk for stroke.[83] It requires no sedation and can be performed portably even on unstable infants. Coronal and sagittal views of the supratentorial brain can be achieved rapidly, but imaging of the posterior fossa is more limited in cranial ultrasound. Parenchymal ischemic injury typically appears as areas of increased. However, ultrasound is less sensitive than CT and MRI in the detection of cerebral ischemic lesions. Doppler sonography shows changes in cerebral blood flow velocities in infants with moderate and severe hypoxic ischemic encephalopathy. No deleterious effects have been detected or reported in the use of transcranial ultrasound in infants.[84,85] Cranial ultrasound is useful for interventricular and germinal matrix hemorrhage, but is inadequate for identifying ischemic stroke, particularly cortically based or posterior infarcts. The lack of sensitivity of cranial ultrasound in the detection of cerebral ischemia limits its overall usefulness, however transcranial ultrasound is useful for identification of parenchymal hemorrhage and IVH in neonates and gross anatomic evaluation of the cerebrum alone.

Nuclear Medicine: SPECT uses tomographic acquisition techniques for detecting the radioactive isotope to generate planar and 3-dimensional images. Because of the short half-life and low energy of the compounds used for diagnostic nuclear medicine imaging, the actual radiation dose to any individual child is quite low. Perfusion techniques can be used to quantify relative cerebral blood volume and flow. PET scan data are generated as planar and 3-dimensional images, and fusion techniques can be used to superimpose physiological information acquired with SPECT and PET onto anatomic data acquired with CT or MR. The availability of combined PET-CT scanners allows acquisition of data in a single procedure. Use of these techniques in children has been limited thus far.

MANAGEMENT

Children with stroke require immediate, specialized attention and if possible should be stabilized and transferred to an institution able to provide pediatric neurology and neurosurgical expertise. The treatment and prevention of stroke in children is not well studied, and most recommendations are based on adult studies, non-randomised trials, or expert opinion. The management options are listed in Box 45.3, and details of drugs used for antithrombotic and antiplatelet therapies are provided in Box 45.4.

Box 45.3: Management Options for Pediatric CVD

Treatment

I. Arterial Ischemic Stroke

1. Thrombolytic agents
   - Intravenous and intra-arterial tPA
2. Antithrombotic and antiplatelet therapies
   - Heparin
   - Low molecular weight heparin
   - Warfarin
   - Aspirin
3. Interventional and surgical procedures

II. Cerebral Venous Thrombosis

III. Hemorrhagic Stroke

Prevention

A. Acute Ischemic Stroke

Management of ischemic stroke involve both initial treatment of the acute stroke event to preserve neurological function and long-term efforts to prevent a second stroke, which occurs in 10% to 25% of children with stroke however in children with high-risk conditions such as sickle cell disease and congenital heart disease, efforts to prevent a first stroke also are important. The emergency department management of stroke can be categorized into general supportive measures, diagnostic modalities, and treatment appropriate to the type of stroke identified.

General: Experimental data from animals and clinical data from studies of stroke in adults suggest beneficial effect of aggressive treatment of infection, fever, blood pressure, hypo/hyperglycemia and seizures. This seems to be equally applicable in children. Routine monitoring of BP, blood sugar, temperature and identification and treatment of infections is therefore essential. Efforts should be made to ameliorate increased intracranial pressure (ICP), treat dehydration, and correct anemia. Control of systemic hypertension is recommended, but caution should be used as rapid reduction of blood pressure has been associated with worse neurological outcomes and larger infarcts in adults. The optimum BP level to be aimed for in children after stroke is not known. An alternative end-point is to keep the cerebral perfusion pressure above 40 mm Hg,[86] which is recommended in children with traumatic brain injury, as lower levels are associated with increased mortality. Correction of hypoxemia is appropriate in all children; also it might be even more important to correct hypoxemia in individuals with an ischemic stroke because of the ischemic penumbra concept but oxygen

Box 45.4: Drugs Used for Antithrombotic and Antiplatelet Therapies in Children

Heparin

- Loading dose not recommended in children with AIS
- 28 U/kg/hour in infants (0-1 year), 20 U/kg/hour in young children, 18 U/kg/hour in older children (adult dose)
- During maintenance treatment, the dose must be carefully monitored and adjusted according to the APTT. The target APTT is 60-85 seconds or 1.5 to two times the baseline value
- *Side-effects:* Hemorrhagic conversion, systemic bleeding, thrombocytopenia
- *Contraindication:* Actual or potential hemorrhagic states, thrombocytopenia, HS, advanced renal or hepatic disease

Low-molecular-weight heparin

- More expensive
- Two preparations are available, used subcutaneously in different doses
- *Contraindication/Side-effects:* Same as above

Warfarin

- Initial dose of 0.2 mg/kg. Titrate subsequent doses to INR values of 2-3
- Infants typically require 0.33 mg/kg, older children 0.99 mg/kg
- *Side-effects:* Fatal or non-fatal hemorrhage, Hemorrhagic conversion, warfarin tissue necrosis
- *Contraindication:* Actual or potential hemorrhagic states, HS, recent or planned surgery of the CNS or eye, and lumbar puncture or other diagnostic procedures with potential for uncontrolled bleeding

Aspirin

- 1-5 mg/dl kg/day
- *Contraindication:* Allergy or hypersensitivity to aspirin, active bleeding
- *Side-effects:* GI upset, systemic bleeding, Reye's syndrome
- Thrombolytic agents and drugs that affect platelet function can increase the risk of hemorrhage

Other antiplatelet agents

- Aggrenox, clopidogrel, ticlopidine
- Being used in adult patients. Limited data on their use in children
- Clopidogrel may be used for stroke at dosages of approximately 1 mg/kg/day in children unable to take aspirin

supplementation is not beneficial in individuals who are not hypoxemic as per available evidence. Hyperglycemia has been found to be associated with a poorer clinical outcome in adult patients with stroke[87] and normoglycemia should be aimed for in pediatric patients as well. Animal studies show that seizures exacerbate ischemic brain injury and therefore early use of anticonvulsants after a seizure prevents recurrence and likely minimizes ischemic damage. There is however no evidence for use of prophylactic anticonvulsants. However, anticonvulsants may be considered in children with hemorrhagic strokes and cerebral venous sinus thrombosis (CVST). Induced hypothermia is not recommended.

As per the American Heart Association Stroke Council and the Council on Cardiovascular Disease in the Young guidelines[88] Antithrombotic and antiplatelet therapy is indicated as below:

LMWH and UFH

For acute anticoagulation, LMWHs offer several potential advantages over UFH, including reproducible pharmacokinetics and fewer monitoring tests. On the other hand, effects of LMWHs cannot be completely reversed within minutes with protamine sulfate or fresh-frozen plasma which acts as a potential disadvantage for LMWH where there is need for its rapid reversal and in such situations it is appropriate to use UFH.

Anticoagulation with LMWH is useful for long-term anticoagulation of children with a substantial risk of recurrent cardiac embolism, CVST, and selected hypercoagulable states.

A protocol for the initiation and adjustment of LMWH in children is provided in Table 45.1.

Table 45.1: Protocol for Using LMWH in Children

Preparation	Initial treatment dose	Initial prophylactic dose
Reviparin, body weight-dependent dose, units/kg per 12 hours		
< 5 kg	150	50
> 5 kg	100	30
Enoxaparin, age-dependent dose, mg/kg per 12 hour		
< 2 months old	1.5	0.75
> 2 months old	1.0	0.5
Dalteparin, all-age pediatric dose, units/kg per 24 hours	129 ± 43	95 ± 52
Tinzaparin, age-dependent dose, units/kg		
0 to 2 months old	275	
2 to 12 months old	250	
1 to 5 years old	240	
5 to 10 years old	200	
10 to 16 years old	275	

The administration of LMWH or UFH may be considered in children for upto 1 week after an ischemic stroke pending further evaluation to determine the cause of the stroke. A child is more likely to benefit from anticoagulation is higher than in adults. The likelihood of stroke resulting from CCAD, vasculopathy, unrecognized cardiac disease, or a coagulopathy is relatively higher in children than in older adults. For these reasons, it may be reasonable to initiate LMWH or UFH in children with AIS pending completion of the diagnostic evaluation. Both LMWH and UFH are commonly used for short-term anticoagulation. For anticoagulation lasting weeks or months, the alternatives include LMWH and oral vitamin K antagonists such as warfarin. LMWH can be administered via a subcutaneous catheter that is replaced weekly, further reducing the number of needles required. Warfarin is orally administered and cheaper. LMWH is given to children subcutaneously at doses of 1 mg/kg every 12 hours (or in neonates, 1.5 mg/kg every 12 hours). Anti-factor Xa levels are used to monitor LMWH because the activated partial thromboplastin time does not reflect LMWH activity. The therapeutic range for anti-factor Xa levels is 0.5 to 1.0 U/ml in a sample drawn 4 to 6 hours after the subcutaneous dose.[88] Once an initial therapeutic level is attained, a weekly anti-factor Xa level is usually adequate during hospitalization, with the frequency reduced to every 3 to 4 weeks in stable outpatients receiving long-term LMWH. Because LMWH is cleared renally, its use in patients with renal failure requires close monitoring.

Warfarin

Anticoagulation with warfarin is reasonable for the long-term anticoagulation of children with a substantial risk of recurrent cardiac embolism, CCAD, CVST, or selected hypercoagulable states.[88] The anticoagulant effect of warfarin typically occurs within 36 to 72 hours after administration. Accurate dosing of warfarin may be more difficult in breast-fed infants due to low levels of vitamin K in breast milk. Warfarin is selected for children requiring prolonged anticoagulation, although LMWH by subcutaneous injection is an alternative option.

Information on the effectiveness or optimal dosing of warfarin for the treatment of CVST or AIS in children is sparse. However, most centers aim for a target international normalized ratio of 2.0 to 3.0 on the basis of data from adult studies and studies of pediatric patients with systemic thrombosis. Several studies have provided data on the safety of warfarin use in children with cerebral and noncerebral thromboses. The risk of major hemorrhage is 3.2% per patient-year in children receiving warfarin for mechanical heart valves.[91] However, in children with arterial stroke receiving warfarin, the risk of major hemorrhagic complications has not been established. With long-term use, monitoring for bone demineralization may be worthwhile. The guidelines for warfarin dosing are illustrated in Table 45.2.[92]

Table 45.2: Warfarin Anticoagulation Protocol for Children*[92]

Stage	INR	Action
Day 1	1.0-1.3	0.2 mg/kg orally
Day 2-4	1.1-1.3	Repeat day 1 loading dose
	1.4-1.9	50% of day 1 loading dose
	2.0-3.0	50% of day 1 loading dose
	3.1-3.5	25% of day 1 loading dose
	>3.5	Hold dosing until INR is < 3.5, then restart according to stage III guidelines
Maintenance	1.1-1.4	Increase by 20% of dose
	1.4-1.9	Increase by 10% of dose
	2.0-3.0	No change
	3.1-3.5	Decrease by 10% of dose
	>3.5	Hold dosing until INR is < 3.5, then restart at 20% less than last dose

Role of Aspirin

Aspirin is a reasonable option for the secondary prevention of AIS in children whose infarction is not due to SCD and in children who are not known to have a high risk of recurrent embolism or a severe hypercoagulable disorder. A dose of 3 to 5 mg/kg per day is a reasonable initial aspirin dose for stroke prevention in children. If dose-related side effects occur with this aspirin dose, a dose reduction to 1 to 3 mg/kg may be considered.[88] In children taking aspirin for stroke prevention, it is reasonable to vaccinate for varicella and to administer an annual influenza vaccine in an effort to reduce the risk of Reye's syndrome. It is reasonable to withhold aspirin during influenza and varicella infections. Because of concern about Reye's syndrome, some members of the group recommend that aspirin be discontinued or its dose halved during febrile illness; others favor continuation of aspirin during most febrile illnesses, given both the lack of evidence for Reye's syndrome in this setting and the apparent increased risk of stroke during such illnesses. In children unable to take aspirin, clopidogrel has been used occasionally for stroke at doses of 1 mg/kg per day; in children. However, adequate data on the use of ticlopidine, clopidogrel, or the combination of low-dose aspirin plus extended-release dipyridamole are lacking.

As per the guidelines from The Royal College of Physician, Pediatric Stroke Working Group and the American College of Chest Physicians 2004 on antithrombotic and thrombolytic therapy use of these agents in AIS is recommended.[89,90] ACCP recommends anticoagulation with low-molecular weight (LMW) heparin or unfractionated heparin for 5-7 days and then aspirin (3-5 mg/day) for children with non-sickle cell-related AIS. Those with dissection-related or cardioembolic AIS should receive anticoagulation with heparin for 3-6 months and then switched to aspirin (3-5 mg/day). Low-molecular weight heparins are preferable to heparin in children because of less frequent monitoring required and lack of interactions. Anti-factor Xa levels are used for monitoring and a weekly monitoring is sufficient once therapeutic levels of 0.5-1 U/ml have been achieved. The Royal College of Physicians however recommend that children with non-sickle cell-related AIS should receive aspirin, children with extra-cranial dissection related AIS should receive anticoagulation, and children with cardioembolic AIS should be treated in consultation with a pediatric cardiologist. Warfarin therapy should be considered in children with AIS caused by cardiac disease, arterial dissection, and hypercoagulable states. There is limited information regarding long-term anticoagulation with warfarin for stroke prophylaxis in children. It is recommended that such children avoid activities that carry an especially high risk of injury. Nevertheless, warfarin can be used with reasonable safety for prolonged anticoagulation in children. Children with sickle cell-related AIS should receive emergent exchange transfusion to reduce the hemoglobin S concentration below 30% while not increasing blood volume (which is increased at baseline in patients with SCD). Children with AIS and increasing ICP and neurological worsening should be evaluated for neurosurgical intervention.

Thrombolytic Agents

Tissue plasminogen activator: Although there are many reports of use of intravenous and intrarterial thrombolytic agents for AIS; these drugs are not approved or evaluated in children with stroke. Children with stroke rarely present within six hours of onset of symptoms[93] and also, strokes are a less common cause of acute neurological symptoms in children. Therefore, these agents have limited use in pediatric stroke patient. In general, thrombolytic therapy is not recommended in children. Thrombolytic therapy with tPA may be considered in selected children with CVST. Until there are additional published safety and efficacy data, tPA generally is not recommended for children with AIS outside a clinical trial. However, there was no consensus about the use of tPA in older adolescents who otherwise meet standard adult tPA eligibility criteria.[88]

B. Cerebral Venous Thrombosis

Treatment of CVST includes supportive or symptomatic measures such as hydration, appropriate antimicrobials, control of seizures with anticonvulsants, and control of intracranial pressure. Children with CVST should have a complete blood count. Those with a CVST and a suspected bacterial infection should receive appropriate antibiotics, periodic assessments of the visual fields and visual acuity should be done given the potential for visual loss owing to severe or long-standing increased intracranial pressure in children with CVST, and appropriate measures to control elevated intracranial pressure and its complications should be instituted. Children with CVST may benefit from a thorough thrombophilic screen to identify underlying coagulation defects, some of which could affect the risk of subsequent re-thromboses and influence therapeutic decisions. Monitoring the intracranial pressure may be considered during the acute phase of CVST. It is reasonable to repeat the neuroimaging studies in children with CVST to confirm vessel recanalization or recurrence of the thrombus. Given the frequency of epileptic seizures in children with an acute CVST, continuous electroencephalography monitoring may be considered for individuals who are unconscious and/or mechanically ventilated.

Anticoagulation: Anticoagulation is the specific treatment and has been found to be safe in this group. Guidelines on the management of stroke recommend anti-coagulation with either intravenous UFH or subcutaneous LMWH in children with CVST, whether or not there is secondary hemorrhage, followed by warfarin therapy for 3 to 6 months. In infants and children with local hemorrhage, close clinical and neuroimaging follow-up is recommended, and anticoagulation should be considered in cases with evidence of thrombus extension.

Thrombolytic Agents. Due to lack of sufficient evidence, thrombolytic therapy is not considered as first-line treatment. In selected children with CVST, the administration of a thrombolytic agent may be considered. It may be considered for children with CVT who progressively worsen despite adequate anticoagulation.[94]

C. Hemorrhagic Stroke

Children with nontraumatic brain hemorrhage should undergo a thorough risk factor evaluation, including standard cerebral angiography. Children with a severe coagulation factor deficiency should receive appropriate factor replacement therapy, and children with less severe factor deficiency should receive factor replacement after trauma. Congenital vascular anomalies should be identified and corrected whenever it is clinically feasible. Stabilizing measures in patients with brain hemorrhage should include optimizing the respiratory effort, controlling systemic hypertension, controlling epileptic seizures, and managing increased intracranial pressure. It is reasonable to follow up asymptomatic individuals who have a condition that predisposes them to intracranial aneurysms with a cranial MRA every 1 to 5 years, depending on the perceived level of risk posed by an underlying condition. If the patient develop symptoms that could be explained by an aneurysm, CTA or CA may be considered even if the patient's MRA fails to show evidence of an aneurysm. Surgical management is the specific therapy for majority of children with HS. Surgical removal of larger lobar hemorrhages is recommended in children who are clinically worsening.[95] Complete surgical excision of AVMs should be aimed for and is possible in 70-90% children. Embolization and/or radiosurgery are other treatment options. Individuals with SAH may benefit from measures to control cerebral vasospasm Surgical evacuation of a supratentorial intracerebral hematoma is not recommended for most. However, information from small numbers of patients suggests that surgery may help selected individuals with developing brain herniation or extremely elevated intracranial pressure. Although there is strong evidence to support the use of periodic blood transfusions in individuals with SCD who are at high risk for ischemic infarction, there are no data to indicate that periodic transfusions reduce the risk of ICH caused by SCD.[88]

Preventive

Chronic transfusion therapy to maintain HbS levels below

30% is indicated in children with SCD and intracranial stenosis, as evidenced by abnormally increased transcranial Doppler velocity.[96] This should not be stopped in children younger than 16 years.

Acute management of ischemic stroke resulting from SCD should include optimal hydration, correction of hypoxemia, and correction of systemic hypotension. Periodic transfusions to reduce the percentage of sickle hemoglobin are effective for reducing the risk of stroke in children 2 to 16 years of age. Children with SCD and a confirmed cerebral infarction should be placed on a regular program of red cell transfusion in conjunction with measures to prevent iron overload. Reducing the percentage of sickle hemoglobin with transfusions before performing CA is indicated in an individual with SCD. For acute cerebral infarction, exchange transfusion designed to reduce sickle hemoglobin to < 30% total hemoglobin is reasonable. Hydroxyurea may be considered in children and young adults with SCD and stroke who cannot continue on long-term transfusion. Bone marrow transplantation may be considered for children with SCD. Surgical revascularization procedures may be considered as a last resort in children with SCD who continue to have cerebrovascular dysfunction despite optimal medical management.[88]

Different revascularization techniques are useful to effectively reduce the risk of stroke resulting from moyamoya disease. Indirect revascularization techniques are generally preferable and should be used in younger children whose small-caliber vessels make direct anastomosis difficult, whereas direct bypass techniques are preferable in older individuals. Revascularization surgery is useful for moyamoya. Indications for revascularization surgery include progressive ischemic symptoms or evidence of inadequate blood flow or cerebral perfusion reserve in an individual without a contraindication to surgery. Aspirin may be considered in individuals with moyamoya after revascularization surgery or in asymptomatic individuals for whom surgery is not anticipated.

Prognosis

Mortality after stroke depends on the cause, location of the lesion and varies from 20-30%. Hemorrhagic stroke has higher mortality than ischemic stroke. Residual neurologic deficit, most commonly minimal to mild residual hemiplegia is most common deficit in survivors. Speech involvement is common if dominant side is involved. Seizures are not uncommonly seen.

Further studies are needed to evaluate secondary prevention strategies in children with stroke as a significant number go on to have a recurrence. Further evidence also needs to be generated for management of CVT and HS in children. Data on incidence, prevalence and outcome amongst Indian children with CVD is awaited.

Screening Relatives of Children with Stroke. Many thrombophilias are familial. When a child with stroke is found to have a thrombophilic condition, other family members may harbor the same condition and be at risk for early pathological thrombosis. Children with perinatal stroke who do not have a thrombophilic condition may still have affected mothers; perinatal stroke in the neonate has been associated with prothrombotic conditions in both fetus and the mother.[97,98]

Thrombophilia screening may be offered to family members of children with ischemic stroke or CVST and known thrombophilic defects. It is reasonable to counsel family members about the risks and benefits of this screening. Thrombophilia screening may be offered to the mothers of children with ischemic stroke that occurred before, during, or immediately after birth even if thrombophilia screening in the neonate is negative.

Strokes in children are being recognized more frequently as diagnostic aids develop and clinician recognition improves. However, because the incidence is still low relative to adult strokes, and children are distinctly different from adults, it remains a challenge to create evidence based diagnostic and treatment guidelines. Due to the low incidence of this disease, future stroke research needs to be pursued with a collaborative effort both nationally and internationally.

References

1. De Veber GA. Cerebrovascular Disease in Children. In: Swaiman KF, Ashwal S, Ferriero DM (eds), Paediatric Neurology – Principles and Practice. Mosby Publishers, St Louis Philadelphia, Fourth Edition 2006:1759.
2. CJ Earley, SJ Kittner, BR Feeser *et al*. "Stroke in Children and Sickle-cell Disease: Baltimore-Washington Cooperative Young Stroke Study", Neurology, Vol. 51, No. 1, 1998:169-76.
3. KS Carvalho and BP Garg. "Arterial Strokes in Children", Neurologic Clinics, Vol. 20, No. 4, 2002:1079-1100.
4. S Lanthier, L Carmant, M David, A Larbrisseau and G deVeber. "Stroke in Children: The Coexistence of Multiple Risk Factors Predicts Poor Outcome", Neurology Vol. 54, No. 2, 2000:371-78.
5. AR Riela and ES Roach. "Etiology of Stroke in Children", Journal of Child Neurology Vol. 8, No. 3, 1993:201-20.

6. GA DeVeber, D MacGregor, R Curtis and S Mayank. "Neurologic Outcome in Survivors of Childhood Arterial Ischemic Stroke and Sinovenous Thrombosis". Journal of Child Neurology Vol. 15, No. 5, 2000:316-24.

7. G DeVeber. "In Pursuit of Evidence-based Treatments for Paediatric Stroke: The UK and Chest Guidelines". The Lancet Neurology Vol. 4, No. 7, 2005:432-36.

8. B Chung and V Wong. "Pediatric Stroke Among Hong Kong Chinese Subjects". Pediatrics, Vol. 114, No. 2, 2004:e206-e212.

9. BS Schoenberg, JF Mellinger and DG Schoenberg. "Cerebrovascular Disease in Infants and Children: A Study of Incidence, Clinical Features and Survival". Neurology Vol. 28, No. 8, 1978:763-68.

10. J Broderick, GT Talbot, E Prenger, A Leach and T Brott. "Stroke in Children within A Major Metropolitan Area: The Surprising Importance of Intracerebral Hemorrhage". Journal of Child Neurology Vol. 8, No. 3, 1993:250-55.

11. O Eeg-Olofsson and Y Ringheim. "Stroke in Children, Clinical Characteristics and Prognosis". Acta Paediatrica Scandinavica Vol. 72, No. 3, 1983:391-95.

12. JK Lynch, DG Hirtz, G DeVeber and KB Nelson. "Report of The National Institute of Neurological Disorders and Stroke Workshop on Perinatal and Childhood Stroke". Pediatrics, Vol. 109, No. 1, 2002;116-23.

13. JK Lynch. "Cerebrovascular Disorders in Children". Current Neurology and Neuroscience Reports, Vol. 4, No. 2, 2004; 129-38.

14. M Giroud, M Lemesle, JB Gouyon, JL Nivelon, C Milan and R Dumas. "Cerebrovascular Disease in Children Under 16 Years of Age in The City of Dijon, France: A Study of Incidence and Clinical Features from 1985 to 1993". Journal of Clinical Epidemiology Vol. 48, No. 11, 1995;1343-48.

15. DB Zahuranec, DL Brown, LD Lisabeth and L B Morgenstern. "Is It Time for A Large, Collaborative Study of Pediatric Stroke?" Stroke, Vol. 36, No. 9, 2005;1825-29.

16. HJ Fullerton, YW Wu, S Zhao and SC Johnston. "Risk of Stroke in Children: Ethnic and Gender Disparities", Neurology, Vol. 61, No. 2, 2003;189-94.

17. KPJ Braun, LJ Kappelle, FJ Kirkham and G DeVeber. "Diagnostic Pitfalls in Paediatric Ischaemic Stroke", Developmental Medicine and Child Neurology, Vol. 48, No. 12, 2006;985-90.

18. LV Gabis, R Yangala and NJ Lenn. "Time Lag to Diagnosis of Stroke in Children", Pediatrics, Vol. 110, No. 5, 2002;924-28.

19. G DeVeber, ES Roach, AR Riela and M Wiznitzer. "Stroke in Children: Recognition, Treatment and Future Directions", Seminars in Pediatric Neurology, Vol. 7, No. 4, 2000:309-17.

20. de Veber G, Andrew M, Canadian Pediatric Ischemic Stroke Study Group, Cerebral Sinovenous Thrombosis in Children. N Engl J Med 2001;345:417.

21. S Satoh, R Shirane and T Yoshimoto. "Clinical Survey of Ischemic Cerebrovascular Disease in Children in a District of Japan". Stroke, Vol. 22, No. 5, 1991;586-89.

22. D Nagaraja, A Verma, AB Taly, MV Kumar and PN Jayakumar. "Cerebrovascular Disease in Children". Acta Neurologica Scandinavica, Vol. 90, No. 4, 1994:251-55.

23. W Zenz, Z Bodo, J Plotho *et al.* "Factor V Leiden and Prothrombin Gene G 20210 A Variant in Children with Ischemic Stroke". Thrombosis and Haemostasis, Vol. 80, No. 5, 1998:763-66.

24. A Dusser, F Goutieres and J Aicardi. "Ischemic Strokes in Children". Journal of Child Neurology Vol. 1, No. 2, 1986: 131-36.

25. DP Younkin. "Diagnosis and Treatment of Ischemic Pediatric Stroke", Current Neurology and Neuroscience Reports, Vol. 2, No. 1, 2002:18-24.

26. V Ganesan, M Prengler, MA McShane, AM Wade and FJ Kirkham. "Investigation of Risk Factors in Children with Arterial Ischemic Stroke". Annals of Neurology, Vol. 53, No. 2, 2003:167-73.

27. H Bouza, M Rutherford, D Acolet, JM Pennock and LMS Dubowitz. "Evolution of Early Hemiplegic Signs in Fullterm Infants with Unilateral Brain Lesions in the Neonatal Period: A Prospective Study", Neuropediatrics, Vol. 25, No. 4, 1994; 201-07.

28. AD Meyer-Heim and E Boltshauser. "Spontaneous Intracranial Haemorrhage in Children: Aetiology, Presentation and Outcome", Brain and Development, Vol. 25, No. 6, 2003; 416-21.

29. CS Lin, J Tsai, P Woo and H Chang "Prehospital Delay and Emergency Department Management of Ischemic Stroke Patients in Taiwan, ROC", Prehospital Emergency Care, Vol. 3, No. 3, 1999;194-200.

30. A Al-Jarallah, MT Al-Rifai, AR Riela and ES Roach. "Nontraumatic Brain Hemorrhage in Children: Etiology and Presentation," Journal of Child Neurology, Vol. 15, No. 5, 2000;284-89.

31. BJP Delsing, CE Catsman-Berrevoets and IM Appel. "Early Prognostic Indicators of Outcome in Ischemic Childhood Stroke", Pediatric Neurology, Vol. 24, No. 4, 2001;283-89.

32. FJ Kirkham. "Stroke in Childhood", Archives of Disease in Childhood, Vol. 81, No. 1, 1999;85-89.

33. KS Carvalho, JB Bodensteiner, PJ Connolly and BP Garg. "Cerebral Venous Thrombosis in Children", Journal of Child Neurology, Vol. 16, No. 8, 2001;574-80.

34. TF Barron, DA Gusnard, RA Zimmerman and RR Clancy. "Cerebral Venous Thrombosis in Neonates and Children", Pediatric Neurology, Vol. 8, No. 2, 1992;112-116.

35. WK Imai, FR Everhart Jr. and JM Sanders Jr. "Cerebral Venous Sinus Thrombosis: Report of A Case and Review of the Literature", Pediatrics, Vol. 70, No. 6, 1982;965-70.

36. MI Shevell, K Silver, AM O'Gorman, GV Watters and JL Montes. "Neonatal Dural Sinus Thrombosis," Pediatric Neurology Vol. 5, No. 3, 1989;161-65.

37. K Calder, P Kokorowski, T Tran and S Henderson. "Emergency Department Presentation of Pediatric Stroke", Pediatric Emergency Care Vol. 19, No. 5, 2003;320-28.

38. V Ganesan, A Hogan, N Shack, A Gordon, E Isaacs and FJ Kirkham. "Outcome After Ischaemic Stroke in Childhood", Developmental Medicine and Child Neurology, Vol. 42, No. 7, 2000:455-61. Trescher WH. Ischemic Stroke Syndromes in Childhood, Pediatr Ann 1992:21:374.

39. AP Gold and S Carter. "Acute Hemiplegia of Infancy and Childhood", Pediatric Clinics of North America, Vol. 23, No. 3,1976:413-33.

40. S Sen and S Oppenheimer. "Bedside Assessment of Stroke and Stroke Mimics", Annals of Indian Academy of Neurology, Vol. 11, No. 5, 2008;S4–S11.

41. Meyer-Heim AD, Boltshauser E. Spontaneous Intracranial Haemorrhage in Children: Aetiology, Presentation and Outcome, Brain Dev 2003:25:416-21.

42. Jones BV, Ball WS, Tomsick TA, Millard J, Crone KR. Vein of Galen Aneurysmal Malformation: Diagnosis and Treatment of 13 Children with Extended Clinical Follow-up, AJNR Am J Neuroradiol 2002:23:1717-24.

43. Kerr LM, Anderson DM, Thompson JA, *et al.* Ischaemic Stroke in the Young: Evaluation and Age Comparison. J Child Neuro 1993;8:266.

44. De Veber G. Canadian Pediatric Ischemic Stroke Study Group, Canadian Pediatric Ischemic Stroke Registry: Analysis of Children with AIS., Ann Neurol 2000:48:526.

45. Ganesan V, Prengler M, McShane MA, *et al.* Investigation of Risk Factors in Children with AIS, Ann Neuro 2003;53:167.

46. Chabrier S, Husson B, Lasjaunias P, *et al.* Stroke in Childhood: Outcome and Recurrence Risk by Mechanism in 59 Patients, J Child Neuro 2000;15:290.

47. Mas JL, Arquizan C, Lamy C, *et al.* Recurrent Cerebrovascular Events Associated with Patent Foramen Ovale, Atrial Septal Aneurysm, or Both, N Engl J Med 2001;345:1740.

48. Palm, Frederick, Christian Urbanek and Armin Grau. "Infection, Its Treatment and the Risk for Stroke". Current Vascular Pharmacology 7.2, 2009:146-52.

49. Lindsberg Perttu J and Armin J Grau. "Inflammation and Infections as Risk Factors for Ischemic Stroke". Stroke 34.10, 2003;2518-32.

50. Gulati S, Kalra V, Seth R, Seth V. Neurotuberculosis: Clinical Manifestations, Diagnosis and Management. Seth V, Kabra V (eds) Essentials of Tuberculosis in Children, III Edition, Jaypee Brothers Medical Publishers, New Delhi, 2006.

51. Chan AKC. "Prothrombotic Disorders and Ischemic Stroke in Children", Seminars in Pediatric Neurology, Vol. 7, No. 4, WB Saunders, 2000.

52. Bonduel M, Sciuccati G, Hepner M, *et al.* Prothrombotic Disorders in Children with Arterial Ischemic Stroke and Sinovenous Thrombosis, Arch Neurol 1999:56:967.

53. Nowak-Göttl, Ulrike, *et al.* "Lipoprotein (a) and Genetic Polymorphisms of Clotting Factor V, Prothrombin and Methylenetetrahydrofolate Reductase are Risk Factors of Spontaneous Ischemic Stroke in Childhood", Blood 94.11, 1999:3678-82.

54. Strater R, Becker S, von Eckardestein A, *et al.* Prospective Assessment of Risk Factors for Recurrent Stroke During Childhood–A 5-year Follow-up Study, Lancet 2002:360:1540.

55. Barreirinho S, Ferro A, Santos M, *et al.* Inherited and Acquired Risk Factors and their Combined Effect in Pediatric Stroke, Pediatr Neurol 2003:28:134.

56. Pegelow CH. Stroke in Children with Sickle Cell Anemia: Etiology and Treatment, Paediatr Drugs 2001:3:421.

57. Ohene-Frempong, Kwaku, *et al.* "Cerebrovascular Accidents in Sickle Cell Disease: Rates and Risk Factors" Blood 91.1, 1998:288-94.

58. Hartfield DS, Lowry NJ, Keene DL, *et al.* Iron deficiency: A Cause of Stroke in Infants and Children, Pediatr Neurol 1997;16:50.

59. Jayakumar PN, Arya BY, Vasudev MK, Angiographic Profile in Childhood Moyamoya Disease, A Study of 8 Caucasian Indian Children, Actav Radiol 1991:32:488.

60. LE Walsh and BP Garg, "Ischemic Strokes in Children", Indian Journal of Pediatrics Vol. 64, No. 5, 1997;613-23.

61. B Balkaran, G Ghar, JS Morris, PW Thomas, BE Serjeant and GR Serjeant "Stroke in a Cohort of Patients with Homozygous Sickle Cell Disease", Journal of Pediatrics Vol. 120, No. 3, 1992;360-66.

62. GJ Kato, RP Hebbel, MH Steinberg and MT Gladwin, "Vasculopathy in Sickle Cell Disease: Biology, Pathophysiology, Genetics, Translational Medicine and New Research Directions", American Journal of Hematology Vol. 84, No. 9, 2009;618-25.

63. Lynch, John Kylan, *et al.* "Report of the National Institute of Neurological Disorders and Stroke Workshop on Perinatal and Childhood Stroke." Pediatrics109.1, 2002:116-23.

64. Chabrier S, Lasjaunias P, Husson B, *et al.* Ischemic Stroke from Dissection of Craniocervical Arteries in Childhood: Report of 12 Patients. Eur J Paediatr Neurol 2003;7:39.

65. Fullerton HJ, Johnston SC, Smith WS. Arterial Dissection and Stroke in Children, Neurology 2001:57:1155.

66. Borges L Bonilha, SF Santos *et al.* "Thrombosis of the Internal Carotid Artery Secondary to Soft Palate Injury in Children and Childhood: Report of Two Cases", Pediatric Neurosurgery, Vol. 32, No. 3, 2000;150-53.

67. Askalan R, Laughlin S, Mayank S, *et al.* Chicken Pox and Stroke in Childhood: A Study of Frequency and Causation, Stroke 2001:32:1257.

68. YD Park, AL Belman, TS Kim *et al.* "Stroke in Pediatric Acquired Immunodeficiency Syndrome", Annals of Neurology Vol. 28, No. 3, 1990;303-11.

69. DM Moriarty, JO Haller, JP Loh and S Fikrig. "Cerebral Infarction in Pediatric Acquired Immunodeficiency Syndrome", Pediatric Radiology Vol. 24, No. 8, 1994;611-12.

70. JS Hutchison, R Ichord, AM Guerguerian and G DeVeber. "Cerebrovascular Disorders", Seminars in Pediatric Neurology Vol. 11, No. 2, 2004;139-46.

71. MAM Salih, AGM Abdel-Gader, AA Al-Jarallah *et al.* "Infectious and Inflammatory Disorders of the Circulatory

System as Risk Factors for Stroke in Saudi Children". Saudi Medical Journal Vol. 27. Supplement 1. 2006:S41-S52.

72. Lanthier S. Lortie A. Michaud J. *et al.* Isolated Angiitis of the CNS in Children. Neurology 2002:56:837.

73. RJ Wityk. C Zanferrari and S Oppenheimer. "Neurovascular Complications of Marfan Syndrome: A Retrospective. Hospital-based Study". Stroke Vol. 33. No. 3. 680-84.

74. Headache Classification Subcommittee of the International Headache Society (IHS). The International Classification of Headache Disorders. 2nd Edition. Cephalalgia 2004:24 suppl 1:1-160.

75. deVeber G. Andrew M. Cerebral Sinovenous Thrombosis in Children N Engl J Med 2001:345:417-23.

76. Menovsky T. van Overbeeke JJ. Cerebral Arteriovenous Malformations in Childhood: State of the Art with Special Reference to Treatment, Eur J Pediatr 1997:156:741-46.

77. Fults D. Kelly DLJ. Natural History of Arteriovenous Malformations of the Brain: A Clinical Study. Neurosurgery 1984:15:658-62.

78. Sahoo T. Johnson EW. Thomas JW. *et al.* Mutations in the Gene Encoding KRIT1. a Krev-1/rap1a Binding Protein. Cause Cerebral Cavernous Malformations (CCM1). Hum Mol Genet 1999:8:2325-33.

79. Al Jarallah A. Al Rifai MT. Riela AR. *et al.* Nontraumatic Brain Hemorrhage in Children: Etiology and Presentation. J Child Neurol 2000:15:284.

80. Menovsky T. van Overbecke JJ. Cerebral Arteriovenous Malformation in Childhood: State of the Art with Special Reference to Treatment. Eur J Pediatr 1997;156:741.

81. Schlaug G, Benfield A, Baird AE, *et al.* The Ischemic Penumbra: Operationally Defined by Diffusion and Perfusion MRI. Neurology 1999;53:1528.

82. Abboud MR. Cure J. Granger S. *et al.* MRA in Children with Sickle Cell Disease and Abnormal Transcranial Doppler USG Findings Enrolled in the STOP Study. Blood 2004;103:2822.

83. Adams RJ. McKie VC. Carl EM. *et al.* Long-term Stroke Risk in Children with Sickle Cell Disease Screened with Transcranial Doppler. Ann Neurol 1997;42:699-704.

84. Childs AM. Cornette L. Ramenghi LA. Tanner SF. Arthur RJ. Martinez D. Levene MI. Magnetic Resonance and Cranial Ultrasound Characteristics of Periventricular White Matter Abnormalities in Newborn Infants. Clin Radiol 2001:56: 647-55.

85. Ilves P. Talvik R. Talvik T. Changes in Doppler Ultrasonography in Asphyxiated Term Infants with Hypoxic-ischaemic Encephalopathy. Acta Paediatr 1998;87:680-84.

86. Adelson PD. Bratton SL. Carney NA. *et al.* Guidelines for the Acute Medical Management of Severe Traumatic Brain Injury in Infants. Children and Adolescents. Cerebral Perfusion Pressure. Pediatr Crit Care Med 2003:4:S31.

87. Capes Se. Hunt D. Malmberg K. *et al.* Stress Hyperglycemia and Prognosis of Stroke in Non-diabetic and Diabetic Patients: A Systematic Overview. Stroke 2001:32:2426.

88. Roach. E Steve. *et al.* "Management of Stroke in Infants and Children a Scientific Statement from a Special Writing Group of the American Heart Association Stroke Council and the Council on Cardiovascular Disease in the Young". Stroke 39.9. 2008:2644-91.

89. Pediatric Stroke Working Group. Stroke in Childhood: Clinical Guidelines for Diagnosis. Management and Rehabilitation. London: Royal College of Physicians of London; 2004.

90. Monagle P. Chan A. Massicotte P. *et al.* Antithrombotic Therapy in Children: The Seventh ACCP Conference on Antithrombotic and Thrombolytic Therapy. Chest 2004:126:645S.

91. Massicotte P. Adams M. Marzinotto V. Brooker LA. Andrew M. Lowmolecular-weight Heparin in Pediatric Patients with Thrombotic Disease: A Dose Finding Study. J Pediatr 1996:128:313-18.

92. Michelson AD. Bovill E. Andrew M. Antithrombotic Therapy in Children. Chest 1995;108(suppl):506S-22S.

93. Gabis LV. Yangala R. Lenn NJ. Time Lag to Diagnosis of Stroke in Children. Pediatrics 2002;110:924.

94. Shroff M. deVeber G. Sinovenous Thrombosis in Children. Neuroimaging Clin N Am 2003;13:115.

95. Broderick JP. Adams HP. Barsan W. *et al.* Guidelines for the Management of Spontaneous Intracerebral Hemorrhage. Stroke 1999;30:905.

96. Adams RJ. McKie VC. Hsu L. *et al.* Prevention of A First Stroke by Transfusions in Children with Sickle Cell Anemia and Abnormal Results on Transcranial Doppler Ultrasonography. New Engl J Med 1998;339:5.

97. Golomb MR. The Contribution of Prothrombotic Disorders to peri- and Neonatal Ischemic Stroke. Semin Thromb Hemost 2003;29:415-24.

98. Curry CJ. Bhullar S. Holmes J. Delozier CD. Roeder ER. Hutchison HT. Risk Factors for Perinatal Arterial Stroke: A Study of 60. Mother-Child Pairs. Pediatr Neurol 2007:37: 99-107.

46 Chapter

NEUROCUTANEOUS SYNDROMES

Sharmila B Mukherjee, Satinder Aneja

Neurocutaneous syndromes are a heterogeneous group of unrelated disorders except for the common characteristic of predominant involvement of the nervous system and skin. Its nomenclature has been constantly changing with evolution of scientific knowledge. The term 'phakomatosis' had its origin from the Greek word 'phakos' (lens) due to the retinal hamartomas found in Tuberous Sclerosis Complex (TSC) that were considered pre-malignant. It was replaced by 'Neurocutaneous syndromes' when the repertoire of disorders expanded and it was recognized that all lesions were not potentially malignant. Initially believed to be due to maldevelopment of neuro-epidermal cells with abnormal patterns of cell migration, it is now thought that each disorder originates from the neural crest. Thus, the latest name started to being used is 'Neurocristopathies'.

Given the diversity of disorders included in this group there is considerable variability in many aspects; presentation, inheritance (sporadic, mendelian, unknown), age of onset (infancy, childhood, adolescence, adulthood or geriatric), clinical manifestations (primary or associated lesions), natural course of disease (indolent to rapidly progressive) and prognosis (good to fatal). There is no established classification system being used. In this chapter we will discuss the clinical approach followed by a brief description of the more common conditions seen in children.

Clinical Approach

The approach varies according to the clinical situation. The establishment of diagnosis begins with visual recognition of skin lesions or other associated clinical stigmata, further clinical exploration of the phenotype, substantiation with relevant investigations, application of diagnostic criteria (wherever available) and genetic confirmation (if known). If a neurocutaneous disorder is suspected based on a pathognomic clinical clue detected on preliminary evaluation, history and examination can be tailored according to the suspected individual disorder. If clinical clues are common to multiple conditions (i.e., café-au-lait macules) the evaluation should be aimed at arriving at the most suitable diagnosis. If the child has a nervous system disorder and a neurocutaneous etiology needs to be ruled out, a systematic evaluation will be required to detect clinical findings that may be suggestive. The clinician must actively look for the following manifestations related to the nervous system involvement, skin lesions, eye and associated comorbidities.

(1) The central nervous system can be affected directly or indirectly due to the presence of cerebrovascular lesions (Table 46.1). Common presentations are seizures (epilepsy), age inappropriate development and behavior (Global developmental delay, Autism spectrum disorder), scholastic underperformance (Intellectual disability, epilepsy, effect of anti-convulsants) and neurological impairment (ataxia, stroke).

Table 46.1: Various Cerebrovascular Lesions Seen in Neurocutaneous Disorders

Cerebrovascular lesion	Neurocutaneous disease
Venous malformation	Blue rubber bleb nevus syndrome
Premature atherosclerosis	Cerebrotendinous xanthomatosis
Aneurysm	Ehlers-Danlos disease
Vasculopathy	Menkes kinky hair disease
Angiomas	Sturge-Weber disease
Arterial and venous thrombosis	Homocystinuria
Moya-moya disease	Neurofibromatosis I
Cerebral infarction	Fabry's disease

(2) Peripheral neuropathy is seen in a few disorders including Neurofibromatosis (NF) 1 and 2, Ataxia-telangiectasia and Fabry's disease. These can manifest as sensory, autonomic and motor manifestations, palpable nerves, carpal tunnel syndrome or sensorineural deafness.

(3) Skin lesions are always present which includes abnormalities of the skin appendages (blood vessels, hair). Examples of these are given in Tables 46.2 and 46.3. Some of these are very obvious and may cause cosmetic disfigurement. Others may be subtle and actively looked for. The parents may not consider certain lesions significant enough to be commented upon or pointed out (even on asking), especially if there are similarly affected family members.

Table 46.2: Various Skin Lesions Seen in Neurocutaneous Disorders

Type of lesion	Neurocutaneous disorder
Hypopigmented	Tuberous Sclerosis Complex, Hypomelanosis of Ito, Xeroderma pigmentosum, Chediak Higashi syndrome
Hyperpigmented	Neurofibromatosis I, Epidermal Nevus syndrome, Incontinentia pigmenti, Basal cell nevus syndrome, Neurocutaneous melanosis
Skin tumours	Epidermal Nevus syndrome, Neurofibromatosis 1 and 2, Tuberous Sclerosis Complex, Fabry's disease
Vascular	Sturge-Weber syndrome, Ataxia-telangiectasia, Blue rubber bleb nevus syndrome, Neurocutaneous angiomatosis, Xeroderma pigmentosum
Hyperkeratotic	Refsum disease, Sjögren Larsson disease
Rashes	Incontinentia pigmenti, Xeroderma pigmentosum
Skin laxity	Ehlers-Danlos syndrome, Pseudoxanthoma elasticum

Table 46.3: Hair Abnormalities Seen in Neurocutaneous Disorders

Abnormal growth	Alopecia: Multiple Carboxylase deficiency, Incontinentia pigmenti, Hypomelanosis of Ito Hypertrichosis: Ataxia-telangiectasia
Abnormal texture	Friable and thin: Adrenoleukodystrophy Kinky: Menkes disease, Giant axonal neuronopathy, Epidermal Nevus syndrome
Abnormal color	Poliosis (white): Tuberous Sclerosis Complex Silvery: Chediak Higashi syndrome Hypopigmented: Incontinentia pigmenti, Homocystinuria, Hypomelanosis of Ito

(4) **Ocular manifestations:** Recognition of characteristic eye lesions is critical since most conditions affect the eye and can lead to serious morbidity. These include structural abnormalities of various components (orbit, lids, conjunctiva, sclera, anterior segment, media, choroid, retina, optic nerve), glaucoma and dysfunction (strabismus, nystagmus) resulting in considerable functional impairment.

(5) Miscellaneous systematic involvement is disease specific and must be actively looked for. The cardiovascular and gastrointestinal systems are commonly involved. Cardiac manifestations include arrhythmias (Refsum disease, TSC), cardiomyopathy (Fabry's disease, Pseudoxanthoma elasticum), mitral valve prolapse (Pseudoxanthoma elasticum) and cardiac rhabdomyoma (TSC). Gastrointestinal manifestations are bleeding (Blue rubber bleb nevus syndrome, Pseudoxanthoma elasticum), sigmoid polyp (TSC) and chronic diarrhea (cerebrotendinous xanthomatosis).

Another important aspect to delve into is the family history. Most of the conditions are hereditary and constructing a third degree family tree may suggest the mode of inheritance if it is Mendelian. TSC and NF are autosomal dominant. Ataxia-telangiectasia, Chediak Higashi syndrome, Cockayne syndrome are autosomal recessive. Fabry's disease, Menkes kinky hair disease and Incontinentia pigmenti are X-linked recessive. Some disorders have a variable phenotype caused by the same gene (due to variable penetrance and expressivity) while different genes can cause the same clinical phenotype (genetic heterogeneity).

The clinical information derived from a detailed history and examination should be synthesized to arrive at a clinical diagnosis. Once this is done investigations should be planned to detect associated medical conditions. In quite a few conditions like TSC and NF international expert groups have laid down diagnostic criteria that make establishment of the diagnosis easier. A schematic representation related to the clinical approach in Neurofibromatosis is given in Figure 46.1. Counseling of the patient and family involves explaining the nature, natural course and prognosis of the disease as well as planning of further management and follow-up. Recent advances in genetic testing have lead to the discovery of mutations in many of the disorders that help in genetic counseling and reproductive options.

NEUROFIBROMATOSIS

Neurofibromatosis (NF) is a group autosomal dominant disorders that have protean manifestations but share the presence of multiple tumors of the peripheral and central nervous system. Eight types of NF have been described in literature, each caused by mutations of different genes. This section focuses on the two commonly known ones; NF 1 (peripheral NF or von Recklinghausen disease) and NF 2 (central NF).

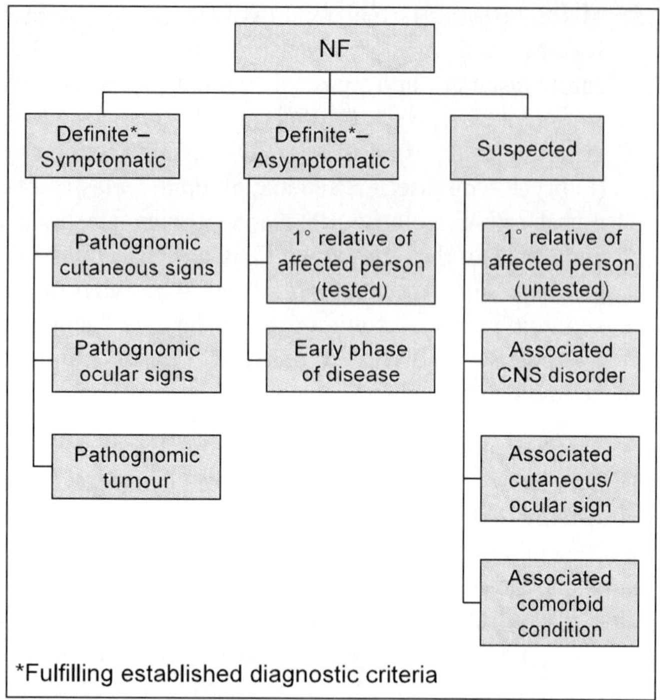

Fig. 46.1: Clinical approach to a case of neurofibromatosis (NF)

Neurofibromatosis 1

Etiopathogesnesis: NF1 is the most common neurocutaneous disorder occurring in 1 per 3000 to 4000 individuals. It results from mutations of the NF1 gene that has been mapped to the locus 17q11.2. It encodes Neurofibromin that functions as a tumor suppressor protein by virtue of its similarity with GTPase-activating proteins that down-regulate the proto-oncogene, p21-*ras*. Neurofibromin is predominantly expressed by neurons, oligodendrocytes, astrocytes and schwann cells. It causes aggregation of melanoblast precursors or schwann cells during neural crest migration and hence its loss may lead to uncontrolled cell growth and tumor formation (hamartomas and schwannomas). More than 200 mutations have been identified out of which almost 50% are *de novo*.

Clinical Manifestations and Diagnosis: The clinical manifestations primarily affect the skin, eyes, central nervous system and bone. At least two of the diagnostic criteria listed in (Table 46.4) must be present to establish a diagnosis. A description of each has been given along with age of appearance, as all are not present at birth, but gradually evolve with age.

(1) *Skin:* The characteristic lesions of NF1 are Café-au-lait macules (CLAM). These may be the only sign present in infancy which progressively increase in number, size and pigmentation. By 5 years of age they are found in almost 99% cases of NF1. The distribution is generalized with a predilection for the extremities and trunk and sparing of the face. Inguinal and axillary freckling are smaller CLAMS that are considered pathognomic of NF1. Neurofibromas are dysplastic tumours that are formed from axonal processes, Schwann cells, fibrobalsts, perineural and mast cells. They can be solitary or multiple. Apart from cosmetic disfigurement they can occasionally be itchy painful and sensitive to touch. Though they typically involve the skin they can also be found along the peripheral nerves, blood vessels and within viscera. Their size is known to increase during puberty

Table 46.4: Diagnostic Criteria of Neurofibromatosis-1
Note the presence of any two is mandatory for establishing diagnosis

Diagnostic criteria	Description of lesion	Age of appearance		
		0 – 2 yr	2 – 6 yr	≥ 6 yr
Café-au-lait macules (≥ 6)	Brownish macules Prepubertal: ≥ 5 mm* Postpubertal ≥ 15 mm*	+	+	+
Axillary/inguinal freckling	Multiple hyperpigmented 2 – 3 mm sized macules	-	+	+++
Neurofibromas (≥ 2) OR	Small rubbery cutaneous lesions with discolored overlying skin	+/-	+	+++
1 Plexiform neurofibroma	Diffuse thickened nerve trunks with overlying hyperpigmented skin	+/-	+	+++
Lisch nodules (≥ 2)	Yellow to brown gelatinous dome shaped projections on the iris	+/ -	+	+++
Optic gliomas	Benign tumors consisting of glial cells and mucinous material	+	+	++
Distinctive osseous lesion	Sphenoid dysplasia or cortical thinning of long bones with or without pseudoarthrosis	+	+	+
First-degree relative with NF-1	Diagnosis based on these criteria	+/-	+/-	+/-

* Greatest diameter, yr - years

or pregnancy. Plexiform neurofibromas may produce limb overgrowth with or without bony deformity and are frequently seen in the orbital or temporal regions.

(2) *Ocular*: Lisch nodules are asymptomatic hamartomas of the iris that can be detected by slit-lamp examination. Hamartomas can also be found in the choroid and retina. Optic gliomas usually develop by 6 years. Symptoms are location dependent though a large number can be asymptomatic. Orbital gliomas cause proptosis, visual field defects and impaired vision. Chiasmatic gliomas can cause hydrocephalus or precocious puberty. Glaucoma may be present due to infiltration and obstruction of the aqueous pathways.

(3) *Neurologic*: Manifestations include macrocephaly, seizures, headache, transient ischemic attacks, stroke, cognitive defects (30-40%), learning disabilities, attention deficit hyperactivity disorder and speech abnormalities.

(4) *Skeletal:* These manifestations include sphenoid wing dysplasia that leads to proptosis and pulsating exophthalmos. The spine can develop scoliosis, kyphosis and vertebral erosion that may result in intrathoracic meningocoeles and short stature. Pseudoarthrosis of the long bones (especially tibia), subperiosteal proliferation, genu valgum or varum and pectus excavatum are also seen.

(5) *Gastrointestinal*: Affected individuals may have abdominal pain, vomiting, constipation and diarrhea.

Majority of affected individuals have a benign course. Poorer prognosis with decreased life expectancy is seen with development of malignancies. Neurofibromas and plexiform neurofibromas may transform into malignant peripheral nerve sheath tumor (MPNST) in 5%. Others include malignant schwannoma, CNS tumors (meningiomas, astrocytomas and neurilemmomas) leukemia, pheochromocytoma, rhabdomyosarcoma, juvenile xanthogranuloma and Wilms' tumor.

Investigations: The focus of clinical assessment is age dependent. In the first 2 years of life plexiform neuromas, glaucoma, sphenoid wing dysplasia, and pseudoarthroses should be actively looked for. Screening magnetic resonance imaging (MRI) of the brain may detect asymptomatic optic nerve gliomas in 15% children with NF1. Other MRI abnormalities found are gliomas in the brainstem or craniocervical junction, plexiform neurofibromas, sphenoid wing dysplasias and lambdoid bone defects. Abnormal signals known as NF spots or unidentified objects (UNO) are seen in the globus pallidus, thalamus, and internal capsule. These are believed to be low-grade gliomas or hamartomas and are not detected by computerised tomographic (CT) scanning. Occasionally cerebral vessels may develop aneurysms, or stenosis resulting in moyamoya disease. An electroencephalogram (EEG) is indicated only when seizures are present. Psychometric evaluation is warranted in preschool children with developmental delay so that strengths and weaknesses can be identified for planning of early intervention. Genetic studies have limited value due to the large number of mutations and absence of affected parents in 50%. When the family history is positive linkage studies may prove to be beneficial making prenatal diagnosis a possibility if the underlying mutation can be identified.

Management: Asymptomatic patients require screening of young children (discussed earlier) and monitoring. Monitoring includes annual expert ophthalmologic examination and tracking for hypertension (due to renal artery stenosis or pheochromocytoma). When symptomatic, treatment is planned according to the specific clinical problem. CLAMs that are cosmetically disfiguring can be treated by dermabrasion, though the chance of recurrence is high. Tumors that cause functional impairment or disfigurement may be treated with judicious surgical excision or debulking. Neurofibromas causing pruritis may benefit from ketotifen. Optic gliomas are usually treated conservatively. Only aggressive and complicated cases are treated with radiation, chemotherapy and surgical excision. Since brain tumors are usually indolent they are not managed aggressively. Orthopedic management includes braces and spinal fusion for kyphoscoliosis and braces for tibial bowing. Intervention programs and special education is indicated for children with cognitive impairment. Genetic counseling is indicated for all.

Neurofibromatosis 2

Etiopathogenesis: NF2 is less common with a prevalence of 1 in 33,000 to 40,000. This is caused by a mutation in the neurofibromin 2 gene located at 22q12.2. Nearly 200 mutations (deletions, nonsense and frameshift) have been discovered that explain the wide variability in symptoms. This gene is a tumor suppressor with the gene product 'Merlin' or 'schwannomin' involved in linking the actin cytoskeleton to glycoproteins in the cell membrane. Since it is important in cell growth and remodeling, tumour formation ensues when it gets inactivated. Mosaicism is known that results in segmental, unilateral or milder presentations.

Clinical Manifestations and Diagnosis: The diagnosis is often difficult in childhood due to the absence of external stigmata of disease and late CNS involvement. Though present since conception, the presentation is usually in the second or third decade though the onset can occur anytime between infancy and old age. If the onset is in childhood manifestations are usually more severe and involve visual symptoms, skin manifestations and mononeuropathy. The diagnostic criteria of NF-2 are given in (Table 46.5). The characteristic bilateral acoustic neuromas occur in 95% cases. They remain asymptomatic until young adulthood after which the symptoms occur depending on size and location. These include unilateral or bilateral progressive hearing loss, tinnitus, headache, ataxia and cranial nerve compression (6th cranial nerve leading to diplopia, 5th nerve facial sensory loss and 7th nerve lower motor facial palsy respectively). In young adults, they can also manifest as space occupying lesions of the cerebellopontine angle.

Table 46.5: Diagnostic Criteria of Neurofibromatosis-2
Diagnostic criteria (presence of one mandatory)
Bilateral eighth nerve masses (consistent with acoustic neuromas by neuroimaging)
A parent, sibling or child with NF-2 and/or unilateral 8th nerve masses or any two of the following: neurofibroma, meningioma, glioma, schwannoma, or juvenile posterior subcapsular lenticular opacities

Ocular signs are extremely important to recognize because these may be the initial presenting manifestations of affected children that may even precede the symptoms related to hearing. Visual disturbance is caused by posterior subcapsular and posterior cortical cataracts, loss of vision by retinal hamartomas, epiretinal membranes, and optic disc meningiomas, papilledema with secondary optic atrophy due to intracranial tumors and ocular motility disturbances due to 3rd, 4th and 6th cranial nerve involvement. Cutaneous signs like CLAMs and neurofibromas are less common. Children can present with mononeuropathy that result in 7th nerve palsy or limb wasting while adults have symptomatic polyneuropathy (3 - 10%) or abnormal nerve conduction studies (40%). The exact pathogenesis is unclear. The hypotheses put forth include intra-axonal Schwann cell proliferation without tumour formation, local toxicity of the tumour cells or cellular dysfunction resulting from Merlin deficiency.

Other tumours are also seen in NF2 besides acoustic neuromas. Schwannomas may involve any or all cranial nerves and the spine. Meningiomas are common with NF-2 accounting for 25% of all childhood meningiomas. Optic nerve sheath meningiomas (ONSM) are common and are more invasive than in adults. These present with progressive visual loss, visual field defects, proptosis, and restriction of upgaze.

NF2 is associated with significant morbidity and reduced life expectancy. Prognosis depends upon the age of onset of symptoms, degree of hearing deficit, and number and location of various tumors. Poor prognosis is associated with early onset (< 20 years) and presence of intracranial meningiomas. Prognosis is better with slice-site or missense mutations and mosaic patients compared to truncating mutations and non-mosaic patients respectively.

Investigations: These are planned according to the clinical situation; establishing of diagnosis in a case with suspected NF2, monitoring an affected case or screening a child of an affected parent (at risk).

(A) **Suspected NF2:** In this situation investigations aim at establishing diagnosis, assessing associated conditions and assisting in genetic counseling.

MRI with and without gadolinium enhancement remains the mainstay for diagnosis of CNS, cranial nerve, and spinal cord tumors. Small intracanalicular tumors may not be seen on standard 5 mm slice thickness through the posterior fossa. Optimal imaging includes 3 mm cuts overlapping by 1.5 mm on both axial and coronal post contrast enhancement views through the internal auditory canals or the use of 3 dimensional volumetric MRI. CT scan can visualize large vestibular schwannomas and meningiomas. Spinal cord MRI imaging is indicated when motor or sensory symptoms are present.

Brainstem auditory-evoked response (BAER) may detect latency abnormalities and early sensorineural hearing loss before a mass is detectable on MRI. Similarly juvenile cataracts may also be detected before evidence of vestibular schwannomas. Dilated eye examinations are warranted to look for additional retinal hamartomas, or epiretinal membranes. Once clinical diagnosis is established direct molecular analysis can be used to identify mutations. The detection rate is reportedly 72% in non-familial cases and 93% in familial cases. If the testing is inconclusive molecular testing of tumor tissue, linkage analysis or indirect genetic testing methods may be considered. If a mutation is found asymptomatic family members may benefit from presymptomatic testing. When a parent has NF2, prenatal testing can be done on amniocytes or chorionic villi, either through direct gene mutation analysis (if mutation known) or by linkage analysis. If the mutation is known, pre-implantation genetic diagnosis may be a suitable option.

(B) **Monitoring of Affected Individuals:** An in-depth clinical examination (dermatological, neurological and ophthalmologic) should be done annually to detect any change in status. Annual cranial MRI focuses on early detection of potential CNS complications. Spinal cord screening is not indicated in the absence of motor or sensory symptoms. Auditory screening with BAER should be done annually. If a vestibular schwannoma is identified acoustic reflex testing should also be included for monitoring disease progression. An annual ophthalmic examination is also recommended since worsening of symptoms and signs can indicate disease progression.

(C) **Screening High Risk Children:** If asymptomatic first degree relatives of affected individuals are found to carry the mutation or mutational analysis results are unavailable, a detailed clinical examination (dermatological, neurological and ophthalmologic) needs to be performed annually. Cranial MRI should be done annually to screen for intracranial tumours, starting at 10-12 years and continuing till the 5th decade. Spinal cord screening is not indicated if the individual is asymptomatic.

Management: This involves treatment of symptomatic tumours and hearing problems in addition to the aforementioned monitoring of affected individuals and genetic counseling. Surgery is the most common approach for clinically significant lesions. Resections of acoustic neuromas are planned according to size and location. Radiation therapy may be considered when surgery is not possible. Small vestibular schwannomas warrant surgical resection and stereotactic radiosurgery, which help to preserve hearing and facial nerve function. If large an educated decision has to be taken between debulking (that preserves hearing) and complete resection (that results in irreversible hearing loss). The options for jugular foramen schwannomas, which are indolent, include surgery, radiation therapy, and watchful waiting. Pharmacotherapy with inhibitors that act on epidermal growth factor receptors (Erlotinib) and monoclonal antibodies that inhibit angiogenic effects of Vascular epidermal growth factor (Bevacizumab) are being explored for unresectable, progressive vestibular schwannomas. Non-vestibular cranial nerve schwannomas are treated with microsurgery and radiosurgery. Radiation and/or chemotherapy are recommended for disabling ependymomas and only palliative chemotherapy for ependymomas that are still unresectable following radiation. Since most intracranial meningiomas are also indolent, surgery is only indicated in cases with serious, disabling symptoms. Orbital surgery is indicated for ONSM when there is progression or development of pain or proptosis. Since the resection of spinal cord tumors is difficult, the risks and benefits of surgery need to be individualized. Cutaneous or subcutaneous growths can be surgically removed.

Auditory brainstem implants are being used with some success in patients with hearing loss secondary to vestibular schwannomas and those with no cochlear nerve function. Hearing augmentation with cochlear implants may also improve quality of life. There is no available treatment for the neuropathies.

TUBEROUS SCLEROSIS COMPLEX (TSC)

The name of this disorder originates from the characteristic firm swellings found on the surface of the brain. Tuber is derived from the Latin word '*tumere*', which means to swell, while 'sclerosis' refers to palpable firmness of the tuber caused by central gliosis. It is also known as 'Bourneville Disease' after the author Desire–Magloire Bourneville who described the clinical phenotype in depth for the first time.

Etiology: TSC is inherited as an autosomal dominant disorder with complete penetrance but variable expressivity. The estimated prevalence is 1 in 6000. More than 100 mutations have been identified in the TSC1 gene, which are either small deletions or insertions. At least half of the cases are sporadic due to new mutations. The same clinical phenotype is due to the TSC1 gene linked to chromosome 9q34 and TSC 2 located at 16p13. The gene product of the former is 'hamartin' and of the latter 'tuberin.' These two proteins probably function together as a protein complex that helps regulate cell growth and size. Alterations produce an abnormal version of hamartin that cannot form a complex with tuberin, leading to overgrowth of cells that grow too large and/or divide too often, which result in noncancerous tumors. It has been observed that individuals with TSC2 have more severe. The ratio of mutations due to TSC1 and TSC2 is 1: 5 in sporadic cases and 1:1 in inherited cases.

Figure 46.2 depicts the physiological role of the Tuberin-Hamartin complex in normal cell growth and metabolism and what happens when there is any disruption of this process. The pathognomic lesions of TSC are tubers in the brain, typically located in the subependymal region of the cerebral hemispheres. These cause expansion of the gyri and distort the cerebral architecture. When they calcify and project into the ventricular cavity they produce a characteristic 'candle-dripping' appearance. Tubers in the

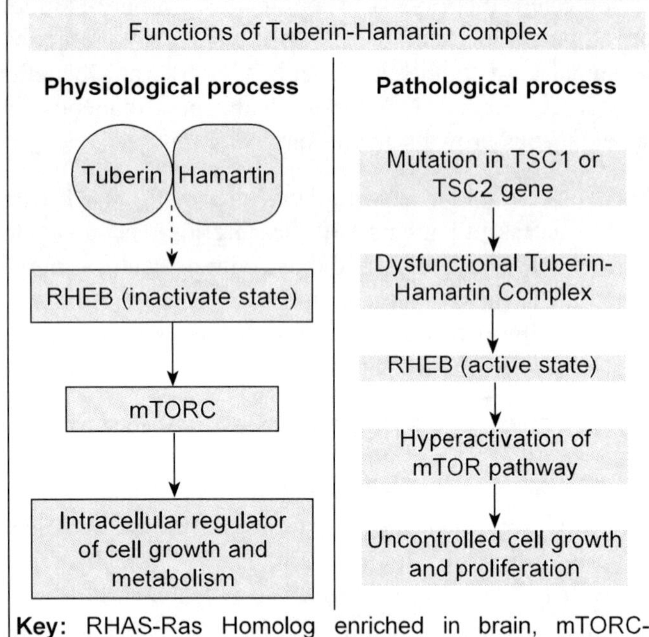

Fig. 46.2: Functions of the Tuberin-Hamartin complex

region of the foramen of Monro may lead to obstruction and the development of a non-communicating hydrocephalus. Microscopic examination of the tubers reveals decreased neurons, proliferation of astrocytes and multinucleated giant neurons and loss of the six layered architecture of the cerebral cortex. Other intracranial lesions seen are white matter abnormalities like subependymal nodules (SEN) and subependymal giant cell astrocytomas (SEGA).

Clinical Manifestations and Diagnosis: TSC is an extremely heterogeneous disease with a wide clinical spectrum within the same family. The clinical manifestations depend on the number and location of the tubers (skin, brain, eyes, heart, kidney and lungs). The diagnostic criteria are given in (Table 46.6).

Table 46.6: Revised Diagnostic Criteria of Tuberous Sclerosis Complex (TSC)

Major Features	Facial angiofibromas or forehead plaque
	Non-traumatic ungual or periungual fibroma
	Hypomelanotic macules (more than three)
	Shagreen patch (connective tissue nevus)
	Multiple retinal nodular hamartomas
	Cortical tuber[a]
	Subependymal nodule
	Subependymal giant cell astrocytoma
	Cardiac rhabdomyoma, single or multiple
	Lymphangiomyomatosis[b]
	Renal angiomyolipoma[b]

Contd.

Contd.

Minor Features	Multiple randomly distributed pits in dental enamel
	Hamartomatous rectal polyps[c]
	Bone cysts[d]
	Cerebral white matter migration lines [a,d,e]
	Gingival fibromas
	Non-renal hamartoma[c]
	Retinal achromic patch
	"Confetti" skin lesions
	Multiple renal cysts[c]
Definite TSC	Either 2 major features or 1 major feature with 2 minor features
Probable TSC	One major feature and one minor feature
Possible TSC	Either 1 major feature or 2 or more minor features

[a] When cerebral cortical dysplasia and cerebral white matter migration tracts occur together, they should be counted as one rather than two features of TSC.

[b] When both lymphangiomyomatosis and renal angiomyolipomas are present, other features of TSC should be present before a definitive diagnosis is assigned.

[c] Histologic confirmation is suggested.

[d] Radiographic confirmation is sufficient.

[e] One panel member recommended three or more radial migration lines constitute a major feature.

(1) *Cutaneous manifestations*: These are the most common manifestation of TSC though not the most common presenting problem as often the pathognomonic external stigmata are disregarded as insignificant by affected individuals. Hypopigmented macules are the most common skin lesions that occur at any age (95%). These are more frequent in TSC2. These are called 'ash-leaf macules when they are lance shaped. Generalized confetti like macules (1-3 mm in size) are also frequently seen. Facial angiofibromas (also called sebaceous adenomas) are tiny red nodules distributed over the nose and cheeks in a butterfly wing distribution. These usually develop between 4 and 6 years of age and are seen in 75% cases. They may enlarge, coalesce, and become fleshy later. Forehead or scalp plaques are skin colored or brownish fibrous lesions that can appear in infancy and seen in 48%. A shagreen patch consists of a raised lesion with a rough orange-peel consistency located primarily in the lumbosacral region is seen in around 19%. Subungual or periungual fibromas may develop in the fingers and toes in 15% which become fleshy during adolescence.

(2) *Central nervous system*: This involvement is the second most common manifestation and the number of tubers is directly proportionate to the degree of neurological impairment. Seizures are the most common presenting symptom since the tubers act as epileptogenic foci. The dysplastic neurons have reduced inhibitory action due to imbalance of GABA receptors and hyperexcitation due to molecular changes in the glutamate receptors. The semiology is usually infantile spasms with hypsarrhythmic EEG pattern and unilateral tonic or clonic seizures. The younger the age of presentation, the greater is the likelihood of epileptic encephalopathy and resultant developmental delay and subsequent intellectual disability. Seizures may be absent or refractory and difficult to treat. Generalized seizures may be difficult to control, and may develop into myoclonic epilepsy later. Poor prognostic factors are onset in infancy, multiple types of seizures coexisting together and multifocal EEG spikes.

Cognitive and behavioral manifestations are seen in a third of affected individuals. These are referred to as TSC associated neuropsychiatric disorders (TAND). Intelligence may range from normal to severe intellectual disability or specific problems in memory, attention or executive skills. Neuropsychiatric disorders commonly seen in children include Autism Spectrum disorder, Attention deficit and hyperactivity disorder, learning disability and Intellectual disability whereas mood disorder, anxiety disorder, obsessive-compulsive behavior, schizophrenia, and bipolar disease are seen in adolescents and adults. Autism, severe cognitive impairment and infantile spasms are associated with TSC2.

Tubers occasionally differentiate into malignant astrocytomas, with the peak age of presentation 8 to 16 years of age. They are benign, slow growing, noninvasive tumors, which may present with features of increased intracranial pressure. SEN can convert into SEGA.

(3) *Renal manifestations*: Though this is the 3rd most common manifestation they are usually asymptomatic. The renal disorders include Angiomyolipomas (seen in 55-70% by adolescence), isolated renal cyst, autosomal dominant polycystic kidney disease and renal cell carcinoma. Symptoms comprise flank pain, acute severe bleeding due to rupture of blood vessel in the angiomyolipoma, hematuria and renal failure.

(4) *Ocular manifestations*: Retinal lesions are mulberry tumors arising from the nerve head or round, flat lesions in the region of the disc, known as phakomas. These are seen in 50% and at any age. They are usually asymptomatic and cause visual impairment only when they impinge on the optic nerve.

(5) *Cardiovascular manifestations*: Approximately 50-60% children have multiple benign rhabdomyomas in the ventricles that may develop in intrauterine life and undergo spontaneous resolution by childhood. They may present as outflow tract obstruction, interference with valvular function, congestive heart failure and arrhythmias.

(6) *Pulmonary manifestations*: These are usually seen in adulthood and mostly in women, though symptomatic in just 1%. The pulmonary abnormalities include multifocal micronodular pneumatocytes, pulmonary cysts and lymphangioleiomyomatosis (LAM) that are lung tumour with abnormal smooth muscle proliferation and cystic changes.

Investigations: TSC is suspected in children with external stigmata, epilepsy especially infantile spasms, unexplained developmental delay or first degree relatives of affected individuals. A careful search for the typical skin and retinal lesions of TSC should be performed in all these cases. Visualization of the hypopigmented lesions can be enhanced using a Wood's ultraviolet lamp. As depicted in Table V the diagnosis is established on satisfaction of diagnostic criteria (two major or 1 major and 2 minor criteria). The extent and severity of organ involvement needs to be ascertained by baseline workup. This includes an MRI of the brain and CT (for calcifications), electrocardiogram, echocardiogram, renal ultrasound and detailed ophthalmologic evaluation. An EEG is indicated in the presence of seizures, unexplained acute regression or change in sleep pattern. Development and neuro-behavioral assessments are required when indicated. Adult women need to get a lung CT scan done. Mutational analysis can detect mutations in 60% clinical phenotypes of TSC1 and 80% TSC2. Genetic counseling needs to be done in all cases. Prenatal diagnosis has been made with genetic tests and identification of characteristic cerebral tubers and cardiac lesions by fetal MR and echocardiogram respectively. After diagnosis affected cases need to be monitored regularly. This includes clinical assessment and neuroimaging and renal ultrasounds every 1 to 3 years even when asymptomatic.

Treatment

This entails monitoring (described above), symptomatic treatment, early detection of complications and genetic counseling. Achieving seizure control is frequently difficult in TSC.[10] Since Vigabatrin is an inhibitor of GABA transaminase it is the anticonvulsant of choice. Adrenocorticotropic hormone is used in Vigabatrin resistant spasms. Neurosurgery is indicated for increased intracranial pressure or hydrocephalus. Early intervention and special education are helpful in children with cognitive impairment. Periungual fibromas that bleed or get infected are managed with laser, phenolization and excision. If facial angiofibromas are disfiguring modalities of treatment include surgical excision, dermabrasion, laser therapy or topical mTOR inhibitors (Rapamycin 1%). Retinal phakomas require surgery only if symptomatic. Renal AML with hemorrhage require embolization followed by steroids. Medical treatment with mTOR inhibitors (Everolimus, Rapamycin) are indicated in the following situations: (i) SEGA and cerebral tubers that are increasing in size but remains asymptomatic; (ii) Asymptomatic growing renal AML that are >3 cm in diameter; (iii) Symptomatic cardiac rhabdomyomas; and (iv) Women with moderate to severe respiratory compromise due to pulmonary LAM. Severe respiratory compromise may warrant a lung transplant.

STURGE-WEBER SYNDROME (SWS)

This disease consists of a characteristic clinical constellation comprising facial nevus (port-wine stain), seizures, hemiparesis, intracranial calcifications and (usually) cognitive impairment. It is named after two British clinicians, WP Sturge (a physician who described an epileptic patient with hemiplegia and the typical cutaneous and ocular manifestations) and FP Weber (a dermatologist who noted the significance of the calcification pattern seen on plain radiographs). It is also known as encephalofacial angiomatosis or craniofacial or trigeminocranial angiomatosis with cerebral calcification.

Etiology: Most cases occur with a frequency of approximately 1/50,000 without any particular gender predilection. It was initially believed to be sporadic, though increased prevalence was reported among relatives of affected individuals. It has recently been discovered that SWS occurs due to a somatic activating mutation of the GNAQ gene. This encodes the protein Guanine nucleotide-binding protein G(q) subunit alpha is involved I intracellular signaling pathways. During normal embryogenesis a vascular plexus develops around the cephalic portion of the neural tube in the 6th week of intrauterine life that undergoes regression by the 9th week. Anomalous development of this primordial vascular bed during the early stages of cerebral vascularization, when the blood supply to the brain, meninges, and face is undergoing reorganization leads to the clinical features. The brain (particularly the molecular layer of the cortex) becomes atrophic and calcified, while the overlying leptomeninges are richly vascularized. It is believed that the primitive ectoderm covering the vascular plexus develops into the skin of the upper face. If the GNAQ mutation occurs early it results in SWS and if it occurs late it results in non-syndromic port-wine stains.

Clinical Manifestations and Diagnosis: The presence of the typical facial port-wine stain warrants further exploration for the possibility of SWS. The skin, eye and CNS are characteristically affected. SWS is referred to as complete when both CNS and facial angiomas are present and incomplete when only one area is affected. According to the Roach classification, Type I has facial and leptomeningeal angiomas and glaucoma, Type II has facial angioma and glaucoma, without inter-cranial involvement and Type III has isolated leptomengingeal angioma and absence of glaucoma. The clinical manifestations are given below:

(1) *Cutaneous:* The deep red, irregular-shaped macule or port-wine stain of variable size is present since birth, usually unilateral (75%) and involves the ophthalmic (V1) and maxillary (V2) division of the trigeminal nerve. The distribution usually includes the upper face and eyelid, but may also be evident over the lower face, oral and pharyngeal mucosa and rarely the trunk, abdomen and limbs.

(2) *Ocular:* This is seen in 30-60% patients. The most common manifestation is diffuse ipsilateral choroidal angioma that appears as a red elevated mass on fundus examination (tomato ketchup appearance). This may give rise to congenital ipsilateral glaucoma in about 33-50% that manifests with buphthalmos and pain. Eyelid, conjunctival and episcleral hemangioms are often seen. Upper eyelid lesions always indicate the presence of cerebral lesions. Optic disc colobomas, heterochromia iridium and cataracts have also been reported.

(3) *Central Nervous System*: Seizures are seen in 75-85% patients due to leptomeningeal angioma. The commonly occur during the 1st year of life and can be difficult to control. These are usually focal tonic-clonic in nature, contralateral to the nevus though infantile spasms have also been reported. The state of constant hypoperfusion and increased oxygen extraction leads to cerebral atrophy and subsequent calcification. Development is usually normal during the 1st year of life but subsequently global developmental delay,

intellectual disability and learning disabilities are seen in a large proportion. This is multifactorial; refractory seizures, adverse effects of multiple anticonvulsants and cerebral atrophy. Other neurologic complications are focal neurological deficits that are contralateral to the nevus (hemiparesis, sensory defects and homonymous hemianopia). Headaches and migraine can occur due to increased vasogenis leakage of plasma and neuropeptides into the vascular space.

(4) *Oral:* These include hemangiomas of the oral mucosa of the lips, gums, floor of the mouth, palate, inner cheeks and tongue that appear reddish and hypertrophic. Maxillary hypertrophy leads to dental malocclusion. Clinically these appear as facial asymmetry, poor oral hygiene and dental problems.

Poor prognostic factors include increasing duration of postictal deficits, increasing atrophy or calcifications, new onset of hemiparesis and deterioration in cognitive functioning.

Investigations: The PWS needs to be evaluated within the first week of life to distinguish whether it is isolated or SWS. The leptomeningeal angioma, ipsilateral cortical atrophy and ex-vacuo dilatation of the lateral ventricle can be detected by MRI with gadolinium contrast. Plain radiographs and CT of the cranium (better option) show characteristic double-lined serpentine intracranial calcification in the occipitoparietal region (railroad-track appearance) by 6-7 years of age. Detailed ophthalmological examination is warranted whenever the V1 distribution is involved. This includes fluorescein angiography (for detection of early filling with late staining) and measurement of intraocular tension. Detailed oro-dental evaluation must be done periodically. EEG and psychometric testing should be done for evaluation of cognitive impairment.

Management: This is a combination of medical and surgical modalities. Anticonvulsants are used for seizure control. If they remain well-controlled seizures the impact on cognitive function is minimized. Patients with medically refractory epilepsy may benefit from vagal nerve stimulation, focal cortical resection, hemispherectomy, corpus callosotomy, or lobectomy in the 1st year of life, to prevent deterioration in development. Early intervention should be started for children with developmental delay and special education for older children. Latanoprost, a prostaglandin, may be used initially to reduce the intraocular pressure but surgical therapy is considered to be the mainstay of treatment since the medical action is short-lived. Standard symptomatic and prophylactic therapy is used for headache. The port-wine stain is treated by multiple sessions of cosmetic laser treatment (flashlamp-pumped pulsed-dye laser) that should be started as soon as possible. The earlier the onset the lesser the number of sessions required. It prevents the development of complications like soft tissue swelling and hypertrophy.

Many neurocutaneous disorders are associated with predominant vascular lesions besides the usual cutaneous, neurological and ocular involvement. The salient features of these syndromes have been briefly described in (Table 46.7). There are many others besides the ones that have been detailed in this chapter. With further evolution of scientific knowledge and advances in molecular genetics and neuroimaging techniques a better understanding of these disorders can be expected.

Table 46.7: Neurocutaneous Syndromes with Vascular Predominance

Syndrome and Prevalence	Inheritance and Gene	Clinical Manifestations				Investigations
		Cutaneous	Neurological	Ocular	Others	
Von Hippel-Lindau disease 1: 36,000	Autosomal dominant (AD) VHL gene 3p25.23	Hemangio-blastoma (HB)	Brain and spine HB, Cerebellar signs, increased ICT	Retinal HB with retinal detachment, vision loss, glaucoma	Pheochromocytoma, cystic lesions in liver, kidneys and pancreas. Endolymphatic cell tumour middle ear Malignancy-renal cell carcinoma	Ophthalmic, CNS abdominal and renal imaging: Screening for Pheochromocytoma Molecular genetic testing
Ataxia-Telangiectasia 1:40,000 to 1:100,000	Autosomal recessive (AR) ATM gene 11q22–23	Telangiectasias-nasal bridge, ear and extremities, loss of skin elasticity, granulomas, café au lait macules	Progressive Spinocerebellar degeneration, motor neuron disease, SMA, Peripheral	Telangiectasias-bulbar conjunctiva	Susceptibility to sino-pulmonary infections Immunodeficiency-absence of helper T cells, IgA, IgE and	Neuroimaging, Chromosomal breakage studies-increased breaks, elevated AFP and CEA, Molecular

Contd.

Contd.

			neuropathy dementia		low IgG. risk of lymphoreticular malignancy. progeria	genetic testing. Immunoblot for ATM protein
Incontinentia Pigmenti Uncommon	X-linked dominant. IKBKG gene Xq28	4 stages-bullous, verrucous, hyperpigmented (linear/ whorled) and atretic lesions. Hair alopecia and nail dystrophy	Seizures. microcephaly GDD/ ID. cortical blindness and hemiparesis	Poor vision. strabismus. cataracts. RD. OA retrolental mass. and vitreous hemorrhage	Teeth affected (small. loss)	MRI brain. dental and ophthalmologic exam Molecular genetic testing
Osler-Weber-Rendu disease/ Hereditary Hemorrhagic Telangiectasia 1: 100.000	AD. Most in ENG gene (9q33-34) and ALK-1 gene (12q13)	Piebaldism-white forelock	Cerebellar ataxia, Strokes GDD/ID. hearing loss		Multiple A-V malformations and telangiectasias. Nasopharynx (epistaxis) and viscera	Imaging. Molecular genetic testing
Klippel-Trenaunay-syndrome 1: 100.000	Sporadic Mutations in PIK3CA gene may be seen	Port-wine hemangioma (One of the triad), varicose veins	Seizures, GDD/ ID, migraine/ headaches microcephaly, macrocephaly		Osseous and soft tissue hypertrophy and deep vascular malformation (rest of triad), polydactyly, syndactyly	MRI: cerebral AVM hemimegalencephaly, orbitofrontal varices, brainstem angiomas, ICA aplasia malformed circle of Willis, EEG
Linear Nevus Syndrome 1:1000 to 1: 10,000	Sporadic	Midline nevus with hyperplasia of epidermis and dermis Subcutaneous hemangiomas	Epilepsy GDD/ ID hemiparesis, homonymous hemianopia	Strabismus, retinal anomalies, coloboma, cataracts,	Coarctation of aorta skeletal (dysplasia, hypoplasia, VDRR kyphoscoliosis), horseshoe kidney, lipomas	Multi-systemic imaging, skin biopsy, ophthalmologic evaluation, EEG
PHACE syndrome Unknown	Unknown	Facial hemangiomas (> 5 mm)	GDD/ID, neurological deficits	Persistent hyperplastic primary vitreous, AbN post. seg. retina, optic disc and nerve staphyloma Coloboma	Cerebrovascular, cardiovascular, midline defects	Neuroimaging, Echocardiography, Ophthalmologic

KEY: AbN-abnormal, AFP-alpha-fetoprotein, AVM-Arteriovenous malformation, CEA-carcinoembryonic antigen, GDD-Global developmental delat, ID-Intellectual disability, Ig-Immunoglobulin, ICA-Internal Carotid Artery, OA-optic atrophy, PHACE(S): **p**osterior fossa brain malformations, **h**emangiomas of the face (large or complex), **a**rterial anomalies, **c**ardiac anomalies, **e**ye abnormalities, **s**ternal clefting/supraumbilical raphe, RD-retinal detachment, VDRR-Vitamin D refractory rickets

Suggested Reading

- Altman N. Neuroimaging of Phakomatoses. Int Ped 2000: 15(1):4-14.
- Antônio JR, Trídico LA, Goloni-Bertollo EM. Neurofibromatosis: Chronological History and Current Issues. An Bras Dermatol 2013;88(3):329-43.
- Braffman B, Naidich TP. The Phakomatoses: Part I. Neurofibromatosis and Tuberous Sclerosis. Neuroimaging Clin N Am 1994;4:299-324.
- Chan JW. Neuro-ophthalmic Features of the Neurocutaneous Syndromes. Int Ophthal Clin 2012;52(3):73-85.
- Cheadle JP, Reeve MP, Sampson JR, Kwiatkowski DJ. Molecular Genetic Advances in Tuberous Sclerosis. Hum Genet 2000;107:97-114.
- Cheng TS. Tuberous Sclerosis Complex: An Update. Hong Kong J. Dermatol, Venereol 2012;20:61-67.
- Comi AM, Weisz CJ, Highet BH. Sturge-Weber Syndrome: Altered Blood Vessel Fibronectin Expression and Morphology. J Child Neurol 2005;20(7):572-77.

- Comi AM. Advances in Sturge-Weber syndrome. Curr Opin Neurol 2006;19(2):124-28.
- DeBella K, Szudek J, Friedman JM: Use of the National Institutes of Health Criteria for Diagnosis of Neurofibromatosis 1 in Children. Pediatrics 2000;105:608-14.
- Gutmann DH, Aylsworth A, Carey JC, *et al.* The Diagnostic Evaluation and Multidisciplinary Management of Neurofibromatosis 1 and Neurofibromatosis 2. JAMA 1997; 278(1):51-57.
- Maher ER, Bentley E, Yates JR, *et al.* Mapping of von Hippel-Lindau Disease to Chromosome 3p Confirmed by Genetic Linkage Analysis. J Neurol Sci 1990;100:27-30.
- Metry DW, Dowd CF, Barkovich AJ, Frieden IJ. The Many Faces of PHACE Syndrome. J Pediatr 2001;139(1):117-23.
- Perlman S, Becker-Catania S, Gatti RA: Ataxia-Telangiectasia: Diagnosis and Treatment. Semin Pediatr Neurol 2003;10(3): 173-82.
- Roach ES, Gomez MR, Nothrup H. Tuberous Sclerosis Complex Consensus Conference: Revised Clinical Diagnostic Criteria. J Child Neurol 1998;13:624-28.
- Ruggieri M. The Different Forms of Neurofibromatosis. Childs Nerv Syst 1999;15(6):295-308.
- Shovlin CL, Guttmacher AE, Buscarini E, *et al.* Diagnostic Criteria for Hereditary Hemorrhagic Telangiectasia (Rendu-Osler-Weber syndrome). Am J Med Genet 2000;91(1):66-67.
- Siddeswari R, Manohar S, Abhilash T. Sturge-Weber Syndrome. J Med Allied Sci 2014;4(2):88-90.
- TS Thiele EA. Managing Epilepsy in Tuberous Sclerosis Complex. J Child Neurol 2004;19(9):680-86.
- Wilson CL, Song LM, Chua H, *et al.* Bleeding from Cavernous Angiomatosis of the Rectum in Klippel-Trenaunay Syndrome: Report of Three Cases and Literature Review. Am J Gastroenterol 2001;96(9):2783-88.

47 Chapter

NEURODEGENERATIVE DISEASES IN CHILDREN: CLINICAL APPROACH

D Meikandan

INTRODUCTION

Neurodegenerative disorders are complex diverse diseases resulting in agonising incapacitation to children or ultimate early fatality. Diagnosis by history alone will give maximum clue by the following:

1. Global developmental arrest in all domains with complete absence of any milestone acquisition.
2. Delayed acquisition of milestone with loss of the same lates.
3. Progressively worsening cognitive, motor and special sensory skills.
4. Progressive different pattern of seizures and abnormal movements and complete loss of posture and motor skills.

Though the ultimate diagnosis and management of neurodegenerative disorders depends upon the underlying genetic mutations, but neuroimaging especially MRI over the years has somewhat simplified the approach of clinician as imaging characteristics narrows down the list of differential diagnosis and thus guides further clinical, laboratory, metabolic and genetic work up. CSF is also useful in selected cases.

Early features of gray matter diseases are personality changes, seizures and dementia. Characteristics of white matter disease are focal neurological deficits, spasticity and blindness.

Whether the process begins in the gray matter or the white matter eventually clinical features of dysfunction develop in both. The electro encephalogram (EEG) is usually abnormal early in the course of gray matter disease and late in the course of white matter disease. MRI shows cortical atrophy in gray matter disease and progressive subcortical demyelination in white matter disease.

Visual somatosensory, auditory evoked responses and motor conduction velocities are useful in documenting demyelination, even sub clinical, in the optic and peripheral nerves, respectively.

Classification of Neurodegenerative Disorders

There are various ways of classifying them.

1. Anatomical gray and white matter.
2. Metabolic and non-metabolic.
3. Progressive encephalopathies.
   Before and after 2 age of years.
4. Infective and non-infective encephalopathies like HIV, encephalopathy, SSPE, progressive multifocal leukoencephalopathy (PML).

Hence, it is better to know the types of disorders which can all produce neurodegeneration generally clinical deterioration, occurs however much be, try, through various known modern techniques.

They are as follows:

1. **Lysosome Storage Disorder.**
2. **Peroxisomal Disorder.**
3. **Mitochondrial Disorders:**
   In all these diseases, apart from brain, involvement (central and peripheral CNS) also nerves and muscles are also affected.
4. **AIDS Encephalopathy and SSPE:**
   Subacute Sclerosing Panencephalitis are commonly seem neuro infective degenerative disorders, we have so far seem as frequently an PML in AIDS.
5. **Progressively Working Autistic Spectral Disorders:**
   After the age of 1½ to 2 years are another common

entity we see as neurodevelopmental pervasive disorder with classical language impairment both verbal and non verbal. Communication skills, repetitive behaviours, restricted activities and interests along with inexplicable social activities they may or may not have epilepsy as a comorbid condition.

6. **Various Metabolic Disorders:**
Neurocutanous syndromes can involve both gray and white matter of the CNS commonly associated with:
    1. Amino Acid Metabolism.
    2. Urea Cycle.
    3. Carbohydrate Cycle.
    4. Fatty Acid Oxidation.
7. **Neurotransmitter Related Disorders:**
In these groups if enzyme identified apart from classical clinical features these children may be saved with prepared dietetic changes through with no promising value to the life.
8. Classically described leucodystrophies, hypomyelination and demyelination disorders after the advent of MRI and MRS studies.
9. Basal ganglia and cerebellar disorder.
10. Neuronal storage disorders with or without megalencephaly disorders of metal metabolism, Wilson, Menkes and a few.
11. Neuronal ceroid lipofuscinoses are classically with refractory epilepsy, and visual impairment and dementia with remarkable accumulation of autofluorescent material in brain, retina and other tissues.
12. **Peroxisomal Biogenesis Disorders:**
Mitochondrial leucoencephalitis and electron transfer disorder have all been added in this innumerable long list of disorders.

As we seen, more and more genetic mutations and subtybes have been identified and neuro disorder included, the list become, extensive and exhaustive. Hence, learning, about a few, and the rest the nerve. These disorders can be identifial and further plan may be evaluated.

It is useful to classify these disorders radiologically also depending upon the side and pattern of involvement. These investigations are most useful in the early stages of metabolic disorders as the end stage of most of these disease have near similar appearances.

I. Radiological Classification

Disorders involving in the gray matter only (Reviews in Neurology 2008).

1. **Deep Gray Matter:**
    (a) Leigh disease.
    (b) MELAS and a few mitochondrial disorders.
    (c) Juvenile Huntington's disease.
2. **Eye of Tiger Signs:**
    Hypointense signals in striatum______________
    Hallervorden Spatz disease.
3. **Braigh Signel in Pallidum:**
    (a) Methylmelonic academia.
    (b) Carbon monoxide poisoning.
    (c) Kernicterus.
4. **Cortical Gray Matter:**
    (a) Neuronal ceroid lipofuscinoses.
    (b) Mucolipidoses type I.

II. Subcortical White Matter–Early

1. **Large Head**
    (a) Alexander disease.
    (b) Van der Knaap disease, Subcortical white matter with multiple cysts formation.
    (c) Canavan disease.
2. **Normal Head Size**
    (a) Galactosemia.
    (b) Abnormal thalami – Krabbe's disease.
    (c) Normal thalami.
    - Pons medulla corticospinal tract involvement.
    - Peroxisomal disorders.
3. **Posterior Parieto Occipital White Matter**
    (a) Adreno leukodystrophy.

4. **Multiple White Matter Lesions**
   (a) Metachromatic leukodystrophy (inverter pinetree appearance).
   (b) Phenylketonuria.
5. **Lack of Myelination**
   Pelizaeus – Merzbacher disease.
6. **Non-Specific White Matter Pattern**
   (a) Nonketotic hyperglycinemia.
   (b) Urea cycle disorders.
   (c) Collagen vascular disease
7. **Cortical Gray Matter**
   (1) *Normal facies (appearances)*
      (a) Cortical dysplasia
         - Fukuyama congenital muscidas dystrophy.
         - Walker-Warburg syndrome.
         - Muscle-eye-brain disease.
   (2) *Abnormal facies*
      (a) Mucopolysaccharidoses
      (b) Lipid storage disorders
      (c) Peroxisomal disorders
8. **Deep Gray Matter Involvement**
   (1) *Primary thalamic involvement*
      (a) Krabbe's disease
      (b) GM_2 gangliosidosis
      (c) GM_1 gangliosidosis
   (2) *Primary globus palladus involvement*
      (a) Canavan's disease
      (b) Methylmalonic academia
      (c) Maple syrup urine disease
   (3) *Primary striatal involvement*
      (a) Leigh syndrome
      (b) MELAS
      (c) Wilson's disease

Subacute Sclerosing Panencephalitis (SSPE) (Fenichel 2009)

The pathogenesis of subacute sclerosing panencephalitis although still obscure reflects defective replication of the measles virus in neural tissues patients with subacute sclerosing panencephalitis have elevated CSF immunoglobulin levels. Gligoclonal bands and increased IgG synthesis rates indicating massive production of measles specific IgG. High CSF titers of measles specific IgG establish the diagnosis of subacute sclerosing panencephalitis and measles virus RNA can be detected in CSF of plasma by reverse transcriptions PCR. EEGs show bilaterally synchronous spike wave or slow wave bursts that assume a suppression burst pattern over time. MRI commonly exhibits T2 Prolongation of subcortical and periventricular white matter and eventually cortical atrophy SSPE is one condition where brain biopsy is done to establish. The diagnosis typical histologic findings in and / or isolation of virus or viral antigen from brain tissue obtained by biopsy or postmortem examination.

Cerebrospinal fluid analysis reveals normal cells but elevated IgG and IgG antibody titers in dilutions > 1:8. Electroencephalographic patterns are normal in stage 1 but in the myoclonic phase suppression burst episodes are seen that are characteristic but not pathognomonic for SSPE. Brain biopsy is no longer routimely indicated for diagnosis of SSPE.

Management of SSPE is primarily supportive and similar the care provided to patients with other neuro-degenerative diseases clinical trials using Isoprinosine with or without interferon suggest significant benefit (30-34% remission rate) compared to patients without treatment (5-10% with spontaneous remission).

Virtually all patients eventually succumb to SSPE most die within 1-3 years of onset from infection or loss of autonomic control mechanisms prevention of SSPE depends on prevention of primary measles infection through vaccination. SSPE has been described in patients who have no history of measles infection and only exposure to the vaccine virus. However of measles infection and only exposure to vaccine virus however wild type virus not vaccine virus has been found in brain tissue of at least some of these patients suggesting that they had subclinical measles previously.

A review of the effect of measles vaccination on the epidemiology of SSPE has demonstrated that measles vaccination protects against SSPE and does not accelerate the course of SSPE or trigger the disease in those already infected with wild measles virus.

Staging of SSPE is done according to modified Jabbour classification as follows stage I mental and behavioural changes forgetfulness, irritability and lethargy. Stage II myclonic jerks dyskinesia, choreoathetosis, afaxia, Stage II decerebrate rigidity and decorticate rigidity and stage IV severe loss of all cortical function. Flexion posturing of limbs and mutism.

WILSON DISEASE

Clinical Features

Wilson disease can present with hepatic, neurological or psychiatric disturbances, alone or in combination. The age at onset ranges from 3 to older than 50 years. Hepatic failure is the prominent clinical feature in children younger than 10 years of age, usually without neurological symptoms or signs. Neurological manifestations with only minimal symptoms of liver disease are more likely when the onset of symptoms is in the second decade. A single symptom such as a disturbance of gait or speech is often the initial features and may remain unchanged for years. Eventually the initial symptoms worsen and new features develop (dysarthria, dystonia, dysdiadochokinesia, rigidity, gait and postural abnormalities, tremor and drooling).

Dystonia of bulbar muscles is responsible for three prominent features of the disease, dysarthria, a fixed pseudosmile (risus sardonicus), and a high-pitched whining noise on inspiration.

Psychiatric disturbances precede the neurological abnormalities in 20% of cases. They range from behavioral disturbances to paranoid psychoses. Dementia is not an early feature of the disease.

The Kayser-Fleischer ring a yellow brown granular deposit at the limbus of the cornea is a certain indicator of the disease. The causes is copper deposition in the descement membrane. It is present in almost all patients with neurological manifestations, although it may be absent in children with liver disease alone.

Diagnosis

Hepatolenticular degeneration is a consideration in any child with dysarthria and dystonia. The association of chronic liver disease with the neurological disturbances increase the probability of hepatolenticular degeneration.

The detection of low serum copper and ceruloplasmin concentrations and increased urinary copper excretion or the demonstration of a Kayser-Fleischer ring by slit-lamp examination establishes the diagnosis. Ninety-six percent of patients will have a serum ceruloplasmin concentration of less than 20 mg/dl corresponding to less than 56 g/dl of ceruloplasmin copper. Molecular genetics testing of the ATP7B gene (Chromosomal locus 13q14.3-q21.1) is clinically available.

MENKES SYNDROME TRICHOPOLIO-DYSTROPHY OR OCCIPITAL HORN SYNDROME

Menkes syndrome has low tissue concentrations of copper due to impaired intestinal copper absorption, accumulation of copper in other tissues, and decreased activity of copper dependent enzymes such as dopamine p-hydroxylase and lysyl oxidase. The defect maps to chromosome xq(B) (Kaler, 2005).

Clinical Features

Affected infants are healthy until age 2 months of age and then show loss of developemental milestone, hypotonia and seizures. The appearances of the scalp hair and eyebrows is almost pathognomonic. The hair is sparse, poorly pigmented and wiry. The shafts break easily, forming short stubble (kinky hair). Radiographs of the long bones suggest osteogenesis imperfecta other facial abnormalities include abnormal fullness of the cheeks, a high-arched palate and micrognathia. Temperature instability and hypoglycemia may be present in the neonatal period. Death usually occurs by 3 years of age.

Occipital horns, are distinctive, wedge shaped calcifications at the sites of attachment of the trapezius muscle and the sternocleidomastoid, muscle to the occipital bone. Occipital horns may be clinically palpable or observed on skull imaging. Other features of the syndrome are lax skin and joints, bladder diverticula, inguinal hernias, and vascular tortuosity. Intellect is normal or slightly reduced.

Autonomic dysfunction, including temperature, instability and hypoglycemia, may be present in the neonatal period. Death occurs by age 3 years. Infants with occipital horn syndrome show developmental arrest and regression by age 3 months. The infant becomes lethargic and less reactive. Myoclonic seizures, provoked by stimulation, are an early and almost constant feature. By the end of the first year, infants are in a chronic vegetative state, and most die before 18 months of age.

Diagnosis

Low plasma concentrations of ceruloplasmin and copper suggest the diagnosis. A protocol of mutation analysis, mutation scanning, and sequences analysis detects mutations in more than 95% of patients. Such testing is clinically available. Prenatal diagnosis is possible.

Neurological and Systemic Features of Infantile Menkes-Onset Kinky Hair Syndrome

- Premature birth
- Low birth weight
- Neonatal jaundice
- Hypothermia
- Decreased facial expression
- Prominent forehead
- Full cheeks
- Narrow palate
- Hypopigmented skin
- Cutis laxa
- Pilitorti
- Inguinal hernia
- Hepatomegaly
- Deafness
- Bladder diverticula
- Joint laxity

Skeletal Anomalies

- Pectus excavatum
- Wormian skull bones
- Metaphyseal spussing of long bones
- Ataxia
- Seizures
- Intracranial hemorrhage

Neuroimaging Findings

- Cerebellar and cerebral atrophy.
- White matter abnormalities.
- Subdural fluid collections.

Dilated and tortuous intracranial and extracranial blood vessels cerebral edema.

NEUROMETABOLIC DISORDERS (MC Kusick,1991)

Disease Category	Estimated Number
Organic acidurias	50
Aminoacidopathies	20
Lysosomal storage disorders	20
Fatty acid oxidation disorders	9
Congenital lactic acidoses	6
Peroxisomal disorders	6
Urea cycle disorders	5
Neuronal ceroid lipofuscinoses	3

Includes sphingolipidoses, mucopolysaccharidoses and glycoprotein degradation disorders.

PROPORTION OF METABOLIC ABNORMALITIES DETECTED DURING A 3-YEAR PERIOD (Borden, M-1984)

Disease Category	No. of Patients	Parent
Organic acidurias	112	50
Amino acidopathies	72	32
Purine and pyrimidine disorders	25	11
Miscellaneous	18	7
Total	**227**	**100**

URINE SCREENING TESTS FOR NEUROMETABOLIC DISORDERS (Menkes, 1990)

Disorder	Ferric Chloride	DNPH	Reducing Substances	Nitroprusside	CTAB/ Berry Spot
PKU	+	+	–	–	–
Galactosemia	–	–	+	–	–
Organic aciduria	+	+	–	–	–
Amino aciduria	–	+	–	–	–
Homocystinuria	–	–	–	+	–
Mucopolysaccharidosis	–	–	–	–	+

CTAB = Cetyl trimethylammonium bromide.
DNPH = Dinitrophenyl hydrazine.
PKU = Phenylketonuria.

FIVE TYPES OF INHERITED NEUROMETA-BOLIC DISORDERS (Saudubray, 1989)

Group	Acidosis	Ketosis	Lactate	Ammonia	Diagnosis
I	–	+	–	–	MSUD
II	+	+	–	–	Organic aciduria
III	+	+	+	–	Lactic acidosis
IV	–	–	–	+	Urea cycle disorder
V	–	–	–	–	NKH. Sulfite oxidase. Peroxisomal. respiratory chain

MSUD = Maple syrup urine disease

NKH = Nonketotic hyperglycinemia.

Clinical Features of Organic Acidurias

Disorder	Vomiting	Poor Feeding	Respiratory Problems	Encelphalopathy	Urine Odor
Methylmalonic aciduria	+	+	+	+	+
Propionicaciduria	+	+	+	+	–
Isovaloric aciduria	+	+	+	+	+
Multiple carboxylase deficiency	+	+	+	+	–

Clinical Syndromes Associated with Congenital Lactic Acidosis

Disorder	Encephalopathy	Recurrent Vomiting	Respiratory Abnormalities	Liver Failure	Myopathy
Leigh diseases	+	–	+	–	–
Alpers diseases	+	+	–	+	–
Kearns Sayre syndrome	+	–	–	–	+
MERFF	+	–	–	–	+
MELAS	+	+	–	–	+

Alpers disease = Progressive neuronal degeneration with liver diseases; Kearns Sayre syndrome = Progressive external ophthalmoplegia; Leigh disease = subacute neurotizing encephalopathy.

MELAS = Mitochondrial encephalopathy with lactic acidosis and stroke-like episodes.

MERFF = Mitochondrial encephalopathy with ragged – red fibers.

Laboratory Study	CDSD0	OTCD	Reye	LPL	Organic aciduria
Acid-base status	Respiratory	Respiratory	Respiratory	Respiratory	Metabolic
Plasma	Alkalosis	Alkalosis	Alkalosis	Alkalosis	Acidosis
Glucose	Normal	Normal	Normal/low	Normal	Low
Urine orotate	Normal	High	Normal	High	Normal
Plasma glycine	Normal	Normal	Normal	Normal	High
Plasma lysine	Normal	Normal	Increased	Low-Normal	–
Urine-lysine	Normal	Normal	Normal	High	Normal
Urine oranic acids	Non-specific	Non-specific	Non-specific	Non-specific	Specific abnormalities

LABORATORY VALUES USEFUL IN DIFFERENTIATING DISEASES PRESENTING WITH HYPER-AMMONEMIA AFTER THE NEONATAL PERIOD

Clinical Features of Peroxisomal Disorders

Disorder	Encephalopathy	Dysmorphic features	Hypotonia	Seizure	Dearness	Blindness
Adrenoleukodystrophy (X-linked)	+	–	–	+	–	–
Zellweger Syndrome	+	+	+	+	+	+
Neonatal adrenoleukodystrophy	+	+	+	+	+	+
Adrenomyeloneuropathy	–	–	–	–	–	–
Infantile Refsum	+	+	+	+	+	+
Rhizomelic Chondrodysplasia punctata	+	+	–	–	–	+

CLINICAL FEATURES OF THE MUCOPOLYSACCHARIDOSES (Nyhan WL 1987)

Eponym/MPS Number	Mental Retardation	Coarse Facies	Hepatosplenomegaly	Dysostosis Multiplex	Corneal Clouding
Hurler/IH	+	+	+	+	+
Hunter/II	+	+	+	+	–
Sanfilippo/III	+	–	–	–	–
Morquio/IV	–	–	–	+	+
Maroteauxlamy/VI	–	–	–	+	+
Scheie/IS	–	–	–	–	+
Sly/VII	–	–	+	+	–

CLINICAL FEATURES OF THE NEURONAL CEROID LIPOFUSCINOSES (Menkes JH 1990)

Disorder	Mental Retardation	Myoclonic Seizures	Loss of Vision	Inclusions	Ataxia
Early Infantitle (Santavuorihaltia)	+	+	Early	Granular	Marked
Late Infantile (Jansky-Bielschouski)	+	+	Late	Curvillinear Fingerprint	Marked
Juvenile (Spielmayer Vogt)	+	Occasional	Early	Fingerprint	Marked

Diagnosis is by demonstration of typical inclusion bodies by electron microscopic examination OR vacuolated. Lymphocytes in skin or Conjunctival biopsy.

DISEASES DISPLAYING A CHERRY-RED MACULAR SPOT (Bradley 2012)

1. GM1 gangliosidosis.
2. GM2 gangliosidosis (Tay Sachs and Sandhoff type) Sialidosis.
3. Niemann-Pick disease types A to D (not E and F); ring may be diffuse and indistinct.
4. Farber lipogranulomatosis.
5. Matachromatic leukodystrophy.
6. Neuronal ceroid [lipofuscionosis, late infantile form ('blue eye', maculopathy) not true Cherry-red spot)].

PELIZAEUS-MERZBACHER DISEASE

Clinical Features

- Disorders related to PLP1 are a continuum of neurological findings from severe central nervous system involvement (Pelizaeus-Merzbacher Disease) to spastic paraplegia.
- Disease characteristics are usually consistent within families. The first symptoms of the neonatal form suggest spasmus nutans. The neonate has an intermittent nodding movement of the head and pendular nystagmus chorea or athetosis develops, psychomotor development arrests by the third month and regression follows.
- Limb movements become ataxic and tone becomes spastic, first in the legs and then in the arms. Optic atrophy and seizures are late occurrences. Death occurs by 5 to 7 years of age.
- The later the disease onset is the slower the progression of the disease and the more prolonged the course. Survival to adult life is relatively common.

Diagnosis

MRI shows diffuse demyelination of the hemispheres with sparing of scattered small areas. Molecular genetic testing is available for diagnosis and carrier detection.

CANAVAN DISEASE (ASPARTOACYLASE DEFICIENCY)

Clinical Features

Psychomotor arrest and regression occur during the first 6 months postpartum.

Clinical features include decreased awareness of the environment difficulty in feeding, irritability and hypotonia.

Eventually, spasticity replaces the initial flaccidity.

A characteristic posture, with leg extension, arm flexion, and head retraction, occurs, especially when the child is stimulated.

Macrocephaly is evident by 6 months of age. The head continues to enlarge throughout infancy, and this growth reaches a plateau by the third year. Optic atrophy leading to blindness evolves between 6 and 10 months. Life expectancy is the second decade.

Diagnosis

Molecular genetic testing is not commercially available. Abnormal excretion of N-acetylaspartic acid is detectable in the urine, and aspartoacylase activity in cultured fibroblasts is less than 40% of normal. MRI shows diffuse symmetrical leukoencephalopathy even before neurological symptoms are evident. Demyelination of peripheral nerves does not occur, and the CSF is normal. Molecular genetic diagnosis is available for the mutation is Ashkenazi jews.

GM1 GANGLIOSIDOSIS

It occurs due to deficiency of the enzyme acid β-galactosidase resulting in defect in ganglioside degradation and its accumulation in neurons leading to neurodegeneration. The gene is located in chromosome 3p22.3.

In infantile form, that is present at birth, there are feeding problems, rash, hepatoplenomegaly, psychomotor regression, seizures, rigidity, deafness and also skeletal abnormalities. Hurler like feature is common. Anterior beaking of vertebral bodies can occur. Fundus may show cherry-red spots. In juvenile form the onset is late, by about 1 year and there is ataxia, dysarthria, spasticity, blindness. Diagnosis is established by detection of the deficient enzyme through enzyme assay in leucocytes and cultured fibroblasts. Transmission is autosomal recessive. There is no treatment.

GM2 GANGLIOSIDOSIS (TAY-SACHS DISEASE)

It occurs from deficiency of the enzyme hexosaminidase A resulting in abnormal accumulation of ganglioside in CNS and subsequent neurodegeneration. There is mutation in the HEXA gene in chromosome 15q23.

The onset is usually between two and six months in an otherwise normal infant. Exaggerated startle reaction to noise is common and often characteristic. Facies is often doll like. The baby loses interest in the surroundings and there is loss of acquired motor functions and visual ability. Progressive spasticity, decerebrate posture and seizures soon develop. Macrocephaly develops soon. A bright cherry-red spot in fundus is a common finding. Diagnosis is established by determination of the deficient enzyme in leucocytes and cultured fibroblasts. Transmission is autosomal recessive. There is no therapy. The disease is common in Ashkenazi jews. Currently accurate carrier detection has been successful in marked reducing the incidence of the disease.

JUVENILE GM2 GANGLIOSIDOSIS

Develops in mid-childhood. Important features are clumsiness, ataxia, followed by spasticity, athetosis, seizures. Cherry-red spot may be seen in fundus, Deficiency of hexosaminidase is variable.

SANDHOFF DISEASE

It is similar to Tay-Sachs disease and results from deficiency of the enzymes hexosaminidase A and B. Mutation in the HEXB gene, seen in this disorder, is located on chromosome 5q13. Psychomotor retardation, seizures, macrocephaly and splenomegaly occurs. Diagnosis is established by deficient levels of the enzymes hexosaminidase A and B in serum and leukocytes. BERA and also VEP may be abnormal later.

METACHROMATIC LEUCODYSTROPHY (MLD)

It is a relatively common form of leukodystrophy seen in India. The basic defect in metachromatic leucodystrophy is the deficiency of the enzyme aryl sulfatase A in brain and other tissues resulting in accumulation of cerebroside sulphate in white matter causing demyelination. It is transmitted as an autosomal recessive trait. The ARSA gene is located in chromosome 22q13.33.

Clinical manifestations usually appear by about 1 year of age, but the onset may be much later in childhood. Initially, there is disturbance in gait, frequent falls, progressive impairment in locomotion. Child becomes dull and apathetic, develops dysarthria and diminished visual fixation. Examination usually reveals hypotonia, weak to absent deep tendon reflexes, nystagmus, optic atrophy, decorticate posture and pseudobulbar palsy. Occasional case may show spasticity with hyperreflexia and extensor plantar response. As the disease progresses there is flaccidity with atrophy of distal muscles. Eventually the child becomes bedridden and demented and mostly succumbs before tenth birthday. In the juvenile type, onset of symptoms is delayed to 5-10 years of age. Deterioration in school performance, and gradual ataxia dysarthria, spasticity, dystonia and seizures develop. Diagnosis is confirmed by demonstration of reduced or absent aryl sulfatase A in one or more body tissues. Metachromatic granules in urinary sediment stained by toluidine blue can be used as a screening test. CSF protein is often raised. Nerve conduction study, BERA and VEP may show abnormality. Intrauterine diagnosis is possible by estimation of the enzyme aryl sulfatase A in the cultured cells of the amniotic fluid. Neuroimaging studies with MRI or CT scan show characteristic diffuse symmetric attenuation of cerebral and cerebral white matter. There is no specific treatment; bone marrow transplant and also stem cell therapy under trial seems to be promising.

KRABBE DISEASE (GLOBOID CELL LEUKODYSTROPHY)

It is due to the deficiency of the enzyme galactocerebroside β-galactosidase resulting in accumulation of galactocerebroside in white matter, commonly myeline sheath, with subsequent destruction. Transmission is autosomal recessive.

The child presents in infancy with irritability, hyperpyrexia, feeding difficulty, seizures, gradual onset of rigidity, hyperreflexia, visual impairment, and optic atrophy. Enlargement of the head is common. Degeneration of peripheral nerves may lead to hypotonia. death usually occurs within 2 years. Late onset KD have visual disturbance, optic atrophy, rigidity, spasticity, ataxia cortical blindness. Diagnosis is established by detecting the deficient enzyme by assay leucocytes and cultured fibroblasts. CSF protein is often elevated. Intrauterine diagnosis is possible by culture of amniotic fluid. Neuroimaging studies like CT and MRI show demyelination in white matter. Stem cell transplant has shown promise if done before symptoms appear. There is no specific treatment.

VAN DER-KNAPP DISEASE

Clinical Features

- Age at onset is between 2 months and 3.5 years. The initial features are episodes of irritability or focal neurological deficits. Steady clinical deterioration follows, often with spasticity and bulbar dysfunction leading to death.

Diagnosis

MRI shows a patchy leukoencephalopathy with cavity formation first affecting the corpus callosum and centrum semiovale. Later, large cystic lesions appear in the brain and spinal cord. Elevated levels of lactate in the brain, blood, and CSF suggest a mitochondrial disturbances.

MUCOPOLYSACCHARIDOSIS (TYPE I) (HURLER SYNDROME)

Clinical Features

- MPS type I (MPS I) is a progressive multisystem disorder with mild to severe features. The traditional classification of Hurler Syndrome. Huler-Scheie Syndrome or Scheie Syndrome, has been discarded in favor of the terms severe MPS I or attenuated MPS I. Individuals with MPS I appear normal at birth. Coarsening of the facial features occurs within the first 2 years. Progressive skeletal dysplasia (dysostosis multiplex) involving all bones occurs in all children develop progressive and profound mental retardation. Death, caused by cardiorespiratory failure, usually occurs within the first 10 years of life.
- The greatest variability occurs in individuals with the attenuated MPS I. Onset is usually between ages 3 and 10 years. Although psychomotor development may be normal in early childhood, individuals with attenuated MPS I may have learning disabilities.
- The rate of disease progression and severity ranges from death in the second to third decades to a normal life span with significant disability from motion of all joints. Hearing loss and cardiac vascular disease are common.

Diagnosis

The physical and radiographic appearance suggests the deiagnosis. Deficiency of the enzyme $\alpha - \mathrm{L} -$ iduronidase in peripheral blood leukocytes (or) cultured fibroblasts establishes the diagnosis. Mutation analysis is used for prenatal diagnosis.

MUCOPOLYSACCHARIDOSIS (TYPE II) (HUNTER SYNDROME)

Clinical Features

Patients with the Hunter Syndrome have a Hurler phenotype but lack corneal clouding. Iduronate sulfatase is the deficient enzyme: dermatan sulfate and heparan sulfate are stored in the viscera and appear in the urine.

The Hurler phenotype may develop rapidly or evolve slowly during childhood and go unrecognized until the second decade or later.

A prominent feature is the appearance of a nodular ivory-colored lesion on the back, usually around the shoulders and upper arms. Affected children have short stature and macrocephaly, with or without communicating hydrocephalus, macroglossia, hoarse voice, conductive and sensorineural hearing loss, hepatomegaly and/or splenomegaly, dysostosis. Multiplex, and joint contractures that include ankylosis of the temporomandibular joint, spinal stenosis, and carpal tunnel syndrome.

Mental regression caused by neuronal storage of gangliosides is slowly progressive, but many patients come to medical attention because of chronic hydrocephalus.

Affected children survive into adult life. The accumulation of storage materials in collagen causes the entrapment of peripheral nerves, especially the median and ulnar nerves.

Diagnosis

The presence of mucopolysacchariduria, with equal excretion of dermatan sulfate and heparan sulfate suggests the diagnosis.

Establishing the diagnosis requires showing enzyme deficiency in cultured fibroblasts or serum. The detection of iduronate sulfatase activity in amniotic fluid is useful for prenatal diagnosis.

MUCOPOLYSACCHARIDOSIS (TYPE VII) (SLY DISEASE)

Clinical Features

The patient has an incomplete Hurler phenotype, with hepatosplenomegaly, inguinal hernias, and dysostosis multiplex as the major features. Corneal clouding does not occur, and the face, although unusual, is not typical of the Hurler phenotype. Psychomotor retardation develops after age 2 but not in all cases.

Diagnosis

Both dermatan sulfate and heparan sulfate are present in the urine, causing a screening test to be positive for mucopolysacchariduria.

Specific diagnosis requires the demonstration β of glucuronidase deficiency in leukocytes or cultured fibroblasts.

MUCOPOLYSACCHARIDOSIS (TYPE III) (SANFILIPPO SYNDROME)

Clinical Features

The Hurler phenotype is not prominent, but hepatomegaly

is present in two thirds of cases. Dwarfism does not occur. The major features is neurological deterioration characterized by delayed motor development beginning toward the end of the second year, followed by an interval of arrested mental development and progressive dementia. Hyperactivity and sleep disorders are relatively common between the ages of 2 and 4 years.

Retardation in most affected children is severe by age 11, and death occurs before age 20. However, considerable variability exists, and MPS type III is a consideration even when the onset of mental regression occurs after age 5.

Diagnosis

Suspect the diagnosis in infants and children with progressive psychomotor regression and a screening test positive for mucopolysacchariduria. The presence of heparan sulfate but not dermatan sulfate, in the urine is presumptive evidence of the disease. Definitive diagnosis requires the demonstration of enzyme deficiency in cultured fibroblasts.

NIEMANN-PICK DISEASE TYPE-C (SPHINGOMYELIN LIPIDOSIS)

Clinical Features

Age at onset and predominant symptoms distinguish three phenotypes. Characteristic of the early – onset form is organomegaly and rapidly progressive hepatic dysfunction during the first year, often in the first 6 months. Developmental delay occurs during the first year, and neurological deterioration (ataxia, vertical gaze apraxia and dementia): occurs between 1 and 3 years of age.

The delayed–onset form is more common than the other two and has the most stereotyped clinical features. Early development is normal. Cerebellar ataxia or dystonia is the initial feature (mean age, 3 years), and apraxia of vertical gaze and cognitive difficulties follow (mean age, 6 years).

Oculomotor apraxia, in which the eyes more reflexively but not voluntarily, is unusual in children.

Vertical gaze apraxia is particularly uncommon and always suggests Niemann-Pick disease type C. Progressive neurological degeneration is relentless. Dementia, seizures and spasticity cause severe disability during the second decade. Organomegaly is seldom prominent early in the course.

The late – onset form begins in adolescence or adult life. It is similar to the delayed – onset form except that the progression is considerably slower.

Diagnosis

Biochemical testing that demonstrates impaired cholesterol esterification and positive filipin staining in cultured fibroblasts confirm the diagnosis.

ADRENOLEUKODYSTROPHY (ALD)

It is a sex-linked disorder associated with leukodystrophy because of accumulation of VLCFA due to disruption of transport of saturated fatty acid into peroxisome resulting in continued elongation of progressively longer fatty acids chain.

The disease usually presents around 5 years of age. Clinically the childhood cerebral form presents with hyperactivity, deterioration in school performance. Gradually affection of auditory discrimination, disturbance in vision, poor handwriting strabismus, ataxia, seizures start manifesting. In some cases, intracranial hypertension, mass lesion, impaired cortical response to stimulation and mild pigmentation occur. Ultimately progressive encephalopathy occurs leading to a vegetative state. MRI characteristically shows symmetric involvement in periventricular white matter in posterior parietal and occipital lobe also corpus callosum. Abnormally high levels of VLCFA in plasma, RBC and cultured fibroblasts is found. Impaired adrenal function is common in about 80% of cases. Treatment consists of treatment of adrenal insufficiency other supportive therapy. BMT and stem cell therapy seems promising. Some cases present late, around adolescence, by about 10 years of age. A predominant feature in them is long tract signs, often paraparesis (Adrenomyeloneuropathy).

ALEXANDER DISEASE

Alexander disease is a rare disorder caused by a mutations in the gene encoding, reduced nicotinamide adenine dinucleotide ubiquinone.

Oxidoreductase flavoprotein – 1 disease transmission is autosomal dominant most affected newborns represent new mutations.

The abnormal gene maps to chromosome 17q21 and encodes glial fibrillary acidic protein.

Rosenthal fibres, the pathological hallmark of disease, are rod-shaped or round bodies that stain red with hematoxylin and eosin and black with myelin stains. They appear as small granules within the cytoplasm of astrocytes. Rosenthal fibers are scattered diffusely in the cerebral cortex and the white matter but they have a predilection for the subpial, subependymal and perivascular regions.

Clinical Features

Diagnosis formerly depended on autopsy. Clinical features expanded with the accuracy of antemortem diagnosis.

Infantile, juvenile and adult forms are recognized. The infantile form is the most common. It accounts for 70% of cases with an identifiable glial fibrillary acidic protein mutation.

The onset is anytime from birth to early childhood. Affected infants, show arrest and regression of psychomotor development, enlargement of the head secondary to megalencephaly, spasticity and seizures.

Megalencephaly, may be the initial features, optic atrophy does not occur. Death by age 2 or 3 years is the rule.

Diagnosis

Four of the five following criteria establish an MRI – based diagnois of Alexander disease.

1. Extensive cerebral white matter abnormalities with a frontal preponderance.
2. A periventricular rim of decreased signal intensity on T2-weighted images and elevated signal intensity on T1-weighted images.
3. Abnormalities of the basal ganglia and thalami.
4. Brainstem abnormalities, particularly involving the medulla and mid brain; and
5. Contrast enhancement of one or more of the following ventricular lining periventricular rim; frontal white matter, optic chiasm, basal ganglia, thalamus, dentate nucleus, brainstem. Genetic testing confirms the diagnosis.

PEROXISOMAL DISORDERS

Clinical Features

Affected newborns respond poorly and have severe hypotonia, arthrogryposis and dysmorphic features. Sucking and crying are weak. Tendon reflexes are hypo active or absent.

Characteristic craniofacial abnormalities include a pear-shaped head owing to a high forehead and an unusual fullness of the cheeks, widened sutures, micrognathia, a high-arched palate, flattoning of the bridge of the nose and hypertelorism. Organ abnormalities include biliary cirrhosis, polycystic kidneys, retinal degeneration and cerebral malformations secondary to abnormalities of neuronal migration. Limited extension of the fingers (camptodactyl) and flexion deformities of the knee and ankee characterize the arthrogryposis.

Neonatal seizures are common. Bones stippling (chondrodysplasia punctata) of the patella and other long bones may occur.

Older children have retinal dystrophy, sensorineural hearing loss, developmental delay with hypotonia and liver dysfunction.

Infants with Zellweger syndrome are significantly impaired and usually die during the first year of life, usually having made no developmental progress. The clinical courses of neonatal adrenoleukodystrophy and infantile Refsum's disease are variable; some children can be very hypotonic and others learn to walk and talk. These conditions are often slowly progressive. Difficult-to-control seizures often begin shortly after birth but may commence any time during infancy. Death from aspiration, gastrointestinal bleeding, or liver failure usually occurs within 6 months to 1 year.

Diagnosis

Diagnosis is established definitely by biochemical assay. Confirm biochemical abnormalities detected in blood and or using with cultured fibroblasts.

Measurement of plasma very-long-chain fatty acid levels is the most commonly used and most informative increases in c26:0 and c26:1 and the ratios c24/c22 and c26/c22 are consistent with a defect in peroxisomal fatty acid metabolism.

HALLERVORDEN-SPATZ SYNDROME

Pantothenate kinase–associated neurodegeneration, previously called Hallervorden-Spatz Syndrome is neurodegeneration with brain iron accumulation. It is a genetic disorder transmitted as an autosomal, recessive trait. The abnormality is in the pank 2 gene; the chromosome locus is 20p13. Two other genetic disorders causing iron deposition in the globus pallidus are aceruloplasminemia and neuroferrifinopathy.

Clinical Features

The characteristic features of pantothenate kinase associated neurodegeneration are progressive dystonia and basal ganglia iron deposition. The disorder becomes symptomatic between 2 and 10 years of age in more than half of patients, but may appear as late as the third decade.

Other features are choreoathetosis, rigidity and dysarthria. Two thirds of patients have a pigmentary retinopathy. Mental deterioration and spasticity follow, with progression to spastic immobility and death within 5 to 10 years.

Diagnosis

The MRI features and molecular genetics testing are the basis for antemortem diagnosis. T2-weighted MRI shows low-intensity signal images from the globus pallidus, with a central area of increased signal intensity, the eye-of-the-tiger sign postmortem examination shows degeneration of the pallidum and substantia nigra with deposition of iron containing material.

LEIGH DISEASE

Clinical Features

Onset of subacute necrotizing encephalomyelopathy is typically between 3 and 12 months of age.

Decompensation, often with lactic acidosis, occurs during an intercurrent illness. Features may include psychomotor regression with hypotonia, spasticity, movement disorders (including chorea), cerebellas ataxia and peripheral neuropathy. Extra neurological manifestations may include hypertrophic cardiomyopathy.

Most individuals have a progressive course with episodic deterioration interspersed with variable periods of stability during which development may be quite stable or even show some progress. Death typically occurs by 2 to 3 years of age, most often due to respiratory or cardiac failure. The features of neurogenic muscle weakness, ataxia and retinitis pigmentosa are neuropathy, ataxia and pigmentary retinopathy. Episodic deterioration interrupts periods of stability, often in association with illnesses.

Diagnosis

Lactate concentrations increase in blood and/or CSF. Lactic acidemia is usually more common in postprandial samples. An oral glucose load causes blood lactate concentrations to double after 60 minutes and is more consistent in CSF samples than blood samples. Blood concentrations of lactate and pyruvate are usually increased and increase even more at the time of clinical exacerbation. MRI greatly increases diagnostic accuracy.

MRI features include bilateral symmetrical hyperintense signal abnormality in the brainstem and/or basal ganglia on T2-weighted images. Approximately 10% to 20% of individuals with subacute necrotizing encephalomyelopathy have detectable abnormalities on molecular genetic testing.

Conclusion

Neurodegenerative diseases can also include: progressive myoclonic encephalopathies and epileptic encephalopathies, and neuromuscular deterioration disorder, but this description of them, it will be beyond the scope of this chapter.

BIOTINIDASE DEFICIENCY

Clinical Features and Diagnosis

The initial features in untreated infants with profound deficiency are seizures and hypotonia. Ketoacidosis, hyperammonemia and organic aciduria are present–Showing biotinidase deficiency in serum, during newborn screening, establishes the diagnosis, in profound biotinidase deficiency, mean serum biotinidase activity is less than 10% of normal. In partial biotinidase deficiency, serum biotinidase activity is 10% to 30% of normal. Recurrent myclopathy and spinal cord involvement are described as the child grows up infancy.

POMPE DISEASE (ACID MALTASE DEFICIENCY)

Clinical Features and Diagnosis

- Infants with acid maltase deficiency have glycogen storage in both skeletal and cardiac muscles. Tendon reflexes are hypoactive or unobtainable. Measuring acid maltase activity cultured skin fibroblasts establishes the diagnosis of acid maltase deficiency. This disease though come under progressive neuromuscular disorder, this should be thought in case of hypotonic infant and cognitive decline.

GLUTARIC ACIDEMIA TYPE I

Clinical Features and Diagnosis

- Megalencephaly is usually present at birth. Neurological findings may be otherwise normal. Affected infants are at first hypotonic and later have mild developmental delay and dyskinesias, and seizures. Metabolic acidosis may be present. Abnormal urinary concentration of glutaric, 3-hydroxyglutaric, 3-hydroxybutyric and acetoacetates are detectable.

GLUCOSE TRANSPORTER PROTEIN DEFICIENCY (DE VIVO DISEASE)

- A defect of glucose transporter protein (GLUT1) leads to impaired glucose transport into the brain and a disease that usually starts in infancy with severe seizures, typically resistant to conventional anticonvulsant medications. This condition is caused by a spontaneous dominant mutation in the gene coding GLUT1 on chromosome 1.
- At a later age, the child exhibits signs of mental retardation, motor delay, impaired language development. The ketogenic diet effectively controls the seizures and other paroxysmal activities in patients with GLUT 1 deficiency, but it has less effect on the cognitive symptoms.
- There is reduced CSF glucose and lactate, and CSF/blood glucose ratio is low (0.33+ 0.07).

REFSUM'S DISEASE (PHYTANIC ACID STORAGE DISEASE)

- Refsum's disease, **heredopatia atactica pyneuritiformis,** is a rare autosomal recessive disorder of phytanic acid metabolism. The gene defect has been localized to chromosome 10 and encodes the peroxisomal enzymes, phytanoyl–CoA hydroxylase.
- The defect in the enzyme that initiates the alpha–oxidation pathway of β-methyl substituted fatty acids leads to phytanic acid accumulation in serum and tissues. Phytanic acid is derived exclusively from dietary sources, mainly chlorophyll, dairy products, meats and fish oils.
- Progressive sensorineural hearing loss, anosmia, cardiomyopathy, and ichthyosis are common. CSF protein is increased in the range of 100 to 700 mg/dl.
- Docosahexaenoic acid has been found to be deficient in peroxisomal disorders, but supplementation does not lead to clinical improvement even though docosahexaenoic acid plasma levels do increase.

SOME CLINICAL CLUES

Conditions showing progressive ataxias:

Abetaliproteinemia. Ataxia telangiectasia. Friedreich ataxia. Maple syrup. Urine disease. Juvenile GM2 gangliosidosis. Pyruvate dehydrogenase deficiency. Refsum's disease. Marinesco-Sjögren's syndrome. Respiratory chain disorders.

Fundus changes in neurodegenerative disorders:

Cherry red spots – Cherry red spot myoclonus syndrome. Farber's lipogranulomatosis. GM1 Gangliosidosis. GM2 gangliosidosis. Metachromatic leucodystrophy. Neimann-Pick disease. Sialidosis type III retinal degeneration–Pigmentary–Refsum's disease.

Causes of Corneal Clouding:

Cerebrohepatorenal syndrome (Zellweger syndrome). Fabry's disease. Tangier's disease. Juvenile MLD.

- **Dysmorphic features** are seen in mucopolysaccharidosis and chromosomal disorders. Facial dysmorphism is also seen in infantle neuroaxonal dystrophy which has pathological features of Hallervorden Spatz disease.
- **Organomegaly** is seen in neuro visceral storage disorders. Both type II and type III Gaucher disease will have predominant splenomegaly along with features of hypersplenism. Sandhoff's disease will have hepatosplenomegaly with Tay-Sach's features.
- **Megalencephaly:** Alexander's disease, Van der Knaap disease, MLD, MPS, MSUD, glutaric aciduria type I, globoid leucodystrophy, galactosemia.
- **Progressive chorea** with intellectual deterioration along with cardiomyopathy is a features of Leigh's disease.
- **Progressive dystonia** is seen in Hallervorden-Spatz disease.
- **Microcephaly** is usually a common features of neurodegenerative disease. Characteristic acquired. Microcephaly is a feature of Rett's syndrome and AIDS encephalopathy.

SUMMARY

1. Neurodegenerative disorders in children form a heterogeneous group of disorders that result in a progressive deterioration of acquired skills which is the hallmark.
2. Grey matter involvement produces seizures, progressive cognitive impairment and loss of speech and vision.
3. Mitochondrial disorders are to be suspected in presence of exercise intolerance with raised serum lactate.
4. Moya moya, as a progressive vasculopathy, cause recurrent strokes and pseudobulbar signs with end stage incapacitation.
5. SSPE and AIDS encephalopathy are infective cause of progressive encephalopathies.
6. DNA mutational analysis is useful in diagnosing many disorders including mitochondrial disorders apart from muscle biopsy.
7. Neuroradiological investigation has made a major breakthrough in the diagnosis of many leucoencephalopathies along with MRS peaks.

Suggested Reading

- Adams RD. Lyon G. Neurology of Hereditary Metabolic Diseases of Children. New York. McGraw-Hill. 1982.
- Ampola MG. Organic Acid Disorder in Metabolic Diseases in Pediatric Practice. Boston. Little Brown. 1982.
- Bodensteimer JB. Guest Editor. The Pediatric Clinics of North America (Pediatric Neurology) 1992 Volume 39–Number 4.
- Borden M. Screening for Metabolic Disease. In Nyhan WL (ed). Abnormalities in Aminoacid Metabolism in Clinical Medicine Norwalk CT. Appleton–Century–Crofts 1984:401.
- Borrett D. Becker LE. Alexander's Disease: A Disease of Astrocytes 1985:108:367-85.
- Brusilow SW. Horwich AL. Urea Cycle Enzymes. The Metabolic Basis of Inherited Disease. in Scriver CR. Beaudet AL. Sly Ws. New York. Mc Graw Hill 1989:629.
- Burri BJ. Sweettnan L. Nyhan WL. Mutant Holocarboxylase Synthetase J. Clin Invest 1981:68(6):1491-95.
- Carballo EC. McKusick V. Detection of Inherited Neuro-metabolic Disorders (A Practical Clinical Approach): Mendelian Inheritance in Man. ed 9. Baltimore. Johns Hopkins University Press. 1991.
- Clarke LA. Mucopolysaccharidoses Type I: In Gene Clinics: Medical Genetics Knowledge Base. http://www.geneclinics.org University of Washington. 2007: September 21.
- Dahipale R. Jain S. Agarwal M. Biotimdase Deficiency Indian Pediatr 2008:45:777-79.
- Daroff RB *et al.*. Principles of Diagnosis and Management. Neurology in Clinical Practice (Bradley's). Sixth edition. Volume 1. 2012.
- Daroff RB *et al.*. Principles of Diagnosis and Management. Neurology in Clinical Practice (Bradley's). Sixth edition. Volume 2. 2012.
- Enrique Chaver E. Carballo MD. McKusick V. Detection of Inherited Neurometabolic Disorders (A Practical Clinical Approach). Mendelian Inheritance in Man. ed 9. Baltimore. Johns Hopkins University Press. 1991.
- Fenichel GM. Clinical Pediatric Neurology: A Signs and Symptoms Approach. Sixth edition. 2009.
- Frank Y. Ashwal S. Neurologic Disorders Associated with Gastrointestinal Disease. Nutritional Deficiencies and Fluid Electrolyte Disorders. In: Pediatric Neurology: Principles and Practice. 4th Edition. Swaiman K.
- Garbern J. Krajewski K. Hobson G Pelizaeus – Merzbacher Disease: In Gene Clinics: Medical Genetics Knowledge Base. http://www.geneclinics.org University of Washington. 2006: September 15.
- Goraspe JR Alexander Disease: in Geneclinics. Medical Genetics Knowledge Base. http://www.geneclinics.org Seattle. University of Washington 2007: March 9.
- Gregory A. Pantothenate Kinase-Associated Neuro-degeneration. University of Washington 2009: January 9.
- Kaler SG ATP7A - Related Copper Transport Disorders: In Geneclinics: Medical Genetics Knowledge Base. http://www.geneclinics.org Seattle. University of Washington 2005:July 13:28.
- Kaler SG. ATP7A - Related Copper Transport Disorders. In Gene Clinics: Medical Genetic Knowledge Base [database online] Seattle. University of Washington 2007:November 6. at http://www.geneclinics.org.
- Kendall BE. Disorders of Lysosomes. Peroxisomes and Mitochondria. Am J Neuroradiol 1992:13:621-53.
- Kennard C. Clinical Neurology. Number Seven. Sep 1994 (Recent Advances in Clinical Neurology) 1994.
- Kliegman Stanton. St Geme Schor. Textbook of Pediatrics (Part I to XV) (Volume 1). First South Asia Edition 2015 (Nelson).
- Kliegman Stanton. St Geme Schor. Textbook of Pediatrics (Part XVI to XXI) (Volume 2). Copyright © 2016. 2015 (Nelson).
- McKusick V. Mendelian Inheritance in MA John Hopkins. Baltimone. University Press. 1991.
- Menkes JH. The Textbook of Child Neurology Metabolic Disease of the Nervous System: Lea and Febiger 1990: P28.
- Metalon R. Canavan Disease In: Geneclinics: Medical Genetics Knowledge Base. http://www.geneclinics.org University of Washington 2006:March 15.
- Naidu S. Bibat G. Lin D. Progressive Cavitating Leuko-encephalopathy: A Novel Childhood Disease. Ann Neurol 2005:58:929-38.
- Naidu S. Moser HW. Peroxisomal Disorder: Pediatric Clinic North America 1990:8:507-20.
- Nyhan WL. Sakati NO. Screening for Metabolic Disease: Diagnostic Recognition of Genetic Disease. Philadelphia. Lea and Febiger. 1987.
- Pascual JM. Wang D. Engelstad K. Saxena LM. Glucose. Supply and the Syndrome of Infantile Neuroglycopenia. Arch Neurol 2007: April 64:507-13. Epub 2007. February 12.
- Pascual JM. Wang D. Lecumberri B. Yang H. Maox. Yang R. De Vivo DC.GLUT1. Deficiency and Other Glucose Transporter Disease: Eur J Endocrinol 2004:May:L50(5):627-33.
- Patterson MC. Niemann-Pick Disease. Type C: In Gene Clinics: Medical Genetics Knowledge Base. http://www.geneclinics.org University of Washington 2007: November 1.
- Phelan JA. Lowe LH. Glasier C. Pediatric Neurodegenerative White Matter Processes: Leukodystrophies and Beyond. Pediatr Radiol 2008:38:729-49.
- Prabhakar S. Alexander M. SSPE Trophical Neurology Eds Shakir RA. Newman P. Poser LM. London: W.B. Saunders. Co 1995:77-95.
- Prabhakar S. Taly AB. Reviews in Neurology Continuing Medical Education Program of Indian Academy of Neurology. 2008.
- Roberts EA. Wilson Disease COXDW. In Geneclinics: Medical Genetics Knowledge Base. http://www.geneclinics.org University of Washington 2006: January 24.
- Robinson BH. Lactic Academia. The Metabolic Basis of Inherited Disease: Scriver CR. Beaudet AL–Sly WS *et al.* (eds): New York. McGraw-Hill 1989:869.
- Saha V. John TJ. Mukundan P. Gnanamuthu C. Prabhakar S. Arjundas G. High Incidence of Subacute Sclerosing Panencephalitis in South India1990:104:151-56.
- Saudubray JH. Ogier H. Bonnefont JP. Clinical Approach to Inherited Metabolic Disease in the Neonatal Period: A 20-Year Survey. 1989.
- Swaiman KF. Ashwal S. Ferriero DM. Schor NF. Pediatric Neurology. Fifth Edition. Principles and Practice (Swaiman's 2014) (Part X to XVII) (Volume 2). 2014.
- Swaiman KF. Ashwal S. Ferriero DM. Schor NF. Pediatric Neurology. Fifth Edition (Volume 1) (Part I and X). Swaiman's Child Neurology. 2014
- Sworeland PT. Johnson KP. SSPE (Subacute Sclerosing Panencephalitis and Other Paramyxovirus Inflections Vol. 12. (56) Holland Publishing Company 1989:417-37.
- Throburn DR. Rahman S. Mitochondrial DNA-Associated Leigh Syndrome and NARP University of Washington. 2006: September 22.
- Van Dor Knaap MS. Valk J. Barth PG. Leukoencephalopathy with Swelling in Children and Adolescents: MRI Patterns and Differential Diagnosis 1995:679-86 (Neuroradiology).
- Wolf B. Worldwide Survey of Neonatal Screening for Biotinidase Deficiency. J. Inherit Metab Dis 1991: 14(6): 923-27.

48 Chapter

HYDROCEPHALUS

Rajeev Kulshrestha

Excessive accumulation of cerebrospinal fluid in the ventricles of the brain associated with ventriculomegaly, thinning of the cortical mantle, and increased intracranial pressure is defined as hydrocephalus (Fig. 48.1 and B).

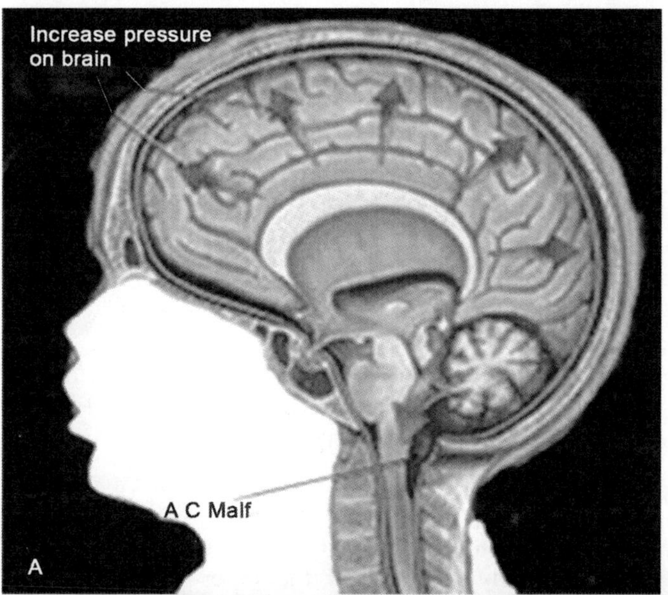

Hydrocephalus is the most common cause of large head in a child, which is a multifaceted problem. The pediatrician, by virtue of being the first contact, is the pacesetter and the coordinator for the long-term management plan of the hydrocephalus, in liaison with the surgeon, which includes comprehensive medical, social, occupational and economic rehabilitation of the affected child and the family. Therefore, it is mandatory that the pediatrician should be aware of the recent advances in the field of diagnosis and management of the hydrocephalus.

Now the first contact is ultrasonologist and obstetrician. Antenatal maternal ultrasonography confirms the presence of hydrocephalus in the first trimester. There are several options following antenatal detection of hydrocephalus. The options are:

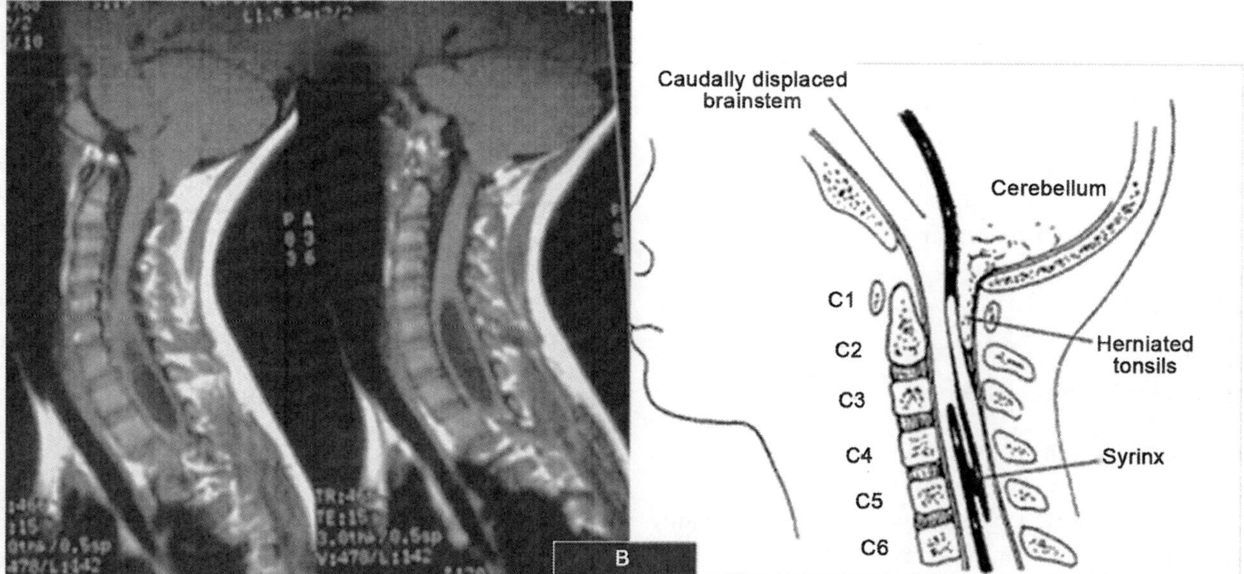

Fig. 48.1A and B: Arnold-Chiari Malformation (marked as AC Malf) showing extension of cerebellum and medulla into upper cervical canal

(a) Fetal intervention.

(b) Pregnancy to be continued if there are no other major associated anomalies.

(c) Termination of pregnancy if associated with anomalies, which are incompatible with life.

The decision making should be without any bias or on strong parental wishes. A multidisciplinary team consisting of obstetrician, ultrasonologist, pediatric geneticist and pediatric surgeon should review the antenatal diagnosis and management plan. Various studies have confirmed the alteration in the management, after the earlier decision was reviewed by the team, in large percentage of the cases.[1]

Incidence

The reported incidence of hydrocephalus is approximately 0.9-1.8 per 1000 live births. The incidence of hydrocephalus associated with spina bifida is approximately 1-3 per 1000 live births. Hydrocephalus is associated in almost 80-90% of the babies born with open neural tube defect.[2] However, the last decade has witnessed steady decline in the incidence of neural tube defects and hydrocephalus.

Family History

2% of all the cases of isolated hydrocephalus may occur as X-linked recessive condition. The overall risk of recurrence in other sibs is 1 in 65 (1.5%). It is about 15-30 times the risk in general population.

Antenatal Diagnosis

Hydrocephalus can be identified as early as 12th week of gestation on routine maternal ultrasonography. The incidence is 0.5 to 2 per 1000 fetuses. The criteria to define ventriculomegaly in the fetus is measurement of ventricles in the region of atria, which is 7.6 mm + 0.6 mm. A measurement above 10 mm suggests ventriculomegaly.

A thorough search of associated anomalies must be made with antenatal diagnosis of ventriculomegaly, as in approximately 70% cases there are associated CNS anomalies.[3]

Pathophysiology

The ventricular system consists of two lateral ventricles, one-third ventricle and one-fourth ventricle. All the four ventricles are connected by narrow pathways. Normally CSF flows through the ventricles, exits at the base of brain into cisterns, which are closed spaces and acts as reservoir. CSF then flows towards surface of the brain and spinal cord and is absorbed into blood stream.

CSF has many putative functions, which are as follows:

a. CSF keeps the brain tissue buoyant, thus provides mechanical protection.

b. It helps in distribution of neuroendocrine factors.

c. It also acts as the carrier for delivering nutrients to the brain cells and also in removing the waste.

d. It facilitates pulsatile cerebral blood flow. CSF flows between the cranium and spine to compensate for changes in the intracranial blood volume.

CSF movement allows arterial expansion and contraction by acting like a spring, which prevents wide changes in the intracranial blood flow. When disorders of CSF flow occur, it may also affect intracranial blood flow and subsequent neuronal and glial vulnerabilities.[4]

a. Cerebrospinal Fluid (CSF) Formation

Formation of CSF is at following sites:

i. Choroidal

Choroid plexus is the major site of CSF formation. Most of the choroid plexus is situated in the medial wall of the lateral ventricles.

ii. Extrachoroidal

Secretions from brain parenchyma across ependymal cells is the other source of CSF formation.

Exact mechanism of CSF formation is not known. Average rate of CSF formation is 0.35 ml/minute, i.e., approximately 500 ml in 24 hours. Choroid plexus in lateral, third and fourth ventricles produces 50-80% of CSF remaining CSF is produced by ventricular ependyma and brain parenchyma as a byproduct of cerebral metabolism.

b. Cerebrospinal Fluid Absorption

CSF flows in caudal direction through the ventricular system and exits by way of foramina Luschkae and Magendie into cortical and subarachnoid space. CSF then travels through tentorial incisura, passes over the convexity of cerebral hemisphere and is absorbed into the venous system at the level of arachnoid villi, which is a collection of mesothelial cells, which invaginates the dura mater in the lateral lacunae of the superior sagittal sinuses.

Rate of CSF absorption depends on pressure gradient from the subarachnoid space across the arachnoid villi to the venous space in the dural venous sinuses.

The balance between production and absorption of CSF is critically important. Hydrocephalus is invariably due to:

i. Obstruction in the CSF pathways. This is the most common cause of hydrocephalus.
ii. Impaired absorption.
iii. Rarely there may be overproduction of CSF, e.g., in papilloma of choroid plexus.

Pathological effects of the obstruction in the CSF pathway or impaired CSF absorption generates increased intracranial pressure, resulting in:

i. Ventricular dilatation, which is often more pronounced in the occipital horns.
ii. Thinning of the cerebral mantle.
iii. Disruption of the ependymal membrane.
iv. Transependymal absorption of the CSF into the periventricular white matter.
v. White matter injury, edema and scarring.

In some children CSF absorption can occur through alternate pathways, resulting in stabilization of ventricular enlargement. This in turn leads to arrested hydrocephalus. Arrest of the progressive enlargement of the ventricles occur in approximately 45% of the cases. These children should be closely monitored and regularly followed up for any changes in the clinical status.

CLASSIFICATION

Broadly Hydrocephalus is classified[5] as:

A. Communicating

CSF pathways are obstructed in the region after it exits from ventricles, i.e., basal cisterns, arachnoid villi or subarachnoid spaces. CSF leaves the ventricular system through patent foramina in the roof of 4th ventricle. The term communicating relates to the fact that the CSF can still flow between the ventricles, which remain open.

B. Non-Communicating

It occurs when the CSF flow is blocked along one or more of the narrow pathways, which connect the ventricles. This type is called as non-communicating or obstructive type, because blockage of the CSF pathway is proximal to foramina of 4th ventricle, which prevents the CSF from reaching the subarachnoid spaces.

ETIOLOGY

A. Congenital

Congenital hydrocephalus is present at birth. The incidence is gradually declining due to antenatal diagnosis and termination of pregnancy. Congenital hydrocephalus is caused by a complex interaction of genetic predisposition and environmental factors. Following are some of the common causes of congenital hydrocephalus.[6,7]

a. Aqueduct Obstruction:

Non-hereditary aqueductal obstruction is the most common cause and accounts for 70% cases. Most common causes of aqueductal obstruction are:

i. **Forking:** Two or more channels replaces single channel.
ii. **Gliosis:** Overgrowth of subependymal neuroglia.
iii. **Narrowing:** Narrowing or septa formation can be a rare cause.

In approximately 2% cases aqueductal obstruction could be sex linked with recessive inheritance. Affected children have following features:

i. Only male babies are affected.
ii. Occasionally other sibs or some family members without hydrocephalus may be mentally retarded.
iii. Mental retardation is severe, which is disproportionate to ventriculomegaly.

Placement of shunt does not improve mental retardation.

b. Obstruction at Foramina of Monroe:

It results in ventriculomegaly of lateral ventricles.

c. Obstruction at the Outlet of IVth Ventricle:

Congenital atresia of foramina of Magendie and

Luschkae causes hydrocephalus. Agenesis of corpus callosum is very commonly associated with this and may be responsible for poor overall intelligence.

d. *Dandy-Walker Syndrome Consists of:*

i. Posterior fossa cyst.

ii. Hypoplasia of cerebellar vermis.

iii. Associated ventriculomegaly of variable degree.

e. *Myelodysplasia:*

70-80% cases of spina bifida have associated ventriculomegaly of variable grades. Associated Arnold-Chiari's malformation has causative role in development of hydrocephalus of some degree in almost every case of spina bifida.[8]

The deformity consists of displacement of the following in the region of cervical canal (Fig. 48.1):

i. Tongue of tissue from inferior vermis of the cerebellum.

ii. Elongated medulla oblongata.

Due to above there is crowding in the region and adhesions forms between tongue of cerebellum and roof of IVth ventricle, resulting in obstruction of the outlet of 4th ventricle. The outcome is mild to moderate. Hydrocephalus in significant percentage of the cases.

Despite high percentage of associated hydrocephalus with spina bifida, only about 20% have evidence of ventriculomegaly at birth. It becomes appreciably apparent during the first few weeks of postnatal period.

Thoracolumber spina bifida is associated with highest incidence of ventriculomegaly (95%), while lowest (65%) is associated with lumbosacral myelomeningocele.

f. *Intrauterine Infection:*

Toxoplasma infection usually occurs in second trimester of pregnancy and causes hydrocephalus by vascular occlusion as well as by obliteration of aqueduct of sylvius. Cytomegalovirus causes severe meningoencephalitis resulting in basal adhesive arachnoiditis. Other viral infections causing intrauterine infection are lymphocytic choriomeningitis and group B Coxsackie virus.

g. *Encephalocele:*

It may have associated hydro-cephalus due to obstruction to CSF pathways or may be associated with distorted ventricular anatomy.

h. *Intracranial Cysts:*

It may cause ventriculomegaly due to obstruction of the CSF pathways.

i. *Skull Base Anomalies:*

It may result in ventriculomegaly.

B. Acquired

a. *Infection:*

Perinatal and postnatal infections *viz.* leptomeningeal inflammation or meningitis can cause obstruction at the aqueduct, or at basal cisterns. The important causes of infection are:

i. **Viral infections:** Toxoplasma or cytomegalic virus.

ii. Pyogenic or tubercular meningitis.

b. *Intraventricular Hemorrhage (IVH):*

In premature neonates IVH usually occurs during severe respiratory distress at the time of delivery or during postnatal period. IVH can occur *in utero* also. Site of IVH is usually subependymal germinal matrix of the lateral ventricles. Hemorrhage may extend later in the ventricles or in brain parenchyma in severe cases. Factors, which precipitate intraventricular hemorrhage, are:

i. Cerebral hypoxia.

ii. Systemic blood pressure changes with severe fluctuations.

iii. Coagulopathies.

Hydrocephalus develops due to obliterative arachnoiditis within posterior fosse as a sequel of hemorrhage. Severe hemorrhage may sometimes causes aqueductal blockage also.

In large majority of cases IVH is mild to moderate and there is tendency to resolve. However, in some cases it may lead to progressive hydrocephalus with elevated intracranial pressure and deteriorating clinical status. Surgical interference is indicated in these situations.

c. *Trauma:*

There may be intracranial bleeding in head trauma, which may result in adhesive arachnoiditis of basal and subarachnoid spaces. Bleeding may also result in blockage of the aqueduct.

d. *Neoplasm:*

Neoplasm causes hydrocephalus either due to obstruction of the CSF pathways or as a result of hemorrhage in the ventricles. Some examples are:

i. Posterior fossa tumors *viz* medulloblastoma, cerebellar astrocytoma or ependymoma, which may obstruct either aqueduct or outlet of 4th ventricle.

ii. Tumors in pineal region block aqueduct.

iii. Hypothalamic or thalamic glioma block 3rd ventricle.

iv. Anterior ventricular glioma or giant subependymal astrocytoma typically obstructs foramen of Monroe.

Preoperative shunting or endoscopic third ventriculostomy is indicated when hydrocephalus is life threatening and/or tumor removal is delayed.

e. *Cranioskeletal Anomalies:*

Macrocephaly or large head is usually associated with achondroplasia, the presenting features of which are as follows:

i. Mild to moderate enlargement of ventricles.

ii. Subarachnoid space of cerebral convexities is prominent.

iii. Associated with mental retardation.

iv. Hydrocephalus tends to arrest spontaneously. Shunting is rarely necessary.

PRESENTING FEATURES

Hydrocephalus is detected in large majority of cases before birth of the baby. Due to routine antennal ultrasonography. However, it must be emphasized that not in all the cases, ventriculomegaly is progressive. Therefore, after birth these babies must be evaluated and followed up to confirm the diagnosis.

The clinical manifestations of hydrocephalus are diverse. It is mandatory to detect hydrocephalus in early stage so as to prevent cerebral parenchymal damage. Hallmark of the diagnosis is an inordinate rate of head growth with macrocephaly.[9,10]

Enlargement of Head

In the early postnatal period head circumference even in congenital hydrocephalus may be normal but later it increases. The cardinal signs of hydrocephalus is:

i. **Large Head:** Head circumference more than 90th percentile for the age.

ii. Abnormal increase of head circumference on serial measurements.

Normal head circumference at birth is 33-35 cms. As an approximate calculation, in normal babies it increases by 2 cms every month for the first 3 months. From 3rd to 6th month of age, head circumference increases by approximately 1.5 cms every month. From 7th to 9th month it increases by one cm every month and than 1.5 cms every 2 months.This method is just an approximate calculation for knowing the head circumference of the baby at the particular age (Fig. 48.2).

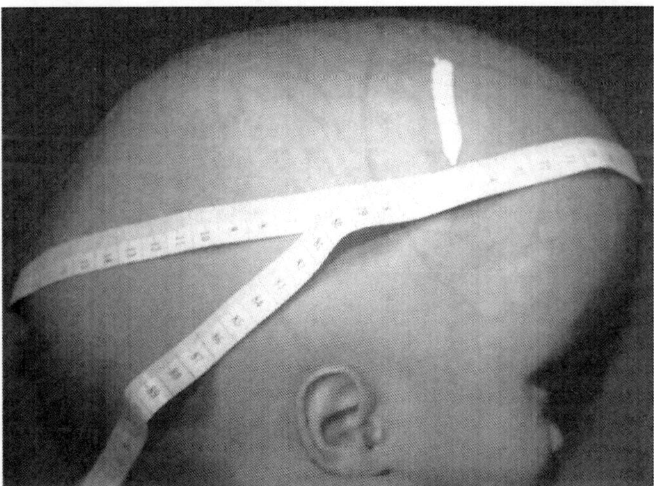

Fig. 48.2: Measurement of head circumference by measuring tape. The tape must be over both parietal and occipital prominence

For accurate information head circumference charts are available. The markings of serial measurements indicate the normal or abnormal head.

Clinical manifestations of hydrocephalus vary depending on the patient's age, cause of obstruction and the extent of brain tissue damage. The presenting features are divided as follows:

I. NEONATES AND INFANTS

A. Early Clinical Features

a. Large head.

b. Progressive head circumference.

c. Bulging fontanelle.

d. Sutural separation of the skull.

e. Vomiting.

B. Continued Features

a. Continued features are due to raised intracranial pressure, which are as follows:

   i. Infant is irritable, cries excessively, and refuses to accept feeds.

   ii. Later baby starts vomiting resulting in failure to thrive.

b. Muscle spasticity.

c. Poor temperature control.

C. Late Clinical Features

Abnormal Size and Shape of Head

i. Head circumference progressively increases more rapidly as compared to normal growth.

ii. Anterior fontanelle is wide, and may be bulged out. Normal pulsations at fontanelle are absent.

iii. There is frontal bossing. Face appears smaller in comparison to large head.

iv. Skull bones are thinned out. There is sutural separation. Due to both, on percussion of skull there is crackpot sign (Mc Ewan's sign).

v. Skin of the scalp is thin and the scalp veins are full and prominent (Fig. 48.3).

vi. Eyeballs are rolled down (sunset sign) (Fig. 48.4). This is probably due to pressure of dilated 3rd ventricle on oculomotor nerve.

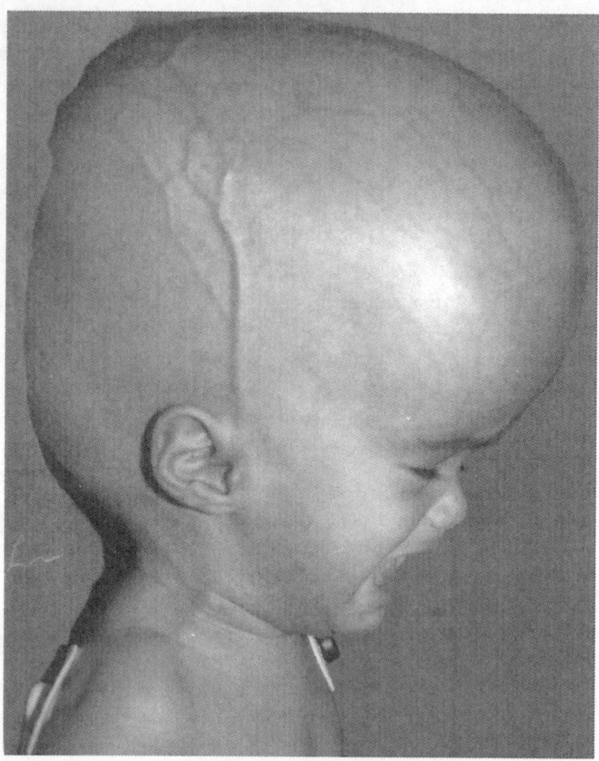

Fig. 48.3: Large head, prominent anterior cranial fosse, frontal bossing and prominent scalp veins

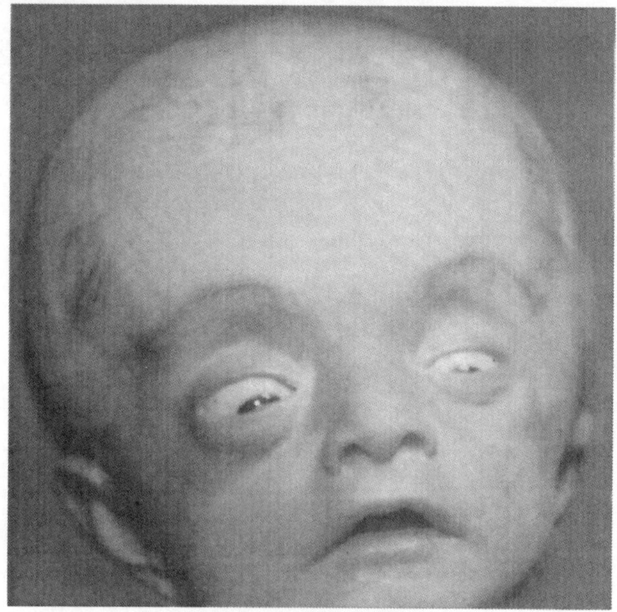

Fig. 48.4: Sunset sign

vii. Shape of the head becomes abnormal depending on the site of obstruction.

   1. If the obstruction is at aqueduct of sylvius, lateral and 3rd ventricles are dilated. Anterior fossa is large and posterior fossa is small. The head is

enlarged with prominent head and flat occiput.

2. When obstruction is at outlet of 4th ventricle, posterior fossa is large due to dilatation of 4th ventricle. Head is large with prominent occiput and flat forehead (Fig. 48.6).

   These features are visible on clinical examination as well as on X-ray skull lateral view.

a. *Neurological Signs:*

Neurological signs due to hydrocephalus per se are unusual. Some of the important neurological features are:

i. Internal strabismus may appear due to pressure on 6th cranial nerve.

ii. Increased extensor tone with spasticity of the lower limbs may be present, if there is pressure on the brainstem.

b. *Delayed Development:*

Due to atrophy of the cerebral cortex and progressive hydrocephalus following features are present:

i. Milestones are delayed. Early hydrocephalus influences the development and intelligence unevenly. Nonverbal capabilities are affected more than the verbal capabilities.

ii. Abnormalities of the eye movement, binocular vision, and acuity in conjunction with impaired motor and coordinated skill adversely influences nonverbal intelligence.

iii. Motor functions and language performance are retarded.

iv. Slow or restricted movements.

v. Feeding is difficult.

II. OLDER CHILDREN

As the skull suture are fused and fontanelle are closed the symptoms are due to raised intracranial pressure, which includes:

a. Headache.

b. Nausea and vomiting.

c. Lethargy.

d. Vision changes. Uncontrolled eye movements.

e. Loss of coordination. Difficulty in walking.

f. Mental aberration such as confusion or psychosis.

g. Decrease in mental abilities.

h. No appreciable enlargement of head circumference.

i. Retinal venous engorgement is a reliable early manifestation. Later papilledema may be evident.

DIFFERENTIAL DIAGNOSIS

One of the most important causes of large head is hydrocephalus. Other causes of large head are:

a. Subdural Hygroma:

There is fluid collection in the subdural region. Clinically appears as large head with frontal prominence.

b. Thickened Skull Bone:

Cranioskeletal dysplasia, e.g., osteoporosis, Russel's dwarfism.

c. Megalencephaly:

i. **Benign:** Familial or constitutional scaphocephaly.

ii. Familial large head.

iii. **Pathological:**

- Gigantism.
- Dwarfism.
- Lysozymal disorders viz. polysaccharide deficiency.

d. Hydranencephaly:

Transillumination of the skull in a dark room confirms the diagnosis.

INVESTIGATION

Clinical examination, neurological evaluation and cranial imaging techniques confirm the diagnosis of hydrocephalus. The pediatrician selects the appropriate diagnostic tool based on patient's age, clinical presentation and presence of known or suspected anomalies of the brain or spinal cord.

Abnormally increasing head circumference plotted on the head circumference chart is one of the very useful and reliable diagnostic tools.

Transillumination of the head should be done routinely in all the neonates with large head to detect hydranencephaly, subdural hygroma, porencephalic cyst, or hugely dilated ventricles.

X-Ray Skull

X-ray skull in AP and lateral views are done. It reveals:

i. Size of head .

ii. Sutural separation.

iii. Thinning of vault.

iv. Shape of the head which indicates site of obstruction.

v. Presence of calcification, which may indicate tumor.

a. *Ultrasonography:*

Antenatal:

Its role in antenatal diagnosis is very important. Hydrocephalus can be diagnosed at 10-12 weeks of intrauterine life.

Postnatal:

Postnatally, ultrasonography is possible only, if anterior fontanelle is open. It has important role in confirmation of the diagnosis and to monitor the intracranial changes. Ultrasonography gives valuable information on:

i. Ventriculomegaly: Sonographic criteria of early detection of hydrocephalus have been identified using precise measurements of occipital horns and lateral ventricular dimensions.

ii. Thickness of cerebral cortex.

iii. Intracranial pathology, viz., intracranial hemorrhage or brain tumors.

iv. Monitors the efficacy of the therapy.

b. *CT Scan:*

It gives detailed information of the size of ventricles, brain parenchyma and intracranial pathology (Figs. 48.5 and 48.6). It also helps with operative planning, as ventricles are usually dilated, proximal to the point of obstruction.

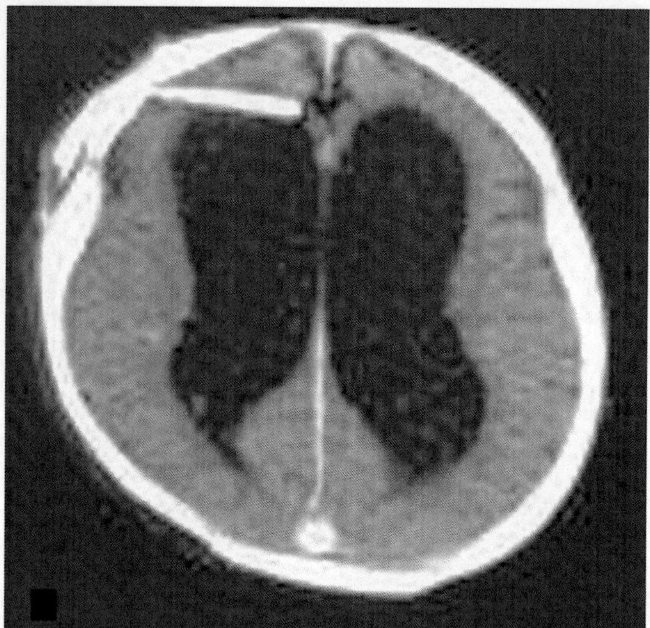

Fig. 48.5: CT scan showing enlarged lateral ventricles and tip of shunt seen at upper end

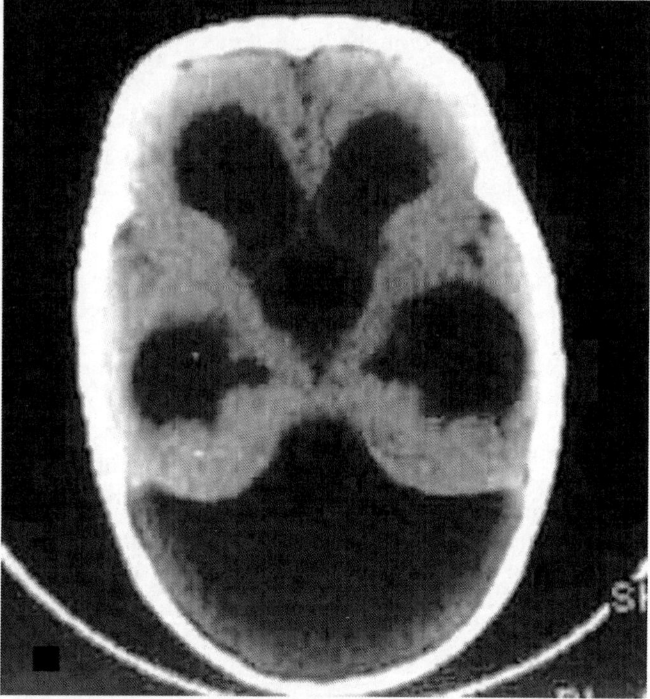

Fig. 48.6: CT scan showing enlarged 4th ventricle with dilatation of lateral and 3rd ventricle

c. *MR Imaging:*

MR imaging should be definitely done in cases of congenital hydrocephalus. MR scan delineates the associated anomalies in the brain such as corpus callosum agenesis, Arnold-Chiari malformation, and vascular malformations. T2-weighted images can show transependymal flow of cerebrospinal fluid.

CSF Dynamic Scan, Ventriculogram and Pneumoencephalogram, Intracranial Pressure (ICP) monitoring were done earlier, but now these investigations are not done due to invasive nature and inherent risk involved

MANAGEMENT

Presence of merely enlarged ventricles is not an indication for treatment per se. The indications for intervention are:

a. Progressive ventricular enlargement reflected as increased head circumference or on ultrasonographic examination.

b. Clinical evidence of adverse effects of raised intracranial pressure or neuronal deficiencies.

Aims of management are:

a. Achieve optimum neurological functions.

b. Prevent or reverse neurological damage due to ventriculomegaly and raised intracranial pressure.

I. NONOPERATIVE MANAGEMENT

Medical Treatment:

Medical therapy is usually a temporizing measure. In mild hydrocephalus or transient conditions it may be effective. Sometimes it is used to tide over crisis. It is mandatory to closely monitor the progress both clinically and ultrasonographically. Clinical and biochemical parameters should be carefully evaluated. If there is any deterioration in the clinical status, surgical intervention should be planned. Following drugs are used:

i. **Isosorbide:** The dose is 2 gms/kg every 6 hourly. It is not used due to very high dose and side effects.

ii. **Diuretics:** Furosemide (1mg/kg/day) interferes with chloride transport in the apical cells of the choroids plexus and can reduce CSF production by as much as 50% of the normal production. Mannitol can also be used.

iii. **Acetazolamide:** It seems to reduce secretion of CSF from choroid plexus. Dose is 25-100 mg/kg/day in two or three divided doses. It is useful in mild hydrocephalus.

II. OPERATIVE TREATMENT

A. Endoscopic Third Ventriculostomy (ETV)

This can be performed in certain types of obstructive hydrocephalus such as primary untreated aqueductal stenosis from tectal plate and pineal region tumours.[11]

Endoscopic third ventriculostomy is contraindicated in patients with communicating hydrocephalus.

Success rate is poor in patient with less than one year of age, and also in patients with preexisting pathology *viz* tumour, previous shunt surgery, prior subarachnoid hemorrhage etc.

ETV is done through a small hole made in the floor of 3rd ventricle by the endoscope. This allows CSF to bypass the obstruction and flow towards the site of resorption around the surface of brain. An ETV is a safe procedure with few complications and a high success rate. It eliminates the risk of CSF infection related to external drainage. It also minimizes the risk of over drainage as it provides more physiological drainage as compared to shunt placement.[12,13,14]

B. Endoscopic Aqueductoplasty and Placement of Stent

This procedure is useful in selected cases of symptomatic isolated fourth ventricle and membranous aqueductal stenosis. Endoscopic placement of a stent in aqueduct is more effective in preventing repeated occlusion of the aqueduct.[15,16]

New optics and smaller size endoscopes have revolutionized the treatment plan specially in noncommunicating hydrocephalus and obviates the need of shunt placement.

C. Placement of Shunt

Ventriculoperitoneal Shunt (VP Shunt) placement is the mainstay of the management of the hydrocephalus (Fig. 48.7A and B).

VP shunt tube is made of silastic material. It has two valves, which allows unidirectional flow of CSF from ventricles to peritoneum. One end of the tube (ventricular end) is put in the anterior

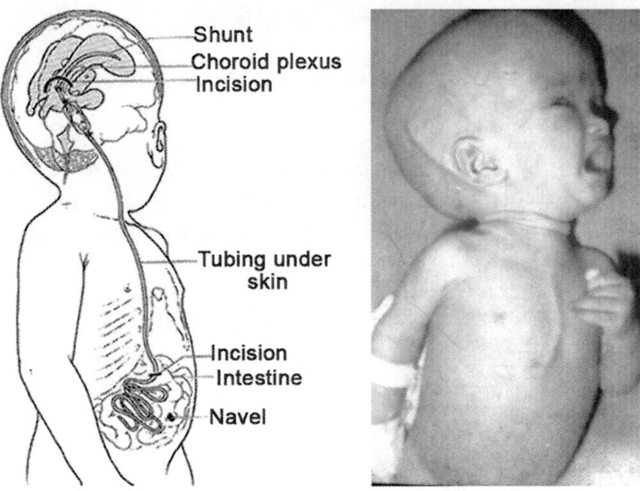

Fig. 48.7A and B: Ventriculoperitoneal shunt

horn of the lateral ventricle. Shunt tube is put in a skin tunnel from scalp, behind the ear to upper abdomen. After giving a small incision in right hypochondrium, peritoneum is opened and lower end of the shunt is placed between diaphragm and liver.

COMPLICATIONS

The incidence of shunt complications is approximately 25-30% over 1 year. They are maximum in first few months after shunt placement (Table 48.1).

Main complications after the shunt surgery are as follows:

Table 48.1: Complications of V-P Shunt

Early Complications	Late Complications
A. ***Mechanical:***	a. Seizures
a. Proximal shunt block	b. Slit ventricle syndrome
b. Malposition of ventricular end	c. Cranial synostosis
c. Block at peritoneal end of shunt	d. Visual changes, i.e., optic atrophy
d. Displacement of shunt tube at the site of connector	
e. Migration of shunt tube	
B. ***Infection:***	
a. Wound infection	
b. Shunt colonization	
c. Peritonitis	
d. Pseudocyst in peritoneal cavity	
C. ***Neurological:***	
a. Seizures	
b. Acute subdural hygroma	
c. Chronic subdural hygroma	

A. Shunt Block

Either ventricular or peritoneal end of the tube may get blocked due to cell debris. Due to block there is raised intracranial pressure with reappearance of sign and symptoms of hydrocephalus. Shunt block is confirmed by:

a. Clinical Examination:

The examination of the reservoir of the shunt, which lies behind the ear on the mastoid bone, gives clue to the site of obstruction.

In normally functioning tube, on compressing the reservoir, it empties and immediately fills on removing the finger pressure over it. The clue to the site of block is as follows:

i. Upper End Block

Reservoir remains flat after removal of the finger pressure on the reservoir of the shunt. It does not refill due to blockage of the ventricular end.

ii. Lower End Block

On pressing the reservoir, it does not empty out easily, instead remains turgid due to block of the peritoneal end.

b. Investigations:

The site of block can be confirmed by doing the dye study after shunt puncture.

B. Shunt Infection

The chances of shunt becoming infected are 3%-15%. Infections most often occur within first 3 months after shunt placement. Shunt gets colonized by the microorganisms *viz.* Staphylococcus.[17,18] The shunt colonization presents with pyrexia with rigors, signs and symptoms of raised intracranial pressure.

Investigations include blood culture and CSF cultures from shunt reservoir to guide antibiotic therapy. Treatment is to start broad spectrum antibiotics and the infected shunt tube is removed and is replaced by new shunt tube after 48-72 hours. Infected shunt must be removed. Endoscopic third ventriculostomy is emerging as an alternate option after shunt infection or malfunction. Infected shunt is removed and ETV is done. High success rate has been reported.[13]

Treatment of infected shunt with antibiotics alone is not recommended, as bacteria can be suppressed for extended periods. Once the antibiotics are discontinued, the bacteria can resurface.

C. Shunt Displacement

Shunt tube may get disconnected at the connector site and may get dislodged. The reappearance of symptoms of raised intracranial pressure and investigations confirms the diagnosis. Treatment is removal of the tube and placement of a new shunt tube.

D. Subdural Hygroma

Subdural hygroma may develop following sudden decompression after the placement of the shunt. The diagnosis is suspected when there is reversal of signs and symptoms of raised intracranial pressure and are confirmed by CT scan.

If subdural hygroma is small then repeated aspirations may be done. Subdural-peritoneal shunt is placed if the subdural hygroma is large.

E. Pseudocyst in the Abdomen

Abdominal pseudocyst is synonymous with low-grade shunt infection. A cyst develops around the lower end of shunt. Despite functioning shunt on clinical examination, symptoms of raised intracranial pressure may develop. Ultrasonography reveals pseudocyst. The treatment is removal of the shunt assembly and placement of a new shunt.

F. Migration of the Shunt

Commonly peritoneal end migrate to other parts of the peritoneal cavity. Hydrocele has been reported if there is associated patent processus vaginalis. Lower end has been reported to penetrate rectum and seen coming out through anus. In these cases lower end of shunt is removed and a new shunt assembly is put in either as an open operation or guided through laparoscope.

G. Slit Ventricular Syndrome (SVS)

SVS is a rare condition, in which brain compliance is unusually low. It mostly occurs in setting of prior ventriculitis or shunt infection. Typically it manifests as headache and other features of raised intracranial pressure.

On investigations, small ventricles are seen. When mechanical obstruction develops in SVS, ventriculomegaly is revealed on diagnostic imaging. Etiology is unknown. The treatment options are:

i. Subtemporal decompression that creates an artificial pressure reservoir and induces slight reenlargement of the slit ventricles.

ii. Replace low-pressure shunt valve with high resistance valve.

Prognosis

Prognosis is assessed in terms of physical, mental and intellectual development and depends to a large extent on the cause of hydrocephalus and duration of illness before the treatment.

Hydrocephalus diagnosed early and treated promptly has a good chances of achieving normal or near normal intelligence.

The children after the treatment should be regularly followed up for the development and shunt complications.

The expected overall survival rate in children is more than 80%.The intelligence quotient (IQ) of approximately half of the shunted children, with infantile hydrocephalus is near normal. Verbal intelligence is better developed than nonverbal functions.

Children's paced auditory serial addition tests have concluded that children with shunted hydrocephalus display deficit in working memory and information processing speed.[19]

References

1. Luks FI, Carr SR, Feit LR *et al.* Experience with a Multidisciplinary Antenatal Diagnosis and Management Model in Fetal Medicine. J. Matern Fetal Neonatal Med 2003:14;333-37.

2. Partington MD. Congenital Hydrocephalus, Neurosurg. Clin. N. Am 2001;36:737.

3. Prockop LD. Hydrocephalus in Merritt's Neurology Eds. LP Rowlands Pub. Lippincot Williams and Wilkins 11th Edition 2005:349-56.

4. Milhort TH, Hammock MK *et al.* Cerebrospinal Fluid Production by the Choroids Plexus and Brain. Science 1997:173:330.

5. Aronyk KE. The History and Classification of Hydrocephalus. Neurosurg. Clin N. Am 1993:4(4):599-609.

6. Chumas P *et al.* Hydrocephalus–What is New. Archives of Diseases in Childhood: Fetal and Neonatal Edition 2001:85(3): F149-54.

7. Seiff ME. Hydrocephalus: In Section of Developmental, Neurocutaneous and Genetic Metabolic Disorders. Manuals of Neurologic Practice. Eds. R W Evans. Pub. Saunders. Philadelphia 2003;889-95.

8. Fishman MA. Hydrocephalus in Section of Disturbances of Neural Tube Closure and Spine. In Rudolph's Pediatrics. Eds. Rudolph CD Pub. Mc Graw Hill. New York. 21st Edition 2003:2180-84.

9. Johnston MV. Kinsman S. Hydrocephalus in Section of Congenital Anomalies of Central Nervous System. In Nelson Textbook of Pediatrics. Eds. RE Behrmanel *et al*. Pub. Saunders Philadelphia 175th Edition 2004;1989.

10. Kulshrestha R. Hydrocephalus in Common Problems in Pediatric Surgery. Eds. R Kulshrestha. Pub CBS Publishers and Distributors. New Delhi. 2nd Edition 2006;340-47.

11. Smith JL. Management of Neural Tube Defects and Hydrocephalus. Refractory Epilepsy and CNS Infections. Pediatric Surgery Edition. Coran AG *et al.* Pub Elsevier Saunders 2012;1673-97.

12. Hayashi N . Hamada H *et al.* Transparent Endoscopic Sheath and Rigid Rod Endoscope Used in Endoscopic Third Ventriculostomy in the Presence of Deformed Ventricular Anatomy. J.Neurosurg 2006:104:321-25.

13. O'Brien DF. Javadpour M *et al.* Endoscopic Third Ventriculostomy: An Outcome Analysis of Primary Cases and Procedure Performed after VP Shunt Malfunction J. Neurosurg 2005:103:393-400.

14. Ruggiero C. Cinalli G *et al.* Endoscopic Third Ventriculostomy in Treatment of Hydrocephalus in Post Fossa Tumors. Childs Nerv. Syst 2004:20(11-12):828-33.

15. Cinalli G. Spennato P. Savareses L *et al.* Endoscopic Aqueductoplasty and Placement of Stent in the Cerebral Aqueduct in the Management of Isolated Fourth Ventricle in the Children J. Neurosurg 2006:104(1 suppl):21.

16. Ersahin Y. Endoscopic Aqueductoplasty With or Without Stent. Minim. Invasive Neurosurg 2006:49(2).124-25.

17. Kulkarni AV *et al.* Cerebrospinal Fluid Shunt Infection: A Prospective Study of Risk Factors. J. Neurosurg 2001;94(2): 195-201.

18. Vinchon M, Dhellemmes P. Cerebrospinal Shunt Infection: Risk Factors and Long-term Follow-up. Childs Nerv. Syst 2006:22(7).692-97.

19. Boyer KM. Yeates KO *et al.* Working Memory and Information Processing Speed in Children with Shunted Hydrocephalus: Analysis of Children's Paced Auditory Aerial Addition Test. J. Int Neuropsycol. Soc 2006:12(3):305-13.

49 Chapter

DRUGS AND DOSES

Devendra Mishra

Entails information on drugs used in some important Pediatric Neurological Disorders, their doses and important side effects, based on standard textbooks of pediatrics, textbooks of pharmacology and relevant literature.

Drugs	Indications	Doses (Post Neonatal)	Important Side Effects
Antiepileptics			
Diazepam	Controlling acute convulsion	0.3 mg/kg/dose, IV, slowly over 2-3 minutes; additional one bolus may be given after 5 min, if needed	Respiratory arrest, hypotension, bradycardia, cardiac arrest
Lorazepam	Do	0.1 mg/kg/dose, IV, over 2-5 min., additional one bolus, if needed, 0.05 mg/kg in 10-15 min	Tachycardia, drowsiness, depression, paradoxical excitement
Midazolam	Do	0.15 mg/kg loading followed by continuous IV infusion of 1 µg/kg/min	Respiratory depression, apnea, amnesia, paradoxical excitation
Phenytoin	Do	15-20 mg/kg/dose, IV, infusion: rate- 1mg/min	Hypotension, bradycardia, extravasation may cause tissue necrosis
Fosphenytoin	Do	15-20 PE/kg/dose, IV, slowly, infusion can be given at 2 PE/kg/min	Same as above but lesser cardiotoxicity
Phenobarbitone	Do	15-20 mg/kg/dose, IV, slowly, rate- 1 mg/min	Hypotension, bradycardia, arrhythmia, respiratory depression
Sodium valproate	Do	20 mg/kg, IV bolus over 10 min	Rash
Carbamazepine	AED prophylaxis of focal seizure, GTS, GTCS, dystonia, SSPE	10-30 mg/kg/day, PO, q-bid/tid, (therapeutic concentration 3-12 µg/ml)	GI disturbance, drowsiness, rash (can be severe simulating Stevens-Johnson Syndrome), diplopia, ataxia, leukopenia
Clobazam	AED prophylaxis of focal seizure, atypical absence, GTCS, myoclonic seizure, LGS (adjunctive therapy)	0.5-1 mg/kg/d, PO, q-od/bid	Dizziness, vomiting, sedation, somnolence, fatigue, behavior problems, suicidal ideation, ataxia, rash, leukopenia
Clonazepam	AED prophylaxis of LGS, myoclonic, akinetic, absence, infantile spasm	0.05-0.2 mg/kg/day, PO, q- bid/tid	Tachycardia, drowsiness, irritability, sedation, behavior disturbance, G.I. disturbances
Corticotrophin (ACTH)	AED prophylaxis of infantile spasms; also multiple sclerosis, severe myasthenia gravis	IS-150 u/m^2/day IM div. bid (75 units /m^2/dose), titrate according to response-tapering gradually; for immunosuppression 1.6 u/kg/day (aqueous) or 50 u/m^2, IM, IV, SC, q 6-8 hrs	Hypertension, opportunistic infection, epistaxis, pancreatitis, esophagitis, insomnia, mood disturbance

Contd.

Contd.

Felbamate	AED prophylaxis of focal seizure, GTCS, (adjunctive therapy) LGS	15-45 mg/kg/day, PO, q-tid	GI disturbance, headache, insomnia, ataxia, behavior and mood disturbance, leucopenia, thrombocytopenia, hepatotoxicity, aplastic anemia
Gabapentin	AED prophylaxis of focal seizure, focal to GTCS (adjunctive therapy)	30-60 mg/kg/day, PO, q-tid	Somnolence, dizziness, headache, tremor, behavior disturbance, GI disturbance, constipation, weight gain diplopia, nystagmus
Lacosamide	AED prophylaxis of focal seizure (adjunctive therapy)	4-12 mg/kg/d div q-bid	Being evaluated, reported are– irritability, tics, excessive crying, cardiac arrhythmia
Lamotrigine	AED prophylaxis of focal seizure, atypical absence, GTCS, LGS	2-15 mg/kg/day, PO q-od/bid; 1-5 mg/kg/d bid with enzyme inducers like valproate	Anorexia, nausea, dizziness, sedation, photosensitivity, shin rash (could be severe like Stevens-Johnson syndrome), diplopia, nystagmus.
Levetiracetam	AED prophylaxis of focal seizure, GTCS, Rolandic epilepsy, LGS, JME	10-60 mg/kg/day, PO, q-bid/tid	Anorexia, headache, somnolence, insomnia, behavior problems
Oxcarbazepine	AED prophylaxis of focal seizure, focal to GTCS	10-30 mg/kg/day, PO, q-bid	Headache, dizziness, ataxia, hyponatremia, diplopia, skin rash, GI disturbance, hyponatremia
Phenobarbitone	AED prophylaxis for GTS, GTCS, focal seizure	3-8 mg/kg/day, PO, q-od/bid, (therapeutic concentration 15-40 μg/ml)	Behavior disturbance (irritability, hyperactivity, lethargy), cognitive disfunction, rash
Phenytoin	AED prophylaxis of GTS, GTCS, focal seizure	3-8 mg/kg/day, PO, q-od/bid, or <3 yr: 8-10mg/kg/d >3 yr: 4-7 mg/kg/d (therapeutic conc. 10-20 μg/ml)	Gum hyperplasia, acne, hirsutism, lymphadenopathy, nystagmus, ataxia, anemia
Prednisolone	AED prophylaxis of infantile spasms, tapering doses after methylprednisolone	2 mg/kg/day, PO, q 6 hr (may use upto 4 mg/kg/d)	Hypertension, psychosis, cushingoid facies, peptic ulcer, opportunistic infection
Rufinamide	AED prophylaxis of focal seizure, LGS (adjunctive therapy)	30-45 mg/kg/d, q- bid	Being evaluated, reported are: nausea, vomiting, somnolence, headache, dizziness, contraindicated in familial short QT interval
Sodium valproate	AED prophylaxis of absence seizure, GTS, GTCS, focal seizure, JME, myoclonic, atonic, akinetic seizures, Infantile spasms, LGS	10-60 mg/kg/day, PO, q-tid/bid (therapeutic concentration 50-100 μg/ml)	GI disturbance, drowsiness, sedation, rash, weight gain, stomatitis, alopecia, tremor, thrombocytopenia, hepatitis, pancreatitis, coma
Stiripentol	AED prophylaxis of Dravet Syndrome (above 2 yeas of age) (adjunctive therapy)	50 mg/kg/d, div, q- bid/tid; max dose 3000 mg/d	Somnolence, anorexia, weight loss, agitation, nausea, vomiting, tremor, dysarthria
Tiagabine	AED prophylaxis of focal seizure (adjunctive therapy)	1.5 mg/kg/day, PO, q-bid/tid	Dizziness, drowsiness, ataxia, tremor, asthenia, nervousness, poor attention span
Topiramate	AED prophylaxis of focal seizure, seizures w LGS, (adjunctive therapy) infantile spasm	1-9 mg/kg/day, PO, q-bid/tid	Mental slowing, anorexia, weight loss, metabolic acidosis, hyperthermia, nephrolithiasis
Vigabatrin	AED prophylaxis of Infantile spasm, focal seizure (adjunctive therapy)	50-150 mg/kg/day, PO, q-bid	Visual field defect– bilateral constriction (persists even after withdrawal), behavior problems, GI disturbance, weight gain

Contd.

Contd.

Zonisamide	AED prophylaxis of focal seizure, GTS, GTCS, atonic myoclonic, absence (adjunctive therapy), infantile spasm	4-8 mg/kg/day, PO, q-bid	Anorexia, somnolence, dizziness, ataxia, weight loss, rash, hypohydrosis fever, renal stone, psychomotor slowing
Analgesics			
Acetaminophen	Pain from neurological disorders like spinal trauma, localized pain and inflammation, diskitis, sciatica, polyneuritis, headache	10-15 mg/kg/dose, PO, q 4-6 hrs or as needed – max dose 60 mg/24 hours	Hepatic toxicity, rash, rare hematologic dysfunction, overdosing may cause FHF
Diclofenac sodium	Do	2-3 mg/kg/day in divided doses, PO	Dizziness, headache, gastric upset, renal impairment
Ibuprofen	Do	8-10 mg/kg/dose, PO	Gastric upset, GI bleed, perforation, renal dysfunction
Gabapentin	Neuropathic pain	15-50 mg/kg/day q tid, PO; max 3600 mg/day	Somnolence, weight gain, GI upset, diplopia, ataxia, behavioral changes
Anti-Infective Agents (Antibacterial)			
Ampicillin (ß-lactam antibiotic)	Acute bacterial meningitis	200-400 mg/kg/day divided 4-6 hrly, IV	Hypersensitivity and drug rash, pseudomembranous colitis
Amikacin sulphate (aminoglycoside)	Acute bacterial meningitis, sp gram negative bacteria	15-22.5 mg/kg/day, div. 8-12 hly, IV	Nephrotoxicity and ototoxicity
Cefotaxime (3rd generation cephalosporine)	Acute bacterial meningitis	100-200 mg/kg/d divided 6-8 hrly, IV	Drug rash, eosinophilia, leucopenia, thrombocytopenia
Ceftazidime (3rd generation cephalosporine)	Acute bacterial meningitis sp from pseudomonas inf	100-150 mg kg/day divided 8 hrly, IV	Drug rash, eosinophilia, leucopenia, thrombocytopenia
Ceftriaxone sodium (3rd generation cephalosporine)	Acute bacterial meningitis	75 mg/kg stat, then 80-100 mg/kg/ day, divided 12-24 hrly, IV, IM	Drug rash, diarrhea, pseudomembranous colitis, hypoprothrombinemia, blood dyscrasia, raised liver enzyme, pancreatitis, oliguria, hematuria, biliary precipitates, bronchospasm
Chloramphenicol	Acute bacterial meningitis	75-100 mg/kg/day, divided 6 hrly, IV	Leucopenia, bone marrow suppression, grey baby syndrome, optic neuritis
Gentamicin (aminoglycoside)	Acute bacterial meningitis	2.5-5 mg//kg/day, divided 8-12 hrly, IV can go upto 7.5 mg/kg/day	Nephrotoxicity and ototoxicity
Meropenem (carbapenem antibiotic)	Acute bacterial meningitis, sp resistant bacteria	120 mg/kg/day, divided 8 hrly, IV	CNS excitation
Nafcillin sodium (penicillinase-resistant penicillin)	Acute bacterial meningitis specially resistant staph infection	100-200 mg/kg/day, divided 6 hrly, IV	Rash
Oxacillin	Acute bacterial meningitis specially resistant staph infection	200 mg/kg/day, IV, divided 6 hrly Also 50-100 mg/kg/day	Similar to penicillin
Penicillin G	Acute bacterial meningitis	300,000 units/kg/day, divided 4-6 hrly, IV	Hypersensitivity and drug dash, anaphylaxis, diarrhea, leucopenia, thrombocytopenia, eosinophilia, elevated liver enzyme

Contd.

Contd.

Vancomycin (glycopeptide antibiotic)	Acute bacterial meningitis specially for staph infection	45-60 mg/kg/day, divided 8-12 hrly, IV	Ototoxicity, nephrotoxicity, hypersensitivity reaction, neutropenia, eosinophilia
Anti-Infective Agents (Antifungal)			
Amphotericin B (desoxycholate form)	Fungal meningitis	0.8-1.2 mg/kg/day, od, IV 1-5 mg/kg/day for liposomal form	Several systemic side effects including nephrotoxicity
Amphotericin B (lipid complex formulation)	Fungal meningitis	5 mg/kg/day, od, IV	Do
Flucytocine	Fungal meningitis	50-150 mg/ kg/day, 6 hrly, IV	Insufficient data in pediatrics
Fluconazole	Fungal meningitis	6-12 mg/kg/day for prolonged period, 28 days for candida, 10-12 weeks for cryptococcal meningitis, PO	Headache, rash, angioedema, anaphylactic rash
Voriconazole	Fungal meningitis (histoplasmosis)	6 mg/kg/dose IV 12 hrly for 2 doses, then 4 mg/kg/dose 12 hrly	Insufficient data in pediatrics
Anti-Infective Agents (Anti-Tubercular)			
Ethambutol	Tuberculous meningitis	15-25 mg/kg/day PO, od-bid	Optic neuritis, impaired colour vision, G.I. upset, hypersensitivity
INH (Isoniazid)	Tuberculous meningitis	10-15 mg/kg/day, PO, od-bid	Hepatotoxicity, rash, peripheral neuritis, hypersensitivity
Pyrazinamide	Tuberculous meningitis	20-40 mg/kg/day, PO, od-bid	Hepatotoxicity, arthralgia, hyperuricemia, GI upset
Rifampicin	Tuberculous meningitis	10-20 mg/kg/day od, PO, early morning empty stomach	Hepatotoxicity, GI upset orange discoloration of secretions, thrombocytopenia, flu like reaction
Streptomycin	Tuberculous meningitis (resistant)	20-40 mg/kg/day, IM, od	Auditory and vestibular toxicity, nephrotoxicity
Miscellaneous Drugs			
Acetazolamide	Intracranial hypertension (chronic), i.e., hydrocephalus, benign intracranial hypertension; intractable epilepsy	25 mg/kg/day, PO, q t.i.d., can increase up to 100 mg/24 hr, Max. 2g/24 hr	Metabolic acidosis, hypokalemia, muscle weakness, aplastic anemia, decreased urate secretion, renal calculi, polyuria, GI irritation
Acetazolamide	Intractable epilepsy	8-30 mg/kg/day, PO, q-t.i.d.	Metabolic acidosis, hypokalemia, muscle weakness, as above
Alprazolam	Panic attacks	0.005-0.02, mg/kg/dose, PO, -t.i.d.	Drowsiness, confusion
Aspirin	Pain, fever from diverse neurologic disorders	10-15 mg/kg/dose, q 4-6 hr	Bleeding, ototoxicity; flue like symptoms, liver toxicity, allergic reactions
Baclofen	Spasticity associated with cerebral palsy, spinal cord lesion	0.2-2 mg/kg/d, q-bid/tid, max dose usually 80 mg; alternatively <8 yr: 60 mg/24 hr; 8-16 yr: 80 mg/24 hr; >16 yr: 120 mg/24 hr; Intrathecal dose 25-50 µg: <12 y: 274 µg/24 hr >12 yr:300-800 µg/24 hr	Drowsiness, ataxia, hypotonia, nausea, vertigo, rash, urinary frequency
Calcium gluconate (elemental calcium 89 mg or 4.46 meq+ /gm of salt)	Hypocalcemic seizure 1-2 ml/kg slow IV push with cardiac monitoring	10 mg/kg over 5-10 min. IV, followed by infusion of 200 mg/ kg/day	Bradycardia, arrhythmia, hypotension (with IV), IV leak-tissue necrosis

Contd.

Contd.

Chloral hydrate	Sedative, hypnotic – short-term management	Sedative: 25-50 mg/kg/24 hr PO/ PR q 6-8 hrly For procedures: 50-75 mg/kg/ dose PO/PR, 30-60 min prior to procedure	GI irritation, hypotension, myocardial/ respiratory depression, paradoxical excitement
Chlorpromazine	Tourette syndrome, nausea and vomiting, behaviour disorders, mania, psychosis, Sydenham chorea	0.5-1mg/kg/dose, q 4-6 hr (antiemetic): 2.5-6 mg/kg/day, q 4-6 hrly (Psychosis)	Dystonia, hypotension, dyskinesia
Clonidine	ADHD (experimental)	0.05-0.4 mg/day, PO, bid-qid	Drowsiness, dry mouth, hypotension
Cyproheptadine hydrochloride	Migraine prophylaxis	2-6 yrs 2 mg/dose, 8-12 hrly; >7 yrs 4 mg/dose, PO, bid-tid (max. 0.5 mg/kg/day)	Drowsiness, appetite stimulation, bronchospasm
Dantrolene sodium	Spasticity associated with cerebral palsy, spinal cord lesion, multiple sclerosis	0.5-10 mg/kg/d, q- bid	Drowsiness, blurred vision, seizures, G.I. disturbance, incontinence, enuresis
Desipramine hydrochloride	ADHD (experimental), depression	1-5 mg/kg/day	Drowsiness, headache, blurred vision, G.I. disturbance, arrhythmia, hypotension
Dexamethasone	Cerebral edema	Loading dose 1-2 mg/kg IV, followed by 1-1.5 mg/kg/day div 6 hrly, tapered over 1-2 weeks	Similar to ACTH and prednisolone (see above)
Dextroamphetamine	ADHD, narcolepsy, exogenous obesity	ADHD: 3-5 yr: 2.5 mg/24 hr, max 40 mg/ 24 hr q OD-TID; >6 yr: 5 mg/24 hr, max 40 mg/24 hr q OD-TID Narcolepsy: 6-12 yr: 5 mg/d, max 60 mg/24 hr; >12 yr: 10 mg/day, max 60 mg/day	Anorexia, G.I. disturbance, headache, insomnia, tremor, agitation, hypertension, arrhythmia, palpitation
Diazepam	Sedation	0.3 mg/kg/dose (max 10 mg), IV, PO	No important report
Diphenhydramine	Vertigo, excessive emesis	5 mg/kg/day, divided 3-4 doses	Drowsiness, dry mouth, blurred vision, CNS effects > GI effects
Furosemide	Raised ICP	1-3 mg/kg IV 6-12 hrly, 1-4 mg/kg oral 12-24 hrly	Dyselectrolytemia (hypokalemia, alkalosis), hyperuricemia, dehydration
Imipramine	Enuresis	10-25 mg at bed time, PO; max dose: 6-12 year-50 mg/24 hr 12-14 yr-75 mg/24 hr	Dry mouth, constipation, urinary retention, blurred vision, insomnia, tremor, palpitation, fatigue, ataxia, sweating, weakness
IVIG	Guillain-Barré syndrome, demyelinating polyneuropathy	0.4 g/kg/day for 5 days	Tachycardia, dyspnea, fever, hypersensitivity reaction
Haloperidol	Tourette syndrome, psychosis, serious behaviour disorder, dystonia, chorea	0.25-0.5 mg/d, PO, titrated to response (max dose 0.15 mg/kg/d)	Dyskinesia, sedation, irritability, withdrawn behavior, cardiac side effects
L-dopa	Dopa responsive dystonia	0.5-2 mg/kg/d, or 50-250 mg/day, PO	G.I. disturbance, insomnia, cardiac disturbances
Mannitol	Raised ICP	0.5-1g/kg IV in 30 mins, maintenance, if needed, 0.25-0.5 g/ kg 4-6 hrly	Excessive diuresis and dehydration
Methylphenidate	ADHD	0.5-1.5 mg/kg/day, PO (max 2 mg/ kg/d), q-od; start with low dose	Loss of appetite, withdrawal, irritability

Contd.

Contd.

Methyl prednisolone	ADEM, SLE, neuromyelitis optica, autoimmune encephalitis	20-30 mg/kg/d, IV, (Max1000 mg/d), 3-5 d	Hypertension
Neostigmine	Myasthenia gravis	0.01-0.04 mg/kg/dose, SC, IM, IV, titrate 4-6 hrly; oral dose 0.4 mg/kg/dose, q- 4-6 hrly	Bradycardia, abdominal cramp, increased urinary frequency
Methyl prednisolone	Immunosuppression	0.5-2 mg/kg/day, IV div 6-12 hrly	Hypertension
Sodium nitroprusside	Hypertensive encephalopathy	0.5-10 μg/kg/min	
Olanzapine	Antipsychotic, severe behaviour disorder, ADHD (experimental)	2.5-10 mg/day, PO	Increased appetite, weight gain, sedation, tremor, hypotension
Phenobarbitone	Sydenham chorea	As above	As above
Propranolol	Migraine	0.6-2 mg/kg/day div 6-8 hrly (maximum dose 4 mg/kg/day), PO, also 10-20 mg TDS	Hypotension, bradycardia, bronchospasm, G.I. upset,
Promethazine	Sedation, nausea, vomiting, motion sickness	0.25-1 mg /kg/dose PO, IV, IM, q 4-6 hrs or as needed	Sedation, hypotension, extrapyramidal symptoms
Pyridostigmine	Myasthenia gravis	0.05-0.15 mg/kg/dose IM, IV, (maximum 10 mg); PO 7 mg/kg/day in 5-6 divided doses	Nausea, increased salivation, colic, increased bronchial secretion, increased peristalsis, diarrhea
Pyridoxine	Pyridoxine dependent and deficiency seizures	50-100 mg/dose PO, IV, IM; maintenance dose 50-100 mg/day; 15 mg/kg/day for pyridoxine dependency life-long	
Risperidone	Autism spectrum disorder (5-16 years), for aggression, self-injury, tantrum	0.25-3 mg/d, PO, q-bid; start with low dose <20 kg: 0.25-3 mg/d >20 kg: 0.5-3 mg/d	Weight gain, tremor, excessive salivation, sedation, extrapyramidal symptoms, prolonged QT interval
Sertraline	Depression, obsessive compulsive disorder, post traumatic stress, ADHD (experimental)	25-100 mg/day, PO 25 mg OD, increase dose by 25 mg every 3-4 days to mx of 200 mg/day	Insomnia, G.I. disturbance
Sodium valproate	Sydenham chorea	As above	As above
Sumatriptan	Migraine	5 mg in wt <25 kg, 10 mg (2 sprays) for wt. 25-50 kg, 20 mg for wt. > 50 kg as nasal spray, orally or subcutaneously	Hot flashes, nausea, vomiting, drowsiness
Thiamine	Wernicke encephalopathy	10-50 mg/kg/d × 2 wk then 5-10 mg/dose for 1 month	Insufficient data in pediatrics
Trihexyphenidyl	Dystonia	0.25 mg/day, divided, q-bid/tid, increasing slowly to 60-80 mg/day, PO or until excessive side effects like urinary retention, confusion, blurred vision	Dryness of mouth, dizziness, constipation, urinary retention, tachycardia, headache, blurring of vision, tachycardia, headache
Rizatriptan	Acute treatment of migraine attack (children > 6 years)	<40 kg: 5 mg PO q-od; >40 kg: 10 mg PO q-od; Maximum: 1 dose in any 24-hour period	Avoid in basilar or hemiplegic migraines

INDEX

E

F

G

H

I

J